The Author

ROBERT M. YOUNGSON, OStJ, MB, ChB, DTM&H, DO, FRCOphth, is a medical graduate of Aberdeen University and has postgraduate qualifications from the Royal College of Surgeons of London, the Royal College of Physicians of England, and from the Royal College of Ophthalmologists. He has worked as a doctor in Singapore, Malaysia, Nepal, Hong Kong, Cyprus, Gibraltar, Germany and the United Kingdom. In a varied career, he has been a general practitioner, a medical administrator, a public health medical officer and, for a number of years, was responsible for investigating Ministerial enquiries on medical matters for the Army. As a serving officer he qualified as an ophthalmic surgeon and eventually became Consultant Adviser and Head of Ophthalmology in the Army Medical Services, in the rank of Colonel. He has been the chairman of various committees concerned with medical research, clinical instruction, medical libraries, and computerization in medicine. Dr Youngson is now a full-time medical writer, and has, to date published 37 books. He is the author of the *Royal Society of Medicine Encyclopedia of Family Health*, the *Royal Society of Medicine Health Encyclopedia*, the *Guinness Encyclopedia of the Human Being*, *The Guinness Encyclopedia of Science*, the *Royal Society of Medicine Dictionary of Symptoms* and the NHS Direct *Medical Encyclopedia* on the Internet. He has also written the Collins Gem *First Aid*, *Women's Health* and *Prescription Drugs* for HarperCollins.

Collins dictionary *of*
Medicine

William Collins' dream of knowledge for all began with the publication of his first book in 1819. A self-educated mill worker, he not only enriched millions of lives, but also founded a flourishing publishing house. Today, staying true to this spirit, Collins books are packed with inspiration, innovation, and practical expertise. They place you at the centre of a world of possibility and give you exactly what you need to explore it.

Collins. Do more.

Collins
dictionary *of*
Medicine
fourth edition

Robert M. Youngson

Collins

HarperCollins Publishers
Westerhill Road, Bishopbriggs,
Glasgow G64 2QT

www.collins.co.uk

First published 1992
Second edition published 1999
Third edition published 2004
Fourth edition published 2005

Reprint 10 9 8 7 6 5 4 3 2 1 0

A catalogue record for this book is available from the British Library

ISBN 0 00 720709 3

Typeset by Davidson Pre-Press Graphics Ltd, Glasgow
Printed and bound in Great Britain by Clays Ltd, St Ives plc.

Contents

Preface   ix

Dictionary of Medicine   1

Illustrations
  Skeleton   660
  Muscle system (front)   661
  Muscle system (back)   662
  Circulatory system   663
  Respiratory system   664
  Brain and spinal cord   665
  Autonomic nervous system   666
  Dental system   667
  Digestive system   668
  Urinary system   669
  Reproductive system   670
  Endocrine system   671
  Lymphatic system   672
  Immune system   673
  Visual system   674
  Lacrimal system   675
  Auditory system   676
  Olfactory system   677
  DNA structure   678
  Skin structure   679

Internet links   682

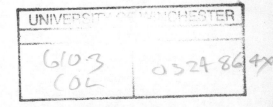

To Elaine

Preface to the Fourth Edition

The number of possible headwords and phrases from which a selection
can be made for a medical dictionary is very large and one of the chief
difficulties is to decide on the criteria for selection. The first requirement
is that the book should be useful, so it must contain a large number of
basic definitions that will find a place in any medical dictionary, however
modest. It must also reflect current medical interest and thus contain
many words and phrases that are of fairly recent coinage; these should
be more than passing verbal fads although it is not always easy to judge
whether an 'in' word or phrase will last. The dictionary must also try to
reflect the weight of medical importance between the many disciplines
and basic sciences that compete with each other for attention.

Medical terms are delightfully logical. Almost the whole vocabulary
is formed by various combinations of a comparatively small number of
roots and combining forms, often of Greek origin. Study of the classical
languages has become uncommon but most people with a serious
interest in English now derive their etymological knowledge by an
almost unconscious recognition of classical elements in familiar words.
To assist readers in this valuable exercise, I have included all important
combining forms used in medical language as well as many prefixes and
suffixes. I have also included derivations whenever these seem to illuminate
meanings. As always, many difficulties reside in nothing more frightening
than terminology. The elucidation of the meaning of a single term can
throw a flood of light on a whole page of text.

This dictionary is unusual in that many entries are expanded well
beyond simple definitions. The motive is to minimize the frustration
felt by many who consult a dictionary and fail to find the depth of
explanation they need. The book also contains many entries of such
public interest that they scarcely require definition. These entries,
however, contain a great deal of much-needed basic information that
may be hard to find elsewhere.

Modern medicine, with its enormous emphasis on science and
technology, is badly in need of humanizing. One sign of this need is
the perennial call to abandon eponymous titles for diseases, syndromes,
instruments, techniques, and so on. But the study of medical history is a
great antidote to the hubris that is liable to spring from academic merit
and professional success, and I think the practice of honouring those
responsible for medical advances should be encouraged. So to help to
promote this interest I have included names, dates and achievements of
hundreds of people whose dedicated work has made the existence of this
dictionary possible.

Many terms and concepts that were in existence at the time of compilation of the earlier editions, but were then thought too specialized or obscure to be included have, in the intervening years, become so important that exclusion is no longer possible. Genetics and molecular biology are now the great peaks in the profile of the sciences basic to medicine. Since the completion of the human genome project, genetics is rapidly taking over control of the direction of medical advance and this is reflected in the balance of entries on genetic matters.

Medical concepts are so elaborately inter-related that the problem of cross-referencing in a dictionary is an embarrassment. In many entries it would be possible to cross-reference, to other entries, a dozen or more of the terms used. This would make tedious reading especially for those to whom elementary terms are familiar. So I have deliberately avoided mechanical cross-referencing of every term that is defined elsewhere. The ardent but puzzled seeker after truth should not, therefore, be discouraged from looking elsewhere for a definition of any term used that is not immediately clearly understood. There are, however, many thousands of cross-references.

Directive 92/27/EEC required that names of medicinal substances should conform in spelling to the recommended International Non-proprietary Name (rINN) list. Fortunately, the majority of British Approved Names (BAN) of drugs are the same as those on the International list, but many have had to be changed wherever they occur. But because many readers will be long familiar with the earlier names I have, in most cases, provided both names. Brand names that have been withdrawn from the UK lists have, however, often shown wonderful persistence in Australia and New Zealand, in various European countries, in South Africa and in the USA, and many of these have been retained alongside their successors.

It is no part of the function of a dictionary complier to comment on the material that has been included or to indicate humour. But here and there the temptation has been irresistible and I have occasionally, and I hope gently, relaxed the gravitas traditionally required of a lexicographer. Undue solemnity seems both inappropriate and unnecessary these days.

The single-handed complication and updating of a dictionary is a daunting undertaking, barely to be contemplated without the support of the other people involved. So once again it is a great satisfaction to be able to acknowledge the help and support of my friends at HarperCollins in Glasgow. I am most grateful to Christopher Riches, the head of the reference department and the fons et origo of this work. Peter Harrison, James Carney and Edwin Moore have, successively over the years, striven mightily to bring this project to such a gratifying state.

Elizabeth McLachlan, the editorial assistant, has also been a firm friend, an invaluable help, and, as the recipient of most of my anxious telephone calls, has invariably been capable, in an instant, of raising my work-depressed spirits with her cheerful good humour.

Robert Youngson
Blandford Forum, April, 2005

a

a- *prefix denoting* not, without or the absence of a quality or object.

AA *abbrev. for* Alcoholics Anonymous, an organization founded in 1935 and dedicated to the control of alcoholism by mutual support, group therapy and self-help.

AAA, throat spray a brand name for a spray containing AINE.

AASH adrenal androgen-stimulating hormone.

ab- *prefix denoting* from, outside, away from. From the Latin *ab*, from.

abacavir a nucleoside reverse transcriptase inhibitor drug used in combination with other anti-HIV drugs to treat AIDS. A brand name is Ziagen. In combination with lamivudine and zidovudine it is marketed as Trizivir.

abacterial 1 not caused by bacteria.
2 without, or in the absence of, bacteria.

abacteruria the absence of bacteria in the urine. The term is used when symptoms suggest a urinary infection but organisms cannot be demonstrated either by microscopy or by culture. See SYMPTOMATIC ABACTERURIA.

Abadie sign a once classical indication of the syphilitic complication TABES DORSALIS. The patient is insensitive to tight squeezing of the Achilles tendon. (Joseph Louis Irénée Jean, 1873–1946. French surgeon).

abalienation a somewhat archaic term meaning any form of mental derangement.

abarognosis the inability to appreciate the weight of an object or to distinguish between objects of different weight. The symptom suggests a lesion in the parietal lobe of the brain.

abasia a disorder of coordination affecting the ability to walk, but not caused by paralysis. It is often associated with the inability to stand upright (astasia). People with abasia–astasia retain the full use of the legs while lying in bed, but when placed upright take a few steps then crumple to the ground. The condition is usually a manifestation of HYSTERIA.

Abbocillin-VK a brand name for PHENOXYMETHYLPENICILLIN.

Abbot pump a portable mechanical device that controls the precise dosage of a drug delivered intravenously through a catheter.

ABC genes genes that code for the ATP-binding cassette transporter proteins that carry compounds across biological membranes. Fourteen different ABC genes are known to be associated with human genetic diseases.

ABCA3 gene a gene that codes for a 1704-amino-acid protein found in the limiting membrane of lamellar bodies. Mutations of this gene cause fatal SURFACTANT deficiency in newborn babies.

ABCA4 gene a gene that codes for a transporter protein found in the photoreceptor membrane disks in retinal rod cells. Mutations cause retinal degenerative diseases such as Stargardt's macular dystrophy, cone-rod dystrophy and some recessive forms of RETINITIS PIGMENTOSA.

ABCG5 genes genes coding for transporter proteins found in the liver and intestines. Mutations cause local accumulations of cholesterol and other sterols (sitosterolaemia).

ABCG8 genes genes with a function similar to that of ABCG5 GENES.

ABC transporter proteins a large and diverse family of cell membrane transport proteins with two transmembrane domains and two ATP-binding regions within the cytosol. The transmembrane domains provide a controllable pathway for transported substance to pass through the cell membrane into or out of the cell.

ABCB1 member 1 of the B subfamily of ABC TRANSPORTER PROTEINS. Also known as MDR1. Polymorphism of the gene for ABCB1 is associated with multi-drug resistance in the treatment of a range of diseases including epilepsy, various cancers, rheumatoid arthritis and inflammatory bowel disease. Clinical experience has shown that several drugs used to treat cancer may become ineffective simultaneously in spite of having unrelated chemical structure. This multi-drug resistance was shown to be due to enhanced expression of ABCB1 which was using ATP-derived energy to *export* drugs from the cytosol to the extracellular fluid.

abciximab a monoclonal antibody drug that inhibits the platelet glycoprotein IIb/IIIa receptor and is used as an adjunct to heparin and aspirin in patients undergoing coronary angioplasty. It is also used for the short-term protection of patients with unstable angina. The drug has been found valuable in coronary stenting. A brand name is Reopro.

abdomen the part of the trunk below the chest. The abdominal cavity lies between the DIAPHRAGM, above, and the pelvic floor, below. It contains the LIVER and most of the digestive system, comprising the STOMACH, the DUODENUM, the JEJUNUM, the ILEUM, the CAECUM with the APPENDIX, the COLON, the RECTUM and the ANAL CANAL. Other abdominal organs include the KIDNEYS, the ADRENAL GLANDS, the SPLEEN, the PANCREAS and some large and important blood vessels, such as the AORTA and the inferior VENA CAVA, around which are many chains of LYMPH NODES. The intestines are hung from the back wall of the abdomen by a much-folded membrane, the MESENTERY, and are covered by the OMENTUM. The lower part of the abdomen, the pelvic cavity, contains the BLADDER. In women, the pelvic cavity also contains the womb (UTERUS), the FALLOPIAN TUBES and the OVARIES; in men, the central PROSTATE GLAND and the VAS DEFERENS, on each side. The wall of the abdomen consists of overlapping layers of muscle and sheets of fibrous tissue. The organs and the interior of the walls are covered with PERITONEUM. See also ABDOMINAL REGIONS.

abdominal 1 pertaining to the ABDOMEN. 2 of a surgical operation performed through an incision in the wall of the abdomen, which could be performed via a different route, e.g. an abdominal hysterectomy.

abdominal apoplexy obstruction to the blood flow and bleeding into an abdominal organ, such as the INTESTINE, or bleeding into the PERITONEAL CAVITY.

abdominal aura a state of hunger, nausea and abdominal pain that may provide warning of an impending epileptic seizure.

abdominal breathing respiration in which most of the work is done by the muscles of the abdominal wall in compressing the abdominal contents and elevating the diaphragm so as to compress the lungs and push out air. The method may be helpful in patients with breathing difficulties.

abdominal delivery see CAESARIAN SECTION.

abdominal gestation a type of ECTOPIC PREGNANCY in which a FETUS develops outside the womb but in the abdominal cavity. This is a dangerous state of affairs liable to lead to profuse internal bleeding.

abdominal hysterectomy surgical removal of the womb (UTERUS) by way of an incision made in the front wall of the ABDOMEN. This method allows excellent access, not only to the uterus but also to the surrounding structures so that they can be examined for disease. Compare VAGINAL HYSTERECTOMY.

abdominal pregnancy a rare form of ECTOPIC PREGNANCY in which the fetus develops outside the womb but within the abdominal cavity. The placenta is attacked to a vascular structure such as the bowel and there is a grave risk of severe haemorrhage.

abdominal quadrant any one of the four areas on the front of the abdomen formed by two imaginary lines, one vertical and one horizontal intersecting at the navel. They four quadrants are called upper and lower right and upper and lower left, as seen from the patient's point of view.

abdominal reflex a reflex muscular contraction caused by firmly stroking each side of the skin of the abdomen in turn with a blunt point. In the normal response the umbilicus moves slightly toward the side stroked.

abdominal region any one of the nine areas into which the surface of the abdomen is divided for descriptive purposes. Centrally, from above down, are the epigastric, umbilical and hypogastric (pubic) regions, and on either side, from above down, are the hypochondriac, lateral and inguinal regions.

abdominal respiration breathing inhalation effected mainly by downward movement of the diaphragm with protrusion of the front wall of the abdomen.

abdominal rigidity a sometimes board-like firmness of the abdominal wall caused by rigid contraction of the muscles. Rigidity is usually a reaction to internal inflammation and suggests PERITONITIS. It may, however be a conscious reaction to pain, especially following surgery, when it is often referred to as abdominal splinting. This may restrict breathing and cause respiratory problems.

abdominal thrust an alternative to the HEIMLICH MANOEUVRE when a patient is unconscious or lying down. With the patient on his or her back, the heel of the hand is placed just above the navel, the free hand is paced on top of the other hand, the arms are kept straight and four rapid thrusts are made downwards and in the direction of the head.

abdominocentesis a procedure in which a needle is passed into the abdomen so that fluid may be removed, either to relieve discomfort or to obtain a sample for diagnosis. AMNIO-CENTESIS is a form of abdominocentesis in which the needle enters the womb.

abdominoperineal relating to the ABDOMEN and to the PERINEUM. The term is used especially of abdominal surgical procedures that also involve the anal region, as in the case of a total removal of the lower part of the COLON and RECTUM for a low cancer of the large intestine.

abdominoplasty an operation to remove excess skin and fat from the abdomen for cosmetic reasons. Large flaps of redundant tissue are cut away and the free edges stitched together. Cosmetic surgeons, who are not noted for their respect for the language, call this procedure an apronectomy. Unless that patient modifies eating habits, the effect of the operation is temporary.

abdominous having a large belly. Pot-bellied.

abducens nerves the sixth of the 12 pairs of cranial nerves. Each abducens nerve supplies the tiny muscle on the outer side of the eye that moves the eye outwards (the lateral rectus muscle). Paralysis of the abducens nerve causes a slight convergent squint with no outward movement of the eye beyond the central position. Also known as abducent nerve.

abducent causing a separation. The word derives from the Latin *ab*, from, and *ducere*, to draw or lead. See also ABDUCTION.

abduction a movement outwards from the mid-line of the body or from the central axis of a limb. The opposite, inward, movement is called ADDUCTION.

abductor muscle a muscle which moves a part away from the mid-line.

Abelcet a brand name for the antifungal drug AMPHOTERICIN B in a liquid complex. It is given by injection.

aberrant deviating from the normal. The term may be applied to variations in the fine detail of body structure, such as the size and position of small arteries, or to modes of behaviour not generally considered acceptable. See also ABNORMAL.

aberration a deviation from normal. The term derives from the Latin *aberrare*, to wander off. See also ABNORMAL.

abetalipoproteinaemia a rare AUTOSOMAL RECESSIVE inherited disorder due to a mutation on chromosome 4 causing failure to synthesize the substance apolipoprotein-B (beta-lipoprotein) present in LOW DENSITY LIPOPROTEINS (LDLs). Cholesterol, fats (triglycerides), lipoproteins and CHYLOMICRONS are almost absent from the blood and there is a consequent impairment of fat supply and of the transport of the fat-soluble vitamins. The result is failure to thrive, neurological abnormalities probably from vitamin deficiency, impairment of vision from retinal degeneration, and usually death before the age of 40. The condition is almost confined to Ashkenazi Jews.

Abidec a brand name for a multivitamin preparation for children containing vitamin A, calciferol, thiamine, riboflavine (riboflavin), pyridoxine, nicotinamide and vitamin C.

Abilify a brand name for the antipsychotic drug ARIPIPRAZOLE, used to treat SCHIZOPHRENIA.

-ability *combining form denoting* power or capacity to do something.

abiogenesis the theory of 'spontaneous generation' – the long-discarded notion that living organisms can be formed from non-living matter. Louis Pasteur's work (see PASTEURIZATION) did much to overthrow this idea which was based largely on the observation that maggots often appeared on rotting meat.

abiotic non-living.

abiotrophy a general and inexact term referring to the effects of ageing, or to any degenerative process of unknown cause affecting tissue, especially nerve tissue. As knowledge extends the need for such terms diminishes.

ablatio an obsolescent term meaning separation.

ablation deliberate removal or separation, especially by surgery.

ablepharia a rare term for a rare condition – the absence of the eyelids. From Greek, *a*, not and *blepharon*, an eyelid.

abnormal deviating from the observed rule or from the consensus opinion of what is acceptable. ABERRANT. See also ABNORMALITY.

abnormality the condition of not conforming to standard recognized patterns of structure, function, behaviour or phenomenon. In some social contexts, normality is no more than a statistical concept, and may be entirely relative. What is normal in one population or group may be abnormal in another. See also ABERRATION.

abnormal psychology a branch of psychology dealing with disorders of behaviour and mental disturbance, and with certain normal phenomena not clearly understood, such as dreams and altered states of consciousness. See also ABERRATION.

abnormal retinal correspondence (ARC) an ocular condition in which one eye uses the sensitive centre of the RETINA, while the other uses a more peripheral part, thereby conferring a crude form of binocular vision with a persistent AMBLYOPIA in the deviating eye that is harder to correct than amblyopia in the absence of ARC. The diagnosis and correction of ARC is undertaken by an ORTHOPTIST.

ABO blood groups a system of blood grouping developed from the discoveries of Karl Landsteiner (1868–1943) in 1900. The designations are arbitrary and the four groups are A, B, AB and O. These represent the antigenic differences in the red cells, the ANTIGEN being present on the red cell membranes. Group A, B and AB people have A, B and A and B antigens, respectively, on their red cells. Group O people have no antigens and are known as universal donors, whose blood, other things being equal, may safely be transfused into anyone. Group A people (about 26% in Europe) have antibodies (agglutinins) to B in their serum and must not be given blood with B antigens. Agglutinins cause red cells with the same letter antigens to clump together and to become useless. Group B people (about 6%) have antibodies to A in their serum and must not be given blood with A antigens. Group O people (about 68%) have both A and B antibodies, so must not be given either A or B blood. Group AB people have no ABO blood group antibodies in their serum and are known as universal recipients. See also RHESUS FACTOR DISEASE and KELL BLOOD GROUP SYSTEM.

abortifacient a drug used to cause ABORTION. Many substances have been reputed to cause abortion and many have been tried in an attempt to procure abortion illegally, mostly without effect. In clinical practice abortion is chiefly induced with one of the PROSTAGLANDINS. Other drugs, such as mifepristone (see ABORTION PILL) and OXYTOCIN, are also used to induce labour.

abortion loss of the FETUS before it is able to survive outside the womb (UTERUS). The term abortion covers accidental or spontaneous ending, or MISCARRIAGE, of pregnancy as well as deliberate termination, whether for medical reasons or as a criminal act. At least 1 in 10 pregnancies ends in abortion, the great majority of these being spontaneous. Deliberate termination of pregnancy is called induced abortion. When this is legal it is called 'therapeutic abortion'. Abortion may be performed legally under certain circumstances and in approved hospitals or clinics. Two doctors, who have seen the patient, must agree that continuation of the pregnancy would be detrimental to her or her baby, or her existing children's, physical or mental health. The term derives from the Latin *aborior*, to set, as of the sun.

abortion pill a drug, RU486 or mifepristone, that acts by blocking the action of PROGESTERONE which is essential to maintain pregnancy. A second drug, one of the PROSTAGLANDINS, has to be taken within 48 hours to complete the expulsion of the fertilized egg. The method is said to be 95% effective. See also ABORTION.

abortionist a person who performs criminal abortions. See also ABORTION.

abortus fever see BRUCELLOSIS.

ABPSS *abbrev. for* Associate of the British Psychological Society.

abrachia absence of arms, usually from birth. For a time, abrachia was commonly caused by the drug THALIDOMIDE acting on the fetus in early pregnancy.

abrasion wearing away of tissue by sustained or heavy friction between surfaces. Abrasion of the biting surfaces of teeth is common. Skin abrasions are among the commonest of all minor injuries. Deliberate abrasion in the cosmetic treatment of ACNE scars or other disfigurement is called dermabrasion.

abreaction a process used in PSYCHOTHERAPY in which repressed thoughts and feelings are brought into consciousness and 'relived'. Abreaction is, it is hoped, followed by CATHARSIS and is most readily achieved when the trouble arises from a recent traumatic event.

abrin an anticancer drug derived from the jequirity bean *Abrus precatorius*. Abrin contains toxic LECTINS that are more effective in inhibiting protein synthesis in some cancers than in normal cells.

abruptio separation. From Latin *abruptus*, broken off.

abruptio placentae premature detachment of the PLACENTA from the wall of the womb (UTERUS).

abruption a tearing away or separation.

abscess a cavity full of PUS surrounded by inflamed or dying tissue, or by dense fibrous tissue which cuts off the blood supply to the centre. Abscesses are nearly always caused by INFECTION and the organisms concerned often persist within the tissue. Some, however, become sterile. They can seldom be effectively treated with antibiotics and must be opened and the contents drained surgically for proper resolution. See also ANTIBIOMA.

abscission the act of cutting off.

abscopal referring to a reaction in body tissue in an area outside an irradiated zone.

absence the state of brief incommunicability and unresponsiveness which occurs repeatedly in the minor form of EPILEPSY known as PETIT MAL or which may occur in conjunction with

other epileptic manifestations, or as a result of HYPERVENTILATION.

absence seizures PETIT MAL attacks. See also EPILEPSY.

Absidia a genus of fungi that can cause MUCORMYCOSIS. *Absidia* species may be thermophilic and can survive high temperatures in composting enclosures.

absolute alcohol alcohol from which all water has been removed.

absolute hypermetropia HYPERMETROPIA of a degree, relative to age, in which clear vision cannot be achieved by accommodation. Thus, a child of 5 with, say, 4 dioptres of hypermetropia may easily see clearly by accommodating; but an adult of 50 with the same refraction could not see clearly without glasses, and would have an absolute hypermetropia of about 3 dioptres.

absolute refractory period the period during which no stimulus, however strong, is able to evoke a response from an excitable tissue. The absolute refractory period follows immediately after a prior response and is brief.

absolute temperature temperature expressed in the Kelvin scale with absolute zero as 0 kelvin. The magnitude of the kelvin is the same as that of the degree Celsius and any Celsius temperature can be represented as an absolute temperature by degrees – 273.15 °C. The term 'degree kelvin' is no longer used; absolute temperatures are shown in kelvins (K) (William, Lord Kelvin, British physicist, 1824–1907).

absorbable sutures see SUTURE.

absorption 1 the movement of liquids and of dissolved substances across a membrane, from one compartment of the body to another or into the blood.

2 the assimilation of digested food material into the blood from the small intestine. Compare ADSORPTION. See also DIGESTION.

abulia loss or impairment of the ability to act decisively, make decisions, or perform actions. Abulia may be caused by DEPRESSION, TUMOUR or other disorders of the frontal lobes of the brain, PREFRONTAL LEUCOTOMY, STROKE or intoxication with NEUROLEPTIC drugs.

abuse incorrect, improper or excessive use or treatment.

abzyme an antibody that has an enzyme-like (catalytic) action.

A.C. before food. A Latin abbreviation for *ante*

cibos, still sometimes used in a prescription.

acalculia total or partial loss of the ability to perform even simple arithmetical calculations. This may rarely be a specific developmental disorder, but is more often acquired as a result of brain damage, usually to the PARIETAL LOBE, in the course of a STROKE. In this case, the acalculia is a kind of APHASIA. Acalculia without obvious cause may be a herald of DEMENTIA.

acamprosate a drug used to assist in the control of alcoholism. Acamprosate has been found to be an effective and well-tolerated adjunct to the management of alcoholism. A brand name is Campral EC.

acanth-, acantho- *combining form denoting* spine or the prickle cell layer of the skin.

acanthamoeba infection infection, with various species of the genus *Acanthamoeba*. *Acanthamoeba culbertsoni* is a ubiquitous soil AMOEBA that may cause infection in people who have suffered facial injuries or who have DIABETES or LYMPHOMAS. Abscess-like masses occur in the skin, lungs, middle ear and even the brain. Infection of the CORNEA can also occur in contact lens wearers, usually from *Acanthamoeba polyphaga*. *Acanthamoeba* cysts are impervious to chlorine in concentrations up to 50 parts per million. They may therefore survive in domestic water supplies. Treatment is with AMPHOTERICIN-B.

acanthocephalid an obligatory parasitic worm of the phylum *Acanthocephala*, having a ring of hooked spines around its head.

acanthocheilonemiasis parasitic INFECTION with the filarial worm *Acanthocheilonema perstans*. The adult worm is found mainly in body cavities or in or under the skin. See FILARIASIS.

acanthocytosis a disorder of red blood cells (erythrocytes) in which the cell surfaces show multiple spine-like projections. This occurs in ABETALIPOPROTEINAEMIA, severe liver disease, vitamin E deficiency (see VITAMINS) and other conditions.

acanthoid resembling a thorn or spiny process.

acantholysis splitting apart of layers of cells in the epidermis often to form a blister.

acanthoma a tumour of cells from the prickle-cell layer of the epidermis. Acanthomata may be benign or malignant.

acanthosis a disease process in the skin featuring overgrowth and thickening of the prickle-cell layer of the EPIDERMIS. This layer lies above its parent layer, the BASAL cell layer, and local overgrowth results in raised, roughened areas such as warts or the lesions of PSORIASIS or ECZEMA.

acanthosis nigricans black or brown pigmented warty areas overlying patches of ACANTHOSIS. These occur in the armpits and other body folds and may sometimes be associated with ACROMEGALY, ADDISON'S DISEASE, POLYCYSTIC OVARY, intestinal CANCER or the INSULIN RESISTANCE SYNDROME.

acapnia absence of CARBON DIOXIDE in the BLOOD or tissues. This cannot occur in life and the term is usually applied imprecisely to a reduced level of CO_2.

acarbose an oral hypoglycaemic drug. A brand name is Glucobay.

acardia congenital absence of the heart. In a single individual this is incompatible with survival beyond the early stages of development, but cases have been reported in which joined twins share a heart present in only one.

acariasis 1 infestation with mites.
2 the effects, on the SKIN, of mite infestation.

acaricide a drug used to kill mites.

acarid a member of the very large order *Acarina*, which includes the mites and ticks. Some are parasitic, some free-living. *Trombiculid* mites are vectors of scrub TYPHUS, and *Sarcoptes scabiei* causes mange in animals and SCABIES in humans.

acarinophobia an abnormal fear of mites or ticks, especially of mites causing SCABIES.

acaro- *combining form denoting* mite.

acarodermatitis skin inflammation caused by mites.

acarophobia see ACARINOPHOBIA.

Acarus a genus of small mites causing itching and DERMATITIS. The flour mite, *Acarus siro*, is the principal culprit.

acatalasia an AUTOSOMAL RECESSIVE enzyme deficiency disease due to low levels of the ENZYME catalase in the red blood cells. This enzyme protects against damaging FREE RADICAL products such as hydrogen peroxide produced by radiation, various drugs and other agencies. The disorder features ulcers of the gums and gangrene of the tooth sockets with loss of the teeth. Some bacteria present in PERIODONTAL DISEASE produce hydrogen peroxide. Also known as Takahara disease.

acatamathesia impairment of understanding or perception, as occurs in sensory APHASIA.

acceleration stress the effects on body function and behaviour of periods of exposure to increased gravitational forces ('g') such as are experienced by fighter pilots or astronauts.

acceptor sites 1 DNA base sequences that bind transcription regulators during protein synthesis.
2 Molecules that bind other chemical groups.

accessory muscle any muscle whose action reinforces that of any other muscle.

accessory nerve one of the eleventh of the 12 pairs of cranial nerves which arise directly from the BRAIN. The accessory nerve also has a spinal root. Fibres from the root from the brain join the vagus nerve. The accessory nerve supplies many muscles in the PALATE, throat, LARYNX, neck, back and upper chest. Damage to an accessory nerve in the neck may cause difficulty in speaking and in swallowing.

accident-prone unusually liable to suffer accidents. Liability to accidents is probably no more than an effect of carelessness and lack of imaginative foresight or sometimes aggression or non-conformity.

acclimatization 1 physiological adaptation to a new environment or situation. Acclimatization to a hot environment may take as long as three weeks, during which undue exposure to heat, or strenuous exercise, may cause HEAT EXHAUSTION.
2 an environmentally-induced functional improvement in a genetically-determined physiological system.

accommodation the automatic process by which the eyes adjust their focus when the gaze is shifted from one point to another at a different distance. Accommodation is achieved by changing the degree of curvature of the internal crystalline lenses of the eyes. In youth, these are naturally elastic and become more curved when the pull on the ligament by which they are suspended is reduced by contraction of the surrounding muscle ring (CILIARY MUSCLE). This allows focusing on near objects. The elasticity of the lenses drops progressively with age so the power of accommodation lessens. In middle age PRESBYOPIA becomes apparent in all but the near-sighted.

accommodative asthenopia a relative weakness of the focusing power of the eye resulting from a refractive error that imposes the need to make unusually strong accommodative effort. There is a sense of eye-tiredness and discomfort and occasionally headache from sustained narrowing of the eyes.

accommodative insufficiency inability to focus the eyes sufficiently to see near objects clearly. Short-sighted people need less than normal accommodation for near; long-sighted people need more. Accommodative power declines almost linearly with age so that about age 45 most people with normal refraction suffer a degree of accommodative insufficiency. Age-related accommodative insufficiency is also known as PRESBYOPIA.

accommodative squint accommodative strabismus, a convergent squint in young children with uncorrected HYPERMETROPIA who are forced to exert accommodation in order to see distant objects clearly and stronger than normal accommodation to see near objects clearly. Physiologically, accommodation is linked to convergence. This mechanism is the commonest cause of squint in children and the consequent AMBLYOPIA.

accouchement an old-fashioned term for childbirth or delivery. From the French verb *coucher*, to lie down.

accoucheur a person who assists at a birth. A lady obstetrician or midwife is sometimes honoured with the title of accoucheuse.

Accupro a brand name for QUINAPRIL.

Accuretic a brand name for the thiazide diuretic HYDROCHLOROTHIAZIDE formulated with the ANGIOTENSIN–CONVERTING ENZYME inhibitor drug QUINAPRIL.

ACE see ANGIOTENSIN-CONVERTING ENZYME.

acebutolol a beta-blocker drug commonly used to treat high blood pressure (HYPERTENSION), ANGINA PECTORIS, heart failure and heart irregularities (arrhythmias). A brand name is Sectral. Formulated with HYDROCHLOROTHIAZIDE it is marketed as Secadrex.

aceclofenac phenylacetoxyacetic acid, an NSAID drug used in the treatment of OSTEOARTHRITIS. A brand name is Preservex.

ACE inhibitors see ANGIOTENSIN-CONVERTING ENZYME INHIBITORS.

A cells 1 the GLUCAGON-secreting cells of the ISLETS OF LANGERHANS in the PANCREAS. Also known as alpha cells to distinguish from the beta cells that secrete INSULIN.

2 the cells of the adrenal medulla that secrete adrenaline.

acellular devoid of cells. Some connective tissues incorporate acellular areas.

acemetacin a non-steroidal anti-inflammatory drug used in the treatment of RHEUMATOID ARTHRITIS. A brand name is Emflex.

acephalocardia congenital absence of both head and heart.

acephalous headless.

acephalus a fetal organism lacking a well-defined head. The term ANENCEPHALY has a similar meaning.

Acepril a brand name for CAPTOPRIL.

acerbation making more severe, sharp or painful. The commoner term, in medicine, is EXACERBATION.

acet- *combining form denoting* acid. From the Latin *acetum*, vinegar.

acetabulum the socket in the side of the bony pelvis into which the spherical head of the thigh bone (FEMUR) fits. The word is derived from the Latin *acetum*, vinegar and *abulum*, the diminutive of *abrum*, a container. The acetabulum was thought to resemble a small vinegar cup.

acetaldehyde a product of the metabolism of large amounts of alcohol. The reaction is catalyzed in the liver by the enzyme alcohol dehydrogenase. The principal cause of the toxic effects of strong drink.

acetaminophen see PARACETAMOL.

acetazolamide a drug that inhibits the enzyme carbonic anhydrase in the kidney tubules, thus acting as a diuretic. In the eye it acts similarly to reduce the rate of secretion of aqueous humour and is useful in the treatment of GLAUCOMA when the intraocular pressure rise cannot be controlled with eye drops alone. The drug is also used in the treatment of EPILEPSY. A brand name is Diamox.

Acetest a brand name for a tablet used to test for ketones in urine and other fluids.

acetoacetic acid a KETONE body occurring in the urine in uncontrolled DIABETES or starvation. See ACETONE BODY.

acetonaemia excessive quantities of acetone bodies in the blood. This may occur in uncontrolled DIABETES or in starvation. A commoner term is KETOSIS; the condition is the cause of diabetic coma. See also ACETONE BODY.

acetone a KETONE body derived from acetyl

coenzyme A in untreated DIABETES or starvation. See also ACETONE BODY.

acetone body a KETONE body. One of the three compounds, acetoacetic acid, 3-hydroxybutanoic acid or acetone, produced when, in the absence of adequate available glucose, fatty acids are used for fuel. Acetone bodies are produced in large quantity in severe untreated DIABETES and are the cause of ACIDOSIS and dangerous diabetic COMA.

acetylcholine the acetic acid ester of choline, an important NEUROTRANSMITTER acting at cholinergic synapses to propagate nerve impulses. It occurs in both the brain and the peripheral nervous system and is the neuro-transmitter at neuromuscular junctions. Acetylcholine is inactivated by the enzyme ACETYLCHOLINESTERASE, and drugs, such as physostigmine (Eserine) and edrophonium (Tensilon), that inhibit this enzyme, prolong the action of the neurotransmitter.

acetylcholine receptor an ion channel that opens when acetylcholine binds to it, so converting chemical diffusion into an electrical signal. Also known as the nicotinic acetylcholine receptor.

acetylcholinesterase an ENZYME that rapidly inactivates ACETYLCHOLINE by breaking it down to acetic acid and choline. Also known as cholinesterase.

acetylcholinesterase inhibitors drugs that block the action of the enzyme ACETYLCHOLINESTERASE which quickly breaks down the neurotransmitter acetylcholine. This neurotransmitter is the linking agent between nerve cells in the outer layer (cortex) of the brain. The early impairment of cognitive function found in a common forms of dementia known as dementia with Lewy bodies (DLB) is associated with a reduction in acetylcholine levels. These drugs, by inhibiting, acetylcholine breakdown, have been found helpful in reducing the severity of the early stages of dementia. They cannot be expected to cure or even delay progress of the dementia. The drug group includes DONEPEZIL, GALANTAMINE and RIVASTIGMINE.

acetylcholine sweat test a test of the function of the sympathetic nervous system. A marked area of the skin is painted with iodine and then with an emulsion of starch in oil. A very small dose of acetylcholine solution is injected. If the local sympathetic system is intact a black dot will appear at each sweat pore. The test can be quantified by counting the dots in a given area.

acetyl coenzyme A an important metabolic agent that transfers acetyl groups to the KREBS CYCLE and to various synthesizing pathways. Usually abbreviated to acetyl CoA.

acetylcysteine a drug used to reduce the stickiness and viscosity of MUCUS. A mucolytic. It is useful for freeing sputum in bronchitis and in liquefying mucus in CYSTIC FIBROSIS. It is also used to improve eye comfort in KERATOCONJUNCTIVITIS SICCA. Acetylcysteine has recently been found to be effective in reducing the risk of kidney damage from X-ray contrast media (contrast nephropathy). A brand name is Parvolex. Formulated with hypromellose it is marketed as Ilube.

acetylsalicylic acid the common analgesic and antiprostaglandin drug Aspirin.

acetylserotonin a product formed as an intermediate in the synthesis pathway for MELATONIN from SEROTONIN.

Acezide a brand name for HYDROCHLOROTHIAZIDE formulated with the ANGIOTENSIN CONVERTING ENZYME inhibitor drug CAPTOPRIL.

achalasia failure of a muscle ring (SPHINCTER) to relax when it should. Achalasia most commonly affects the sphincter at the bottom of the gullet (OESOPHAGUS). See also ACHALSIA OF THE CARDIA.

achalasia of the cardia inability of the lower end of the gullet (oesophagus) to relax, because of spasm. The cause is unknown. There may be regurgitation of food, inhalation of swallowed material, with pneumonia and severe loss of weight. The condition is sometimes complicated by cancer of the oesophagus. Also known as cardiospasm.

ache a persistent dull pain.

achievement motivation the persistent impulse to attain a high standard of performance in any activity.

Achilles reflex the ankle jerk. Sudden contraction of the calf muscles when the ACHILLES TENDON is struck with a tendon hammer. A test of the integrity of the reflex arc involving the first and second sacral segments of the spinal cord.

Achilles tendon the prominent tendon just above the heel by means of which the powerful muscles of the calf are attached to the large heel bone. Contraction of the prominent calf muscles pulls the Achilles tendon upwards so that the ankle is straightened and the heel leaves the ground. The Achilles tendon is essential in walking and running and is easily strained or torn. (Named after Achilles, son of Peleus and Thetis, who, as a baby, was said to have been held by his heel and dipped in the river Styx by his mother to make him invulnerable. He died from a heel wound).

achlorhydria absence of the normal hydrochloric acid in the stomach as a result of wasting (atrophy) of the acid-secreting cells in the lining. Achlorhydria is commonly found in PERNICIOUS ANAEMIA when autoimmune damage to the stomach lining is associated with loss of secretion of an intrinsic factor in the stomach that leads to failure of vitamin B_{12} absorption.

acholia absence of bile secretion into the small intestine. In acholia, the stools are clay-coloured. Because bile is also needed to emulsify dietary fat before it can be absorbed, the stools are also fatty and may be difficult to flush away.

acholuria absence of bile pigments from the urine in a condition in which this might be expected.

acholuric jaundice jaundice without bile pigments in the urine. There are excessive amounts of unconjugated BILIRUBIN in the blood. Unconjugated bilirubin is water-insoluble and is bound to albumin. Conjugated bilirubin is water-soluble and can appear in the urine.

achondroplasia a dominant genetic defect that interferes with the growth of the cartilage at the growing sites at the end of long bones, resulting in a characteristic form of dwarfism. Achondroplasia has no effect other than on growth.

achondroplastic dwarf a person with very short arms and legs as a result of ACHONDROPLASIA. Many circus dwarfs are achondroplastic.

achromatopsia a rare but severe defect of colour vision in which the world is perceived almost in monochrome.

Achromycin a brand name for TETRACYCLINE.

achylia absence of CHYLE.

aciclovir a drug highly active against the herpes simplex virus which causes COLD SORES and

GENITAL HERPES and against the closely similar varicella-zoster virus which causes CHICKENPOX and SHINGLES. Early treatment with the drug, taken by mouth, can greatly reduce the severity of shingles. Brand names are Zovirax and Soothelip,

acid 1 any compound capable of releasing hydrogen ions when dissolved in water.
2 a solution with a hydrogen ion concentration greater than that of pure water.
3 having a pH of less than 7. pH is the common logarithm of the reciprocal of the hydrogen ion concentration.

acidaemia a condition of raised blood acidity. The state in which the pH of the blood has fallen below normal.

acid-base balance the effect of mechanisms that operate to ensure that the body fluids remain nearly neutral, being neither significantly acidic nor alkaline. This balance is maintained, in spite of the acids produced in metabolic processes, by the controlling action of the kidneys, by breathing out increased or decreased quantities of carbon dioxide as required and by the chemical buffering effect of bicarbonate in the blood. See also ACIDOSIS.

acid fast of a stained tissue or organism, retaining the stain even in the presence of acid. Acid-fastness is a feature of certain organisms, such as the tubercle bacillus *Mycobacterium tuberculosis*, that have wax and fat in their cell walls. The fact is used as an aid to identification.

acidic hydrolases enzymes that break down molecules in an acidic environment at an optimum pH of about 5. They include acid phosphatases, lipases, proteases, glycosidases and nucleases. Many of the acid hydrolases are held in LYSOSOMES.

acidophilic 1 readily stained with acid dyes.
2 thriving in an acid environment.

acidosis a serious condition in which the acidity of the blood rises (pH falls). The blood acidity is normally kept within narrow limits by automatic, feedback mechanisms, and acidosis occurs only in extreme and unusual circumstances such as severe untreated DIABETES (when acid ketone bodies are produced) or advanced kidney disease. Also called acidaemia.

acid reflux the cause of the symptom of HEARTBURN. The stomach is protected against strong ACID, but the gullet (OESOPHAGUS) is not.

So when acid regurgitates upwards into the oesophagus, there is a burning pain in the centre of the lower part of the chest. Acid reflux commonly occurs in HIATUS HERNIA.

acid-sensitive ion channels voltage-insensitive protein cell-membrane sub-units which are activated and open when the pH falls below about 7.0. The activation of neuronal acid-sensitive channels can lead to neuronal death by excessive loading of the neurons by calcium. Many other calcium-permeable channels are inhibited as pH falls. Ischaemic tissue such as the surroundings of brain infarcts are at reduced pH.

acinar pertaining to an ACINUS or acini. Grape-shaped or sac-like.

acinus 1 the part of the air passage of the lung beyond each of the smallest (terminal) bronchioles. There are about 12,000 acini in each lung. The lung ALVEOLI arise from the acini.
2 any terminal sac-like process of a compound gland.

acipimox a nicotinic acid derivative drug used in the treatment of certain types of raised blood cholesterol. A brand name is Olbetam.

acitretin 10 a retinoid drug used to treat psoriasis, seborrhoea and icthyosis. A brand name is Neogaston.

Ackee poisoning vomiting sickness of Jamaica. This is caused by ingestion of the unripe fruit of the tree *Blighia sapida* which contains a poison capable of interfering with glucose formation in the liver. This can cause HYPOGLYCAEMIA, vomiting, convulsions and loss of consciousness.

aclasis deformation or abnormal moulding of a structure, such as a bone, during fetal development or growth.

acne acne vulgaris, a common skin disease of adolescence and early adult life, affecting white people and featuring blackheads (COMEDONES), PUSTULES and scarring. It is a disorder of the oil-secreting (SEBACEOUS) glands of the skin originating at puberty when androgens stimulate sebaceous secretion, and normal skin flora, especially *Propionibacterium acnes*, use these triglycerides as nutrition and increase greatly in number. Large populations of *P. acnes* attract lymphocytes and neutrophils to the follicle. Acne is also a feature of CIRRHOSIS of the liver, cyanotic congenital heart disease and excess ANDROGEN production, or androgen treatment, in women. Severe acne is sometimes associated with muscle and joint pain and even joint swelling from fluid collection (effusion). Treatment is by retinoids to combat the aberrant keratinization that causes impaction in the follicles; antibiotics such as tetracyclines to reduce *P. acnes* populations and specifically combat inflammation by their non-antibiotic action; and the use of 585 nanometre pulsed-dye laser light.

Acnecide a brand name for BENZOYLE PEROXIDE in a preparation used to treat ACNE.

Acnegel a brand name for BENZOYL PEROXIDE in a preparation used to treat ACNE.

acne rosacea an obsolescent term for ROSACEA.

Acnidazil a brand name for MICONAZOLE formulated for external use with benzoyl peroxide for the treatment of ACNE.

Acnisal a brand name for SALICYLIC ACID.

aconite a poisonous mixture of alkaloids derived from the roots of the plant *Aconitum napellus*. Also known as Wolf's bane, Monkshood and Friar's cowl. Aconite is no longer used in medicine.

acou- *combining form denoting* hearing. From Greek *akouein*, to hear.

acoustic nerve the short, eighth, cranial nerve connecting each inner ear to the brain and carrying nerve impulses subserving hearing and balance. Also known as the auditory nerve. The acoustic nerve is sometimes the seat of a non-cancerous but dangerous tumour, an ACOUSTIC SCHWANNOMA, which can cause much local damage by compression and which is not readily accessible for removal.

acoustic schwannoma a non-malignant but hardly benign tumour of the cells of the sheath of Schwann on the acoustic nerve. The tumour causes one-sided deafness and tinnitus and eventually expands inwards into the cranial cavity to occupy the space between the cerebellum and the pons of the brainstem (the cerebello-pontine angle). Surgical approach is difficult but untreated growing tumours are liable to prove fatal. Also known as acoustic neuroma or vestibular schwannoma. (Theodor Schwann, 1810–82, German anatomist).

acoustic trauma the often damaging effect of loud noise on the inner ear. The degree of damage is related to the intensity multiplied by the time. A nearby explosion may cause as much damage as years of exposure to noise of lower amplitude. The hair cells in the ORGAN OF CORTI are injured by excessive movement and the higher pitched sounds are the first to be lost.

acquired characteristics features of an organism, such as the human being, arising from environmental influences or bodily functioning, rather than from heredity of genes.

acquired immune deficiency a group of disorders, including acquired AGAMMAGLOBULINAEMIA, protein-losing immunodeficiency, nutritional immunodeficiency and AIDS (ACQUIRED IMMUNE DEFICIENCY SYNDROME) in which the natural resistance to infection is greatly reduced.

acquired immune deficiency syndrome (AIDS) a disease caused by the human immunodeficiency virus (HIV) and transmitted by sexual contact or by blood spread on infected needles and other implements. AIDS is not a specifically homosexual disorder. Rather it is a disease of populations that harbour large numbers of HIV. The virus attacks a particular group of white cells of the immune system (helper T lymphocytes) causing a severe reduction in the ability of the body to resist infection and certain forms of cancer. The resulting recurrent infections, often with organisms not normally causing disease (opportunistic infectors), can usually be treated, but, to date, no wholly effective treatment for the underlying HIV infection has been developed. Combinations of drugs, including protease inhibitors, reverse transcriptase inhibitors, fusion inhibitors and DNA polymerase inhibitors, can, however, greatly prolong life and have virtually converted AIDS from an inevitably fatal, to a potentially serious chronic disease. The condition may involve many different disorders including a form of pneumonia caused by *Pneumocystis carinii*, CYTOMEGALOVIRUS infections, widespread herpes simplex infections, widespread thrush (CANDIDIASIS), KAPOSI'S SARCOMA and other malignancies, and brain damage from direct infection of neurons by HIV. The presence of the AIDS virus can be detected by the ELISA and other tests.

acrania partial or complete absence of the skull bones and sometimes of other head bones at birth. See also ANENCEPHALY.

acridine a dye molecule capable of causing a FRAME-SHIFT MUTATION in DNA by interposing between adjacent base pairs. Acridine orange stains nucleic acid so that under ultraviolet light DNA appears green and RNA appears orange.

acriflavine an orange powder derived from acridine and used, in solution, as an antiseptic for skin cleansing and wound irrigation.

acrivastine an ANTIHISTAMINE drug used in the treatment of allergies. A brand name is Benadryl.

acro- *combining form denoting* outermost, at the tip or extremity. From Greek *akros*, an extremity.

acroagnosia absence of perception of the position of a limb, or even of its existence.

acrocephalosyndactylism a congenital malformation consisting of a pointed head and fusion of the fingers and toes. The condition is also known as Apert's syndrome. (Eugène Apert, French paediatrician, 1868–1940).

acrocephaly see OXYCEPHALY.

acrocyanosis blueness, coldness and sweating of the hands and feet in cold weather, due to spasm of small blood vessels. Acrocyanosis is a feature of RAYNAUD'S DISEASE.

acrodermatitis enteropathica a rare genetic skin inflammation (DERMATITIS), affecting mainly the extremities, with reddening, ulceration and pustule formation. The condition is caused by the inability to absorb zinc from the diet and can be treated by zinc supplements.

acrodynia pink disease. A now rare, severe childhood illness formerly caused by mercury poisoning from teething powders. Acrodynia features pink, itching extremities, sweating, floppiness, loss of appetite, insomnia and low blood pressure. The disease was also caused by local applications of mercury-containing medication.

acromegaly a serious disorder resulting from overproduction of growth hormone by the pituitary gland during adult life, after the growing ends of the bones (the epiphyses) have fused and the normal growth process is complete. The condition is usually the result of a benign tumour of the pituitary gland. There is no change in body height, but gradual enlargement of the jaw, tongue, nose, ribs, hands and feet occurs. There is also CUTIS VERTICIS GYRATA. If excessive growth hormone production occurs before the epiphyses have fused the result is gigantism. Acromegaly is treated by removing the cause.

acromicric dysplasia see MOORE-FEDERMAN SYNDROME.

acromioclavicular joint the joint between the outer end of the collar-bone (clavicle) and the ACROMION process on the shoulder-blade (scapula).

acromion the outermost extremity of the spine of the shoulder-blade. The acromion is joined to the outer tip of the collar bone (clavicle) in the acromioclavicular joint.

acroparaesthesia extreme sensitivity at the tips of the fingers or toes. Tingling or numbness in the extremities. The symptom may be a feature of POLYNEURITIS or of nerve compression.

acrosome a tiny sac or double membrane in the head of a SPERMATOZOON that contains the digestive enzymes needed to break down the protective cell membrane of the egg (OVUM) and allow penetration. Release of these enzymes is called the acrosome reaction.

acrosome stabilizing factor a glycoprotein substance derived from the EPIDIDYMIS that inhibits the release of acrosomal enzymes and may thus prevent fertilization.

acrylamide a substance used in the plastics industry that is toxic to nerve fibres. Inhalation of the vapour from the crystalline substance can cause nerve degeneration and permanent paralysis.

ACTG *abbrev. for* AIDS Clinical Trials Group. This is a large US government-sponsored organisation dedicated to research into the treatment of AIDS.

ACTH adrenocorticotropic HORMONE. This hormone is produced by the pituitary gland, on instructions from the hypothalamus (the part of the brain immediately above the gland) when a stressful situation arises. ACTH is carried by the blood to the adrenal glands and prompts them to secrete the hormone cortisol into the bloodstream. ACTH is sometimes used as medication.

Actifed a brand name for TRIPROLIDINE and PSEUDOEPHEDRINE.

Actilyse a brand name for the fibrin-dissolving (fibrinolytic) TISSUE PLASMINOGEN ACTIVATOR drug ALTEPLASE.

actin a contractile protein in MUSCLE, found in

the thin filaments, to which the myosin cross-bridges bind. Actin filaments are also abundant inside all nucleated cells where they form the cytoskeleton, determining cell shape and, in the case of amoebic cells, cell movement. An actin contractile ring forms around the equator of a dividing cell at the end of MITOSIS and tightens so as to pinch the two daughter cells apart.

actin binding proteins a large collection of different proteins that function by binding to ACTIN as part of the cytoskeleton. They include EF1 in pseudopodia; fascin in stress fibres, microvilli, and acrosomal process; scruin in acrosomal process; villin in microvilli; dematin in the red cell cortical network just under the plasma membrane; fimbrin in microvilli and adhesion plaques; spectrin in cortical networks; dystrophin in muscle cell cortical networks; and filamin in pseudopodia, stress fibres and filopodia.

acting out impulsive, irrational actions that may display previously repressed feelings or emotions or unconscious wishes. The term may be applied to uncontrollable outbursts in children or neurotic adults.

actinic pertaining to radiation from the sun or to the biological effects of sunlight. Public awareness of the dangers of actinic radiation, and especially of its role in the production of BASAL CELL CARCINOMA (rodent ulcer), SQUAMOUS CELL CARCINOMA, MALIGNANT MELANOMA and PTERYGIUM has been growing in recent years and has somewhat diminished enthusiasm for sunbathing.

actinic keratosis local overgrowth and thickening of the EPIDERMIS of the skin caused by sunlight. This condition can progress to a form of skin cancer (SQUAMOUS CELL CARCINOMA) and is usually treated by freezing.

actino- *combining form denoting* light, having rays, radiational. From the Greek *aktinos*, a ray.

actinomycetoma a tumour-like collection of fungus-like bacterial colonies in the tissues, often involving the lower limbs, and caused by ACTINOMYCOSIS. This essentially tropical condition arises from a thorn injury, often to barefoot people, and is sometimes called 'madura foot'.

actinomycin D Dactinomycin, an antibiotic derived from *Streptomyces pavullus* which causes breaks in DNA. This side effect renders it unsuitable as an antibacterial drug, but makes

it useful as an anti-cancer drug. A brand name is Cosmegen Lyovac. There are other actinomycins in the group produced by *Streptomyces chrysomallas*.

actinomycosis a persistent disease caused by filamentous, branching bacteria such as *Actinomyces israelii* whose colonies resemble those of a fungus. The organism exists in the mouth, especially around the teeth and may be transmitted by bites or knuckle injuries by teeth. The disease features multiple abscesses, often around the jaws or in the abdomen or lungs, which discharge thin pus, containing yellow 'sulphur granules'. It has been reported in women fitted with intrauterine contraceptive devices (IUCDs). Treatment is with benzylpenicillin or other antibiotics.

actins filamentary contractile proteins forming the cytoskeleton of cells. Actins contribute to cell shape, cell motility and to some internal cell functions.

action potential the electrical signal propagated in nerve and muscle cells. It consists of a zone of reversal of the normal charge on the membrane so that the outside briefly becomes negative relative to the inside, instead of vice versa. This zone of depolarization, which is caused by the opening of ion channels, then moves along the fibre at a rate very much slower than the speed of normal electrical conduction along a wire. Action potentials operate according to an 'all-or-none' law. They function fully or not at all.

activated cells cells that have changed in response to a stimulus. Examples are macrophages, oocytes and neutrophil polymorphs.

activated charcoal a highly absorbent form of carbon used to absorb gas, to deodorize and to inactivate a number of ingested poisons.

activated protein C resistance an abnormality in the regulation of blood clotting often found in patients with an unexplained THROMBOSIS. It is associated with a mutation in the gene for the clotting factor, Factor V, and may provide an explanation of the common genetic predisposition to thrombosis (thrombophilia).

activated partial thromboplastin time a measurement of the time taken for the clotting system of the blood to produce the clot protein known as fibrin. The time is generally 25 to 39 seconds. This measurement is a general test of the system and is also used to assess the effectiveness of the anticoagulant drug HEPARIN. It may also be used as the basis of a test for ACTIVATED PROTEIN C RESISTANCE.

activation energy the energy needed to form chemical bonds during a chemical reaction or to break existing ones.

Active a brand name for testing strips for blood glucose in the range 0.6 to 33.3 mmol per litre.

active hyperaemia the increase in blood flow though a tissue or organ occurring during, and as a necessary part of, increased metabolic activity.

active immunity immunity to disease resulting from infection with the disease or immunization with a vaccine. In both cases there is active production of ANTIBODIES.

active site 1 the region of an ENZYME to which the substance being affected binds so as to undergo a catalyzed reaction. 2 the localized part of a protein to which a substrate binds.

active transport the movement of dissolved substances across a membrane in the direction opposite to that of normal diffusion. Active transport operates against gradients of chemical concentration, electrical charge of electro-chemical state. It requires the expenditure of energy.

Actrapid a brand name for INSULIN. Both human and porcine varieties are available.

Actuss a brand name for PHOLCODEINE.

acu- *combining form denoting* a needle. From the Latin *acus*, a needle.

acuity keenness of sense perception, especially in relation to vision and hearing.

Acular a brand name for the non-steroidal anti-inflammatory drug KETOROLAC.

Acupan a brand name for the non-opioid pain-killing drug NEFOPAM.

acupressure an offshoot of ACUPUNCTURE in which finger pressure is used instead of needles.

acupuncture a branch of Chinese medicine, now also used by some Western doctors, in which needles are inserted into the skin at certain points to produce ANAESTHESIA and, it is claimed, to treat disease by a process described as 'unblocking' of bodily meridians. These meridians, however, have no physical existence and the process does not appear to have any scientific or logical basis as a form of therapy.

The psychological and suggestional effects of such a procedure may, however, be considerable and the occurrence of temporary changes is to be expected in some patients. There are more substantial grounds for the use of acupuncture as an anaesthetic agent as it is known to cause a release of ENDORPHINS. But it is an unreliable method of inducing anaesthesia and is not used when conventional scientific methods are available. Acupuncture has acquired a reputation as a treatment for headache, especially migraine. A difficulty in testing this is that trials that appear to support the hypothesis cannot easily include comparable sham acupuncture and are thus uncontrolled. See also ALTERNATIVE MEDICINE.

acute short, sharp and quickly over. Acute conditions usually start abruptly, last for a few days and then either settle or become persistent and long-lasting (CHRONIC). From the Latin *acutus*, sharp.

acute abdomen a semi-formal term for a surgical emergency involving the abdominal contents in which the patient is suffering severe pain and often SHOCK. Common causes of acute abdomen include PERITONITIS from ruptured APPENDIX following appendicitis or perforated PEPTIC ULCER, and ruptured spleen or liver following injury. Urgent operative treatment is almost always required.

acute appendicitis see APPENDICITIS.

acute brain syndromes severe confusional states of sudden onset caused by any circumstance that leads to an inadequate supply of oxygenated blood to the brain. Such causes include HEART FAILURE, coronary thrombosis, severe chest infection, toxic states or severe metabolic disorders. There is clouding of consciousness, disorientation, defects of time perception, failure of logic, delirium, hallucinations and often delusions of persecution. The treatment is that of the underlying cause. Full recovery is common.

acute phase proteins a large number of proteins released into the blood by the liver during infections and which exert a wide range of effects on the inflammatory process, on the function of immune cells and on tissue repair. Acute phase proteins appear in the bloodstream in the early stages of an inflammation or tissue injury as a result of the production of CYTOKINES such as INTERLEUKIN-1 and

INTERLEUKIN-6. They include C-REACTIVE PROTEIN, mannose-binding protein, serum amyloid P, fibrinogen, ceruloplasmin, alpha$_1$ antitrypsin, ANGIOTENSIN, haptoglobin and fibronectin.

acute rheumatism see RHEUMATIC FEVER.

acute tubular necrosis a severe kidney disorder featuring patchy damage to the fluid-reabsorbing tubules. Many of the lining cells of the tubules are destroyed and many of the tubules blocked. The condition may be due to inadequate blood supply or to various toxic effects including those of certain drugs such as the aminoglycoside antibiotics. There is a rapid decline in kidney function and patients usually require to be maintained on dialysis while recovery is taking place.

acute yellow atrophy a serious disorder involving widespread liver damage following exposure to toxic substances, such as chloroform, or to liver viruses.

acyl-CoA dehydrogenases enzymes that activate the first stage of the oxidation of fatty acids.

ad- *prefix denoting* to, towards.

Adalat a brand name for NIFEDIPINE. Beta-Adalat also contains the beta-blocker ATENOLOL.

adalimumab a human tumour necrosis factor-alpha monoclonal antibody used to treat severe active RHEUMATOID ARTHRITIS in cases in which treatment with methotrexate fails to produce an adequate response. The antibody binds to TNF-alpha and blocks its interaction with cell surface TNF receptors. This reduces chronic inflammation and cartilage destruction. A brand name is Humira.

Adam's apple the popular name for the voice box (LARYNX) at the upper end of the windpipe (TRACHEA). The larynx is larger and more protuberant in men than in women and contains longer vocal cords, which is why men have deeper voices than women.

ADAM software Animated Dissection of Anatomy for Medicine. A CD-ROM program designed to assist in the learning of anatomy.

Adams-Stokes attacks see STOKES-ADAMS ATTACKS.

ADAM33 an enzyme of the metalloprotease-disintegrin family found mainly on the surface membranes of airway smooth muscle cells. There has been speculation that this enzyme may be involved in the remodelling of airway muscle layers that occurs in severe chronic ASTHMA.

adapalene a retinoid-like drug used externally in the treatment of ACNE. The drug should not be used during pregnancy. A brand name is Differin.

adaptation 1 adjustment of sensitivity, usually in the direction of reduction, as a result of repeated stimulation. 2 the adjustment of an organism, including man, in part or in whole, to changes in environment or to external stress. Adaptation is an essential feature of all living things and the likelihood of survival often depends on how effectively it operates.

adaptation syndrome the psychological and hormonal responses to acute stress, such as severe injury, or to prolonged stress. The immediate shock reaction, featuring release of cortisols and adrenaline, is followed by a phase of increasing adaptation to the injured state and then either by healing or by bodily decline.

ADC see AIDS DEMENTIA COMPLEX.

Adcortyl a brand name of the steroid drug TRIAMCINOLONE.

Adcortyl in Orabase a brand name for TRIAMCINOLONE in an oral base formulation suitable for the treatment of mouth ulcers.

addiction dependence for comfort of mind or body on the repeated use of a drug such as nicotine, alcohol or heroin. In some cases, the addiction is physiological – that is, the use of the drug has led to persistent changes in the way the body functions, so that its absence causes physical symptoms (withdrawal symptoms). In others, the dependence is psychological only. Research on rats has indicated that strong conditioned reflexes are often associated with drug addiction and that these make relapses more likely. The nucleus accumbens, linking the dopamine system with the limbic system appears to be importantly involved in addiction.

Addisonian pernicious anaemia a form of ANAEMIA caused by the failure of the stomach to secrete a necessary factor called the intrinsic factor. As a result the body is unable to absorb vitamin B$_{12}$ and it is the absence of this vitamin that causes the anaemia. Red cells are larger than normal, irregular in shape and size and reduced in number. Untreated pernicious anaemia leads to neurological damage, which can be severe, including SUBACUTE combined degeneration of the spinal cord. Treatment is with hydroxycobalamin injections. (Thomas Addison, English physician, 1793–1860).

Addison's disease a disorder of the adrenal glands leading to a deficient output of cortisol and aldosterone. There is weakness, tiredness, pigmentation of the skin, low blood pressure, intestinal disorders and inability to cope with injury or surgical stress. Treatment is by steroid replacement, usually with hydrocortisone. (Thomas Addison, 1793–1860, English physician).

additive any substance added to something, especially a food, in order to improve or preserve it. Additives are of economic and nutritional importance but some people may display allergic sensitivity to some of them.

addressins components in cell membranes that mediate adhesion to particular molecules on the surfaces of other cells. They function to effect cell-to-cell interactions and to help in the distribution of cells within an organism.

adduction a movement towards the centre line of the body. Muscles which adduct are called adductors. The term derives from the Latin *ad*, to and *ducere*, to draw. Compare ABDUCTION.

adefovir dipivoxil an antiviral drug used to treat chronic HEPATITIS B. A brand name is Hepsera.

adenectomy surgical removal of a GLAND.

adenine a purine base. One of the four key biochemical units from which genes are formed in DNA and by which the two helical halves of the DNA molecule are linked together. Adenine pairs with thymine in DNA, but in RNA it pairs with uracil.

adenine arabinoside ARA-A or vidarabine. An antiviral drug active against several DNA viruses.

adenitis inflammation of a LYMPH NODE or any GLAND. The usage, lymphadenitis, reflects the persistence of the effect of the earlier erroneous belief that lymph nodes were glands.

adeno- *combining form denoting* gland or glandular.

adenoacanthoma a type of cancer (an ADENOCARCINOMA) affecting the lining of the womb (ENDOMETRIUM), in which the normally columnar cells are replaced by flattened (SQUAMOUS) cells.

adenocarcinoma a cancer arising from gland tissue in a lining membrane (EPITHELIUM) and

usually showing the glandular features of the original tissue. Most cancers of the breast and large intestine (COLON) are adenocarcinomas.

Adenocor a brand name for ADENOSINE.

adenohypophysis the front lobe of the PITUITARY GLAND. This is structurally and functionally distinguishable from the rear lobe (posterior pituitary).

adenoid 1 gland-like.
2 one of the ADENOIDS.

adenoidectomy surgical removal of the ADENOIDS. This is a comparatively minor operation in which the adenoid tissue is scraped off the back wall of the nose with an instrument inserted through the mouth.

adenoids collections of overgrown gland-like tissue, present on the back wall of the nose above the tonsils in children, which shrivel and disappear in adolescence or early adult life. The adenoids contain LYMPHOCYTES and are part of the body's defence (immune) system.

adenoma a benign (non-malignant) and relatively common TUMOUR arising from lining tissue that contains glands. The glandular structure is retained in the tumour which may continue to secrete, and often over-produce, the original product.

adenoma sebaceum a feature of TUBEROUS SCLEROSIS. Multiple, small, reddish-yellow, waxy-looking PAPULES appear on the face.

adenomatosis an abnormal overgrowth of, or TUMOUR formation in, two or more of the ENDOCRINE glands, usually the THYROID, the ADRENALS or the PITUITARY.

adenomatous goitre see NODULAR GOITRE.

adenomyoma a benign tumour of smooth muscle and glandular tissue occurring mainly in the womb (UTERUS) and RECTUM.

adenomyosis a benign condition, affecting most often the womb (UTERUS), in which glandular lining tissue occurs within the muscular wall. A form of ENDOMETRIOSIS.

adenopathy any inflammation, abnormal enlargement or other disorder of LYMPH NODES. The term literally means any disease of GLANDS, and lymph nodes are not glands, but common usage restricts the meaning to lymph node disease or affection.

adenosine a purine NUCLEOSIDE consisting of one molecule of adenine and one molecule of d-ribose. It is formed in the body by the enzymatic breakdown of adenosine triphosphate (ATP). Adenosine is a NEUROTRANSMITTER, a HORMONE, and a NEUROMODULATOR. It is also a potent blocking agent for the atrioventricular node of the heart and is used by injection as a drug to correct irregularities in the action of the heart. A brand name is Adenocor.

adenosine deaminase inhibitor a drug that interferes with the action of the enzyme adenosine deaminase necessary for the irreversible conversion of adenosine to inosine. Failure to form inosine leads to abnormalities in purine nucleoside metabolism that are toxic to the cell concerned. This provides the opportunity to use adenosine deaminase inhibitors as anticancer drugs. The very expensive drug pentostatin (Nipent) is used to treat hairy cell leukaemia in adults.

adenovirus early region genes genes that are activated in the early stages of an adenovirus infection and that change the transcription mechanisms of the host cell, and activate host genes that code for metastasis-inhibiting proteins.

adenosine monophosphate (AMP) a derivative of ADENOSINE TRIPHOSPHATE (ATP).

adenosine triphosphate (ATP) a compound found in cells, consisting of the NUCLEOSIDE adenosine attached to three molecules of phosphoric acid. Adenosine triphosphate is the main energy-releasing entity of the cell. While it is being formed from adenosine diphosphate (ADP), ATP accepts energy from the breakdown of fuel molecules. During its breakdown to ADP or AMP it donates the energy to cell functions. As the energy source for the entire body, ATP is constantly being formed and broken down. At rest, a human consumes about 40 Kg of ATP per day. During strenuous exercise the rate of ATP cycling may reach half a Kg per minute.

adenosis excessive growth of GLANDS. The term is also used for any disease of glands.

adenovirus one of a family of over 30 different DNA viruses which infects man, causing colds, sore throat, CONJUNCTIVITIS and sometimes PNEUMONIA and GASTROENTERITIS.

adenylate cyclase the enzyme that converts ADENOSINE TRIPHOSPHATE (ATP) to cyclic AMP.

adenylosuccinase deficiency an AUTOSOMAL RECESSIVE inherited ENZYME deficiency disease that features AUTISM, mental retardation and a tendency to self-mutilation. CT SCANNING shows defective development of the CEREBELLUM.

ADH *abbrev. for* ANTIDIURETIC HORMONE.

adherens junction a point of junction between cells at which ACTIN filaments from inside the cells pass across the adjacent cell membranes. A broad, belt-like adherens junction is called an adhesion belt.

adhesins proteins on the outer surfaces of micro-organisms that allow them to bind to cells they are attacking.

adhesion 1 abnormal union between body surfaces or other tissues. Adhesions do not occur if tissues are healthy and retain intact epithelial coverings. But if the 'non-stick' surfaces are deficient or diseased, the underlying tissue will readily heal together. Adhesions between peritoneum and bowel are common following abdominal surgery. These are the result of failure of physiological removal of fibrin (fibrinolysis) following injury to the mesothelial cell monolayer forming the peritoneum.
2 a fibrous band holding together normally separate bodily parts.

adhesion molecule CD31 a clinically important minor histocompatibility antigen in humans that, when mismatched, has been implicated in GRAFT-VERSUS-HOST DISEASE. This may occur in the recipients of bone marrow from unrelated donors of even apparently identical HLA type.

adiadochokinesia the inability to perform alternating movements, such as rotating a closed fist, at a reasonably rapid rate. Adiadochokinesia is a sign of cerebellar malfunction. A lesser degree of such inability is called dysdiadochokinesia. See also CEREBELLAR ATAXIA.

Adie's pupil an apparently spontaneous abnormality of the pupil of the eye mainly affecting women. One pupil is larger than the other and does not show the normal brisk constriction on exposure to bright light or during near focusing. The condition is not of great medical importance but may, at first, arouse medical concern because of the often serious neurological significance of a fixed dilated pupil. (William John Adie, Australian-born British neurologist, 1886–1935).

Adipine MR a brand name for NIFEDIPINE.

adipo- *combining form denoting* fat.

adipocere a wax-like substance, consisting

mainly of fatty acids, into which the soft tissues of a dead body, buried in moist earth, are converted.

adipocyte a fat cell. A cell that synthesizes and stores neutral fats (triacylglycerols or TRIGLYCERIDES). Human fat is a liquid at body temperature, so adipocytes are normally filled with oil. Adipocytes develop from adipoblasts, which derive from fibroblasts.

adiponecrosis neonatorum localized areas of death of fat cells occurring under the skin of healthy large babies born after prolonged labour.

adipose tissue fat cells held together, in large masses, by delicate connective tissue. Adipose tissue is both an insulant and a long-term fuel store, in which food in excess of requirements is converted to neutral fat (see TRIGLYCERIDE) and deposited. The term is derived from the Latin *adeps*, lard.

adiposis dolorosa a rare form of OBESITY in which the fat deposits under the skin are painful and tender. The condition is also known as neurolipomatosis.

adiposogenital dystrophy see FROHLICH'S SYNDROME.

adipsin an enzyme secreted by fat cells, and also present in the Schwann cells of nerve fibres, that is thought to regulate fat metabolism. It acts on free lipoproteins and is concerned with fat oxidation. Its levels are markedly reduced in genetically obese mice. The full function of adipsin remains unclear.

Adizem a brand name for DILTIAZEM.

Adizem-XL a brand name for DILTIAZEM in a controlled-release formulation.

adjuvant 1 any substance added to a drug to increase its effect.
2 any substance which, added to an ANTIGEN, non-specifically increases its power to stimulate the production of antibodies (see ANTIBODY).

Adlerian theory a school of psychological thought which maintains that much of our behaviour is a response to subconscious efforts to compensate for inferiority. (Alfred Adler, German psychiatrist, 1870–1937).

ADMS *abbrev. for* Assistant Director of Medical Services.

adnexa adjoining parts of the body. The adnexa of the eyes are the lacrimal glands, the eyelids, and the lacrimal drainage system. The uterine adnexa are the FALLOPIAN TUBES and the OVARIES. The term is derived from the Latin *annexere*, to tie on.

A DNA one of the three forms of DNA. This form is found in DNA gels with relatively little water. It is a right-hand helix with about 11 bases per turn.

ADNS *abbrev. for* Assistant Director of Nursing Services.

adolescence the period of life from PUBERTY to maturity.

ADP adenosine diphosphate. See ADENOSINE TRIPHOSPHATE.

adrenal apoplexy acute catastrophic failure of the adrenal glands often resulting from massive bleeding into the glands with destruction of gland tissue. The condition is usually a response to severe bodily injury or systemic infections but may result from heart disease, acute alcoholic poisoning, anticoagulation treatment or coagulation disorders. In adrenal apoplexy the output of cortisol is very low, far lower than the shock situation requires, and the danger to the patient correspondingly high. In those who survive, long-term hormone replacement therapy is necessary.

adrenal cortex the outer zone of the ADRENAL GLAND that secretes CORTISOL, sex hormones (ANDROGENS) and ALDOSTERONE. See also ADRENAL MEDULLA.

adrenal cortical insufficiency failure of the ADRENAL CORTEX to secrete adequate hormones. This may be due to congenital deficiency of the enzymes necessary for the synthesis of the adrenal hormones, or to disease of the gland, as in ADDISON'S DISEASE. The condition is treated by long-term steroid replacement therapy.

adrenal glands the small internally secreting (ENDOCRINE) organs which sit like triangular caps one on top of each KIDNEY (hence the name). Each adrenal has two distinct parts, the inner core, which produces ADRENALINE, and an outer layer (the cortex) which produces various steroid hormones. Formerly known as suprarenal glands, which, of course, means the same thing.

adrenal gland hyperplasia see CONGENITAL ADRENAL HYPERPLASIA.

adrenaline epinephrine, a HORMONE secreted by the inner part of the ADRENAL GLANDS. It is produced when unusual efforts are required. It speeds up the heart, increases the rate and ease of breathing, raises the blood pressure, deflects blood from the digestive system to the muscles, mobilizes the fuel glucose and causes a sense of alertness and excitement. It has been described as the hormone of 'fright, fight and flight'. Adrenaline is available for use as a drug. Also known, especially in USA, as epinephrine.

adrenal inhibitors drugs used to treat overactivity of the adrenal cortex that causes hypercortisolism and primary aldosteronism. An example is trilostane (Modrenal).

adrenal medulla the inner part of the ADRENAL GLAND that secretes the hormones ADRENALINE and noradrenaline. The secreting cells are called chromaffin cells. See also ADRENAL CORTEX.

adrenal stimulating hormones drugs used to treat adrenal insufficiency. An example is tetracosactide (Synacthen).

adrenal virilism the appearance of male characteristics in a female as a result of excessive production of male sex hormones by the adrenal gland. This may cause a form of PSEUDOHERMAPHRODITISM.

adrenarche the changes in the outer layer of the adrenal gland that occur at puberty, with the production of male sex hormones (androgens) in both sexes that bring about some of the external sexual characteristics and the prompting of libido.

adrenergic having effects similar to those of ADRENALINE. Drugs with adrenaline-like action are called adrenergic. A nerve which releases noradrenaline (a substance closely related to adrenaline) at its endings to pass on its impulses to other nerves, or to muscle fibres, is described as an adrenergic nerve.

adrenergic-blocking drugs alpha-adrenergic receptors are in the muscle walls of arteries. Stimulation of these cause the arteries to narrow. Blockage will cause the arteries to widen. Beta$_1$ adrenergic receptors are in the heart. Stimulation causes an increase in heart rate and force. Beta$_2$ adrenergic receptors are in the muscles of the BRONCHI and of the arteries, in both of which stimulation causes relaxation. Blocking drugs that block both fl$_1$ and fl$_2$ slow the heart and cause constriction of the air passages and the arteries. This can be dangerous to asthmatics. Some beta-blockers are relatively selective for the heart and are less likely to constrict the air passages. See also ALPHA-ADRENOCEPTOR BLOCKING DRUGS.

adrenergic neurone blockers drugs used to treat hypertension. An example is guanethidine (Ismelin).

adreno- *combining form denoting* the adrenal gland.

adrenocorticotrophic causing stimulation of the outer layer of the adrenal gland and promoting secretion of the adrenal cortical hormones.

adrenoceptor see BETA-ADRENOCEPTOR.

adrenogenital syndrome now called congenital adrenal hyperplasia, this condition is due to various inherited enzyme defects, such as 21-hydroxylase defect, that interfere with the production of STEROIDS by the adrenals. The low blood steroid levels causes the PITUITARY gland to send out large quantities of the adrenal stimulating hormone ACTH and this results in an abnormally high output of male sex hormones, with virilization at birth and male sexual precocity.

adrenoleukodystrophy an X-linked recessive peroxisome disorder affecting the adrenal glands and the white matter of the central nervous system. The disease features the accumulation of very long-chain fatty acids causing progressive dysfunction of these tissues by demyelinization. The disease usually manifests itself between the ages of 4 and 8 years and often leads to total disability within two years. Adult forms occur but are rare.

adrenolytic drug therapy the use of a drug to reduce the output of hormones from the adrenal glands, in particular the use of the 11-beta-hydroxylase inhibitor, metyrapone, to cut CORTISOL production in CUSHING'S SYNDROME.

Adriamycin doxorubicin. An anticancer drug which acts by interfering with cell division.

adsorption the process by which a substance, such as a gas or dissolved solid, is attracted to, and adheres to, a surface.

adultery voluntary sexual intercourse between a married person and a person who is not the legal spouse. For good reasons, adultery has generally been condemned. It has ethical, theological and legal implications. In some cultures adultery still carries a death penalty.

adult respiratory distress syndrome a severe form of failure of lung function in which the tiny air sacs are damaged and become flooded with a fluid containing protein. There is severe breathlessness and a dangerous reduction in the supply of oxygen to the blood.

advanced trauma life support program
a formal set of procedures recommended for use by doctors dealing with severely injured people or those with catastrophic bleeding from disease. One of the central factors in the program is the treatment of shock from reduced blood volume by the immediate infusion of fluids.

advancement surgical detachment of one end of a muscle or tendon, and its reattachment at a position in front of its normal site, so as to alter or strengthen its action. When the muscle end is moved backwards, this is called recession.

adventitia the outer covering or layer of an organ, especially a blood vessel.

adventitious 1 accidentally acquired or added by chance.
2 occurring in an unusual place or in an irregular manner.

AED *abbrev. for* AUTOMATED EXTERNAL DEFIBRILLATOR.

Aedes a genus of mosquito of which the best know species is *A. aegypti*, which transmits the organisms causing YELLOW FEVER and DENGUE.

aero- *combining form denoting* air or gas.

aeroallergen airborne particles, especially tree and grass pollens, that can induce allergic responses, such as hay fever (ALLERGIC RHINITIS) in sensitized people.

aerobe an organism, especially a bacterium, that requires oxygen or air to live. Some bacteria are ANAEROBIC.

aerobic 1 of a process that requires gaseous oxygen.
2 of an organism that is able to live only in the presence of oxygen. Compare anaerobic.
3 relating to aerobics or AEROBIC EXERCISE.

aerobic exercise a system of physical exercising in which the degree of exertion is such that it can be maintained for long periods without undue breathlessness. The object of aerobic exercise is to increase the efficiency of the heart and lungs and their ability to supply oxygen to the tissues.

Aerocrom a brand name for CROMOGLYCATE.

aerodontalgia tooth pain associated with a marked change in atmospheric pressure, as in high altitude flying.

embolism see AIR EMBOLISM.

Aerolin Autohaler a brand name for an inhaler containing a preparation of SALBUTAMOL.

aeromedicine the study of any medical disorder caused by or made worse by flight in aircraft. The study of the techniques of evacuation of sick or injured by air. See also AEROSPACE MEDICINE.

Aeromonas hydrophilia a VIBRIO-like organism that contaminates water and often causes traveller's diarrhoea. It may also infect wounds and cause SEPTICAEMIA.

aerophagy air swallowing. This is common in people with indigestion whose efforts to bring up wind eventually result in the swallowing of sufficient air to produce a belch. Aerophagy is common in people with peptic ulcers or gallstones.

aerosol a suspension of very small droplets of a liquid or particles of a solid, in air. A range of drugs can be given in aerosol form for inhalation. Many sufferers from ASTHMA rely heavily on inhalers or aerosol dispensers.

aerospace medicine the branch of medicine dealing with the physical and psychological effects and implications of flying and space travel, including those of excessive accelerations, weightlessness, isolation and zero gravity.

aerotitis a general term for symptoms and disorders arising in the middle ears from changes in external pressure. Aerotitis includes the effects of changes in barometric pressure as in aircraft flights, and, by analogy, changes in water pressure experienced by divers.

Aesculapius the Greek mythological son of Apollo. Aesculapius was the God of medicine. His symbol was the snake twined round a staff – now the universal symbol of medicine. His daughters were Hygeia and Therapia, representing, respectively, preventive medicine and medical treatment.

aetiology the cause of a disease. This may involve many factors, including susceptibility arising from a hereditary tendency or genetic cause, environmental factors, previous related illness, unwise or unhealthy lifestyle, exposure to infective agents, and so on. The term is derived from the Greek *aitia*, a cause and *logos*, a discourse. Compare PATHOGENESIS.

afebrile having a normal temperature. The term is usually applied to a patient who has been fevered or who might be expected to be.

affect mood or emotion. The word is often used to describe the external signs of emotion, as perceived by another person.

affection any disorder or disease of the body.

affective pertaining to mood or emotion.

affective disorders abnormalities of mood or emotion, especially DEPRESSION, MANIA, and the MANIC-DEPRESSIVE or bipolar disorder.

affective functions the brain functions concerned with the emotions, especially those of fear, pleasure, gratification of all kinds, sexuality and jealousy. Affective functions are centered in the most primitive parts of the brain, especially the limbic area which we have in common with many of the other animals.

afferent directed toward a central organ or part, as in the case of sensory nerves that carry impulses to the spinal cord and brain.

afferent neurone a nerve cell whose body lies outside the central nervous system and which conveys information to the CNS from sensory receptors at the periphery.

affinity the strength of binding between a receptor, such as an ANTIGEN binding site on an antibody, and a LIGAND, such as an EPITOPE on an antigen.

afibrinogenaemia a disorder of blood clotting due to a genetically induced absence of the fibrin precursor FIBRINOGEN in the blood. There is prolonged bleeding time as the blood is almost incapable of clotting. Bleeding can be controlled by donated fibrinogen present in CRYOPRECIPITATE.

aflatoxins poisonous fungal products produced by *Aspergillus flavus* which grows on peanuts and grains stored in damp conditions. Aflatoxins act by binding to enzymes so that cell metabolism is blocked. If the fungus is eaten by cattle, the toxins can be released in the milk. Aflatoxins are believed to be a cause of primary liver cancer in people, especially those who have had HEPATITIS B.

AFOM *abbrev. for* Associate of the Faculty of Occupational Medicine.

African sleeping sickness see TRYPANOSOMIASIS.

afterbirth the PLACENTA, the umbilical cord and the ruptured membranes which surrounded the FETUS before birth. These parts are expelled from the womb (UTERUS) within an hour or two of birth.

after-effect a delayed effect of some physiological or psychological stimulus.

after-image a visual negative impression of a bright object or light, which persists for a few seconds after the gaze is shifted or the eyes closed. Persistence of a positive image after moving the eyes implies a potentially serious neurological defect.

after-pains pains similar to, but less severe than, those of labour, felt during the few days after childbirth as the uterus contracts to return to its normal size.

agalactia absence of secretion of milk following childbirth.

agammaglobulinaemia complete absence of the normal blood gamma globulin proteins. The gamma globulins are IMMUNOGLOBULINS (ANTIBODIES) their absence leads to a dangerous susceptibility to infection – immune deficiency.

agar a seaweed extract, sometimes called agar-agar, much used in bacteriological laboratories because it forms a convenient gel for the suspension of nutrient culture material, such as blood or broth, on which micro-organisms can be grown in an incubator.

ageing the gradual accumulation of minor bodily injuries or degenerations often associated with a gradual decrease in functional capacity, that affects all human beings, to a greater or lesser degree, after middle age.

ageism in medicine discrimination in the selection or provision of treatment on the grounds of age.

agenesis absence of an organ or part as a result of failure of development in the early stages. The drug THALIDOMIDE caused agenesis of the limbs.

agent orange a defoliant preparation containing the very toxic heterocyclic hydrocarbon DIOXIN. Agent orange was widely used in the Vietnam war and is thought to have been the cause of many cases of cancer and of congenital malformations among the exposed population.

age-related macular degeneration (AMD, ARMD) a disorder affecting the central and most important part of the RETINA in elderly people and causing progressive loss of central vision. Peripheral vision is retained. AMD may be dry or wet. The dry form is due to degenerative changes in the tissues under the retina; the wet form is caused by the development of a CHOROIDAL NEOVASCULAR MEMBRANE which leaks fluid under the retina with progressive destruction of the rods and cones and connecting nerves. Mutation of the gene for complement factor H is an important risk factor. A proportion of cases are thought to be attributable to cigarette smoking. Antioxidant vitamin supplements slightly reduce the risk. The anti-angiogenic drug anecortave acetate, injected close to the posterior sclera, appears to be of value. Progress of the condition can sometimes be stopped by laser burns to seal the leakage, but established disciform degeneration is irremediable, short of MACULAR TRANSLOCATION. See also VASCULAR ENDOTHELIAL GROWTH FACTOR.

age roles certain characteristic patterns of behaviour expected of people of different ages. Age roles, once of central importance, and marked in their transitional stages by formal rites of passage, have become less prominent in modern industrialized society.

agglutination the clumping and sticking together of normally free cells or bacteria or other small particles so as to form visible aggregates. Agglutination is one of the ways in which ANTIBODIES operate. From the Latin *ad*, to and *glutinare*, to glue.

agglutinin a substance that causes cells or other particles to clump together and, usually, to lose their former properties. 'Warm' agglutinins function at normal body temperatures; 'cold' agglutinins do so at lower temperatures. Agglutinins can cause severe ANAEMIA.

agglutinogen an ANTIGEN that stimulates the production of a substance that induces agglutination (an agglutinin).

aggrastat an anticoagulant drug used for the prevention of heart attacks in patients with unstable ANGINA PECTORIS. A brand name is Tirofiban. See SAW-SCALED VIPER VENOM.

aggrecan an extracellular PROTEOGLYCAN that forms exceptionally large aggregates giving cartilage its particular gel-like properties and resistance to deformation.

aggregation factor a protein that forms cross links between the cell membranes of different cells to bind them together to form tissues.

aggression feelings or acts of hostility. Abnormal aggression is often associated with emotional deprivation in childhood, head injury, or brain disease, such as tumour, excessive alcohol intake or the use of drugs such as amphetamines (amfetamines).

agitation a state of mind, usually due to anxiety or tension, which causes obvious restlessness.

agnathia absence of the jaw.

agnosia a disorder of the 'association' areas of the brain, in which the person cannot correctly interpret sensory input. Agnosia commonly follows STROKE.

agonal relating to the events occurring in the last moments of life, such as the cessation of breathing or the heartbeat.

agonist 1 a molecule, such as a HORMONE, NEUROTRANSMITTER or drug, that attaches (binds) to a cell receptor site to produce an effect on the cell. Many drugs are agonists having an effect similar or identical to natural body agonists. Other drugs act on the receptor in a blocking role and are antagonists. An antagonist is a molecule that interferes with or prevents the action of the agonist. 2 a contracting muscle that is opposed by contraction of another associated muscle, the antagonist.

agony 1 intense physical or mental pain. 2 the struggle that sometimes precedes death.

agoraphobia an abnormal fear of open spaces or of being alone or in public places. Agoraphobia may be so severe that the sufferer refuses to leave his or her own home and becomes permanently house-bound. It is the commonest of the phobias. The term derives from the Greek *agora*, an open assembly place or market and *phobia*, fear or horror.

agranulocytosis a condition in which the white cells of the blood are not being produced in adequate quantity by the bone marrow. This is most commonly caused as a toxic side effect on the bone marrow of various drugs such as the sulphonamides, the thiouracil derivatives, PENICILLIN, CHLORPROMAZINE, CHLORPROPAMIDE, PHENINDIONE, AMIDOPYRINE and CHLOROTHIAZIDE. Because of the deficiency or absence of protective white cells, there is severe sore throat, fever, TOXAEMIA and sometimes SEPTICAEMIA. The condition may be fatal.

agraphia acquired inability to exercise the mental processes necessary for writing. There is no disorder of hand or eye function or coordination. In right-handed and many left-handed people, agraphia results from damage in the left parietal lobe of the brain, the part concerned with language.

agrin a protein released by motor neurons that brings about the close aggregation of acetylcholine receptors on muscle cells.

ague a burning fever with hot and cold spells and severe shivering or rigor when the temperature is rising, as is experienced in MALARIA.

AGXT *abbrev. for* alanine glyoxalate aminotransferase, an ENZYME necessary for the metabolism in the liver of the amino acid alanine. The gene that codes for this protein is on the long arm of chromosome number 2. Mutations of this gene results in increased oxalate in the urine with kidney stones and even fatal kidney failure. Prenatal genetic diagnosis is possible.

ahaptoglobinaemia a genetically-induced absence of haptoglobin, one of the blood serum proteins.

AID *abbrev. for* ARTIFICIAL INSEMINATION by an anonymous donor. Compare AIH.

AIDA system *abbrev. for* Automated Insulin Dosage Advisor. This is an experimental computer expert system used to determine optimum insulin dosage for people with DIABETES MELLITUS. Further development is required before such systems can safely be used in clinical practice.

AIDS *acronym for* the ACQUIRED IMMUNE DEFICIENCY SYNDROME.

AIDS-associated malignancies cancers that are caused, promoted or encouraged by AIDS. They include KAPOSI'S SARCOMA, non-HODGKIN'S LYMPHOMA, multiple MYELOMATOSIS, SEMINOMA and brain cancer.

AIDS dementia complex a feature of certain cases of AIDS in which there is so much direct damage to brain cells by HIV that DEMENTIA occurs. The condition occurs in some 20% of people with untreated AIDS in the late stages. The drug ZIDOVUDINE appears to be capable of greatly reducing the likelihood of this effect. Other anti-AIDS drugs may be less useful in preventing ADC.

AIDS enteropathy a form of MALABSORPTION suffered by some people with AIDS. The small intestine lining shows blunting of the villi and a reduction in the rate of reproduction of lining cells. The condition is probably caused by invasion by HIV or by a general immune system dysfunction. About a quarter of all the body's lymphatic tissue is in the intestine.

AIDS phobia a morbid fear, unsupported by any clear evidence, that one is suffering from AIDS. All the features of HYPOCHONDRIASIS are present but with intense concentration on AIDS. Various normal body functions and minor symptoms and signs are interpreted as proof of the presence of the disease.

AIDS-related complex (ARC) a syndrome affecting HIV positive people. There is generalized enlargement of lymph nodes, which contain HIV, vague illness, fever, night sweats, loss of appetite and weight, diarrhoea and THRUSH in the mouth (oral CANDIDIASIS). ARC tends to progress to the fully developed ACQUIRED IMMUNE DEFICIENCY SYNDROME (AIDS).

AIDS-related malignancies see AIDS-associated malignancies.

AIH *abbrev. for* ARTIFICIAL INSEMINATION with semen obtained from the husband or partner.

ainhum fissuring in the fold between the toes or fingers followed by the development of a constricting band around the base of the digit, usually the little toe, which eventually leads to spontaneous amputation. The condition is fairly common in Africa.

air the mixture of gases forming the atmosphere of the earth. It consists of about 78% nitrogen, 21% oxygen, 0.1% argon, 0.03% carbon dioxide and smaller proportions of rare gases and ozone. A continuing adequate supply of oxygen is essential to life.

air bag injuries damage to the body sustained by vehicle air bags which inflate at an almost explosive rate in order to provide protection. Ocular injuries and limb fractures have been described. The distance from the body to the steering-wheel appears to be a critical factor in determining injuries from air bags.

air embolism, bubbles of air in the circulating blood, which cause blockage of small arteries, thereby cutting off supply to important areas, such as parts of the brain.

air hunger deep and rapid gasping respiration of the kind that occurs in severe DIABETIC ACIDOSIS and coma.

Airomir a brand name for an inhaler containing a preparation of SALBUTAMOL.

air sickness a form of MOTION SICKNESS experienced during air travel.

airway 1 the passages from the nose and mouth down to the air sacs in the lungs, by way of which air enters and leaves the body.
2 a curved plastic air tube often used by

anaesthetist to prevent the tongue from falling back and obstructing breathing.

airway hyper-reactivity the strong tendency, in people with ASTHMA, for the air passages to undergo a sudden and abnormal degree of narrowing under the influence of various stimuli such as inhaled pollen grains or house mite droppings, changes of temperature, emotional upset or exercise.

akathisia the inability to sit quietly because of uncontrollable movements caused by drugs, especially the phenothiazine derivatives (see PHENOTHIAZINE DRUGS) used to treat mental disorders.

akinesia loss of the power of voluntary movement. Paralysis of the motor function.

Aknemin a brand name for MINOCYCLINE.

alalia loss of the power of speech.

alariasis an intestinal fluke infestation with *Alaria americana* believed to be acquired by eating raw frogs legs or preparing frogs legs for cooking.

alastrim a mild form of SMALLPOX. Happily, smallpox has been eradicated – an event unique in medical history – and the name is of academic interest only.

albendazole a drug used to get rid of round-worms, hookworms and other worm parasites and to treat HYDATID DISEASE. The drug is on the WHO official list.

Albers-Schonberg disease see OSTEOPETROSIS.

albinism congenital absence of the normal body colouring pigment MELANIN. This is formed from tyrosine by the action of an enzyme tyrosinase present in cells called melanocytes. There are two kinds of albinism, tyrosinase positive and tyrosinase negative, due to mutations in different GENES that are not ALLELES. Albinism is an AUTOSOMAL RECESSIVE inheritance. Because the two mutations are on unrelated genes, people HETEROZYGOUS for both of the abnormal genes have normal colouring. For the same reason, two albino parents do not necessarily have albino children. Tyrosinase negative people are completely free of pigment, have pure white hair, pink-white skin and blue eyes and usually have visual problems. Tyrosinase positive people are less severely affected. Albinos often have defective eyesight from pigment deficiency in the eyes, and usually suffer from NYSTAGMUS.

albino a person with a genetic defect causing absence of the normal body pigment, MELANIN, which gives colour to the hair, eyes and skin. The gene responsible is recessive and the parents usually have normal colouring. The term derives from the Latin *albus*, white. See ALBINISM.

albumen 1 a nutritive substance surrounding a developing EMBRYO, as in the white of an egg. **2** ALBUMIN.

albumin a protein, soluble in water, synthesized in the liver and present in the blood PLASMA. Albumin, the most abundant blood protein, concentrates the blood and attracts water, thereby maintaining the circulating blood volume. Compare GLOBULINS.

albuminuria albumin in the urine. This usually indicates kidney disease such as GLOMERULONEPHRITIS or the NEPHROTIC SYNDROME. In orthostatic albuminuria, albumin is present only after the person has stood for a long time and is absent from the early morning urine. This is not considered dangerous.

albumose of a class of albuminous substances formed by the action of digestive enzymes on proteins.

Albustix a brand name for a urine dip strip test for ALBUMIN.

alclometasone a moderately strong CORTICOSTEROID drug used externally in the treatment of inflammatory skin disorders. A brand name is Modrasone.

Alcobon a brand name for the antifungal drug FLUCYTOSINE in intravenous form.

alcohol a colourless volatile liquid obtained by fermenting sugars or starches with yeast and used as a solvent, a skin cleaner and hardener, and as an intoxicating drink. Also known as ethyl alcohol or ethanol.

alcohol forensic tests tests based on alcohol breakdown products used to reveal recent drinking both in the short term (hours) or the longer term (several months). Levels of ethyl glucuronide in urine or blood reveal drinking after 1 to 5 days; phosphatidyl ethanol levels reveal drinking after one to three weeks; and the combined levels of four fatty acid ethyl esters in hair provide evidence for up to several months after drinking.

alcoholic 1 pertaining to alcohol. **2** containing alcohol.

3 a person who habitually consumes alcoholic drinks to excess or who is addicted to alcohol to the detriment of health. A person suffering from ALCOHOLISM.

alcoholism **1** psychophysiological dependence on ALCOHOL with compulsive consumption of alcohol.
2 damage to the stomach lining, liver, nervous system, heart or voluntary muscles caused by prolonged exposure to high blood levels of alcohol.

alcohology the study of the nature and management of alcohol abuse.

alcohol withdrawal syndrome a group of symptoms and signs that develop within 6–24 hours of taking the last drink in a person suffering from ALCOHOLISM. They include agitation, anxiety, tremors, loss of appetite, nausea, vomiting, sweating, insomnia, disorientation, grand mal seizures and delirium tremens. Treatment involves sedation, counselling, reassurance and social support. Benzodiazepine drugs are currently favoured. Attention is given to nutrition and especially to vitamin B deficiencies. PSYCHOTROPIC ANALGESIC NITROUS OXIDE has been used to good effect in many patients.

alcuronium a neuromuscular blocking drug with an effect similar to that of curare, used by anaesthetists as a non-depolarizing muscle relaxant. The drug is on the WHO official list.

Aldactide a brand name for HYDROFLUMETHIAZIDE with SPIRONOLACTONE.

Aldactone a brand name for SPIRONOLACTONE.

Aldazine a brand name for THIORIDAZINE.

Aldecin a brand name for BECLOMETHAZINE.

aldehyde a product of dehydrogenated (metabolized) alcohol, hence the name. Aldehydes cause most of the toxic effects of bibulous overindulgence (hangover).

aldehyde dehydrogenase inhibitors drugs used as adjuncts in the treatment of alcoholism. An example is disulfiram (Antabuse).

aldesleukin an INTERLEUKIN 2 drug made by genetic engineering. A brand name is Proleukin.

Aldomet a brand name for METHYLDOPA.

Aldomide a brand name for LODOXAMINE.

aldosterone one of the STEROID hormones produced by the outer part of the adrenal gland. Aldosterone is concerned with the control of salt and water loss in the urine.

aldosterone inhibitors drugs used to treat refractory oedema resulting from abnormally raised aldosterone levels and to help in the diagnosis and management of CUSHING'S SYNDROME. An example is metyrapone (Metopirone).

aldosteronism the condition caused by excessive secretion of the adrenal HORMONE aldosterone. It features muscle weakness, high blood pressure (HYPERTENSION), ALKALOSIS, excessive urinary output and thirst.

Aldrich syndrome a sex-linked RECESSIVE bleeding disorder of children featuring DERMATITIS, OTITIS MEDIA, a reduction in blood platelets (THROMBOCYTOPENIA) with intestinal bleeding and black stools and a deficiency of immune GLOBULINS. (Robert Anderson Aldrich, American paediatrician, b. 1917).

alemtuzumab a monoclonal antibody drug used to treat leukaemia. A brand name is Mabcampath.

alendronate a drug used in the prevention and treatment of post-menopausal OSTEOPOROSIS. A brand name is Fosamax.

Alepam a brand name for OXAZEPAM.

Aleppo boil a form of LEISHMANIASIS. A slow-healing ulcer caused by the single-cell parasite *Leishmania tropica*. It is also called Delhi boil, Baghdad boil or oriental sore.

aleukaemic leukaemia a kind of CANCER of the blood, in which abnormal white blood cells are produced in the bone marrow, but do not appear in the blood.

Alexander technique a method of therapy for various physical and psychological disorders said to be caused by faulty posture. The pupil is taught how to break habits of slouching and adopt a new and better bearing, thereby, it is claimed, being relieved of such problems as insomnia, lethargy and chronic ill health.

alexia word blindness. The inability to read, occurring as a result of brain damage, usually from arterial disease. Alexia is common after stroke affecting the left side of the brain with damage to the fibres connecting the visual part of the brain and the part concerned with the function of reading in the left angular gyrus. The word is derived from the Greek *a*, not and *legein*, to speak.

alfacalcidol a synthetic form of vitamin D used to treat low blood calcium and bone softening (OSTEOMALACIA) caused by kidney disease. Brand names are Alfad and One-alpha.

Alfad a brand name for ALFACALCIDOL.

alfentanil a narcotic analgesic drug used before and during anaesthesia. A brand name is Rapifen.

alfuzocin a uroselective alpha-adrenergic blocker drug used to treat benign enlargement of the prostate gland. A brand name is Xatral.

algesia pain. See also ANALGESIC. The term derives from the Greek *algos*, pain.

Algicon a brand name for a mixture of antacid preparations containing Aluminium hydroxide and magnesium carbomate.

algology the study of the nature, causes and management of pain.

alfentanil a narcotic-type pain-killing drug. A brand name is Rapifen.

alfuzosin an alpha-blocker drug used in the treatment of prostate enlargement. Brand names are Xatral and Xatral XL.

algid cold, clammy skin.

algid malaria a dangerous form in which the parasites in the blood cause a condition like bacterial SHOCK, with low blood pressure and cold skin. Urgent treatment to combat shock with transfusions and DOPAMINE, and energetic attack on the infecting malarial parasites, are necessary.

alginic acid an ANTACID drug used in the treatment of stomach ulcer and indigestion. When supplied in combination with other drugs brand names are Gastrocote, Gaviscon and Topal.

algodystrophy a syndrome featuring OSTEOPOROSIS around joints, pain, swelling, excessive sweating, flushing and blanching of the skin and then atrophy, and loss of joint movement. It is probably due to disturbance of the sympathetic nervous system with interference with the small blood vessels. The condition usually clears up within a few months but there may be residual joint contractures.

algometer an instrument for measuring the threshold of perception of touch or pressure stimuli and the strength of such stimuli needed for the perception of pain.

alienation 1 a state of estrangement from, or inability to relate to, other people, concepts, social norms, or even oneself. Alienation, especially of the latter type, may be a feature of psychiatric disorder, but equally it may result from an accurate perception of the social environment.

2 a feeling that one's thoughts and emotions are under the control of someone else or that others have access to one's mind. One of the symptoms of SCHIZOPHRENIA.

alimentary canal the digestive tract, extending from the mouth to the anus, in which food is converted by enzymes to a form suitable for absorption and through which the processed material passes into the bloodstream. The canal includes the PHARYNX, the OESOPHAGUS, the STOMACH and the small and large INTESTINES.

alimentation the act or process of giving or receiving nourishment.

aliphatic of any organic compound in which all carbon atom chains are arranged linearly rather than in rings, or that have rings that do not have the stability of benzene rings (SEE AROMATIC). All non-cyclic organic compounds are aliphatic and cyclic aliphatic compounds are called alicyclic compounds.

alicyclic of any organic compound with closed rings of carbon atoms but that still has aliphatic properties.

aliquot 1 a sample quantity of a larger amount of a substance.

2 an amount that is an exact divisor of the whole quantity of a substance.

alisphenoid the greater wing of the SPHENOID BONE.

alkalaemia an increase in the alkalinity of the blood above normal. ALKALOSIS. A rise in the pH of the blood.

alkaline phosphatases ENZYMES with an optimum pH in the alkaline range, that break down phosphate bonds in compounds. They are widely distributed in the body, and are released into the blood in large quantites in a number of conditions including obstructive JAUNDICE and certain bone diseases. This forms the basis of a common biochemical test.

alkaloids a group of bitter tasting plant poisons, many of which are of medical importance. The alkaloids, which include nicotine, strychnine, morphine, codeine, atropine, caffeine and quinine, have powerful actions on the body. Alkaloids are small, complex, nitrogen-containing molecules often produced by plants as an evolutionary survival characteristic in an environment containing herbivorous animals.

alkalosis an abnormal degree of alkalinity of the blood, usually due to loss of acid by prolonged vomiting or to hysterical over-breathing with abnormal loss of carbon dioxide.

alkaptonuria a genetic disease in which a gene mutation on chromosome 3 results in a defective enzyme that leads to the accumulation of a coloured polymer molecule homogentisic acid. This binds to the COLLAGEN of cartilage, making it brittle and easily worn away. The result is a form of OSTEOARTHRITIS. In alkaptonuria, the urine turns black on exposure to light or alkali.

Alkeran a brand name for the anticancer drug MELPHALAN.

alkylating agent a drug which interferes with DNA synthesis by adding an alkyl group and preventing the uncoiling of the strands. This halts DNA replication so that cells cannot reproduce, an effect useful in the treatment of cancer. Drugs in this group include nitrogen mustard, CHLORAMBUCIL, CYCLOPHOSPHAMIDE, BUSULPHAN (busulfan) and thiotepa.

allantoin a drug used externally in the treatment of ACNE, usually in combination with other drugs.

allantois a membranous sac that develops from the hindgut in the EMBRYO and takes part in the formation of the umbilical cord and the PLACENTA.

Allegron a brand name for NORTRIPTYLINE.

allelo- *combining form denoting* meaning from one to the other, being in a mutual or reciprocal relation.

allele short for allelomorph. 1 genes that occupy corresponding positions (HOMOLOGOUS loci) on homologous chromosomes. Humans have two, usually identical, alleles for each gene, one on each AUTOSOMAL chromosome of a pair. 2 one of the ways in which a gene, at a particular location on a chromosome, may differ in its DNA sequence from the normal or from its fellow at the corresponding location on the other chromosome. If different alleles of a gene occur at the corresponding sites on the pair of chromosomes the individual is said to be HETEROZYGOUS for the gene. If the two alleles are abnormal in the same way, the individual is HOMOZYGOUS and the characteristic determined by the gene defect will be present. Heterozygous individuals will show the features of the DOMINANT gene. The other allele is RECESSIVE. The term derives from the Greek *allos*, another.

allelic exclusion a state in which only one of a pair of ALLELES can be expressed.

Aller-eze a brand name for CLEMASTINE.

allergen any ANTIGEN causing ALLERGY or causing an allergic reaction in a sensitive person.

allergic alveolitis inflammation of the small air sacs in the lungs, usually caused by inhalation of organic dusts. There are various named types, including Bird (or pigeon) fancier's lung, Farmer's lung, Mushroom worker's lung, BAGASSOSIS, Maltworker's lung and Maple bark disease.

allergic dermatitis inflammation of the skin following contact with any substance to which the person is allergic.

allergic rhinitis the more respectable term for hay fever (which is not a fever and is not caused by hay). The susceptibility is often inherited (see ATOPY). A specific IMMUNOGLOBULIN (IgE) coats the MAST CELLS in the nose and air passages. When the specific ALLERGEN – grass or tree pollen etc – reaches the mast cells it combines with the IgE and this triggers the release of granules in the mast cells containing HISTAMINE and other highly irritating substances.

allergy hypersensitivity to body contact with a foreign substance (an ALLERGEN), especially grass or tree pollens, foods, dust, mites or certain metals such as nickel. The effect may take several forms, including weals (URTICARIA), DERMATITIS, ASTHMA or hay fever (ALLERGIC RHINITIS). Allergy is mediated by the E class of antibodies (IgE). An allergic response implies that there has been a prior contact with the allergen during which the immunological processes leading to the hypersensitivity have occurred. Susceptibility to allergy is often of genetic origin. The term derives from the Greek *allos*, other and *ergon*, work. See also ALLERGIC DERMATITIS.

allo- a prefix meaning 1 different, foreign or pertaining or belonging to a different individual, 2 opposed to.

allogeneic 1 pertaining to the range of genetic differences in different individuals of the same species. 2 of a donated graft from a non-identical donor.

allograft a graft taken from a genetically

27

distinct (allogeneic) member of the same species. Also known as homograft or homologous graft.

allopathy a term used by practitioners of homeopathy to refer to conventional medicine, which is based on the assumption that treatment should be directed so as to oppose disease processes – witness the number of 'anti-' entries in this dictionary. Contrast with HOMOEOPATHY, in which. paradoxically, 'like' is claimed to cure 'like'.

allopurinol a drug used to treat gout. Allopurinol is an xanthine oxidase inhibitor which reduces the production of uric acid from nucleic acid breakdown. The drug is on the WHO official list. A brand name is Zyloric.

alloreactive lymphocytes lymphocytes responsible for the strong humoral and cellular responses to non-self antigens. Repeated exposure to the lymphocytes of another person, as occurs in unprotected sexual intercourse, promotes a significant immune response to that person's lymphocytes compared with other person's lymphocytes. This is probably due to exposure to HLA antigens on white cells and epithelial cells in semen. There is evidence that such mucosal alloimmunization may provide some protection against HIV infection.

Allormed a brand name for ALLOPURINOL.

allotype an allelic variant of an antigen which can prove immunogenic in people with a different version of the allele.

all-or-none law the property in muscle and nerve fibres of either responding wholly to a stimulus or not at all. The strength of the stimulus must exceed a particular threshold or there will be no response, but when the response occurs it is total. The law applies to individual fibres and a graded response is obtained by a variation in the number of fibres activated.

allosteric protein a protein that changes from one folding conformation to a different shape when another molecule binds to it. The change in conformation alters the activity or properties of the protein.

allotype an allelic variant of an ANTIGEN. Such a variant may elicit an immune response in an apparently normal person.

all-trans retinoic acid see TRETINOIN.

allylamine antifungals drugs used to treat fungal infections of the skin. An example is terbinafine (Lamisil).

Almacarb a brand name for a mixture of ALUMINIUM HYDROXIDE and MAGNESIUM CARBONATE.

Almodan a brand name for AMOXICILLIN.

almoner a hospital welfare official or medical social worker.

almotriptan a selective serotonin agonist used to treat moderate to severe MIGRAINE. A brand name is Almogran.

Almogran a brand name for ALMOTRIPTAN.

Alodorm a brand name for NITRAZEPAM.

alopecia baldness. The commonest form is hereditary and affects males, but baldness may also be caused by old age, disease, chemotherapy or radiation for cancer and treatment with thallium compounds, vitamin A or retinoids. Alopecia areata features localized patches of complete baldness, usually with regrowth of hair within 9 months. The new hair is often white at first. The cause is unknown. The condition is currently treated with local steroids, MINOXIDIL, PUVA or immunotherapy. Early in 2004 it was reported that implanted stem cells from hair follicles could promote growth of hair and other skin elements.

aloxiprin a non-steroidal pain killing and anti-inflammatory drug (NSAID).

alpha- *combining form denoting* first. Alpha is the first letter of the Greek alphabet.

alpha,-antitrypsin a glycoprotein in the serum which can inactivate protein-splitting enzymes such as TRYPSIN, elastase and collagenase. A HOMOZYGOUS hereditary deficiency of alpha-antitrypsin can cause liver disease in infancy and childhood and, rarely CIRRHOSIS of the liver and emphysema in adults.

alpha,-antitrypsin deficiency a hereditary disorder featuring the deficiency of an enzyme that is protective against a protein-splitting enzyme that can damage the air sacs in the lungs and the cells of the liver. People with alpha 1-antitrypsin deficiency are more prone than normal to EMPHYSEMA and to certain forms of liver disease. It is responsible for 25% of deaths from juvenile liver cirrhosis. A strong case has been made for the proposition that this was the disease suffered by Frédéric Chopin and from which he died.

alpha-2-macroglobulin gene (A2M gene) a gene that codes for a protease inhibitor concerned with the degradation and clearance of beta-amyloid, the protein that accumulates in the brain in ALZHEIMER'S DISEASE. A mutated allele of this gene was reported in 1998 and it has been found that people with Alzheimer's disease are more likely to have a mutated A2M gene than their siblings.

alpha-actinin-3 ACTN3, a group of genes one of which, the R allele, codes for the fast-acting muscle protein ACTIN. The X allele does not produce this protein. Interestingly it has been found that 95% of champion sprinters have at least one copy of the R allele and 50% have two. In controls, 72% have one R allele and only 30% have two.

alpha-adrenoceptor blocking drugs drugs that cause widening of arteries (vasodilatation) by blocking the action of adrenaline-like hormones. They include DOXAZOCIN (Cardura), INDORAMIN (Baratol), PRAZOCIN (Hypovase) and TERAZOCIN (Hytrin). Overdosage causes a severe drop in blood pressure, a fast pulse, nausea, vomiting and diarrhoea, a dry mouth, flushed skin, convulsions, drowsiness and coma.

alphafetoprotein a protein synthesized in the fetal liver and intestine and present in fetal blood and in the uterine fluid. Raised levels may indicate that the fetus has SPINA BIFIDA or ANENCEPHALY and further investigation becomes urgent. Alphafetoprotein is also produced by certain malignant tumours and its estimation is sometimes used as a marker for the diagnosis of these tumours or their recurrence.

alpha-glucosidase inhibitors drugs used to treat Type II (non-insulin-dependent) DIABETES. An example is acarbose (Glucobay).

alpha helix a coiled configuration of the POLYPEPTIDE chain found in many proteins. This is one of the commonest forms of secondary structure in proteins.

alpha-lactalbumin a drug used in a protein-lipid complex with oleic acid to form a compound effective in treating skin papillomas. It functions by killing transformed cells by a mechanism similar to APOPTOSIS.

alpha motor neurones large motor nerve fibres whose cell bodies are in the front 'horn' of the spinal cord and which innervate voluntary muscles.

Alphamox a brand name for AMOXYCILLIN.

Alphaparin a brand name for CERTOPARIN.

alpha rhythm _or_ **alpha wave** the most prominent waveform found in the ELECTROENCEPHALOGRAM – the recording electrical activity of the brain. It is characterized by 8 to 12 oscillations per second when the subject is at rest.

alphatocopherol vitamin E.

alphaviruses a group of 26 viruses transmitted by mosquitoes, eight of which can cause illness, sometimes serious. Alphavirus infections feature fever, muscle and joint pain, a rash and sometimes ENCEPHALITIS. Most cases are mild.

Alphosyl a brand name for ALLANTOIN and COAL TAR, a preparation used in the treatment of PSORIASIS.

Alport's syndrome a rare inherited form of the kidney disease GLOMERULONEPHRITIS often associated with perceptive deafness and sometimes CATARACT. The syndrome is caused by defects in the Type IV collagen of basement membranes due to gene mutations. It usually begins in childhood or early adult life with blood in the urine. There may also be short sight (MYOPIA), RETINITIS PIGMENTOSA and THROMBOCYTOPENIA. (Arthur Cecil Alport, South African physician, 1880–1959).

alprazolam a benzodiazepine anti-anxiety drug. A brand name is Xanax.

Alprim a brand name for TRIMETHOPRIM.

alprostadil a PROSTAGLANDIN drug used by penile injection for the treatment of impotence. An erection lasting for two or three hours is commonly achieved, but sales of alprostadil may be adversely affected by the development of drugs such as VIAGRA. Brand names are Caverject, Muse, and Viridal Duo.

Altacite Plus a brand name for HYDROTALCITE with dimethicone (dimeticone).

alteplase a TISSUE PLASMINOGEN ACTIVATOR drug made by recombinant DNA technology. In mid-2003 the drug was approved for the treatment of ischaemic stroke by experts. It must be given within three hours and cerebral haemorrhage must be excluded. A brand name is Actilyse.

alternative hypothesis the possibility (which should always be borne in mind) that an explanation of a phenomenon or result, however apparently obvious, may not be correct. See also NULL HYPOTHESIS.

alternative medicine forms of medical practice the bases of which have not been, or cannot be, subjected to rigorous scientific scrutiny, or which, when scientifically tested, are not found to be effective. Some forms of alternative medicine do not meet generally accepted criteria of rational validity. They include HOMEOPATHY, ACUPUNCTURE to treat disease, AROMATHERAPY, REFLEXOLOGY and IRIDOLOGY. Alternative medical therapies are commonly successful in the short term because of the therapeutic effect of human interaction and the expectation of results confidently predicted (PLACEBO EFFECT), but seldom have useful long-term effects. The reputation of alternative therapies has much to do with the psychological mechanism by which chance results favourable to a hypothesis are noted and remembered whereas those unfavourable are not. In late 2003 the British Government, alarmed at the proliferation of unqualified alternative practitioners, announced plans to regulate and control the practice of alternative medicine. See also COMPLEMENTARY MEDICINE.

altitude sickness a disorder occurring in unadapted people who proceed rapidly to altitudes above about 4,000 m. There is a sense of fullness in the chest, headache, nausea, loss of appetite and sleeplessness, and the condition may progress, sometimes suddenly, to a malignant and highly dangerous phase. This is a dangerous condition characterized by excess fluid (oedema) in the lungs and the brain. Also known as mountain sickness.

altretamine an anticancer drug used to treat advanced caner of the ovary.

altruism behaviour manifesting unselfish concern for the advantage of others. Much seemingly altruistic behaviour can be shown, on analysis, not to be so, and there are those who hold that altruism is a myth. Most social scientists, however, accept the concept.

Alu-cap a brand name for ALUMINIUM HYDROXIDE.

alu sequence family a family of DNA sequences in the human genome, some 300 base pairs long, that serves no apparent genetic purpose. The alu sequences are found scattered throughout the chromosomes and occur about 500,000 times, constituting about 5% of human DNA. Copies of the alu sequences occur in slightly varying forms and these variations allow DNA FINGERPRINTING of individuals. Alu sequences are mainly of cytosine/guanine and are specific to species and do not code for any product. They cause visible gram-negative

bands when chromosomes are stained with Gram's stain and can be used to identify human DNA for forensic purposes.

Alu-Tab a brand name for ALUMINIUM HYDROXIDE.

Aludrox a brand name for a preparation containing ALUMINIUM HYDROXIDE.

aluminium acetate a drug used externally to treat OTITIS EXTERNA. The solution is commonly applied on gauze wicks inserted into the external ear canal.

aluminium hydroxide an antacid drug. The drug is on the WHO official list. Brand names of preparations containing the drug are Alu-cap, Aludrox, Maalox and Mucogel.

aluminium oxide an abrasive preparation used externally in the treatment of ACNE. A brand name is Brasivol.

aluminosis a rare form of poisoning that may feature DEMENTIA speech difficulties and loss of fine motor abilities in the hands. Aluminosis is no longer thought to be a cause of Alzheimer's disease.

Alupent a brand name for ORCIPRENALINE.

alveolar-capillary block syndrome a condition of inadequate oxygenation of the blood as a result of failure of oxygen to pass across the membranes between the lung ALVEOLI and the blood capillaries.

alveolar dead space the volume of inspired air that fills the tubes leading to the air sacs (alveoli) of the lungs, but which is unable to undergo gas exchange with the blood.

alveolectomy a dental operation to smooth off irregular bone on the edges of tooth sockets so that a better fit may be obtained for dentures.

alveolus 1 one of the many million tiny, thin-walled, air sacs in the lungs.
2 a tooth socket in the jaw bone.
3 any small cavity or sac.

alverine citrate an ANTISPASMODIC drug used in the treatment of menstrual pain. A brand name is Spasmonal.

alymphocytosis absence or severe deficiency of LYMPHOCYTES in the blood. This results in an immune deficiency state.

Alzheimer's disease a brain disorder that is by far the commonest cause of DEMENTIA. A common disorder with important genetic elements featuring severe brain shrinkage from loss of nerve tissue, accumulation of AMYLOID A-beta peptide in the brain cells and plaques and tangled masses of fibres. The A-beta peptide is cleaved from the natural AMYLOID PRECURSOR PROTEIN (APP). A mutation of the gene on chromosome 21 for APP is a cause of Alzheimer's disease. Mutations in the genes for presenilin 1 and 2, which have a role in the cleavage of A-beta peptide from APP can also cause the disease. There is progressively worsening dementia. People with DOWN'S SYNDROME develop this disorder 10 to 30 years earlier than other people. Down's syndrome is caused by an extra chromosome 21 and features slow accumulation of A-beta peptide. Vaccination with A peptide may be a possible preventive. (Alois Alzheimer, German neurologist, 1864–1915).

anakinra a human INTERLEUKIN-1-receptor antagonist used to combat the pro-inflammatory interleukins in RHEUMATOID ARTHRITIS. A brand name is Kineret.

amalgam a dental material consisting of powdered mercury, silver and tin which, when mixed, may be forced into a drilled and cleaned cavity in a tooth where it hardens within a few minutes. Surprisingly, in spite of occasional expressed concern, amalgam does not seem to present the risk of mercury poisoning.

Amanita a genus of mushrooms most of which are extremely poisonous. A common species is *Amanita phalloides*, so named because of its resemblance to a penis.

amantadine an antiviral drug, also used to treat PARKINSON'S DISEASE. Brand names are Lysovir and Symmetrel.

Amaryl a brand name for GLIMEPIRIDE.

amastigotes LEISHMAN-DONOVAN BODIES.

amaurosis an old-fashioned term for blindness. From the Greek *amauros*, dark or obscure. See also AMAUROSIS FUGAX.

amaurosis fugax transient loss of vision, usually for a few seconds or minutes caused by interference to the blood supply to parts of the brain or eye by tiny EMBOLI or by spasm of the arteries supplying the eye. Repeated attacks can damage the RETINA and the condition is a warning of the grave danger of STROKE. Amaurosis fugax is a form of TRANSIENT ISCHAEMIC ATTACK.

amaurotic familial idiocy an out-of-date term for a range of rare hereditary diseases, now known as the GANGLIOSIDOSES. Progressive degeneration occurs in the brain and the retinas.

amber codon the three-nucleotide group UAG (uracil, adenine, guanine) that forms a stop CODON marking the point at which the synthesis of a protein ends. Two other codons, UAA and UGA, have the same function. One of these three codons marks the end of every gene.

amber mutation a mutation that creates an AMBER CODON.

ambidexterity the ability to use either hand with the same facility. True ambidexterity, with no bias to one side, is rare and runs in families.

ambisexual having undifferentiated or ambiguous sexual orientation so that attraction to either sex may be experienced. See also BISEXUAL.

Ambisome a brand name for AMPHOTERICIN.

amblyopia 1 visual defect resulting from failure, from any cause, to form sharp, central retinal images in early life. In most cases the affected eyes appear structurally normal. 2 visual defect resulting from poisoning (toxic amblyopia) or a deficiency of an essential dietary ingredient. The term derived from the Greek *amblus*, dull or blunt and *ops*, an eye.

amblyoscope or **synoptophore** an instrument used in ORTHOPTICS to present to the subject images at different angles of convergence or divergence so that the fusional ability can be tested.

ambulance chaser a slang term for a lawyer who obtains business by encouraging accident victims to sue doctors or others for damages, often on a contingency basis.

ambulatory 1 pertaining to walking. 2 capable of walking and not bedridden.

amelioration a reduction in severity. A partial recovery.

amelo- *combining form denoting* tooth enamel.

ameloblastic odontoma a tumour of tooth-forming tissue. Also known as odontoblastoma.

ameloblastoma a BENIGN tumour arising from the tissue that gives rise to the tooth internal lining. Ameloblastomas usually occur in the lower jaw (mandible) and are also known as adamantinomas.

amelogenesis imperfecta a hereditary defect of the mineralization of tooth enamel which is unusually soft and is rapidly worn away.

amelogenin a structural protein used as a drug to treat PERIODONTITIS. The drug is formulated as a gel that is placed under a flap in the gum surrounding the root of the tooth and promotes regrowth of gum tissue that has been destroyed by the inflammatory process. A brand name is Emdogain.

amenorrhoea the absence of menstruation. This is normal before puberty and after the menopause. During the reproductive years, the commonest causes are pregnancy and LACTATION, but it can be caused by a number of hormonal and other disorders.

ament a person mentally deficient from birth. The term literally means 'without a mind'.

amentia the absence, from failure of development, of the intellectual powers.

amethocaine tetracaine, a local anaesthetic drug which is effective when in contact with surfaces as well as when given by injection. It resembles COCAINE in its action and can readily be absorbed in dangerous amounts from mucous membranes. Brand names are Ametop. Minims Tetracaine.

ametropia any deviation, in the relaxed focus of the eye, from the normal state in which distant objects form sharp and clear images on the RETINA. Ametropia may take the form of HYPERMETROPIA, MYOPIA or the meridional visual defect ASTIGMATISM. The state of normal refraction is called emmetropia.

Amfipen a brand name for AMPICILLIN.

Amias a brand name for the angiotensin II antagonist CANDESARTAN.

amidopyrine aminopyrine. A painkilling drug once widely used as an aspirin substitute but now out of favour because of the risk of inducing a sometimes fatal drop in the number of white cells in the blood (AGRANULOCYTOSIS).

amidotrizoate a substance sometimes used as a contrast medium for X-ray examination. It is on the WHO list of selected drugs.

amifostine a drug used to reduce the side effects of anticancer treatments, especially the dangers of infection and of damage to the kidneys. A brand name is Ethyol.

amikacin an antibiotic drug, one of the AMINOGLYCOSIDES. The drug is on the WHO official list. A brand name is Amikin.

Amil-Co a brand name for a preparation of AMILORIDE and HYDROCHLOROTHIAZIDE.

amiloride a thiazide DIURETIC drug that acts by reducing reabsorption of sodium, and thus water, in the kidneys. A potassium-sparing diuretic used in the treatment of high blood pressure (HYPERTENSION), HEART FAILURE or

other conditions in which excess fluid is retained in the body. The drug is on the WHO official list. Formulated in combination with other drugs under brand names such as Amil-Co, Burinex A, Fru-Co, Frumil, Kalten, Lasoride, Moducren, Moduret 25, Moduretic and Navispare.

amine a class of organic compounds derived from ammonia by replacing one or more of the hydrogen atoms by a member of the paraffin series or by an aromatic group. Amines occur widely in the body, and many drugs are amines.

amine hormone any hormone derived from the amino acid tyrosine. Amine hormones include ADRENALINE, NORADRENALINE and thyroid hormones. These are also called catecholamines.

amine test a for BACTERIAL VAGINOSIS – vaginal infection with *Gardnerella vaginalis* – sometimes called the 'fish' test. A drop of vaginal discharge is mixed with a drop of saline on a slide and a drop of 5% potassium hydroxide added. If positive, a fishy amine smell is at once apparent.

amino acids the basic constituent of protein. Amino acids can be considered to be the 'alphabet' of letters from which proteins are written. Their properties are determined by their side chains. Body protein breaks down into 20 different amino acids. Some of these can be synthesized by the body but some can not. The latter are known as 'essential amino acids' and must be obtained from protein in the diet. Amino acids group together to form peptides. Linkages between amino acids are called peptide bonds. Dipeptides have two amino acids, polypeptides have many. Polypeptides join to form proteins. The reverse process occurs when proteins are digested. Some amino acids, such as glycine, arginine, aspartic acid and glutamic acid, also perform specific biological functions in addition to helping to form proteins. The German organic chemist Emil Fischer (1825–1919) elicited an understanding of amino acids, peptides and proteins which was of fundamental importance in the development of organic chemistry and biochemistry. He was awarded the Nobel Prize in Chemistry in 1902. See also STEREOISOMERS.

aminoaciduria the presence of amino acids in the urine. This occurs in a group of disorders that feature abnormal protein METABOLISM.

aminoacylation the attachment of an amino acid to the acceptor arm of a TRANSFER RNA molecule. This is an essential step in the synthesis of a protein. The attachment is brought about by the appropriate AMINOACYL-TRNA SYNTHETASE.

aminoacyl-tRNA synthetase one of a group of 20 enzymes each of which is specific for the catalyzation of the linkage of a particular AMINO ACID to its own type of TRANSFER RNA during protein synthesis. There are 20 amino acids in body proteins.

aminobenzoic acid a drug used in the treatment of SCLERODERMA and PEYRONIE'S DISEASE. The action is to reduce the tendency to the formation of fibrous tissue. A brand name is Potaba.

aminocaproic acid a drug that reduces the tendency for fibrin in the blood to be broken down. It thus aids in the clotting of blood in wounds.

aminoglutethamide a drug that interferes with the synthesis of STEROIDS, OESTROGENS and ANDROGENS by the ADRENAL GLANDS. It does this by blocking an enzyme that allows the conversion of CHOLESTEROL. A brand name is Ormeten.

aminoglycosides a class of antibiotics which include STREPTOMYCIN, TOBRAMYCIN, KANAMYCIN, AMIKACIN, GENTAMICIN and NEOMYCIN. They act by causing misreading of certain CODONS on messenger RNA and are transported into bacterial cells only if free oxygen is present. The aminoglycosides can cause deafness and TINNITUS if taken in excess or if not excreted normally because of kidney disease. They can also cause damage to the kidneys.

aminopeptidases enzymes that break the peptide bond of the amino acid at the end of a POLYPEPTIDE chain. Aminopeptidases occur in the small intestine and participate in the digestive breakdown of proteins to free amino acids.

aminophylline a THEOPHYLLINE drug in combination with ethylenediamine used in the control of ASTHMA. In acute cases it can be given by intravenous injection but it is also effective by mouth or in a SUPPOSITORY. The drug is on the WHO official list. Brand names are Pecram and Phyllocontin.

aminotransferases enzymes present in liver cells which are released into the blood in liver disease, such as HEPATITIS, that damages liver cells. The most important are aspartate aminotransferase (AST) and alanine aminotransferase (ALT). Measurement of the levels of these enzymes in the blood is a valuable test of liver damage.

amiodarone a drug used to treat heart rhythm irregularities such as paroxysmal ATRIAL FIBRILLATION. There are numerous side effects. A brand name is Cordarone X.

amisulpride a drug used in the treatment of SCHIZOPHRENIA. A brand name is Solian.

Amitrip a brand name for AMITRIPTYLINE.

amitriptyline a tricyclic antidepressant drug. The drug is on the WHO official list. A brand name is Triptafen.

amlodipine a drug used in the treatment of ANGINA PECTORIS and high blood pressure (HYPERTENSION). A brand name is Istin.

ammonia a substance produced when AMINO ACIDS are broken down. Ammonia is converted by the liver into urea and excreted in the urine. Urea can be broken down by bacterial enzymes to release ammonia. This may be a cause of nappy rash in babies.

amnesia loss of memory as a result of physical or mental disease or injury, especially head injury. Amnesia for events occurring before the head injury is called retrograde amnesia. Anterograde amnesia is loss of memory for events occurring after the injury.

amnesic aphasia loss of memory for the names of objects, states or conditions.

amniocentesis a method of obtaining early information about the health and genetic constitution of the growing fetus, by taking a sample of the fluid from the womb (AMNIOTIC FLUID) for analysis usually between the 15th and 18th week of pregnancy. Cellular debris in the fluid provides DNA for chromosome analysis and sex determination and the fluid contains specific substances characteristic of various diseases. The risk of fetal loss from this procedure is estimated to be 0.5% to 1% above the natural level of spontaneous abortion.

amniography radiography of the fetus after injection of radiopaque material into the amniotic sac.

amnion one layer of the fluid-filled double membrane surrounding the fetus before birth. The amnion is the inner of two membranes, the other being the chorion. The membranes normally rupture and release the AMNIOTIC FLUID ('breaking of the waters' before the baby is born).

amnioscopy endoscopic examination of the amniotic cavity.

amniotic pertaining to the AMNION.

amniotic fluid a liquid produced by one of the membranes which surround the fetus throughout pregnancy and by fetal urination, in which the fetus floats. The volume of amniotic fluid at full term is usually about 1 litre.

amniotomy intentional rupturing of the fetal membranes to induce or facilitate labour.

amobarbital amylobarbitone, a barbiturate drug used for the short-term treatment of insomnia. A brand name is Amytal.

amoeba a single-celled microscopic organism of indefinite shape commonly found in water, damp soil and as parasites of other animals. Some amoebae, such as *Entamoeba histolytica* and *Acanthamoeba castellani* cause disease in man, respectively AMOEBIC DYSENTERY and acanthamoebic keratitis.

amoebiasis a group of disorders caused by the amoeba, *Entamoeba histolytica*. It may include AMOEBIC DYSENTERY, widespread damage to the large intestine and abscesses in the liver (AMOEBIC ABSCESS), lungs and brain.

amoebic abscess local destruction and liquefaction of tissue, usually in the liver, as a result of the toxic action of the amoeba, *Entamoeba histolytica*. The affected area becomes walled off by fibrous tissue and the contents are said to resemble anchovy sauce. Amoebic liver abscesses sometimes break though the DIAPHRAGM into the lung and the contents may be coughed up.

amoebic dysentery an acute, inflammatory infection of the COLON caused by the amoeba *Entamoeba histolytica*, characterized by ulceration of the lining with pain and diarrhoea. The amoebae undermine the bowel lining, enter the veins in the wall of the intestine, and are carried to the liver where they may cause large abscesses.

amoebicide a drug used to kill PATHOGENIC amoebae.

amoeboid resembling an amoeba, especially in its method of locomotion. An amoeba is a shapeless, jelly-like, single-celled organism that moves by pushing out a protrusion, a

pseudopodium, in the required direction and then flowing into it.

amok a form of homicidal mania featuring extreme agitation and the attempt to kill as many people as possible. The attack is said to be followed by loss of memory for the event (AMNESIA). Amok was originally described as occurring among Malayan men armed with parangs. The modern form, which is far from unknown in the West, is more likely to feature a Kalashnikov automatic rifle.

Amoram a brand name for AMOXYCILLIN.

amorolfine a drug used externally in the treatment of TINEA infection of the skin. A brand name is Loceryl.

amorphous 1 of no particular shape or form. 2 lacking distinct crystalline structure.

amotivational syndrome an effect of prolonged heavy use of MARIJUANA (cannabis). There is apathy, unwillingness to persist at any task and usually a gain in weight.

amoxapine a tricyclic antidepressant drug similar to IMIPRAMINE. Overdosage may cause acute kidney failure, convulsions and coma. A brand name is Asendis.

amoxicillin amoxycillin, an AMPICILLIN-like penicillin antibiotic, effective in TYPHOID and many other infections. Brand names are Amoxil and Galenamox. Compounded with lansoprazol and clarithromycin it is marketed as Heliclear.

Amoxil a brand name for AMOXICILLIN.

ampakines drugs that act on nerve cell receptors to make them more responsive to the NEUROTRANSMITTER glutamate. A few small clinical trials have suggested that ampakines can significantly improve memory in elderly people. Neuroscientists remain sceptical.

amphetamine amfetamine, a central nervous system (CNS) stimulant drug with few medical uses but commonly abused to obtain a 'high'. Amphetamine use leads to tolerance and sometimes physical dependence. Overdosage causes irritability, tremor, restlessness, insomnia, flushing, nausea and vomiting, irregularity of the pulse, delirium, hallucinations, convulsions and coma. Amphetamine can precipitate a PSYCHOSIS in predisposed people.

amphi- a prefix meaning two, both or either.

amphiarthrosis a type of joint allowing very limited movement because the bones are connected by FIBROCARTILAGE. Such joints occur between adjacent vertebrae or between the ribs and the breast bone.

amphipathic of a chemical structure having both hydrophobic and hydrophilic surfaces as in the case of the phospholipid molecules of the cell membrane. Some proteins have amphipathic regions.

amphotericin an antibiotic produced from *Streptomyces nodosus* used to treat systemic fungal infections. The drug is liable to cause kidney damage. Brand names are Ambisome, Amphocil and Fungizone. Amphotericin B is marketed under the brand name Abelcet.

ampicillin a widely used penicillin antibiotic, effective by mouth and capable of killing many GRAM-NEGATIVE as well as GRAM-POSITIVE organisms. About one third of the dose is excreted unchanged in the urine. The drug precipitates a characteristic rash if given to people incubating GLANDULAR FEVER (infective mononucleosis). The drug is on the WHO official list. A brand name is Penbritin.

Ampicyn a brand name for AMPICILLIN.

amplification the production of extra copies of a DNA sequence. These may be within the chromosomal sequence or outside it.

ampoule a small, hermetically sealed flask, usually containing medicine for administration by injection.

Amprace a brand name for ENALAPRIL.

amprenavir a protease inhibitor drug used to treat HIV infections. A brand name is Agenerase.

ampulla a widened (dilated) segment of a gland or small tube.

ampulla of Vater a small sac-like widening (dilation) at the point of junction of the bile and pancreatic ducts where they enter the DUODENUM. Cancer of the head of the PANCREAS can block the ampulla and cause obstructive JAUNDICE.

amputation removal, by surgical operation or injury, or rarely by disease, of part of the body. From the Latin *ambi*, around and *putare*, to prune.

amputee a person who has suffered an AMPUTATION.

AMQ *abbrev. for* American Medical Qualification.

AMS *abbrev. for* Army Medical Services.

amsacrine a cytotoxic drug used to treat acute myeloid leukaemia. A brand name is Amsidine.

AMWA *abbrev. for* American Medical Women's Association.

Amyand's hernia an inguinal HERNIA containing an acutely inflamed appendix, (Claudius Amyand, 1681–1740, Principal surgeon to Westminster and St George's Hospitals, London and Fellow of the Royal Society).

amygdala an almond-shaped brain nucleus at the front of the temporal lobe. The amygdala is concerned with memory registration.

amygdalin a glycoside found in the stones of bitter almonds, from which LAETRILE was isolated.

amygdalo- *combining form denoting* almond-like, almond-shaped or almond-related.

amygdaloid 1 almond shaped.
2 relating to the AMYGDALA.

amyl- *combining form denoting* starch.

amylaceous starch-like.

amylase an ENZYME that converts starch to simpler carbohydrates such as disaccharides and small polysaccharides.

amyl nitrite a volatile drug used by inhalation in the control of pain in ANGINA PECTORIS. It acts by relaxing smooth muscle and thus dilating arteries, including the coronary arteries. The pain is relieved because of the improved blood supply to the heart muscle.

amylobarbitone amobarbital, a BARBITURATE drug used for the short-term treatment of insomnia. Brand names are Amytal and Sodium Amytal.

amyloid one of a range of proteins deposited in the brain in spongiform encephalopathies such as CREUTZFELDT-JAKOB DISEASE, in other degenerative brain disorders such as ALZHEIMER'S DISEASE, and in the tissues in a wide range of long-term suppurative disorders (see AMYLOIDOSIS). It is a hard, waxy proteinaceous substance in the form of straight, rigid, non-branching fibrils, 10–15 nm in diameter that are insoluble in water and relatively resistant to breakdown by proteolytic enzymes. There is a considerable range of amyloid proteins mainly specific for the different conditions in which amyloid is deposited. From the Latin *amylum*, starch.

amyloidosis a disorder of protein metabolism of multiple origin resulting in localized or generalized deposition of AMYLOID in the tissues. In general (systemic) amyloidosis the organs mainly affected are the liver, kidneys, spleen and heart. Amyloidosis occurs in conditions of chronic inflammation, such as TUBERCULOSIS, leprosy (HANSEN'S DISEASE) and RHEUMATOID ARTHRITIS and in B lymphocyte disorders, such as multiple myeloma. Local amyloidosis of the islets of Langerhans in the pancreas is a feature of maturity onset (Type II) DIABETES. Rarely, no predisposing cause can be identified. In this case the condition is called primary amyloidosis.

amyloid precursor protein a natural brain protein that is coded for on chromosome 21. This protein is related in some way to memory. Point mutations are found in the gene for this protein in people who suffer from a familial form of early-onset ALZHEIMER'S DISEASE. Only a small proportion of cases of Alzheimer's disease, however, are caused in this way. Abnormally folded AMYLOID protein in the form of plaques and tangles occur in brain cells in Alzheimer's disease but also in chronic suppurative states in other parts of the body.

amylum starch.

amyotonia lack of muscle tone. See AMYOTONIA CONGENITA.

amyotonia congenita the 'floppy baby' syndrome, in which the new-born baby's muscles are weak and the limbs floppy. In many such cases the condition is benign and recovery is complete, but some are suffering from spinal muscular atrophy (WERDNIG-HOFFMANN DISEASE).

amyotrophic lateral sclerosis a fatal condition of progressive degeneration of the motor tracts in the spinal cord, brainstem and motor cortex of the brain causing muscle atrophy and increasing weakness. Death usually occurs within five or six years of onset. Toxicity from glutamate, a NEUROTRANSMITTER, is thought to be a possible cause and antiglutamate drugs such as RILUZOLE (Rilutek) have been developed that appear to slow the progress of the disease. A form of motor neurone disease.

Amytal a brand name for AMYLOBARBITONE (amobarbital), a barbiturate hypnotic drug of medium duration of action.

an- *prefix denoting* not, negative. This is the euphonic form of the Greek *a*, not, negative.

ana- *prefix denoting* up, upward, or back, backward.

Anabact a brand name for METRONIDAZOLE

formulated in a gel for external use only.

anabolic 1 pertaining to a chemical reaction in which small molecules, such as amino acids, are combined to form larger molecules, such as proteins.
2 of any substance that increases the rate of metabolism of a cell or organism.
3 of a drug, such as a male sex hormone, that promotes body bulk.

anabolic steroids drugs which promote tissue growth, especially of muscle, by stimulating protein synthesis. Anabolic steroids are synthetic male sex hormones and tend to cause VIRILIZATION. These steroids are sometimes misused by athletes and bodybuilders to gain an unfair advantage. The risks are considerable and include life-threatening varicella-zoster pneumonitis, renal-cell carcinoma, liver damage with jaundice, systemic infection with *Candida albicans* including ENDOPHTHALMITIS, breast enlargement (gynaecomastia), mood swings and aggressiveness ('steroid rage') and induction of psychotic disorders. Women run the additional risks of virilization.

anabolism building up of the tissues. The metabolic process by which the complex biochemical structure of living tissue is synthesized from simple nutritional elements such as sugars, amino acids and fatty acids. Contrast with CATABOLISM, which is the break-down of complex tissues to simpler, consumable, substances. The term is derived from the Greek *anabole*, to build up or throw up.

anaemia a reduction in the amount of HAEMOGLOBIN in the blood. There are several different kinds of anaemia including simple iron deficiency anaemia, haemolytic anaemia, pernicious anaemia, and aplastic anaemia.

anaemic suffering from anaemia.

anaerobic living and being capable of reproducing in the absence of free oxygen. Only certain very simple organisms, such as some bacteria, are capable of complete anaerobic existence.

anaesthesia loss of the sensations of touch, pressure, pain or temperature in any part of, or in the whole of, the body. This may be due to injury or disease of nerves or brain, or to deliberate medical interference. Drugs are commonly used to effect either general or local anaesthesia.

anaesthetic 1 insensitive.

2 relating to anaesthesia.

3 causing anaesthesia.

4 a drug used to cause unconsciousness or insensitivity to pain.

anaesthetist a doctor skilled in the administration of all forms of local and general anesthetics for surgical, obstetrical and other purposes, and in the techniques of life support for the critically ill or injured.

anaesthetization the induction of anaesthesia.

Anafranil a brand name for CLOMIPRAMINE.

anakinra a human INTERLEUKIN-1-receptor antagonist used to combat the pro-inflammatory interleukins in RHEUMATOID ARTHRITIS. A brand name is Kineret.

anal 1 relating to the anus, the controlled terminus of the digestive tract.

2 concerning the putative stage of psychosexual development of the child in which pleasure is obtained from sensations associated with the anus. See FREUDIAN THEORY.

anal atresia a congenital condition in which the anus is imperforate. There is often an associated ANAL FISTULA.

anal canal the 5 cm-long terminal portion of the intestine that lies immediately below the RECTUM. The anal canal contains two muscular rings (SPHINCTERS) that can close it tightly and seven or more longitudinal pads of MUCOUS MEMBRANE that contain veins and press together to act as an additional sealing mechanism.

anal dilatation the forcible manual enlargement of the anal canal to 'four fingers' done under general anaesthesia for the treatment of piles (HAEMORRHOIDS) of any degree.

anal dilatation test a test used along with other signs to help in the detection of anal sexual abuse in children. The buttocks are gently parted and, after a short time, the anus opens (reflex dilatation). This effect, alone, provides no conclusive evidence and occurs in up to 14% of children who have never been abused. Other signs of anal sexual abuse include anal tears (fissures), loss of SPHINCTER control, shortening and eversion of the ANAL CANAL, vein congestion and reddening in the area and thickening of the surrounding tissues.

analeptic 1 any drug, such as doxapram, that stimulates the central nervous system.

2 generally restorative.

3 stimulating to the breathing.

analeptic drugs drugs that stimulate the nerve centres in the brain responsible for breathing and increase the strength of the nerve impulses to the respiratory muscles.

anal-expulsive a term applied by some psychoanalysts to people who show certain personality traits such as ambition, conceit or suspicion. These traits are said to manifest habits, attitudes and values associated with the infantile pleasure in the expulsion of faeces. See also ANAL-RETENTIVE, FREUDIAN THEORY.

anal fissure sometimes called fissure-in-ano, this is a longitudinal tear in the wall of the anus, usually directly backwards. There is inevitable infection and a swollen skin tag, called a sentinel pile forms at the site. There is burning pain on defaecation. Surgical treatment is effective but about 10% of patients suffer anal incontinence, mainly for flatus. BOTULINUM TOXIN has been used.

anal fistula a persistent discharging track between the anus and the exterior, opening on the skin near the anus. Fistula is usually associated with an abscess in the tissues surrounding the anal canal.

analgesic 1 pain-relieving.

2 a pain-relieving drug.

analgesic drugs the important group of pain-killing drugs that ranges from the mild and comparatively safe, such as paracetamol, to the powerful and dangerous, such as morphine and heroin.

anal incontinence the inability to retain faeces voluntarily in the rectum. It is due to sphincter injury, often from obstetrical tears, to neurological or psychological disturbances, to prolapse of the rectum, to constipation with faecal impaction or to dementia.

anal intercourse a form of sexual intercourse, usually homosexual, in which the anus performs the sexual function of the vagina.

anal-retentive a psychoanalytic term indicating traits such as miserliness, obsessiveness, obstinacy and meticulousness. These characteristics are said to originate in values formed during the 'anal stage' of development when particular pleasure was taken in the retention of faeces. See also FREUDIAN THEORY.

anal sphincter the double muscular ring surrounding the anal canal which, in conjunction with the thick, well-vascularized lining of the canal, produces a watertight seal except during defaecation.

anal stage a stage in the psychosexual development, proposed by Sigmund Freud, in which the child's preoccupation is with the anal region and the faeces.

anal stricture an abnormal narrowing of the anus or anal canal as a result of disease.

analysand a person undergoing psychoanalysis.

analysis the determination of the constituents of which anything is composed. Compare synthesis. See also PSYCHOANALYSIS.

anamnesis the complete clinical case history of a patient. From the Greek *anamnesis*, a reminiscence.

anamnestic of an immunological reaction that is enhanced by a repeated exposure to an ALLERGEN.

Anamorph a brand name for MORPHINE.

anaphase a stage in cell division (MITOSIS) in which the separated individual chromosomes migrate to opposite ends of the cell in preparation for the division of the cell into two new individuals.

anaphrodisia absence of sexual desire or interest.

anaphylactic pertaining to ANAPHYLAXIS.

anaphylatoxin any substance that can directly cause degranulation of MAST CELLS thereby bringing about an acute allergic reaction.

anaphylaxis a severe, often fatal, form of hypersensitivity allergic reaction most commonly provoked by drugs such as penicillin, intravenous iron or procainamide, but also brought on by allergy to foods, vaccines, insect bites or snake bites and contact with latex rubber. There is always a history of a previous reaction to the ALLERGEN. The effects are a drop in blood pressure (hypotension), local swelling of the skin (angio-oedema) and mucous membranes, narrowing of the air tubes (bronchi), itching, vomiting and abdominal pain. The sooner the onset after exposure to the allergen, the more severe the reaction. Anaphylactic shock is a serious, widespread allergic attack which may cause death by AIRWAY obstruction from swelling of the lining of the LARYNX.

anaplasia loss of the cellular microscopic features which distinguish one type from another. Anaplastic cells become smaller and simpler in structure and no longer combine to form recognizable tissues. Anaplasia is a common feature of cancer and, in general, the greater the anaplasia the more malignant and dangerous the tumour.

anasarca an old-fashioned term for fluid accumulation in the tissues (OEDEMA).

anastomosis a direct surgical connection formed between two tubular structures by stitching or a communication between an artery and a vein without intervening smaller vessels.

anastrozole an anti-oestrogen drug. Anastrozole is an aromatase-inhibitor anti-estrogen drug used in the treatment of advanced breast cancer in post-menopausal women. An aromatase is an enzyme that promotes the conversion of testosterone to the aromatic compound oestradiol (estradiol). This process occurs in women, and its inhibition can reduce oestrogen levels which can be helpful in the control of oestrogen-dependent tumours. The side effects may include any of those due to oestrogen deficiency. A brand name is Arimidex.

Anatensol a brand name for FLUPHENAZINE.

anatomical 1 pertaining to the structure of the body (the ANATOMY or to dissection.
2 structural, as distinct from functional (PHYSIOLOGICAL).

anatomy 1 the structure of the body, or the study of the structure. See illustrations at the back of the book.
2 a textbook or treatise on anatomical science. The list of entries that follows highlights the key entries in this dictionary related to anatomy: adrenal gland, alimentary canal, aorta, artery, bone, brain, bladder, bronchus, cardiovascular system, circulation, circulatory system, colon, diaphragm, digestive system, duodenum, Fallopian, tube, gastrointestinal tract, heart, muscle, ileum, islets of Langerhans, jejunum, kidney, ligament, liver, lungs, lymphatic, system, lymph node, oesophagus, organ, ovary, pancreas, penis, peritoneum, pituitary gland, rectum, skeleton, skin, small intestine, spleen, stomach, tendon, testicle, thymus, thyroid gland, uterus, vein, vena cava, ventricle, vertebra, vulva.

ANCA *abbrev. for* Anti Neutrophil Cytoplasmic Antibodies. ANCA specific for proteinase 3 or myeloperoxidase are features of VASCULITIS and WEGENER'S GRANULOMATOSIS.

ancestral genes DNA sequences in animal species that lived millions of years ago but that, although much modified by mutation and rearrangement are still present in whole or in part in the contemporary human genome. Some distinct and separate human genes share sequences that suggest they may have had a common ancestry.

anchorage dependence a property of cells that can grow and proliferate only if fixed to a substrate. Many cancer cells do not show anchorage dependence and can be grown in a liquid culture.

Ancotil a brand name for FLUCYTOSINE.

ancrod a protease occurring in the venom of the Malaysian pit viper *Agkistrodon rhodostoma*. The enzyme removes fibrinogen from the circulating blood without converting it to fibrin. It does not cause platelet aggregation and is used by Chinese doctors to treat stroke.

Ancylostoma duodenale the common nematode hookworm, causing infestation in Europe, Mediterranean areas and Asia. It is the cause of ANCYLOSTOMIASIS.

ancylostomiasis the disease caused by, or the effects of, heavy hookworm infestation. The main features are ANAEMIA and loss of weight. Treatment is with one of the range of ANTHELMINTIC drugs.

Anderson-Fabry disease an X-LINKED RECESSIVE genetic disorder which is therefore fully expressed in the male, who has only one X CHROMOSOME. Females are either carriers or show a partial form. There is abnormal deposition of a substance ceramide trihexoside in the cell LYSOSOMES leading to widespread damage to blood vessels in most of the organs in the body. The disease features tingling and severe burning pain in the extremities, nausea, vomiting, abdominal pain, muscle and joint pain, RAYNAUD'S PHENOMENON, slightly raised, scaly, bright red to blue-black spots on the skin, corneal changes, cataract, deafness, a tendency to heart attack and heart valve disease and kidney failure. The location of the mutated gene for the deficient enzyme, alpha-galactosidase A, is now known and the prospects for treatment have improved. (W. Anderson, English surgeon and dermatologist, 1842–1900, and Johannes Fabry, German physician, 1860–1930).

Andriol a brand name for TESTOSTERONE.

andro- *combining form denoting* man-like, male, pertaining to man in the sense of a male person.

Androcur a brand name for CYPROTERONE ACETATE.

androgen receptor gene a gene on the X chromosome that codes for the receptors for male sex hormones. Mutations in this gene have been found in men with the rare condition of familial cancer of the breast.

androgenic alopecia male-pattern baldness in a woman caused by abnormal male sex hormone output from congenital adrenal hyperplasia or other causes.

androgens male sex hormones. Androgens are STEROIDS and include testosterone and androsterone. As drugs, they are used to stimulate the development of sexual characteristics in boys when there is inadequate output from the testicles and to stimulate red cell formation in APLASTIC ANAEMIA. See also ANABOLIC STEROIDS. The term androgen derives from the Greek *andros*, a man and *gennao*, to make.

androgenous pertaining to the birth or preferential production of male offspring.

androgen receptors molecules on the surface of cells that bind androgens and bring about their effects within the cells. They are specific GLYCOPROTEINS coded for by genes on the X chromosome.

androgynous hermaphroditic. Exhibiting both male and female characteristics. From the Greek *andros*, a man and *gune*, a woman.

android 1 a non-biological organism having human characteristics. A synthetic person or humanoid robot.
2 man-like, male-like, as of the pelvis. Compare gynaecoid.

Andropatch a brand name for TESTOSTERONE formulated in a transdermal patch.

andropause the period, usually occurring between the ages of 45 and 55, during which a man's testosterone levels may fall, leading to a reduction in vigour and sexual drive. The term is rarely used, the etymologically-shaky term 'male MENOPAUSE' being commonly preferred.

androsterone a metabolite of the male sex hormone TESTOSTERONE, excreted in urine of both men and women.

Anectine a brand name for SUXAMETHONIUM CHLORIDE.

anencephaly absence of the greater part of the brain and of the bones (ACRANIA) at the rear of the skull. Anencephaly is a defect of development arising from a severe NEURAL TUBE DEFECT early in the development of the embryo and is incompatible with life. Anencephalic babies are born dead or die soon after birth. The term derives from the Greek *an*, not and *encephalon*, a brain. See ACEPHALUS.

anergy specific immunological tolerance in which T cells and B cells fail to respond normally by producing an immune response to antigens. The state can be reversed.

Anethaine a brand name for AMETHOCAINE.

anethol an ingredient in a mixture of essential oils used in the treatment of kidney stones. A brand name is Rowatinex.

aneuploidy an abnormality in the number of CHROMOSOMES by loss or duplication. The number may be smaller or greater than the normal diploid constitution. The loss of a whole chromosome is lethal. A chromosome extra to one of the pairs is called TRISOMY. Trisomy 21, for instance, causes DOWN'S SYNDROME. DNA aneuploidy refers to abnormal quantities of DNA in a nucleus. See also MOSAICISM.

aneurin vitamin B1, thiamin. This is plentiful in cereals and fresh vegetables, legumes, fruit, meat and milk, but there is very little in refined foods, fat, sugar or alcohol. Deficiency causes BERI-BERI in 12 months. Also known as thiamine.

aneurysm a berry-like or diffuse swelling on an artery, usually at or near a branch, and caused by localized damage or weakness to the vessel wall. Aneurysms can also involve the heart wall after a section has been weakened. See also BERRY ANEURYSM. The term derives from the Greek *anaeurusma*, a widening.

Anexate a brand name for FLUMAZENIL.

angel dust a slang term for the powerful analgesic and anaesthetic drug Phencyclidine commonly abused for recreational purposes. It is also known by the abbreviation PCP. Abuse of this drug can lead to muscle rigidity, convulsions and death.

anger a strong emotion aroused by a sense of wrong, whether justified or not.

angiitis inflammation of a blood vessel.

Angilol a brand name for PROPRANOLOL.

angina 1 a sore throat severe enough to cause a sensation of choking.
2 ANGINA PECTORIS.

3 one of a number of conditions featuring painful spasms.

angina pectoris the symptom of oppression, pain or tightness in the centre of the chest which occurs when the CORONARY arteries are unable to provide an adequate blood supply to meet the immediate demands of the heart muscle. Angina is almost always related to exercise or emotion and is relieved by rest. It is worse in cold conditions and after a meal. The symptom is often described as of a tight band round the chest. The pain may radiate down the arms, especially the left, or up into the neck or jaw. There may be associated breathlessness. Rapidly worsening angina, induced by ever-lessening amounts of exertion, is called unstable angina and requires urgent attention. Angina can be controlled with nitrates, especially nitroglycerine which is best taken in a tablet held under the tongue. The term derives from the Latin *angere*, to strangle and *pectus*, the breast. See also CORONARY SYNDROME.

Anginine a brand name for GLYCERLY TRINITRATE.

angio- *combining form denoting* a blood vessel. From the Greek *angeion*, a vessel.

angioblasts cells in the embryo that give rise to blood capillaries.

angiodysplasia abnormal blood vessel formation. Angiodysplasia of the intestinal lining is one of the causes of bleeding into the bowel.

angiogenesis the origination and development of new capillary blood vessels in normal or malignant tissue. Angiogenesis is necessary so that a growing or enlarging tissue, with its increasing metabolic needs, obtains an adequate blood supply providing oxygen, nutrients and waste drainage. Various angiogenetic factors are secreted by blood-deprived (ischaemic) cells and these operate on the inner lining (endothelium) of existing blood vessels to cause the budding out of new capillaries.
Angiogenesis can be exploited in two ways in medicine – it can, in theory be inhibited in the treatment of CANCER, DIABETIC RETINOPATHY, OBESITY, ENDOMETRIOSIS and ATHEROSCLEROSIS; or it can be encouraged to treat heart attacks, ununited fractures, neurodegenerative disease, peripheral blood circulation deficiencies and baldness.

angiogenesis inhibitor one of a range of

substances that block the development of new blood vessels (angiogenesis) and show promise as anticancer drugs. Cancers cannot grow beyond microscopic size unless they develop new blood vessels. If this is prevented they will regress or remain dormant and harmless. Research has shown that the angiogenesis inhibitors endostatin and angiostatin are capable of eliminating cancers of the breast, colon, prostate and brain in mice and can do so without undesirable side effects in the short term. These two drugs act in different ways and research on humans with cancer was started in mid-1998. The drugs are believed not to induce drug resistance in mice.

angiogenic growth factors promoters of the production of new small blood vessels. They include VASCULAR ENDOTHELIAL GROWTH FACTOR (VEGF); acidic and basic fibroblast growth factor; transforming growth factor alpha and beta; tumour necrosis growth factor-alpha; platelet-derived growth factor; angiogenin; and interleukin-8.

angiography a form of X-ray examination using a CONTRAST MEDIUM which renders the blood visible in blood vessels into which it has been injected. Angiography does not show the vessels themselves, but outlines the shape of the blood column. A fine tube (catheter) is used to direct the contrast medium to the required place. See also DIGITAL SUBTRACTION ANGIOGRAPHY.

angiology the study of blood and lymph vessels. From the Greek *angeion*, a vessel and *logos*, a discourse.

angiomyofibrosarcoma a very rare sarcomatous tumour that probably arises from a pre-existing ANGIOMYXOMA. It has been found in the ischiorectal fossa of a woman.

angioma a benign (non-malignant) tumour of blood vessels.

angiomyxoma a rare, slow-growing, and non-metastasizing tumour mainly affecting women and occurring in the anogenital region.

angioneurotic oedema a form of allergy in which contact with certain foodstuffs, plants, drugs or pollens or an insect sting causes swelling of the lining of the nose, mouth, throat or digestive tract. The main danger is from ASPHYXIA from oedema of the LARYNX.

angio-oedema an acute, painless blistering of the skin or swelling of the underlying tissues, with fluid collection, due to food or drug allergy, infection or emotional stress.

angiopathy any disease of the blood or lymph vessels.

Angiopine MR a brand name for NIFEDIPINE.

angioplasty a method of widening the bore of an artery narrowed by disease, usually ATHEROSCLEROSIS. A surgical procedure to promote the normal flow of blood to an important part, such as the heart muscle or the brain. A common technique is BALLOON ANGIOPLASTY.

angiosarcoma a rare malignant tumour of the lining cells of small blood vessels that often occurs in several places at once and may affect the liver as a complication of CIRRHOSIS. It is known to occur in people who were exposed to the medical contrast medium thorotrast up to 25 years before and has been found in workers with vinyl chloride. The tumour is highly malignant and treatment is rarely effective.

angioscope an optical instrument used to examine the interior of blood vessels.

angioscopy direct visual examination of the inside of a blood vessel during life. Modern angioscopes are fine, fibre-optic catheters capable of passing into the coronary arteries so that the state of their inner walls may be ascertained. This procedure, however, is not without risk.

angiospasm temporary closure or partial closure of a section of an artery as a result of contraction of the circularly placed muscle in its wall.

angiostatin a degradation product of PLASMINOGEN that interferes with the development of blood vessels (angiogenesis) and offers promise as an anticancer agent. Growth of tumours beyond about 3 cu. mm. depends on the development of a good blood supply by the growth of small blood vessels. This applies both to the primary tumour and to any remote deposits (mestastases) of spread cancer. Trials have shown that angiostatin can cause early tumours to die from lack of a blood supply. See also ENDOSTATIN.

angiostrongyliasis infestation with the rat worm parasites *Angiostrongylus cantonensis* and *A. costaricensis* usually acquired by eating snails, shrimps or fish, the intermediate hosts. The former parasite can affect the brain causing eosinophilic MENINGITIS or the eyes causing visual loss. *A. costaricensis* causes eosinophilic GASTROENTERITIS.

angiotensin the vasoconstrictor polypeptide hormone, angiotensin II, which is released by the action of the enzyme renin. Its precursor, angiotensin I, is inactive until acted on by the angiotensin-converting enzyme, mainly in the lungs. Angiotensin II has a powerful effect on raising the blood pressure. It binds to angiotensin receptors and constricts the circular smooth muscle of blood vessel walls. It prompts cells of the adrenal cortex to secrete the hormone ALDOSTERONE. It modulates blood flow through the kidneys and acts directly on the heart muscle. By promoting raised blood pressure it encourages the development of the arterial disease ATHEROSCLEROSIS.

angiotensin II antagonist one of a range of drugs that act directly on angiotensin at its receptor sites so as to block its action. These drugs include CANDESARTAN, IRBESARTAN, LOSARTAN, VALSARTAN, telmisartan (Micardis), Olmesartan (Olmetec) and eprosartan (Teveten).

angiotensin-converting enzyme the (ACE) enzyme that converts angiotensin I to the active form angiotensin II. The gene for this enzyme has two alleles, the *I* allele and the *D* allele. Research has shown that the *I* allele is associated with significantly better physical performance, endurance and response to physical training than the *D* allele. The difference is especially marked if the *I* allele is present at both loci and compared with people with the *D* allele at both loci.

angiotensin-converting enzyme inhibitors a class of drugs used in the treatment of raised blood pressure and to assist in the management of heart failure. They act by preventing the conversion of ANGIOTENSIN I to angiotensin II. The term is usually abbreviated to ACE inhibitors. They include ENALAPRIL, RAMIPRIL, QUINAPRIL, CAPTOPRIL, LISINOPRIL, PERINDOPRIL and TRANDOLAPRIL.

Angitil SR a brand name for DILTIAZEM.

angle-closure glaucoma an acute or subacute condition of raised pressure within the eye due to an obstruction to the normal outflow of aqueous humour from the eye. This may be due to structural factors such as undue narrowness of the angle between the back of the cornea and the iris or to inflammatory adhesions. The condition can usually be corrected by an operation to make a small opening in the periphery of the iris (a peripheral iridectomy or iridotomy). This may be done with a LASER.

Ångstrom unit a unit of very small size appropriate to the measurement of molecules and atoms. It is equal to one tenth of a nanometer (0.1 nm).

anhidrosis absence of sweating or inadequate secretion of sweat.

anhidrotic tending to cause absence of sweating. The term is also applied to any drug or skin application which reduces or prevents sweating.

anhydraemia a deficiency of water in the blood.

anilinctus oral sexual stimulation of the anus.

animal cloning the artificial production of one or more apparently perfect copies of an existing animal by inserting a copy of its DNA into an ovum from which the nuclear genetic material has been removed and then persuading the ovum to function as a ZYGOTE. There are indications that the process, as currently used, may in some way damage the genome. Many of the mammalian clones so far produced show defects that appear to reduce the normal life span.

animism the belief held by many primitive peoples that a spirit resides within every object, controlling its existence and influencing events in the natural world.

anion a negatively charged ion that is attracted to an anode (positively-charged electrode), in electrolysis. Anions are usually shown as the second group in simple inorganic molecules, thus Cl^- is the anion when common salt (NaCl) is dissociated in solution. Na^+ is the CATION.

aniridia absence of the iris of the eye. This may be CONGENITAL or, more commonly, the result of injury.

anis-, aniso- *combining form denoting* unequal.

anisakiasis herring worm disease caused by the larvae of worms of the *Anisakidae* family. A parasitic infection acquired by eating raw herrings. A fibrous mass (granuloma) forms in the intestine causing fever, colic and intermittent obstruction. Surgical treatment may be needed.

aniseikonia an ocular defect in which the size or shape of the retinal images are different in the two eyes. This is often the result of ANISOMETROPIA. From the Greek *an*, not *iso*, equal and *eicon*, an image.

aniso- a prefix meaning unequal.

anisocoria inequality in the size of the pupils of the eye.

anisocytosis inequality in the size of red blood cells found in many kinds of ANAEMIA but especially in MEGALOBLASTIC anaemia.

anisometropia the condition in which the focus is different in the two eyes. One eye may be normal and the other MYOPIC or HYPERMETROPIC, or one eye may be ASTIGMATIC. From the Greek *an*, not *iso*, equal and *metron*, a measure.

anistreplase a clot-dissolving drug used to try to re-establish blood flow in the heart muscle in the early treatment of heart attacks. A brand name is Eminase.

ankle the joint between the lower ends of the TIBIA and FIBULA and the upper surface of the talus bone of the foot. The talus sits on top of the heel bone (calcaneum).

ankle clonus a rhythmical, sustained series of flexion movements at the ankle. This is produced in people with damage to the nerve pathways in the spinal cord or brain (an upper motor neurone lesion), by a deliberate rapid, stretching of the ACHILLES TENDON, by forcibly flexing the foot. The spinal reflex arc is intact but the normal control on it, from above, is defective.

ankylo- *combining form denoting* stiff, fused or fixed.

ankyloglossia tongue-tied condition due to an unduly tight central fold of mucous membrane connecting the under side of the tongue to the floor of the mouth (FRENULUM). This is easily relieved by snipping the frenulum with scissors.

ankylosing spondylitis a chronic inflammatory disease of the spinal column leading to stiffening and fixity of the ligaments and bones, so that, eventually, almost all movement is lost.

ankylosis fixation and immobilization of a joint by disease which has so damaged the bearing surfaces that the bone ends have been able to fuse permanently together. Sometimes ankylosis is deliberately performed, as a surgical procedure, to relieve pain. From the Greek *ankylos*, bent.

anlagen a localized cell cluster in an embryo that develops into a particular body part in the mature organism.

Ann Arbor classification a method of deciding on the stage to which any case of HODGKIN'S DISEASE has progressed. Staging is important in deciding the best treatment and in determining the outlook (prognosis). In Stage I only one lymph node or one extra-lymphatic site is involved. In Stage IV, tissues such as bone marrow and liver are affected.

annealing the joining-up of complementary single strands of DNA that have been separated by heat, or the joining of parts of separate strands that have complementary base sequences, to form a double helix.

annexin one of a family of over 20 proteins first described in 1990, that include vascular anticoagulant proteins, placental proteins, placental anticoagulant proteins, lipocortins and endonexins. Annexins have similar structures, usually with four domains of 70 amino acids, and all are capable of binding calcium and phospholipids. They are present in a wide variety of cell types. Annexin II acts to bind plasminogen and TISSUE PLASMINOGEN ACTIVATOR to the endothelial cell surface. Annexin V forms an antithrombotic shield around procoagulant phospholipids.

annexinopathies diseases caused by abnormalities in an ANNEXIN. An abnormally high level of Annexin II, for instance, causes a bleeding disorder with excessive fibrinolysis. Annexin V deficiency causes accelerated blood coagulation in the antiphospholipid syndrome (HUGHES' SYNDROME).

annular ring-shaped. Mainly used to refer to anything that encircles a hollow tube of organ as in the case of an annular cancer of the colon.

annular ligament a fibrous band that surrounds the ankle joint and the wrist joint, acting to retain in position the ligaments passing across the joint.

annulus any ring-like structure.

annulus fibrosus the tough fibrous outer zone of the intervertebral disc that normally retains the soft inner nucleus pulposus. Weakness of the annulus fibrosus allows prolapse of the pulpy centre in the condition inaccurately known as 'slipped disc'.

anodontia partial or total congenital absence of the teeth.

anodyne 1 pain-relieving or relaxing.
2 a drug or other agency that relieves pain.

anogenital pertaining to the anus and to the genitalia.

anomaly anything differing from the normal.

anomia inability to name things, usually the result of a neurological defect.

anomic dysphasia a form of DYSPHASIA in which the affected person is able to recognize objects but cannot name them; or a dysphasia in which there is inability to relate a name to its particular object.

anomie lack of moral principle, whether in an individual or in a society.

Anopheles a genus of mosquito containing a number of species that transmit the malarial parasite from person to person when feeding on blood. Species commonly transmitting malaria include *A. gambiae* (Africa), *A. stephensi* (Middle east), *A. culicifacies* (India), *A. maculatus* (Far East) and *A. punctulatus* (Australasia).

Anpec a brand name for VERAPAMIL.

anopheline pertaining to the ANOPHELES genus of mosquitoes.

anorchism congenital absence of testicles from the scrotum. This is usually due to undescended testicle (CRYPTORCHIDISM) but may be due to injury or infection or may occur without obvious cause, when it is sometimes called the 'vanishing testes syndrome'. Treatment is by the use of male sex hormones or a plastic prosthetic testicle implant.

anorectic, anoretic, anorexic 1 featuring or causing loss of appetite.
2 a drug that suppresses appetite.

anorectic drugs drugs that suppress appetite and may be useful in the management of OBESITY. They include AMPHETAMINE (amfetamine) and its derivatives, mazindol (Teronc), phentermine (Duromine) and fenfluramine. These drugs have lost status since it became apparent that addiction is possible and that fenfluramine and phentermine can cause valvular heart disease.

anorexia loss of appetite, especially as a result of disease. From the Greek *an*, not and *orexis*, appetite.

anorexia nervosa a serious disorder of perception causing the sufferer, almost always a young woman, to believe that she is too fat, when, in fact, she may be very thin. Food intake is drastically reduced and emaciation results. Treatment is difficult and the best efforts of those trying to help are often frustrated by the determination of the sufferer to avoid eating. Hospital treatment is usually necessary as there is a real risk of a fatal outcome, often from suicide.

anorgasmia the inability to achieve an orgasm. Apart from those cases associated with IMPOTENCE, this is commoner in women than in men and is seldom an organic disorder. Anorgasmia may be due to various psychosexual factors and can often be corrected by skilled counselling.

anorthopia see METAMORPHOPSIA.

anoscope see PROCTOSCOPE.

anosmia loss of the sense of smell. This often results from injury to the delicate fibres of the OLFACTORY NERVE as they pass through the bone above the nose (the cribriform plate).

anovulation failure of the ovaries to produce eggs so that conception is impossible. This may result from low levels of gonadotrophin-releasing hormone, excess prolactin, pituitary failure, excessive exercise, ANOREXIA NERVOSA, stress, KALLMAN'S SYNDROME, SHEEHAN'S SYNDROME, pituitary tumours, excess radiation to the brain, or from natural states such as pregnancy and lactation. Anovulation is also caused by oral contraceptives.

anoxaemia an abnormal or extreme reduction in the oxygen content of the blood. Literal anoxaemia is incompatible with life and, as commonly used, the term is incorrect.

anoxia local absence of oxygen, usually as a result of interference with the blood supply. Complete anoxia is rare, the more usual condition being a relative insufficiency, which is known as hypoxia.

ansa an anatomical structure, especially neurological, in the form of a loop or arc. From the Latin *ansa*, the handle of a jug.

ansamycins drugs used to treat TUBERCULOSIS. An example is rifabutin (Mycobutin).

Antabuse disulfiram. A drug sometimes used in the management of alcoholism, which causes severe nausea and vomiting, sweating, breathlessness, headache and chest pain if any alcohol is taken after it has been given. Disulfiram inhibits the enzyme aldehyde dehydrogenase that breaks down acetaldehyde, a toxic metabolite of alcohol, so that this accumulates. The method is a form of aversion therapy and is not without danger of collapse and death from the toxic effects.

antacid a drug used to combat excess stomach acid or to treat the symptom of ACID REFLUX.

Antacid drugs are often compounds of magnesium or aluminium. Antacids may also provide a protective coating to the lining of the stomach and DUODENUM.

Antadine a brand name for AMANTADINE.

antagonist 1 a muscle that acts to oppose the action of another muscle (the agonist).
2 a drug that counteracts or neutralizes the action of another drug. The antonym of antagonist is agonist.

antazoline an ANTIHISTAMINE drug that also has weak local anaesthetic and ANTICHOLINERGIC effects. A brand name is Otrivine-Antistin.

ante- *prefix denoting* before, either in time, order or position. From the Latin *ante*, before.

anteflexion a forward bending of an organ such as the womb. Compare ANTEVERSION.

antegrade, anterograde proceeding in the normal or usual direction. The antonym of antegrade is retrograde.

ante mortem before death.

antenatal before birth. Prenatal.

antenatal care medical surveillance and review performed during pregnancy for the early detection of possible complications of pregnancy, especially pre-eclamptic toxaemia (see PRE-ECLAMPSIA) and uterine and fetal abnormalities. Antenatal care includes general examination, abdominal examination, vaginal examination, regular tests to monitor the progress of the pregnancy, ultrasound scanning, checks of weight gain, blood checks, tests of HORMONES and ENZYMES to assess the efficiency of the PLACENTA, and frequent tests of the blood pressure and urine. See also ANTENATAL SCREENING.

antenatal screening a part of ANTENATAL CARE often involving ultrasound imaging of the uterus and fetus, and sometime AMNIOCENTESIS or CHORIONIC VILLUS SAMPLING. Antenatal screening can detect multiple pregnancies, abnormally placed placentas, excess uterine fluid (HYDRAMNIOS) and fetal abnormalities such as SPINA BIFIDA, ANENCEPHALY, congenital heart disease, polycystic kidneys and bowel and urinary tract obstruction.

Antenex a brand name for DIAZEPAM.

antepartum before a baby is delivered.

antepartum haemorrhage bleeding occurring in pregnancy after about the 24th week. There may be a risk to the baby, which might be in

danger of inadequate blood supply, and to the mother.

anterior at or towards the front of the body.

anterior commissure a nerve fibre bundle running across the midline of the brain from one hemisphere to the other, just in front of the THIRD VENTRICLE.

anterograde amnesia loss of memory for a variable period following a head injury or an epileptic seizure. The length of the period of AMNESIA following a head injury is usually proportional to the severity. Compare RETROGRADE AMNESIA.

anthelmintic a drug used to kill or drive out parasitic worms from the intestines. From the Greek *anti*, against and *elmins*, a worm.

anthracosis a chronic lung disease resulting from repeated inhalation of coal dust. Inflammation of the lungs with extensive fibrous tissue formation leads to a reduction in lung function and sometimes severe disability.

Anthisan a brand name for MEPYRAMINE.

anthracycline derivatives drugs used to treat metastatic cancer. An example is mitoxantrone (Novantrone).

anthracycline glycoside antibiotics drugs used to treat relapsed LEUKAEMIA. Examples are aclarubicin, doxorubicin (Caelyx), daunorubicin (Daunoxome), epidubicin (Pharmorubicin) and idarubicin (Zavedos).

Anthranol a brand name for DITHRANOL.

anthraquinone glycosides an anti-inflammatory group of drug used in the treatment of mouth ulcers. A brand name is Pyralvex.

anthrax a serious infection of skin, intestine or lungs caused by spores of Bacillus anthracis which can be transmitted to man from infected animals or animal products. There are large and damaging BOILS, severe GASTROENTERITIS and an often fatal PNEUMONIA. Anthrax has been intensively investigated as a bacteriological weapon and concern has been expressed over its suitability as a terrorist weapon. From the Greek *anthrax*, coal, possibly because of the black centre and the surrounding redness of the skin lesions.

anthropo- *combining form denoting* human or man.

anthropoid resembling man.

anthropology the science of humankind, and of human cultural differences, from the earliest times to the present. Anthropology is thus a very wide subject, concerned not simply with the less familiar human groups but with every aspect of humankind in a social context. Increasingly, anthropology overlaps the social sciences, but, at the same time, preserves a certain detachment from concern with the more utilitarian aspects of such studies, as befits one of the basic sciences. Cultural anthropology, or ethnology, is a comparative study of cultural systems and includes concern with early archeology, religion, myth, political and economic systems and language. Other branches of cultural anthropology include psychological, legal and urban anthropology. The observation, recording and analysis of anthropological data in the course of 'field work' is called ethnography. Physical anthropology is the study of human evolution, including recent diversification of humans. Social anthropology covers the whole field of humans in their social context.

anthropometry human body measurement and weighing for scientific purposes such as anthropological or nutritional research or as an aid to clinical assessment.

anthropomorphism attributing human characteristics to the diety, to inanimate objects, animals, or phenomena. Due to our experiential limitations and need to find explanations, however unsatisfactory, we commonly resort to an anthropomorphic concept of anything transcendental.

anthropophagous man-eating. Cannibal.

anti- *prefix denoting* against, opposite, counteractive.

anti-amoebic able to destroy or suppress amoebae of medical importance.

anti-androgen drugs drugs given to sexually criminal men to inhibit male sex hormone action and dampen down their urges. These include cyproterone acetate, CIMETIDINE and SPIRONOLACTONE. Anti-androgen drugs may cause breast enlargement (gynaecomastia).

anti-angiogenic drugs a group of currently experimental anticancer drugs that act by inhibiting the growth of the small blood vessels on which cancers depend for their growth. The group includes ANGIOSTATIN, ENDOSTATIN, THALIDOMIDE, SQUALAMINE, 2-methoxy-oestradiol (estradiol), vitaxin and marimastat.

anti-arrhythmic drugs drugs used to correct

irregularity of the heart beat. They include DIGOXIN, VERAPAMIL, AMIODARONE, QUINIDINE, procainamide, LIGNOCAINE (lidocaine), flecainide and CALCIUM CHANNEL BLOCKERS.

antibacterial effective against bacteria.

antibioma a hard swelling containing sterile pus caused by the long-term use of antibiotics to treat an abscess that should have been opened and emptied. Such a lump may mimic a cancer and often required surgical exploration and drainage.

antibiotic drugs a very extensive range of drugs able to kill or prevent reproduction of bacteria in the body without killing the patient. Antibiotics were originally derived from cultures of living organisms, such as fungi or bacteria, but, today, many are chemically synthesized. The antibiotics have enormously extended the scope and effectiveness of medical therapy against bacterial infection, but have not succeeded in eliminating any bacterial diseases. The extensive, and not always judicious, use of antibiotics has led to widespread evolutionary changes in bacteria in response to their new environment, manifested by the acquisition, by natural selection, of resistance to these drugs. This forces researchers to produce ever new and more effective antibiotics. The antibiotics include such classes as the aminoglycosides, amphenicols, ansamycins, lincosamides, macrolides, polypeptides, tetracyclines and beta-lactams. The beta-lactams include groups such as carbapenems, cephalosporins, cephamycins, monobactams, oxacephems and penicillins.

antibiotic-associated colitis inflammation of the colon, with diarrhoea, as a result of the change in the normal bacterial flora of the colon from the use of broad-spectrum antibiotics. Many cases are due to the overgrowth of *Clostridium difficile* an organism that produces an irritating toxin.

antibiotic resistance the natural tendency for bacteria, under the processes of natural selection in an antibiotic-rich environment, to evolve in such a way as to become capable of surviving in spite of these drugs. Antibiotic resistance is a rapidly increasing problem largely as a result of worldwide misuse and overuse of antibiotics in conditions that do not require them. See also ANTIBIOTIC-RESISTANT STAPHYLOCOCCI.

antibiotic-resistant staphylococci
organisms that continue to multiply and cause
disease in people treated with a range of wide-
spectrum antibiotics including methicillin.
Methicillin has been used for years in cases of
infections with staphylococci that produce the
penicillin-destroying enzyme penicillinase.
Some staphylococci have, however, evolved that
can survive in an environment of methicillin
and these germs are now endemic in many
hospitals.

antibody a Y-shaped protein molecule, called
an IMMUNOGLOBULIN, produced by the B group
of lymphocytes in response to the presence of a
ANTIGEN. An appropriate B lymphocyte is
selected from the existing repertoire. This then
produces a clone of PLASMA CELLS each capable
of synthesizing large numbers of specific
antibodies to combat the infection. The B cells
also produce memory cells. Subsequent
infection with the same antigen prompts the
memory cells to clone plasma cells and produce
the correct antibodies without further delay.
This is an important way in which an infection
leads to subsequent immunity. Antibodies are
able to neutralize antigens or render them
susceptible to destruction by PHAGOCYTES in
the body. The basic structure of an antibody
consists of four polypeptide chains linked by
disulphide bridges, two larger structures called
HEAVY CHAINS and two smaller called LIGHT
CHAINS.

antibody-deficiency syndromes conditions
such as hypogamma-globulinaemia,
AGAMMAGLOBULINAEMIA and dysgamma-
globulinaemia, in which there is defective
production of IMMUNOGLOBULINS.

**antibody-dependent cell-mediated
cytotoxicity** the killing of a target cell,
which has been coated with an antibody, by a
MACROPHAGE, neutrophil or natural killer cell
that carries the surface receptor that binds to
the particular antibody.

anticarcinogen any agent that interferes with
the action of a cancer-producing effect.

anticardiolipin antibodies see
ANTIPHOSPHOLIPID SYNDROME.

anticholinergic antagonistic to the action of
acetyl choline or to the parasympathetic or
other CHOLINERGIC nerve supply. Acetyl choline
stimulates muscle contraction in the intestines
and elsewhere and slows the heart.

Anticholinergic substances, such as ATROPINE,
relieve muscle spasm, dilate the pupils and
speed up the heart.

anticholinesterase any substance opposing
the action of the enzyme cholinesterase,
which breaks down the NEUROTRANSMITTER
acetylcholine, releasing the inactive choline
for further synthesis to acetylcholine. An
anticholinesterase agent thus potentiates the
action of acetylcholine, a major neurotransmitter carrying nerve impulses across
synapses and from nerves to muscles. Continued
action causes serious effects. A number of
organophosphorus insecticides and some nerve
gases are anticholinesterases. Poisoning
produces nausea, vomiting, sweating, salivation,
restlessness, tightness of the chest, blurred
vision, diarrhoea convulsions and death.

anticipation the occurrence of a hereditary
disease at progressively earlier ages, and in
progressively more severe form, in successive
generations. This is a feature of a range of
conditions that includes myotonic dystrophy,
the fragile X syndrome and Huntington's
disease.

anticoagulant a drug used to limit the normal
clotting processes of the blood. Anticoagulants
are used in conditions in which dangerous clots
can form in blood vessels. Anticoagulant drugs
include HEPARIN, LOW MOLECULAR WEIGHT
HEPARIN and WARFARIN. Anticoagulant
treatment carries its own dangers, specifically
those related to internal bleeding. The principal
danger is of bleeding within the skull and
resultant STROKE. The danger is greatest in
elderly people with high blood pressure. This
may be spontaneous or may follow quite minor
trauma to the head. Careful control of dosage
with regular blood checks of PROTHROMBIN
TIME, and the avoidance of head injury,
minimize the risk.

anticodon a sequence of three nucleotides in
transfer RNA complementary to the three
nucleotides in a codon on messenger RNA.
The anticodon specifies a particular amino acid
which is selected and assembled for protein
synthesis.

anticonvulsant a drug used to prevent or
reduce the severity of epileptic attacks, or to
prevent dangerous muscle contraction in
electroconvulsive therapy. Anticonvulsant drugs
include PHENYTOIN (Epanutin),

PHENOBARBITONE (phenobarbital) (Luminal), ETHOSUXIMIDE (Zarontin), CARBAMAZEPINE (Tegretol), SODIUM VALPROATE (Epilim) and CLONAZEPAM (Rivotril).

anticytokine therapy treatment by interference with the function of CYTOKINES. Tumour necrosis factor, for instance, is an inflammatory cytokine involved in the pathogenesis of RHEUMATOID ARTHRITIS. The use of a TUMOUR NECROSIS FACTOR ANTAGONIST has led to significant improvement in this disease.

anti-D immunoglobulin a preparation of human ANTIBODY (immunoglobulin) used to prevent a rhesus-negative woman from forming antibodies to fetal rhesus-positive red blood cells. The immunoglobulin is given after birth, miscarriage or abortion of a rhesus-positive fetus with the object of protecting any subsequent baby against attack by maternal antibodies. The drug is on the WHO official list. A brand name is Partobulin.

antidepressant one of the large range of drugs used to treat depression. Classes of antidepressant drugs include bicyclics, tricyclics, tetracyclics, monoamine oxidase inhibitors (MAOIs) and selective serotonin re-uptake inhibitors. Some of the most commonly used drugs are lithium (Camcolit), nortriptyline (Allegron), amoxapine (Asendis), citalopram (Cipramil), protriptyline (Concordin), flupenthixol (flupentixol) (Fluanxol), maprotiline (Ludiomil), tradozone (Molipaxin), fluphenazine (Modecate, Moditen), phenelzine (Nardil), tranylcypromine (Parnate), dothiepin (dosulepin) (Prothiaden), promazine (Sparine), thioridazine (Melleril), imipramine (Tofranil), perphenazine (Fentanyl), prochlorperazine (Stemetil), trifluoperazine (Stelazine), amitryptyline (Triptafen), clomipramine (Anafranil), doxepin (Sinequan), isocarboxazid (Marplan), tranylcypromine (Parnate), fluoxetine (Prozac) and tryptophan (Optimax).

antidiuretic hormone vasopressin. The hormone released by the rear part of the PITUITARY gland which acts on the kidneys to control water excretion. In the absence of this hormone, large quantities of urine are produced, as in DIABETES INSIPIDUS.

antidopaminergics see ANTIEMETICS.

antidote a drug or other agent which neutralizes or counteracts the action or effect of a poison. There are few specific antidotes. These include NALOXONE for narcotic opiate poisoning, desferrioxamine for iron poisoning, cobalt edetate for cyanide poisoning and n-acetylcysteine for paracetamol poisoning. Activated charcoal may be valuable to absorb poisons.

antiemetics drugs used to prevent vomiting. Antiemetic drugs include metoclopramide (Maxolon) and domperidone (Motilium).

antiendotoxin antibodies IMMUNOGLOBULIN against the core region that all ENDOTOXINS have in common. Anticore antibody is effective against endotoxin from a wide range of organisms including GRAM NEGATIVE bacteria.

antienzyme a substance that interferes with the action of, or counteracts, an ENZYME.

antiepileptic drugs drugs used to prevent, or reduce the liability to, epileptic seizures. They include SODIUM VALPROATE, CARBAMAZEPINE, ACETAZOLAMIDE, LAMOTRIGINE, PHENOBARBITONE (phenobarbital), CLONAZEPAM, PHENYTOIN, CLOBAZAM and GABAPENTIN.

antifibrinolysis the prevention of the breakdown of fibrin which is a major element in the formation of a blood clot. Drugs such as aminocaproic acid and tranexamic acid inhibit fibrinolysis.

antifibrinolytics drugs used to treat excessive bleeding as in menorrhagia or to help in the control of bleeding during surgery. Examples are tranexamic acid (Cyklokapron) and aprotinin (Trasylol).

antifibrotics drugs used to treat disorders due to abnormal scar formation such as PEYRONIE'S DISEASE or SCLERODERMA. An example is potassium para-aminobenzoate (Potaba).

antifungal effective in the treatment or control of fungus infections.

anti-GAD antibodies antibodies to the enzyme glutamic acid decarboxylase. These antibodies are present in DIABETES MELLITUS and appear before the disease become clinically manifest. They may be useful predictors of the condition, but are also found in the STIFF MAN SYNDROME and other conditions.

antigen any molecule recognized by the immune system of the body as signalling 'foreign', and which will provoke the production of a specific ANTIBODY. Antigens include molecules on the surfaces of infective viruses, bacteria and fungi, pollen grains and donor body tissue cells.

antigen/antibody complex the association of an ANTIGEN with its resulting ANTIBODY to form a molecular group which can be damaging to tissues, especially to the lining of blood vessels. More usually called an immune complex. A growing number of diseases is recognized as being caused by antigen/antibody complexes. See also IMMUNE COMPLEXES.

antigenicity the power, or degree of power, to act as an ANTIGEN.

antigenic determinant a cluster of EPITOPES.

antigen-presenting cell a cell, such as a macrophage, a B cell or a dendritic cell, that presents processed antigenic peptides and MHC class II molecules to the T cell receptor on CD4 T cells.

antihaemophilic globulin the blood coagulation factor, Factor VIII, which is deficient in people suffering from HAEMOPHILIA.

antihelminthic ANTHELMINTIC.

antihistamine one of a group of drugs which act against histamine – a powerful and highly irritant agent released in the body by MAST CELLS, after contact with certain ALLERGENS. Antihistamine drugs fall into two groups – those that block H_1 receptors and act mainly on blood vessels, and those that block H_2 receptors and act mainly on the secretion of acid in the stomach. H_1 receptor blockers include diphenhydramine, chlorpheniramine (chlorphenamine) (Piriton), terfenadine (Triludan), promethazine (Phenergan), cyproheptadine (Periactin), mequitazine (Primalan) and phenindamine (Thephorin). H_2 receptor blockers are not usually referred to as antihistamines, although this is what they are. They include CIMETIDINE (Tagamet), and RANITIDINE (Zantac).

antihypertensive 1 acting against high blood pressure (HYPERTENSION).
2 a drug used in the treatment of high blood pressure.

antihyperlipidaemia drugs drugs that reduce the levels of cholesterol and fats (triglycerides) in the blood. They include statin drugs (see STATINS) such as SIMVASTATIN, ATORVASTATIN, PROVASTATIN, ROSUVASTATIN and FLUVASTATIN that block the synthesis of cholesterol; bile acid sequestrants such as CHOLESTYRAMINE

(colestyramine) and COLESTIPOL that bind and remove from the intestine bile acids which are derived from cholesterol; fibrates such as CIPROFIBRATE, BENZAFIBRATE and GEMFIBROZIL that interfere with cholesterol synthesis; and nicotinic acid derivatives that interfere with the release of fats from body fat stores and increase the activity of fat-splitting enzymes.

anti-inflammatory acting against inflammation. The main anti-inflammatory drugs are the CORTICOSTEROIDS but these must always be used with caution as inflammation is usually beneficial.

antileprotics drugs used to treat HANSEN'S DISEASE (leprosy). Examples are dapsone and clofazimine (Lamprene).

antileukotreines drugs that blocks the action of certain natural LEUKOTRIENES which cause the air passaged to tighten and narrow in ASTHMA. Some of them, like montelukast and zafirlukast are LEUKOTRIENE RECEPTOR ANTAGONISTS. Others inhibit the synthesis of leukotrienes.

antilymphocyte antibodies antibodies that have developed to the human leucocyte (HLA) antigens on B and T cells. Monoclonal antilymphocyte antibodies have been used to prevent graft rejection but are dangerously liable to lead to severe infection from the resulting acquired immune deficiency.

antimalarial 1 effective in the treatment or prevention of malaria.
2 an antimalarial drug.

antimalarials drugs used to prevent and treat MALARIA. They include chloroquine (Avloclor), dapsone, pyrimethamine (Daraprim), mefloquine (Lariam), atovaquone with proguanil hydrochloride (Malarone), proguanil (Paludrine) and artemether with lumefantrine (Riamet).

antimetabolite an anticancer, or CYTOTOXIC, drug which acts by combining with essential enzymes within cancer cells so as to interfere with their metabolism and growth. To be useful, antimetabolites must be significantly more toxic to cancer cells than to normal cells.

antimicrobial able to destroy microorganisms.

antimitotic 1 anything which interferes with cell division.
2 an anticancer drug, or agency, which acts by interfering with the reproduction of cancer cells.

antimonials antimony-containing drugs,

especially the pentavalent group such as sodium stibogluconate (Stibophen) and meglumine antimoniate, used in the treatment of KALA-AZAR (LEISHMANIASIS).

antimony a brittle, flaky metal, many of the compounds of which are poisonous.

antimuscarinics drugs used to treat reversible airway obstruction as in ASTHMA and chronic BRONCHITIS. Examples are ipratropium bromide (Atrovent), oxitropium (Oxivent) and tiotropium (Spiriva).

antimycotic a drug used in the treatment of fungus infections.

antimyelin antibodies antibodies against myelin oligodendrocyte glycoprotein (MOG) and mylein basic protein (MBP) that are commonly found in people who have had an isolated episode suggesting MULTIPLE SCLEROSIS. Research has shown that people with anti-MOG and anti-MBP antibodies are liable to have relapses of the disease more often and earlier than those without the antibodies. Only 23% of those without the antibodies have the relapse, while 95% of those with the antibodies develop established MS.

antineoplastic able to control the growth or spread of cancers (neoplasms).

antineoplaston a peptide derivative that was the occasion of a major legal action in 1997 when a Texas doctor was indicted for criminal contempt and fraud for allegedly violating federal court orders not to treat cancer patients with this drug. The case stirred up the perennial controversy between those who believe that all patients are entitled to seek alternatives to orthodox scientific medicine and those who believe that in serious conditions this can be dangerous.

antinuclear factor antibodies directed at elements in the nuclei of cells, such as DNA. Low levels are present in most people, but significantly high levels are found in RHEUMATOID ARTHRITIS, SJOGREN'S DISEASE, fibrosing alveolitis, persistent liver disease, ADDISON'S DISEASE, MYASTHENIA GRAVIS, LEUKAEMIA and systemic LUPUS ERYTHEMATOSUS.

antioxidants substances that inhibit oxidative changes in molecules. Many oxidative changes are destructive and this applies as much to the human body as to non-biological chemistry. Recognition that many of the fundamentally

damaging processes in disease are oxidative in nature and result from the action of oxygen FREE RADICALS has raised interest in the possibility of using antioxidants to minimize such damage. The most popular choice for this purpose are the antioxidant vitamins C and E. There is evidence that, taken in adequate dosage, these vitamins act synergistically to reduce free radical effects. See also FLAVONOIDS and FRENCH PARADOX.

antiparallel of two structures that lie parallel to each other but that run in opposite directions. The best-known example of antiparalellism is that of the two strands in the DNA molecule.

antiparkinsonism drugs drugs used to control the effects of PARKINSON'S DISEASE. They include levodopa (Sinemet), amantadine (Symmetrel), bromocriptine (Parlodel) and selegilene (Eldepryl).

antiperspirant a drug or skin preparation used to inhibit perspiration or prevent excessive perspiration.

antiphospholipid syndrome see HUGHES' SYNDROME.

antiplatelet antibodies antibodies that attack blood PLATELETS. Most are formed as a result of an AUTOIMMUNE process but some cases result from passage of maternal antibodies through the placenta before birth, or from platelet transfusion. Autoantibodies are common in SYSTEMIC LUPUS ERYTHEMATOSUS or HUGHES' SYNDROME. The effect of antiplatelet antibodies is to produce a drop in the number of platelets (THROMBOCYTOPENIA).

antiprotozoals drugs used to treat infections with protozal organisms. Examples are tinidazole (Fastigyn) for amoebiasis, giardiasis, ulcerative gingivitis and trichomoniasis; and pentamidine (Pentacarinat) and atovaquone (Wellvone) for *Pneumocystis carinii* pneumonia.

antipruritic any drug or other treatment effective in relieving itching.

antipsoriatics drugs used to treat PSORIASIS. They include coal tar (Clinitar, Exorex, Pentrax, Psoriderm); coal tar extract with allantoin (Alphosyl); coal tar with cade oil and arachis oil (Polytar); salicylic acid (Capasal); and dithranol (Dithrocream).

antipsychotic a drug used in the treatment or control of severe mental illness such as SCHIZOPHRENIA. The antipsychotic drugs include such groups as the benzamides

(Amisulpride, Dolmatil, Solian); benzisoxzoles (Risperidal); butyrophenones (Anquil, Dozic, Droleptan, Haldol, Serenace); phenothiazines (Fentazin, Largactil, Melleril, Modecate, Moditen, Neulactil, Nozinan, Stelazine); and thioxanthines (Clopixol, Depixol).

antipyretic a drug or other measure which lowers a raised body temperature.

antirabies serum serum containing specific antibodies against rabies, used to prevent the development of the disease in those who have been bitten by a rabid animal.

antirachitic acting against rickets or the development of rickets.

antirheumatic any treatment for, or prophylaxis against, any form of rheumatism.

anti-Ro a non-organ specific IgG (IMMUNOGLOBULIN G) autoantibody directed against a soluble ribonucleoprotein. It is associated with SJÖGREN'S SYNDROME and other connective tissue disorders. Maternal anti-Ro can reach the fetal heart via the placenta during pregnancy and cause damage to the conducting system, resulting in congenital heart block.

antiscorbutic tending to prevent, or able to cure, SCURVY. The antiscorbutic substance is vitamin C (ascorbic acid).

antisense RNA RNA molecules transcribed, not from DNA in the usual manner, but from DNA strands complementary to those that produce normal messenger RNA. Antisense RNA occurs in nature and is inhibitory on gene action. It can be produced synthetically and offers such therapeutic possibilities as turning off viral genes.

antisepsis the use of strong poisons to kill bacteria and other dangerous microorganisms. Antisepsis is still used in the cleansing of wounds and skin and for the sterilization of surgical instruments, but modern surgery would not be possible using antisepsis alone. See also ASEPSIS.

antiseptic 1 pertaining to, or able to produce, ANTISEPSIS.
2 any substance capable of killing infective micro-organisms.

antiserum animal or human blood serum which contains ANTIBODIES to infective organisms or to the TOXINS produced by organisms. The serum donor must previously have been infected with the organisms concerned.

antisocial personality disorder a condition of defective capacity for affection or for feeling for others. Affected people are conscienceless and seemingly unaware of the destructive effects of their behaviour on others. They cannot form satisfactory relationships in marriage or at work and often manifest uncontrolled aggression. Stealing, gambling, drug-taking, alcoholism, fire-raising and assault are common features. Such people do not respond to punishment and are a source of much trouble to society. It is questionable whether there is any effective treatment, but see THERAPEUTIC COMMUNITY.

antispasmodic a drug which relieves sustained contraction in muscle, whether voluntary or otherwise.

antistreptolysin titre the level, in the blood, of antibodies to STREPTOCOCCI. A high or rising titre indicates a recent streptococcal infection.

antitetanus immunoglobulin a preparation of antibodies against TETANUS used to protect people who have suffered penetrating wounds that may have been contaminated with tetanus spores. It is used in conjunction with careful surgical toilet and the drug METRONIDAZOLE. The immunoglobulin is also used in cases of established tetanus. The drug is on the WHO official list.

antitetanus serum a serum containing specific antibodies against TETANUS, usually obtained from a horse which has been inoculated with tetanus organisms and has developed immunity to the disease. Because of the possible allergic dangers of anti-tetanus serum it has been largely replaced by ANTITETANUS IMMUNOGLOBULIN.

antithrombin a plasma protein that diminishes the activity of THROMBIN, or the amount of thrombin produced during or following coagulation of the blood.

antithrombin III deficiency an inherited deficiency of certain protein-splitting enzymes (proteases) which normally participate in the blood clotting cascade sequence. Women with this deficiency are at serious risk of developing THROMBOEMBOLISM in pregnancy and HEPARIN treatment is necessary.

antitoxin an ANTIBODY formed by the immune system in response to the presence of TOXIN, produced by bacteria.

antitragus the small projection on the free

border of the external ear above the centre of the lobe. The tragus is the more prominent triangular projection on the front of the ear, immediately above the front edge of the lobe.

antitrypsin see ALPHA-ANTITRYPSIN.

antitussive 1 preventing or relieving cough. 2 a drug used to relieve or abolish coughing.

antivenene an ANTISERUM containing specific antibodies to the venom of poisonous snakes, scorpions or spiders.

antivenom see ANTIVENENE.

antiviral acting against viruses.

antivitamins substances that antagonize or break down vitamins, such as the ENZYME thiaminase present in raw fish. Antivitamins are sometimes used in the treatment of cancer.

antrostomy a surgical operation for SINUSITIS, in which an opening is made into one of the antrums (sinuses) around the nose so as to allow infected material to drain away.

antrum a hollow cavity or sinus in a bone. The maxillary antrums (or antra) are the cavities in the cheek bones. The mastoid bones, below and behind the ears, contain the mastoid antrums (antra). From the Latin *antrum*, a cave.

anuresis see ANURIA.

anuria cessation of the production of urine by the kidneys. Anuria is always very serious, unless of brief duration. Uncorrected anuria leads to a build-up of toxic waste material in the blood and eventual death.

anus the short terminal portion of the ALIMENTARY CANAL which contains two SPHINCTERS by means of which the contents of the RECTUM are retained until they can conveniently be discharged as faeces. Between the sphincters are 6 to 10 vertical columns of mucous membrane containing plexuses of veins. These press together to form watertight seals.

anxiety the natural response to threat or danger, real or perceived and characterized, in its extreme form, by a rapid heart rate, tremulousness, a dry mouth, a feeling of tightness in the chest, sweaty palms, weakness, nausea, bowel hurry with diarrhoea, insomnia, fatigue, headache, and loss of appetite. Anxiety is a response to stress and is a concomitant of a wide spectrum of diseases. But it is also a vital motivating factor causing us to respond constructively to dangers of all kinds and to make greater efforts in all kinds of situations.

Anxiety disorders include PANIC DISORDERS, OBSESSIVE-COMPULSIVE DISORDERS, PHOBIAS, POST-TRAUMATIC STRESS DISORDER and GENERALIZED ANXIETY DISORDER.

anxiolytic 1 operating to relieve ANXIETY or to treat an anxiety disorder. 2 a drug used to treat anxiety.

aorta the main, and largest ARTERY of the body which springs directly from the lower pumping chamber on the left side of the heart and gives off branches to the heart muscle, the head, arms, trunk, chest and abdominal organs and legs.

aortic aneurysm a dangerous sac-like widening (dilation) of the wall of the AORTA. Aortic aneurysm was once most commonly caused by SYPHILIS but is now usually the result of ATHEROSCLEROSIS.

aortic body chemoreceptor groups of nerve cells in the arch of the AORTA that are sensitive to, and respond to changes in the concentration of hydrogen ions, oxygen and carbon dioxide in the blood.

aortic dissection a dangerous and painful disorder in which blood under pressure is forced into a plane within the wall of the largest artery in the body and causes a splitting effect. The condition pre-supposes some structural weakness of the wall of the artery. In about 10% of cases the condition results from spontaneous rupture of one of the tiny arteries (vasa vasorum) that supply the arterial wall with blood. There is a risk of complete rupture which is usually fatal. Improved surgical management, including replacement of the aorta, has reduced the overall in-hospital death rate to below 30%.

aortic incompetence leakiness of the aortic valve of the heart, with regurgitation of blood through the closed valve.

aortic regurgitation abnormal back flow of blood from the aorta through the aortic valve. In developing countries the valvular defect is mainly due to as complication of rheumatic fever; in Western countries the defect is usually congenital.

aortic stenosis narrowing of the aortic valve of the heart.

aortic arch syndrome pulseless disease or TAKAYASU DISEASE. There is narrowing of the arch of the main artery of the body and its major branches. The pulses in the arm, head and neck are greatly diminished. Fainting, headache, defective vision and muscle wasting occur.

aortic valve the three-cusp valve at the origin of the AORTA that allows easy movement of blood from the left VENTRICLE of the heart into the aorta but prevents its backward flow.

aortitis inflammation of the aorta. This is now uncommon and is usually due to GIANT CELL ARTERITIS or occurs as a complication of ANKYLOSING SPONDYLITIS or REITER'S SYNDROME. Aortitis was once commonly due to SYPHILIS.

aortography X-ray examination of the AORTA after injection of a radio-opaque contrast medium into the bloodstream.

APACHE score *acronym for* Acute Physiology and Chronic Health Evaluation. A scoring method of determining the probable outcome in critically ill patients. The factors used include age, physiological abnormality, current diagnosis, presence of other disorders, prior functional disability and treatment given. In most cases the results are comparable with the prognosis given by experienced doctors. The current version is APACHE III.

APC resistance *abbrev. for* activated protein C resistance, an abnormal tendency to blood clotting caused by a mutation in the gene for blood clotting Factor V. This mutation is known as the FACTOR V LEIDEN MUTATION. APC resistance is the commonest cause of inherited THROMBOPHILIA.

aperient a laxative or mild purgative.

Apert's syndrome see ACROCEPHALOSYNDACTYLISM. (Eugène Apert, French paediatrician, 1868–1840).

apeu virus a species in the *Bunyavirus* genus that may cause fever, headache, muscle and joint pain and a reduction in the white cells in the blood.

apex the tip of an organ with a pointed end. The apex of the heart is at the lower left side and the apex of the lung is at the top. The tooth apex is at the tip of each root.

apex beat the furthest outward and downward point at which a finger laid on the chest is lifted with each heart beat. Displacement to the left usually indicates enlargement of the heart.

Apgar score a numerical index used to assess the state of well-being of a new-born baby. The figures 0, 1 or 2 are assigned to each of five variables – the heart rate, the breathing, the muscle tone, the reflex irritability and the skin colour, and added. A normal baby will score 7 to 10. (Virginia Apgar, American anaesthetist, 1909–74).

aphagia inability to swallow. See also DYSPHAGIA.

aphakia absence of the internal crystalline lens of the eye. Aphakia results either from surgical removal or from penetrating injury, which may be followed by absorption. An aphakic eye is severely out of focus and requires a powerful lens for clear vision. Such a lens may be provided as a contact lens, so as to avoid the undue magnification and distortion of glasses. In some cases a lens implant within the eye may be considered feasible.

aphasia an acquired speech disorder resulting from brain damage which affects the understanding and production of language rather than the mechanical aspects of articulation. Aphasia is a common feature of STROKE affecting usually the left side of the brain. In sensory aphasia the essential problem is in understanding information input as in speech, writing or gesture. In motor aphasia, reception of input information may be normal but the ability to express thoughts, which may be entirely normal, is lost or defective both in speech and in writing. Various combinations of disability occur. Names may be forgotten while relationships or functions may be retained. Vocabulary may be severely reduced and circumlocution engaged in. Speech may be hesitant or confined to expletives. Motor aphasia often causes depressing frustration.

apheresis a separating out of a component, usually from the blood. See also PLASMAPHERESIS.

aphonia loss of voice, usually as a result of disorder of the LARYNX or VOCAL CORDS.

aphrodisiac 1 promoting sexual desire or performance.
2 a drug purporting to stimulate sexual interest or excitement or enhance sexual performance. The general medical consensus is that there is no such thing as an aphrodisiac. But any agency, such as Viagra, that can improve confidence in the anticipated performance, can act as an aphrodisiac. From the Greek *Aphrodite*, the goddess of love and beauty.

aphthae small, superficial, and often painful ulcers of the inside of the mouth and

sometimes of the skin of the genitals. See also
APHTHOUS ULCERS.

aphthous ulcers a term which, although
tautological, is in common use. Aphthous ulcers
are very common, small, painful mouth ulcers,
affecting people between the ages of 10 and 40,
females more than males. They are a few
millimetres in diameter and up to five in
number and occur on the insides of the lips and
cheeks and on the edges of the tongue. They last
for 414 days.

apicectomy the removal of the tip of a tooth
root. This is done if root canal treatment has
been unsuccessful or is inappropriate.

aplasia failure of the development of an organ
or tissue or its congenital absence.

aplastic unable to form new cells or tissue.

aplastic anaemia a serious form of anaemia
in which no new blood cells are formed in the
bone marrow. About 30% of cases follow virus
infections, especially MEASLES, MUMPS and
HEPATITIS or are induced by drugs such as
BUTAZOLIDINE, SULPHONAMIDES,
CHLORAMPHENICOL or dipyrone. The condition
results from damage to the haemopoietic stem
cells often from an autoimmune process that
can be checked by immunosuppressive drug
treatment. Blood transfusions are often
necessary to maintain life.

apneustic breathing prolonged breath-
holding occurring during inspiration or, less
often, during expiration and followed by rapid
breathing. This phenomenon is caused by
brainstem damage in the PONS.

apnoea absence of breathing for short periods.
This may be a pre-AGONAL effect or may result
from forced overbreathing which reduces the
blood levels of carbon dioxide and hence a
major stimulus to respiration.

apo- a prefix denoting separate or derived from.

apocrine pertaining to glands that give off some
of their intracellular contents as part of their
secretion.

apocrine glands the type of sweat glands
found in the hairy parts of the body, especially
in the armpits and the groin. Apocrine sweat
contains material that is broken down by skin
bacteria to substances responsible for
unpleasant body odour.

apoenzyme a protein substance which can act
as an ENZYME in the presence of a coenzyme.

apoferritin a substance with which absorbed

iron may be complexed in the body to form a
ferritin store. Ferritin is one of the two forms
of iron store in the cells of the body. The other
is haemosiderin.

apolipoprotein one of a number of
glycoproteins forming part of the surface
of LIPOPROTEIN particles in the blood.
Apolipoproteins are polar structures which
provide structural stability to the lipoprotein
and act as receptors that help to determine the
fate of the particle. Some act as cofactors for
enzymes involved in lipid and lipoprotein
metabolism. The level of apolipoprotein-A is
genetically induced and a high level is a strong
risk factor for premature coronary heart
disease. It is a feature of FAMILIAL
HYPERCHOLESTEROLAEMIA. Apolipoprotein-B
is the binding site of low-density lipoproteins
(LDL) to cellular LDL receptors and is
concerned in the movement of CHYLOMICRONS
from the intestine. Apolipoprotein-C is present
on chylomicrons, high-density lipoproteins and
very low-density lipoproteins. Apolipoprotein-
E genotyping has been used to predict the
likelihood of ALZHEIMER'S DISEASE.

apomorphine a morphine derivative used as
an expectorant, emetic, and hypnotic. In large
doses it promotes severe vomiting. Used in the
treatment of Parkinson's disease. Brand names
are Apo-go and Uprima.

aponeurosis a thin flat sheet of tendinous
tissue which covers a muscle or by which broad,
flat muscles are connected to bone.

apophyseal joints joints between bony
protrusions, as in the spinal column.

apophysis any natural protrusion forming part
of a bone, such as a tubercle or tuberosity.

apoplexy an old-fashioned term for STROKE.
From the Greek *apoplexia*, a striking down.

apoptosis cell 'suicide'. A form of programmed
cell death, by endonuclease digestion of DNA.
Apoptosis is necessary to make way for new cells
and occurs constantly in the growing fetus and
elsewhere. The p53 gene can induce an
organismally-protective apoptosis in cells whose
DNA has been dangerously damaged to the point
where cancerous change is liable to occur.

apothecary an old-fashioned term for a
pharmaceutical chemist. Apothecaries used to
prepare their own medicines but this practice
has now largely died out.

appendage a part or organ of the body joined

to another part. A protruding part of the body.

appendicectomy the surgical operation for the removal of the vermiform appendix.

appendicitis acute inflammation of the blind-ended 'vermiform' APPENDIX. The condition usually starts with central abdominal pain and slight fever. Vomiting may occur. The pain then shifts to the lower right corner of the abdomen and increases in severity. It is made worse by movement or coughing. There is considerable local tenderness and either constipation or slight diarrhoea may occur. The main danger is rupture of an obstructed appendix, release of the contents into the abdominal cavity, and PERITONITIS. Treatment usually involves an operation to remove the inflamed appendix, but conservative management is sometimes appropriate. The diagnosis is not always easy. CT scanning has been found helpful.

appendicular skeleton the bones of the shoulder girdle and arms and of the pelvic girdle and legs. Compare AXIAL SKELETON.

appendix 1 the worm-like structure attached to the CAECUM at the beginning of the large intestine and known as the vermiform appendix.

2 an APPENDAGE.

appetite desire, whether for food, drink, sex, work or anything else that humans can enjoy. Lack of appetite for food is called anorexia, of which a particularly dangerous kind is ANOREXIA NERVOSA.

appetite suppressants drugs used to reduce the urge to eat and to help in the control of obesity.

applanation tonometry a standard method of measuring the pressure of the fluids within the eye by determining the force necessary to flatten a standard area of the CORNEA. Unduly raised pressure is the hallmark of GLAUCOMA.

apposition a placing of structures side by side. The term is often used in relation to the edges of wound, as in SUTURING.

apraclonidine a drug used in the treatment of GLAUCOMA. A brand name is Iopidine.

apraxia loss of the ability to carry out skilled movements with control and accuracy. Apraxia is a common manifestation of STROKE.

aprepitant a neurokinin receptor antagonist drug to prevent the nausea and vomiting, whether current or delayed, associated with cisplatin-based anticancer therapy. Aprepitant

is an orally active antagonist of substance P neurokinin-1 receptors and is the first of a new class of antiemetic drugs.

Apresoline a brand name for HYDRALAZINE.

Aprinox a brand name for BENDROFLUAZIDE (bendroflumethiazide).

aproctous having an imperforate ANUS.

aprotinin a drug used in the treatment of bleeding resulting from the excessive breakdown of the fibrin that forms blood clots. An antifibrinolytic. A brand name is Trasylol.

Aprovel a brand name for IRBESARTAN.

aptyalism absence of saliva.

APUD acronym for amine precursor uptake (and) decarboxylation.

APUD cell tumour a tumour, consisting of APUD cells, found most commonly in the intestines but sometimes in the pancreas, adrenals, thyroid or pituitary glands. APUD cell tumours often secrete powerful hormones.

APUD hypothesis the hypothesis that cells of the nervous system and cells that produce peptide hormones (APUD cells) might have a common embryonic origin and that the progenitors migrate to the gastrointestinal tract and the endocrine organs where they differentiate. This idea has been shown to be of only limited application, causing the originator, Professor Anthony Pearse (1916–2003) to suggest that the acronym should stand for 'Anthony Pearse's Ultimate Delusion'. See also APUD CELL TUMOUR.

apyrexial free from fever. No longer feverish.

aqua water.

Aquasept a brand name for TRICLOSAN.

aqueduct a channel carrying water or other liquid. There are a dozen named aqueducts in the body. The aqueduct of the midbrain (aqueduct of Sylvius) is a narrow channel for cerebrospinal fluid lying between the third and fourth VENTRICLES of the brain.

aqueduct stenosis narrowing of the aqueduct of Sylvius between the two central fluid spaces of the brain, the third and fourth ventricles. This is the cause of 'water on the brain' (HYDOCEPHALUS) in about one third of cases. There are many causes including ENCEPHALITIS, MENINGITIS, TOXOPLASMOSIS, NEUROFIBROMATOSIS and the Chiari malformation, and it may be genetically induced.

aqueous humour the watery fluid filling the

front chamber of the eye between the back of the CORNEA and the front of the IRIS.

ARA *abbrev. for* Area Health Authority or associate of the Institute of Hospital Administrators.

ara-A adenine arabinoside or vidarabine. This is an analogue of adenine and acts by inhibiting DNA polymerase so that viral DNA synthesis is inhibited. It is effective against herpes viruses, varicella-zoster virus, vaccinia and hepatitis B viruses.

arachidonic acid an unsaturated fatty acid, formed from LINOLENIC acid, and a precursor of prostaglandins and thomboxanes.

arachis oil an oil used as an ingredient in various preparations such as ear wax softeners, enemas and skin medications.

arachnid any of the eight-legged arthropods of the class *Arachnida*, including spiders, scorpions, mites, and ticks. From the Greek *arachne*, a spider.

arachno- *combining form denoting* a spider, spider-like or resembling a spider's web.

arachnodactyly having abnormally long, spider-like hands and fingers. Arachnodactyly is a feature of MARFAN'S SYNDROME.

arachnoid the delicate middle layer of the three MENINGES covering the spinal cord and brain, lying between the pia mater and dura mater. Unlike the pia mater, the arachnoid bridges over the grooves (sulci) on the surface of the brain and covers many large blood vessels lying in the sulci. Bleeding from any of these vessels causes a subarachnoid haemorrhage. From the Greek *arachne*, a spider.

arachnoidal granulations projections of the middle (ARACHNOID) layer of the MENINGES through the dura mater into the cerebral veins. The arachnoid granulations are the site of reabsorption of cerebrospinal fluid (CSF) into the blood. Failure of CSF to reach them leads to HYDROCEPHALUS. They are also known as arachnoid villi or Pacchionian bodies.

arachnoiditis inflammation of the arachnoid mater.

arachnoid mater see ARACHNOID.

arbo- *combining form denoting* a tree or tree-like.

arboviral encephalitis brain inflammation caused by an arthropod-borne virus (ARBOVIRUS).

arbovirus any of the hundred or so viruses

transmitted by an arthropod vectors such as mosquitoes, bugs, lice, ticks and mites. The group includes viruses that cause various forms of ENCEPHALITIS, haemorrhagic fevers, YELLOW FEVER, DENGUE, Kyasanur Forest disease, Rift Valley fever and Chikungunya Forest fever.

ARC *acronym for* 1 AIDS-RELATED COMPLEX. A lesser form of AIDS, often preceding the fully developed condition.
2 ABNORMAL RETINAL CORRESPONDENCE.

archenteron the embryonic digestive tract.

archetypes a term used by the Swiss psychiatrist and mystical thinker Carl Jung (1875–1961) to characterize some of the features of the 'collective unconscious' he believed common to all humankind. Archetypes were, he believed, inherent tendencies to experience and symbolize the many different and important human situations in particular ways. Jung pointed out that all the great mythological and religious systems display these archetypes in common.

Arcoxia a brand name for ETORICOXIB.

arcuate bowed, arched or curved. From the Latin *arcus*, a bow.

arcus juvenilis a condition identical to ARCUS SENILIS but occurring in young people. Sometimes called embryotoxon. Arcus juvenilis may be associated with a familial disorder featuring high blood cholesterol levels (hyperlipidaemia).

arcus senilis a white ring near the outer margin of the CORNEA. This is a normal feature of age and is of no significance. Vision is never affected.

ARDS *abbrev. for* adult RESPIRATORY DISTRESS SYNDROME.

Aredia a brand name for PAMIDRONATE.

areflexia absence of tendon jerk reflexes.

arenavirus any of the family of *Arenaviridae* of viruses which includes those causing LASSA FEVER and LYMPHOCYTIC CHORIOMENINGITIS. The name derives from the sand-like appearance of the internal granules seen on electron microscopy.

areola the pink or brown area surrounding the nipple of the female breast. It contains tiny protuberances under which are the areolar glands which lubricate the skin to protect it during suckling. From areola, the diminutive of the Latin *area*, a courtyard or space.

argemone poisoning epidemic dropsy

(oedema), a condition caused by mustard oil contaminated with extracts of the seeds of the poppy weed *Argemone mexicana*. There is fever, vomiting, diarrhoea, fluid retention, HEART FAILURE and GLAUCOMA.

arginine vasopressin VASOPRESSIN, one of the two hormones from the rear lobe of the PITUITARY GLAND.

argipressin a vasopressin analogue drug used to treat diabetes insipidus and bleeding from oesophageal varices. A brand name is Pitressin.

argon laser a low-powered LASER widely used in ophthalmology.

Argyll Robertson pupil a pupil which contracts normally when the eye focuses on a near object, but does not constrict when a bright light is shone into the eye. This indicates damage to part of the mechanism controlling the pupil reaction to light and was, at one time, taken to be an invariable indication of SYPHILIS affecting the nervous system. (Douglas Moray Cooper Lamb Argyll Robertson, Scottish ophthalmic surgeon, 1837–1909).

argyria a permanent gray staining of the CONJUNCTIVA or skin resulting from prolonged exposure to silver salts, as in silver nitrate eye drops.

Aricept a brand name for DONEPEZIL.

Arimidex a brand name for ANASTROZOLE.

aripiprazole a dopamine partial agonist drug used to treat SCHIZOPHRENIA. Aripiprazole is a member of a new class of antipsychotic drugs with agonist properties in parts of the brain in which the local concentrations of dopamine are abnormally low and antagonist action in parts in which levels of dopamine are abnormally high. Extrapyramidal effects are said to be avoided. A brand name is ABILIFY.

arithmetical mean the total of all values divided by the number of observations. If the distribution of the values is skewed, the arithmetical mean is a misleading figure. In such a case the GEOMETRIC MEAN is appropriate.

Arixtra a brand name for FONDAPARINUX.

ARMD see MACULAR DEGENERATION.

Arnold-Chiari syndrome a group of disorders in which the lower part of the brain and sometimes the CEREBELLUM are forced through the bony opening for the spinal cord in the base of the skull (the foramen magnum). This commonly causes 'water on the brain' (HYDROCEPHALUS). (Julius A. Arnold,

German pathologist, 1835–1927, and Hans von Chiari, Austrian pathologist, 1851–1916).

aromatases a class of enzymes that can act on steroids to produce aromatic rings. All the sex hormones are four-ring structures. The first of the four rings of an oestrogen steroid (the A ring) is aromatic; that of the androgens is not. Aromatases catalyze the desaturation of steroid A rings, so can convert androgens to oestrogens. See also AROMATASE INHIBITOR.

aromatase hypothesis the widely accepted proposition that male sex hormones (androgens) are converted to oestrogens by aromatase enzymes before they can act on certain target cells such as those in the hypothalamus concerned with reproductive functions. In females aromatases convert adrenal androgens to oestrogens in the ovaries, skin and elsewhere.

aromatase inhibitors a group of anti-cancer drugs that act by preventing the enzymatic conversion of androgens to oestrogens. These drugs are used especially in post-menopausal women with breast cancers that are being encouraged by oestrogens but that fail to respond to drugs such as tamoxifen. The third-generation aromatase inhibitors, developed in the early 1990s, which include anastrozole (Arimidex), letrozole (Femara) and exemestane (Aromasin), are now challenging tamoxifen as the treatment of choice in post-menopausal women with oestrogen-receptor-positive breast cancers.

aromatherapy a form of alternative therapy in which essential oils from herbs, flowers and spices are selected according to the nature of the problem and are massaged into the skin and then inhaled. The procedure is claimed to be especially effective for anxiety and depression but is also used to treat various skin disorders. See also ALTERNATIVE MEDICINE.

aromatic of a class of chemical compounds originally so named because many of them have a fragrant smell derived from benzene. Today, by extension, the term is used to refer to compounds containing one or more structures of the pattern of benzene – a ring of six carbon atoms with alternate single and double bonds. The female sex hormones and many drugs contain aromatic rings. Compounds that contain no rings or rings that are not benzene rings are said to be aliphatic.

aromatic amines a group of chemical compounds some of which are known to be capable of causing cancer. They include benzidine, B-naphthylamine and 4-amino diphenyl. Many industrial workers exposed to these chemicals, especially in the rubber industry, developed bladder cancer.

arousal the state of heightened awareness and alertness caused by a strong external stimulus such as danger or sexual interest.

Arpicolin a brand name for PROCYCLIDINE.

Arpimycin a brand name for ERYTHROMYCIN.

ARRC *abbrev. for* Associate, Royal Red Cross.

arrest cessation of normal action, especially of the heart.

arrhenoblastoma a tumour of the ovary which secretes both male and female sex hormones and which may cause VIRILIZATION in women or children and may lead to precocious puberty. Also called an androblastoma.

arrhythmia any abnormality in the regularity of the heart beat. Arrythmia is caused by a defect in the generation or conduction of electrical impulses in the heart.

arsenic a metallic element some of whose compounds are violently poisonous. Formerly widely used in insecticides and weed killers and in various industrial processes.

arsphenamine an organic arsenical compound formerly used to treat syphilis. Treatment with arsenical drugs was called arsenotherapy.

Artane a brand name for BENZHEXOL.

artefact dermatitis see DERMATITIS ARTEFACTA.

artemether a semi-synthetic derivative of ARTEMISININ. The drug is on the WHO official list.

artemisinin an antimalarial drug derived from *Artemisia annua*. The drug is claimed to be effective in treating cerebral malaria and is active against chloroquine-resistant *P. falciparum* and chloroquine-sensitive *P. falciparum* and *P. vivax*. The drug is a traditional Chinese remedy. See also QUINGHAO.

arterial relating to arteries.

arterio- *combining form denoting* artery.

arteriography X-ray examination of arteries following injection of a radio-opaque dye. The same as ANGIOGRAPHY.

arteriole a small terminal branch of an artery, intermediate in size between an artery and a CAPILLARY.

arteriolosclerosis a disease featuring hardening of ARTERIOLES. There is little deposition of CHOLESTEROL but often serious reduction in the bore of the vessels by deposition of fibrous tissue in the walls and thickening of the lining (intima).

arteriosclerosis hardening of the arteries. The term, once ubiquitous, has become imprecise and has virtually fallen out of use because pure arteriosclerosis is rare. It has been replaced by the term ATHEROSCLEROSIS, which more accurately describes the common degenerative disease of arteries. Pure arteriosclerosis may occur as a result of calcium deposition in the middle coat (media) of arteries, reducing their elasticity.

arteriotomy cutting or opening into an ARTERY.

arteriovenous aneurysm see ARTERIO-VENOUS FISTULA.

arteriovenous fistula an abnormal communication between an artery and a vein. It may be congenital or the result of injury or disease. Blood is shunted at high pressure into the vein causing it to enlarge and become thickened and arterialized.

arteriovenous malformation an abnormal, congenital network or clump of blood vessels linking an artery and a vein. These may occur anywhere in the body but are especially dangerous within the skull. The commonest presentation is a SUBARACHNOID HAEMORRHAGE. Blood flow though an arteriovenous malformation is often rapid and may be audible through the skull with a stethoscope.

arteritis one of a number of inflammatory diseases of small arteries characterized by swelling, tenderness and possible obstruction to the blood flow. See TEMPORAL ARTERITIS.

artery an elastic, muscular-walled tube carrying blood at high pressure from the heart to any part of the body. From the Greek *arteria*, an air duct. It was once believed that, in life, arteries contained air.

artesunate a drug used to treat difficult cases of *Falciparum* malaria. The drug is on the WHO official list.

arthralgia pain in a joint. From the Greek *arthron*, a joint and *algos*, pain.

Arthrexin a brand name for INDOMETHACIN.

arthritis inflammation in a joint, usually with swelling, redness, pain and restriction of movement. The main kinds are OSTEOARTHRITIS, RHEUMATOID ARTHRITIS, septic or infective arthritis and GOUT, but arthritis can be caused by many other disease processes and may occur in conditions such as GONORRHOEA, ACROMEGALY, AMYLOIDOSIS, BRUCELLOSIS, HYPERLIPIDAEMIA, LEPROSY, SARCOIDOSIS, PSORIASIS and SYPHILIS.

arthritis mutilans severe deformities especially of the hands and wrists, resulting from long-term untreated or inadequately treated rheumatoid arthritis. There is extensive reabsorption of bones with collapse of soft tissue resulting in gross mutilation.

arthro- *combining form denoting* a joint or articulation.

arthrocentesis puncturing a joint with a needle to withdraw fluid.

arthrodesis the fusion of the bones on either side of a joint so that no joint movement is possible. This may occur spontaneously, as a result of disease processes, or may be a deliberate surgical act done to relieve pain and improve function.

arthrography X-ray examination of a joint after injection of a radio-opaque fluid or a gas.

arthrogryposis congenital fixation of the limb joints, usually in an extended position. The condition is probably due to a destructive disorder of the motor nerves to the muscles around the affected joints during the pregnancy.

arthropathy any disease of a joint.

arthroplasty the surgical creation of a new joint or the insertion of an artificial joint. Total hip joint replacement is a common example of arthroplasty. The operation is done to restore mobility, and relieve pain and deformity. Problems may arise from loss of firm fixation and mechanical wear of the prosthetic parts.

arthropod any one the phylum *Arthropoda*, which includes all the insects, the crustaceans and arachnids. As the name implies, arthropods have jointed legs.

arthropod-borne fevers a very large range of infections transmitted by insects (ARTHROPODS) such as house flies, mosquitoes, tsetse flies, biting black flies, sandflies, ticks, mites, lice and fleas. They include the arbovirus infections, DENGUE, various dysenteries, FILARIASIS, LYME DISEASE, MALARIA, PLAGUE, Q FEVER, RELAPSING FEVER, Salmonella infections, TRYPANOSOMIASIS, TULARAEMIA, TYPHUS and YELLOW FEVER.

arthroscopy examination of the inside of a joint by an optical device, usually a fine bore fibreoptic endoscope.

arthrosis 1 any abnormal connection or joint occurring between bones.
2 any degenerative process in a joint.

Arthus reaction Arthus phenomenon, a local necrotic reaction that occurs when an ANTIGEN is injected into the skin of a person previously sensitized to it. The preformed antibody combines with the injected antigen causing a high local concentration of immune complexes and severe tissue damage. (Nicholas Maurice Arthus, French physiologist, 1862–1945).

articular pertaining to a joint.

articulation a joint.

artificial chromosome the result of a biotechnology still at an experimental stage. Human chromosomes, consisting of a centromere of highly repetitive DNA sequences, telomeric DNA, a marker gene and some random sequences of genomic DNA, have been successfully prepared. When these ingredients were introduced into a human cell line they became coated with histone proteins and formed highly coiled structures. They also replicated and passed on copies to daughter cells through more than 200 cell divisions.

artificial eye a plastic shell simulation of the visible part of the eye, used for cosmetic purposes when an eye has been removed or is greatly shrunken. Some artificial eyes are capable of a wide range of realistic movement by virtue of an implant in the tissues behind. Pupil responses to changing light intensity are also possible using a liquid crystal display.

artificial heart a mechanical pumping device intended to maintain the blood circulation of a person whose heart is no longer able to do so. Heart-lung machines can maintain an effective circulation for many hours while a heart operation is performed, but to date, no artificial heart has been shown capable of doing this indefinitely. The main complications including infection, bleeding at connections and blood clotting (thrombosis) with the production of many dangerous emboli. Artificial hearts have, however, been successful in keeping patients alive until a heart transplant can be done. Implantable artificial hearts have functioned for up to about eight months in patients awaiting cardiac transplantation.

artificial insemination a method of achieving pregnancy when normal sexual intercourse is impossible, or when the male partner is sterile.

Fresh semen is taken up in a narrow syringe or pipette and injected high into the vagina or into the mouth of the womb. The success rate is high. An example of positive EUGENICS is artificial insemination with sperm from anonymous donors guaranteed to be of high mental or physical calibre. The frozen sperm of certain Nobel Prize winners is stored, for this purpose, by the Repository for Germinal Choice, founded in 1979. See AID, AIH.

artificial intelligence the characteristics of a machine designed to perform some of the perceptive or logical functions of the human organism in a manner appearing to be beyond the merely mechanical. AI is largely a matter of computer programming, in which stored records of past experience are made to modify future responses, but it also encompasses research into humanoid methods of data acquisition, the use of fuzzy logic and of artificial neural networks.

artificial kidney a dialysis machine in which the patient's blood is exposed to one side of a membrane of large surface area, on the other side of which is a fluid into which the unwanted waste materials in the blood can pass by natural diffusion. People undergoing dialysis must have a permanent shunt formed between an artery and a vein, usually in the arm, so that they can readily be connected to the machine. Dialysis sessions last for 26 hours and must be repeated up to three times a week. See also PERITONEAL DIALYSIS.

artificial limb a PROSTHESIS designed to replace an amputated arm or leg. Artificial limbs may perform a purely supportive function or may simulate, to varying degrees, some of the functions of the part.

artificial liver an as yet unrealized entity that is, nevertheless, the subject of promising research and development. Current ambitions are to produce extracorporeal devices that will enable patients with liver failure to be kept alive until regeneration of transplantation is achieved. The principal difficulty arises from the large number of different metabolic functions performed by the liver. A promising approach is the use of cloned human liver cells grown around numerous fine semipermeable tubules through which the patient's blood is passed.

artificial lungs experimental devices for maintaining the oxygenation of the blood and the removal of carbon dioxide. Considerable research has shown that, in theory, such devices can be made small enough for implantation in the human body. New polymer membranes, using polyimide material with added fluorine have been developed, that, compared with previous materials, improve oxygen transfer 70 times and carbon dioxide transfer 100 times.

artificial muscles electroactive polymers (EAPs), plastic substances that move in response to electrical stimulation. These are dielectric elastomers which, when in sheet form and sandwiched between compliant electrodes to which a voltage is applied, contract in the direction of the electric field line and expand perpendicularly to that direction. The effect is the result of a simple attraction between opposite charges. Artificial muscles are a recent technological advance in mechanical actuation likely to be widely exploited in medicine and in other fields as replacements for bulky and unsuitable electric motors.

artificial oxygen carriers synthetic solutions capable of carrying and unloading oxygen, that can safely be administered intravenously to improve the oxygenation of tissues. Substances such as perfluorocarbons can be emulsified and infused and are capable of working in the manner of haemoglobin. When the technology and safety has been fully established, artificial oxygen carriers are expected to make an important contribution to solving the discrepancy between demand and supply of blood for transfusion.

artificial pacemaker see PACEMAKER.

artificial respiration an emergency procedure calculated to save life when normal breathing is absent or insufficient, as in partial drowning, poisoning or head injury. The most effective form of artificial respiration is the mouth-to-mouth method in which the lungs of the victim are repeatedly inflated by blowing into the mouth while pinching the nose.

artificial saliva drugs used to treat dry mouth. Examples are xylitol and mucin (As Saliva Orthana), carboxy-methylcellulose (Glandosane) and malic acid (Salivix).

artificial tears bland solutions designed to maintain the wetness of the cornea in conditions of abnormal dryness from inadequate tear secretion. Methylcellulose is a common ingredient.

aryepiglottic pertaining to the ARYTENOID cartilages and to the EPIGLOTTIS.

arytenoid ladle-shaped. Pertaining to the two small cartilages attached to the vocal cords at the back of the LARYNX or to the arytenoid muscles of the larynx. From the Greek *arutaina*, a pitcher or ladle, and *eidos*, like.

Arythmol a brand name for PROPAFENONE.

Asacol a brand name for MESALAZINE.

asbestosis a chronic lung disease caused by inhaling asbestos dust over a period. Thickening and scarring of the lung tissue occurs with reduced efficiency of oxygen and carbon dioxide interchange with the blood. The resulting breathlessness may progress to respiratory failure.

Ascabiol a brand name for BENZYL BENZOATE.

ascariasis infestation with the roundworm *Ascaris lumbricoides* which lives, often in considerable numbers, in the small intestine.

ascending aorta the first part of the aorta, extending upwards from its origin in the upper surface of the heart to the aortic arch.

ascending colon the part of the large intestine on the right side, running up from the CAECUM to the bend near the liver.

Ascensia a brand name for testing strips for blood glucose in the range 0.6 to 33.3 mmole per litre.

Aschoff nodule a specific microscopic sign of RHEUMATIC FEVER. An area of dead tissue (necrosis) is surrounded by lymphocytes, scavenging cells (histiocytes) and giant cells. (Karl Albert Ludwig Aschoff, German pathologist, 1866–1942).

ascites a collection of fluid in the peritoneal cavity – the space in the ABDOMEN surrounding the internal organs. Ascites occurs in HEART FAILURE, the NEPHROTIC SYNDROME and in CIRRHOSIS of the LIVER.

ascorbic acid vitamin C. A white, crystalline substance found in citrus fruits, tomatoes, potatoes, and leafy green vegetables. Small doses are needed to prevent the bleeding disease of SCURVY and regular large doses are useful as an antioxidant in combatting dangerous FREE RADICALS. The drug is on the WHO official list. A brand name is Redoxon.

-ase *suffix denoting* an enzyme. In most cases the suffix is added to a term for the substance acted upon or to the biochemical action promoted by

the enzyme. Thus a lipase is an enzyme that acts on fats and a reverse transcriptase is an enzyme that promoted the transcription of DNA from RNA (which is the reverse of the usual direction). The suffix originated in the ending of the term diastase, a polysaccharide-splitting enzyme named in 1838.

Asendis a brand name for AMOXAPINE.

asepsis the complete absence of all bacteria or other microorganisms capable of causing infection. Asepsis, as distinct from antisepsis, is the concept that made modern surgery possible.

aseptic meningitis 1 inflammation of the MENINGES resulting from contact with various toxic or irritating substances such as blood, air, drugs or chemical irritants but not bacteria. 2 an obsolescent term for MENINGITIS caused by organisms that do not produce pus, or for viral meningitis.

Aserbine a brand name for a preparation of MALIC ACID, BENZOIC ACID, SALICYLIC ACID and propylene glycol.

asexual characterizing a simple form of binary, or budding, reproduction in which only a single individual organism is involved. Reproduction without male and female GAMETES.

Asian flu an acute viral INFLUENZA caused by the influenza A-2 virus.

Asiatic cholera a common form of cholera caused by the organism Vibrio cholerae.

Asilomar conference a meeting, in 1975, of genetic engineers who had become alarmed at the possibility of creating potentially dangerous new micro-organisms by recombinant DNA techniques. The scientists agreed to call for a world-wide moratorium on certain classes of experiment.

Asilone a brand name for ALUMINIUM HYDROXIDE, MAGNESIUM OXIDE and DIMETHICONE (dimeticone).

Asmanex Twisthaler a breath-actuated inhaler containing the steroid drug MOMETASONE as a dry powder for the treatment of ASTHMA. The drug is poorly absorbed from the lungs but this preparation is not recommended for children.

Asmasal a brand name for SALBUTAMOL.

asomatognosia the inability to recognize the presence of part of the body affected by sensory paralysis. This is common following a STROKE.

asparaginase an ENZYME that destroys one of the 20 AMINO ACIDS from which proteins are formed. It is used in the treatment of LEUKAEMIA.

The most useful are L-asparaginases which split an amino group from L-asparagine, converting it to aspartic acid. Tumour cells require asparagine which they cannot synthesize as normal cells can. The drug is on the WHO official list.

aspartame an artificial sweetener derived from aspartic acid and phenylalanine.

aspartate aminotransferase one of the enzymes released into the blood when tissue, such as liver or heart muscle, is damaged. Measurement of the level of such enzymes gives a useful indication of the extent of the damage.

aspartic acid an AMINO ACID which the body can synthesise. It is found in sugar cane and sugar beet and in asparagus.

aspartylglycosaminuria a disease due to deficiency of the enzyme aspartylglycosaminidase which splits acetylglucosamine from the polypeptide chain of glycoproteins. Aspartylglucosamine is excreted in large quantities in the urine. Affected children are short, with coarse features, cataracts, over-mobile joints and mental retardation. Most of the reported cases have been in Finland.

Aspav a brand name for PAPAVERETUM combined with ASPIRIN and PAPAVERINE.

Asperger's syndrome a condition similar to, but usually less severe than AUTISM, that affects about 1–2 persons in 1000, males more often than females. Affected people, who are normally intelligent, are physically clumsy, have unusual narrow interests and great difficulty in managing social relationships and are often considered simply as eccentric loners. Special training in social skills can be valuable.

aspergilloma a tumour-like mass that can form in the lungs in the course of the disease ASPERGILLOSIS. This can cause coughing of blood and may be mistaken for BRONCHIAL CARCINOMA. The condition is common in people with healed tuberculous cavities in the lungs. Surgery to remove that affected parts of the lung may be necessary.

aspergillosis a disease caused by infection with, or hypersensitivity to, fungi of the genus *Aspergillus*, especially *Aspergillus fumigatus* and *Aspergillus niger*. It often affects the skin of the external ear and may affect the lungs or other parts of the body. Infections are treated with azole antifungal drugs especially vorconazole.

aspermia the absence of spermatozoa in the semen or the inability to ejaculate semen. Obstructive aspermia is due to the blockage of the VAS DEFERENS on both sides. This may be congenital or acquired from infection or injury, or from VASECTOMY. CYSTIC FIBROSIS causes aspermia as a result of failure of development of the vas or associated structures.

asphyxia suffocation by interference with the free AIRWAY between the atmosphere and the air sacs in the lungs. Asphyxia is usually the cause of death in drowning, choking, strangling, inhalation of a gas which excludes oxygen, foreign body airway obstruction and OEDEMA of the LARYNX.

asphyxiation the process of causing, or suffering, ASPHYXIA.

aspiration drawing out of fluid by suction, usually by syringe and needle, but sometimes by mouth or pump suction through a plastic or rubber tube.

aspiration pneumonia pneumonia caused by the inhalation of infected or irritating material, such as vomited stomach contents.

aspirator any device used to remove liquid from a body space by suction.

aspirin acetylsalicylic acid. A drug used as a painkiller, to reduce fever, as an antiplatelet agent to reduce the tendency of blood to clot within the circulation, and as a means of reducing the likelihood of heart attack, stroke, diabetic retinopathy, migraine and colon cancer. Aspirin is an inhibitor of the cyclo-oxygenase (COX) class of enzymes which form PROSTAGLANDINS. This accounts for the wide range of its actions. Daily aspirin is recommended for people at risk of coronary events, and complications commonly have been shown often to arise in those on long-term aspirin who stop the therapy for any reason. Aspirin also has a growing reputation as an anticancer drug possibly by its action in promoting apoptosis (cell suicide) in cancer cells. There is some evidence that aspirin may reduce the risk of developing ALZHEIMER'S DISEASE. There is no doubt that it reduces the risk of dementia caused by repetitive small episodes of brain damage by thrombosis. See also CYCLO-OXYGENASE and COX-2 INHIBITORS.

aspirin sensitive asthma an acute sensitivity to small amounts of ASPIRIN that affects about 3% of asthmatics, causing severe attacks, both immediately and later. Some of those who react in this way also do so to tartrazine and other azo food dyes.

Aspro a brand name for ASPIRIN.

assassin bug a blood-sucking insect of the family *Reduviidae*. The insect transmitter of South American Trypanosomiasis (CHAGAS' DISEASE).

assay qualitative or quantitative analysis of a substance such as a drug.

assigned sex the nominal sex or gender assumed or decided upon when a baby has genitals of ambiguous appearance. The assigned sex may or may not correspond to the actual chromosomal sex. Sometimes assigned sex has to be changed later in life and this may lead to TRANSSEXUALISM.

assimilation the process of incorporating nutrient material into cells after digestion and absorption.

association areas areas of the outer layer of the brain concerned with the integration of sensory and other data with other aspects of brain function, and the elaboration of them into the complex processes underlying higher mental functions such as language, imagination and creativity. Thus, damage to the visual association area, while not in any way affecting the primary function of vision, might lead to an inability to recognize or interpret what is seen.

association fibres nerve fibres running just under the surface (CORTEX) of the brain and connecting adjacent parts of the cortex.

AST ASPARTATE AMINOTRANSFERASE.

astasia inability to stand upright because of lack of muscular coordination, not because of paralysis.

asteatotic eczema a kind of dermatitis associated with the drying out of the skin characteristic of the elderly or the malnourished and especially those in conditions of low atmospheric humidity and excessively in contact with detergents and soaps. There is cracking and fissuring. Rehydration of the skin with water-based creams is effective.

astemizole an ANTIHISTAMINE drug used in the treatment of hay fever and allergic skin disorders. A brand name is Hismanal.

astereognosis the inability to recognize the shape of objects by touch. This is a fairly common consequence of STROKE.

asterixis a recurrent flapping tremor of the arms, like the action of a bird's wings. Asterixis

is characteristic of the brain disorder associated with liver failure – hepatic encephalopathy.

asteroid hyalitis an eye condition in which many small, white bodies become suspended in the vitreous humour. In the light of the ophthalmoscope these gleam in a strikingly star-like manner. Also known as steroid hyalosis.

asthenia lack or loss of strength or energy. Tropical anhidrotic asthenia results from the inability to sweat over large areas of skin following PRICKLY HEAT. From the Greek *asthenes*, weak.

asthenic a slender, lightly muscled physique. One of the recognized SOMATOTYPES.

asthenopia 'eyestrain', headaches or visual difficulty attributed to misuse of the eyes. A vague and, in the absence of refractive error, often imaginary entity. The term is not now generally used by ophthalmologists. See also ACCOMMODATIVE ASTHENOPIA.

asthma a disease in which the circular smooth muscles of the branching air tubes of the lungs are liable to go into a state of spasm so that they are narrowed and the passage of air is impeded. Equally important is the inflammatory swelling of the lining of the air tubes. The principal signs are wheezing and cough. The bronchospasm and swelling may be induced by a variety of stimuli, but sensitivity to an allergy-causing substance (ALLERGEN) is amongst the commonest. Asthma can also be brought on by infection, emotion and exertion. Genetic susceptibility to asthma may involve the prostaglandin D2 receptor gene. Asthma is not a minor disorder and claims around 2000 lives a year in Britain. Treatment is by inhalation of bronchodilator drugs such as SALBUTAMOL. The important role of inhaled steroids to reduce inflammatory effects has been increasingly recognized in recent years. The asthmatic should be able to recognize when the condition is going out of control, in spite of treatment, and should seek urgent medical advice. See also BRITTLE ASTHMA and CHITIN.

astigmatic of a lens, unable to focus a point image from a point object. Having ASTIGMATISM.

astigmatism an optical error in which objects in the same plane, but of different orientation, are brought to a focus in different planes at the back of the eye. Thus, vertical objects may be seen in focus while horizontal objects may be out of focus. Astigmatism is usually due to a lack of sphericity in the outer surface of the CORNEA, one meridian being more steeply curved than the others. An astigmatic lens cannot produce a point image of a point object. The defect can be corrected by cylindrical spectacle lenses. From the Greek *a*, not and *stigma*, a spot or point.

astragalus the talus bone. The upper bone of the foot, on which the tibia rests.

astringent 1 a drug that shrinks cells and tightens surfaces by denaturing cell protein. 2 having the property of tightening surfaces.

astro- *combining form denoting* a star.

astrocytes star-shaped connective tissue cells of the nervous system that link nerve cells to blood vessels and, by wrapping round brain capillaries, help to form the BLOOD-BRAIN BARRIER. Neurological connective tissue (neuroglial) cells.

astrocytoma a tumour derived from the supporting tissue of nerve cells (neuroglia). The astrocytoma varies widely in malignancy and rate of growth.

astrovirus a virus that causes diarrhoea in children and may be present in large numbers in the stools of adults without causing ill effects. Most adults have antibodies to the virus.

asylum a once compassionate but now pejorative term for a psychiatric hospital or an institution for the care of the elderly and infirm.

asymbolia a form of APHASIA in which there is inability to interpret or use symbols such as words, gestures, numbers, diagrams, musical notation or any form of writing. See APHASIA.

asymptomatic free of symptoms or not causing symptoms.

asynergia a severe movement disorder due to faulty coordination of groups of muscles normally acting in conjunction. Asynergia involves the breaking down of movements into their component parts so that movements become jerky and sequential. It is due to dysfunction of the CEREBELLUM.

asystole the form of CARDIAC ARREST in which there is no heart beat and the electrocardiogram tracing is straight. This is in contrast with the other form, ventricular fibrillation, in which the heart muscle is twitching rapidly.

A.T. 10 a brand name for DIHYDROTACHYSTEROL.

Atarax a brand name for HYDROXYZINE.

ataraxia tranquillity or peace of mind.

atavism the reappearance of a genetic characteristic after generations of absence.

This may be caused by the coincidence of two recessive genes, by recombination, or by mutation. The organism or individual so produced is often called a 'throwback'.

atavistic featuring characteristics not seen for many generations, or of a more primitive evolutionary form of the organism.

ataxia unsteadiness in standing and walking from a disorder of the control mechanisms in the brain, or from inadequate information input to the brain from the skin, muscles and joints. From the Greek *a*, not and *taxis*, order or arrangement.

ataxia-hypogonadism a genetically induced deficiency of the sex-gland stimulating hormone gonadotrophin in males with CEREBELLAR ATAXIA.

ataxic showing ATAXIA. A person suffering from ataxia.

atazanavir an azapeptide HIV protease inhibitor that selectively inhibits virus-specific processing of *gag* and *gag-pol* polyproteins in HIV-infected cells. Once-daily dosage is adequate but the drug is used in combination with other anti-HIV agents. A brand name is Reyataz.

atelectasis failure of the normal expansion of part or all of a lung. This is a feature of the RESPIRATORY DISTRESS SYNDROME of premature babies. The term may be used more generally to refer to failure of dilatation of a part that normally dilates.

ateleiosis DWARFISM caused by a deficient output of anterior pituitary hormones in childhood. The secondary sexual characteristics are normal as are the thyroid and adrenal functions.

atenolol a beta adrenoceptor blocker drug that acts mostly on the heart and has a long action. It slows the heart and corrects irregularities of rhythm. It is used to treat high blood pressure (HYPERTENSION) and ANGINA PECTORIS. The drug has been found to have a significant protective effect against heart attacks during the two years or so after non-cardiac surgery. The drug is on the WHO official list. Brand names are Tenormin, Tenoret 50 and Totamol.

Atensine a brand name for DIAZEPAM.

atheroma the material containing CHOLESTEROL, degenerate muscle cells, blood clot, blood PLATELETS and fibrous tissue, which forms on the inner surface of arteries in the disease of ATHEROSCLEROSIS and which promotes THROMBOSIS and obstruction to the blood flow. From the Greek *athara*, gruel or porridge, and *oma*, a lump.

atherosclerosis a degenerative disease of arteries in which fatty plaques of ATHEROMA develop on the inner lining of arteries so that the normal flow of blood is impeded. The cause of atherosclerosis is not clearly understood but it is related to diet, especially one high in saturated fats and to the resulting concentration of low density LIPOPROTEINS in the blood. Interaction of antibodies with heat-shock protein 60 leading to endothelial damage seems to be a probable mechanism. Smoking is a major risk factor for the disease. High blood pressure (HYPERTENSION) is also damaging to arteries and encourages atherosclerosis. This, in turn, encourages hypertension. Atherosclerosis affects most of the arteries in the body but is especially dangerous when it narrows the CORONARY ARTERIES that supply the heart muscle with blood, or the CAROTID and VERTEBRAL arteries and their branches, that supply the brain. Coronary narrowing causes ANGINA PECTORIS and heart attacks and narrowing of the brain arteries causes STROKE and DEMENTIA. Atherosclerosis may also interfere with the blood supply to the limbs and often causes GANGRENE. It is the major cause of death in the Western world and is responsible for more deaths than any other single condition. Worldwide, many more women die from heart attacks and strokes than from breast cancer.

atherothrombosis clotting of blood within an artery at the site of an atheromatous plaque. Atherothrombosis is the principal cause of death in the Western world because of its complications – heart attack, stroke, limb gangrene, and ischaemic organ disease including dementia. Antiplatelet therapy to prevent atherothrombosis can reduce vascular disease mortality by 15% and non-fatal vascular events by 30%.

athetosis a neurological disorder featuring involuntary, slow writhing movements of the hands, arms, face and tongue caused by a form of CEREBRAL PALSY. The commonest causes are ERYTHROBLASTOSIS FETALIS from rhesus incompatibility and brain lack of oxygen during birth. Intelligence may be unaffected but there is usually severe speech difficulty and the appearance suggests mental retardation to the observer. Seizures are common.

athlete's foot a popular term for the fungus infection commonly occurring between the toes. The medical term is TINEA PEDIS.

Ativan a brand name for LORAZEPAM.

atlanto-axial instability abnormal mobility of the articulation of the ATLAS BONE with the AXIS BONE. This is demonstrable on X-ray by a separation of more than 3 mm, at the front, between the body of the atlas and the odontoid process of the axis. People with this abnormality should avoid activities that could bring about dislocation (subluxation) of the bones and serious risk to the spinal cord. Atlanto-axial instability is found in about 20% of people with Down's syndrome because of laxity in the ligaments between the skull and the spine.

atlas see ATLAS BONE.

atlas bone the uppermost, or first, vertebra of the spinal column. The atlas is unique in having no body or spinous process. In head nodding, the skull moves on the atlas, but in head rotation the atlas locks with the skull and both rotate on the second vertebra, the AXIS.

atomoxetine a highly selective inhibitor of the pre-synaptic noradrenaline transporter used to reduce the signs and symptoms of ATTENTION DEFICIT HYPERACTIVITY DISORDER (ADHD) in children over six years of age. A brand name is STRATTERA.

atony sustained abnormal relaxation of muscle. Lack of muscular tone or contractile tendency. Atony of the uterus prevents its normal reduction in size after delivery of the baby and placenta and leads to bleeding which is often serious.

atopic eczema a common form of dermatitis caused by allergy to an ALLERGEN operating at a site remote from the affected area. See also ATOPY.

atopy a state giving rise to an allergy in which the reaction occurs at a different site from that of contact with the causal ALLERGEN. Atopy is an immediate hypersensitivity reaction associated with IMMUNOGLOBULIN E (IgE) and is a maternally transmitted genetic disorder due to mutations in a gene on chromosome 11. This gene codes for the IgE receptor on MAST CELLS. Atopy causes a proneness to ASTHMA, HAY FEVER and ECZEMA (atopic DERMATITIS). The term is derived from the Greek *a*, not and *topos*, a place.

atorvastatin a cholesterol-lowering drug.

A brand name is Lipitor. See STATINS.

atosiban a competitive OXYTOCIN receptor antagonist used to quieten a uterus contracting at an undesirably early stage of gestation and allow greater maturation of the fetus before birth. A brand name is Tractocile.

Atovaquone a drug used in the treatment of MALARIA and TOXOPLASMOSIS. Brand names are Wellvone and, in combination with proguanil, Malarone.

ATP ADENOSINE TRIPHOSPHATE.

ATPase an enzyme that hydrolyses ATP to ADP and inorganic phosphate. See ADENOSINE TRIPHOSPHATE.

atractaspididae bites bites by the African burrowing asp or mole viper *Atractaspis engaddensis* that strikes sideways with a long fang. The result is pain, swelling, local tissue death, nausea, vomiting, diarrhoea, difficulty in breathing and sometimes respiratory failure.

atrabilious of a peevish or melancholy disposition.

atracurium a muscle relaxant drug used in anaesthesia. A brand name is Tracrium.

atresia 1 developmental failure of the formation of the lumen of a normally hollow organ or duct.
2 the absence of an opening in a natural channel of the body.

atrial fibrillation a heart defect involving the upper chambers in which the rate at which they contract is chaotically irregular both in force and speed. It may be caused by heart muscle damage from RHEUMATIC FEVER or ATHEROSCLEROSIS or by thyroid overactivity. A new focus in the muscle may set up its own rhythm and this may compete with the normal rhythm. Only some of the irregular beats are transmitted down to the lower chambers (ventricles) and the pulse is correspondingly irregular. Atrial fibrillation is common and accounts for one third of all strokes in people over 65 years of age. A rare familial form has been recognized. Treatment by radio frequency ablation using a catheter in a pulmonary vein is usually effective in controlling the disorder. Fibrillation of recent onset can usually be stopped by a single oral dose of flecainide or propafenone.

atrial flutter an abnormality of heart rhythm affecting the upper chambers of the heart which beat at an abnormally rapid rate of between 240

and 400 per minute. It is believed to be a form of oscillation caused by a feed-back loop of impulses within the heart muscle and independently of the natural pace-maker – the sino-atrial node. These impulses are transmitted to the lower chambers and the result is a grossly irregular pulse with a heart rate of 60 to 180 beats per minute.

atrial natriuretic peptides see ATRIOPEPTIN.

atrial septal defect a hole in the wall between the upper two chambers of the heart.

atrichia absence of hair.

atrio- *combining form denoting* a chamber or ATRIUM.

atriopeptin a hormone stored in the muscle cells of the atria of the HEART and released into the blood when the blood volume increases beyond the optimum. Atriopeptin increases the rate of urine production and salt excretion. The discovery of atriopeptin led to the realization that this was one of a family of small peptides, called the atrial natriuretic peptides (ANPs), with receptors in the heart, lungs, kidneys, bone marrow, thymus and brain. ANPs have amino acid sequences from 28 to 53 moieties.

atrioventricular pertaining to the association of the upper and lower chambers of the heart – respectively, the atria and the ventricles. It often implies progression from an atrium to a ventricle.

atrioventricular node a 'junction-box', between the upper and lower chambers of the heart, in the band of specialized heart muscle fibres which conduct the electrical impulses controlling the contraction of the heart. It assists in the correct timing of the contractions, first of the atria and then of the ventricles.

atrioventricular valves the valves lying between the atria and the ventricles of the HEART that ensure movement of the blood from the former to the latter only. They are, on the right side, the tricuspid valve, and on the left, the mitral valve.

atrium one of the thin-walled upper chambers of the heart which receive blood from the veins and pass it down to the lower, more powerful, pumping chambers (the ventricles).

atrophic gastritis long-term (chronic) inflammation of the stomach with atrophy of the lining mucous membrane and poor or absent secretion of acid, PEPSIN and the INTRINSIC FACTOR. Loss of the intrinsic factor leads to PERNICIOUS ANAEMIA.

atrophic rhinitis an unpleasant condition affecting the inner lining of the nose which becomes dry and crusty and produces a foul odour. There is loss of the sense of smell and frequent nose-bleeds.

atrophy wasting and loss of substance due to cell degeneration and death. This may be a natural ageing process or it may be due to simple disuse. From the Greek *atrophia*, hunger or want of food.

atropine a bitter, poisonous alkaloid obtained from the plant *Atropa belladonna* ('deadly nightshade') and the seeds of the Thorn-apple. It blocks acetyl choline receptors and is used to relax spasm in smooth muscle in the intestines and other organs. It is also extensively used by ophthalmologists to dilate the pupil of the eye in the treatment of inflammatory disease and sometimes to facilitate examination. The drug is on the WHO official list. The generic term derives from the Greek *a*, not, and *tropos*, turning. Atropos was one of the three fates noted for her inexorable tendency to cut the thread of life.

atrotoxin a component of rattlesnake venom.

Atrovent a brand name for IPRATROPIUM BROMIDE in inhaler form or as a liquid for nebulization.

attention the direction of some of the channels of sensory input to a restricted area of the environment. Since the number of possible sources of information in the environment is so great, attention, which selectively directs and concentrates awareness and controls input, is of the first importance. Attention is seldom continuous for long and is determined mainly by the degree of interest in the source of the information. Attention is closely related to effectiveness in memory storage. It is no accident that people with a wide range of strong interests tend to have well-stocked minds. Motivation, as towards learning or achieving qualification, is a less powerful stimulus to attention than interest. Fortunately, interest grows with knowledge. Attention can be objectively demonstrated by such methods as electro-encephalography or PET scanning, which show special activity in the parts of the brain most employed at the time.

attention deficit hyperactivity disorder (ADHD) a childhood disorder affecting boys ten times as often as girls and featuring constant excessive physical activity, restlessness, unthinking impulsiveness, short span of attention and concentration, lack of responsiveness and unwillingness to participate with others in normal childhood activities. An MRI study published in late 2003 showed that children and adolescents with ADHD had reduced brain volume in the dorsal prefrontal cortices and in the anterior temporal corices. Even so, the condition is believed to be grossly over-diagnosed. In some areas in the USA 5% of boys aged 10-11 are being treated for this condition, mostly with methylphenidate (Ritalin). The drug ATOMOXETINE, which is neither a psychostimulant nor an amphetamine derivative, was introduced in mid-2004.

attenuated weakened or reduced, and so altered in characteristics so as no longer to be dangerous. The term is applied to organisms that have been specially cultured so as to reduce their virulence and make them suitable for use in vaccines.

audio- *combining form denoting* hearing.

audiogram a record of the sensitivity, or threshold, of hearing at different frequencies.

audiolingual pertaining to hearing and speaking in the process of learning a language.

audiologist a specialist in the diagnosis and treatment of defects of hearing.

audiology the scientific study of hearing and of the medical management of hearing defects.

audiometer an instrument for measuring the lowest levels at which pure tones can be heard at each of a range of frequencies, either by air or by bone conduction. The results are recorded as an AUDIOGRAM.

audiometry measurement of the sensitivity, or threshold, of a person's hearing at different pitches (frequencies). Hearing loss is never uniform over the whole range of sounds, from low to high pitch, so it is necessary to test the hearing with sounds of different pitches. In people with a hearing defect, audiometry can give warning of factors causing hearing loss so that these can be avoided. It also helps to determine the suitability, and best kind, of a hearing aid and helps in decisions about surgery.

auditory pertaining to hearing or to the organs of hearing.

auditory evoked responses subtle electrical changes in the brain waves, demonstrable on the ELECTROENCEPHALOGRAM, which are induced by loud noises. The method provides only a crude estimate of the hearing ability but gives some objective proof of hearing without the cooperation of the subject.

auditory nerve the acoustic or vestibulocochlear nerve. The 8th cranial nerve.

auditory ossicles the chain of three tiny bone in the middle ear which acts as an impedance transformer, efficiently coupling the relatively large low-impedance movement of the ear drum to the smaller, high-impedance movement of the fluid in the cochlea of the inner ear.

aura the symptoms providing a warning of an impending attack of some kind, such as an epileptic seizure or a migraine episode. These may take the form, respectively, of a feeling of coldness and the perception of sparkling lights.

aural pertaining to, or perceived by, the ear.

auranofin a gold preparation that can be taken by mouth for the treatment of RHEUMATOID ARTHRITIS. A brand name is Ridaura.

Aureomycin a brand name for the antibiotic CHLORTETRACYCLINE.

auri- *combining form denoting* the ear.

auricle 1 the pinna, or external ear.
2 an obsolescent term for one of the upper chambers of the heart (atrium).

auricular 1 pertaining to the ear or to hearing.
2 pertaining to an auricle, or atrium, of the heart.

auricular fibrillation see ATRIAL FIBRILLATION.

auricularis any of the three small flat muscles attached to the cartilage of the external ear. These are the vestigial remnants of the muscle still highly functional in other mammals, such as cats.

auriscope an instrument used for examining the interior of the tube leading from the outside to the ear drum (the external auditory meatus).

auscultation the act of listening with a stethoscope to the sounds made by the heart, lungs, blood passing through narrowed vessels, the movement of fluid or gas in the abdomen, and so on. The doctor listens for changes in the normal sounds and for new (adventitious) sounds. Heart specialists become skilled in the interpretation of subtle sounds inaudible to the novice. From the Latin *auscultare*, to listen attentively.

Australia antigen the hepatitis B virus surface ANTIGEN (HBsAg).

Austramycin a brand name for TETRACYCLINE.

Austrapen a brand name for AMPICILLIN.

aut-, auto- *prefix denoting* self. From the Greek *autos*, self.

autacoid a hormone or other substance produced in an organ and released into the blood to be carried to other parts of the organism to produce various effects.

autism a serious childhood disorder of higher brain function in which the child is withdrawn, self-absorbed, aloof, interested in objects but not in people, prone to repetitive movement and sometimes self-injury, and often unable to communicate by normal speech. Autism is now regarded as a spectrum disorder with mild ASPERGER'S SYNDROME at one end and grossly disabling autism at the other. There are growing indications that it is the result of organic brain abnormalities leading to the inability to distinguish between the recognition of people and the recognition of inanimate objects. The single most consistent physical sign of autism is abnormal enlargement of the head. This is strongly associated with polymorphism of the HOXA1 gene. No association has been demonstrated between autism and the use of MMR VACCINATION. The incidence of autism appears to be about 2.6 cases per 1000 live births. The condition can be reliably diagnosed between the ages of 2 and 3 and must be distinguished from simple mental retardation, emotional deprivation, early onset epilepsy, Rett syndrome and various neurodegenerative disorders.

autoagglutination the spontaneous clumping together of red blood cells. This is a feature of the AUTOIMMUNE DISEASE haemolytic anaemia

autoanalysis an attempt to perform PSYCHOANALYSIS upon oneself.

autoantibody an antibody derived from the immune system, which then acts against body tissues or constituents.

autochthonous native to a particular place, thus a term sometimes used to describe an AUTOGRAFT.

autoclave a strong sealed chamber in which surgical instruments, towels, dressings, and other items can be sterilized by steam under raised pressure.

autocrine 1 of a substance secreted by a cell and released into the extracellular fluid, that then acts on the cell.

2 of a cell responding to such chemical messengers.

autoeroticism 1 the deliberate arousal of sexual feeling in the absence of a sexual partner. **2** the satisfaction of sexual desire by MASTURBATION.

autogamy self-fertilization. This can occur by the fusion of two split nuclei.

autogenous originating within the self, as in a vaccine prepared from a person's own bacteria. Compare EXOGENOUS.

autograft tissue transplanted from one site in an individual to another in the same person. No immunological problems arise with autografts.

autohaemotherapy treatment of disease using the patient's own blood, which is withdrawn from a vein and then injected intramuscularly.

autoimmune disease one of a wide range of conditions in which destructive inflammation of various body tissues is caused by antibodies produced because the body has ceased to regard certain cells of the affected part as 'self'. Autoimmune diseases include ADDISON'S DISEASE, AUTOIMMUNE ENTEROPATHY, primary biliary cirrhosis, Goodpasture's syndrome, HASHIMOTO'S THYROIDITIS, MYASTHENIA GRAVIS, MYXOEDEMA, PEMPHIGOID, RHEUMATOID ARTHRITIS, SJOGREN'S SYNDROME, SYMPATHETIC OPHTHALMITIS, both forms of LUPUS ERYTHEMATOSUS, THYROTOXICOSIS, ULCERATIVE COLITIS and possibly MULTIPLE SCLEROSIS.

autoimmune enteropathy a disorder of the small intestine featuring severe atrophy of the absorptive VILLI and circulating antibodies against the cells that form the lining of the intestine (enterocytes). The condition does not respond to a gluten-free diet but there is a good response if this is combined with treatment directed against the immune system process that produces the enterocyte autoantibodies.

autoimmunization the process that leads to AUTOIMMUNE DISEASE.

autoinfection infection with bacteria or viruses surviving on or in the body, or transferred from one part of the body to another.

autoinoculation 1 inoculation with a vaccine derived from substances from the same person's body. **2** a secondary or recurrent infection by organisms already in the body.

autointoxication poisoning by substances produced in the body either as a result of

infection, or from damaged tissue or the products of abnormal metabolic processes.

autologous derived from the same person, as in the case of transfusions or transplantation.

autologous blood donation transfusion of a person's own blood. Blood may be taken some time prior to surgery, stored and then used, if necessary during or after surgery. Alternatively, one or two units of blood may be taken immediately before surgery and replaced by a non-blood infusion. This dilutes the patient's blood so that fewer red cells are lost in bleeding. The blood is then re-transfused at the end of surgery when no further blood loss is anticipated. The method became popular among patients when concern about HIV contamination of donated blood was at its height, but interest declined when HIV antibody testing was incorporated into donor screening and stringent criteria were required for donors. Studies have shown that autologous blood transfusion is uneconomical as a routine procedure.

autolysis the destruction of tissues or cells by substances, such as ENZYMES, present in the same body.

automated external defibrillator a device intended for use by non-medical persons trained in CARDIO-PULMONARY RESUSCITATION (CPR) for the emergency treatment of cardiac arrest caused by ventricular fibrillation especially in out-of-hospital situations.

automatism the quality of acting in a mechanical or involuntary manner. A feature of some forms of SCHIZOPHRENIA.

autonomic nervous system the part of the nervous system controlling involuntary functions, such as the heart beat, the secretion of glands and the contraction of blood vessels. It is subdivided into the SYMPATHETIC and the PARASYMPATHETIC divisions which are, in general, antagonistic and in balance. The term autonomic derives from the Greek *autos*, self, and *nomos*, a law (see Fig. 7).

Autopen a brand name for a reusable insulin injection pen that uses standard dose cartridges.

autopsy a postmortem pathological examination done to determine the cause of death or past medical history or to assist in medical research.

autoradiography a method of producing a permanent record of a pattern of molecules to which radioactive tracers have been attached, by laying a photographic film in close contact with the medium containing the molecules. Autoradiography is commonly performed following ELECTROPHORESIS of molecules.

autosomal of any chromosome other than the sex chromosome pair.

autosomal disorders genetic disorders caused by defective genes carried on chromosomes (AUTOSOMES) other than the sex chromosomes. Compare SEX-LINKED DISORDERS.

autosomal polycystic kidney disease a genetic kidney disorder featuring numerous kidney cysts, pain, bleeding into the urine, fever, kidney stones, high blood pressure and ultimately kidney failure between the ages of 40 and 60. The disease may be dominant or recessive. The dominant form affects 1 child in 1000 and is one of the commonest genetically-determined diseases. The gene for this form has been cloned and is on the short arm of chromosome 16.

autosome any one of the ordinary paired CHROMOSOMES other than the sex chromosomes.

autosuggestion a form of self-conditioning involving repeated internal assertion of positive and helpful propositions.

autotomy 1 fission of an organism, such as a bacterium or other cell.
2 surgical removal of a part of one's own body.

autotopagnosia inability of a person to identify his own body parts, such as nose, ear, chin, etc. This is usually the result of a neurological defect. From the Greek *auto*, self and *topos*, place.

autotransfusion a transfusion with one's own blood. The blood may be collected early, in anticipation of need, or may be salvaged from internal bleeding and returned to the circulation, during a surgical operation. See also AUTOLOGOUS BLOOD DONATION.

autumn crocus a plant, *Colchicum autumnale*, from which the valuable gout remedy colchicine is derived.

avascular lacking blood vessels.

avascular necrosis death of a tissue, especially bone, as a result of deprivation of its blood supply. Avascular necrosis of bone is often referred to as osteonecrosis.

Avelox a brand name for MOXIFLOXACIN.

aversion therapy a form of treatment for addiction or antisocial behaviour in which

the undesirable activity is forcibly associated in the mind of the subject with an unpleasant experience. It is not widely used. See also ANTABUSE.

avian influenza 'bird 'flu' caused by the H5N1 virus that caused epidemics in poultry in Japan, Korea, Thailand, China and Vietnam early in 2004. The virus is capable of spreading from birds to humans. By early 2005 there had been 44 known cases of H5N1 infection in humans with 32 deaths. There is serious concern that recombination with human influenza viruses may already have occurred, raising the danger of human-to-human infection.

aviation medicine the branch of medicine concerned with the medical hazards of atmospheric and space flight and with the special problems of aeromedical evacuation of the sick and wounded.

avirulent not highly infective or likely to cause disease.

avitaminosis the state of vitamin deficiency or a disorder caused by a deficiency of one or more vitamins.

Avloclor a brand name for CHLOROQUINE.

AV node see ATRIOVENTRICULAR NODE.

Avodart a brand name for DUTASTERIDE.

avoidant personality disorder a disorder characterized by a persistent and excessive shrinkage from contact with unfamiliar people, of such degree as to interfere with normal social functioning. A pathological degree of shyness.

Avomine a brand name for PROMETHAZINE.

Avonex a brand name for INTERFERON BETA-1a.

AVP *abbrev. for* arginine vasopressin, a hormone secreted by the rear lobe of the pituitary gland, usually called vasopressin. It is also known as the ANTIDIURETIC HORMONE.

avulsion forcible tearing off, or separation, of part of the body usually in the course of major injury. From the Latin *avulsio*, to separate by force.

avulsion fracture a fracture in which a strong tendon pull tears off a part of a bone at the site of the tendon attachment. Avulsion fractures of the HUMERUS are common at the upper and lower ends.

axial skeleton the skull and spine (vertebral column).

axial musculature the muscles connecting the head to the spine and those lying along the long axis of the spine.

Axid a brand name for NIZATIDINE.

axilla the armpit.

axillary pertaining to all the structures lying in the AXILLA, such as the axillary lymph nodes.

axis 1 the second of the vertebrae of the spine, upon which the skull and first vertebra (ATLAS) can rotate. The axis bone has a short, stout vertical peg called the odontoid process around which the atlas can rotate.
2 an imaginary central line of a part or of the body.
3 the meridian in a CYLINDRICAL LENS that possesses no optical power. The curve of maximal power is at right angles to the axis.

axon the long fibre-like process of a nerve cell which, bundled together with many thousands of other axons, forms the anatomical structure known as a nerve. The axon conducts nerve impulses away from the nerve body.

axonotmesis a severe injury to a peripheral nerve without severance of the sheath, so that, although the nerve fibres may have degenerated, regeneration and ultimate recovery of function is possible. Regeneration, if it occurs, does so at a rate of somewhat less than 1 mm per day.

ayurvedism an ancient Hindu system of medicine contained in the Ayur Veda, a treatise on the art of healing and prolonging life.

Azactam a brand name for AZTREONAM.

azapropazone a non-steroidal anti-inflammatory (NSAID) drug used in the treatment of conditions such as RHEUMATOID ARTHRITIS. A brand nameis Rheumox.

azatadine an ANTIHISTAMINE and SEROTONIN antagonist drug used in the treatment of allergic conditions.

azathioprine a drug used to suppress the immune system so as to avoid rejection of donor transplants. Immune suppression may have serious side effects such as the flare-up

of latent infections and an increased risk of malignant tumours such as lymphomas, but azathioprine is safer than other immunosuppressive drugs. Also used to treat rheumatism. The drug is on the WHO official list. A brand name is Imuran.

azelaic acid an antibacterial drug used externally in the form of a skin cream. A brand name is Skinoren.

azelastine an ANTIHISTAMINE drug used in the treatment of hay fever. Brand names are Optilast and Rhinolast.

azithromycin an ANTIBIOTIC drug used in the treatment of a range of infections including genital Chlamydia. A brand name is Zithromax.

azlocillin an acylureidopenicillin effective against the organism *Pseudomonas aeruginosa*, otherwise difficult to attack effectively. A brand name is Securopen.

azoospermia absence of spermatozoa from the seminal fluid, a cause of male sterility. Sperms may still be being produced in the testes.

azotaemia URAEMIA. The clinical syndrome resulting from failure of the kidneys.

AZT *abbrev. for* azidothymidine or Zidovudine. A drug used in attempts to control AIDS. The drug is toxic but does seem to be able to prolong life. A short course of AZT has been shown to be capable of halving the incidence of transmission of HIV from mother to baby. AZT is now commonly used in combination with other anti-HIV drugs especially protease inhibitors.

aztreonam a BETA-LACTAM antibiotic effective against aerobic GRAM NEGATIVE organisms. A brand name is Azactam.

azygous occurring singly rather than in pairs. From the Greek *azugos*, unyoked.

azygous vein one of the three unpaired veins of the ABDOMEN and THORAX.

b

B the symbol for the element barium.

babesiosis a disease spread by hard-bodied (*Ixodid*) ticks. The organism responsible, *Babesia bigemina*, invades the red blood cells causing them to rupture. There is fever, muscle aches, spleen enlargement and anaemia and the condition is sometimes fatal, especially if the spleen has been removed. There is no specific treatment. Babesiosis was the first disease shown to be transmitted by an ARTHROPOD.

Babinski's sign an extension and fanning out of the toes when the sole of the foot is stroked firmly with a pointed object. This reaction, instead of the normal curling up of the toes, indicates damage to the motor system above the level of the spinal nerves and is common in STROKE. (Joseph François Babinski, 1857–1932, French neurologist).

baby blues an Americanism for the fleeting episodes of misery and tearfulness which affect about half of all pregnant women, especially those having their first baby.

Bac *abbrev. for* Bachelor of Acupuncture.

bacillary 1 rod-shaped.
2 relating to, or caused by, a bacillus.

bacillary dysentery an acute infection of the bowel, mainly caused by the organism *Shigella sonnei*, and, in severe cases, featuring diarrhoea, colicky abdominal pain, fever, blood and pus in the stools and dehydration. Many cases are mild.

bacilliform rod-shaped. Shaped like a BACILLUS.

bacillophobia an abnormal fear of bacilli.

bacilluria bacilli in the urine.

bacillus 1 a bacterium of the genus *Bacillus*, such as *Bacillus anthracis*, *Bacillus cereus* or *Bacillus subtilis*. These bacteria tend to form long chains.
2 any bacterium, especially if rod-shaped.

bacitracin an antibiotic derived from the bacterium *Bacillus subtilis*. It acts by interfering with the formation of the bacterial cell membrane and is highly effective against many organisms especially the HAEMOLYTIC streptococcus. Unfortunately, it is so liable to damage the kidneys that it must be confined to external use. Brand names of preparations containing bacitracin are Cicatrin and Polyfax.

backache pain or discomfort in the area of the spine.

backbone the vertebral column or spine.

back mutation the return of a gene to its original nucleotide sequence after a mutation.

baclofen a drug derived from the NEUROTRANSMITTER GABA that interferes with nerve transmission in the spinal cord and relaxes muscle spasm. It is used to alleviate the effects of conditions such as STROKE and MULTIPLE SCLEROSIS. A brand name is Lioresal.

bacteraemia bacteria in the circulating blood. This is often transient and is not necessarily serious. See also the more significant condition of SEPTICAEMIA.

bacteraemic shock a state of shock occurring during the course of, and usually as a result of, the circulation of bacteria in the blood. Bacteraemic shock is especially associated with gram-negative organisms.

bacteria single-celled, microscopic, living organisms occurring in countless numbers almost everywhere. Most are harmless; only a small proportion cause disease. Bacteria may be cocci which are spherical and usually about 1000th of a millimetre (1) in diameter. These include bunched staphylococci and single-strand grouped streptococci. Bacilli are straight rod-shaped organisms; vibrios are curved; and spirilla (including spirochaetes) are wavy. Bacteria reproduce rapidly with a generation time, under ideal conditions, of about 20 min. Those that cause human disease reproduce best at human body temperature (37 °C). Some of them are unable to synthesize DNA at 42 but will do so readily at 37. Bacteria produce powerful poisons (toxins) which are among the most poisonous substances known. It is the toxins that cause disease by binding on to body cells, gravely affecting their function or even survival.

bacterial bronchopneumonia a patchy form of PNEUMONIA caused by bacterial infection of the lung, usually secondary to infection in the bronchi.

bacterial conjugation a kind of sexual intercourse between bacteria in which, after close contact between them, DNA is transferred from one to the other. Some bacteria have a tubular structure on the external surface known as a sex pilus. This is believed to be the route of transfer of DNA during conjugation.

bacterial culture the growing of micro-organisms on a culture medium, such as agar, in an incubator kept at body temperature, for purposes of identification.

bacterial colony a discrete accumulation of a very large number of bacteria, usually occurring as a CLONE of a single organism or of a small number. Colonies grow best on selected media.

bacterial encephalitis inflammation of the brain caused by bacteria.

bacterial endocarditis see INFECTIVE ENDOCARDITIS.

bacterial meningitis see MENINGITIS.

bacterial vaginosis a very common condition featuring a frothy, greyish vaginal discharge without irritation caused by the organism *Gardnerella vaginalis* and other bacteria. The condition is commoner in women who have sex with women than in those who are exclusively heterosexual. It is present in up to half of women who regularly have sex with women. It is treated with METRONIDAZOLE, but as about half the sexual partners also carry the organisms, they, too, must be treated. See also AMINE TEST.

bactericidal able to kill bacteria.

bactericidal permeability-increasing protein a protein that acts on bacteria, especially meningococci, to increase their membrane permeability and so kill them.

It also binds to and clears bacterial toxin. The substance has been proposed as a one of the modalities for treating bacterial MENINGITIS.

bacteriology the scientific study of bacteria. Medical bacteriology is the study of organisms that can cause disease or which are normally present, harmlessly or beneficially, in the body.

bacteriophage phage, a virus that infects bacteria. Most bacteriophages are simple organisms consisting of a DNA or RNA core and a protein coat, but some are more complex. Phages incorporate their genetic material into the host genome and replicate. Some cause the death of the cell; some do not.

bacteriostatic able to restrain or control the multiplication of bacteria, without actually killing them. When a bacteriostatic effect is achieved organisms are more susceptible to destruction by the immune system.

bacterium the singular of BACTERIA.

bacteriuria bacteria in the urine. The presence of 100,000 or more disease-producing bacteria per millilitre of urine indicates a urinary tract infection.

Bacteroides a genus of GRAM NEGATIVE, non-motile, ANAEROBIC bacteria normally occurring in the mouth and digestive tract. Some species can cause disease.

Bactroban cream *or* **ointment** a brand name for MUPIROCIN for external use.

Bactroban nasal a brand name for a MUPIROCIN ointment for nasal use.

bad breath malodorous exhalation. Halitosis. The mouth is the chief source of the odour, but this may also come from the nose, the lungs and, rarely, the stomach.

bad cholesterol an informal term for the cholesterol carried in low density LIPOPROTEINS (LDLs).

bad trip a popular expression for a highly unpleasant reaction to a hallucinogenic drug. Such reactions may recur months later without further exposure to the drug.

bagassosis a lung disease caused by allergy to inhaled dust from sugar cane waste (bagasse). There is persistent lung inflammation (PNEUMONITIS) with progressive replacement of functioning lung with scar tissue.

Baker's cyst a painless swelling occurring behind the knee when there is escape of joint fluid (synovial fluid) through the capsule of the joint as a result of excessive production.

(William Morrant Baker, English surgeon, 1838–1896).

baker's itch dermatitis caused by flour mites of the *Pyemotes* genus.

BAL *abbrev. for* British antilewisite, or DIMERCAPROL.

Balamuthia mandrillaris infection a disease, first described in 1990, caused by the amoebic protozoal organism *Balamuthia mandrillaris*. It is a granulomatous encephalitis that can affect both humans and animals. The granulomas can affect the face as well as the brain, and those in the brain cause space-occupying symptoms and signs. Diagnosis is by identifying the amoebae and cysts. There is no known effective treatment.

balanced anaesthesia a commonly employed form of general anaesthesia in which two or more anaesthetic agents are used in small doses to provide a summed effect.

balanitis inflammation of the bulb (GLANS) of the penis, usually the result of neglect of personal hygiene in the uncircumcized but sometimes from infection with THRUSH (candidiasis).

balanoposthitis inflammation of the glans of the penis and of the foreskin (prepuce).

balanopreputial pertaining to the GLANS and the foreskin.

balantidiasis a kind of DYSENTERY caused by infection with the ciliated protozoan *Balantidium coli*, an organism that is often present in the bowels of people with no symptoms. This is the largest protozoan parasite of humans. The condition resembles AMOEBIC DYSENTERY and large ulcers form in the lining of the colon. Severe attacks are commoner in poorly nourished people. The condition is treated with TETRACYCLINE or METRONIDAZOLE.

baldness premature hair loss. Male baldness is common and is thought to be due to an AUTOSOMAL gene that behaves in a DOMINANT manner in males and in a RECESSIVE MANNER in females. This is called a sex-influenced trait.

Balkan beam an orthopaedic appliance set up above a bed to allow balanced traction in the management of a fractured thigh bone (femur).

Balkan grippe see Q FEVER.

Balkan nephropathy a type of chronic NEPHRITIS occurring in certain rural populations in the central Danube basin on the borders of Bulgaria, Yugoslavia and Romania and affecting 10% to 75% of families. The onset is insidious with protein in the urine, gradual impairment of kidney function, coppery discolouration of the skin and anaemia. The outlook is poor and most affected people die within three years. The cause is unknown but the condition may be due to a toxic fungus that grows on wet maize and other grains.

ballism an extreme form of CHOREA in which the limbs are flung about violently. It is a disorder of the EXTRAPYRAMIDAL SYSTEM of the brain. STEREOTACTIC SURGERY may be helpful.

balloon angioplasty the use of a BALLOON CATHETER to restore more normal width to an artery narrowed by ATHEROSCLEROSIS. The catheter is threaded along the artery to the site of the narrowing and the balloon is then inflated, crushing the atherosclerotic plaque into the wall.

balloon catheter a fine double tube, with an expandible cylindrical inflatable portion near one end. A balloon catheter can be passed along an artery to an area partially blocked by disease and then inflated so as to stretch and widen the vessel. The device is also used to treat narrowing of the heart valves and, sometimes, narrowing of the URETHRA from enlargement of the PROSTATE GLAND.

balloon valvuloplasty the use of a balloon catheter to overcome narrowing (stenosis) of a heart valve.

ballottement a physical sign of a solid organ, a fetus or a suspected mass, lying within fluid. The area is given a sharp push with the tips of the fingers and the mass swings quickly away and then back again to strike the fingertips and confirm its presence. Ballottement may thus show either fluid or an internal mass.

balm 1 an old-fashioned term for anything believed to sooth and heal.

2 an aromatic, oily resin exuded by various trees and shrubs and sometimes used in medicine as an ointment or inhalant.

balneology the study of balneotherapy – medical treatment employing mineral baths. There is grave doubt as to whether balneology can be classified as a science.

Balnetar a brand name for a COAL TAR preparation.

balsalazide a drug used in the treatment of ULCERATIVE COLITIS. A brand name is Colazide.

balsam an oily or gummy resin, usually containing benzoic or cinnamic acids, obtained from various trees and used to flavour medicines or as an inhalant.

bambuterol a selective beta-agonist drug used in the treatment of ASTHMA. A brand name is Bambec.

bandage a binder. A strip of woven cotton, wool, plastic, rubber or other material wrapped firmly round any part of the body for a variety of reasons. Bandages may be non-stretch or elastic, conforming or otherwise, adhesive or plain.

bandage contact lens a very thin, high water content CONTACT LENS used to protect the cornea from abrasion with the eyelids in various conditions, such as corneal ulcer or corneal dystrophies.

banding patterns transverse stripes visible on stained chromosomes that vary with different kinds of stain.

Bang's disease BRUCELLOSIS.

Banocide a brand name for DIETHYLCARBAMAZINE.

Banti's syndrome enlarged spleen, overactivity of the spleen in destroying red blood cells (hypersplenism) and enlarged liver due to a rise in the blood pressure in the portal vein system (portal hypertension) or to an obstruction in the splenic vein. (Guido Banti, Italian physician, 1852–1925).

Bantu siderosis excessive iron stores in the body due to a large intake of beer prepared in iron pots. The condition can lead to CIRRHOSIS of the liver.

BAO *abbrev. for* Bachelor of the Art of Obstetrics.

baragnosis inability to estimate the weight of an object.

Baratol a brand name for INDORAMIN.

barber's itch an old-fashioned and non-specific term for one of a variety of skin eruptions or infections involving the shaving area and purported to be spread by the barber. Also known as sycosis barbae.

barbiturates sedative drugs derived from barbituric acid. The barbiturates are classified into three groups according to their duration of action – short, medium and long. Few barbiturates are now widely used, the main exceptions being the very short acting drug thiopentone (thiopental) (Pentothal), which is still used to induce anaesthesia, and the long acting phenobarbitone (phenobarbital) which

is used to control some forms of EPILEPSY. The first barbiturate was synthesized from urea in urine provided by a young woman called Barbara, hence the name.

barbiturism the toxic state of coma or delirium following an overdose of barbiturates. Poisoning with any barbiturate drug.

Barbloc a brand name for PINDOLOL.

barbotage a method of pain control designed to interrupt the pain pathways in the spinal cord. 20 ml of cerebrospinal fluid are repeatedly withdrawn and reinjected from the space surrounding the cord. Most patients enjoy relief of pain for up to seven months.

bare lymphocyte syndrome a rare autosomal recessive immunodeficiency genetic disorder that results in the absence of the class 2 MAJOR HISTOCOMPATIBILITY COMPLEX glycoprotein molecules. Children with this mutation are extremely susceptible to infection with all kinds of organisms and seldom survive for more than four years from birth.

bariatric pertaining to obesity and weight control.

bariatric surgery surgery aimed at combating obesity. Procedures include various methods of reducing the volumetric capacity of the stomach by banding or stapling. The method seems, currently, to be the most successful way of avoiding the complications of severe obesity.

barium enema the instillation of a liquid paste of barium sulphate into the rectum and lower colon for the purposes of contrast X-ray examination.

barium meal an X-ray examination enhanced by the use of the insoluble barium sulphate, usually in the form of a liquid suspension. Barium is opaque to X rays and will thus reveal the internal structure of a hollow organ. Barium X rays are useful in the investigation of any part of the digestive tract. They can reveal out-pouchings from the lower part of the throat (PHARYNGEAL POUCH), narrowing (stenosis or stricture) of the gullet (oesophagus), swallowing disorders, HIATUS HERNIA, stomach and duodenal ulcers, tumours or POLYPS anywhere in the bowel but especially in the colon, abnormal pouches (diverticula) in the colon, CROHN'S DISEASE (regional ileitis) and COELIAC DISEASE.

barium sulphate an insoluble substance used as a contrast medium for X-ray examination.

The drug is on the WHO official list.

barium swallow an X-ray examination of the gullet (OESOPHAGUS) performed while a solution of barium is being swallowed. This may reveal abnormal narrowing.

Barker hypothesis the proposition that a baby's nourishment *in utero* and during infancy determines the subsequent development of risk factors such as high blood pressure, blood clotting biochemistry and glucose intolerance and is thus a major determinant of coronary heart disease later in life.

baroreceptor a nerve ending which produces an output when there is a change in ambient pressure. Also known as baroceptor.

barosinusitis sinus inflammation with symptoms induced by changes in atmospheric pressure. Also called sinus barotrauma.

barotrauma injury resulting from changes in atmospheric (barometric) pressure as in aircraft flight. Barotrauma mostly affects the ear drums when there is obstruction to the EUSTACHIAN TUBES. The most serious forms of barotrauma result from explosive noise which can literally shake the delicate hair-cell transducers in the middle ear to pieces.

Barr body a condensed clump of CHROMATIN occurring in the nucleus of cells in normal females and corresponding to an inactive X chromosome. The Barr body also occurs in males with two or more X chromosomes an addition to the Y chromosome. See also X-INACTIVATION. (Murray Llewellyn Barr, Canadian anatomist, b. 1908).

bar reader a device used in ORTHOPTICS consisting of a narrow opaque strip fixed between the reader's eyes and the printed page so that different parts of the page are occluded from each eye. The method is used to promote single binocular vision.

barrel chest the characteristic appearance of a person suffering from EMPHYSEMA.

barren sterile. Incapable of producing offspring.

Barrett's oesophagus a gullet (oesophagus) in which long-standing inflammation (oesophagitis) has led to a change in the nature of the lining mucus membrane to a columnar form. An ulcer may develop (Barrett's ulcer) and lead to narrowing (stricture) or possibly cancer. (Norman Rupert Barrett, Australian-born English surgeon, 1903–1979).

barrier contraceptive any contraceptive, such

as a condom or a diaphragm shield, that imposes a barrier between the spermatozoa and the ovum. See also CONTRACEPTION.

barrier creams creams used to protect the skin against environmental hazards. Most of them are based on the water-repellant and biologically inert range of silicone compounds and are not particularly effective.

barrier nursing local isolation of a patient with an infectious disease so as to avoid spread. The 'barrier' takes the form of gowns, caps, overshoes, gloves and masks which are donned by staff and visitors before approaching the patient and discarded before returning to the normal environment.

Bartholinitis inflammation, sometimes with abscess formation, in one of the BARTHOLIN'S GLANDS.

Bartholin's cyst an accumulation of mucin secretion causing expansion of one of the BARTHOLIN'S GLANDS to form a swelling to one side of the vaginal entrance.

Bartholin's glands mucus-secreting glands lying between the back part of the vaginal orifice and the lesser lips (labia minora) on either side. They secrete under the influence of sexual excitement and facilitate sexual intercourse. (Carpar Secundus Bartholin, 1655–1738, Danish surgeon).

bartonellosis a South American infectious disease, spread by sandflies and affecting the blood cells. It is caused by the organism *Bartonella bacilliformis* which is found in or on the red blood cells. The major form, Oroya fever, features high temperature, anaemia, and enlargement of the spleen and lymph nodes but responds well to antibiotics. Sometimes the nervous system is involved. The condition is also known as Carrion's disease, verruga fever and Guaitara fever.

basal pertaining to, situated at, or forming, an anatomical base of any kind.

basal cell a cell of the single-cell-thick lowest layer of epithelia, such as the epidermis of the skin, from which all the more superficial layers are derived by MITOSIS.

basal cell carcinoma rodent ulcer. A skin cancer which can be very destructive locally if neglected, but which very rarely spreads to other parts of the body. It is related to ultraviolet light damage from sunlight.

basal ganglia the discrete, grey nerve cell

masses lying deep in the lower part of the brain within the white matter. They consist, on each side, of the caudate nucleus, the putamen and the globus pallidus. They receive numerous connections from the outer layer (cortex) of the CEREBRUM, above, and from the CEREBELLUM, behind. They are concerned with the control of motor function.

basal meningitis MENINGITIS affecting primarily the membranes covering the base of the brain. This tends to be a feature of the less acute forms, of tubercular meningitis and of inadequately treated bacterial meningitis.

basal metabolic rate the rate at which energy is used by a person at rest. The BMR is measured in terms of the heat given off in a given time.

basal metabolism the minimum amount of energy needed to maintain the vital functions – heart beat, respiration and digestion – in a person at complete rest.

basal narcosis premedication with narcotic drugs to reduce anxiety and post-operative shock.

base a chemical compound that combines with an acid to form a salt and water. A term applied in genetics to one of the four nitrogenous bases of DNA and RNA. In DNA the bases are adenine, thymine, guanine and cytosine. Guanine and adenine are purines and cytosine and thymine are pyrimidines. In RNA, the pyrimidine base uracil replaces thymine. (See also BASE PAIR).

base analogue any compound structurally similar to a DNA BASE that can substitute for a base and thus cause a mutation.

base pair two linked molecules, one a purine the other a pyrimidine, that lie across the two strands of the DNA double helix. The bases are linked by easily-broken hydrogen bonds and the linkage occurs only in a particular, complementary, way – adenine with thymine and guanine with cytosine. This is the essence of DNA replication, which starts with the separation of a length of the two strands at bonds. In RNA, uracil replaces thymine and adenine links with it. Distance along a DNA sequence is measured as the number of base pairs.

basement membrane a thin lamina, consisting of collagen, glycosaminoglycans, fibronectins and other substances, on which one or more layers of cells, especially epithelial cells, rest. Basal membranes are double-layered,

the outer layer being secreted by the epithelial cells and the inner layer by connective tissue.

basidiobolomycosis an infection with a zygomycetous mould fungus, *Basidiobolus haptosporus*. This is seen mainly in children in Africa and Indonesia. There are localized, hard, woody swellings under the skin. The condition responds to treatment with potassium iodide.

basilar relating to, or situated at or near a base, especially the base of the skull or of the brain.

basilar artery an important artery formed from the junction of the two vertebral arteries that run up through the side processes of the vertebrae of the neck. The basilar artery runs up in a groove on the front surface of the PONS to supply most of the BRAINSTEM and CEREBELLUM and then joins the arterial circle, the circle of Willis, on the base of the brain.

basilar membrane the membrane in the COCHLEA of the inner ear which supports the ORGAN OF CORTI – the mechanism by which sound vibrations are converted to nerve impulses. The basilar membrane vibrates sympathetically in different parts under the influence of vibrations of different frequencies causing the stimulation of different groups of hair cells.

basilar meningitis see BASAL MENINGITIS.

basilic BASILAR.

basiliximab a chimeric monoclonal antibody to the alpha chain (CD 25), one of the three transmembrane protein chain receptors of INTERLEUKIN 2R. This interleukin plays an important role in T lymphocyte proliferation. On resting T cells the level of expression of CD 25 is low but allogenic stimulation after organ grafting causes it to rise. This provides specificity for a means of control of graft rejection. Trials have suggested that basiliximab can reduce graft rejection by one third. A brand name is Simulect.

basket forceps surgical forceps designed to grasp, and retain for removal, an object such as a small stone.

basophil having an affinity for alkali. The term is used conveniently to refer to the group of blood white cells (leukocytes) whose internal granules take up an alkaline stain. The granules in basophils are mainly histamine and it is the release of this powerful chemical that causes most of the trouble in allergy. Basophils closely resemble tissue MAST CELLS.

basophilia a rise in the proportion of BASOPHIL white cells in the blood. Punctate basophilia is a disorder of young red cells which show several deep blue dots on Romanowsky staining. This is a feature of any severe ANAEMIA but especially of BETA-THALASSAEMIA and lead poisoning.

basophilic staining readily with basic dyes.

basophobia abnormal fear of standing upright or walking. See also ABASIA.

BAT *abbrev. for* brown adipose tissue.

bat ear a minor disfigurement of childhood in which the ears are larger and more protruding than usual.

bathophobia abnormal fear of depths.

Batista procedure SEE HEART REDUCTION.

battered-baby syndrome the clinical condition of a baby or young child who has been assaulted. The child is often malnourished. There may be multiple bruising, including finger marks, X-ray indication of healed fractures, tearing of the central fold behind the upper lip, cigarette burns, bite marks, and sometimes indications of bleeding inside the skull or brain. See also SHAKEN BABY SYNDROME.

battle fatigue a stress syndrome, now usually called post-traumatic stress disorder, caused by prolonged exposure to the trauma of warfare. There is repetitive reliving of the painful experience, nightmares, persistent anxiety, over-alertness, irritability, restlessness, jumpiness and insomnia.

Battle's sign discolouration behind the ear in fracture of the middle part of the base of the skull. (William Henry Battle, English surgeon, 1855–1936).

Baxan a brand name for CEFADROXIL.

BC, BCh, BChir *abbrev. for* Bachelor of Surgery. An alternative is ChB.

B cells B LYMPHOCYTES, one of the two main classes of lymphocytes, white cells found in the blood, lymph nodes and tissues which, with other cells, form the immune system of the body. B lymphocytes form CLONES of plasma cells which manufacture antibodies (IMMUNOGLOBULINS).

BC, Bch *abbrev. for* Bachelor of Surgery.

BCG vaccine a vaccine containing Bacille Calmette-Guerin, an attenuated strain of the bovine tubercle bacillus. The vaccine is used to confer a measure of immunity on people who, on Mantoux or Heaf testing are shown not to have had a primary infection with tuberculosis. It is equally effective in giving protection against leprosy. BCG vaccine is available in a freeze-dried form. The drug is on the WHO official list. (Leon Charles Albert Calmette, 1863–1933, French surgeon, and Camille Guerin, 1872–1961, French veterinary surgeon).

BChD *abbrev. for* Bachelor of Dental Surgery.

Bchir *abbrev. for* Bachelor of Surgery.

bcl-1 proto-ONCOGENE concerned with the persistence of LYMPHOCYTES. Mutations can cause various kinds of lymphocytic lymphom as and chronic lymphocytic leukaemia. bcl-1 genes are situated at chromosome sites that break easily.

bcl-2 proto-ONCOGENE. This gene is over-expressed in various tumours, especially non-Hodgkin lymphoma, resulting in resistance to APOPTOSIS (programmed cell death) with encouragement of tumour growth. Antisense nucleotide sequences (oligonucleotides) targeted at BCL-2 messenger RNA reduces the expression of BCL-2 and increases apoptosis in these tumours with clinical improvement.

BDA *abbrev. for* British Dental Association.

B DNA one of the three forms of DNA. It is a right-hand helix with about 10 bases per turn, and is the commonest form of chromosomal DNA.

BDS *abbrev. for* Bachelor of Dental Surgery.

BDSC *abbrev. for* Bachelor of Dental Science.

BdentSc *abbrev. for* Bachelor of Dental Science.

bearing down 1 the pains experienced in the second stage of labour.

2 the expulsive effort made by a woman in contracting the abdominal muscles and diaphragm in labour.

3 a sense of something descending in the pelvis experienced by women with PROLAPSE of the womb.

becaplermin recombinant human platelet-derived growth factor used to promote the healing of leg ulcers, especially in diabetics. A brand name is Regranex.

Becloforte a brand name for BECLOMETHAZONE.

beclometasone beclomethasone, a drug widely used by inhalation to treat ASTHMA that is not controlled by bronchodilating drugs or that is deemed necessary to control the inflammatory element in the disease. The drug is on the WHO official list. Inhalers include Aerobec, Asmabec, Beclazone, Becloforte, Becodisks, Beconase

Becotide, Filair, Pulvinal Beclometazone and Qvar. Other forms include Nasobec and Propaderm.

Beconase a brand name for BECLOMETHAZONE.

Becotide a brand name for BECLOMETHAZONE.

Becquerel a unit of the strength of radioactivity from a particular source. A Becquerel is defined as one nuclear disintegration per second.

bed bath a method of washing a patient who is too weak or frail to be taken to a bathroom. Waterproof sheets are used and one side is sponged at a time.

bed-blocking the use of hospital beds by elderly patients who cannot leave hospital because they are unfit to look after themselves and have no place in a residential care home.

bedbug *Cimex lectularis*, a blood-sucking insect that feeds on mammals. It is a broad, reddish, flat parasite of man, found all over the world in human habitations. It does not transmit any important disease.

bedpan a receptacle, of stainless steel, plastic or disposable moulded paper, for the excreta of those unable easily to get out of bed.

bedlam the slang term for the Bethlehem Royal Hospital in London, the first psychiatric hospital, founded around 1400. Visits to observe the noisy madmen became a popular entertainment and the term soon came to be used for any uproar. The site of Bedlam was moved several times and it is now associated with the Maudsley Hospital.

bedridden forced, by severity of illness or psychological misfortune, to remain permanently in bed.

Bedsonia an obsolete term for organisms of the genus *Chlamydia*, including those that cause trachoma and psittacosis.

bed sores ulcers of the skin, and, in some severe cases, of the underlying muscles also, caused by local deprivation of blood supply as a result of sustained pressure. Bed sores are sometimes called decubitus ulcers or pressure sores. They can be avoided by regular changes of position and by skilled nursing.

bedwetting see ENURESIS.

beer drinkers' cardiomyopathy enlargement and defective functioning of the heart muscle with congestive HEART FAILURE in heavy drinkers of beer. Some cases were found to be due to the toxic effect of cobalt added to beer.

behaviour therapy a method of treating neurotic disorders and modifying unacceptable patterns of behaviour by establishing CONDITIONED REFLEXES, using positive and negative reinforcement, by reward and punishment, respectively. Behaviour therapy has been shown to be effective in obsessive-compulsive disorders, phobias, sexual dysfunction, aggressive conduct in SCHIZOPHRENIA and in some cases of so-called MYALGIC ENCEPHALOMYELITIS. In general, it is more useful in treating circumscribed conditions than in dealing with widespread personality disorders.

Behçet's syndrome a persistent (chronic) disease of obscure origin, causing painful, recurrent ulcers of the mouth and genital area, internal inflammation of the eyes (UVEITIS), ARTHRITIS and blisters, pustules and inflammatory bumps on the skin. (Halushi Behçet, 1889–1948, Turkish dermatologist).

bejel a non-venereal form of SYPHILIS affecting mainly children and occurring principally in the Eastern Mediterranean. The condition is becoming rare.

belching bringing up gas (eructation), which is usually air, swallowed during the attempts to achieve the relief of a belch or during greedy eating. It is uncommon for gases to be formed in the stomach or intestines as a result of dyspeptic conditions. In most cases, persistent belching can be prevented by taking account of these facts. See also FLATULENCE.

belladonna a crude form of ATROPINE derived from the leaves and roots of the poisonous plant, *Atropa belladonna*. The term derives from the cosmetic use of the alkaloid to widen the pupils. Bella donna is Italian for beautiful woman.

belle indifference an inappropriate lack of emotional response to claimed severe disablement or incapacitating symptoms in HYSTERIA.

Bell's palsy paralysis of some or all of the muscles on one side of the face, so that the corner of the mouth droops, the lower lid falls away, and the affected side of the face becomes flattened and expressionless. Many cases of Bell's palsy are due to herpes simplex virus infections. Polymerase chain reaction amplification has shown the herpes simplex virus genome in a high proportion of cases.

A faster and more complete recovery can often be achieved by treatment with the anti-herpes drug aciclovir (Zovirax). The early use of steroids such as prednisolone also improves the prognosis. (Sir Charles Bell, 1774–1842, Scottish surgeon).

Bell's phenomenon a protective effect seen in BELL'S PALSY. The attempt to close the eyes tightly causes the exposed eye on the paralysed side of the face to roll upwards. This protects the eye by helping to keep the cornea moist.

belly a common name for the ABDOMEN.

belly button an informal term for the navel (UMBILICUS).

Benadryl a brand name for DIPHENHYDRAMINE.

Bence Jones protein a MONOCLONAL immunoglobulin formed in excess by B lymphocytes and found in the serum and urine in cases of multiple myeloma. (Henry Bence Jones, 1818–1873, English physician).

Bence Jones proteinuria the presence of BENCE JONES PROTEIN in the urine.

bendrofluazide bendroflumethazide, a thiazide DIURETIC drug used to treat high blood pressure (HYPERTENSION) and HEART FAILURE. Brand names are Aprinox, Centyl K and Neo-Naclex. Formulated with beta-blockers it is marketed under the brand names Corgaretic, Prestim, Inderetic and Inderex.

bends decompression sickness. The effect of the release of dissolved nitrogen in the form of bubbles in the blood. These can block small arteries, causing pain, especially in the joints, but having their most dangerous effect in the brain.

benefix a brand name for recombinant human Factor IX formulated as a drug.

benign not MALIGNANT. Mild, and of favourable outlook. Not usually tending to cause death. A benign tumour is a local growth, from an increase in the number of cells, which has no tendency to invade adjacent tissues or to seed out to remote parts of the body. Benign tumours are commonly enclosed in a definite capsule. They can, however cause trouble by local pressure effects, especially in confined spaces such as the inside of the skull.

benign familial neonatal convulsions a rare autosomal dominant disorder due to a gene on the long arm of chromosome 20. The condition features brief CLONIC seizures occurring within a few days or a week or two of birth. Longer-term follow-up, however, suggests that the adjective 'benign' might be inappropriate. A number of cases have been described in which STATUS EPILEPTICUS and death have occurred.

benign intracranial hypertension a syndrome of raised pressure within the skull in the absence of a brain tumour, HYDROCEPHALUS or other obvious cause. The condition is only relatively benign as it often leads to visual loss from compression damage to the optic nerves. It occurs most often in women below the age of 40 and causes severe headache and nausea but no deterioration of intellect or consciousness. Obesity is a common association. Ophthalmoscopic examination shows striking swelling of the optic discs (papilloedema).

benign paroxysmal positional vertigo a very common cause of dizziness precipitated by head movements or by lying down or turning over in bed. There is a typical circular movement of the eyes (rotational nystagmus) when the head is inclined and turned to the affected side. The disorder is due to debris in the semicircular canals that moves with head movement causing a current of endolymph and stimulation of the position sense mechanism. In nearly 80% of cases the condition resolves spontaneously in a few days or weeks. The condition can be corrected by a sequence of movements of the head and truck that rotates the posterior semicircular canal in a plane so that debris is moved into the utricle (Epley manoeuvre).

Benoral a brand name for BENORYLATE (benorilate).

benorylate benorilate, a drug derived from ASPIRIN and PARACETAMOL which is less irritating to the stomach than aspirin, but equally effective as a painkiller and non-steroidal anti-inflammatory drug in the treatment of arthritic pain. A brand name is Benoral.

Benoxyl a brand name for BENZOYL PEROXIDE.

benserazide a dopamine precursor drug given in conjunction with LEVODOPA in the treatment of PARKINSON'S DISEASE to prevent the break-down of levodopa in the body. A brand name is Madopar.

bentiromide test a test of the secretory output of the PANCREAS other than of insulin and glucagon. The test depends on the breaking-down effect of pancreatic digestive enzymes on a marker given by mouth.

benperidol a drug with phenothiazine-like properties used in the treatment of socially unacceptable sexual deviant behaviour. A brand name is Benquil.

Benylin a brand name for DIPHENHYDRAMINE with other ingredients.

Benzac a brand name for BENZOYL PEROXIDE.

Benzagel a brand name for BENZOYL PEROXIDE.

Benzamycin a brand name for ERYTHROMYCIN formulated with BENZOYL PEROXIDE for external use only.

benzalkonium chloride an antiseptic used in solution for skin and wound cleansing, as a means of sterilizing eye drops and contact lens solutions and as an ingredient in throat lozenges. Allergic reactions occur. Benzalkonium is included in Bradosol lozenges and, for external use only, in Conotrane, Dermol, Drapolene, Emulsiderm and Oilatum Plus.

benzathine penicillin an early, long-acting penicillin that must be given by injection.

Benzedrine a now historic brand name for AMPHETAMINE (amfetamine).

benzene poisoning poisoning with the widely used industrial solvent and raw material benzene. There is dizziness, EUPHORIA, headache, weakness, trembling, clumsiness, tightness in the chest, coma and convulsions. Long-term, small-dose poisoning causes loss of appetite, irritability, severe ANAEMIA, LEUKAEMIA and LYMPHOMAS.

benzhexol trihexyphenidyl, an anticholinergic drug that blocks the action of ACETYLCHOLINE in the nervous system. It is used to treat the symptoms of PARKINSON'S DISEASE. A brand name is Broflex.

benzidine a yellowish or reddish crystalline powder used in a test to detect small quantities of blood.

benznidazole an antiprotozoal drug used mainly to treat South American trypanosomiasis (Chagas' disease). The drug is on the WHO official list.

benzocaine a tasteless white powder with powerful local anesthetic properties. Often used in lozenges in combination with antiseptics. The drug is an ingredient in AAA Spray, Intralgin, Merocaine and Tyrozets.

benzodiazepine drugs a range of sedative and muscle relaxant drugs which have largely replaced the BARBITURATES as being allegedly safer, but now beginning to be regarded with much the same critical attitudes. The range includes diazepam (Diazemuls), chlordiazepoxide (Librium), lorazepam (Ativan) and nitrazepam (Mogadon and Somnite). Long-acting benzodiazepines include flurazepam (Dalmane), clobazam (Frisium), dipotassium clorazepate (Tranxene) and alprazolam (Xanax). Addiction to the benzodiazepine drugs is common.

benzoic acid a drug used externally, often in combination with SALICYLIC ACID, to assist in the healing of leg ulcers by the removal of superficial dead tissue (sloughs). The drug is on the WHO official list. A brand name is Aserbine.

benzopyrine a yellow, crystalline, aromatic CARCINOGEN found in coal tar and cigarette smoke.

benzoyl peroxide a drug used externally to treat ACNE. It acts to peel off surface layers of skin and unblock skin pores. The drug is on the WHO official list. Brand names are Acnecide, Benzamycin, Brevoxyl, Panoxyl and Quinoderm.

benzthiazide a diuretic drug used in the treatment of excess fluid accumulation in the body (oedema). A brand name for a preparation containing this drug is Dytide.

benztropine benzatropine, an anticholinergic drug used to control the symptoms of PARKINSON'S DISEASE. A brand name is Cogentin.

benzydamine hydrochloride a drug used as an oral rinse in the treatment of painful inflammatory mouth disorders. A brand name is Difflam.

benzyl benzoate an oily liquid used as a lotion for the treatment of SCABIES. The drug is on the WHO official list. A brand name is Ascabiol.

benzylpenicillin Penicillin G. The original highly active penicillin. An antibiotic that remains useful although less effective than formerly against many strains of bacteria. It is inactivated by bacterial beta-lactamases. It is destroyed by the digestive system and must be given by injection. The drug is on the WHO official list.

beractant a SURFACTANT drug used in the treatment of the RESPIRATORY DISTRESS SYNDROME. A brand name is Survanta.

bereavement serious loss, usually of that of a beloved person, but also of any valued thing, including health and wealth. Bereavement gives rise to a characteristic pattern of psychological reaction involving various recognizable stages, known as mourning. The strength of the reaction varies with the perceived value of what is lost.

beri-beri a deficiency disease caused by inadequate intake of vitamin B1 (Thiamine) and featuring widespread nerve degeneration with damage to the brain, spinal cord and heart. There is severe fatigue, loss of memory, irritability, insomnia, burning pain in the feet, foot drop, confusion and paralysis. In 'wet' there is damage to the heart muscle and widespread fluid retention in the tissues (OEDEMA).

Berkatens a brand name for VERAPAMIL.

Berocca a brand name for a mixture of B VITAMINS and vitamin C.

Berotec a brand name for FENOTEROL.

berry aneurysm a berry-like swelling at the branching point of an artery under the brain, especially on the Circle of Willis, due to a congenital weakness, the rupture of which causes an often-fatal subarachnoid haemorrhage. (Sir James Berry, 1860–1946, Canadian surgeon).

berylliosis disease caused by contact with the poisonous metal element beryllium found in fluorescent light tubes and TV tubes. It is a persistent form of pneumonia caused by inhaling dust or fumes containing the metal. Severe lung damage may result.

bestiality sexual intercourse with an animal other than a human.

beta the second letter of the Greek alphabet, often used to denote the order in a sequence.

beta-adrenergic pertaining to the class of receptors for ADRENALINE and NORADRENALINE known as the beta receptors.

beta-adrenoceptor one of the many the receptor sites at which noradrenaline and other hormones act to cause muscle to contract or relax. Beta-adrenoceptors occur in blood vessels, in the heart, in the bronchi, in the intestines, in the bladder, in the womb and elsewhere. The effect of the hormones at these sites can be prevented by beta-blocker drugs.

beta-adrenoceptor blocking drugs beta blockers. Drugs that selectively block the action of adrenaline on the BETA ADRENOCEPTORS. Beta adrenoceptors speed the heart and increase its contractility. Beta blockers have the opposite effect. They are used to treat HEART FAILURE, ANGINA PECTORIS, high blood pressure, heart irregularities, ANXIETY and MIGRAINE.

Overdosage causes a very slow pulse, low blood pressure, convulsions and coma. Up to 35% of patients have genetic mutations that affect their response to these drugs. This large class of drugs includes atenolol, propranolol, sotalol, levobunolol, metoprolol, timolol, betaxolol, esmolol, celiprolol, nodolol, carvedilol, bisoprolol, pindolol, oxprenolol, acebutolol, etc. Beta blockers were developed by the Scottish-born pharmacologist Sir James Whyte Black (1924) who also developed the drug cimetidine that has revolutionized the treatment of stomach and duodenal ulcers. See also ADRENERGIC-BLOCKING DRUGS.

beta blocker see BETA-ADRENOCEPTOR BLOCKING DRUGS.

Beta-Cardone a brand name for SOTALOL.

beta carotene a precursor of vitamin A.

beta cells 1 the cells in the islets of Langerhans in the PANCREAS that produce insulin. 2 the basophil cells of the front lobe of the PITUITARY GLAND.

Betadine the brand name for POVIDONE IODINE, a mild antiseptic, which is used as a surgical scrub or as a lotion, ointment, mouthwash or gargle.

beta-endorphin one of the body's own substances with morphine-like actions. It is part of the precursor molecule of ACTH.

Betaferon a brand name for INTERFERON BETA-1b.

Betagan a brand name for LEVOBUNOLOL.

betahistine a drug used to control the symptoms – vertigo and nausea – of MÉNIÈRE'S DISEASE. A brand name is Serc.

beta-lactam antibiotics an important group of drugs that includes the penicillins and the cephalosporins. All have a 4-membered beta-lactam ring as part of the basic structure. Many organisms produce beta-lactamase enzymes that can destroy these antibiotics. This is a common cause of bacterial resistance to antibiotics. Certain molecules called BETA-LACTAM INHIBITORS, however, can bind to beta-lactamase enzymes and inactivate them.

beta-lactam inhibitors a range of drugs that block the action of the bacterial enzymes that break down the beta-lactam structure in penicillins and cephalosporins. These inhibitors, which include clavulanic acid, are used in conjunction with antibiotics. Brand names are Augmentin and Timentin.

beta-lipotrophin part of the ACTH precursor

pro-opiocortin. It is a pro-hormone for the ENDORPHINS, the ENKEPHALINS and the MELANOCYTE stimulating hormone.

Betaloc a brand name for METOPROLOL.

betamethasone a corticosteroid drug used directly on the skin to treat ECZEMA and PSORIASIS, by inhalation to treat ASTHMA, by mouth for more severe allergic conditions and by injection to reduce brain swelling in head injuries, tumour and infections. The drug is on the WHO official list. Brand names are Betnelan, Betnesol, Betnovate, Bettamousse and Vista-Methasone.

Betamin a brand name for THIAMINE.

Beta-Prograne a brand name for PROPRANOLOL.

beta rhythm the electrical brain wave on the ELECTROENCEPHALOGRAM associated with a state of alertness and having a frequency of 18 to 30 Hz.

beta-thalassaemia a form of THALASSAEMIA caused by failure to synthesize the beta chains of HAEMOGLOBIN.

betaxolol a BETA-BLOCKER drug used in the treatment of high blood pressure (HYPERTENSION) and, in the form of eyedrops, GLAUCOMA. Brand names are Kerlone and Betoptic.

betel an Indian climbing plant, *Piper betle*, the leaves of which are wrapped round the nut of the Areca palm and chewed with lime for their salivatory effect. Betel is chewed by a tenth of the world's population. The chief alkaloid is arecoline, a PARASYMPATHOMIMETIC drug. Betel itself is probably harmless but the lime used with it causes cancer of the mouth. In some areas betel chewing accounts for 20% of all cancers.

bethanechol a CHOLINERGIC drug which acts mainly on the bowel and bladder, stimulating these organs to empty. It is used to treat reflux oesophagitis and urinary retention. A brand name is Myotonine.

Betim a brand name for TIMOLOL.

Betnelan a brand name for BETAMETHASONE.

Betnesol a brand name for BETAMETHASONE.

Betnesol-N a brand name for NEOMYCIN with BETAMETHASONE, for external use in the form of eye or ear drops.

Betnovate a brand name for BETAMETHASONE for external use on the skin.

Betz cells the large pyramidal cells of the motor cortex of the brain. The medical student joke that equates 'abetzia' with lack of intellectual capacity is based on inaccurate knowledge of the function of these cells. (Vladimir Aleksandrovich Betz, 1834–1894, Ukrainian anatomist).

bevacizumab the first anti-angiogenesis drug to be shown effective in treating metastatic cancer. Bevacizumab is a recombinant humanized monoclonal antibody that attacks the protein that promotes growth of blood vessels, the vascular endothelial growth factor. Used in combination with standard anticancer chemotherapy the drug shrinks tumours and extends the life of affected patients.

bexarotine an antineoplastic retinoid drug used to treat the skin complications of T cell lymphoma. A brand name is Targretin.

Bextra a brand name for VALDECOXIB.

bezafibrate a cholesterol-lowering drug. Brand names are Bezalip, Bezalip Mono and Zimbacol XL.

Bezalip a brand name for bezafibrate, a drug used to lower blood cholesterol levels.

bezoar a ball of hair and other material forming in the stomach or intestine and rare in the psychologically normal. In more gullible times bezoars have been valued for their magical properties.

bhang *or* **bang** the dried leaves of Cannabis sativa, the hemp plant from which MARIJUANA is derived.

BHy *abbrev. for* Bachelor of Hygiene.

BHyg *abbrev. for* Bachelor of Hygiene.

bicalutamide an anti-androgen, antineoplastic drug used in the treatment of advanced prostate cancer. A brand name is Casodex.

biceps muscle the prominent and powerful muscle on the front of the upper arm which bends the elbow and rotates the forearm outwards, as in using a screwdriver.

Bicillin a brand name for benzathine PENICILLIN.

bicipital pertaining to the biceps.

Bicnu a brand name for CARMUSTINE. The name is derived from the chemical name 1,3-bis (2-chloroethyl)-1-nitrosourea.

bicornuate having two horns or horn-like projections, as in bicornuate uterus.

bicuspid having two cusps, or projections, as on the biting surface (crown) of a PREMOLAR tooth. One of the valves in the heart, the mitral valve, is bicuspid.

B.I.D. *abbrev. for* brought in dead.
bifid divided into two parts. Forked or cleft.
bifocal having two different foci. In bifocal spectacles each lens has a lower segment of greater power for convenience in reading.
bifurcation a fork or double prong. Bifurcations are very common in blood vessels and in the bronchial 'tree' of the lungs. At a bifurcation the sum of the cross-sectional area of the two branches usually exceeds that of the parent branch. Since this happens many times, there is a progressive increase in the unit volume of the system.
bigeminy the occurrence of events in pairs. The term is applied expecially to coupled heart beats, suggesting heart disease.
biguanides drugs, such as METFORMIN and PHENFORMIN used to treat Type II DIABETES. They are part of the group of oral hypoglycaemic drugs. Biguanides act by reducing the efficiency of ION movement across cell membranes thus interfering with the production of glucose by the liver and reducing the energy yield from glucose used as fuel.
bikini incision an abdominal surgical incision so placed as to be concealed by the most exiguous of swimwear.
bilateral involving or affecting both sides. In the case of paired organs, bilateral means affecting both of them.
bile the dark greenish-brown fluid secreted by the LIVER, stored and concentrated in the GALL BLADDER, and ejected into the DUODENUM to assist in the absorption of fats. Bile contains bile salts which help to emulsify fats, bile pigments derived from the breakdown of red blood cells, cholesterol, lecithin and traces of various minerals and metals.
bile acids cholic and chenodeoxycholic acids. These are produced in the liver from cholesterol, linked with glycine or taurine to form BILE SALTS and passed into the small intestine in the bile.
bile acid sequestrant a drug that binds to bile acids that have entered the intestine via the bile duct, so altering them that they cannot be absorbed back into the bloodstream in the usual way and are excreted in the faeces. Cholesterol is converted to bile acids by the liver. Loss of bile acids means more conversion of cholesterol and a lowering in total body cholesterol.

bile duct the narrow tube which carries BILE from the liver to the bowel. The bile collecting tubules in the liver join up to form a main tube called the hepatic duct. Just under the liver, this gives off a branch, the cystic duct, to the gall bladder. The duct continues down, as the 'common bile duct' to run into the DUODENUM.
bile duct cancer this may be an actual ADENOCARCINOMA of the duct but is more often a cancer of the head of the pancreas involving the point at which the bile duct enters the DUODENUM. The result is blockage of the duct and obstructive JAUNDICE.
bile duct obstruction most cases are caused by gallstones or by cancer of the head of the PANCREAS. Signs are pale stools, dark urine, progressive yellow colouring of the skin by deposition of bile pigments (JAUNDICE), itching and loss of appetite and weight.
bile salts the sodium salts found in bile. Sodium taurocholate and sodium glycocholate. These salts act as emulsifying agents to assist in the absorption of dietary fats.
bilharzia a parasitic tropical disease caused by one of the blood flukes of the *Schistosoma* genus. A synonym for SCHISTOSOMIASIS. (Theodor Maximilian Bilharz, 1825–1862, German physician and anatomist).
biliary atresia a congenital disorder in which the larger branches of the bile ducts are so narrowed that the bile cannot escape and the baby becomes severely jaundiced with enlargement of the liver. Recent studies suggest that defects in expression of the villin gene may be implicated.
biliary cirrhosis a slowly developing liver disease in which a widespread inflammation of the small internal bile ducts causes a gradual replacement of functioning liver with scar tissue. It may be an AUTOIMMUNE disorder, secondary to obstruction to the outflow of bile from the liver, or of unknown cause (primary biliary cirrhosis).
biliary colic severe pain caused by the attempts of the gall bladder or bile duct to overcome the obstruction of a gallstone by contraction of the muscle fibres in the wall.
biliary dyskinesia a tendency to spasm of the outlet of the BILE DUCT (sphincter of Oddi) so that the movement of bile into the duodenum is impeded.
biliousness an inaccurate term for the feeling

of nausea and flatulence associated with minor dyspepsia or any other mild stomach upset.

bilirubin a coloured substance in bile derived from the breakdown of haemoglobin in effete red blood cells at the end of their 120 day life. Bilirubin is conjugated with glucuronic acid in the liver and excreted in the bile, giving the stools their characteristic colour. When it cannot escape freely into the bowel it accumulates in the blood, staining the skin to cause JAUNDICE. The stools become pale and the urine dark. Conjugated bilirubin is water-soluble.

Billroth's operation surgical removal of the part of the stomach (partial gastrectomy) with stitching of the remainder to the DUODENUM, or to the JEJUNUM just below the duodenum, in the treatment of stomach ulcer. (Christian Albert Billroth, 1829–1894, Prussian surgeon).

Biltricide a brand name for PRAZIQUANTEL.

bimanual performed using both hands. In a bimanual gynaecological or obstetrical examination, one hand is placed on the abdomen and one or two fingers of the other hand are placed in the vagina.

bimatoprost a synthetic PROSTAGLANDIN drug used as eye drops to control raised intraocular pressure in GLAUCOMA. A brand name is Lumigan.

binaural 1 related to two ears.
2 hearing with both ears.

Binet-Simon scales a series of intelligence tests for children. (Alfred Binet, 1857–1911, French psychologist).

binge drinking the practice of drinking excessive amounts of alcohol regularly. A binge has been defined as a pattern of drinking that brings the blood alcohol level to 80 mg per 100 ml (0.08%) or more. A 2003 British Government report indicates that binge drinking in the UK has risen markedly in recent years, especially among young people and that the problem is markedly more severe in the UK than in other European countries. Nearly 20% of the total alcohol taken is consumed by underage drinkers.

binge-purge syndrome BULIMIA. An eating disorder featuring uncontrollable bouts of eating followed by deliberate induction of vomiting and the use of strong laxatives.

binocular pertaining to both eyes or to the simultaneous use of both eyes.

binocular vision simultaneous perception with both eyes.

binovular of twins, derived from two separate eggs and thus non-identical. Compare UNIOVULAR.

Binovum a brand name for ETHINYLOESTRADIOL (ethinylestradiol) formulated with a PROGESTOGEN drug as an oral contraceptive.

Binswanger's encephalopathy a widespread brain disorder caused by severe arterial disease and high blood pressure so that multiple area of sub-cortical white matter (nerve fibres) are deprived of adequate blood supply and die. The result is a rapidly progressive DEMENTIA associated with acute STROKES. Deterioration is usually rapid. (O.L. Binswanger, 1852–1929, German psychiatrist).

bioassay a method of measuring the potency of a drug or other biochemical agent by comparing its effects on animals with those of known preparations of standard strength.

bioavailability the amount of a drug that reaches the blood regardless of how it is given. After intravenous injection bioavailability is 100%, but the bioavailability of drugs given by mouth is often much less, because many drugs are broken down by the digestive enzymes and many are poorly absorbed.

biochemistry the study of the chemical processes going on in living organisms, especially humans. Biochemistry is concerned, among other things, with the acceleration of biochemical processes by ENZYMES; with the chemical messengers of the body (HORMONES); with communication between cells at cell membranes; with the chemical processes which govern cell survival and reproduction; with the production of energy in cells; and with the processes of digestion of food and the way in which the resulting chemical substances are utilized for energy and structural purposes.

bioengineering see BIOLOGICAL ENGINEERING.

bioethics the study of the ethical and moral questions arising from the growing possible application of biological and genetic knowledge, especially in BIOLOGICAL ENGINEERING.

biofeedback the provision, usually in 'real time', of information to a person about the levels of activity of normally unconscious bodily processes. This is done in the hope that some control or adjustment may be exercised. The information is provided in the form of a moving meter needle, a changing sound, a light of varying brightness, or any other form of display. There is evidence that biofeedback methods can lower blood pressure, but only by a small amount. It is probably valuable as an aid to learning how to relax. Most of the popular claims for biofeedback cannot be substantiated.

biofilm a slime-enclosed community of bacterial colonies that is very difficult to eradicate even with the most powerful antibiotics or sterilizing systems. Biofilms can occur on any body surface, on teeth (as dental plaque), medical equipment, medical tubing, contact lenses and elsewhere. They are held together by a matrix produced by the bacteria themselves and within this the bacteria communicate by chemical messengers, and generate proteins including enzymes that inactivate some antibiotics. Biofilms also have major industrial and economic implications and are being intensively studied.

biogenesis the recognition that complex living organisms arise only from other living organisms and do not originate by spontaneous generation, as was once believed.

bioinformatics the branch of information science concerned with large databases of biochemical or pharmaceutical information.

biological containment steps taken to prevent the free replication of laboratory-produced recombinant DNA in the natural environment. A principal method is to use vectors and hosts that have been so modified that they will not survive outside the laboratory.

biological engineering a range of techniques in which biological substances are used, often at an industrial level, for practical purposes. The scope of biological engineering is widening rapidly and includes the extensive use of natural ENZYMES and the application of GENETIC ENGINEERING.

biological marker biomarker, a substance, physiological characteristic, gene, etc. that indicates, or may indicate, the presence of disease, a physiological abnormality or a psychological condition.

biological warfare the use of micro-organisms capable of spreading and causing epidemics of disease, for military purposes.

biological weapons micro-organisms and the means of their deliberate dissemination for the purpose of killing or disabling members of military or civilian populations for warlike purposes. Only a few micro-organisms have

suitable properties for storage and dissemination. These include the ANTHRAX bacillus, the paralyzing toxin of *Clostridium botulinum*, the plague bacillus *Yersinia pestis* and the deadly EBOLA VIRUS.

biology the science of living organisms and life processes.

biomechanical engineering the applications of the principles of mechanical engineering to improve the results of surgical treatment, especially by the design of prosthetic parts and the use of new materials. Engineers have answers to many surgeon's problems; close cooperation is essential.

biomedical engineering the cooperative investigation by engineers and doctors of the effective application of all branches of engineering so as to broaden the scope of medicine. Electronics, robotics, hydraulics, rheology, materials science and software engineering are among the more fruitful branches from which medicine has benefited.

biometrics the statistical study of biological data.

biomicroscopy examination of living structure using a microscope. Biomicroscopy is mainly employed, in a clinical context, by OPHTHALMOLOGISTS. See SLIT LAMP.

bionic relating to a living or life-like system enhanced by, or constructed from, electronic or mechanical components.

bionics biological principles applied to the design of engineering systems, especially electronic systems.

biophysics the physics of biological processes and systems.

biopiracy the use of wild plants by international companies to develop medicines, without recompensing the countries from which they are taken.

Bioplex a brand name for CARBENOXOLONE.

biopsy a small sample of tissue, taken for microscopic examination, so that the nature of a disease process can be determined. Breast biopsies are commonly done to investigate suspicious lumps. Suspicious skin growths are normally biopsied, and in the course of surgery under general anaesthesia, it is common for biopsies to be taken. The tissue obtained is soaked in molten paraffin wax and allowed to harden into a block. Very thin slices are then cut and mounted on glass slides for staining and examination by a histopathologist.

biorhythms the inherent periodicity, or cyclical nature, of many body functions such as the heart beat, respiration, menstruation, sleeping and waking, bowel PERISTALSIS, and body temperature. Some of these cyclical phenomena are under the control of a central biological clock based on a 24 hour 'circadian' rhythm. Melatonin secreted by the pineal gland in a cyclical manner and synchronized by daylight and darkness is the agent of this rhythm.

Biorphen a brand name for ORPHENADRINE.

biosurgery the use of live sterile maggots to clean up and disinfect infected wounds.

biotechnology the use of micro-organisms or biological processes for commercial, medical or social purposes. The earliest known examples of biotechnology are the fermentation of wines and the making of cheese.

biotin a water-soluble B vitamin concerned in the metabolism of fats and carbohydrates. Deficiency causes DERMATITIS, muscle pain, loss of appetite and ANAEMIA.

biparietal relating to both PARIETAL bones of the skull.

biperiden an ANTICHOLINERGIC drug used in the treatment of PARKINSON'S DISEASE. The drug is on the WHO official list. A brand name is Akineton.

Biphasil a brand name for an oral CONTRACEPTIVE.

bipolar disorder formerly called manic-depressive psychosis, this is a severe psychiatric disorder featuring extreme alternations of mood from euphoria and hyperactivity to depression and apathy.

Biquinate a brand name for QUININE.

bird-fancier's lung a form of allergic pneumonia caused by inhaling the dust from dried bird droppings. See also PIGEON-FANCIER'S LUNG.

birefringence splitting of light into two separate beams.

birth the act or process of being born. The expulsion of the baby from the uterus.

birth canal the exit route through which the baby is forced by the contraction of the womb. The canal consists of the widely stretched cervix of the uterus, the vagina, and the small and large external lips – the labia.

birth control a euphemism for CONTRACEPTION. Strictly speaking, the term also includes celibacy, sexual continence, sterilization, castration and abortion.

birthing ball a large soft rubber ball used by women during childbirth to give support and to aid pain relief.

birthing pool a large bath in which a woman can give birth.

birth injury an injury sustained during birth. Such an injury may be caused by the medical attendants (IATROGENIC injury) as a result of difficult delivery by forceps or vacuum extraction, or by attempts to turn the baby into a better position for delivery.

birthmarks benign tumours of skin blood vessels, including the temporary strawberry marks, portwine stains (capillary haemangiomas) and the conspicuous cavernous haemangiomas which are raised, lumpy and highly coloured and consists of a mass of medium-sized blood vessels and blood spaces.

bisacodyl a drug used in the treatment of constipation. A brand name is Dulco-Lax.

bisexual 1 pertaining to BISEXUALITY.
2 a person who manifests bisexuality.

bisexuality the inclination for, or capability of, sexual intercourse with either men or women. Bisexual behaviour is relatively common; genuine emotional neutrality in the choice of sex objects is very rare.

BIS monitor a device used to give warning that a patient under general anaesthesia might be in a state of awareness or feeling pain. The device is a single electrode ELECTROENCEPHALOGRAM that performs bispectral analysis of the complex waveforms from the brain to produce an index of awareness on a scale in which 100 is full wakefulness.

bismuth a drug that reacts with the stomach secretions to form a protective coat over the inner lining (mucous membrane) and especially over the floors of peptic ulcers. Bismuth also has a specific effect against the organism *Helicobacter pylori* which is implicated in the production of peptic ulcers, but has been superceded in this role by more effective drugs such as metronidazole or clarithromycin.

Bisodol a brand name for a mixture of sodium bicarbonate, chalk (calcium carbonate) and magnesium carbonate.

bisoprolol a drug used in the treatment of ANGINA PECTORIS and high blood pressure (HYPERTENSION). Brand names are Cardicor, Emcor and Monocor.

bisphosphonate one of a class of drugs that resemble pyrophosphate but are not readily hydrolysed. They interfere with the action of OSTEOCLASTS and thus prevent bone reabsorption in conditions such as PAGET'S DISEASE and OSTEOPOROSIS.

bite a dental term describing the relationship of the teeth of the lower jaw (MANDIBLE) to those of the upper and how they come together (the occlusion).

bite-wing a dental X-ray film used within the mouth and having a paper projection that can be held between the teeth to secure it in place during the exposure.

bithionol a bacteriostatic agent useful against many organisms. It was formerly incorporated in medicated soaps. It is also used in the treatment of parasitic diseases such as PARAGONIMIASIS.

Bitot's spots foamy white patches in the CONJUNCTIVA at the corners of the eyes, strongly suggestive of vitamin A deficiency. (Pierre Bitot, 1822–1888, French physician).

black box epidemiology a derogatory term for the tendency to assume that a causal relationship exists between a factor and a disease simply because both are known to be increasing or decreasing. A 'black box' is a system of which the input and the output are known but of which nothing is known about what happens inside.

black death the bubonic PLAGUE that devastated parts of Europe and Asia around 1350 and recurred at intervals for 300 years until the pandemic of 1664–5.

black eye a collection of blood released into the tissues around the eye, just under the thin, and relatively transparent, eyelid skin. The medical term is rather more impressive – periorbital haematoma.

black fly one of various small, hump-backed, dark coloured biting flies of he family *Simuliidae*. The black fly *Simulium damnosum* transmits ONCHOCERCIASIS.

blackhead an accumulation of fatty sebaceous material in a sebaceous gland or hair follicle, with oxidation of the outer layer, causing a colour change from white to dark brown or black. Blackheads, or comedones, occur in the skin disorder ACNE.

black lung PNEUMOCONIOSIS caused by long term inhalation of coal dust.

blackout a common term for a temporary loss of vision or consciousness. This may be a harmless fainting attack or a brief period of visual loss caused by standing up suddenly. Both are due to transient shortage of blood to the brain (cerebral ischaemia).

black stools an appearance with various causes, the most important being the release of blood into the intestine at a high level, often into the stomach. The blood is altered and turns black. This is called melaena and may be a sign of stomach or duodenal ulcer or stomach cancer.

black tongue a fungus infection of the tongue, parasitic glossitis, featuring black or brown furry patches and local enlargement of the tongue papillae. Sometimes called 'black hairy tongue', the condition is easily treated.

black vomit vomited altered blood that has been acted on by the stomach acid.

blackwater fever a popular term for a dangerous complication of the type of MALARIA caused by the parasite *Plasmodium falciparum*. The malarial parasites break down red blood cells in such numbers that freed haemoglobin passes through the kidneys and darkens the urine.

bladder see URINARY BLADDER.

bladder stone a calculus or hard collection of crystallized mineral salts, forming in the urinary bladder.

Blalock's operation a palliative operation performed for the relief of FALLOT'S TETRALOGY in very young babies. One of the SUBCLAVIAN arteries is joined to the artery to the lungs (pulmonary artery). (Alfred Blalock, 1899–1964, American surgeon).

blast cell an immature or primitive cell from which mature, differentiated cells are derived. The term refers mainly to the progenitors of blood cells (haemopoietic cells). The presence of these in the circulating blood is a feature of acute leukaemia.

blastocyst the state of the development of the embryo at about eight days after fertilization, when implantation in the wall of the womb occurs. At this stage it consists of a double-layered sphere full of fluid. The outer layer, the trophoblast, forms the placenta, the inner layer forms the future fetus.

-blastoma *suffix denoting* a tumour of cells microscopically resembling the embryonic state of the tissue from which the tumour arises.

blastomere the cell produced when a zygote has completed its first division.

blastomycosis a fungus disease caused by Blastomyces dermatitidis affecting the lungs, the lymph nodes at the roots of the lungs, and sometimes the skin, bones and genitourinary system. The disease resembles TUBERCULOSIS. It occurs in North America and Africa.

bleb a blister-like collection of fluid, within or under the epidermis of the skin, usually containing serum or blood.

bleeder 1 a person with HAEMOPHILIA or other bleeding disorder.

2 a person unduly prone to bleed.

3 a surgeon's term for an artery cut during an operation.

bleeding haemorrhage.

bleeding time the time from the infliction of a very small wound, such as a prick, and the cessation of bleeding. Bleeding time is increased in PLATELET deficiency and after taking aspirin or other PROSTAGLANDIN inhibitors.

blennorrhoea inflammation of the transparent membrane covering the white of the eye (the conjunctiva) and of the eyelids, usually caused by the organism Chlamydia trachomatis.

bleomycin a toxic glycopeptide antibiotic that interferes with the synthesis of DNA and is used as an anticancer drug, usually in combination with other drugs. It has some value in HODGKIN'S DISEASE, other LYMPHOMAS and squamous cell cancers of the skin. Side effects include FIBROSIS of the lungs, drying and discoloration of the skin over the back of joints. The drug is on the WHO official list.

blephar- *combining form denoting* eyelid.

blepharectomy surgical removal of part or all of an eyelid.

blepharitis inflammation of the eyelids. Blepharitis features redness of the lid margins, some greasy scales on the lashes, and a constant, annoying irritation. It is often associated with dandruff.

blepharochalasis baggy eyelids caused by the abnormal forward protrusion of fat from the eye sockets.

blepharoconjunctivitis inflammation of the eyelids and of the associated conjunctiva.

blepharoplasty 1 any plastic operation on the eyelids.

2 cosmetic plastic surgery for baggy eyelids.

blepharoptosis see PTOSIS.

blepharospasm uncontrollable winking or sustained tight closure of the eyes caused by involuntary contraction of the flat eyelid muscle under the skin. Blepharospasm may result from a sharp foreign body in the eye or a corneal ulcer, but also occurs as a psychologically induced TIC. Botulinum toxin has been found useful in this condition.

blind loop syndrome an uncommon disorder caused by stagnation of bowel contents as a result of adhesions, constrictions, pouches or other similar abnormalities. It features diarrhoea, fatty stools, abdominal pain, loss of weight, anaemia and vitamin deficiency.

blind spot the projection into space of the optic nerve head (optic disc) on the RETINA. This consists solely of nerve fibres and has no receptor elements (rods or cones). The blind spot lies about 15 to the outer side of whatever point we are looking at because the optic disc lies about 15 to the inner side of the macula.

blister a fluid-filled swelling occurring within or just under the skin, usually as a result of heat injury or unaccustomed friction. The fluid is serum from the blood and is usually sterile.

Blocadren a brand name for TIMOLOL.

blockade the use of a drug to occupy, seal, or otherwise render inoperative, a receptor for natural hormones or neurotransmitters.

blocking 1 the injection of a local anaesthetic around a nerve to prevent the passage of sensory impulses.

2 involuntary interruption of a train of thought by emotional upset or psychotic disorder.

blood a complex fluid vital to life and circulated by the pumping action of the heart. The average blood volume is 5 litres. It is a transport medium, especially for oxygen, which it carries in the red blood cells linked to the HAEMOGLOBIN with which they are filled. It also transports dissolved sugars, dissolved proteins such as ALBUMIN and GLOBULIN, protein constituents (AMINO ACIDS), fat-protein combinations (LIPOPROTEINS), emulsified fats (TRIGLYCERIDES), vitamins, minerals and hormones. Blood also carries waste products such as carbon dioxide, urea, lactic acid, and innumerable other substances. In addition to the countless red cells the blood carries enormous numbers of uncoloured cells most of which are concerned in the defence of the individual against infection and cancer.

It also contains large numbers of small non-nucleated bodies called PLATELETS which are concerned with BLOOD CLOTTING (coagulation).

blood agar a bacterial culture medium of AGAR to which whole blood has been added. Blood agar selectively encouraged the growth of certain bacteria.

blood alcohol the amount of alcohol in the blood expressed as a quantity per given volume of blood. Blood alcohol levels are often expressed in milligrams of alcohol per 100 millilitres of blood.

blood bank a refrigerated store where donated blood is kept until required for transfusion. Blood can be kept for 3 weeks, at which time 20% to 30% of the red cells are non-viable and the levels of the clotting factors are low.

blood blister a blister filled with blood.

blood—brain barrier the effective obstruction to the passage of certain drugs and other substances from the blood to the brain cells and the cerebrospinal fluid. The basis of the blood-brain barrier is that the endothelial cells comprising the walls of the brain capillaries are more tightly joined together than elsewhere and their gaps are further occluded by ASTROCYTES. In other part of the body the capillary endothelial cells have gaps between them through which quite large molecules can pass. Substances in the brain blood can reach the brain cells or the cerebrospinal fluid only by passing though the plasma membranes of the endothelial cells. The blood-brain barrier protects the brain against many dangers, but can interfere with attempts at treatment of brain conditions.

blood casts moulds of the kidney tubules, cast in clotted blood, and found in the urine in certain kidney diseases.

blood cells any of the formed elements in the BLOOD which constitute about half the blood volume.

blood cholesterol the level of CHOLESTEROL circulating in the blood in combination with other fats and proteins in the form of low and high density LIPOPROTEINS. Cholesterol levels vary with sex, age, diet and hereditary factors. In people who get most of their energy from carbohydrates cholesterol levels are low. The blood cholesterol varies considerably from time to time, so a single uncontrolled reading is of little significance.

blood clotting the cascaded sequence of changes which occur when blood comes in contact with damaged tissue and which culminates in the production of a solid seal in the damaged vessel. At least 13 factors are consecutively involved in a process that culminates in the conversion of the protein fibrinogen to the fibrin that forms the main constituent of the clot. This last stage is catalyzed by the enzyme thrombin. The smooth endothelial lining of the blood vessels normally prevents clotting within the circulation, but damage to this lining may allow THROMBOSIS to occur.

blood count determination of the number of red and white blood cells per millilitre of blood. The white cell count usually includes a differential count, in which the percentages of the different kinds of white cells is estimated.

blood crisis the sudden appearance of large numbers of immature nucleated red cells in the circulating BLOOD.

blood culture incubation of a sample of blood in a suitable culture medium so as to encourage reproduction of bacteria, which are possible causes of disease, for purposes of identification.

blood dyscrasia any abnormality of the blood cells or of the clotting elements.

blood electrolytes simple inorganic compounds in solution in the blood that form charged particles called IONS. The concentration of ions is critical for normal body function and the movement of ions is fundamental to much of the basic functioning of all the cells of the body. Measurement of blood electrolytes is therefore an important investigation in many conditions.

blood enzyme tests measurement of the presence and quantities of ENZYMES released from cells damaged by disease processes. Enzymes are released especially from the liver, in HEPATITIS and other disorders, from the heart muscle damaged by MYOCARDIAL INFARCTION in a heart attack. The more extensive the area of damage, the higher will be the levels of these enzymes in the blood.

blood gas analysis an invaluable investigation providing information of literally vital importance. Arterial oxygen saturation (PaO_2) and carbon dioxide levels ($PaCO_2$) indicate any inadequacy of oxygenation and of breathing. See also OXIMETER.

blood glucose the levels of sugar in the circulating blood. Blood glucose is of critical importance in DIABETES in which the ideal of treatment is to keep the levels within the normal range of 3.5 to 5.2 mmol/l – an ideal seldom achieved.

blood groups see ABO BLOOD GROUPS, KELL BLOOD GROUP SYSTEM and RHESUS FACTOR.

blood in urine see HAEMATURIA.

blood letting the removal of a quantity of blood for therapeutic purposes. Also called venesection or phlebotomy. The procedure is rarely needed and is confined to conditions such as POLYCYTHAEMIA, HAEMOCHROMATOSIS, PORPHYRIA and sometimes HEART FAILURE.

blood poisoning a common term for SEPTICAEMIA or TOXAEMIA.

blood pool scanning a method of measuring the efficiency of the left VENTRICLE of the heart and of detecting ballooning (aneurysm) of the ventricle. A RADIONUCLIDE is injected into the blood and measured with a GAMMA CAMERA.

blood pressure the pressure exerted on the artery walls and derived from the force of the contraction of the lower chambers of the heart (the VENTRICLES). Blood pressure changes constantly. Peak pressure is called the systolic pressure and the running pressure between beats is called the diastolic pressure. Blood pressure in measured in millimetres of mercury. A typical normal reading is 120/80. See also HYPERTENSION and KOROTKOFF SOUNDS.

blood sedimentation rate the rate at which the red cells settle when a column of blood is held vertically in a narrow tube. Also called the erythrocyte sedimentation rate (ESR). A rapid rate is a non-specific indicator of the presence of some inflammatory disease process.

blood serum the liquid part of the blood (blood plasma) with the protein which forms during clotting (fibrin) removed. Serum remains liquid.

blood substitute any fluid substance used for transfusion that can perform one or more of the functions of blood. Blood substitutes include PLASMA solutions, dextran solutions and saline and other electrolyte solutions. Genuine blood substitutes that can transport oxygen are still in the experimental stages.

blood sugar see BLOOD GLUCOSE.

blood transfusion the administration of blood, by instillation into a vein, to replace blood lost or to treat a failure of blood production. Before transfusion, the blood group of the recipient must be known and serum from the blood to be transfused is cross-matched with the recipient's blood cells to confirm compatibility. Sometimes the patient's own blood, collected at operation or obtained earlier, is used.

blood urea the levels of UREA in the blood. Normal kidney function keeps the blood urea levels low by excreting it in the urine. A high blood urea suggests kidney failure.

blood vessel any artery, arteriole, capillary, venule or vein.

blowfly a fly of the family Calliphoridae that deposits its eggs in wounds or open sores. A few days later the area is infected with maggots, but these remove dead tissue and do little harm.

BLS, *abbrev. for* basic life support.

blue baby a baby with an inadequate amount of oxygen in the blood, resulting in CYANOSIS. This is usually due to congenital heart disease of a type in which the blood returning to the heart from the body is not wholly passed to the lungs to be reoxygenated.

blue bloater a medical slang term for a person with CYANOSIS and OEDEMA. Both can be caused by lung diseases such as chronic bronchitis or emphysema which impede movement of oxygen from atmosphere to blood, causing cyanosis, and increase the strain on the heart leading to failure and an accumulation of fluid in the tissues (oedema).

blue scleras an appearance caused by undue thinness of the scleral coats of the eyes so that the underlying blood vessel layer shows through. Blue scleras are a feature of the brittle bone disease OSTEOGENESIS IMPERFECTA.

blunt dissection a technique in surgery or anatomical dissection in which tissue planes are separated or opened and underlying structures exposed without cutting. Blunt dissection often involves the use of scissors in an opening, rather than a closing, mode. The closed tips are pushed into tissue and then separated so as to split tissue planes.

blunt end an ending in DNA in which both strands of the molecule stop at the same base-pair so that no single strand protrudes.

blushing a transient reddening of the face, ears and neck, often spreading to the upper part of the chest, caused by a widening (dilatation) of small blood vessels in the skin so that more blood flows.

BM *abbrev. for* Bachelor of Medicine. An alternative is MB.

BMA *abbrev. for* British Medical Association.

BmedBiol *abbrev. for* Bachelor of Medical Biology.

BmedSc, BmedSci *abbrev. for* Bachelor of Medical Science.

BMI *abbrev. for* body mass index. This relates weight to height and is used to assess the nutritional state. BMI = the weight (in kg) divided by the height (in m) squared. The acceptable normal range is 20–25. A figure of 30 indicates obesity and 40 gross obesity.

BMJ *abbrev. for British Medical Journal.*

BMR *abbrev. for* BASAL METABOLIC RATE.

BN *abbrev. for* Bachelor of Nursing.

Bocasan a brand name for SODIUM PERBORATE.

body and soul a duality that has been accepted, largely without question, since the earliest times. The term soul is, however, indefinable in scientific terms but is taken to be an entity associated with the body but clearly distinguished from it. Various accounts of the properties of the soul have been asserted from time to time by theologians, but such assertions are not of a nature as can be verified.

body bag a plastic bag for transporting a human corpse.

body contour surgery a form of cosmetic plastic surgery involving the removal of excess fat deposits under the skin by suction or by surgical excision.

body image the mental picture of the body provided by the association connections between the part of the brain concerned with body sensation (the sensory CORTEX in the postcentral GYRUS) and those parts concerned with the special senses. Body image is distorted in various conditions, especially ANOREXIA NERVOSA.

body language the communication of information, usually of a personal nature, without the medium of speech, writing or other agreed codes. Body language involves a range of subtle or obvious physical attitudes, expressions, gestures and relative positions. It can, and often does, eloquently reflect current states of mind and attitudes towards others, whether positive or negative. Body language is often at variance with explicit verbal statement

and in such cases is often the more reliable indicator.

body louse the human ectoparasite, Pediculus humanus.

body mass index (BMI) the weight in kilograms divided by a number obtained by taking the height in metres and multiplying it by itself (kg/m^2). The BMI is a more satisfactory way of determining the risk of obesity than simple weight. The normal range of BMI is 19 to 25. Obesity is defined as a BMI of 27 or over. People with this figure show a significant excess of illness over those in the normal range.

body odour a socially unacceptable smell usually caused by the action of bacteria on the sweat produced by the sweat glands of the armpits and the groin areas (apocrine glands).

body packer a slang term for a person who smuggles narcotics in the intestines, usually contained in condoms. This is a dangerous trade with a high mortality from poisoning.

body piercing body decorations in the form of metal rings or studs applied to any part of the body especially the external ears, nose, lips, tongue, nipples, umbilicus, and genitalia. Body piercing is being adopted by an increasing number of people in the Western world, exposing them to a range of health risks including hepatitis and HIV infection, bleeding, shock, allergies, interference with surgery, burns from electrosurgical instruments, and interference with X ray and MRI investigations.

bodywork an informal term for any claimed therapy, such as massage, in which parts of the body are manipulated.

boil an infection of a hair follicle which has progressed to abscess formation. Most boils are caused by STAPHYLOCOCCAL infection. A stye is a small boil in a lash follicle.

bolus 1 a chewed-up quantity of food in a state ready to be swallowed.
2 the dose of a drug injected as rapidly a possible into a vein so as to be diluted as little as possible.

bomb a radioactive source held in a container for the purpose of RADIOTHERAPY.

bomb calorimeter a small insulated chamber in which a carefully weighed sample of food can be burnt and the amount of heat derived from the combustion calculated from the measured rise in temperature. The device is used to measure the calorific value of various foodstuffs. See also CALORIE.

bonding the formation of a strong relationship, particularly that between a mother and her new-born child. Bonding is believed to be important for the future psychological well-being of the infant.

bonding, dental the application of strongly adhesive cosmetic or protective surface material to a tooth. Bonding material is often applied in a plastic state and smoothed off before hardening.

Bondronat a brand name for IBANDRONIC ACID.

bone the principle skeletal structural material of the body. Bone consists of a protein, type 1 COLLAGEN scaffolding impregnated with calcium phosphate hydroxyapatite crystals. As bone grows new bone is laid down immediately under the bone-covering membrane (periostium) and is absorbed from the inner surface. Oestrogens inhibit periosteal bone formation in women but promotes internal bone formation; androgens promote periosteal bone formation in males. The marrow of the flat bones are the sites of blood production. See also BONE MARROW.

bone abscess a persistent local infection of the bone marrow with inflammation (osteomyelitis) and sometimes a track to the exterior (a sinus).

bone cancer primary bone cancers are called osteogenic sarcomas and are comparatively rare. Secondary bone cancer, occurring as a remote spread (metastasis) from a primary cancer elsewhere, are much more common. See also OSTEOSARCOMA.

bone conduction the transmission of sound to the inner ear hearing mechanisms by way of bone rather than by the normal air, eardrum and middle ear route.

bone cyst a local thinning and expansion of bone with a fluid-filled centre. Solitary bone cysts sometimes occur during the growth period. They may also be caused by tumours, especially the benign OSTEOCLASTOMAS. Bone cysts are usually unsuspected until the bone suddenly breaks on the application of a minor force.

Bonefos a brand name for SODIUM CLODRONATE.

bone fractures bone breaks may be partial (greenstick), with intact skin (simple), with penetration of the skin (compound) or

with involvement of blood vessels or nerves (complicated). They may be transverse, oblique or spiral or the bone may be shattered (comminuted).

bone-growth stimulators devices used in an attempt to promote healing of ununited fractures or fractures unduly slow to unite. They subject the fracture site to pulsed electromagnetic fields or to ultrasound and appear, in some cases, to have a useful effect. Many different factors determine failure of normal bone healing, however, and not all are aided by molecular vibration.

bone imaging methods of investigating bone diseases. These include X rays and the use of radioactive isotopes (radionuclides) which concentrate in bone, giving off radiation that can be detected. Modern techniques of radionuclide scanning, using a GAMMA CAMERA can be more sensitive, and safer, than X-rays. See also BONE SCANNING.

bone marrow the substance contained within bone cavities. This is red in the flat bones and the vertebrae, and yellow from fat in adult long bones. The volume of the red marrow in young adults is about 15 l. The basic marrow stem cell differentiates into HAEMOGLOBIN-carrying red blood cells, the white blood cells of the immune system and the blood PLATELETS which are essential for BLOOD CLOTTING.

bone marrow biopsy a sample of marrow usually taken from the crest of the pelvis at the back under local anaesthesia using a broad stout needle attached to a syringe. Marrow biopsies allow diagnoses of the various forms of ANAEMIA, of failure of red cell production (aplastic anaemia), of reduced white cell production (AGRANULOCYTOSIS) and of the various kinds of white cell cancer (LEUKAEMIA).

bone marrow transplant a means of providing a recipient with a new set of blood-forming cells from which a continuing supply of healthy new red and white blood cells can be derived. Marrow is sucked out of the marrow cavity of the pelvis or breastbone of the donor and injected into one of the recipient's veins.

bone scanning a method of diagnosis in which various diphosphonate substances labelled with a radioactive isotope of technetium are injected into the bloodstream. Within three hours about half of the material injected has been deposited in the bones, the highest concentration being in those areas in which bone blood flow and new bone formation are greatest. The whole body is then examined with a GAMMA CAMERA. A range of bone diseases can be detected early by this means and the method is highly sensitive to the presence of cancer that has spread to the bones from other parts of the body.

Bonnevie-Ullrich syndrome a condition similar to TURNER'S SYNDROME but affecting males. The chromosome constitution (karyotype) is often normal. There is short stature, webbing of the neck, an abnormally broad face with wide-set eyes (hypertelorism), drooping lids (ptosis), low-set ears, LYMPHOEDEMA and malformation of the urinary system. (K. Bonnevie, 1872–1950, American geneticist; and O. Ullrich, 1894–1957 German paediatrician).

Bonney's blue a preparation of crystal violent with brilliant green used by surgeons as a skin marking ink to outline proposed areas to be removed or to show the line of incisions. The dye is non-tattooing. (William Francis Victor Bonney, 1872–1953, English gynaecologist).

booster a dose of a vaccine, given at an interval after the primary vaccination, to increase the effect. Once ANTIBODIES have been produced in response to any particular infectious disease agent (ANTIGEN), the reappearance of this agent will provoke a large new production of antibodies.

borborygmi bowel noises caused by the gurgling of gas through the almost liquid contents of the small bowel as they are passed along by the process of PERISTALSIS.

borderline personality disorder a psychiatric disorder intermediate between normality and genuine psychiatric illness. A person with a borderline disorder is impulsive, often aggressive, with unexpected swings of emotion from depression to elation and a tendency to regard others as enemies.

Bordetella a genus of coccobacilli that have an affinity for the respiratory system and includes *Bordetella pertussis* the organism responsible for whooping cough. These organisms are sensitive to various antibiotics including TETRACYCLINE, ERYTHROMYCIN and CHLORAMPHENICOL. (Jules Bordet, 1870–1961, Belgian bacteriologist).

boric acid a mildly antiseptic drug used externally as a constituent of various skin preparations.

Bornholm disease an infection with a COXSACKIE VIRUS which causes sudden attacks of pain in the central lower chest and upper abdomen, with headache, fever, sore throat and general upset. These attacks may occur repeatedly over a period of several weeks. There is no specific treatment. (First reported on Bornholm island off the Danish coast.).

Borrelia a genus of spiral-shaped bacteria that includes the organism *Borrelia burgdoferi* responsible for LYME DISEASE and Borrelia recurrentis that causes RELAPSING FEVER. (Amedee Borrel, 1867–1936, Strasbourg bacteriologist).

bortezomib the first of a new class of anticancer drugs that act by inhibition of the action of PROTEASOMES. When proteasomes in tumour cells are inhibited, these cells become greatly sensitized to the action of cytotoxic drugs. The drug has been found to produce a 35% response rate in patients with relapsed and refractory multiple MYELOMATOSIS. A brand name is Velcade.

bosentan an ENDOTHELIN-1 receptor antagonist drug used to treat pulmonary hypertension. A brand name is Tracleer.

bot an informal term for a mild illness in humans.

bot flies flies of the genera *Gasterophilus*, *Oestrus* or *Dermatobia* whose larvae can burrow into human skin, eyes or nasal openings. Parasitization by fly larvae is called myiasis.

Botox a brand name for a powder used to reconstitute a solution of botulinum A toxin complexed with haemagglutinin. This is used to treat a wide and increasing range of conditions. See BOTULINUM TOXIN.

bottle-feeding the popular alternative to breast-feeding for babies. Formula milk cannot be made identical to human milk and the bottle-fed baby is deprived of many valuable antibodies present in the mother's milk. The risks of contamination of the feed are also greater with bottle than with breast-feeding.

botulinum toxin a powerful EXOTOXIN produced by the organism *Clostridium botulinum* which, in carefully controlled minute dosage, has been found useful in the treatment of an increasing range of conditions. It is given, often with excellent effect in squint (STRABISMUS) caused by overactive eye muscles; uncontrollable spasm of the eyelid muscles (blepharospasm); NYSTAGMUS; sixth nerve palsy; hyperlacrimation;

drooling; spastic club foot (dynamic equinus foot deformity) in children with cerebral palsy; tennis elbow; facial spasm; excessive sweating of the armpits and palms; gustatory sweating; vaginismus; post-stroke spasticity; TORTICOLLIS; WRITER'S CRAMP; other occupational cramps; essential hand tremor; BRUXISM; tics; swallowing difficulty (dysphagia); tension headaches; MIGRAINE; backache; and anal fissure. The toxin can also be used to cause a temporary deliberate drooping of the upper lid (blepharoptosis) as an alternative to sewing the lids together (tarsorrhaphy) for the treatment of corneal ulceration and other conditions. The preparations has also become a popular and, for the providers, lucrative remedy for the cosmetic removal of the appearance of wrinkles.

botulism food poisoning by the toxin of the organism *Clostridium botulinum* which may contaminate homemade meat pastes and tinned foods. The toxin causes vomiting, abdominal pain and severe muscle paralysis, including paralysis of the respiratory muscles. A small dose may be fatal.

bougie a smooth, often flexible, round-ended instrument used to widen abnormal narrowing (strictures) in a body passage, such as those in the URETHRA or OESOPHAGUS.

Bourneville's disease a dominant genetic disease of the nervous system causing growths which lead to epilepsy, paralysis, mental retardation and personality disorders. It is also called epiloia and tuberous sclerosis. (D. M. Bourneville, 1840–1909, French neurologist).

bouton a swelling or thickening, especially on the skin.

bovine somatotrophin a growth hormone given to cattle to increase their size. Doubts have been expressed as to the risks of the hormone, or some of its products, appearing in the milk.

bovine spongiform encephalopathy (BSE) a PRION DISEASE of cattle similar to, possibly identical to, CREUTZFELDT-JAKOB DISEASE in humans. The first cases appeared in 1985 believed to be the result of the feeding of calves in 1981–82 with meat-and-bone meal from infected animals. Only a few animals in each herd were affected; in more than one third of farms with BSE only one animal developed the disease. The question of whether new-variant CJD was acquired by eating beef products

from infected animals has not been positively answered.

bowel the intestine. A tube, about 8 m long, which extends from the throat to the anus and consists of the oesophagus, stomach, duodenum, jejunum, ileum, colon, sigmoid colon, rectum and anal canal.

bowel lengthening a surgical operation used to treat the SHORT-BOWEL SYNDROME in children as an alternative to bowel transplantation. The procedure involves freeing a length of intestine from the mesentery, dividing it longitudinally, converting each half into a tube and connecting these end to end. The blood supply to each half must be carefully maintained.

bowel movement DEFAECATION. The normal frequency of bowel movement varies between three times a day and three times a week.

bowel sounds the noise made by the movement of the bowel contents, under the influence of PERISTALSIS which, although normally almost silent, can easily be heard through a stethoscope. Bowel sounds become much louder if there is any intestinal obstruction and are abolished in the condition of paralytic ileus. See also BORBORYGMI.

bow legs bandy legs or GENU VARUS.

Bowen's disease a cancer of surface cells (squamous epithelium) which does not extend into the deeper layers but often occurs in several places simultaneously. An intra-epidermal carcinoma. (John Templeton Bowen, 1857–1941, American dermatologist).

Bowman's capsule the filtering unit in the kidney by which urine is formed from the blood. Sometimes called the malpighian corpuscle. (Sir William Bowman, 1816–1892, English surgeon and ophthalmologist).

BP *abbrev. for* British Pharmacopoeia. This is an official list of drugs with their properties, functions, side effects and dosage.

BPharm *abbrev. for* Bachelor of Pharmacy.

brace 1 an ORTHODONTIC appliance used to correct malposition of the teeth by exerting pressure in the desired direction. Sustained pressure on a tooth causes bone absorption on the side opposite that on which pressure is applied and bone growth on the same side. **2** an externally worn leg support needed when a leg is unstable from muscle weakness or joint disease, or a spinal support used to correct deformity such as SCOLIOSIS.

brachial pertaining to the arm.

brachial artery the main artery supplying the arm with blood.

brachial plexus the complicated rearrangement of spinal nerves arising from the spinal cord in the neck and in the upper back, which occupies the armpit (axilla), and supplies the many muscles of the arm.

brachy- *combining form denoting* short.

brachycephalic having a short, wide, almost spherical head.

brachydactyly abnormally short fingers or toes.

brachytherapy a form of RADIOTHERAPY in which sealed sources of radioactive material are inserted for various periods into body cavities or directly into tumours, so as to lie as close as possible to the area to be radiated.

bracken food poisoning poisoning with the fiddleheads of the ostrich fern (*Matteuccia struthiopteris*), a delicacy popular in maritime Canada and Northeast USA. This food appears to contain a heat-labile toxin that can be destroyed by boiling for 10 minutes. Microwave cooking for short periods may not inactivate the toxin. Other common ferns are known to be either poisonous or carcinogenic.

BRCA genes tumour suppressor genes, the mutation of which is responsible for an inherited predisposition to breast and ovarian cancer. In 1990 BRCA1 was found to be on the long arm of chromosome 17, and it was cloned in 1994. It is involved in about 5% of all breast cancers. In these cases, and in many cases of invasive breast cancer, there is decreased expression of BRCA1. A considerable number of FRAMESHIFT or NONSENSE MUTATIONS have been found that confer high risk of cancer. BRCA2, located on chromosome 13, is less commonly a cause of inherited breast cancer.

brady- *combining form denoting* slow.

bradycardia a slow heart rate. In the healthy this often indicates a high degree of fitness, but bradycardia can be a sign of heart disease, such as heart block, an effects of digitalis or beta-blocker overdosage or the result of thyroid underaction (MYXOEDEMA).

bradykinesia abnormal slowing of voluntary movement, usually with a diminished range of movement. Bradykinesia is a feature of PARKINSON'S DISEASE.

bradykinin a peptide that widens blood vessels (vasodilatation) and lowers blood pressure, increases capillary permeability and the secretion of saliva and mediates pain associated with inflammation. Bradykinin is inactivated by the angiotensin-converting enzyme.

braille a method of coding information using groups of six raised spots embossed on paper, to enable the blind to read through touch. (Louis Braille, 1809–1852, French school teacher).

brain the central organ of the body, to the maintenance, supply, transport and protection of which all the remainder of the body is dedicated. The brain contain more than 100 billion nerve cells with more than 10^{15} synapses. There are two main parts to the brain, the cerebrum and the cerebellum. The larger part, the cerebrum, initiates and coordinates all voluntary and most involuntary functions and is the seat of emotion, memory and intelligence. It is the medium by which all sensation, and the results of the mechanisms underlying all satisfaction, are conveyed to consciousness. It is essentially concerned with the collection, processing and storage of information, with the correlation of new data with stored data and with the organization and control of resulting responsive action. Response to stimulus is of the essence of brain function. Much is known, from the effects of disease and injury, of the localization of functions, in the brain, such as movement, sensation, vision, hearing, smell and speech. The location of areas responsible for registration and recall of memory is known, but the physical basis of memory storage remains obscure. Memory is not, like some other functions, located in a single definable area but is probably dispersed into all areas concerned with functions which may involve it. The cerebellum, the smaller part, is concerned mainly with the complex computations necessary to organize the muscle contractions needed to maintain the balance of the body and to allow walking and other movements. More than one tenth of the cardiac output is required to maintain brain function. See also BRAINSTEM.

brain abscess the serious consequence of access of pus-forming organisms to the inner parts of the brain, by spread through the bone following middle ear infection (OTITIS MEDIA and MASTOIDITIS) or severe sinusitis, by spread by the blood, or as a result of a penetrating injury of the brain by an infected object or missile.

brain damage a term applied more often to the physically subtle, but functionally serious, injury sustained from temporary oxygen and sugar deprivation, than to gross and obvious injury from direct violence. Brain damage also commonly results from sudden local haemorrhage or THROMBOSIS, causing STROKE, and from toxic substances especially alcohol. Bacterial toxins released in the course of meningitis and brain abscess and inflammation caused by viruses are also damaging. Diseases such as multiple sclerosis can cause brain damage, as can the repeated multiple small haemorrhages sustained in boxing. Brain damage often affects the areas of higher function in a patchy way with loss of certain functions and retention of others. There may be paralysis and loss of sensation on one side of the body, epileptic fits, speech disturbances or loss of word comprehension (APHASIA), loss of certain learned voluntary skills (APRAXIA), or loss of part of the field of vision. Alternatively, brain damage may have a diffuse effect causing, in addition to focal effects, interference with conscious thought, memory and judgement. Loss of memory (amnesia) is a common feature. A proportion of brain-damaged people end up in a state of almost complete loss of the higher mental functions (AMENTIA).

brain death the absence of any signs of brain function. The state in which there are no reflex responses above the neck, there is no spontaneous breathing, and the ELECTROENCEPHALOGRAM shows no sign of electrical activity in the brain. This definition does not apply unless it can also be shown that a cause such as deep intoxication, or paralysing drugs, can be completely ruled out, and the effect of lowered body temperature (HYPOTHERMIA) eliminated.

brain fever a common term for ENCEPHALITIS.

brain haemorrhage see CEREBRAL HAEMORRHAGE.

brain imaging the demonstration of details of brain structure by such means as X-rays, ANGIOGRAPHY, DIGITAL SUBTRACTION ANGIOGRAPHY, CT SCANNING, magnetic resonance imaging (MRI) or positron emission tomography (PET) scanning.

brain sand X-ray opaque calcified granules in the pineal gland commonly present in adult life. The condition is harmless and may prove clinically useful as it may demonstrate shifting of the pineal to one side as a result of a space-occupying condition on the other. Also known as acervulus cerebri.

brainstem the part of the brain consisting of the medulla oblongata and pons, which connects the main brain (cerebrum) to the spinal cord. The brainstem contains the 'vital centres' for respiration and heart-beat and the nuclei of most of the CRANIAL NERVES as well as massive motor and sensory nerve trunks passing to and from the cord.

brain tumour secondary spread of cancer to the brain, from a primary tumour elsewhere in the body is common. Primary tumour, originating in the skull is less common. Primary tumours arise from the brain coverings (MENINGIOMAS), the neurological supportive tissue (GLIOMAS), the blood vessels (HAEMANGIOMAS), the bone (OSTEOMAS) or the pituitary gland (PITUITARY ADENOMAS). Some are of congenital origin (CRANIOPHARYNGIOMAS, TERATOMAS) and are due to abnormal development.

brainwashing concentrated and sustained indoctrination designed to delete a person's fundamental beliefs and attitudes and replace them with new, imposed data. It is questionable whether this intention can ever be fully realized.

brain wave one of many periodic electric potentials generated in the brain and detectable by the ELECTROENCEPHALOGRAM. Some of the brain waves are dominant and of recognizable frequency.

bran the fibrous outer coat of wheat grain normally removed in milling to make the flour more attractive to many palates. Bran is valuable in the treatment of constipation and other disorders of the large bowel.

branchial cyst a soft swelling on the side of the neck arising from the persistence of a track left when a developmental cleft (branchial cleft) fails to close during fetal life.

branchial fistula a small midline opening in the neck connecting to the pharynx and present at birth. This results from a minor developmental defect during fetal life. See also BRANCHIAL CYST.

Brasivol a brand name for ALUMINIUM OXIDE used as an abrasive.

Braxton-Hicks' contractions the common, irregular, painless and harmless contractions of the womb which occur throughout pregnancy. (John Braxton-Hicks, 1825–1897, English gynaecologist).

BRCS *abbrev. for* British Red Cross Society.

breakbone fever DENGUE.

breakthrough bleeding menstrual bleeding occurring in the course of hormone treatment to suppress the menstrual cycle.

breast abscess local inflammation in the breast with pus formation. Infection is commonly acquired during breast feeding because of nipple abrasion. There is painful swelling, redness, tenderness, tension and inability to pass milk.

breast augmentation a procedure in cosmetic plastic surgery designed to increase the size of the female breast usually by implanting a silicone oil-filled silicone rubber bag.

breastbone the STERNUM.

breast cancer the commonest form of cancer in women, affecting about 1 in 12 women in Britain. Early breast cancer hardly ever causes pain and the only sign is a slowly growing lump. Later signs are distortion of the normal breast contour by skin dimpling, indrawing of the nipple, bleeding from the nipple, an orange-skin appearance (peau d'orange) of the breast skin, and rubbery, firm, easily felt lymph nodes in the armpit.

breast enlargement this may occur in both sexes in the first week or so after birth, from maternal sex hormones acquired in the womb. In girls, the breasts enlarge at puberty under the influence of hormones. Breast enlargement is normal in pregnancy and especially during milk production (LACTATION). Adolescent boys may suffer breast enlargement (see GYNAECOMASTIA).

breast-feeding the normal, and best, method of providing baby nutrition. The chemical constitution of breast milk is attuned to the digestive capacity of the baby and the nutritional balance is exactly what is required.

breast plastic and reconstructive surgery this includes BREAST ENLARGEMENT (augmentation mammoplasty), breast reduction, and breast reconstruction for women who have had to have a breast removed.

breast pump a device used to relieve engorged and painful breasts of excess milk, or to remove milk for use later.

breast self-examination an important method of screening for breast cancer, which should be performed regularly by every woman. It includes a visual check, using a mirror, for any change in the appearance, and careful palpation for lumps, with the flat of the hand.

breath-holding attacks a form of infantile blackmail imposed on indulgent parents by determined and manipulative young children. The attacks superficially resemble epileptic seizures, but, although the child may turn purple and even appear to lose consciousness, they are harmless.

breathing the automatic, and usually unconscious, process by which air is drawn into the LUNGS for the purpose of oxygenating the blood and disposing of carbon dioxide. Breathing involves a periodic increase in the volume of the chest occasioned by the raising and outward movement of the ribs and the flattening of the domed DIAPHRAGM. This is an active process involving muscle contraction and results in air being forced into the lungs by atmospheric pressure. Expiration is passive, the air escaping as a result of elastic recoil of the lungs and relaxation of the respiratory muscles.

breathlessness an automatic increase in the rate of respiration in response to a reduction in the levels of oxygen, and an increase in the levels of carbon dioxide, in the blood. Undue breathlessness, inappropriate to the degree of exertion, is an important sign of possible HEART FAILURE or of any other condition that leads to inadequate oxygenation of the blood. Breathlessness should be distinguished from hyperventilation which is usually either a response to acute anxiety or a voluntary activity. The medical term for breathlessness is dyspnoea.

breech delivery buttock-first birth.

bregma the point on the top of the skull at which the irregular junction lines of the bone (the coronal and sagittal sutures) meet. Also known as sinciput.

bretylate a brand name for BRETYLIUM TOSYLATE.

bretylium tosylate a drug used to help to restore normal heart rhythm in the form of cardiac arrest known as VENTRICULAR FIBRILLATION. A brand name is Bretylate.

Brevinor a brand name for ETHINYLOESTRADIOL (ethinylestradiol) formulated with a PROGESTOGEN drug as an oral contraceptive.

Brevital a short-acting barbiturate drug, methohexital sodium, used as an induction agent in general anaesthesia.

Bricanyl a brand name for TERBUTALINE sulphate.

bridge a fixed support for false teeth which bridges across the gap between surviving natural teeth.

Bright's disease an old-fashioned term for the kidney disease GLOMERULONEPHRITIS. (Richard Bright, 1789–1858, English physician).

Brill's disease a mild relapse of epidemic, louse-borne TYPHUS occurring many years after the initial attack. The organism Rickettsia prowazekii can be isolated from the blood. (Nathan Edwin Brill, 1860–1925, American physician).

brimonidine a drug used in the form of eyedrops in the treatment of GLAUCOMA. The drug may be used when beta-blocker eyedrops are medically undesirable or when they are inadeqately effective in controlling the glaucoma. A brand name is Alphagan.

brinzolamide a carbonic anhydrase inhibitor drug used in the form of eye drops to control GLAUCOMA. A brand name is Azopt.

Britaject a brand name for APOMORPHINE.

British antilewisite (BAL) see DIMERCAPROL.

BritLofex a brand name for LOFEXIDINE.

brittle asthma a rare form of ASTHMA affecting mainly females and featuring sudden, very severe, often life-threatening attacks. Those affected have a mild degree of immune deficiency, with poorly-controlled asthma in spite of substantial doses of inhaled steroids and wide diurnal swings in their peak flow meter readings. The term is also applied to people whose asthma is normally well controlled but who, nevertheless, suffer occasional sudden severe attacks.

brittle bones a popular term usually applied to bones liable to fracture on minimal force because of loss of structural strength from conditions such as OSTEOPOROSIS or the hereditary disease OSTEOGENESIS IMPERFECTA.

broad ligaments double folds of PERITONEUM hanging over the womb (uterus) and FALLOPIAN TUBES to form a partition in the pelvis.

broad-spectrum a term most commonly applied to antibiotics implying that the drug is effective over a wide range of organisms. Widely applicable or effective. Prolonged use of broad-spectrum antibiotics, such as AMPICILLIN or the CEPHALOSPORINS, will usually destroy most of the normal organisms of the bowel and these will tend to be replaced by resistant species. It is therefore considered better practice to use narrow-spectrum drugs so long as these are known to be effective against the organism concerned.

Broca's expressive aphasia a speech defect that commonly follows STROKE. There is loss of fluency but not comprehension and separation of words in a telegraphic manner with omission of inessential words such as prepositions, articles and conjunctions. See also APHASIA. (Pierre Paul Broca, 1824–1880, French neurosurgeon).

Broca's area an area of the surface layer of the brain (cortex), on the left side near the front, concerned with speech.

Brodie's abscess a persistent OSTEOMYELITIS, usually of a long bone, featuring a cavity of dead tissue surrounded by fibrous tissue and small blood vessels (granulation tissue). In the pre-antibiotic era Brodie's abscess was common, persistent and disabling. The condition is now rare. (Sir Benjamin Collins Brodie, 1783–1862, English surgeon).

broken neck fracture, often with dislocation, of any of the bony vertebrae of the neck. The importance is not so much the bony injury as the probable injury to the spinal cord lying within the bony canal. Such injury is likely to be serious and may be fatal. Survivors often suffer permanent paralysis below the level of the injury. Neurological damage can be increased by moving a person with a broken neck.

broken veins an inaccurate popular term applied to the condition of TELANGIECTASIA which is a localized dilatation of blood vessels near the surface of the skin. This is one of the natural features of the ageing skin and results from loss of collagen support. Actual breaks in the veins would result in extensive bruising.

Brolene a preparation of propamidine isetionate used as eye drops to treat infective conjunctivitis. See also GOLDEN EYE OINTMENT.

bromazepam a BENZODIAZEPAM drug used in the treatment of anxiety and insomnia.

bromhidrosis profuse odorous sweat, especially from the feet, caused by the breakdown of short-chain FATTY ACIDS, especially isovaleric acid.

bromism poisoning with bromides. These cause headache, apathy muscle weakness and a skin rash.

bromocriptine an ERGOT derivative drug with DOPAMINE-like effects. It is used in the treatment of PARKINSON'S DISEASE and ACROMEGALY and given to prevent LACTATION by inhibiting the secretion of the hormone prolactin by the pituitary gland. A brand name is Parlodel.

bromphenyramine an ANTIHISTAMINE drug used in the sympomatic treatment of hay fever and other allergic conditions. A brand name is Dimotane.

bromsulphthalein a substance used in a liver function test. The rate of clearance of bromsulphthalein from the blood, after injection, is a measure of liver efficiency. The test is now largely replaced by enzyme tests.

Brompton cocktail a mixture of alcohol, morphine and cocaine given for intractable pain in terminally ill people, especially those dying of cancer. The mixture was evolved at the Brompton Hospital, London.

bronch- *combining form denoting* the air tubes of the lung (bronchi).

bronchial pertaining to any part of the branching system of breathing tubes (the bronchial tree).

bronchial asthma a tautological term; all ASTHMA is bronchial.

bronchiectasis permanent areas of local widening of the smaller air tubes of the lung (the bronchi) with persistent infection and a tendency to retention of local infected secretions. There is profuse sputum.

bronchiole one of the many thin-walled, tubular branches of the bronchi, which extend the airway to the terminal air sacs (alveoli). Bronchi have cartilaginous rings, bronchioles do not.

bronchiolitis a development of severe acute BRONCHITIS in which the inflammation spreads to the smaller bronchioles. If this happens the state is indistinguishable from BRONCHOPNEUMONIA.

bronchitis ACUTE or CHRONIC inflammation of the lining of a BRONCHUS. Acute bronchitis commonly follows a cold or influenza, usually in winter. There is a cough with increasing production of sputum, fever, breathlessness, wheezing and sometimes pain in the chest. Chronic bronchitis may be caused by breathing a polluted atmosphere or by smoking. There is constant sputum production and acute infective flare-ups occur. Repeated attacks of winter bronchitis are an early feature of chronic bronchitis.

broncho- *combining form denoting* a major air tube (BRONCHUS).

bronchoconstriction contraction of the circular muscles in the walls of the bronchi, so narrowing the bore of the tubes and restricting air entry. See also BRONCHOSPASM.

bronchoconstrictor a drug or other agent which causes BRONCHOCONSTRICTION.

bronchodilatation widening of the bore of a bronchus by relaxation of the circular muscles in its wall. Bronchodilator drugs are used in the treatment of ASTHMA.

bronchogram an X ray of the bronchial tree taken during BRONCHOGRAPHY.

bronchography an X-ray examination in which the branches of the bronchi are made conspicuous by lining them with an inhaled or injected material opaque to X-rays. Bronchography is especially useful in the diagnosis of BRONCHIECTASIS, but is giving way to fibreoptic BRONCHOSCOPY and less invasive methods such as refined CT or MRI scanning.

bronchopneumonia an acute infection of the lung substance, usually by organisms such as STREPTOCOCCUS, Haemophilus, Klebsiella or Legionella. It can also be caused by the inhalation of irritant substances, especially vomit (aspiration pneumonia).

bronchopulmonary dysplasia a chronic lung disorder affecting premature babies who need supplementary oxygen and artificial ventilation. There is acute and chronic lung damage with inflammation, fibrosis and remodelling.

bronchoscopy direct visual inspection of the insides of the air tubes (bronchi), either through a hollow metal tube or by means of a fibre optic ENDOSCOPE.

bronchospasm tight contraction of the smooth circularly-placed muscles in the walls of the air tubes (bronchi) in the lungs with resulting severe narrowing. Bronchospasm is the main feature of, and cause of the symptoms in, asthma, and is often the result of an allergy.

bronchus a breathing tube. A branch of the windpipe (TRACHEA) or of another bronchus. The trachea divides into two main bronchi, one for each lung, and these, in turn, divide into further, smaller bronchi. See also BRONCHIOLES.

bronchus, cancer of this is the commonest site of lung cancer, more properly described as bronchial carcinoma.

bronzed diabetes see HAEMOCHROMATOSIS.

brown fat a kind of animal body fat more readily available for rapid conversion to heat than is normal yellow fat. It is believed that hibernating animals use their brown fat in the recovery from the winter state. Small human babies have deposits of brown fat around the spine.

brown induration a pathological description of lung tissue featuring acute congestion and water-logging (oedema) with blood in the air sacs (alveoli).

Brown-Sequard syndrome a neurological disorder, caused by compression of one side of the spinal cord in the lower back, featuring paralysis on the injured side and loss of sensation on the other side. (Charles Edouard Brown-Sequard, 1817–1894, Mauritian physician).

brucellosis an infectious disease, caused by bacteria of the genus *Brucella*, and contracted by eating infected meat and dairy products, or by contact with the secretions of sheep, goats or cows. The disease is characterized by lethargy, general MALAISE, aches and pains and fever. The fever lasts for a week or so, settles for a few days, then returns (undulant fever). Sometimes these recurrences persist for months or years, usually becoming progressively milder. (Major-General Sir David Bruce, 1855–1931, British Army pathologist).

Bruch's membrane an insulating membrane that separates the RETINA from the underlying CHOROID. In older people, Bruch's membrane is liable to develop splits or cracks through which blood vessels branching from the choroidal fine vessels may pass. This can lead to AGE-RELATED MACULAR DEGENERATION.

Brufen a brand name for IBUPROFEN.

Brugia filariasis a parasitic disease caused by infection with *Brugia malayi*, a microscopic worm similar to *Wuchereria bancrofti* which is the cause of the commonest type of FILARIASIS. It is spread by mosquitoes and can lead to ELEPHANTIASIS.

bruise the appearance caused by blood released into or under the skin, usually as a result of injury, but sometimes occurring spontaneously in case of bleeding disorders or disease of the blood vessels.

bruits abnormal sounds or murmurs heard with a stethoscope and usually caused by the flow of blood past some obstruction or narrowing. They may be caused by heart valve abnormalities with turbulence or regurgitation

of the blood flow, or they may be heard over major arteries, such as those of the neck (carotids), narrowed by ATHEROSCLEROSIS.

Brulidine a brand name for DIBROMOPROPAMIDINE.

bruxism habitual grinding or clenching of the teeth, often to the point of wearing away the enamel and eroding the crowns. The habit is often unconscious. Bruxism is also common during sleep.

bryostatin-1 a drug with a unique action against cancer cells, that is being used in trials of treatment of leukaemia and malignant melanoma. Bryostatin is formed by a bacterium *Endobugula sertula* that parasitizes the boat-fouling marine animal *Bugula neritina*. The drug also shows promise as a stimulant of the immune system against breast cancer.

BS *abbrev. for* Bachelor of Surgery.

BSc *abbrev. for* Bachelor of Science.

BSc (MedSci) *abbrev. for* Bachelor of Science (Medical Sciences).

B-type natriuretic peptide see NATRIURETIC PEPTIDE.

bubo a swelling in the groin, or in the armpit, from enlargement of one or more lymph nodes as a result of infection. Buboes occur in many infections including PLAGUE, CHANCROID, SYPHILIS, GONORRHOEA, LYMPHOGRANULOMA VENEREUM and TUBERCULOSIS.

bubonic plague a highly infectious disease caused by the organism Yersinia pestis, spread by rat fleas. There is high fever, severe headache, pain and swelling in the groin, severe TOXAEMIA and mental confusion. Antibiotics are effective.

buccal relating to the cheek.

buccal smear a convenient way to obtain cells for chromosomal and other studies and to obtain a sample of DNA. The inside of the cheek is gently scraped with a spatula and the cells spread on a glass slide.

Buccal Sustac a brand name for GLYCERYL TRINITRATE.

Buccastem a brand name for PROCHLORPERAZINE.

buck teeth undue protrusion of the central upper teeth. This can readily be put right by orthodontic treatment.

Bucky grid an assembly of lead strips resembling an open venetian blind, placed between a patient being X-rayed and the screen or film, to improve the collimation and reduce scatter of radiation on the film. (Gustav P. Bucky, 1880–1963, German-born American radiologist).

buclizine an ANTIHISTAMINE drug used in the treatment of MIGRAINE. A brand name in a preparation also containing PARACETAMOL and CODEINE is Migraleve.

Budd-Chiari syndrome a rare condition of clotting of the blood (thrombosis) in the large veins of the liver from excessive numbers of blood red cells (POLYCYTHAEMIA), myeloproliferative disorders, SICKLE CELL ANAEMIA, PAROXYSMAL NOCTURNAL HAEMOGLOBINURIA, the antiphospholipid syndrome, deficiencies of protein C, protein S and antithrombin III, injury or other causes. There is pain, liver enlargement, yellowing of the skin (JAUNDICE), liver failure, a collection of fluid in the abdomen (ascites) and, unless a porto-systemic shunt or liver transplant is done, usually death within a year. (George Budd, 1808–1882, English physician, and Hans von Chiari, 1851–1916, Austrian pathologist).

budesonide a corticosteroid drug used in a nasal spray for hay fever (allergic rhinitis) or as an inhalant for ASTHMA. Brand names are Entocort, Pulicort and Rhinocort. With EFORMOTEROL (formoterol) it is marketed as Symbicort.

Buerger's disease an arterial disease of male smokers featuring obstruction of arteries, especially those supplying the legs, followed by gangrene necessitating amputation. It is also called thromboangiitis obliterans. Sufferers often continue to smoke. (Leo Buerger, 1879–1943, American physician).

buffers chemical substances in the blood, such as lactic acid or bicarbonate, which act to limit changes in the composition, especially the acidity, by binding hydrogen ions. Buffers are important in maintaining constancy when acids are added or removed.

buffy coat the creamy layer of white blood cells that forms between the PLASMA and the column of packed red cells when anticoagulated blood is centrifuged. Practical use is made of this layering in the production of buffy coat-poor red cell transfusion fluids in cases in which it is considered that the risk of post-operative infection from the immunosuppressive effect of white cells in transfused blood is excessive.

bug one of various wingless or four-winged insects of the order *Hemiptera* and especially of the suborder *Heteroptera*, with piercing and sucking mouth parts. The bugs of medical importance include the cone nose (*Reduviid*) 'assassin' or 'kissing' bugs which transmit CHAGAS' DISEASE, and the bed bug, *Cimex lectularis*, which cause painful bites.

buggery see sodomy.

bulbar palsy a neurological disorder causing progressive paralysis of the tongue, throat and voice box (larynx) so that swallowing and speaking become difficult or impossible. Bulbar palsy is a feature of MULTIPLE SCLEROSIS, AMYOTROPHIC LATERAL SCLEROSIS, MOTOR NEURONE DISEASE, and POLIOMYELITIS.

bulbo-urethral glands two small glands that open into the URETHRA just below the bladder in the male, and secrete a clear lubricant fluid that facilitates sexual inter-course. Also known as COWPER'S GLANDS.

bulimia an uncontrollable, compulsive eating disorder, usually affecting young women who regularly eat to the point of bloating and nausea. 15,000 calories may be taken in a few hours. Binges are followed by induced vomiting and deliberate purgation. People with this disorder often show damage to the teeth from stomach acid and scars on the fingers from tooth trauma occurring while inducing vomiting. The most effective treatment, as recommended by NICE, is cognitive behaviour therapy. Compare ANOREXIA NERVOSA.

bulla a large blister or vesicle. A thin-walled abnormal cavity filled with liquid or a gas.

bullet-proof vest a term that seems to promise more than it can fulfil. No wearable vest is completely bullet-proof. The 'proofing' is relative but is often life-saving. Modern protective vests are made of a nylon-like polymer called Kevlar in which aromatic rings replace the nylon hydrocarbon structure. The difference increases the stiffness 16 times over that of earlier nylon protective vests, and a garment made from 20 fine layers of this material can prevent a 9 mm bullet moving at 270 metres per second from depressing the skin more than 45 mm.

bullous emphysema acute overinflation of the lungs with breakdown of the alveoli to form larger air spaces, often due to strong inspiratory efforts to overcome obstruction in the air passages (bronchi).

bullous pemphigoid a skin disease of elderly

people that features large tense blisters. The condition is caused by an immunological disorder and usually responds well to steroids or immunosuppressive treatment.

bumetanide a quick-acting DIURETIC drug used to relieve the fluid retention (OEDEMA) occurring in HEART FAILURE, kidney disease such as the NEPHROTIC SYNDROME and liver CIRRHOSIS. A brand name is Burinex.

BUN acronym for blood urea nitrogen. This is estimated when kidney function is in question.

bundle branch block functional obstruction to one or other branch of the specialized muscle fibre conducting tissue of the heart (the bundle of His) which controls the timing of the contraction of the lower chambers (the ventricles). Bundle branch block usually implies that the heart muscle, generally, has been damaged, often by an inadequate blood supply from the coronary arteries. In extensive block, the outlook is poor.

bunion inflammation of the protective, fluid-filled tissue bag (BURSA) overlying the main joint of the big toe. This is due to wearing pointed shoes which lever the big toes outward and exert pressure on the prominent joint.

bunyavirus any one of the *Bunyaviridae* family of over 250 viruses that cause a variety of mosquito transmitted (ARBOVIRUS) fevers including California ENCEPHALITIS. Most of the bunyavirus infections are mild feverish illnesses, with headache and joint pain and sometimes with a rash. Full recovery is usual.

buphthalmos enlargement of the corneas resulting from abnormally raised pressure within the eyes at birth (congenital GLAUCOMA). The eyes appear unnaturally large because of the greater corneal diameter. Early detection and treatment can save sight. From the Greek *bous*, an ox and *ophthalmos*, an eye.

bupivacaine a long-acting local anaesthetic drug often used for nerve blocks, especially in epidural anaesthesia during childbirth and for the control of postoperative pain. The drug is on the WHO official list. A brand name is Marcaine.

buprenorphine a powerful painkilling drug that binds to the body's opioid receptors. It acts for 6–8 hours. Brand names are Subutex, Temgesic and Transtec.

bupropion a drug used in the treatment of tobacco, drug and alcohol dependency.

Bupropion reacts adversely with a wide range of other drugs and may induce seizures in sensitive persons. When used, a strict regime is necessary. A brand name is Zyban.

Burinex A, Burinex K brand names for BUMETANIDE.

Burkitt's lymphoma a tumour of B lymphocytes occurring mainly in Central Africa and New Guinea and associated with the Epstein Barr virus, spread by insects. It affects mainly the lower and upper jaws of young children but can affect most parts of the body. Burkitt's lymphoma was one of the first human tumours to be shown to be caused in this way. The tumour commonly spreads to the abdomen where large secondary masses may form, affecting the bowel. Immunosuppressive chemotherapy with cyclophosphamide or METHOTREXATE is apparently curative in 80% of early cases and about 40% of those with advanced, widespread disease. (Dennis Parsons Burkitt, 1911–93, English medical researcher, bran apostle, and Fellow of the Royal Society).

burns the damage response of the skin and underlying tissues to high temperature from any source. Burns may be partial or full thickness, the latter requiring grafting.

burning feet syndrome a symptom complex due to a combined deficiency of B vitamins.

burp a belch.

burr hole a small circular hole drilled in bone, usually the skull, by means of a drill (burr). Burr holes are often made as a preliminary to raising a flap of bone to get access to the brain.

bursa a small fibrous sac lined with a membrane which secretes a lubricating fluid (synovial membrane). Bursas are efficient protective and friction-reducing structures and occur around joints and in areas where tendons pass over bones.

bursa of Fabricius an organ in the cloacal-hind gut junction birds found to be important in the maturation of B lymphocytes (B for bursa). The equivalent in humans is probably the tonsils or lymphoid tissue in the intestine.

bursiform pouch-like.

bursitis inflammation of a BURSA. Bursitis is commonly due to excess local pressure or undue friction, but it may also result from rheumatic disease or infection. Common examples are HOUSEMAID'S KNEE, TENNIS ELBOW and BUNION.

Buscopan a brand name for HYOSCINE.

buserelin a gonadothropin-releasing hormone drug used in the treatment of ENDOMETRIOSIS and INFERTILITY. Brand names are Suprecur and Suprefact.

Buspar a brand name for BUSPIRONE.

buspirone a non-benzodiazepine antianxiety drug with slow onset of effect. A brand name is Buspar.

busulphan busulfan, an alkylating anticancer drug used especially in the treatment of chronic granulocytic LEUKAEMIA. It is very toxic and can destroy the function of the BONE MARROW unless its use is carefully monitored. It can also cause widespread FIBROSIS of the lungs. A brand name is Myleran.

Butacote a brand name for PHENYLBUTAZONE brand.

Butazolidin a historic brand name for the powerful, but now little-used, NSAID drug PHENYLBUTAZONE.

Buteyko method a complementary medicine breath control technique used to prevent hyperventilation and which is claimed to be able to treat asthma without drugs. Unscientific treatment of asthma involve real potential dangers to life.

butobarbitone butobarbital, a barbiturate hypnotic drug of medium duration of action. A brand name is Soneryl.

buttock one of the twinned masses of powerful muscle at the base of the trunk, behind. Each buttock consists of three muscles – the gluteus maximus, gluteus medius and gluteus minimus. These muscles arise from the back of the bony pelvis and run into the upper end of the back of the thigh bone (femur) and act to straighten the flexed hip joint.

butyric pertaining to butter or derived from BUTYRIC ACID.

butyric acid a water-soluble saturated FATTY ACID occurring in animal milk fats. It has a strong rancid odour.

butyrophenones a group of phenothiazine derivative drugs used in the treatment of SCHIZOPHRENIA. The group includes HALOPERIDOL, triperidol and benperidol.

BVMS *abbrev. for* Bachelor of Veterinary Medicine & Surgery.

bypass operations a surgical procedure to restore continuity of flow of blood, intestinal contents, cerebrospinal fluid, urine, etc, when a body tube or conduit is obstructed. Arterial bypass operations on the coronary arteries have saved many lives and relieved much distress.

byssinosis an allergic PNEUMONITIS, similar to BAGGASOSIS and bird-fancier's lung, caused by dust inhalation. Byssinosis is caused by the dust produced in the manufacture of cotton, flax or hemp goods. There is breathlessness, chest tightness and cough becoming progressively worse as exposure continues.

C

CAB *abbrev. for* cellulose acetate-butyrate, a plastic widely used to make one form of gas-permeable hard CONTACT LENS.

Cabaser a brand name for CABERGOLINE.

cabergoline a dopamine agonist drug used to treat breast disorders and to stop LACTATION soon after delivery. A brand name is Dostinex.

CABG *abbrev. for* CORONARY ARTERY BYPASS graft.

Cache Valley virus infection a disease, caused by one of the viruses of the *Bunyaviridae* family, featuring severe fever, muscle ache, headache, vomiting and a rash, and progressing to brain inflammation (encephalitis), muscle necrosis and multi-organ failure. The disease is not uncommon in livestock and other large mammals but is very rare in humans.

cachexia, a state of severe muscle wasting and weakness occurring in the late stages of serious illnesses such as cancer. The usual condition of bodily decline in those dying after long debilitating illnesses. Cachexia is not due to malnutrition and research findings suggest that an important element in the causation may be selective depletion of the myosin heavy chain in myofibrillary proteins.

Cacit D3 a brand name for a mixture of calcium carbonate and vitamin D3 (CHOLECALCIFEROL) (colecalciferol).

cacosmia a HALLUCINATION of an unpleasant smell.

cadaver a corpse. The term may correctly be applied to any corpse, but tends to be confined to corpses used for anatomical dissection.

cadaverine an AMINE found in decomposing body tissue.

cadexomer iodine a drug used externally in preparations to absorb discharge from skin ulcers and wounds. Brand names are Iodoflex and Iodosorb.

cadherins a family of calcium-dependent adhesion molecules found on the surface of cells. Cadherins are trans-membrane glycoproteins that mediate cell to cell junctions and contribute to the maintenance of cell shape. Cadherins differ in molecular weight at different locations, ranging from 120 to 135Kd.

cadmium a poisonous metal sometimes encountered as an air pollutant in industrial processes. Inhaled cadmium dust can cause lung inflammation. Cadmium is also damaging to the kidneys and can cause softening of the bones (OSTEOMALACIA).

caduceus an emblem or symbol consisting of the winged staff of Mercury around which two serpents are entwined in opposite directions. The caduceus appears on the cap badges of members of the Royal Army Medical Corps (RAMC) and is the emblem of the American Army Medical Corps.

caecostomy a surgical connection between the CAECUM and the exterior, by way of an opening in the front wall of the abdomen.

caecum the large blind-ended pouch in the bowel at the beginning of the large intestine (COLON) in the lower right quadrant of the abdomen. The end of the ILEUM joins the caecum at the ileo-caecal valve. From the caecum protrudes the worm-like (vermiform) APPENDIX.

Caelyx a brand name for DOXORUBICIN.

caeruloplasmin a copper-containing globulin formed in the liver. Deficiency causes WILSON'S DISEASE, and blood levels are very low in acute liver failure.

CAESAR an important and historic trial of

multiple therapy for HIV-positive people carried out in Canada, Australia, Europe and South Africa (hence the acronym). CAESAR showed conclusively that the addition of LAMIVUDINE or lamivudine plus loviride to a treatment regimen containing zidovudine can significantly reduce progression to AIDS and death. All routine anti-HIV treatment now involves drug combinations.

Caesarian section an operation to deliver a baby through an incision in the abdomen, performed when natural delivery is impracticable or dangerous or urgency is necessary.

caesium 137 a radioactive ISOTOPE with a half-life of 30 years used as an implant for radiotherapy.

cafe au lait spots milk coffee-coloured oval patches, from one to 15cm or more long, on the skin. If more than five of these occur in childhood, and especially if they extend into the armpit, it is likely that the condition of NEUROFIBROMATOSIS (Recklinghausen's disease) is developing.

Cafergot a brand name for a mixture of ERGOTAMINE and CAFFEINE.

caffeine one of the most popular and widely used drugs of mild addiction. Caffeine is used, in the form of coffee, tea and Cola-flavoured drinks, by about half the population of the world. It elevates mood, controls drowsiness, decreases fatigue and increases capacity for work. Caffeine is incorporated in various drug formulations such as Cafergot and Migril for the treatment of MIGRAINE.

cainotophobia abnormal fear of newness.

caisson disease a disorder affecting divers who return to the surface too rapidly after being under high presure. Nitrogen in solution in the blood and tissues is released as bubbles which block small arteries and cause pains in the joints (the 'bends'), severe cramps, paralysis and even death.

Calabar bean the poisonous seed of the African plant *Physostigma venenosum*, the source of the drug PHYSOSTIGMINE.

Calabar swelling transient inflammatory lumps under the skin caused by the adult worm of the filarial parasite *Loa loa*.

Caladryl a brand name for a mixture of CALAMINE, camphor and DIPHENHYDRAMINE.

calamine zinc carbonate, zinc silicate or zinc oxide. Calamine is widely used as a bland,

mildly astringent, skin lotion. A little phenol (carbolic acid) is often added for its itch-relieving properties. Calamine lotion is on the WHO official list. A brand name for a skin preparation containing calamine is Hydrocal.

calcaneal spur syndrome the effects of a spur of bone (exostosis), readily visible on X-ray, that forms on the inner weight-bearing surface of the heel bone (calcaneus) and extends forward horizontally into the soft tissue (plantar fascia) beneath the skin of the sole. The condition is painful in its early stages but tends to become less so as the spur enlarges. It is treated by injections of steroid mixed with a local anaesthetic.

calcaneus the heel bone, or os calcis.

calcar a spur or spur-like projection from a bone or tendon.

calcareous chalky. Containing, or pertaining to, calcium or lime.

calcarine fissure a conspicuous groove in the visual area of the brain at the back (occipital cortex). Also called the calcarine sulcus.

Calceos a brand name for a preparation of calcium carbonate and vitamin D_3 used to treat OSTEOPOROSIS.

Calcicard a trade name for DILTIAZEM.

calcicosis a form of PNEUMOCONIOSIS caused by long-term inhalation of chalk (calcium carbonate) dust, as from marble cutting or polishing.

Calcichew a brand name for calcium carbonate used to treat OSTEOPOROSIS.

Calcichew D3 a brand name for calcium carbonate and Vitamin D3 used to treat OSTEOPOROSIS.

calciferol vitamin D. A fat-soluble vitamin necessary for the absorption of calcium from the intestine. Deficiency causes RICKETS in infants and OSTEOMALACIA in adults.

calcification deposition of calcium salts, usually calcium hydroxyapatite crystals, in body tissues, especially when there has been prolonged inflammation or injury. Calcification is normal in bones and teeth.

calcific tendinitis an inflammatory disorder of the rotator cuff tendons involving calcification most commonly close to the insertion of the supraspinatus tendon on the greater tuberosity of the humerus. About half of those with the disorder suffer shoulder pain and limitation of movement at the shoulder. The condition is self-limiting but recovery can be hastened by ultrasound treatment.

Calcihep a trade name for HEPARIN.

Calcijex a brand name for CALCITRIOL.

Calcimax a trade name for CALCIUM.

calcinosis abnormal deposition of calcium salts in skin, muscles, or connective tissues in the course of a connective tissue disorder such as SCLERODERMA or DERMATOMYOSITIS.

Calciparine a brand name for HEPARIN.

calcipotriol a vitamin D-analogue drug used in the treatment of PSORIASIS. A brand name for an external preparation is Dovonex. Formulated with betamethasone it is marketed as Dovobet.

Calcisorb a trade name for SODIUM CELLULOSE PHOSPHATE.

Calcitare a trade name for CALCITONIN.

calcitonin salcatonin or calcitonin (salmon), a hormone secreted by the THYROID gland, independently of the thyroid hormones, and concerned with the control of calcium levels in the blood. It acts on bone to interfere with the release of calcium. It is less important in calcium balance than the parathyroid glands. Used as a drug under the brand name Miacalcic.

calcitonin gene-related peptide receptor the receptor for a peptide found in trigeminal nerve sensory neurons which is a powerful dilator of cerebral and dural arteries. An infusion of the calcitonin gene-related peptide will induce MIGRAINE and the specific antagonist BIBN 4096 BS is effective in treating an attack of migraine.

calcitriol a vitamin D analogue drug used in the treatment of low calcium levels resulting from kidney disease. Brand names are Calcijex, Rocatrol and Silkis.

calcium a mineral present in large quantity in the body, mainly in the form of calcium phosphate in the bones and the teeth. Electrically charged calcium atoms (ions) are present in the blood and body fluids and are essential for many physiological processes including cell membrane permeability, cell excitability, the initiation and transmission of electrical impulses, muscle contraction, cell shape and cell motility. Calcium is necessary for blood coagulation, the production of ATP, and enzyme actions. Calcium levels in the blood are kept within narrow limits by feedback mechanisms. Brand names of preparations containing calcium used to treat OSTEOPOROSIS are Ostram and Sandocal.

calcium alginate a drug used externally in the treatment of skin ulcers. A brand name for an alginate dressing is Kaltostat.

calcium antagonists see CALCIUM CHANNEL BLOCKERS.

calcium carbonate chalk. A drug used in the treatment of OSTEOPOROSIS. Brand names of preparations containing calcium carbonate are Adcal, Cacit, Calceos and Calcichew.

calcium channel blockers a range of drugs that block movement of calcium ions across cell membranes and so interfere with the action of the muscle fibres in arteries and elsewhere. They are useful in controlling high blood pressure (HYPERTENSION) and heart irregularity, and are also used to treat angina, heart irregularities and Raynaud's phenomenon. Research has suggested, however, that the risk of heart attacks in people being treated with certain calcium channel blocker drugs may be higher than with other drugs used to control high blood pressure. Examples are nifedipine (Adalat, Angiopine MR, Calcidate MR, Fortipine LA), diltiazem (Adizem, SR, Adizem XL, Angitil SR, Angitil XL), nicardipine (Cardene), nifedipine (Tensipine MR), verapamil (Securon), nisoldipine (Syscor MR), lercandipine (Zanidip).

calcium chloride a calcium salt limited in its usefulness because of its irritating properties. It may be given by very slow intravenous injection and is sometimes used in cases of cardiac arrest.

calcium folinate a drug used to counteract the folate-antagonist action of METHOTREXATE. The drug is on the WHO official list.

calcium gluconate a calcium salt commonly given by mouth as a calcium supplement in the treatment of RICKETS, OSTEOMALACIA and OSTEOPOROSIS.

calcium lactate a calcium salt used as a calcium supplement.

calcium oxalate a calcium salt occurring in the urine, sometimes in such high concentration as to form urinary stones (calculi).

calcium sodium lactate a combination of calcium and sodium lactates used to supplement body calcium.

calculus a stone of any kind formed abnormally in the body, mainly in the urinary system and the gall bladder. Calculi form in fluids in which high concentrations of chemical substances are dissolved. Their formation is encouraged by infection.

calculus (dental) see DENTAL CALCULUS.

caldesmons proteins that bind CALCIUM and CALMODULIN and are involved in cell adhesion, shape and motility.

Caldwell-Luc operation an operation to drain pus from the sinus in the upper jaw (the maxillary antrum) by making an opening though the bone high behind the upper lip. (George Walker Caldwell, 1834–1918, American ENT surgeon; and Henri Luc, 1855–1925, French ENT surgeon).

calendar method a contraceptive idea based on the fact that ovulation occurs 14 days before the onset of the next menstrual period, and on the unreliable assumption that the length of future menstrual periods can be predicted on the basis of previous cycles. See also CONTRACEPTION.

caliper splint an external support for a leg weakened by muscular disorder or ankle or knee instability. It usually consists of a metal rod on either side attached to the heel of the shoe and a strap around the leg.

calisthenics physical exercises to build up muscles and improve the efficiency of the heart and lungs.

calix 1 any cuplike structure.
2 one of the many divisions of the urine collecting structure of the pelvis of the kidney. The plural is calices.

callosity a protective response of the skin to excessive or prolonged friction or pressure, especially over a bony prominence. A common example is the corn on a toe caused by ill-fitting footwear or by an abnormally positioned toe.

callus 1 a collection of partly calcified tissue, formed in the blood clot around the site of a healing fracture. Callus is readily visible on X-ray and indicates that healing is under way.
2 a skin thickening (see CALLOSITY).

calmodulins small intracellular proteins that can bind to one to four calcium ions, producing complexes that can change the configuration of associated proteins such as enzymes. Calmodulins react to changing calcium levels and are involved in such processes as cell proliferation, glucose metabolism and the release of neurotransmitters.

calor the Latin word for heat. One of the 'cardinal signs' of inflammation – rubor, dolor, calor, tumor – respectively, redness, pain, heat and swelling.

caloric pertaining to heat or calories.

caloric test a test of the balancing mechanisms in the inner ear. Instillation of hot and cold water into the ear causes jerky movement of the eyes (NYSTAGMUS) if the vestibular apparatus is functioning normally. If, however, there is disease of the balancing mechanism (semicircular canals) the nystagmus will be absent or much reduced in extent.

calorie the amount of heat needed to raise 1g of water by 1 °C. For nutritional purposes the Calorie (or kilocalorie) is the amount of heat needed to raise 1000 grams of water by 1 °C. The modern unit is the joule. 1 calorie is a little over 4 joules (1 cal = 4.2 J).

calorific anything producing or able to produce heat, or pertaining to heat production.

calorimetry measurement of the energy value of foodstuffs or the energy expenditure of a person. Food is burnt in a special chamber called a BOMB CALORIMETER and the heat rise measured. Human energy expenditure can be measured indirectly by assessing the amount of oxygen consumed.

Calpol paediatric a brand name for PARACETAMOL intended for children.

Caltrate a brand name for CALCIUM with vitamin D3.

calvarium the vault of the skull. The skull less the jaw and facial bones.

Calvita a trade name for a mixture of VITAMINS and minerals.

CAM a brand name for EPHEDRINE in the form of an elixir.

Camcolit 250 a trade name for LITHIUM.

Campral EC a brand name for ACAMPROSATE.

Campto a brand name for the camptothecin drug IRINOTECAN.

camptothecins a new class of cytotoxic anticancer drugs based on the plant alkaloid camptothecin found in the wood, bark and fruit of the tree *Camptotheca acuminata*. Camptothecins attack the enzyme TOPOISOMERASE. The class includes the drugs TOPOTECAN and IRINOTECAN both of which are showing promising results in the treatment of small cell lung cancer and ovarian cancer.

campylobacter enteritis a common type of food poisoning, caused by the organism *Campylobacter jejuni*. Sources of infection include water, raw milk, poultry and dogs.

Campylobacter jejuni the commonest cause of bacterial food poisoning in Britain. See CAMPYLOBACTER ENTERITIS.

Canale-Smith syndrome an AUTOIMMUNE disease caused by mutations of the *Fas* gene, or defects in the *Fas* expression cascade, that leads to defective APOPTOSIS in lymphocytes. The result is a lymphoproliferative disorder with lymphadenopathy, spleen enlargement, possible lymphoma development and other effects including excess gamma globulin production.

canaliculotomy a minor operation to open up a blocked CANALICULUS by removing a small triangular piece from its back wall, thereby allowing tears to pass into the LACRIMAL SAC.

canaliculus a narrow channel in the body, such as a tear duct. The lacrimal canaliculi run fron the inner corner of each eyelid to the LACRIMAL SAC.

canalization forming a channel. A blood vessel blocked by blood clot may, in time, recanalize.

canal of Schlemm a fine, circular, sometimes multi-channel passage, running round the periphery of the CORNEA (limbus) in the SCLERA. Aqueous humour from the eye drains out through the TRABECULAR MESHWORK into the canal of Schlemm. (Friedrich. S. Schlemm, 1795–1858, German anatomist).

cancellous of a spongy, porous, lattice-like structure. A term applied to the inner parts of bone.

cancer a disease of DNA used by the medical profession as a convenient and comprehensive label for all forms of malignant growths. There are two broad classes of cancers—those which arise from surface linings (carcinomas) and those which arise from solid tissues (sarcomas). Cancers spread by local invasion and by lymph and blood spread (metastases) and their degree of malignancy is a measure of the rapidity with which they spread. It has long been believed that cancers start either as the result of small genetic changes to genes called tumour suppressor genes that restrain the ability of cells to divide, or to genes called oncogenes which suffer mutations. Research now suggests that many other abnormalities are probably involved. In early cancers there is much disruption of the chromosomes, some of which are duplicated or lost or truncated and parts

fused together. Chromosomal instability appears to be an important element. It is only a matter of time before cancers are classified by their pattern of gene abnormality. Although some aspects of the biology of cancers remain obscure, recent years have shown remarkable advances in the effective treatment of many cancers. The list that follows highlights the key entries related to cancer in the dictionary: adenocarcinoma, basal cell carcinoma, bile duct cancer, bone cancer, BRCA gene, breast cancer, cancer, cancer screening, carcinoma, carcinoma in situ, carcinomatosis, cervical cancer, colon cancer, gall bladder cancer, kissing cancer, liver cancer, lung cancer, oat-cell carcinoma, precancerous, prostate cancer, rectal cancer, skin cancer, squamous cell carcinoma, sarcoma, stomach cancer, tumour, tumour lysis syndrome, tumour markers, tumour necrosis factor, tumour necrosis factor antagonist, tumour-specific antigens.

cancericidal destructive to cancer cells.

cancerous pertaining to cancer.

cancer phobia, cancerophobia an irrational fear of cancer. Cancer phobia does not prompt rational courses such as regular screening and avoidance of risk factors, but rather compulsively performed rituals such as repeated hand-washing and avoidance of contact with other persons. Minor symptoms are interpreted as signs of cancer and panic attacks may occur. Behaviour therapy is often effective.

cancer screening an attempt to detect cancer early by routine examination of apparently healthy people. Screening methods include the PAP SMEAR TEST, BREAST SELF-EXAMINATION, MAMMOGRAPHY, chest X-ray, sputum tests, and tests for hidden (occult) blood in the stools.

cancroid resembling a cancer.

cancrum oris a disease affecting grossly malnourished and neglected children in which infection, ulceration and progressive tissue destruction occur around the mouth until large areas of both cheeks and nose are eaten away, leaving the cavities of the mouth and nose exposed.

candesartan an ANGIOTENSIN II antagonist drug used in the treatment of high blood pressure (HYPERTENSION). A brand name is Amias.

candida any yeast-like fungus species of the genus *Candida* especially CANDIDA ALBICANS.

Candida albicans the common THRUSH fungus. *Candida* is a yeast-like fungus commonly affecting the mouth, the vagina and the GLANS of the penis and sometimes causing serious infections in immunocompromized people or in the debilitated who have to have heavy or prolonged antibiotic treatment. It is also a common infecting agent in people with DIABETES or CUSHING'S SYNDROME. Also known as monilia.

candidiasis THRUSH. Also known as candidosis.

Canesten a brand name for CLOTRIMAZOLE.

canicola infection a form of LEPTOSPIROSIS caused by *Leptospira canicola* derived from dogs or pigs. It is less severe than WEIL'S DISEASE.

canine tooth one of the two pairs of pointed teeth on either side of the two central pairs of incisor teeth. Canines are tearing teeth; incisors are cutting teeth.

canker sore a small painful mouth ulcer. See also APHTHOUS ULCER.

cannabinols the active ingredients of CANNABIS.

cannabis a drug derived from the hemp plant. Marijuana is the dried leaves, flowers or stems of various species of the hemp grass *Cannabis*, especially *Cannabis sativa*, *Cannabis indica* and *Cannabis americana*. Cannabis resin contains the cannabinoid tetrahydrocannabinol which produces euphoria (the easy promotion of silly laughter or giggling) and an apparent heightening of all the senses, especially vision, with distortion of dimensions. There is slowing of reflexes, distortion of distance and alteration in the sense of responsibility. Driving becomes dangerous. Much valued is an illusory sense of deep philosophical insight or a conviction of omniscience. Panic attacks or acute anxiety may occur, and SCHIZOPHRENIA, MANIA, DEPERSONALIZATION or confusional psychoses have been precipitated. Persistent heavy users may become apathetic and show loss of interest and concern (amotivational syndrome). Cannabis does, however, have some valuable medical uses. It is a sedative that can relieve some side effects of drugs and can help some patients to live more comfortably with some serious illnesses. The former rigidity of official attitude against its therapeutic use is softening, especially since cannabinoid receptors were found to be widely expressed throughout the central nervous system. A number of American States have approved its medical use. See also GLUTAMATE.

cannabism any toxic or other undesirable effect of excessive or habitual use of CANNABIS.

cannibalism the act or practice of eating the flesh of members of the same species.

cannula a hollow surgical tube, into which is inserted a close fitting, sharp-pointed inner stiffener called a trocar. The combination can easily be pushed through the skin or the lining of a blood vessel or other tissue. When in position, the trocar is pulled backwards out of the cannula, leaving the latter in place. Fluids or other materials may then be passed.

cannulation insertion of a CANNULA.

cannon waves occasional high pressure waves seen in the jugular veins when the upper chambers of the heart (atria) are out of sync with the lower chambers (ventricles) and the right atrium contracts against a full ventricle and the valve between the two is closed.

canthariasis any disorder caused by beetles (Coleoptera) or their larvae, especially by *Cantheris* species.

cantharides a poisonous, blistering preparation made from the powdered, dried bodies of the beetle *Cantharis vesicatoria*. Cantharides has been used criminally as an aphrodisiac with grave consequences. Also known as 'Spanish fly'.

canthus the corner the eye where the upper and lower eyelids meet. In epicanthus, the upper lid margin curves over to conceal the canthus.

canthorrhaphy stitching together of the angle of the eyelids so as to narrow the lid opening. Also known as lateral TARSORRHAPHY.

canthotomy slitting of the CANTHUS so as to widen the lid opening.

Cantil a brand name for MEPENZOLATE.

capacitiation changes that occur in the heads of spermatozoa when they are in the uterus or fallopian tube that lead to the release of enzymes that allow penetration of the egg. An oestrogen environment promotes capitation; progestins of the luteal phase of the menstrual cycle oppose it.

Capadex a brand name for a mixture of DEXTROPROPOXYPHENE and PARACETAMOL.

cap binding protein a protein that binds to the ends of messenger RNA molecules and helps to speed up protein synthesis on ribosomes.

cap contraceptive a BARRIER CONTRACEPTIVE

device in the form of a small dome-shaped plastic cup that fits snugly over the cervix of the womb and is usually left in place except during menstrual periods. Accurate fitting is important and the cap may become accidentally displaced. CERVICITIS may occur from infection of retained mucus. The cap is, in general, less satisfactory than the diaphragm contraceptive device. See also CONTRACEPTION.

CAPD *abbrev. for* continuous ambulatory peritoneal dialysis.

CAPE *abbrev. for* Clifton assessment procedure for the elderly. This is a series of tests to assess the mental and behavioural capacity of old people.

capecitabine an anticancer drug used especially in treatment of cancers of the rectum or colon that have been found to have spread. A brand name is Xeloda.

Capgras' syndrome a rare delusional disorder in which the sufferer is convinced that someone emotionally close, has been replaced by an exact double with evil intentions. (Jean Marie Joseph Capgras, 1873–1950, French psychiatrist).

capillariasis an infection with the parasitic worm *Capillaria phillipinensis* which invades the lining of the small intestine causing pain and severe diarrhoea and interfering with the absorption of food.

capillary the smallest and most numerous of all the blood vessels. Capillaries form dense networks between the arteries and the veins, and it is only in the capillary beds that interchange of oxygen, carbon dioxide and nutrients can take place with the cells.

capitellum, capitulum any small rounded prominence or ending on a bone.

Caplan's syndrome a form of coal-worker's PNEUMOCONIOSIS in which progressive FIBROSIS of the lungs, in the form of large nodules, is associated with RHEUMATOID ARTHRITIS. (Anthony Caplan, 1907–76, English physician).

caplet a medicinal tablet, usually oval in shape, coated with a soluble substance.

Capoten a brand name for CAPTOPRIL.

Capozide a brand name for HYDROCHLORO-THIAZIDE formulated with the ANGIOTENSIN CONVERTING ENZYME inhibitor drug CAPTOPRIL.

capreomycin an antibiotic drug derived from Streptomyces capreolus and used in the treatment of TUBERCULOSIS resistant to standard drugs such as RIFAMPICIN, ISONIAZID, ETHAMBUTOL and STREPTOMYCIN. The drug is on the WHO official list. A brand name is Capastat.

capsaicin a pain-killing drug for external application used in the treatment of post-shingles pain and other painful peripheral nerve disorders. Brand names are Axsain and Zacin.

capsicum oleoresin a drug used externally with other ingredients as an embrocation for the relief of rheumatic pain, backache, fibrositis and sciatica. A brand name is Balmosa.

capsid the protein coat that encloses the genome of a virus.

capsule 1 any outer covering such as the tough, protective outer coat of solid organs including the kidneys, liver and spleen or the delicate outer membrane of the internal crystalline lens of the eye. Joints, too, have capsules which contribute to their stability and function.
2 soluble gelatine containers for drugs in powder or liquid form.

capsulectomy surgical removal of a CAPSULE or part of a capsule.

capsulitis inflammation of the capsule of a joint.

capsulotomy cutting a CAPSULE, especially the capsule of the internal lens of the eye.

captopril an angiotensin converting enzyme inhibitor (ACE INHIBITOR) drug used in the treatment of HEART FAILURE and high blood pressure (HYPERTENSION). The drug is on the WHO official list. Brand names are Acepril and Capoten and, with the addition of a thiazide DIURETIC drug, Acezide, Capozide.

Capurate a trade name for ALLOPURINOL.

caput 1 a head.
2 an abbreviation for CAPUT SUCCEDANIUM.

caput medusae a conspicuous whorl of large veins sometimes seen radiating from the navel in CIRRHOSIS of the liver. This is an attempt to provide a shunt (collateral circulation) around obstructed liver veins. The Gorgon, Medusa, had snakes instead of hair, hence the name.

caput succedaneum a boggy (oedematous) swelling of a baby's scalp seen for a period after birth and caused by sustained scalp pressure against the edges of the widened (dilated) cervix. The caput disappears within hours or days.

Carace a brand name for the ANGIOTENSIN CONVERTING ENZYME inhibitor drug LISINOPRIL.

Carace 10 Plus a brand name for the ANGIOTENSIN CONVERTING ENZYME inhibitor drug LISINOPRIL formulated with the diuretic HYDROCHLOROTHIAZIDE.

Carafate a trade name for SUCRALFATE.

carbachol a drug with ACETYL CHOLINE-like properties of stimulating the PARASYMPATHETIC NERVOUS SYSTEM. It is used to stimulate PERISTALSIS in the intestine, to treat retention of urine and sometimes to treat GLAUCOMA.

carbamazepine a drug used in the control of EPILEPSY and especially to relieve or prevent the pain of TRIGEMINAL NEURALGIA. The drug is on the WHO official list. A brand name is Tegretol.

carbaminohaemoglobin a combination of carbon dioxide and haemoglobin by which a proportion of the blood transport of carbon dioxide from the tissues to the lungs is effected.

carbapenems a range of antibiotic drugs that are derivatives of thienamycin produced from *Streptomyces cattleya*. The carbapenems act by inhibiting the synthesis of the bacterial wall and are bactericidal. They have a broad spectrum of action against both Gram-positive and Gram-negative organisms.

carbaryl a carbamate pesticide used to kill caterpillar apple pests and incorporated in lotions and shampoos used to get rid of head and pubic lice. It has an ANTICHOLINESTERASE action. A brand name is Calyderm.

carbenicillin an antibiotic of the penicillin group. Carboxy-benzyl-penicillin.

carbenoxolone a drug used to promote healing in stomach and duodenal ulcers. A brand name is Bioplex. Formulated with magnesium trisilicate it is marketed as Pyrogastrone.

carbidopa a drug that prevents the breakdown of the drug levodopa in the body and thus enhances its action in PARKINSON'S DISEASE. See also BENSERAZIDE. A brand name is Sinemet.

carbimazole an antithyroid drug that interferes with the production of thyroid hormone and is used in the treatment of HYPERTHYROIDISM. A brand name is Neo-Mercazole.

carbimide, calcium a drug that produces very unpleasant symptoms if followed by alcohol. Like DISULFIRAM, it is occasionally used to try to discourage drinking in alcoholics.

carbocisteine a drug used to disperse excess mucus or to treat GLUE EAR in children. A brand name is Mycodyne.

carbohydrates compounds of carbon, oxygen and hydrogen forming an important part of the diet and contributing mainly energy. They include sugars, starches and celluloses and are structurally classified into three groups –

monosaccharides, disaccharides and polysaccharides. Starches and celluloses are polysaccharides.

carbolic acid phenol. A strong acid sometimes used to destroy skin LESIONS or, in a diluted form, as an adjuct to lotions to relieve itching. An example is calamine and phenol. Carbolic acid is sometimes used as a general antiseptic agent.

carbomer an ocular lubricant polyacrylic acid used as eye drops in the treatment of dry eyes. Brand names are Geltears, Liposic and Viscotears.

carbon the non-metallic element on which all organic chemistry is based and which is thus present in all organic matter. A carbon atom is capable of combining with up to four other atoms (tetravalent), including other carbon atoms; it is this property that allows so many compounds to be formed.

carbon cycle the important biological cycle in which carbon in carbon dioxide in the atmosphere is taken up by plants, incorporated, by photosynthesis, into carbohydrates which are eaten by animals, and the carbon then oxidised and finally returned to the atmosphere as carbon dioxide waste gas.

carbon dioxide a compound in which an atom of carbon is linked to two atoms of oxygen (CO_2). Carbon dioxide is a colourless, odourless gas and is one of the chief waste products of tissue metabolism.

carbonic anhydrase an ENZYME that reversibly catalyses the breakdown of carbonic acid into carbon dioxide and water, thus allowing the easy transfer of carbon dioxide from the tissues to the atmosphere via the blood and the lungs. In the stomach a carbonic anhydrase frees hydrogen ions for the formation of hydrochloric acid; and in the pancreas they produce bicarbonate to neutralize duodenal acid from the stomach.

carbonic anhydrase inhibitors a class of drug that act by blocking the action of the enzyme CARBONIC ANHYDRASE. This enzyme greatly speeds up the reaction between carbon dioxide and water to form carbonic acid, a compound needed for the production of many of the body's secretions. Carbonic anhydrase is present in high concentration in the eye, the kidneys, stomach lining and pancreas. Inhibitor drugs reduce the rate of secretion of aqueous humour in the eye and is useful in treating GLAUCOMA.

These drugs are also valuable in treating mountain sickness, periodic paralysis and absence attacks (PETIT MAL). The group includes ACETAZOLAMIDE and DORZOLAMIDE.

carbon monoxide a simple, but poisonous, compound consisting of an atom of carbon linked to an atom of oxygen (CO). It is formed when carbon is oxidized in conditions of limited oxygen, as in the internal combustion engine.

carboplatin an anticancer drug. A brand name is Paraplatin.

carboxyhaemoglobin the stable compound formed between CARBON MONOXIDE and HAEMOGLOBIN that does not readily dissociate. As a result, the oxygen carrying power of the blood is limited. A high level of carboxy-haemoglobin is the cause of death in carbon monoxide poisoning as from car exhaust.

carboxylic acids a group of non-steroidal anti-inflammatory and ANALGESIC drugs that includes aspirin, aloxiprin, mefenamic acid, fenbufen and ibuprofen.

carboxylic acid derivatives drugs used to treat epilepsy. Examples are valproic acid (Convulex) and sodium valproate (Epilim).

carboxymethylcellulose a drug used as artificial saliva in the treatment of dry mouth. A brand name is Glandosane.

carbromal a mild sedative and hypnotic drug. It may cause skin rashes, especially in people sensitive to bromine. The drug is now seldom used.

carbuncle a multiple-headed boil. A severe STAPHYLOCOCCAL INFECTION of several adjacent hair follicles which may be over 5 cm across.

carcinogen any CANCER-producing agency.

carcinogenesis the causation of cancer, whether CARCINOMA or SARCOMA.

carcinogenic 1 causing cancer.
2 capable of causing cancer.

carcinoid syndrome a rare condition in which bowel tumours of cells of endocrine origin spread to other parts of the body and secrete large quantities of highly active substances such as SEROTONIN, HISTAMINE, BRADYKININ, ACTH, INSULIN or growth hormone. These cause symptoms such as flushing, diarrhoea, cramping abdominal pain, serious heart damage, arthritis and asthma. Carcinoid syndrome produces unpredictable and severe swings of blood pressure during general anaesthesia calling for careful anaesthetic management. The SOMATOSTATIN analogue drug octreotide (Sandostatin) is important in this context.

carcinoma any CANCER of a surface layer (EPITHELIUM) of the body. Carcinomas are by far the commonest form of cancer and occur on any epithelium especially those of the glandular tissue of the breast, the skin (epidermis), the large bowel, the air tubes (bronchi) of the lungs, and the womb (uterus). Compare SARCOMA.

carcinoma in situ a cancer that remains wholly at the site of its origin and has not spread to deeper tissues or remotely by METASTASIS.

carcinomatosis the state of widespread distribution of CANCER throughout the body occurring at a late stage in many cancers.

Cardene a brand name for NICARDIPINE.

card-, cardio- *combining form denoting* heart.

cardia the opening of the lower end of the gullet (OESOPHAGUS) into the STOMACH.

cardiac 1 pertaining to the heart.
2 pertaining to the CARDIA.

cardiac achalasia failure of food to pass normally from the gullet into the stomach, without organic obstruction.

cardiac arrest complete cessation of the normal heart contractions so that the pumping of the blood stops. In about 30 percent of cases the heart muscle is motionless (asystolic); in the remainder it is in a state of quivering, ineffectual fluttering (ventricular fibrillation). Asystolic cardiac arrest is treated by intravenous injection of VASOPRESSIN alone or followed by ADRENALINE, ventricular fibrillation is treated by electrical defibrillation.

cardiac asthma attacks of severe breathlessness, often occurring at night, caused by congestion of the lungs from failure of the heart to pump blood away from the lungs fast enough (left HEART FAILURE).

cardiac bypass use of a temporary mechanical pump to maintain the blood circulation during a heart operation or to assist the heart during a period of recovery from heart disease or surgery.

cardiac catheterization the passage of a fine, soft, plastic tube into the heart by way of a vein or artery for the purposes of taking measurements of blood pressure or blood gas concentrations, introducing contrast media for ANGIOGRAPHY, or performing BALLOON VALVOTOMY or ANGIOPLASTY.

cardiac massage deliberate repeated compression of the heart so as to maintain the blood circulation when the heart has stopped beating (CARDIAC ARREST). In external cardiac masssage, the heart is repeatedly compressed between the back of the breast bone and the front of the spine by pressure on the front of the chest. In internal massage, the heart is exposed and squeezed with the hand.

cardiac murmur any abnormal sound arising from the heart. Murmurs are timed according to the phase of the heartbeat in which they occur. They may be may be presystolic, systolic, pansystolic, diastolic or continuous (see SYSTOLE). They are also described according to their character.

cardiac neurosis an unjustified conviction that one is suffering from heart disease. A form of HYPOCHONDRIASIS.

cardiac oedema accumulation of fluid in the dependent parts of the body as a result of HEART FAILURE.

cardiac output the volume of blood pumped by the heart in one minute. It is equal to the stroke volume – the output per beat – multiplied by the number of beats per minute.

cardiac pacemaker see PACEMAKER.

cardiac remodelling see HEART REDUCTION.

cardiac stress test an ELECTROCARDIOGRAM (ECG) test done while the subject is exercising, as on a treadmill. This may reveal evidence of relative insufficiency of coronary blood flow that would not show up on an ECG done at rest.

cardiac syndrome X an informal term for the condition of a patient who suffers chest pain typical of angina but who shows no radiological evidence of coronary artery disease and electrocardiographic changes only on exercise stress testing. Some experts believe that this condition is due to transient narrowing of small coronary artery branches (microvascular spasm).

cardiac tamponade abnormal compression of the heart from outside. This may occur as a result of penetrating injuries or a collection of blood or fluid in the sac surrounding the heart (the PERICARDIUM). Tamponade seriously interferes with heart action and calls for urgent relief.

cardiac troponin I a regulatory protein that has been found to be a sensitive marker for heart damage from heart attack (myocardial

infarction) occurring during surgery, a time when the detection of a heart attack may be clinically difficult. Blood levels of this protein are measured prior to surgery and at intervals of a few hours afterwards. A rise is strongly suggestive of a myocardial infarction. The method does not replace the conventional procedures of creatine kinase measurement, ELECTROCARDIOGRAPHY and ECHOCARDIOGRAPHY.

cardialgia pain in the heart.

cardiectomy surgical removal of the upper part of the stomach (the cardia).

Cardilate MR a brand name for NIFEDIPINE.

Cardinol a trade name for PROPRANOLOL.

cardioactive having an effect on the heart.

cardiogenic originating in, or caused by, the heart or a heart disease.

cardiogenic shock surgical SHOCK due to inadequate blood circulation as a result of HEART FAILURE or PULMONARY EMBOLISM.

cardiogram see ELECTROCARDIOGRAM.

cardiography a study of the heart action and function by means of electronic instruments, such as the electro-cardiogram, or by ultrasound scanning (ECHOCARDIOGRAPHY).

cardioinhibitory retarding the heart's action.

cardiolipin a substance derived from beef heart muscle and once much used in the WASSERMAN REACTION test for SYPHILIS. Current interest is focused on immunoglobulins known as anticardiolipin antibodies.

cardiolith a stone (calculus) inside the heart.

cardiologist a heart specialist, usually a physician concerned with the minutiae of cardiac diagnosis and medical treatment, rather than a heart surgeon.

cardiology the study of the heart and its disorders. The list that follows highlights the key entries related to cardiology in the dictionary: angina pectoris, aortic incompetence, aortic stenosis, cardiogenic shock, cardiogram, cardiography, cardioinhibitory, cardiolipin, cardiolith, cardiologist, cardiology, cardiomegaly, cardiomyopathy, cardiomyoplasty, cardionatrin, cardioneurosis, cardiopathy, cardiotoxic, cardiovascular disease, cardiovascular surgeon, cardioversion, carditis, congenital heart disease, congestive heart failure, diastolic heart failure, echocardiography, ectopic heart beat, heart, electrocardiogram, endocarditis, heart attack, heart block, heart disease, heart enlargement, heart examination, heart failure, heart valve replacement, mitral incompetence, mitral stenosis, pericarditis, valvotomy.

cardiomegaly enlargement of the heart. This is caused by an increase in the bulk of the heart muscle (hypertrophy) or by a ballooning out of the chambers of the heart (dilatation).

cardiomyopathy 1 a disease of heart muscle of unknown cause and classified into thickened (hypertrophic), ballooned (dilated) and unyielding (constrictive) cardiomyopathies. 2 heart muscle damage from alcohol, vitamin deficiency, infections, athletic activity, anabolic steroids, autoimmune disease and sarcoidosis. The term is also sometimes applied to heart muscle damage from an inadequate coronary blood supply.

cardiomyoplasty an experimental method of strengthening the action of the heart in cases of heart failure by wrapping the ventricles with living muscles from the back (latissimus dorsi) and prompting these to contract in synchrony with the heartbeat by means of an artificial pacemaker.

cardionatrin see ATRIAL NATRIURETIC FACTOR.

cardioneurosis an unreasonable and irrational conviction that one is suffering from heart disease, sustained in spite of clear evidence to the contrary. See also DA COSTA'S SYNDROME.

cardiopathy any heart disorder or disease.

cardioplegia deliberate temporary stopping of the heart beat (contractions) in the course of heart surgery, either by cooling or by means of drugs.

cardiopulmonary pertaining to the heart and the lungs.

cardiopulmonary bypass the avoidance of circulation of blood through the heart and lungs by the use of an artificial pumping device (HEART-LUNG MACHINE), so as to allow unimpeded open heart surgery or heart transplantation.

cardiopulmonary resuscitation combined heart compression (CARDIAC MASSAGE) and 'kiss of life' (mouth-to-mouth artificial respiration). Commonly abbreviated to CPR. New guidelines, issued by the International Liaison Committee on Resuscitation (ILCOR) in August 2000, recommend that lay people should no longer check for a pulse before starting chest compressions. If no signs such as breathing, coughing, spontaneous motions, or movements in response to stimulation are present chest compressions should begin. If only one helper is present, chest compression alone, without mouth-to-mouth artificial respiration, is acceptable. Chest compressions generate enough force to clear most obstructions and therefore rescuers are now to begin CPR immediately and let chest compressions clear the airway.

cardiorenal pertaining to the heart and the kidneys.

cardiorespiratory pertaining to the heart and the respiratory system.

cardiorrhaphy stitching (suturing) the heart muscle usually to repair a traumatic wound.

cardiorrhexis rupture of the wall of the heart.

cardiospasm tight contraction and failure to relax (ACHALASIA) of the muscle ring (sphincter) at the lower end of the gullet (the CARDIA). This causes obstruction to the passage of food. Cardiospasm has nothing to do with the heart, but relates to the CARDIA.

cardiothoracic pertaining to the heart and the chest cavity and its contents.

cardiotocography a method of producing a composite recording of the fetal heart rate and the activity of the womb during late pregnancy and labour, by means of a microphone applied to the mother's abdominal wall or by picking up the fetal ELECTROCARDIOGRAPH.

cardiotomy cutting into the heart or into the CARDIA of the stomach.

cardiotomy syndrome fever, inflammation of the heart sac (PERICARDITIS) and collection of fluid betwen the two layers of the lung coverings (PLEURAL EFFUSION) occurring within weeks or months of an operation on the heart.

cardiotoxic having a damaging or poisoning effect on the heart.

cardiovascular relating to the heart and its connected closed circulatory system of blood vessels (arteries, arterioles, capillaries, venules and veins).

cardiovascular disease any disease of the heart or the blood vessels. Cardiovascular disease is by far the commonest cause of death and disability in the Western World. See also ATHEROSCLEROSIS.

cardiovascular surgeon a heart surgeon and specialist in the surgery of blood vessels.

cardioversion the conversion of a dangerously rapid or irregular heart beat to normal rhythm with an electric shock. A common use is in defibrillation for one of the forms of CARDIAC ARREST or in the correction of ATRIAL FIBRILLATION.

carditis inflammation of the heart.

Cardura, Cardura XL brand names for DOXAZOSIN.

care plan a plan for the medical care of a particular patient or the welfare of a child in care.

Carey-Coombs murmur a transient murmur heard between beats (diastolic murmur) in the acute early stages of heart involvement in RHEUMATIC FEVER but not thereafter. (Carey Franklin Coombs, 1879–1932, English physician). The origin of the hyphen remains a mystery.

caries decay of a tooth or a bone.

carina any keel-shaped ridge in the body, especially the ridge formed where the TRACHEA divides into the two bronchi.

cariogenic tending to cause dental CARIES.

carious decayed.

carisoprodol a centrally-acting muscle relaxant drug used in the treatment of muscle spasms. A brand name is Carisoma.

carmellose a substance that can be applied to the skin or to mucous membrances to form a protective film. Brand names are Celluvisc and, with pectin and gelatin, Orabase.

carminative 1 having the power to relax muscle rings (sphincters) so as to release gas and relieve flatulence.

2 A drug having this property.

carmustine an alkylating agent anticancer drug. A brand name is Bicnu.

carnal knowledge sexual intercourse.

carneous mole a flesh-like mass of tissue in the womb consisting of a dead fetus in its AMNION which has become covered with altered blood clot. The effect of long-retained products of conception. See also ABORTION.

Carnitor a brand name for LEVOCARNITINE.

carotene one of a group of orange pigments found in carrots and some other vegetables. Beta-carotene (provitamin A) is converted to vitamin A in the liver. This vitamin is needed for normal growth and development of bone and skin, for the development of the fetus and for the proper functioning of the RETINA.

carotenaemia excessive carotene in the blood, often causing yellowing of the skin.

carotenoids a large group of yellow or orange pigments occurring in plants some of which have antioxidant properties. Some of the carotenoids are carotenes.

carotid artery one of the paired arteries running up on either side of the front of the neck which, together with the two vertebral arteries, provide the whole blood supply to the head, including the brain.

carotid body a chemical receptor, situated at the first branch of each carotid artery, that monitors oxygen levels in the blood and regulates the rate of breathing accordingly.

carotid endarterectomy a surgical procedure to widen the lumen of a carotid artery narrowed by ATHEROSCLEROSIS. Preoperative assessment is by duplex ultrasound, magnetic resonance angiography (MRA) and CT angiography. The vessel is clamped and opened with a longitudinal incision and the atherosclerotic plages removed. The effectiveness of the procedure depends largely on how extensively the state of branches of the carotids higher up towards the brain are affected. Carotid stenosis may be caused by a wafer-thin fibrous diaphragm.

carotid sinus a small widening of the wall of each CAROTID ARTERY, at the first branch (bifurcation), that contains pressure-sensitive nerve endings to monitor blood pressure and provide feedback data for its control.

carotid sinus syndrome a tendency to faint or to suffer convulsions or even CARDIAC ARREST as a result of over-stimulation of the carotid sinus causing extreme slowing of the heart.

carpal pertaining to the wrist or wrist bones (carpals).

carpal tunnel a restricted space on the front of the wrist, bounded by ligaments, through which pass the tendons which flex the fingers and wrist and one of the two sensory nerves to the hand, the median nerve.

carpal tunnel syndrome the result of any swelling occurring within the CARPAL TUNNEL. There is compression of the median nerve causing pain, numbness and tingling in one half of the hand, on the thumb side. The condition is commonest in middle aged women and may require injections of steroids or surgical decompression. Ultrasound treatment has also been used.

carphology aimless plucking at the bedclothes seen in people in delirium, exhaustion or DEMENTIA.

carpometacarpal pertaining to the wrist bones (carpals) and the bones of the palms of the hands (metacarpals), especially to the joints betweem them.

carpopedal pertaining to the hands and feet. The term is most often used in referring to spasm of the muscles affecting the hands and feet (carpopedal spasm) that occurs in TETANY.

carpus the wrist or the bones of the wrist.

carrier 1 a person permanently or temporarily immune to a disease-producing organism (pathogen) which is present in his or her body, and which can be passed on, directly or indirectly, to others. A person who carries infectious organisms without ever having suffered the disease is known as a 'casual carrier'. 2 a person with one normal and one affected gene (heterozygous) for a condition which is expressed only if both genes bear the defect for the condition (recessive inheritance). Such a person does not show the condition but can pass on the gene to an offspring who could inherit the other gene from the other parent. 3 any molecule that, by attaching itself to a non-immunogenic molecule, can provide EPITOPES for helper T cells thus making the second molecule immunogenic. See also TYPHOID CARRIER.

Carrion's disease see BARTONELLOSIS. (Daniel A. Carrion, 1850–86, Peruvian medical student).

car sickness see MOTION SICKNESS.

carteolol a BETA-BLOCKER drug used as eyedrops in the treatment of GLAUCOMA. A brand name is Teoptic.

Cartesian relating to the philosophy, methods or coordinates of Descartes, who proposed the notion of a mind-body dualism ('ghost in the machine') which has haunted medical thought ever since, but which is now beginning to be rejected by many of those with enough interest to consider the matter. (René Descartes, 1596–1650, French mathematician and philosopher)

cartilage gristle. A dense form of connective tissue performing various functions in the body such as providing bearing surfaces in the joints, flexible linkages for the ribs, and a supportive tissue in which bone may be formed during growth.

cartilaginous of, pertaining to, or formed in, CARTILAGE.

caruncle 1 a small fleshy protuberance which may be normal or abnormal depending on its location. 2 the small body at the inner corner of each eye.

carvedilol a drug used in the treatment of HEART FAILURE and ANGINA PECTORIS. A brand name is Eucardic.

Carylderm a brand name for CARBARYL.

cascade a physiological system in which the completion of one event has an outcome that initiates the next successive event. Blood coagulation, for instance, is a cascade involving more than a dozen successive events. In genetics a cascade system controls the order in which genes are expressed.

cascara sagrada the 'sacred bark' of the cascara buckthorn tree *Rhamnus purshiana* formerly popular as a strong laxative, but now seldom recommended.

caseation degeneration of dead tissue into a cheese like material. Caseation was a common feature of TUBERCULOSIS of the lungs and led to cavity formation. Also known as caseous degeneration.

casein a protein derived from CASEINOGEN in milk by the action of renin in the stomach.

caseinogen the principal protein in milk, present in higher proportion in cow's milk than in human milk.

Casoni test a test for tapeworm larval infestation (HYDATID DISEASE). A small quantity of sterile hydatid fluid is injected into the skin and causes a local reaction if positive. (Tomaso Casoni, 1880–1933, Italian physician).

caspases a family of proteases, some of which are involved in APOPTOSIS.

cassava poisoning the effect of the cyanide in unprocessed cassava. There is unsteadiness of gait due to damage to the nerve fibre tracts in the spinal cord (tropical spinal ataxia).

cassette a light-tight container for X-ray film.

cast 1 an abnormal moulded shape, corresponding to the inside of a kidney tubule or a small air tube in the lungs (bronchiole) formed when excreted material such as protein or mucus solidifies in situ. 2 a supportive shell of bandage-reinforced Plaster of Paris used to immobilize fractures during healing.

Castleman's tumour benign, hyaline, giant

lymph node hyperplasia. The condition is frequently associated with the autoimmune mucocutaneous disease PEMPHIGUS and this usually improves markedly if the tumour is removed. It is presumed that the Castleman's tumour secretes autoantibodies against epidermal proteins. (Benjamin Castleman, 1906–1982, American pathologist).

castor oil an oil derived from the poisonous seeds of the plant, Ricinus communis and formerly used to treat CONSTIPATION.

castration the removal of the testicles (orchidectomy or orchiectomy), or, sometimes, of all the male external genitalia. The term is also occasionally used to refer to the removal of the ovaries in women. Castration can be valuable in the treatment of androgen dependent cancer of the prostate gland, even if widespread.

casual carrier see CARRIER.

CAT *abbrev. for* computerized axial tomography (CT SCANNING).

catabolism the breakdown of complex body molecules to simpler forms, as when muscle protein breaks down to amino acids or fats to glycerol and fatty acids. The opposite process is called ANABOLISM and both processes are encompassed in METABOLISM.

catalase an ENZYME found in the microbodies (peroxisomes) of cells that promotes the reaction in which two molecules of hydrogen peroxide are converted to two molecules of water and one molecule of oxygen.

catalepsy muscle rigidity, lack of awareness and the abnormal maintenance, often for long periods, of sometimes bizarre postures or attitudes. This was once a common feature of SCHIZOPHRENIA but seems to have become rare in recent years.

catalyst a chemical substance that promotes or accelerates a chemical reaction without itself being changed. Most biochemical catalysts are ENZYMES and almost all body chemistry depends on the catalytic action of thousands of different enzymes.

catamnesis an old-fashioned term for the medical history following an illness. Doctors can no longer hope to get away with the use of such terms with intent to impress.

cataplasm a poultice.

cataplexy the momentary paralysis, or weakness of the limbs, that sometimes affects

people surprised by a strong emotion such as, anger, fear, jealousy, happiness or hilarity.

Catapres a brand name for CLONIDINE, a drug used to treat high blood pressure (HYPERTENSION). A stimulator of the alpha$_2$-adrenoceptor sites. See also ALPHA-ADRENOCEPTOR BLOCKING DRUGS.

cataract opacification of the internal focussing lens of the eye (the crystalline lens) due to irreversible structural changes in the orderly arrangement of the fibres from which the lens is made as a result of aggregation of crystallin protein in the lens. These changes may be CONGENITAL, the result of trauma, or, most commonly, an apparently spontaneous age-related effect. Some experts believe that age-related cataract is caused by ultraviolet radiation in sunlight but others disagree.

cataract surgery the operation to remove a cataractous lens and, usually, to replace it with a plastic lens implant. This operation can now be performed through a very small incision. The lens can be emulsified and sucked out and replaced with a flexible plastic implant that is inserted rolled up.

catarrh inflammation of mucous membrane lining of an organ, especially the nose and throat. Catarrhal inflammation results in excess mucus secretion.

catatonia a syndrome of abnormalities of movement or position associated with psychiatric conditions, hysteria or organic brain disease. There may be stereotyped movements, meaningless violence, overactivity, CATALEPSY, negativism or stupor.

cat cry syndrome see CRI DU CHAT SYNDROME.

catecholamines the group of AMINES, which includes adrenaline, noradrenaline, dopamine and chemically related amines. These are derived from the amino acid tyrosine, and act as neurotransmitters or hormones.

categorical variables qualitative variables, variables that cannot meaningfully be expressed in numbers. eg. skin colour.

catgut twisted strips of COLLAGEN prepared from sheep intestine and used as surgical stitches (SUTURES) and ties (LIGATURES). Catgut is absorbable and need not be removed. Chromic catgut is processed chemically to retard the rate of absorption.

catharsis 1 purging of the bowels.
2 a psychoanalytic term meaning the release

of anxiety and tension experienced when repressed matter, which has been 'poisoning' the mind, is brought into consciousness.

cathepsin any ENZYME that acts to split the interior PEPTIDE bonds of a protein, causing its decomposition.

cathepsis protein HYDROLYSIS by CATHEPSINS.

catheter a flexible plastic tube used to empty hollow organs, especially the urinary bladder, or to gain access to inaccessible parts of the body, especially the blood vessels and the heart. Drainage catheters have not changed much in recent years but there has been a revolution in the design and application of catheters for other purposes such as ANGIOGRAPHY and BALLOON CATHETER treatments. See also CARDIAC CATHETERIZATION and URINARY CATHETERIZATION.

catheterization the act of passing a CATHETER into the body for any purpose. See CARDIAC CATHETERIZATION and URINARY CATHETERIZATION.

catheterization, intermittent the passage of a urinary catheter to empty the bladder on an 'as required' basis in cases of outflow obstruction as from prostate gland enlargement. The procedure can be performed by the sufferer himself and may afford great relief. Current medical opinion is that the method is safe, effective and could, with benefit, be more widely used.

cathetron a device for delivering highly radioactive substances into proximity to a tumour and returning them to a shielded safe after use.

cathexis a Freudian concept in which 'emotional energy' is said to be concentrated on, or attached to, an idea, person or object, in much the way, according to Freud, that an electric charge can be retained on insulating material. The investment of 'libidinal' energy in something. See also FREUDIAN THEORY.

cation a positively charged atom, such as Na^+ or K^+, which is attracted towards a negative electrode (cathode). An atom which, in solution, takes a positive charge. Unlike charges attract; like charges repel.

CAT scanning see CT SCANNING.

cat-scratch fever a disease caused by an unknown organism transmitted by the scratch of a cat. A small, red, crusted swelling develops at the site of the scratch, local lymph nodes become swollen and tender and form abscesses, and there is fever, headache and loss of appetite.

caucasian a term commonly used to refer to a person who is neither black, brown, yellow or red. It is based on the anthropologically disreputable theory that humankind can be divided into five ethnic classes – Caucasians, Negroes, Mongols, Malaysians and Americans.

cauda equina the leash of spinal nerves hanging down in the spinal canal below the termination of the SPINAL CORD, at about the level of the first lumbar vertebra.

cauda equina syndrome the result of a central protrusion backwards of the pulpy inner material (nucleus pulposus) of an INTERVERTEBRAL DISC, in the part of the spinal canal below the termination of the spinal cord. A leash of nerves run down in this area and these may be compressed. There is acute back pain, SCIATICA and interference with bladder function.

caudal pertaining to the tail end of the body. Denoting a tailward direction in anatomy. Although not externally visible, the human tail still exists, in a vestigial form, as the COCCYX.

caudate possessing a tail.

caudate nucleus a large collection of grey matter (nerve cell bodies) lying deep in the white matter of the lower part of the CEREBRUM on either side of the midline, and concerned with the control of movement. One of the basal ganglia of the brain.

caul a persistent AMNION membrane covering the baby's head at birth. Normally, the amnion ruptures before birth allowing the baby to pass through.

cauliflower ear the result of repeated blows to the ears with bleeding between the cartilage and the skin, and the subsequent organization of the blood clot into fibrous tissue. One of the least serious occupational hazards of boxing.

causalgia severe and persistent burning pain in a limb caused by partial damage to a nerve trunk, usually from physical injury. The injured nerve spontaneously generates impulses which are interpreted by the brain as pain.

caustic any chemical substance which corrodes and destroys bodily tissue.

cauterization the deliberate destruction of tissue by the local application of heat using an instrument known as a cautery. This may be a simple heated probe, an electrically heated wire loop, a high-frequency electrode or a laser. See also DIATHERMY.

cautery a surgical instrument or agent used to burn, scar or destroy tissue. The electric cautery often consists of a short loop of wire, at the end of an insulated handle, which is made red hot by the passage of an electric current. The actual cautery is a metal rod heated in a flame.

caval pertaining to the great veins, the VENA CAVAE.

Caverject a brand name for ALPROSTADIL.

cavernous sinus the large vein channel, lying immediately behind each eye socket (orbit) and on each side of the PITUITARY GLAND. Through it run a loop of the internal carotid artery, the nerve supplying the central part of the face with sensation, and several nerves supplying the muscles that move the eye. The sinuses receive veins from the face and orbits and communicate with each other and with other large veins surrounding the brain.

cavernous sinus thrombosis a serious condition caused by the backward spread of infection from the veins of the face or eye socket into an important venous channel, the cavernous sinus, within the skull. Intensive antibiotic treatment is necessary to save life.

cavity, dental an area of tooth enamel destroyed by acids formed by the action of mouth bacteria on carbohydrate food particles accumulating around unbrushed teeth.

cavus a foot deformity in which the longitudinal arch is greatly exaggerated. See also, PES CAVUS.

CCFP *abbrev. for* Certificate of the College of Family Physicians.

CCHE *abbrev. for* Central Council for Health Education.

CCN proteins a family of six cellular signalling regulator proteins with a wide range of functions. They are concerned in cell proliferation and differentiation, wound healing, OSTEOGENESIS, CHONDROGENESIS and ANGIOGENESIS.

CCU *abbrev. for* coronary care unit.

CD *abbrev. for* cluster of differentiation (or designation). This is a standard descriptive code applied to antigenic surface molecules on white cells, especially T LYMPHOCYTES, that are identified by a particular group of monoclonal antibodies. Well over 100 CD receptors have been described.

CD1 antigen a cell membrane complex found on THYMUS cells, on some peripheral B cells and on dendritic cells in the skin. They are coded for by five genes on chromosome 1 and are structurally similar to the MAJOR HISTOCOMPATIBILITY COMPLEX.

CD2 antigen a complex found on some bone marrow stem cells and on pre-thymocytes. The genes are on chromosome 1.

CD3 antigen a cell membrane complex of five polypeptide chains that is the signal transduction element of the T cell receptor on helper and cytotoxic T cells. Transduction occurs on interaction with antigen.

CD4 antigen a glycoprotein cell surface molecule on helper T cells (T LYMPHOCYTES) that recognizes major histocompatibility complex (MHC) class II molecules on antigen-presenting cells. Because of this, helper T cells are often referred to as CD4 cells.

CD5 antigen a membrane glycoprotein found on all human T cells, but on greater quantity on helper T cells. Found also on peritoneal and pleural B cells.

CD8 antigen a glycoprotein cell surface molecule on cytotoxic T cells (T LYMPHOCYTES) that recognizes major histocompatibility complex (MHC) class I molecules on target cells. Because of this, cytotoxic T cells are often referred to as CD8 cells.

CD14 antigen a lipopolysaccharide-binding protein found on the cell membranes of macrophages, monocytes, dendritic cells and other cells of the germinal follicles of the spleen. CD14 antigens are thought to be essential for the differentiation of the cells of the monocyte and myelocyte series. The genes are on chromosome 5.

CDH *abbrev. for* 1 congenital dislocation of the hip.
2 congenital disease of the heart.

CEA *abbrev. for* carcinoembryonic antigen. This is a protein material originally isolated from colon cancer cells and used as a marker in the diagnosis and follow-up of cases of cancer.

Cedocard Retard a brand name for ISOSORBIDE DINITRATE.

cefaclor a broad-spectrum antibiotic. One of the CEPHALOSPORINS that can be taken by mouth. Brand names are Distaclor and Keftid.

cefadroxil a CEPHALOSPORIN ANTIBIOTIC drug. A brand name is Baxan

cefamandole a CEPHALOSPORIN ANTIBIOTIC drug. A brand name is Kefadol.

cefixime a CEPHALOSPORIN ANTIBIOTIC drug. A brand name is Suprax.

cefotaxime a third-generation CEPHALOSPORIN antibiotic active against Gram-negative organisms but not staphylococci. A brand name is Claforan.

cefpirome a CEPHALOSPORIN ANTIBIOTIC drug. A brand name is Cefrom.

cefpodixime a CEPHALOSPORIN ANTIBIOTIC drug. A brand name is Orelox.

Cefrom a brand name for CEFPIROME.

ceftazidime a CEPHALOSPORIN ANTIBIOTIC drug. The drug is on the WHO official list. Brand names are Fortum and Kefadim.

ceftriaxone a CEPHALOSPORIN ANTIBIOTIC drug. The drug is on the WHO official list. The drug is on the WHO official list. A brand name is Rocephin.

cefuroxime a second-generation CEPHALOSPORIN antibiotic active against staphylococci and some GRAM-NEGATIVE organisms. It must be given by injection. Brand names are Zinacef and Zinnat.

Celance a brand name for PERGOLIDE.

celebrity worship syndrome a common condition of intense preoccupation with all ascertainable aspects, real or media-contrived, of the life of a current 'star' personality. In severe cases the syndrome amounts to an obsession that may feature stalking and other criminal activity. The syndrome is now taken seriously by psychologists and even by some anthropologists who hold that celebrities have always provided useful role models. Fortunately, for most, celebrity worship is no more than a harmless entertainment.

Celestone a trade name for BETAMETHASONE.

Celevac a brand name for METHYL CELLULOSE.

celiprolol a cardio-selective beta blocker drug. A brand name is Celectol.

cell the structural unit of the body and of all living things, whether plant or animal. Body cells vary in size from one hundredth of a millimetre to about a tenth of a millimetre, in the case of the OVUM. They are structurally complex and are engaged in constant physical, biochemical and genetic activity. The outer cell membrane contains specialized sites for the receipt of chemical information from the external environment and other receptors for the pumping of dissolved substances into and out of the cell. The central nucleus contains the chromatin – the DNA genetic blueprint for the reproduction of the cell and for the synthesis of enzymes. Surrounding the nucleus is the cytoplasm. This contains many important structures (organelles), such as the MITOCHONDRIA (tiny bags containing enzymes needed for the metabolic processes of the cell and for the conversion of glucose and oxygen into energy) and the RIBOSOMES in which proteins are formed.

cell biology the study of cells and their functions. The list that follows highlights the key entries related to cell biology in the dictionary: activated cells, basal cell, B cells, beta cells, Betz cells, blood cells, cell, cell differentiation, cell line, centrioles, cytotoxic T cells, delta cells, dendritic cell, endoplasmic reticulum, extracellular, extracellular matrix, germ cells, giant cell, Golgi apparatus, helper T cell, intercellular, intracellular, killer cells, Langerhans cell, mast cell, lysosomes, membrane-protein ion channels, memory cells, mitochondria, mononuclear cell, nucleus, organelle, peroxisomes, plasma cell, plasma membrane, Purkinje cells, red blood cell, resting membrane potential, ribosomes, Schwann cell, regenerative cell therapy, squamous cell, stem cell, T cell, unicellular, white blood cell.

Cellcept a brand name for MYCOPHENOLATE MOFETIL.

cell differentiation the process by which primitive dividing cells, all of which originally appear identical, alter and diversify to form different tissues and organs. See also HOMEOBOX GENES.

cell-free protein synthesis the artificial production of proteins by the addition of MESSENGER RNA to a medium containing enzymes, amino acids, ribosomes, transfer RNA and cofactors.

cell line the CLONE or clones of cells derived from a small piece of tissue grown in culture.

cell-mediated immunity action by the immune system involving T cells (T LYMPHOCYTES) and concerned with protection against viruses, fungi, TUBERCULOSIS and cancers and rejection of foreign grafted material. Cell-mediated immunity is not primarily effected by ANTIBODIES.

cellular infiltration 1 the movement of inflammatory white cells into tissue.
2 the movement of cancer cells into a tissue.

cellular telephone dangers these include inattention to driving with the risk of traffic accidents, a significant risk of interference with cardiac pacemakers, and a postulated risk to the brain from high-frequency (microwave) electromagnetic radiation. Research suggests that the risk of pacemaker upset is significant only if the telephone is held over the pacemaker site. Scientists agree that the brain heating effect of radiation from phones is negligible. Several major studies of the possible dangers of brain cancer and other diseases have produced no statistically significant findings. Research continues.

cellulite a lay term for the fatty deposits, with connective tissue strand dimpling, around the thighs and buttocks.

cellulitis spreading inflammation of tissue, most commonly the skin, caused by infection with organisms, often streptococci, which secrete enzymes that break down natural defensive planes in the tissue and allow spread of infection. Cellulitis usually responds well to antibiotics.

Cellulone a trade name for METHYL CELLULOSE.

cellulose a complex polysaccharide forming the structural elements in plants and forming 'roughage' in many vegetable foodstuffs. Cellulose cannot be digested to simpler sugars and remains in the intestine.

Celevac a brand name for methyl cellulose, used as a laxative.

Celsius scale a temperature scale in which the freezing point is 0 degrees and the boiling point 100. This corresponds to the old Centigrade scale and is a sensible alternative to the arbitrary Fahrenheit scale, with 32 as freezing point and 212 as boiling point. So the normal body temperature of 98.4 °F has become 37 °C. (Anders Celsius, 1701–1744, Swedish astronomer).

cementum the layer of calcified substance covering the root of a tooth.

cementoblast a cell that actively forms CEMENTUM.

cementocyte a cell found in the tiny spaces (lacunae) in the CEMENTUM and having processes radiating into the cementum CANALICULI.

censor a Freudian idea for the supposed agency that distorts or symbolizes repressed unpleasant material in the unconscious so that it need not be directly recognized either in dreams or in waking awareness. See also FREUDIAN THEORY.

centesis surgical puncture of a membrane or body cavity, usually for diagnostic purposes. See AMNIOCENTESIS, PARACENTESIS.

centigrade this is identical, in every respect, to the CELSIUS SCALE. Centigrade literally means '100 levels' and this is what the Celsius scale contains. The change to Celsius was purely for honorific reasons.

centigray a unit of radioactivity used in RADIOTHERAPY. A gray is the energy absorption of 1 joule per kg of irradiated material. 1 gy is equivalent to 100 rads so 1 centigray is equivalent to 1 rad (radiation absorbed dose).

centiles see PERCENTILE.

centimorgan a unit of distance between two genes on a chromosome, representing a 1% probability of recombination in a single meiotic event. Named after Thomas Hunt Morgan (1866–1945) the American Nobel-prizewinning geneticist often described as the father of modern genetics.

central alpha-agonists drugs used to treat menopausal flushing. An example is clonidine hydrochloride (Dixarit).

central anticholinergic syndrome a form of atropine poisoning in which atropine acts on central nervous system cholinergic receptors to cause neurological disturbances including confusion and even long-lasting coma. The syndrome is occasionally seen after surgical anaesthesia in which atropine premedication has been given or after dobutamine-atropine stress echocardiography. It has also been described after MEFLOQUINE treatment of MALARIA.

central dogma the proposition by Francis Crick (1916–2004) that, in genetics, the only possible progression was from DNA to RNA to protein. The discovery that retroviruses used RNA to make DNA demonstrated the riskiness of pronouncing dogmas in science.

centrally-acting antihypertensives drugs used to treat high blood pressure that act directly on the brain. Examples are methyldopa (Aldomet), clonidine (Catapres) and moxonidine (Physiotens).

central nervous system (CNS) the brain and

its downward continuation, the spinal cord, which lies in the spinal canal within the spine (vertebral column). The central nervous system is entirely encased in bone and is contrasted with the peripheral nervous system, which consists of the 12 pairs of cranial nerves arising directly from the brain, the 31 pairs of spinal nerves running out of the spinal cord, and the AUTONOMIC NERVOUS SYSTEM.

central pontine myelinolysis a rare disorder featuring an area of severe loss of myelin in nerve fibres running through the middle of the PONS in the brainstem. There is progressive failure of verbal articulation (dysarthria) and spastic paralysis in all four limbs (quadriplegia). The condition may occur in alcoholism, liver disease, kidney failure and rapid correction of severe sodium depletion.

central venous pressure the pressure of blood in the right atrium. This is measured by an in-dwelling catheter carrying a pressure transducer. Central venous pressure readings provide valuable diagnostic information in a range of serious heart and lung conditions.

centrifuge a laboratory machine that subjects matter suspended in solution to powerful outward-tending forces by high-speed rotation. This allows particles of different mass to be separated into bands.

centriole a short, hollow, cylindrical ORGANELLE consisting of nine sets of microtubules and usually occurring in pairs set at right angles to each other. Centrioles are responsible for the production of the spindle apparatus that appears just before the separation of the chromosomes into two sets prior to cell division.

centrilobular situated at the centre of a LOBULE of an organ, such as the liver.

centriole one of the two rod-like bodies in cells forming the poles of the spindles during cell division.

centromere the constriction in a chromosome at which the two identical halves (chromatids) of the newly longitudinally-divided chromosome are joined, and at which the chromosome attaches to the spindle fibre during division (mitosis). The centromere contains no genes.

centrosome a small mass of CYTOPLASM, lying near the nucleus of a cell and consisting of a pair of centrioles, which divides into two parts before cell division. These migrate to the poles

of the cell and the spindle develops between them.

cephal-, cephalo- *combining form denoting* head.

cephalad situated towards the head.

cephalalgia headache or pain in the head.

cephalexin cefalexin, a CEPHALOSPORIN antibiotic effective by mouth. Brand names are Ceporex and Keflex.

cephalhaematoma a collection of blood between a baby's skull and the overlying membrane (the PERIOSTEUM) usually resulting from unavoidable injury sustained in the course of a difficult forceps delivery. Cephalhaematoma appearing later in life must be investigated, because it may indicate a fractured skull.

cephalic relating to the head or in the direction of the head.

cephalocele a protrusion of part of the brain through an opening in the skull.

cephalodynia headache.

cephalometry measurement of the various diameters and other dimensions of the head.

cephalosporin one of a range of antibiotics first obtained from a *Cephalosporium* fungus found in the sea near a sewage outflow. Their chemical structure is very similar to that of the penicillins and many semisynthetic forms have been developed. Their toxicity is low and they are effective against a wide range of organisms. Unfortunately, the spelling of cephalosporin drug names shows an apparently arbitrary distribution of 'ceph', 'cep' and 'cef', with a strong tendency to the latter, assisted by the recent requirement to adopt European nomenclature regulations.

cephamandole cefamandole, a cephalosporin antibiotic.

cephazolin cefazolin, a CEPHALOSPORIN antibiotic drug. A brand name is Kefzol.

cephradine cefradine, a CEPHALOSPORIN antibiotic drug. A brand name is Velosef

Ceporex a brand name for cephalexin (cefalexin), a CEPHALOSPORIN antibiotic.

cercaria the tailed, swimming larva of a trematode worm, such as a SCHISTOSOME.

cerebellar ataxia MOTOR incoordination due to disease of the CEREBELLUM.

cerebellum the smaller sub-brain lying below and behind the CEREBRUM. The cerebellum has long been thought to be concerned only with the coordination of information concerned with posture, balance and fine voluntary movement. Recent studies have shown, however, that the cerebellum functions to assist in many cognitive and perceptual processes. The cerebellum may also have a role to play in coordinating sensory input, and even in memory, attention and emotion.

cerebral 1 pertaining to the cerebrum or brain. 2 having the quality of intellectualism.

cerebral activators drugs used in an attempt to improve the condition of people with mild degrees of DEMENTIA. Examples are co-dergocrine (Hydergine) and naftidrofuryl oxalate (Praxilene).

cerebral cortex the grey outer layer of the cerebral hemispheres, consisting of the layered masses of nerve cell bodies which perform the higher neurological functions.

cerebral haemorrhage bleeding within the brain or under the membranes surrounding it. See also SUBARACHNOID HAEMORRHAGE, STROKE.

cerebral hemispheres the two halves of the CEREBRUM joined by the CORPUS CALLOSUM.

cerebral palsy see SPASTIC PARALYSIS.

cerebral thrombosis blockage of an artery supplying the brain with blood so that an area of brain is deprived and suffers injury or tissue death. This is a very common cause of STROKE.

cerebration thinking.

cerebrosides glucolipids present in nerve tissue, especially in myelin sheaths. Their metabolism requires HYDROLASES and it is inherited mutations of the genes for these enzymes that causes conditions such serious as Tay-Sachs, Gaucher's, Fabry's and Niemann-Pick disease.

cerebrospinal pertaining to both the brain and the spinal cord.

cerebrospinal fever see MENINGITIS.

cerebrospinal fluid the watery fluid that bathes the brain and spinal cord and also circulates within the ventricles of the brain and the central canal of the cord.

cerebrospinal meningitis inflammation of the MENINGES of both brain and spinal cord.

cerebrovascular pertaining to the blood vessels supplying the brain.

cerebrovascular accident medical jargon or euphemism for any of the events causing STROKE, such as cerebral thrombosis, cerebral haemorrhage or EMBOLISM of a cerebral artery.

cerebrovascular disease damage to the brain caused by disease of the arteries supplying it with blood, especially ATHEROSCLEROSIS. Arterial disease results in an inadequate blood flow and a reduction in the supply of vital oxygen and sugar. This leads to TRANSIENT ISCHAEMIC ATTACKS and STROKE.

cerebrum the largest, and most highly developed, part of the brain. It contains the neural structures for memory and personality, cerebration, volition, speech, vision, hearing, voluntary movement, all bodily sensation, smell, taste and other functions.

CertAvMed *abbrev. for* Certificate in Aviation Medicine.

certification of insanity a now historic documentary deposition that a person suffering from a mental disorder should be indefinitely physically detained. Certification was abolished in Britain in 1959 and replaced by a Mental Health Act which makes provision for compulsory admission to hospital for periods of observation of up to 28 days (Section 25), or for longer periods, if necessary (Section 26). This is done on application by the nearest relative or by the Mental Welfare Officer supported by the recommendation of two doctors.

certoparin a heparin-like drug used to prevent the formation of blood clots in the veins. A brand name is Alphaparin.

Cerubidin a brand name for DAUNORUBICIN.

cerumen ear wax.

ceruminosis excess ear wax production. This leads to blockage of the external ear canal (the auditory meatus) and readily-remediable deafness.

cerumolytics drugs used to soften ear wax. Examples are urea hydrogen peroxide (Exterol), docusate sodium (Waxsol) and sodium bicarbonate war drops.

cervical pertaining to a neck. This may be the neck of the body or the neck of an organ such as the womb. The noun, from the adjective 'cervical' is 'cervix'.

cervical cancer cancer of the cervix of the womb (uterus). This cancer is the second highest cause of cancer deaths in women worldwide with half a million new cases each year. It is usually associated with the human papillomavirus (HPV) and the strain HPV-16 is present is almost half of all cases of this cancer.

Several trials of vaccines against this strain of HPV have shown that vaccination can significantly reduce the risk of developing cervical cancer.

cervical cap see CAP, CONTRACEPTIVE.

cervical disc syndrome neck and shoulder pain and loss of sensation resulting from protrusion of the pulpy centre of an INTERVERTEBRAL DISC in the neck region. The extruded nucleus pulposus presses on the spinal nerve roots.

cervical erosion an inaccurate term for the normal extension of the inner lining of the womb out on to the usually smooth and lighter-coloured membrane covering the mouth of the cervix.

cervical incompetence the inability of the inner opening of the neck of the womb to remain properly closed. This is a cause of repeated, painless, spontaneous abortions around the fourth or fifth month of pregnancy and affects about one pregnancy in 100. This can be prevented with a temporary encircling stitch (a Shirodkar suture), but the difficulty is to know which women are likely to be affected. Women with a history of mid-term miscarriage are obvious candidates for cerclage. The procedure can be done as an emergency if threatened miscarriage is detected in time.

cervical intraepithelial neoplasia (CIN) a cancer of the cervix that is still confined to the outer layer, the epithelium, and is readily curable. CIN is graded I to III depending on the degree of severity. The principal cause of CIN is the human papillomavirus type 16, and promiscuous sexual intercourse with men is an important risk factor for cervical cancer. But about 1 woman in 5 who have never had heterosexual intercourse carries the papillomavirus.

cervical osteoarthritis a wearing away of the cartilage surfaces of the spinal bones (vertebrae) of the neck. This is commonest in middle age and causes persistent pain, neck stiffness and sometimes tenderness on pressure over the affected area. See also SPONDARTHRITIS, SPONDYLITIS.

cervical rib a short, floating, rudimentary rib attached to the lowest neck vertebra on one or both sides. In about 10% of cases the rib causes compression of arteries or nerves in the neck,

leading to pain and tingling, or sometimes more serious effects, in the arm or hand.

cervical smear test PAP smear. A screening test for cancer of the neck of the womb. Surface cells are scraped off with a wooden or plastic spatula and spread on a slide for microscopic examination. It was developed by George Nicholas Papanicolaou (1883–1962), an American pathologist of Greek origin. Many experts suggest 3-yearly screening for sexually active women over 35 and women who have been pregnant three or more times. The test is also advised for women asking for contraceptive advice. Developments in cervical smear technology include examination by robot.

cervical spondylosis a degenerative condition of the bones of the neck, with backward outgrowth of bone causing narrowing of the spinal canal, and possible compression of the spinal cord. This may lead to muscle weakness and walking disorders.

cervicectomy surgical removal of the neck of the womb (cervix of the UTERUS).

cervicitis inflammation of the neck of the womb. Most cases are caused by sexually transmitted organisms, especially *Chlamydia trachomatis*, causing non-specific urethritis; the gonococcus, causing gonorrhoea; and herpes simplex virus, type II, causing venereal herpes.

cervix the neck of the womb (UTERUS).

cestode a flat worm of the class *Cestoda* which includes the tapeworms.

cetalkonium an antiseptic and analgesic drug used to treat mouth ulcers, discomfort from dentures and infant teething symptoms. A brand name is Bonjela.

Cetavlex a brand name for CETRIMIDE.

cetirizine an ANTIHISTAMINE drug used in the treatment of hay fever and other allergic conditions. A brand name is Zirtek Allergy.

cetrimide a detergent antiseptic and cleaning substance used in solution or as an ointment. A brand name is Cetavlex.

cetylpyridinium chloride an antiseptic drug used in the treatment of throat and mouth infections, usually in the form of lozenges. A brand name is Merocaine.

CFCs see CHLOROFLUOROCARBONS.

Chagas' disease South American trypanosomiasis, a disease spread by the cone-nosed or assassin *reduviid* bug. The organism is *Trypanosma cruzi* and the disease is a major cause of heart damage and HEART FAILURE in endemic areas. (Carlos Chagas, 1879–1934, Brazilian physician).

chain reaction a self-sustaining reaction maintained by producing products that induce it. Neutrons produced by atomic fission in a mass of uranium can induce sustainable further fission of uranium atoms.

chalasia abnormal relaxation or loss of retaining power, especially of the muscle ring at the lower end of the OESOPHAGUS.

chalazion a hard, pea-like swelling in an eyelid, often becoming inflamed, and due to the retention of secretion in a MEIBOMIAN GLAND. Also known as a meibomian cyst.

chalcosis copper poisoning. Abnormal deposition of copper in the tissues.

chalicosis a form of PNEUMOCONIOSIS caused by inhaling stone dust. Also called flint disease.

chalones POLYPEPTIDEs or glycoproteins, released by actively-dividing cells that inhibits chromosomal reproduction (MITOSIS) in cells of the tissue in which they are formed, thus controlling a tendency to HYPERPLASIA.

chamomile a drug used in ointments for the treatment of nappy rash, chapped skin or sore nipples. A brand name is Kamillosan.

chancre the painless, hard-based primary sore of syphilis, which appears on the genitals within four weeks of exposure. It is a shallow ulcer with a base resembling wet wash-leather. This teems with the spirochaetes that cause the disease.

chancroid a sexually transmitted disease of the tropics, often called 'soft sore'. It causes multiple painful ulcers on the genitals and swelling of the groin lymph nodes (buboes).

Chandipura virus a member of the *Vesiculovirus* genus of the Rhabdoviridae family. The virus is a cause of a severe form of acute encephalitis and is thought to be spread by the female sandfly (phlebotomus). At the time of writing, Koch's postulates had not been fulfilled for this virus and encephalitis.

change of life see MENOPAUSE.

chaos theory the mathematical conception that some phenomena that seem random may be of a deterministic order highly sensitive to initial conditions and perturbations. There is a growing appreciation that chaos may be a feature of many biological systems and that chaos theory may prove to have many applications in medicine.

chaperones chaperonins, intracellular proteins that assist in the correct folding of other proteins by means of hydrophobic surfaces that recognize and bind to exposed hydrophobic surfaces on misfolded proteins. Intracellular proteins with these abnormal configurations interact abnormally with other molecules, and many disease processes relate to misfolded proteins. Misfolding of proteins that are regulators of growth and differentiation, for instance, may be an important factor in the causation of cancers. Protein misfolding may be a factor in as many as half of all diseases. Increasing understanding of this phenomenon may lead to new and important therapies.

character disorders see PERSONALITY DISORDERS.

charcoal a black substance formed by heating wood in an atmosphere of restricted oxygen. Charcoal is a powerful adsorber of gases and of fine particulate matter and can be used as an antidote to various poisons, a deodorant, a filter and a remover of intestinal gas. Activated charcoal has been treated to increased its adsorptive properties. It is on the WHO official list.

Charcot-Marie-Tooth disease a hereditary nervous system disorder causing atrophy of the muscles of the lower legs, followed by atrophy of the small muscles of the hands. There is no effective treatment. (Jean-Martin Charcot, 1825–1893, French neurologist; Pierre Marie, 1853–1940, French neurologist; and Howard Henry Tooth, 1856–1926, English physician).

Charcot's joints joints rendered anaesthetic by disease which are, in consequence, vulnerable and suffer damage from repeated injury. Charcot's joints may be caused by many agencies including SYPHILIS, DIABETES, LEPROSY, spinal cord tumour, SYRINGOMYELIA, SUBACUTE COMBINED DEGENERATION OF THE CORD, and steroid injections into the joints. (Jean-Martin Charcot, 1825–1893, French neurologist).

charlatan a person unjustifiably claiming knowledge or skill, especially of medicine or healing. In this age of pseudoscience, it is often difficult to distinguish the charlatan from the merely uninformed.

charleyhorse a popular term for stiffness and cramp of the limbs following unaccustomed or unduly vigorous activity.

CHART *acronym for* Continuous

Hyperfractionated Accelerated Radiotherapy, a form of treatment for non-small-cell lung cancer that has produced a significant improvement in survival compared with conventional radiotherapy.

ChB *abbrev. for* Bachelor of Surgery.

ChD *abbrev. for* Doctor of Surgery.

cheekbiting the undesired interposition of the mucous membrane lining of the cheek between the upper and lower teeth causing pain and local injury.

cheekbone the zygomatic bone.

cheil- *combining form denoting* the lip.

cheilectomy surgical removal of part of the lip, as for a suspected cancer.

cheilion the angle of the mouth.

cheilitis inflammation of the lips from any cause such as sunlight, thrush, vitamin B2 deficiency, streptococcal or staphylococcal infection or constant drooling at the corners.

cheilosis a zone of rawness along the line of closure of the lips that is a feature of vitamin B deficiency diseases such as PELLAGRA.

cheiro- *combining form denoting* the hand.

cheiromegaly enlargement of one or both hands that is not a growth hormone disorder or the result of disease of the pituitary gland. The condition may be caused by SYRINGOMYELIA.

cheiroplasty plastic surgery on the hand.

cheiropompholyx a kind of ECZEMA affecting the palms of the hands in which tiny blisters (vesicles) form. A similar condition of the feet is called podopompholyx.

chelating agents a range of organic compounds that can assimilate and fix metallic ions and thus remove them from the body. They are useful in cases of poisoning and tissue damage from metals. Examples are desferrioxamine (Desferal), dimercaprol, penicillamine (Distamine), deferiprone (Ferriprox), and sodium calcium edetate (Limclair).

chemical castration producing the hormonal effect of castration by means of drugs that block androgen or oestrogen receptors or inhibit the production of natural sex hormones. The term is more often used in a legal than in a medical context.

chemo- *combining form denoting* chemistry or chemical. The term is also used informally as an abbreviation of CHEMOTHERAPY.

chemocautery deliberate tissue destruction by a caustic substance.

chemokines a family of structurally-related protein CYTOKINES that can induce activation and migration of specific types of white cell by chemotaxis. They have a fundamental role in inflammation and are concerned in the immune system protective responses to infecting organisms. Chemokines are also concerned in ANGIOGENESIS.

chemonucleolysis the use of an enzyme injected into the inner pulpy centre of an intervertebral disc so as to break down and liquefy the material. This is done as a treatment for 'slipped disc' (prolapsed intervertebral disc) with pressure on the nerve roots in the spinal canal.

chemopallidectomy injection of a destructive chemical into the GLOBUS PALLIDUM of the brain to relieve the rigidity of PARKINSON'S DISEASE.

chemoprophylaxis the use of drugs or antibacterial chemical agents to prevent the development or spread of infectious diseases.

chemoreceptors nerve endings stimulated to produce nerve impulses by contact with chemical substances or as a result of changes in the local concentration of chemical substances. The receptors for smell and taste, those for oxygen in the carotid bodies and those for glucose in the pancreas are of this type.

chemosis collection of fluid under the CONJUNCTIVA covering the white of the eye so that it balloons forward. Chemosis is an indication of severe inflammation, often from allergy. On resolution of the inflammation, the conjuctiva settles back into place.

chemosurgery the use of chemicals to destroy unwanted tissue.

chemotactic pertaining to CHEMOTAXIS.

chemotaxins agents that promote CHEMOTAXIS.

chemotaxis the movement of a cell or other living organism in a particular direction as a result of attraction by an increasing concentration of a chemical substance. Cells of the immune system find their prey by this means.

chemotherapy the internal use of chemical agents to treat disease, especially infections, infestations and tumours. At one time, the antibiotics were excluded from this group, as being of natural origin, but as many of these have been synthesized this distinction has become too fine. Indeed, since the whole spectrum of pharmacology involves the exhibition of chemical molecules, the term might be thought to have lost all specificity. Commonly-recognized chemotherapeutic agents, however, include drugs used against cancers and leukaemias ('chemo') and those given to kill viruses, microbes, fungi, protozoa, worms and other parasites.

Chemotrim a trade name for a preparation containing SULPHAMETHOXAZOLE and TRIMETHOPRIM.

chenodeoxycholic acid a bile acid with detergent properties. It has been used as a drug to dissolve GALLSTONES, but this takes 6 months to 2 years.

Chenofalk a trade name for CHENODEOXYCOLIC ACID.

Cheyne-Stokes respiration periods of very shallow, almost imperceptible, breathing alternating with periods of deep breathing. This sequence often precedes death (John Cheyne, 1777–1836, Scottish physician; and William Stokes, 1804–78, Irish physician).

chiasma 1 the intersection and partial crossing of the optic nerves behind the eyes within the skull. The fibres on the outer halves of each optic nerve do not cross over; those on the inner halves of each nerve do. Also known as the optic chiasm.
2 the site at which a pair of homologous chromosomes exchange material during MEIOSIS.

chickenpox a usually trivial infectious disease of childhood caused by the varicella-zoster virus which also causes SHINGLES in adults. There is a rash of tiny, flat, red spots which quickly become small blisters (vesicles), turn milky, dry to crusts and then scab off.

chiclero's ulcer a self-healing skin ulcer affecting the sapodilla tree tappers in Mexico, Guatemala and Honduras. It is a form of LEISHMANIASIS of the skin (cutaneous Leishmaniasis) caused by *Leishmania mexicana* and spread by sandflies.

chicungunya fever an ARBOVIRUS haemorrhagic fever caused by a TOGAVIRUS and transmitted by mosquitoes. The name means 'doubled up' and refers to the severe joint pain which is the principal feature. There is usually a second phase of fever and pain, with an itchy rash.

chief medical officer a doctor, appointed by the British Government to monitor the health

of the nation and to determine the factors that influence it; to act as a spokesperson for the medical profession; to ensure that all relevant government departments are kept effectively in touch with the medical profession on all matters of importance to the public weal; and to ensure that the United Kingdom is adequately represented internationally on medical matters. He or she is also chief medical officer to a range of Ministries including the Home Office, the Department of Education, the Social Security Department and the Department of Agriculture, Fisheries and Food. The CMO, who is also prominently involved as chairperson or as a committee member of various Health Department and research national bodies, is roughly the equivalent of the US Surgeon-General.

chigger the harvest mite, commonly encountered in the fields in autumn. The bites cause irritation, a form of SCABIES, and sometimes severe dermatitis. In the Far East chiggers transmit scrub typhus. They can be avoided by the use of insect repellents. Not to be confused with CHIGOE.

chigoe *Tunga penetrans*, sometimes called the 'jigger flea' or chigoe, is common in tropical Africa and tropical America. After mating the female burrows under the skin, often under the big toenail or elsewhere on the feet and grows to the size of a pea because of the enormous swelling of her abdomen from a mass of eggs.

chilblain raised, red, round itchy swelling of the skin of the fingers and toes occurring in cold weather. This and other related disorders, are included in the term 'perniosis'.

child abuse active assault or physical or emotional neglect of a child. Characteristic injuries include finger-shaped bruises, bruises at different stages, mouth injuries especially tearing of the fold of membrane behind the centre of the upper lip and small bruises or burns on the face. Unexplained fractures or X-ray evidence of old, untreated fractures are common, as are injuries which are out of proportion to the claimed cause.

childbed fever infection of the raw inner surface of the womb where the PLACENTA has separated. Also called puerperal sepsis. This once highly dangerous condition is now easily treated with antibiotics.

child guidance the skilled management of

problems such as solitariness, anxiety, PHOBIAS, serious learning difficulties, persistent bedwetting, sleep disturbances or persistently aggressive behaviour.

chill a sudden short fever causing shivering (rigor) and a feeling of coldness. This may be caused by any acute infection.

Chilomastix a genus of protozoal parasite found in the intestines and occasionally causing diarrhoea.

Chimax a brand name for FLUTAMIDE.

chimera an organism that contains a mixture of genetically different cells derived from more than one ZYGOTE. A chimera may, for instance, occur as a result of fertilization by more than one spermatozoon; fusion of two zygotes; an ALLOGENEIC bone marrow graft; cell exchange between dizygotic twin fetuses; or combination of portions of embryos of different species. Compare MOSAICISM. The term derives from the name of a mythical monster with a lion's head, a goat's body, and a serpent's tail.

chimeric DNA recombinant DNA.

Chinese avian influenza a disease caused by the H5N1 influenza virus first isolated in South Africa in the 1960s and which, in early 1997 caused the death of thousands of chickens in Hong Kong and later in the year a small number of human cases with a number of deaths. All the poultry in Hong Kong were destroyed and a serious human epidemic avoided. The influenza A virus exhibits the genetic intermingling of avian and human strains producing new viruses with serious potential for pandemics.

Chinese medicine a traditional system based on the principles of Yin and Yang and involving treatment with ACUPUNCTURE and with a large pharmacopoeia of drugs chosen from vegetable and animal sources on fanciful non-scientific principles.

Chinese paralytic syndrome an acute paralyzing illness affecting children and young adults in Northern China. Doubts have been expressed as to whether this is a distinct condition or a variant of POLIOMYELITIS. It is thought possible that the widespread use of oral polio vaccine may have led to an antigenic change resulting in altered pathogenicity.

Chinese restaurant syndrome headache, nausea, a tight or burning sensation in the face, head and chest and sometimes dizziness and diarrhoea coming on one to two hours after a meal containing a large amount of MONOSODIUM GLUTAMATE. Some critics reject this explanation.

Chinine a trade name for QUININE.

chip blower an instrument used in dentistry to remove debris from a tooth cavity during drilling.

chirality the state of two molecules having identical structure except that they display 'handedness' (as in the right and left hand) and are mirror images of one another. Such pairs of molecules are also known as enantiomers or optical isomers. When dissolved in a fluid they rotate a plane-polarized beam in opposite directions.

chiro an informal abbreviation for a person engaged in CHIROPRACTIC.

chiro- see CHEIRO-.

chiropody a specialty supplementary to medicine devoted to the care of the feet and the treatment of minor foot complaints such as ingrowing toenails, bunions, plantar warts, foot strain, flat feet and the care of the feet of diabetics. In the United States, chiropody is known as podiatry, the other half of the activity being, perhaps, left to manicurists. From the Greek *cheir*, hand, and *podos*, foot.

chiropractic a form of alternative therapy based on the belief that bodily disorders spring from maladjustments of the relationships of the bones of the spine. Chiropractic is often effective in treating back problems but the underlying philosophy has no scientific foundation. See also ALTERNATIVE MEDICINE.

chi squared test a series of statistical procedures used to test how closely the observed result of a trial or a statistical observation corresponds to an expectation, hypothesis or hoped-for result. If, for instance, the expected outcome of a trial is that half the participants will show a particular result, the expected frequency (E) is the total number of participants divided by 2. If Y is the number that show the result and N is the number that do not, then chi squared = $(Y-E)^2/E + (N-E)^2/E$. A low chi squared value supports the expectation or hypothesis; a high value rejects it. Tables relating the value to statistical significance are available.

chitin a carbohydrate polymer (polysaccharide) found in worms, insects, crustaceans and fungi but not in mammals. Mammalian chitinases, however, exist and one has been implicated in allergic ASTHMA. Neutralization of this enzyme reduces airway inflammation and hyperresponsiveness.

Chlamydia a genus of small, non-motile, GRAM NEGATIVE bacteria that occupy cells and were thus once thought to be viruses. They carry both DNA and RNA and multiply by binary fission. They can be destroyed by tetracycline antibiotics.

chlamydial infections infections with organism of the genus *Chlamydia*. *Chlamydia trachomatis* causes pelvic inflammatory disease (PID) including CERVICITIS and SALPINGITIS, URETHRITIS, REITER'S SYNDROME and TRACHOMA. With the exception of the last, these infections are sexually transmitted. *Chlamydia psittaci* causes PSITTACOSIS and is usually acquired from birds.

chloasma a mask-like area of dark coloration (pigmentation) of the skin around the eyes, nose, cheeks and forehead, which often affects women during pregnancy or when taking oral contraceptives. Chloasma is made worse by exposure to sunlight. The pigmentation usually fades in time.

chloracne an ACNE-like skin eruption caused by frequent contact with chlorinated hydrocarbons.

chloral betaine cloral betaine, a sedative drug. A brand name is Welldorm.

chloral hydrate a bitter substance used in solution as a sedative and hypnotic. The drug is on the WHO official list. A brand name is Welldorm elixir.

chlor, chloro- *combining form denoting* 1 that a hydrogen atom in a molecule has been replaced by a chlorine atom.
2 any chlorinated substance.
3 green.

chlorambucil a nitrogen mustard drug used in the treatment of LEUKAEMIA and LYMPHOMAS including HODGKIN'S DISEASE. The drug is on the WHO official list. A brand name is Leukeran.

chloramphenicol an antibiotic originally derived from the soil bacterium *Streptomyces venezuelae*. It is highly effective in many serious conditions but has some dangerous side effects which limit its use mainly to external eye infections. In view of the spread of antibiotic-resistant organisms, however, systemic chloramphenicol is again being used to treat dangerous infections. The drug is on the WHO

official list. Brand names of the eye preparations are Chloromycetin, Kemicetin, Minims chloramphenicol and Sno Phenicol.

chlorbutol chlorobutanol, an antibacterial drug used in mouthwashes and other preparations. A brand name is Frador.

chlordiazepoxide a benzodiazepine sedative and tranquillizer. Millions are dependent on this and other benzodiazepine drugs and their addictive potential is well established. A brand name is Librium.

chlorhexidine a disinfectant agent widely used in surgery for preoperative skin cleansing and for sterilizing instruments by soakage. The drug is on the WHO official list. A brand name is Hibitane.

chlorhydria having acid, or an unusually large quantity of acid, in the stomach.

chlormethiazole clomethiazole, a sedative and anticonvulsant drug related to vitamin B_1 used in the management of the alcohol withdrawal syndrome and especially DELIRIUM TREMENS, in STATUS EPILEPTICUS, in pre-eclampsia and ECLAMPSIA and to sedate patients unfit for general anaesthesia who are having essential surgery under local anaesthesia. A brand name is Heminevrin.

chlormethine an alkylating drug that has been used to treat cancer. It is very toxic and causes severe vomiting. The drug is on the WHO official list.

Chlorocort a trade name for eye drops containing CHLORAMPHENICOL and HYDROCORTISONE.

chloroethane see ETHYL CHLORIDE.

chlorofluorocarbons a range of compounds, composed of chlorine, fluorine, carbon and hydrogen, used as aerosol propellants and refrigerants. CFCs have become discredited because of their effect on the ozone layer.

chloroform a heavy, colourless, volatile liquid once widely used as a pleasant and easy general anaesthetic but now abandoned because of its tendency to cause CARDIAC ARREST and other dangerous complications including delayed liver atrophy.

chloroma a form of acute LEUKAEMIA of granulocyte white cells in which green-coloured tumour masses occur. A kind of granulocytic SARCOMA.

Chloromycetin a brand name for CHLORAMPHENICOL.

chlorophillins substances derived from chlorophyll which can be used as deodorants.

chloropsia green vision. This may result from toxic damage to the CONES of the RETINA as in DIGITALIS poisoning.

chloroquine a drug used in the treatment of MALARIA, RHEUMATOID ARTHRITIS and lupus erythematosus. The drug is on the WHO official list. Brand names are Avoclor and Nivaquine.

chlorosis a greenish tinge to the skin formerly associated with severe iron deficiency anaemia in malnourished young women. It is now almost unknown in developed countries.

chloroxylenol an antiseptic drug used in mouthwashes and other preparations. The drug is on the WHO official list. A brand name is Rinstead.

chlorpheniramine chlorphenamine, an antihistamine drug used for the symptomatic relief of allergic disorders such as hay fever and urticaria. The drug is on the WHO official list. Brand names are Piriton, and, with ephedrine, Haymine and Galpseud Plus.

chlorpromazine a drug derived from phenothiazine used as an antipsychotic, a tranquillizer and to prevent vomiting (antiemetic). Historically, chlorpromazine was the first truly effective anti-psychotic drug. A brand name is Largactil.

chlorquinaldol an antibacterial and antifungal drug used externally in conjunction with a topical steroid. A brand name is Locoid C.

chlortetracycline an antibiotic obtained from the soil bacterium *Streptomyces aureofaciens*. A brand name is Deteclo. With TRIAMCINOLONE it is marketed as Aureocort.

chlorthalidone chlortalidone, a DIURETIC drug of medium potency that increases the output of urine over a period of 48 hours. Brand names are Hygroton, Kalspare, and with ATENOLOL, Tenoretic.

ChM *abbrev. for* Master of Surgery.

choana a funnel-shaped opening, especially one of the internal openings of the nose into the PHARYNX.

chocolate cyst a cyst full of altered blood, usually on an ovary, in ENDOMETRIOSIS.

choking partial or total obstruction of the main air passage (the LARYNX or TRACHEA) by foreign body or external pressure. This induces a protective COUGH response which often clears the obstruction.

chol-, chole- *combining form denoting* BILE.

cholagogue a drug, such as dehydrocholic acid, that promotes the flow of bile.

cholang- *combining form denoting* bile duct.

cholangiectasis local widening of the bile duct.

cholangiocarcinoma cancer of the bile ducts.

cholangiography X-ray or other imaging examination of the bile ducts, usually after a fluid substance opaque to radiation has been introduced. The main object of cholangiography is to show stones in the bile ducts and gall bladder. The method may be done by direct injection through the skin into the liver (percutaneous, transhepatic cholangiography) or, by way of a flexible endoscope, through the bile duct opening in the duodenum (endoscopic retrograde cholangiography).

cholangiolitis inflammation of the bile capillaries.

cholangioma a benign tumour of a bile duct within the liver.

cholangitis inflammation of the bile ducts. This is usually secondary to obstruction by gall stones so that infected material is unable to escape into the bowel.

cholecalciferol colecalciferol, vitamin D_3, the natural form of the vitamin, formed in the skin by the action of the ultra-violet component of sunlight on 7-dehydrocholesterol. As a drug, the vitamin is usually formulated along with calcium for the treatment of calcium deficiency or OSTEOPOROSIS. Brand names are Cacit D3, Calceos and Calcichew.

cholecyst- *combining form denoting* gall bladder.

cholecystectomy surgical removal of the gall bladder.

cholecystitis inflammation of the gall bladder. This common condition is nearly always associated with obstruction to the outflow from the gall bladder, usually by a gallstone but sometimes by thickened mucus or a worm or, rarely, by cancer. There is severe pain under the right lower ribs, fever, shivering, restlessness, pallor, vomiting and sweating. JAUNDICE may occur. Treatment is with antibiotics, bed rest, pain relief and fluids followed by surgical removal of the gall bladder.

cholecystography X-ray of the gall bladder, usually facilitated by the use of a contrast medium, so that gallstones can be readily seen.

cholecystojejunostomy the establishment of continuity between the inside of the gall bladder and the inside of the small intestine.

cholecystokinase an ENZYME that accelerates the breakdown of CHOLECYSTOKININ.

cholecystokinin a HORMONE released into the blood from the lining of the duodenum when fat and acid are present. It causes the gallbladder to contract and the sphincter of Oddi to relax, so sending bile into the duodenum to emulsify the fat, and stimulates the pancreas to secrete fat- and protein-splitting enzymes.

cholecystolithiasis gall stones in the gall bladder.

cholecystostomy an opening made into the gallbladder, usually for drainage of its contents to the exterior by way of a tube passing through the abdominal wall.

cholecystotomy cutting into the gall bladder.

choledocho- *combining form denoting* the common bile duct.

choledocholithiasis stones in the common bile duct.

choledocholithotomy surgical removal of gall stones from a bile duct.

choledochostomy draining of the common bile duct through the abdominal wall.

cholelithiasis the condition of having gallstones.

cholera a highly infectious disease caused by the organism *Vibrio cholerae*, usually acquired in contaminated food or drinking water. 1–3 days after infection there is profuse watery diarrhoea and vomiting and severe, often fatal, dehydration from fluid loss. Timely and effective fluid replacement is life-saving.

cholescintigraphy a method of visualizing the biliary system by the use of a radio-active substance which, when injected into the blood, rapidly concentrates in the gallbladder and bile ducts. Failure of the gallbladder to show up suggests blockage of the cystic duct and support a diagnosis of CHOLECYSTITIS.

cholestasis slowing or cessation of the flow of bile. This may lead, by a damming-back process, to JAUNDICE.

cholesteatoma a tumour-like mass of cells, shed by the outer layer of the skin of an infected eardrum, which relentlessly invades the middle ear through a perforation in the drum, to cause serious internal damage. The condition was once often fatal but advances in microsurgical management with radical clearance of all disease tissue and the use of fibrin glue and

bone paté have greatly improved the outlook.

cholesterol an essential body ingredient found in all human cells, mainly as part of the structure of the cell membranes. It is needed to form the essential steroid hormones, CORTISOL, corticosterone and ALDOSTERONE, the male and female sex hormones and the bile acids. It is synthesized in the liver and a large quantity of cholesterol passes down the bile duct into the intestine every day. Most of it is reabsorbed. A diet high in saturated fats encourages high blood cholesterol levels. Soluble dietary fibre and various drugs can bind intestinal cholesterol and prevent its reabsorption. Cholesterol is carried to the tissues in tiny cholesterol carriers called low density lipoproteins (LDLs). Oxidation of these allows cholesterol to be deposited in the walls of arteries causing dangerous narrowing (ATHEROSCLEROSIS).

cholesterol emboli syndrome a condition resulting from the freeing of cholesterol crystals into the bloodstream from plaques of ATHEROMA in ATHEROSCLEROSIS and the movement of this material with the blood to obstruct small arteries in various parts of the body. Cholesterol emboli can cause TRANSIENT ISCHAEMIC ATTACKS, and damage to the brain, kidneys, spleen, eyes, heart, intestine and skin. Emboli are often released during or after ANGIOGRAPHY.

cholestyramine colestyramine, a drug used in the treatment of HYPERLIPIDAEMIA. It is an anion-exchange resin that binds bile acids so that they cannot be reabsorbed and are lost in the stools. This stimulates the conversion of body cholesterol into more bile acids. A brand name is Questran.

choline one of the B vitamins necessary for the metabolism of fats and the protection of the liver against fatty deposition. The important NEUROTRANSMITTER acetylcholine is formed from it.

cholinergic 1 pertaining to nerves that release ACETYLCHOLINE at their endings, including the nerves to the voluntary muscles and all the PARASYMPATHETIC nerves.
2 having effects similar to those of acetylcholine.

cholinergic crisis a state caused by over-activity of ACETYLCHOLINE due to overdosage of drugs that block the enzyme that inactivates acetylcholine (ANTICHOLINESTERASE drugs).

There is muscle twitching and paralysis, sweating, salivation and pallor and the pupils are very small. These are the effects of military 'nerve gases'.

cholinesterase an enzyme that rapidly breaks down acetylcholine to acetic acid and choline so that its action as a NEUROTRANSMITTER ceases.

cholinesterase inhibitor a drug or agent that blocks the action of CHOLINESTERASE so that acetylcholine accumulates, often dangerously. The insecticides malathion and parathion are cholinesterase inhibitors, as are the drugs physostigmine (eserine), neostigmine, edrophonium, pyridostigmine, tacrine, demecarium and ambendonium. Other cholinesterase inhibitors are the nerve gases sarin, soman and tabun. Sarin has a lethal dose in humans of less than 1 mg.

choluria bile in the urine.

chondral pertaining to CARTILAGE.

chondrification a change to CARTILAGE.

chondritis inflammation of CARTILAGE. This is usually associated with mechanical injury or prolonged wearing stress.

chondro- *combining form denoting* cartilage.

chondroblasts cells that differentiate from fibroblasts and mature into CHONDROCYTES.

chondrocalcinosis the deposition of crystals of calcium pyrophosphate dihydrate in cartilage. Degenerative changes result and, in joints, a form of arthritis, known as PSEUDOGOUT, occurs.

chondrocostal pertaining to the COSTAL CARTILAGES and the ribs. Also known as costochondral.

chondrocytes cells that secrete the non-cellular matrix of cartilage and become trapped in minute spaces within it.

chondrogenesis cartilage formation.

chondroitin a viscous compound of protein and carbohydrate (a GLYCOSAMINOGLYCAN or MUCOPOLYSACCHARIDE) found in crystalline lenses and corneas and in some other connective tissues.

chondroma a benign tumour of CARTILAGE.

chondromalacia patellae a mild form of OSTEOARTHRITIS affecting the CARTILAGE on the back of the knee-cap (patella) and causing pain and stiffness, especially when climbing or descending stairs.

chondromatosis multiple benign cartilage tumours in bone occurring most commonly in

the hands. A spontaneous break (pathological fracture) sometimes occurs from thinning and weakening of bone.

chondrosarcoma a rare malignant tumour of the cartilaginous parts of bone affecting mainly the pelvis, ribs and breastbone (sternum) and causes a slowly expanding swelling. The outlook after surgical removal is usually favourable.

chondrotome a surgical instrument for cutting CARTILAGE.

Choragon a brand name for CHORIONIC GONADOTROPHIN.

chordee angulation of the penis, when erect, usually as a result of a patch of scar tissue on the undersurface, or from the congenital deformity of HYPOSPADIAS. Chordee can seriously interfere with sexual intercourse. See also PEYRONIE'S DISEASE.

chordoma a slow-growing tumour of the spine arising from remnants of the primitive NOTOCHORD. Chordomas rarely spread remotely, but can cause severe local damage.

chordotomy deliberate cutting of a nerve tract in the spinal cord, usually a sensory tract in an attempt to relieve severe and otherwise uncontrollable pain.

chorea an involuntary, purposeless jerky movement, repeatedly affecting especially the face, shoulders and hips and caused by disease of the basal ganglia of the brain. Popularly called St. Vitus' dance. See HUNTINGTON'S CHOREA.

choreiform resembling CHOREA.

chorio- *combining form denoting* CHORION or CHOROID.

chorioadenoma a tumor of the womb (uterus) of intermediate malignancy between a HYDATIDIFORM MOLE and a CHORIOCARCINOMA. The tumour invades the wall of the uterus and may seed off to other sites.

choriocarcinoma a malignant growth arising from the tissues which develop into the PLACENTA. Also known as a CHORION EPITHELIOMA.

choriomeningitis inflammation of the MENINGES with involvement of the CHOROID PLEXUSES. Choriomeningitis is caused by an arenavirus that is endemic in house mice and pet hamsters. There is sudden fever, headache and stiff neck but the condition usually settles in about a week. Many lymphocytes are found in the cerebrospinal fluid. The full name of the condition is acute lymphocytic choriomeningitis.

chorion the outer of the two membranes that enclose the embryo. The inner is called the amnion.

chorion epithelioma a highly malignant tumour of the CHORION usually occurring after a HYDATIDIFORM MOLE has developed instead of a normal fetus. Bleeding may continue after an abortion or the cancer may develop months or years after the start of an unsuspected pregnancy. Multiple CORPUS LUTEUM cysts develop in the ovaries and the cancer spreads rapidly to all parts of the body. In one-fifth of cases the tumour develops following a normal pregnancy. The condition is treated with cancer chemotherapy.

chorionic gonadotrophin a hormone secreted by the placenta, throughout pregnancy, to maintain the CORPUS LUTEUM of the ovary. The corpus luteum produces the steroid hormones oestrogen and progesterone, especially the latter, and this prevents further ovulation and menstruation during the remainder of the pregnancy. At the end of pregnancy, the loss of the placenta allows for eventual resumption of ovulation. The hormone is available as a drug for the treatment of infertility, poor gonadal development and delayed puberty under such brand names as Choragon and Pregnyl.

chorionic villi the finger-like projections from the CHORION into the wall of the womb at the site at which the PLACENTA is developing. Since both the chorionic villi and the embryo are derived from the same fertilized ovum a sample of the former provides material for genetic studies of the latter. Chorionic villus sampling has become an important method of early pre-natal screening for genetic defects.

chorionic villus sampling removal, by way of a fine tube or needle, of a small part of the tissue in process of forming the PLACENTA. This has the same DNA as the embryo so allows gene analysis and may give very early warning of inherited disease. The chorionic villi can be sucked out through a fine flexible tube passed through the vagina and the neck of the womb (cervix) and guided to the site of the placenta under ultrasound scanning control. Sometimes the sample is taken by passing a needle through the abdominal wall. There is some evidence that this procedure is associated with a higher than average incidence of fetal abnormality.

chorioretinitis any inflammatory process involving the CHOROID and the overlying RETINA of the eye.

choroid the densely pigmented layer of blood vessels lying just under the retina of the eye, contributing to its fuel and oxygen supply and optical efficiency.

choroidal neovascular membrane (CNV) a sheet of proliferating tiny new blood vessels from the CHOROID that pushes forward through breaks in BRUCH'S MEMBRANE to lie immediately under the RETINA. It then leaks fluid which pools under, and elevates, the retina locally causing visual loss. This is the mechanism underlying age-related MACULAR DEGENERATION.

choroideraemia a rare genetic disorder featuring progressive degeneration of the CHOROID coat of the eye and leading to progressive visual loss and eventual blindness.

choroiditis inflammation of the choroid coat of the eye. This invariably damages the overlying retina, usually causing localized patches of destruction with corresponding areas of visual loss.

choroid plexus pouch-like, blood-vessel-filled projections of the inner layer of the MENINGES, the PIA MATER, into all four ventricles of the brain. Cerebrospinal fluid is continuously formed, mainly by secretion through the thin walls of the choroid plexuses.

Christmas factor one of the 20 or so factors necessary for the normal clotting of the blood. Christmas factor is Factor IX and its absence causes a form of HAEMOPHILIA sometimes called Christmas disease. (Named after Stephen Christmas, the patient in whom this deficiency was first found).

Christmas disease HAEMOPHILIA caused by absence of Factor IX (CHRISTMAS FACTOR).

chrom- *combining form denoting* colour, pigment or stain.

chromaffin able to be easily stained with coloured chromium salts.

chromatid one of the two duplicated copies of a chromosome produced by replication while still connected at the CENTROMERE before separation at the subsequent cell division. Each chromatid becomes a new chromosome.

chromatin the elongated, fine-stranded

complex of roughly equal quantities of DNA and the protein histone, from which chromosomes are made by condensing into a coil. The individual chromosomes cannot be distinguished in a chromatin strand.

chromatism 1 abnormal pigmentation.
2 CHROMATIC ABERRATION.

chromatic aberration colour fringes around the edge of the image cast by a lens.

chromatocyte a pigmented cell.

chromatography a method of separating the components of a complex mixture, such as a gas, by passing it through selectively adsorbing media.

chromatolysis loss of the ability of a part of a cell to take up a stain from microscopic purposes. Nuclear chromatolysis implies dissolution of the nucleus.

chromatophore a pigment-containing cell.

chromatopsia abnormal perception of colour. This may be due to a toxic effects on the RETINA, developing CATARACT, hallucinogenic drugs or psychiatric disorders.

chromium deficiency a rare condition sometimes occurring in people on long-term intravenous feeding. There is a diabetes-like condition with raised blood sugar (hyperglycaemia).

chromoblastomycosis a deep fungus tropical infection of the skin, usually on the foot, caused by a variety of fungi, and acquired on splinters of decaying wood. There are warty nodules that may ulcerate. The condition is very persistent. It is also known as chromomycosis.

chromogenesis the production of pigment.

chromogranins calcium-binding glycoproteins found in the secretory granules of all endocrine glands. They are cleaved to form biologically-active peptides.

chromophil readily capable of taking up biological stains or dyes. See also CHROMOPHOBE. Chromophil cells are those with granules that readily stain with dyes.

chromophobe resistant to biological stains. This property can be an important distinguishing characteristic in identifying some cells. Chromophobe cells are those with granules that do not take up dyes.

chromosomal sex the gender as determined by the nature of the sex chromosomes – female for two X chromosomes (XX) and male for one X and one Y (XY).

chromosome one of the discrete coiled DNA and protein structures, present in all animal and plant cells, which carry the genetic code for the construction of the body of the organism. Chromosomes are DNA bound to the protein histone in an enormously condensed manner. The packing ratio (DNA length divided by the chromosome length) may be as great as 7000. The code is represented by the GENES, of which there are about 100,000 in humans, strung along the chromosomes. Each normal human body cell contains 46 chromosomes, arranged in 23 pairs. A deficiency of chromosomes is incompatible with life but it is not uncommon for a person to have an extra copy of one of the chromosomes, invariably with undesirable effect. Chromosomes carry most, but not all, of the cell's DNA. Some of it is carried by the MITOCHONDRIA. The term arose when these 'coloured bodies' were first distinguished under the microscope by means of specific stains. So the term 'chromosome' actually refers to a characteristic not present in life.

chromosome analysis examination of stained CHROMOSOMES in a stage at which they are widely separated and easily visualized. The chromosomes are photographed and set out in matching pairs in an orderly arrangement known as a karyotype. The process allows ready diagnosis of a range of conditions known to be the result of gross chromosomal, rather than gene, abnormalities.

chronaxie the minimum time for which an adequate electric current must be applied to a nerve to produce a contraction of the associated muscle. An adequate current is one that is at least twice the threshold value.

chronic lasting for a long time. A chronic disorder may be mild or severe but will usually involve some long-term or permanent organic change in the body. From the Greek *chronos*, time.

chronic fatigue syndrome the currently-preferred name for the condition formerly known, with questionable accuracy, as myalgic encephalomyelitis. This distressing condition predominantly affects women and features severe fatigue, muscle aching and emotional disturbance brought on by exercise, sometimes minimal. This complex is found in many conditions and the diagnosis is usually made by the subject after thorough investigation has proved negative. The medical profession is divided as to whether or not this is an organic entity. There is no evidence that the condition involves inflammation of the brain or spinal cord as the earlier name would imply. There is, however, no doubting the distress and disability of the unfortunate sufferers and their families. Also known as Royal Free disease, epidemic neuromyasthenia, Otago mystery disease, Icelandic disease, institutional mass hysteria, benign myalgic encephalomyelitis and the postviral fatigue syndrome. Graded exercise for the condition has been found helpful. Some cases have responded well to behaviour therapy.

chronic obstructive lung disease
see CHRONIC OBSTRUCTIVE PULMONARY DISEASE.

chronic obstructive pulmonary disease
a condition affecting mainly elderly people who have partial obstruction to the flow of oxygen from the atmosphere to the blood in the lungs that cannot be completely relieved by treatment. COPD may be caused by one of at least three conditions – breakdown of the walls of the tiny lung air sacs (alveoli) leading to EMPHYSEMA, excessive mucus and pus production in the air tubes as in chronic BRONCHITIS, and long-term ASTHMA.

chronic pain syndromes conditions which feature long-term pain that cannot readily be attributed to any known pathological cause. Also known as pain dysfunction syndromes they include such conditions as repetitive strain injury, reflex sympathetic dystrophy and post-traumatic pain.

chronopharmacology the study of DIURNAL variations in drug absorption, distribution and excretion, and in variations in the response of biological systems to drugs at different times.

chrysotherapy treatment with gold salts such as sodium aurothiomalate or auranofin. These are used in RHEUMATOID ARTHRITIS and are effective in slowing or halting the progression of the disease, but have many side effects.

Churg-Strauss syndrome a rare form of blood vessel inflammation (vasculitis) that is almost invariably accompanied by severe ASTHMA. The cause is unknown and although the condition responds well to treatment with steroids or immunosuppressive drugs, the asthma usually persists. The syndrome is distinct from other vasculitides. There are suspicions that it may possibly be caused by

certain drugs used to treat asthma, especially antileukotriene drugs.

Chvostek's sign an indication of the hypersensitivity of muscles occurring in conditions of lowered blood calcium. Tapping the branches of the facial nerve in front of the ear with the finger tip causes twitching of the muscles of the face. This is an indication of latent TETANY. (Franz Chvostek, 1835–84, Austrian surgeon).

chyl-, chylo- *combining form denoting* CHYLE.

chyle a milky alkaline fluid consisting of lymph and emulsified fat that is absorbed into fine ducts called lacteals in the lining of the intestine after a fatty meal. Chyle is carried by lymph vessels into the bloodstream.

chylomicrons microscopic globules, 80 to 1000 nanometres in diameter, of fat, phospholipids, cholesterol, fat-soluble vitamins and other materials. Chylomicrons are formed by the epithelium of the small intestine and are found in the blood during the ingestion of dietary fats, etc. The size of chylomicrons relates to the proportion of fats in the diet, being greatest after high-fat meals. Chylomicrons, and some of their contents are broken don in the liver and the constituents released.

chylothorax a rare condition of accumulation of CHYLE in the space between the lung coverings (pleural cavity). The chyle escapes from the thoracic duct, usually as a result of injury.

chyluria emulsified fat in the urine imparting a milky appearance. This may occur if the lymphatic channels in the abdomen, that normally conduct CHYLE are obstructed in FILARIASIS.

chyme semifluid, partly digested food passed from the stomach into the small intestine for further digestion and absorption.

chymopoiesis conversion of food into CHYME.

chymotrypsin an ENZYME that breaks down (digests) protein to amino acids and simpler substances. It is secreted by the pancreas and released into the DUODENUM. The enzyme is also used to clean wounds and in an earlier form of cataract surgery to cut the suspensory ligament (zonules) of the cataractous lens.

CI *abbrev. for* CONFIDENCE INTERVAL.

Cialis a brand name for the anti-impotence drug TADALAFIL.

Cicatrin a brand name for a preparation for

external use containing BACITRACIN and NEOMYCIN.

cicatrix a scar. Scar tissue.

cicatrization formation of a scar.

cidofovir a DNA POLYMERASE INHIBITOR drug. A brand name is Viside.

Cidomycin a brand name for GENTAMYCIN.

ciguatera poisoning a kind of poisoning common in the Caribbean and Pacific regions acquired by eating fish containing ciguatoxin. This is thought to originate in an alga *Gambierdiscus toxicus*. There is numbness of the mouth and throat, pain in the abdomen, muscles and joints, headache, breathlessness and paralysis.

CIH *abbrev. for* Certificate in Industrial Health.

Cilamox a trade name for AMOXYCILLIN.

cilastatin a drug used in combination with the beta-lactam antibiotic imipenem (carbapenem) to prevent its degradation in the kidneys so that its action can be prolonged. A brand name for the combination is Primaxin IV.

cilazapril an ANGIOTENSIN-CONVERTING ENZYME INHIBITOR drug used to treat HEART FAILURE and high blood pressure (HYPERTENSION). A brand name is Vascace.

Cilest a brand name for ETHINYLOESTRADIOL (ethinylestradiol) formulated with the PROGESTOGEN drug norelgestromin as an oral contraceptive.

cilia 1 the microscopic hairlike processes extending from the surface of certain kinds of lining cells (ciliated epithelium) and capable of a rhythmical lashing motion.
2 eyelashes.

ciliary 1 pertaining to CILIA.
2 pertaining to the CILIARY BODY.

ciliary body the thickened ring of muscular and blood vascular tissue that forms the root of the IRIS and contains the focusing muscle of the eye. It is continuous with the CHOROID.

ciliary movement the rhythmical beating movement of CILIA on the surface of ciliated EPITHELIUM reminiscent of wind blowing across a field of ripe corn.

cilostazol an antithrombotic and vasodialtor drug used to improve blood supply to the extremities in people with peripheral vascular disease and INTERMITTENT CLAUDICATION. A brand name is Pletal.

Ciloxan a brand name for CIPROFLOXACIN.

cimetidine a histamine H-2 receptor antagonist drug used to limit acid production in the stomach in cases of peptic ulcer. The drug is on the WHO official list. Brand names are Tagamet, Dyspamet, Galenamet, and Zita.

CIN *abbrev. for* CERVICAL INTRAEPITHLIAL NEOPLASIA.

cinchocaine a powerful local anaesthetic drug for local application usually in conjunction with a steroid. Brand names for combination preparations are Ultraproct and Uniroid-HC.

cinchona a south American tree, genus *Cinchona*, from the bark of which quinine is derived.

cinnarizine a drug used to treat vomiting and MÉNIÈRE'S SYNDROME. A brand name is Stugeron.

cinoxacin a quinolone antibiotic drug used mainly to treat urinary infections. A trade name is Cinobac.

Cipralex a brand name for ESCITALOPRAM.

ciprofibrate an anti-cholesterol fibrate drug used to treat high blood lipid levels that fail to respond to dietary measures. The drug lowers the levels of low-density lipoproteins (LDLs). A brand name is Modalim.

ciprofloxacin an antibiotic used to treat urinary infections and, as eye drops, for the treatment of corneal ulcers. The drug is on the WHO official list. Brand names are Ciproxin and Ciloxan.

Ciproxin a brand name for CIPROFLOXACIN.

circadian exhibiting a 24 hour periodicity.

circadian rhythm a biological 24 hour cycle that applies to many physiological processes and variables and is synchronized to the day-night cycle occasioned by the rotation of the earth. See also BIORHYTHMS.

circinate ring-shaped.

circulation movement in a circle or around a circuit, especially the movement of the blood through the arteries, capillaries and veins, as a result of the pumping action of the heart.

circumcision surgical removal of the male foreskin (prepuce) or of parts of the female external genitalia. Male circumcision is mostly done for ritual purposes, as in Jews and Muslims, but is occasionally necessary for medical reasons. Female circumcision is a culturally-determined but barbaric practice causing pain, mutilation and distress to millions of women. The procedure may be limited to removal of the clitoris or may also involve removal of all the external genitalia and stitching together of the raw surfaces so that they heal across and make sexual intercourse impossible (infibulation).

circumcorneal around the periphery of the CORNEA.

circumduction the movement of a limb that causes the hand or foot to describe a circle.

circumflex bent into the form of an arc or circle.

circumoral around the mouth.

circumvallate surrounded by a groove or by a raised ring as in the case of the circumvallate papillae on the tongue.

cirrhosis replacement of functional tissue by a network of fine scars (fibrous tissue) so that there is hardening and function is lost.

cirrhosis of the liver the late effects of long-term damage from various toxic or damaging agencies such as alcohol, organic poisons and viruses. Cirrhosis is the replacement of part of the normal tissue of the liver by inert, non-functioning fibrous tissue. It is the end stage of disorders which have been so damaging to the organ that the normal processes of regeneration have been unable to cope. The whole structure of the organ is invaded by fibrous tissue, causing it to become nodular. Within large nodules, some normal liver tissue may survive, but most of the functioning liver tissue is replaced. Blood now unable to pass through the liver has to try to find an alternative route back to the heart. It can do this by way of the veins draining the upper part of the intestine, especially those in the stomach and at the lower end of the gullet (OESOPHAGUS). But, in the process, these veins become greatly enlarged and varicose and one of the most serious complications of cirrhosis is bleeding from these VARICES with vomiting of blood.

cirsoid resembling a varicose vein.

cis 1 in chemistry, being on the same side. Usually refers to two groups being on the same side of a ring or of a double bond. 2 in genetics, describing two sites on the same molecule of DNA. Compare TRANS.

cis- *prefix denoting* that two groups in a molecule are in the CIS CONFIGURATION. The prefix is usually italicized.

cisapride a prokinetic drug that aids in stomach emptying and helps to relieve heartburn (reflux oesophagitis). A trade name is Prepulsid.

cis configuration having both of the dominant ALLELES, of two or more gene pairs, on one chromosome, and the recessive alleles on the other (HOMOLOGOUS) chromosome.

cisplatin an anticancer drug. Like any drug that damages cells it has side effects. Cisplatin can cause progressive kidney impairment. The drug is on the WHO official list.

cisterna an enclosed space acting as a fluid reservoir. The cisterna magna is a space filled with cerebrospinal fluid lying between the CEREBELLUM and the MEDULLA OBLONGATA.

cisternography an obsolescent imaging technique used to investigate pituitary gland tumours. An X-ray contrast medium is injected into the cerebrospinal fluid by passing a needle in between the upper bone of the spine and the under side of the skull.

cistron a short length of DNA that codes for a protein subunit (a polypeptide), together with adjacent sequences that control its expression. It is the smallest unit that transmits genetic information.

citalpram a serotonin reuptake inhibitor drug used as an antidepressant. A brand name is Cipramil.

citric acid an ingredient of various effervescent medications such as urine alkalizing agents.

cladribine an anticancer drug used to treat hairy cell LEUKAEMIA and B cell chronic lymphocytic leukaemia. A brand name is Leustat.

Claforan a brand name for CEFOTAXIME.

clairvoyance the claimed ability to perceive other than by the senses. Most if not all episodes of alleged clairvoyance are either illusory or fraudulent.

CLANZ *abbrev. for* Clinical Leaders Association of New Zealand.

clap a slang term for GONORRHOEA.

clarithromycin a MACROLIDE antibiotic drug. A brand name is Klaricid.

class switching the change, by a B cell, of the class of an antibody it produces (for example from IgM to IgG) without a change in its specificity.

-clast *combining form denoting* anything that breaks up or crushes.

claudication see INTERMITTENT CLAUDICATION.

claustrophobia fear of confined spaces. This is one of the phobic disorders and is usually associated with others such as agoraphobia.

claustrum any structure resembling a barrier.

clavicle the collar-bone, which runs from the upper and outer corner of the breastbone (sternum) to connect to a process on the outer side of the shoulder-blade (scapula).

clavulanic acid a drug that interferes with beta-lactamase enzymes that inactivate many penicillin-type antibiotics, such as AMOXICILLIN. Combined with the antibiotic, this drug can overcome drug resistance.

clavus a corn.

clawfoot see TALIPES.

clearance 1 the removal of a substance from the blood, usually by the kidneys.
2 the rate of such removal.

cleavage 1 the process of splitting, especially the repeated stages of cell division that produce a BLASTULA from an ovum that has been fertilized by a spermatozoon.
2 the breaking down of a complex molecule into smaller parts.
3 the vertical furrow between a woman's breasts visible when low-cut garments are worn. For inscrutable reasons this exerts an irresistible attraction on the gaze of most men.

cleft lip and palate a developmental defect caused by the failure of full fusion together of the processes which grow out from the front end of the primitive tube-like structure of the body to form the face.

cleidocranial dysostosis a congenital disorder featuring defective bone formation in the collar bones (clavicles) and the skull.

clemastine an ANTIHISTAMINE drug used to treat hay fever and other allergic conditions. A brand name is Tavegil.

clenched fist sign pressure of the tightly closed hand against the centre of the chest. This gesture is typical of the patient suffering from ANGINA PECTORIS or the early stages of a heart attack.

clergyman's knee inflammation and swelling of the BURSA in front of the knee cap (patella) allegedly from excessively prolonged pressure during prayer. Prepatellar bursitis is uncommon in these less fervent days.

clergyman's throat hoarseness and pain on speaking due to overuse of the voice and faulty habits of voice production. The condition is due to inflammation of the vocal cords and is nowadays more common in pop singers.

Clexane a brand name for ENOXAPARIN.

climacteric the MENOPAUSE. The time in life after which reproduction is no longer possible. This is an exclusively female phenomenon; the male menopause is a journalistic fiction.

Climaval a brand name for OESTRADIOL (estradiol).

climax 1 a point of maximal intensity in a progression of events.
2 an ORGASM.

clindamycin an antibiotic drug that penetrates well into bone to treat OSTEOMYELITIS. The drug is on the WHO official list. Brand names are Dalacin C and, for external use, Dalacin T.

clinic 1 a medical institution in which a number of specialists work in association, usually dealing with outpatients.
2 a training session in practical medicine for medical students.

clinical 1 concerned with the immediate observation, examination and treatment of patients.
2 relating to a CLINIC.

clinical governance a systematic approach to raising standards of health care and tackling poor performance in hospitals.

clinical pathology the science and practice of medical diagnosis by laboratory examination and analysis of tissue specimens (BIOPSIES), body fluids and other samples. Clinical pathology is subdivided into VIROLOGY, BACTERIOLOGY, clinical chemistry, SEROLOGY and pathological HISTOLOGY.

clinical thermometer one of a variety of devices for measuring and indicating the temperature of the human body. Clinical thermometers may have an analogue or a digital display and cover a short range of temperature around 37 °C.

clinician any doctor, of any speciality, dealing directly with patients.

clinicopathological conference a teaching symposium in which a full account of the clinical aspects of a particular case is given and followed by an account by a pathologist of his or her findings on examination of biopsy tissue or at postmortem examination.

clinistix a narrow strip of card impregnated with an enzyme that produces a purple colour when dipped into urine containing sugar. This is a convenient routine screening test for DIABETES.

Clinitar a brand name for a local cream

preparation containing COAL TAR.

clinitest a method of urine testing for sugar (glucose) using a tablet that is dropped into the urine in a test tube. This method gives a quantitative result by causing colour changes from green (0.5% glucose) to orange (2% glucose).

clinoid resembling a bed.

Clinoril a brand name for SULINDAC.

clioquinol vioform, an antibacterial and antifungal drug commonly formulated in combination with a steroid drug for external use. Brand names are Betnovate C, Locorten-Vioform, Quinaband, Synalar C and Vioform-Hydrocortisone

clitoridectomy see CIRCUMCISION.

clitoriditis inflammation of the clitoris, usually as part of a general VULVITIS.

clitoris the female analogue of the penis. The principle erectile sexual organ in women and the main erogenic centre. It lies under the pubic bone at the front junction of the inner lips (labia minora) and immediately in front of the urethra, to which it is closely applied. The clitoris has a substantial nerve and blood supply. From the Greek *kleitoris*, little hill.

clitoromegaly abnormal enlargement of the CLITORIS.

clobazam a long-acting BENZODIAZEPINE drug used to treat anxiety or to control epilepsy. A brand name is Frisium.

clobetasol a powerful steroid drug used for external application in severe dermatological disorders. Brand names are Dermovate and Eumovate.

clobetasone a steroid drug used externally for skin and non-infective eye inflammation. A brand name is Cloburate and, in conjunction with an antibitic and an antifungal drug, Trimovate.

cloaca the combined urinary and faecal opening in the embryo before the two become separated. The term derives from the Latin *cloaca* a sewer.

clofazimine a drug used to treat LEPROSY. It is effective in controlling the ERYTHEMA NODOSUM reaction. The drug is on the WHO official list. A brand name is Lamprene.

Clomid a brand name for CLOMIPHENE (clomifene).

clomiphene clomifene, an anti-oestrogen drug used to treat INFERTILITY by virtue of its ability

to stimulate the production of eggs from the ovaries (ovulation). Multiple pregnancies often result. The drug is on the WHO official list. A brand name is Clomid.

clomipramine a tricyclic antidepressant drug useful, also, in phobic anxiety and obsessive states. The drug is on the WHO official list. A brand name is Anafranil.

clonal selection the production by an antigen of an expanding CLONE of lymphocytes from a single cell bearing a receptor complementary to the antigen.

clonazepam a BENZODIAZEPINE drug used to control EPILEPSY and TRIGEMINAL NEURALGIA. The drug is on the WHO official list. A brand name is Rivotril.

clone 1 a perfect copy, or a population of perfect copies, of any organism. Cloning occurs when an organism reproduces non-sexually, so that the genetic content (genome) of each is identical. 2 a number of identical cells derived from a single cell by repetitive division. 3 a perfect copy, or any number of copies, of any DNA sequence, such as a gene, or any other nucleotide sequence.

clonic pertaining to CLONUS.

clonidine an alpha$_2$ adrenoreceptor stimulator (AGONIST) that is effective in lowering blood pressure and controlling some cases of MIGRAINE and postmenopausal flushing. Stopping treatment may produce a dangerous rise in blood pressure. Brand names are Dixarit and Catapres.

cloning animals see ANIMAL CLONING.

clonorchiasis a parasitic infection, common in the Far East, acquired by eating raw fish containing the trematode worm *Clonorchis sinensis*.

clonus repetitive contraction and relaxation of stretched muscles which have been deprived of the smoothing and controlling influence of higher centres in the nervous system, in conditions such as STROKE. A feature of an 'upper motor neurone lesion'. Clonus is also a feature of GRAND MAL epilepsy.

clopamide a thiazide diuretic drug. Formulated with the BETA BLOCKER drug PINDOLOL it is marketed under the brand name Viskaldix.

Clopixol a brand name for ZUCLOPENTHIXOL.

clorazepate a long-acting BENZODIAZEPINE drug used to treat anxiety. A brand name is Tranxene.

closed reduction realignment of a fracture or restoration of dislocation by manipulation only and without open surgery.

Clostridium any bacterium of the genus *Clostridium*. These are rod shaped and spore-forming and mostly able to reproduce in the absence of free oxygen (anaerobic). The genus includes *Clostridium welchii* which causes gas gangrene, *Clostridium tetani* which causes TETANUS and *Clostridium botulinum* which causes BOTULISM.

Clostridium difficile a fecal organism endemic in hospitals and responsible for the majority of hospital-acquired cases of diarrhoea in elderly patients. Its prevalence in hospital is largely due to the high levels of antibiotic usage. Bowel infection can be cleared by oral treatment with the antibiotic vancomycin which is not appreciably absorbed into the bloodstream.

clot a thick, coagulated, viscous mass, especially of blood elements.

Clotam a brand name for TOLFENAMIC ACID.

clotrimazole a drug effective against a wide range of fungi. It is used in the form of creams, for local application. Brand names are Canesten and Masnoderm. Formulated with BETAMETHASONE it is marketed under the brand name Lotriderm.

clotting see BLOOD CLOTTING.

clove oil an aromatic oil distilled from the flower buds of the clove tree, used mainly by dentists as a mild antiseptic and toothache reliever. Mixed with zinc oxide, it forms a widely used temporary dressing for a tooth cavity.

cloxacillin a semisynthetic penicillin antibiotic that resists the destructive penicillinase enzymes that some staphylococci produce. The drug also resists degradation by stomach acid and so can be taken by mouth. The drug is on the WHO official list. A brand name of a preparation combined with ampicillin is Ampiclox.

clozapine an antipsychotic drug notable for its absence of side effects such as tremors and repetitive movements (dyskinesias). It does, however, tend to affect white blood cell production and regular blood checks are necessary. Between 1 and 2% of those taking the drug suffer a drop in white cell count. This returns to normal within a month of stopping the drug. Clozapine can restore people to an almost normal life after years

of intractable SCHIZOPHRENIA. A brand name is Clozaril.

clubbing see FINGER CLUBBING.

clubfoot see TALIPES.

clumping aggregation or clustering and adhering together.

cluster B personality a narcissistic, histrionic, changeable personality that over-reacts to external circumstances, suffers frequent frustration, is often unhappy, angry and resentful and inclined to blame others for the unhappiness. People with cluster B personality often seek psychotherapy but seldom derive permanent benefit from it.

cluster headache a migrainous type of headache, usually centred around one eye, and occurring in clusters often several times daily for weeks, then ceasing for periods of weeks or months.

Clutton's joints painless swellings of the long bones near the joints caused by a congenital syphilitic involvement of the growing areas (EPIPHYSES). (Henry Hugh Clutton, 1850–1909, English surgeon).

clysis infusion of fluid into the body.

clyster an archaic term for an ENEMA.

CM *abbrev. for* Master of Surgery.

CMB *abbrev. for* Central Midwives' Board.

CMF *abbrev. for* Christian Medical Fellowship.

CMV *abbrev. for* CYTOMEGALOVIRUS, one of the herpes group.

CNO *abbrev. for* Chief Nursing Officer.

CNS *abbrev. for* the central nervous system.

co- prefix signifying with, together, jointly.

coagulase an enzyme secreted by the micro-organism *Staphylococcus aureus* that causes clotting in blood plasma by converting prothrombin to thrombin. This ability probably contributes to the tendency of the organism to form abscesses.

coagulation, blood see BLOOD CLOTTING.

coagulum a clot.

coal tar a complex mixture of organic substances, especially polycyclic hydrocarbons, derived from the distillation of coal. Although the action of this mixture is not well understood, coal tar preparations are used empirically to treat various skin disorders such as ECZEMA and PSORIASIS. The drug is on the WHO official list. It is contained in numerous trade preparations such as Baltar, Capasal, Carbo-Dome, Gelcotar, Pentrax, Polytar,

Psoriderm and Tar Band.

coarctation a constriction or narrowing, especially of a blood vessel.

coarctation of the aorta a congenital narrowing of a short section of the main artery of the body, the aorta, usually just beyond the point at which the arteries to the head and arms are given off. The pulses in the arms are much stronger than those in the legs.

cobalamine vitamin B$_{12}$. The specific treatment for PERNICIOUS ANAEMIA.

cobalt an element in the vitamin B$_{12}$ molecule. The isotope Cobalt-60 is a powerful emitter of gamma rays and is used as a radiation source for sterilizing medical materials and in the treatment of cancer.

Cobalin-H a brand name for HYDROXOCOBALAMIN.

Co-Betaloc a brand name for METOPROLOL formulated with the diuretic HYDROCHLOROTHIAZIDE.

co-phenotrope a mixture of DIPHENOXYLATE hydrochloride and atropine in a ratio of 100 to 1 used to control diarrhoea. A brand name is Lomotil.

Co-proxamol a brand name for a painkilling mixture of PARACETAMOL and DEXTROPROPOXYPHENE. Also known as Distalgesic.

cocaine the main alkaloid of the bush *Erythroxylon coca*, introduced to medicine by Sigmund Freud. Cocaine was the first effective local anaesthetic drug, but is now little used in medicine, having been replaced by safer and less damaging analogues. It is a major 'recreational' drug, producing a euphoria similar to that of AMPHETAMINE (amfetamine) and has many undesirable behavioural and social effects. Recent research indicates that regular use of cocaine inhibits the ability of brain cells to form new dendrites and synaptic connections with other cells under conditions of normal physiological stimulation. This occurs because cocaine and amphetamines (amfetamines) cause dendrites to grow in a similar way without the appropriate stimuli. The suggestion is that cocaine use may interfere with the ability to formulate original ideas. Psychological testing indicates that some users suffer persistent cognitive loss. See also CRACK.

co-carcinogen a substance, not in itself capable of causing cancer, that, operating in conjunction with other agents, promotes the development of cancer.

coccidioidomycosis a fungus infection caused by inhalation of the wind-borne spores of the fungus *Coccidioides immitis*. The disease occurs in the Southern States of America and in South America and features an influenza-like illness followed, weeks or months later, by fever, loss of weight, breathlessness and coughing of blood.

coccidiosis a tropical parasitic disease caused by the accidental eating of the egg cysts of the PROTOZOA *Isospora belli*. It features fever, abdominal pain and watery diarrhoea and usually settles in a week or two.

coccobacillus a short, oval BACILLUS.

coccus a common type of spherical or spheroidal bacterium. Cocci connected in line are called STREPTOCOCCI; those in bunches are called STAPHYLOCOCCI.

coccydynia persistent pain in the tail region of the spine, usually following a fracture of the small bones of the coccyx from a fall or a kick.

coccygeal pertaining to the COCCYX.

coccyx the rudimentary tail bone, consisting of four small vertebrae fused together and joined to the curved SACRUM. From the resemblance of the bone to a cuckoo's beak.

cochlea the structure in the inner ear containing the coiled transducer, the organ of Corti, that converts sound energy into nerve impulse information. The cochlea resembles a snail shell.

cochlear implant a device designed to stimulate the acoustic nerve so as to produce some form of hearing in people wholly deaf from inner ear disease. Although there have been great advances in multichannel implants, the results still cannot be said to compare with natural hearing. But cochlear implants can make a substantial difference to children born deaf or becoming totally deaf before 3 years of age, so long as the implant is inserted before the age of five. Most of the children who receive such implants are able to develop intelligible speech.

cochlear nerve the branch of the 8th cranial nerve (ACOUSTIC NERVE) concerned with hearing.

cockroach allergy a previously unsuspected cause, or precipitant of ASTHMA in inner-city children. In one large group of inner-city children with asthma, 36.8% were found to be allergic to cockroach allergen. Research showed that more of these children were allergic to cockroaches than to house dust mite droppings or to cat dander.

Codalgin a trade name for CODEINE and PARACETAMOL.

Codate a trade name for CODEINE.

codeine an alkaloid derived from opium, used to control moderate pain, to relieve unnecessary coughing and to check diarrhoea. Codeine is not a drug of addiction and is available without prescription. The drug is on the WHO official list. It is contained in various branded preparations such as Co-Codamol, Codafen Continus, Galcodine, Kapake, Migraleve, Solpadol, Tylex and Zapain.

Codelix a trade name for CODEINE.

coding strand the single strand of a separated double helix of DNA that has the same base sequence as the MESSENGER RNA (mRNA) formed from the complementary DNA strand. The coding strand is not used to form mRNA.

Codiphen a trade name for a mixture of ASPIRIN and CODEINE.

Codis a trade name for a mixture of ASPIRIN and CODEINE.

codliver oil an extract of the liver of the codfish, rich in vitamins A and D.

codominant alleles a pair of ALLELEs both of which contribute to the phenotype, neither being dominant over the other.

codon a sequence of three consecutive nucleotides (a triplet) along a strand of DNA or messenger RNA that specifies a particular AMINO ACID or a stop signal during protein synthesis. The order of the codons along the DNA molecule determines the sequence of particular amino acids in the protein produced.

coelenterata jellyfish, corals, hydroids and sea anemones, some of which can cause painful stings. The sting of the jellyfish *Chironex fleckeri* is sometimes fatal. Coelenterate toxins can cause damage to the blood cells, the heart and the skin.

coeliac pertaining to the cavity of the abdomen.

coeliac disease an intestinal disorder caused by intolerance to gluten proteins the gliadins, hordeins and secalins in wheat, barley and rye. The intestinal mucosa becomes infiltrated with CD8 and CD4 lymphocytes (T cells) leading to crypt hyperplasia and atrophy of the absorbing VILLI. The result is MALABSORPTION, especially of fats, with fat excretion in the stools (STEATORRHOEA). The condition is also called 'gluten-induced enteropathy'.

coenzymes small organic molecules, acting as cofactors that must bind to an enzyme before it can function properly. Tightly-bound coenzymes are called prosthetic groups; loosely-bound coenzymes are more like cosubstrates. Most of the B vitamins are coenzymes.

coffee a mildly stimulating drink made from the roasted and ground seeds or beans of one of several trees of the genus Coffea, which grows in East Asia and Africa. The active element is CAFFEINE and medical scientists have been arguing for years whether or not coffee, in moderation, is harmful.

coffee grounds vomit vomit containing blood that has been in the stomach and has been acted on, and partially digested by stomach acids and enzymes, so as to resemble wet coffee grounds.

Cogentin a brand name for BENZTROPINE (benzatropine).

cognition the mental processes by which knowledge is acquired. These include perception, reasoning and possibly intuition.

cognitive behaviour therapy a method of psychotherapy that concentrates on effects, and the individual's thoughts about them, rather than hypothetical causes – on actual behaviour and its immediate motivation rather than on theories of causation and the unconscious mind. It is the first form of psychotherapy to show substantial improvement in conditions such as obsessive-compulsive disorder, panic states, eating disorders, hypochondriasis and chronic fatigue syndrome. It has also been found useful in managing attempted suicide, unexplained physical symptoms and even unemployment. Research suggests that it is a potentially useful additional treatment in cases of chronic SCHIZOPHRENIA.

cognitive dissonance a psychological term meaning conflict resulting from inconsistency between beliefs and actions, as of a person professing an ethical code but cheating at the Customs.

cohort a group of persons all born on the same day. Cohort studies are valuable in medical and epidemiological research.

coil, contraceptive, a plastic or metal device worn semi-permanently in the womb which acts to prevent implantation of the fertilized ovum, probably by inducing a low-grade local inflammation. One of several forms of intra-uterine contraceptive device (IUCD/IUD). See also CONTRACEPTION.

coitus copulation or the physical act of sex.

coitus interruptus withdrawal of the penis from the vagina after copulation has been in progress for some time, but before the male orgasm and ejaculation, occur. An unreliable method of contraception, liable to let couples down in more ways than one.

colchicine an alkaloid derived from bulbous plants of the genus *Colchicum*, such as the autumn crocus, used to treat GOUT and to induce chromosome doubling. The drug is on the WHO official list.

cold an inflammation of the nose and throat lining caused by one of more than 200 different kinds of viruses. Infection is by touch rather than by droplet inhalation and virus access is often via the CONJUNCTIVA. The medical term is coryza.

cold agglutinin a substance found in blood serum that causes red blood cells to clump together (agglutination) if the blood is kept at low temperatures.

cold injury frostbite. Death of tissue, usually at the extremities, by freezing.

cold sores a flare-up of a herpes simplex infection, featuring tense, painful and crusting small blisters (vesicles) at the junction of the skin and mucous membrane of the lips and sometimes the nose.

colectomy surgical removal of the large intestine (COLON). When this is done, a new outlet must be made for the lower end of the remaining intestine, in the form of a COLOSTOMY or ILEOSTOMY.

Colestid a brand name for COLESTIPOL.

colestipol a BILE ACID SEQUESTRANT drug used to treat abnormally high levels of lipoproteins. A brand name is Colestid.

colic periodic spasms of pain caused by stretching of the walls of a hollow organ undergoing powerful contraction, often in the attempt to overcome a partial obstruction or to move a hard object, such as a stone.

colic, infantile excessive crying and an appearance of distress in a healthy young baby. This may be due to air swallowing, milk intolerance or natural hyperactivity but is seldom due to colic.

Colifoam a brand name for HYDROCORTISONE.

coliform of, or pertaining to, the bacterium *Escherichia coli*, which is present in countless numbers in the colon.

colistin sulphomethate sodium colistimethate sodium, an antibiotic effective against *Pseudomonas aeruginosa* infections of the lung. A brand name is Promixin.

colistin an antibiotic produced by the bacterium *Bacillus colistinus* and effective against *Pseudomonas aeruginosa*. It is used to sterilize the inside of the bowel and bladder and on the skin and external ear. A brand name is Colomycin.

colitis inflammation of the COLON. See ULCERATIVE COLITIS.

collagen an important protein structural element in the body. Collagen fibres are very strong and, formed into bundles which are often twisted together, make up much of the connective tissue of the body. Bones are made of collagen impregnated with inorganic calcium and phosphorus salts. Vitamin C is necessary for the cross-linking and full strength of the collagen molecule.

collagenases enzymes that can break down COLLAGEN and gelatin.

collagen disease a term formerly, and erroneously, applied to such conditions as rheumatic fever, ankylosing spondylitis, polyarteritis nodosa, lupus erythematosus, rheumatoid arthritis and dermatomyositis but now applied to those known to be caused by defects in the chemical structure of collagen and its distribution and quantity. The collagen diseases include solar and senile elastosis, SCURVY, STRIAE, KELOIDS, PEYRONIE'S DISEASE, PSEUDOXANTHOMA ELASTICUM and the EHLERS-DANLOS SYNDROME.

collapse an abrupt failure of health, strength or psychological fortitude. The term is used more by the laity than by the medical profession.

collapsing pulse a sharply rising and suddenly dropping pulse wave characteristic of leakage of the aortic valve of the heart (AORTIC INCOMPETENCE).

collar-bone the CLAVICLE. This comparatively delicate bone is readily fractured either by direct violence or by a force applied indirectly, as in a fall on the outstretched arm.

collar, orthopaedic see ORTHOPAEDIC COLLAR.

collateral circulation the opening up of small

shunting vessels around the site of blockage of an artery that helps to compensate for the loss of direct blood supply.

collective unconscious an entity, deemed to be a kind of storehouse of ancestral memory, proposed by the Swiss psychiatrist and philosopher Karl Gustav Jung (1875–1961) to explain similarities in symbolism among disparate peoples.

Colles' fracture a common fracture of the forearm bones at the wrist, usually caused by a fall on to the outstretched hand. The break results in a typical 'dinner-fork' deformity with the bones of the wrist forced backwards. Treatment consists in reducing the fracture by strong traction on the hand under anaesthesia and enclosing in a cast. (Abraham Colles, 1773–1843, Irish surgeon).

collimator 1 a shield, shutter or cone, usually of lead, attached to an X-ray tube to limit the width of the beam.
2 a thick perforated lead plate designed to allow passage only of parallel radiation, as in a GAMMA CAMERA.

colliquative 1 featuring a turning to liquid of solid tissue, often after death.
2 denoting excessive watery discharge.

collodion an inflammable, syrupy solution of pyroxylin in ether and alcohol, used as a surgical dressing or to hold dressings in place. When painted on the skin, collodion dries to form a flexible cellulose film.

colloid a substance in which particles are in suspension in a fluid medium. The particles are too small to settle by gravity or to be readily filtered. The colloid state lies between that of a solution and that of an emulsion.

coloboma a congenital gap in a part, especially in the IRIS or CHOROID of the eye or in an eyelid.

colocynth a drastic purgative drug, no longer in use.

Colofac a brand name for MEBEVERINE.

Colomycin a brand name for COLISTIN.

colon the large intestine. It is called 'large' because of its diameter. Its main function is to conserve water by absorption from the bowel contents. It also promotes the growth of bacteria which synthesize vitamins.

colon cancer this is very common and increases in frequency with age. Colon cancers may cause obstruction, a change in the shape of the stools and blood in the stools. Treatment is

by surgical removal of the affected length of bowel and the results depend on the stage reached.

colon, irritable see IRRITABLE BOWEL SYNDROME.

colonization the establishment of a colony of micro-organisms at a particular site, such as inside the nostrils or in the large intestine.

colonoscopy an important method of examination of the inside of the COLON, using a steerable, flexible, fibreoptic endoscope which allows meticulous inspection, the taking of biopsies, and, in some cases, treatment.

colon, spastic see IRRITABLE BOWEL SYNDROME.

colony a local growth of large numbers of micro-organisms derived from one individual (a clone) or from a small number. A visible growth of bacteria or other microorganisms on a nutrient medium in a culture plate.

colony stimulating factor one of a number of glycoprotein factors that allow and promote the reproduction and differentiation of blood cells and their precursor cells.

colorectal pertaining to the COLON and the RECTUM.

colostomy an artificial anus on the front wall of the abdomen, formed when the cut upper end of the colon is brought to the exterior. This is often necessary when the colon has to be cut through, as in the treatment of cancer. Evacuated bowel contents are collected in a waterproof bag. Colostomies are often temporary.

colostrum the yellowish, protein-rich, milk-like fluid secreted by the breasts for the first two or three days after the birth of a baby. Colostrum contains large fat globules and a high content of antibodies.

colotomy a surgical cut (incision) into the COLON.

colour blindness an inaccurate term for a lack of perceptual sensitivity to certain colours. Absolute colour blindness is almost unknown. Most colour perception defects are for red or green or both. About 10% of males have a colour perception defect, but this is rare in females.

colour power angiography (CPA) doppler ultrasound imaging a method of displaying in remarkable detail any part of the vascular system of the body. The method has been used to demonstrate maldevelopment of the placental villi which can compromise the development of the fetus and the future health of the individual.

colpagia pain in the vagina.

colpatresia occlusion of the vagina.

colpitis inflammation of the vagina. VAGINITIS.

colpo- *combining form denoting* the vagina.

colpocentesis see CULDOCENTESIS.

colpocoele a HERNIA, of either the bladder or the rectum, into the vagina.

colpohysterectomy surgical removal of the womb through the vagina. A vaginal HYSTERECTOMY.

colpoperineorrhaphy a gynaecological operation to tighten a lax vaginal opening or to repair a tear in the PERINEUM.

colporrhaphy repair of a torn or lax vagina, especially if there has been herniation of the bladder or rectum.

colposcopy optical examination of the vagina and the neck of the womb (cervix). The modern colposcope is a low-power binocular microscope with a long focus. The vagina is held open with a SPECULUM. Colposcopy provides a detailed view of the structure of the surface lining and suspicious areas, from which samples can be taken, are easily seen. Colposcopy is the routine next step after a cervical smear (Pap smear) has shown some abnormality.

colpospasm sustained contraction of the muscular wall of the vagina.

colyones natural inhibitors of cell growth and proliferation. Colyones are coded for by colygenes.

coma a state of deep unconsciousness from which the affected person cannot be aroused even by strong stimulation. Coma can result from head injury, oxygen lack, interruption of the blood supply to the brain, poisoning and various disease states such as those occurring in uncontrolled diabetes, liver failure and kidney failure.

comatose in, or resembling, a state of coma.

combination therapy treatment, especially for cancer, in which various different modalities, such as surgery, radiotherapy or chemotherapy, are used together or sequentially.

combined immune deficiency disease a condition in which both main classes of immune system cells, the T cells and the B cells, are absent. The effect is a severe and usually fatal inability to resist infection.

combined oral contraceptive a hormonal contraceptive containing both an oestrogen and a PROGESTOGEN drug. See also CONTRACEPTION.

comedo, comedone a BLACKHEAD. See also ACNE.

comedocarcinoma an ADENOCARCINOMA of the breast in which the milk ducts are filled with cancer cells forming COMEDO-like bodies.

commensal a micro-organism that lives continuously on, or in certain parts of, the body, without causing disease. Commensals sometimes exclude more dangerous organisms, but may cause disease if they gain access to parts of the body other than their normal habitat.

comminuted broken in several places, especially of a bone fracture; shattered.

commissure 1 a line or point at which two things are joined.
2 a nerve fibre bundle passing from one side of the brain or spinal cord to the other to connect similar structures.

commissurotomy cutting of any COMMISSURE, especially the midline transverse nerve tract bundle that connects the two halves of the CEREBRUM.

Committee on Safety of Medicines an official body that receives reports of adverse side effects of drugs, vaccines, X-ray contrast media, blood products, materials IUCDs or contact lens fluids from doctors, dentists and pharmacists by way of the Medicines Control Agency. Prescribers are provided with prepaid yellow cards with they are urged to complete and send in whenever adverse effects are noted.

commode a bedside chair with a cut-away seat under which is placed a receptacle for urine and faeces.

common bile duct the final duct carrying bile from the liver and the gall bladder, to the duodenum.

common cold see COLD.

communicable disease an infectious disease. A disease capable of being transmitted, by any means, from one person to another.

comparative anatomy the study of the similarities and differences between the body structure of different animals. Although external appearances may vary considerably, in many cases the similarities are much greater than the differences. This observation has been one of the principal reasons for the belief that we have evolved from common ancestors.

compartment syndrome the effects of tissue swelling within a compartment of the body, usually the forearm or the lower leg. There is compression of the blood vessels and resulting muscle atrophy. Operation to open up the tissue planes and relieve the pressure may be urgently needed.

compatibility able to be safely mixed, as in the case of blood for transfusion or drugs for simultaneous administration.

compensation neurosis an inappropriate concern with real or imaginary disability following an industrial accident or civil injury, and with the assumed right to financial compensation. The condition often clears up after a satisfactory settlement.

compensatory hypertrophy an increase in the size of an organ or volume of a tissue following loss or malfunction of the paired organ or loss of functioning tissue.

complement a collection of about 20 serum proteins involved in the immune system process by which the action of antibodies against the invading agent (the ANTIGEN) is completed. Complement combines with antigen-antibody complexes to bring about the breakdown of the antigen-bearing cell or molecule. Some of the serum proteins form enzyme-activated cascades to produce molecules involved in INFLAMMATION, PHAGOCYTOSIS and cell rupture.

complementary of a NUCLEOTIDE or nucleotide sequence the base, or bases, of which can link to one or more other bases to form a BASE PAIR or a sequence of base pairs.

complementary base pairs see BASE PAIRs.

complementary DNA a sample of DNA that has been produced from MESSENGER RNA after conversion into double-strand DNA.

complementary feeding bottle feeding of a baby primarily nourished from the breast.

complementary genes genes which, although not alleles, perform similar or opposing functions. Complementary genes may cooperate in the production of an effect or they may tend to oppose its production.

complementary medicine a better term than the designation ALTERNATIVE MEDICINE, in view of the fact that no informed medical scientist believes that any of the existing therapies outside the range of orthodox medicine offer an alternative to evidence-based scientific medical practice. The use of the title 'complementary'

should not, however, be taken to imply that, when tested disinterestedly, such therapies are effective. Several well-designed, randomized controlled trials reported in 2002 failed to prove the value of, or to validate the claimed effectiveness of, acupuncture for cocaine addiction; St John's Wort or sertraline for severe depression; chelation therapy for coronary artery disease; homoeopathy for asthmatic adults with house dust mite excreta allergies; vitamin and mineral supplements to prevent respiratory infections; ginkgo for memory loss; or prayer for the outcome of myocardial infarction.

complementary pairs the pairs of bases that link together, like the rungs of a ladder, along the length of the DNA molecule. The whole process of DNA replication depends on the fact that, in DNA, adenine can only link to thymine and guanine can only link to cytosine

complement fixation the taking up of COMPLEMENT by antigen-antibody complexes. This process forms the basis of a number of tests to confirm infection with particular organisms.

complete linkage the location of genes sufficiently close to each other in a chromosome that they are always transmitted together to daughter cells. In the phenotype, the effects of such genes always occur together in the same individual.

complex a psychoanalytic term defining a group of tendencies, with strong emotional associations, but which is socially unacceptable and therefore repressed – with dire consequences. Freudians lay great emphasis on the Oedipus complex, which is said to be based on the desire for sexual access to the mother and the wish to dispose of the father. See also FREUDIAN THEORY.

complicated fracture a fracture of bone associated with significant injury to other structures such as arteries, nerves or muscles.

complication an additional disorder, or new feature, arising in the course of, or as a result of, a disease, injury or abnormality.

compos mentis literally, of composed mind. Sane.

compound fracture a bone break with perforation of the skin so that the fracture site has been in contact, however briefly, with the outside environment or the surface of the skin. Such a fracture is infected and requires different management from a non-compound (simple) fracture.

Compazine a trade name for PROCHLORPERAZINE.

compress a pad of gauze or other material firmly applied to a part of the body to apply heat, cold or medication or to control bleeding (haemorrhage).

compulsion 1 an irresistible, or near-irresistible, impulse to perform an action, even if irrational or against the interests of the actor. 2 an act performed in response to such an impulse. See also COMPULSIVE BEHAVIOUR.

compulsive behaviour behaviour resulting from an abnormal and uncontrollable need to perform a particular action. If the impulse is resisted, there is intense anxiety. The action is often repetitive and ritualized. A manifestation of an obsessive-compulsive disorder.

computerized axial tomography see CT SCANNING.

computers in medicine see MEDICAL COMPUTING.

conation the mental processes characterized by aim, impulse, desire, will and striving. The functioning of the active part of the personality. Compare COGNITION and AFFECT.

conception 1 penetration of an OVUM by a SPERMATOZOON, with the initiation of a new individual and the state of pregnancy. The formation of a ZYGOTE. 2 the individual zygote or embryo so formed.

conceptus the product of CONCEPTION.

concha the visible, external part of the ear. Also known as the pinna or auricle.

concretion a solid mass of chalky or inorganic material formed in a cavity or tissue of the body. A CALCULUS.

concussion a 'shaking-up' of the brain, from violent acceleration or deceleration of the head, causing unconsciousness lasting for seconds to hours. The injury is probably associated with some bleeding inside the brain and in many cases actual destruction of nerve tissue occurs. People who have suffered concussion require expert clinical observation in hospital for at least 24 hours.

condenser 1 a device in which gas is cooled to a liquid. 2 an optical device that concentrates light on an object to be examined by microscopy. 3 a dental instrument for compressing filling material into a prepared tooth cavity.

conditional lethal mutation a mutation that will kill a cell under certain conditions but not under others.

conditioned reflex an automatic response to a stimulus which differs from that initially causing the response but which has become associated with it by repetition. The sight of food causes a dog to salivate. If a bell is rung every time the food appears, the bell alone will, in time, cause salivation.

conditioning an important element in human programming and behaviour. Conditioning is a form of learning in which a particular stimulus will eventually and reliably elicit a particular behavioral response.

condom a barrier contraceptive of thin rubber worn on the erect penis. The condom also offers significant protection, in either direction, against sexually transmitted diseases, including AIDS. Research has shown that condom failure is on the increase. The female condom was an excellent idea that, for inscrutable reasons, seems never to have caught on. See also CONTRACEPTION.

conduct disorders patterns of behaviour that consistently violate the rights of others or the accepted norms of society. The effects equate closely with criminal behaviour and include burglary, fire-raising, destroying property, cruelty and physical aggression with weapons.

conduction defect a failure of the normal passage of controlling electrical impulses through the specialized conduction muscle fibres of the heart. Conduction defects lead to various forms of HEART BLOCK.

conductive deafness a hearing defect caused by a disorder in any part of the ear between the external acoustic canal (auditory meatus) and the fluid in the COCHLEA. Compare SENSORI-NEURAL DEAFNESS.

conductive paste 1 a jelly-like substance capable of effecting a low electrical contact resistance between the skin and an electrode, as used in electrocardiography. 2 a gel used between the skin and an ultrasound transducer so as to reduce energy losses and improve the scanning performance.

condyle a rounded prominence at the end of a long bone that gives attachment to tendons and articulates with the adjacent bone.

Condyline a brand name for PODOPHYLLOTOXIN.

condylitis inflammation of a CONDYLE, as in TENNIS ELBOW.

condylomata acuminata soft, pinkish, cauliflower-like warts on the genitals caused by papovaviruses – the same viruses that cause other kinds of warts – and spread by sexual intercourse.

condylomata lata flat, moist, red or gray masses occurring on the glans of the penis or on the vulva in secondary SYPHILIS. They swarm with spirochaetes and are highly infectious.

cone biopsy the removal of a cone-shaped segment of tissue from the inside of the neck of the womb to provide material for positive microscopic diagnosis. This is done under general anaesthesia when a cervical smear test suggests that cancer may be present.

cones the tiny light-sensitive transducers of the RETINA that are present in greatest concentration in the central part, the macula. Cones are less sensitive than the more peripherally placed, colour-blind rods, but are capable of distinguishing three primary colours.

cone shell stings a toxic injection from the dart of the colourful coneshell mollusc. The effect is muscular paralysis which may be so widespread as to affect the breathing and cause death. Expert resuscitation in hospital is necessary.

confabulation the recounting of fictitious and repetitive, but often plausible, detail of past events to cover gaps in the memory. This is common in various forms of dementia and is most characteristic of the alcohol-induced KORSAKOFF'S SYNDROME.

confidence interval (CI) a statistical term that quantifies uncertainty. In a clinical trial, the 95% confidence interval (the interval usually employed) for any relevant variable is the range of values within which we can be 95% sure that the true value lies for the entire population of people from which those patients participating in the trial are taken. The greater the number of patients on which the confidence interval is based the narrower it becomes.

confidentiality the principle which protects the right of patients to expect that details of their medical conditions should be divulged only to those who need to know them for medical purposes.

confinement the period from the start of labour to the delivery of the afterbirth (placenta).

conflict the effect of the presence of two mutually incompatible wishes or emotions. Unacceptably unpleasant conflict leads to REPRESSION and this may be manifested as NEUROSIS.

conformational epitope adjacent amino acid strings at different points in a folded protein, making a complex site to which an antibody can bind. Conformational epitopes are less stable than LINEAR EPITOPES, a fact that explains why some allergies are outgrown in time. Allergies, such as peanut allergy, in which the antibody (IgE) binds to a linear epitope tend to persist.

conformational exposure a technique of identification of abnormal proteins in which conformational epitopes that become exposed when a protein is misfolded are identified. The most impressive recent use of this technique was revealed in late 2003 when a method of detecting the protease-resistant prion protein PrP^{Sc} was published. Researchers found three amino acid residues, Arg-Arg-Tyr, that occurred twice in this protein. Rabbits were immunized with peptides based on this motif and were used to generate a polyclonal antibody that was able to identify PrP^{Sc}, in vitro, from cows, sheep and humans.

conformer a mould placed in a cavity to preserve its shape and prevent shrinkage.

confrontation 1 insistence by one person that another person should give due attention and weight to data asserted or opinions expressed. 2 a rough method of visual field testing in which the examiner compares the extent of the area of the patient's visual perception with his or her own, while sitting face to face and with opposite eyes mutually fixated.

confusion a state of DISORIENTATION from disturbance of memory, loss of contact with reality, HALLUCINATION or DEMENTIA. Confusion is often temporary and the result of brain disorder from toxic influences, EPILEPSY or head injury.

congeal to clot or coagulate.

congener one of a group of chemical compounds with a common parent substance or derived from a common basic formula.

congenic of organisms that differ only at a single genetic locus.

congenic strains strains of animals, such as rats, that are genetically identical except for a single chromosome segment. If such strains show differences in disease or other characteristics, the locus for these features must be within that segment. Important genetic research can be done using congenic strains.

congenital present at birth and resulting from factors operating before birth. A congenital disorder need not be hereditary, although many are. Conditions acquired during fetal life are congenital as are those acquired during the process of birth.

congenital adrenal hyperplasia an autosomal recessive disorder, featuring enlargement of the ADRENAL GLANDS, that results from a deficiency of one of the five enzymes needed to synthesize cortisol. The absence of this hormone causes the pituitary to secrete abnormally high quantities of ACTH (corticotropin) which overstimulates the adrenals, causing enlargement. More importantly, the precursors of cortisol are overproduced and some of these are converted to sex hormones especially androgens. This can cause ambiguous genitalia in baby girls. This is also aldosterone deficiency with excessive sodium loss and abnormally raised potassium levels.

congenital anomaly any abnormality present at birth.

congenital dislocation of the hip an abnormal relationship, present at birth, of the head of the thigh bone (femur) to the socket (acetabulum) in the pelvis. The condition is commoner in girl babies and requires early treatment if a severe walking defect is to be avoided.

congenital heart disease a range of heart disorders, of varying degrees of severity, present at birth. Congenital heart disease affects about one live baby in 120 and is caused by factors operating early in pregnancy. These include virus infections, especially RUBELLA, drugs, DIABETES and SYSTEMIC LUPUS ERYTHEMATOSUS in the mother. Congenital heart disease is a feature of DOWN'S SYNDROME and other chromosomal defects, including TRISOMY 13 and TRISOMY 18. The diseases include 'hole in the heart' (SEPTAL DEFECTS), PATENT DUCTUS ARTERIOSUS, pulmonary valve narrowing (stenosis), AORTIC STENOSIS and FALLOT'S TETRALOGY.

congenital syphilis SYPHILIS acquired by the fetus from the mother during pregnancy and present at birth. Congenital syphilis may feature severe early skin rashes, often occurring in the first 10 weeks of life, bone and cartilage defects, liver and kidney disturbances, damage to the corneas (interstitial keratitis), deafness, peg teeth, saddle-shaped nose and scars at the angles of the mouth. Treatment is with penicillin.

congestion an abnormal collection of fluid, often blood, causing engorgement in an organ or part. Congestion is the result of some other disease process, such as infection or HEART FAILURE, and will usually settle when the cause is removed.

congestion, nasal see NASAL CONGESTION.

congestive heart failure see HEART FAILURE.

coniosis any disorder caused by dust.

conization removal of a cone-shaped segment from the inside of the cervix of the womb, as in CONE BIOPSY.

conjugate coupled or joined in pairs or groups. Of co-valently linked complexes of two or more molecules.

conjugate measurements measurements of distances between bony points, especially various measurements of the inlet and outlet of the female pelvis in connection with prospective childbirth.

conjugated protein a compound of a protein with a nonprotein.

conjugation 1 chemical combination or linkage of chemical groups to organic molecules, often to produce a water-soluble form and allow more ready excretion. 2 the exchange of genetic material between paired single-cell organisms, such as bacteria.

conjunctiva the transparent membrane attached around the CORNEA, covering the white of the eye and reflected back over the inner surfaces of the eyelids.

conjunctivitis inflammation of the CONJUNCTIVA. This is most commonly caused by infection but may result from ALLERGY, chemical irritation from dusts, gases, industrial vapours or injudicious medication and radiation of various kinds, including sunlight.

connectin a protein found on the surface of some cancer cells that binds to cytoskeleton ACTINS and glycoproteins on other cells.

connective tissue loose or dense collections of COLLAGEN fibres and many cells, in a liquid, gelatinous or solid medium. Connective tissue participates in the structure of organs or body tissue or binds them together. It includes cartilage, bone, tooth dentine and lymphoid tissue.

connective tissue diseases this is a large group which includes RHEUMATOID ARTHRITIS, STILL'S DISEASE (juvenile rheumatoid arthritis), infective ARTHRITIS, SYSTEMIC LUPUS ERYTHEMATOSUS, PROGRESSIVE SYSTEMIC SCLEROSIS, various forms of ARTERITIS, POLYMYOSITIS and DERMATOMYOSITIS.

connexin-26 one of a number of gap junction connexin proteins. Gap junctions between cells allow the passage of ions and small molecules from one cell to another. The gene for connexin-26 has been located and is situated on chromosome 13. A single base deletion mutation of this gene results in the complete absence of this connexin, and the only effect detected to date is a recessive form of sensorineural deafness.

Conn's syndrome a rare condition caused by a tumour of the cells in an adrenal gland which secrete the hormone ALDOSTERONE. The result is over-production of this hormone with salt and water retention and a resulting excess of fluid in the tissues (OEDEMA), and high blood pressure (HYPERTENSION). (Jerome William Conn, American physician, b. 1907).

conotruncal facial anomaly a genetic condition featuring abnormally wide separation of the eyes with narrowed lid openings and puffy lids; misshapen nose that appears to be divided into an upper and a lower part; and low-set ears with lobe anomalies. The condition is nearly always associated with abnormalities in the internal structures of the neck. It is caused by CONTIGUOUS GENE SYNDROME involving 24 to 30 genes on chromosome 22. See also DI GEORGE SYNDROME and T-BOX GENE SYNDROME.

consanguinity blood relationship. The term does not imply any particular degree of closeness and ranges from identical twin to remote cousin.

conscious awareness of one's existence, sensations, and environment. Capable of thought and perception.

consciousness full awareness of self and of one's environment. The conviction that it is possible to explain the sources of consciousness has spawned a small library books purporting to do so.

consciousness, grades of a scale of degrees useful in clinical practice. Grade 0 = fully conscious; 1, responds to voice; 2, unconscious but reacts to minor applied pain; 3, unconscious but shows some reaction to a strong painful stimulus; 4, no response to any stimulus.

consensual 1 pertaining to the reflex response of an organ to the reflex action of another, usually paired, organ. For example, the constriction response of one pupil to light is accompanied by the constriction of the other. This is a consensual reflex.
2 involving common consent, as in the consent of both parties to an act of sexual intercourse.

consent the implicit or explicit agreement to medical or surgical treatment or physical examination. Civil rights against personal interference are retained, however, and anything done against a person's will may be deemed an assault in law.

conservative recombination recombination of broken segments of DNA without the synthesis of any new sequences.

conservative treatment treatment that avoids extreme or radical measures but that aims to maintain or improve the state of the patient.

conserved of genetic entities that remain unchanged between individuals of a species or between different species or over a period of time. The adjective is often qualified as in 'highly conserved'.

consolidation 1 becoming, or having become, solid, especially in the case of lung tissue affected by LOBAR PNEUMONIA.
2 the conversion of short-term into long-term memory.

constipation unduly infrequent and difficult evacuation of the bowels. This disorder is often due to deliberate suppression of the desire to defaecate. It is almost unknown in people whose diet is largely vegetable with a high fibre content.

constitutive mutation a mutation whose effect is to cause a normally regulated gene or group of genes to express themselves continuously.

constrict 1 to narrow or make smaller, to shrink or contract.
2 to squeeze or compress.

constriction 1 a narrowing.
2 the act or process of narrowing.

constrictive pericarditis inflammation and thickening by fibrous tissue of the outer covering of the heart (pericardium) that prevents normal relaxation and filling of the heart chambers. Also known as Pick's disease (F.J. Pick, 1867–1926, German physician).

constrictor a muscle that contracts, narrows or compresses a part or organ of the body.

consultant a highly qualified and selected specialist doctor who practices without supervision. A doctor who gives expert professional advice. A person at the apex of the medical hierarchy.

consultation a clinical occasion on which the advice and medical care of a doctor is sought.

consummation the first act of sexual intercourse after marriage. Nowadays, this has mainly legal significance.

consumption an obsolete term for pulmonary TUBERCULOSIS.

Contac 400 a trade name for a mixture of ATROPINE, HYOSCINE, HYOSCYAMINE and PSEUDOEPHEDRINE.

contact dermatitis skin inflammation (ECZEMA) caused by an allergic reaction to a substance that has been in contact with the skin.

contact inhibition the control or cessation of cell growth and reproduction due to contact with adjacent cells. This important restraint is lost in cancer.

contact lens an optical correction worn in contact with the cornea and taking the place of spectacles. Most contact lens wearers are shortsighted (myopic) and enjoy a generally better standard of vision than with glasses. Hard contact lenses are made of acrylic PMMA (poly-methyl-methacrylate or 'Perspex') or CAB (cellulose acetate-butyrate) or co-polymers of various plastics. Soft lenses are mostly made of HEMA (hydroxy-ethyl-methacrylate). Hard lenses are always of smaller diameter than the cornea, soft lenses are usually of greater diameter.

contact tracing a public health measure designed to limit the spread of infectious disease, especially sexually transmitted diseases and conditions, such as typhoid, in which transmission by healthy carriers can occur.

contagious the literal meaning – spread by touch or direct contact – has given way to a looser usage and the term is now used simply to mean 'infectious'. Chickenpox, once thought contagious is now known to be spread by droplets; the common cold, once thought to be spread by droplets is now known to be literally contagious.

contiguous gene syndrome a syndrome featuring a range of apparently unrelated clinical defects that are actually due to deletion of a length of DNA containing adjacent genes the loss of each of which causes a specific defect.

continence self-control or restraint, especially in relation to sexual activity. The antonym, incontinence, seems, nowadays, to be applied mainly to urination and defaecation.

contraception the prevention of CONCEPTION by avoiding fertile periods; by imposing a barrier between the sperms and the egg; by killing sperms; or by preventing the release of eggs from the ovaries. Intrauterine contraceptive devices (IUCDs) act by preventing implantation of fertilized ova but are also usually considered a form of contraception. Testosterone and progestagens are being investigated as hormonal contraceptives for men. See also BARRIER CONTRACEPTIVE, CAP CONTRACEPTIVE, COITUS INTERRUPTUS, COMBINED ORAL CONTRACEPTIVE, CONDOM, CONOVA 30, DIAPHRAGM CONTRACEPTIVE, FOAM CONTRACEPTIVE.

contractile capable of contracting or of causing contraction.

contractile ring a ring of actin filaments around the equator of a cell formed at the end of MITOSIS. Tightening of this ring lead to the separation of the two daughter cells.

contracted pelvis a pelvis with an abnormal reduction in one or more of the internal dimensions. This can interfere with the passage of the baby's head during childbirth (parturition) so that birth is obstructed and CAESARIAN SECTION may be necessary.

contraction the primary function of muscle by which a change of shape brings the ends closer together. By contracting, muscles bring about movement of bones or other parts.

contractions a term usually applied to the periodic tightening and shortening of the muscle fibres in the womb (uterus) during labour which gradually bring about the expulsion of the baby. All muscles act by contraction.

contracture permanent shortening of tissue, such as muscle, tendon or skin, as a result of disuse, injury or disease. Contracture leads to the inability to straighten joints fully and to permanent deformity and disability. Skin contractures often follow burns.

contraindication anything which makes a proposed or possible form of medical treatment undesirable or dangerous.

contralateral pertaining to the opposite side. The term ipsilateral is used in referring to the same side.

contrast medium any substance offering greater resistance to the passage of X rays than soft tissues that can be introduced into a hollow organ so as to outline its interior during radiology. Contrast media include a suspension of a barium salt for the intestine (barium meal or enema) and iodine-containing fluids for the blood vessels and urinary tract.

contre coup damage occurring at a point opposite the point of impact, especially of injury to the brain against the inside of the skull. A sudden force applied to the skull may cause brain bruising at the opposite pole.

contusion a bruise.

convalescence 1 the period of recovery following an illness, injury or surgical operation.
2 the process of such recovery.

convergent evolution 1 the process in which phylogenetically distinct lineages acquire similar characteristics.
2 evolutionary changes in which descendants resemble each other more closely than their progenitors did.

convergent squint SEE STRABISMUS.

convergent thinking analytical thinking that follows a set of rules, as in arithmetic, or in which the logical validity of the thought processes is checked and verified. Compare divergent or creative 'lateral' thinking, characterized by unorthodox mental processes but often productive of a number of different and sometimes valuable solutions.

conversion disorder a psychological conflict that manifests itself as an organic dysfunction or physical symptom. Formerly known as HYSTERIA.

convolutions the folded elevations, or gyri, of the brain into which the surface layer (cortex) is thrown so as to accommodate its great area.

Convulex a brand name for VALPROIC ACID.

convulsion a fit or seizure. A convulsion may involve the whole body (grand mal) or part of the body (focal seizure). Convulsions are a feature of EPILEPSY but may occur in high fever (FEBRILE CONVULSIONS), brain tumour, ENCEPHALITIS, head injury, stroke and various kinds of poisoning.

convulsion, febrile see FEBRILE CONVULSIONS.

Cooley's anaemia an inherited abnormality of haemoglobin which causes breakdown of red blood cells and anaemia. The condition is usually called THALASSAEMIA major. (Thomas Benton Cooley, 1871–1945, American paediatrician).

Coombs' test a test for the type of anaemia in which the red cells are unduly fragile and break down easily, as a result of an immune disorder (autoimmune HAEMOLYTIC ANAEMIA). The test uses rabbit serum containing antihuman globulin antibodies obtained by injecting rabbits with human globulin. Such serum will cause the patient's red cells to clump together (agglutinate) if they are already coated with antibodies (IMMUNOGLOBULIN) as in autoimmune haemolytic anaemia. (Robin Royston Amos Coombs, English Professor of Biology, b. 1921).

Copaxone a brand name for GLATIRAMER.

COPD *abbrev. for* CHRONIC OBSTRUCTIVE PULMONARY DISEASE.

copolymer a POLYMER consisting of repeated units of two or more subunits.

copolymer-1 a mixture of synthetic random polypeptides made from the amino acids alanine, glutamic acid, lysine and tyrosine that has been found to reduce the relapse rate in MULTIPLE SCLEROSIS. Research suggests that the drug can reduce the relapse rate, in patients subject to relapses, from 75% to 66%. The drug is believed to act on helper T cells so as to promote cloning of those whose CYTOKINES are mainly B cell antibody-stimulating (Th-2) rather than those whose cytokines have a mainly inflammatory and destructive effect (Th-1). A brand name for copolymer-1 is Copaxone.

copper deficiency this rare condition occasionally affects young children, causing retardation of growth, rarefaction of bones and anaemia.

copro- *combining form denoting* faeces.

coprolalia sustained obscenity of speech.

coprolith a faece hardened like stone. A faecalith.

coprophilia abnormal attraction to faeces.

copulation a joining together in the act of COITUS. The physical element in sexual intercourse.

cor the heart.

coracoid a bony process on the outer side of the shoulder-blade (scapula) which projects forward under the outer end of the collar-bone (clavicle).

Coracten a brand name for NIFEDIPINE.

Corbeton a trade name for OXPRENOLOL.

Cordarone a brand name for AMIODARONE.

Cordilox a brand name for VERAPAMIL.

cordotomy partial severing of some of the nerve tracts in the spinal cord performed for the relief of severe and otherwise uncontrollable pain.

corectopia positioning of the pupil other than in the centre of the iris.

core octamer an elongated structure of four pairs of histone protein subunits forming a core around which DNA is wound. Histones are strongly basic proteins that show little variation in sequence from one species to another.

Corgard a brand name for NADOLOL.

corium the layer of living skin under the mainly dead outer layer. The 'true' skin, containing nerve endings, sweat glands, and blood vessels.

Corlan a brand name for HYDROCORTISONE.

corn a protective response to local skin pressure in the form of an increased production of flattened, horny cells (cornified epithelium). The local pressure forces these hard cells further into the skin and stimulates further production.

cornea the outer, and principle, lens of the eye through which the coloured iris with its central hole (the pupil) can be seen. The cornea performs most of the focusing of the eye. Fine adjustment (ACCOMMODATION) is done by the internal crystalline lens.

corneal abrasion local loss of the outer layer (epithelium) of the cornea, so that the sensory nerves are exposed to stimulation by movement of the lids. This may be exquisitely painful. The epithelium usually regrows in a day or two.

corneal dystrophy one of a range of conditions in which any of the three main layers of the cornea may be affected by a disorder of growth or development. Dystrophies usually interfere with the transparency or optical efficiency of the cornea and commonly damage vision. A few are very painful but most are painless. Some dystrophies can be readily treated by CORNEAL GRAFT.

corneal epithelium the thin, layered, outer 'skin' of the cornea. Advances in cell culture techniques have made it possible to grow complete sheets of viable corneal epithelium from a tiny sample taken from the edge of the patient's cornea. This is an important advance in the management of conditions featuring corneal epithelial disorders.

corneal graft replacement of a central disk of opaque CORNEA, usually about 7 mm in diameter, with a clear disc of exactly the same size from a donated eye. The clear disc is held in place with a very fine zig-zag stitch.

corneal reflex 1 automatic blinking on light touch to the cornea. The reflex is sometimes used by anaesthetists and others as a test of the level of consciousness.

2 the position of the reflection of a small light on the cornea when it is directly regarded by the subject. If mid-pupillary in one eye and eccentric in the other, the subject has a squint.

corneal transplant a CORNEAL GRAFT.

corneal ulceration an area of tissue destruction and cratering on the CORNEA. Corneal ulcers are almost always caused by infection, the commonest agent being Herpes simplex, the cold sore virus.

corona any structure resembling a crown.

coronal relating to the crown of the head.

coronal plane a vertical anatomical plane that divides the standing body into front and rear halves. A plane lying in the direction of the side-to-side CORONAL SUTURE of the skull.

coronal suture the irregular line of junction of the paired parietal bones of the skull with the frontal bone.

corona radiata 1 the radiating 'crown' of nerve fibre bundles running up from the INTERNAL CAPSULE of the brain to all parts of the CORTEX. 2 a layer of cells radiating outwards from the maturing OVUM and which persist for a time after ovulation.

coronary pertaining to a crown. The CORONARY ARTERIES arise from the main artery of the body immediately above the heart, and give off branches which spread like a crown, over the surface of the heart.

coronary angioplasty BALLOON ANGIOPLASTY performed in a CORONARY ARTERY. This is normally performed as an elective procedure after angiography demonstrates a local obstruction in the coronary blood flow. It has recently been shown, however, that primary coronary angioplasty is a more effective and more often life-saving procedure for the treatment of acute myocardial infarction (heart attack) than attempts to break down the obstructing blood clot by enzymatic treatment (fibrinolysis). A critical factor is the length of time elapsing between the blockage and the angioplasty. This is necessarily longer than the time to fibrinolysis. See also BALLOON CATHETER.

coronary artery one of two important branches of the AORTA that supply the heart muscle with blood. The left coronary artery divides almost at once into two main trunks, so it is common for surgeons to refer to the three coronary arteries. Smaller branches of the coronary arteries spread over the surface of the heart and send twigs into the heart muscle. Obstruction of a coronary artery branch, by ATHEROSCLEROSIS and subsequent THROMBOSIS, is commoner than blockage of one of the main trunks. Such obstruction causes a heart attack by depriving a part of the heart muscle of its blood supply to cause local death of muscle tissue (myocardial infarction).

coronary artery bypass the use of a short length of vein to connect the AORTA to a point on a CORONARY artery beyond a narrowing or obstruction. A triple bypass is often performed at the same operation. The veins soon thicken and become arterialized. Alternatively, an internal mammary artery can be disconnected and sewn into the coronary artery beyond the obstruction.

coronary artery disease any disease of the CORONARY ARTERIES, but particularly ATHEROSCLEROSIS or other arteropathy that prejudices the flow of blood and hence the blood supply to the heart muscle. See also CORONARY SYNDROME.

coronary artery ectasia abnormal widening of a coronary artery or branch that affects about 2% of the general population. The cause is unknown but is thought possibly to be due to excessive local production of NITRIC OXIDE as a result of the use of nitrites.

coronary care unit a hospital department or ward set aside for the monitoring and intensive care management of people who have suffered attacks of CORONARY THROMBOSIS and are in an unstable condition.

coronary insufficiency a reduction in the coronary blood flow of such degree as to limit the full action of the heart muscle on demand. Coronary insufficiency commonly causes ANGINA PECTORIS.

coronary occlusion complete obstruction of blood flow in a CORONARY artery.

coronary restenosis the recurrence of narrowing of coronary arteries after treatment by balloon angioplasty or other means. STENTING is reliably capable of preventing restenosis especially if antiproliferative-drug-eluting stents are used. In-stent restenosis is treated by intracoronary gamma and beta irradiation. Antisense therapies or gene therapy may prove important im managing restenosis.

coronary stenting see STENTING.

coronary syndrome a general term for any condition caused by disease of the coronary arteries, in particular ATHEROSCLEROSIS. The most important of these diseases are stable or unstable ANGINA PECTORIS and HEART ATTACK. An appreciation of coronary syndromes has gone well beyond that of simple mechanical blockage by an atheromatous plaque and overlying blood clotting. The plaque is now known to be a complex active entity containing, besides other ingredients, inflammatory cells, endothelial cells and smooth muscle cells. These components are in active communication with each other by way of CYTOKINE signalling systems. Chlamydial and other infections may also be involved in atherogenesis and plaque instability.

coronary thrombosis a heart attack caused by clotting of blood at the site of narrowing of a coronary artery, so that the heart muscle is locally deprived of blood and part of the muscle dies. Coronary narrowing is almost always caused by ATHEROSCLEROSIS. See also CORONARY SYNDROME.

coronary veins the vessels that drain blood from the heart muscle, joining to form a vein that empties into the right ATRIUM.

coronavirus one of the many types of virus that can cause the common cold. The virus has attracted much recent attention since it was discovered that a new strain of coronavirus was the cause of SARS.

coroner a barrister, solicitor or doctor, appointed by the County authorities mainly for the purpose of enquiring into the cause of death in cases in which this is not immediately apparent or in which death cannot be certified by an attending doctor.

Coro-Nitro a brand name for GLYCERYL TRINITRATE (nitroglycerine).

corpulence obesity. Being excessively fat.

cor pulmonale a heart disorder caused by a rise in the resistance to the passage of blood through the lungs from conditions such as chronic bronchitis, EMPHYSEMA, SILICOSIS or INTERSTITIAL FIBROSIS. The result is enlargement of the main pumping chamber (ventricle) on the right side and often right HEART FAILURE.

corpus albicans the white fibrous tissue body remaining in an ovary after the CORPUS LUTEUM has regressed.

corpus callosum the wide curved band of nerve fibres (white matter) that connects the two cerebral hemispheres.

corpuscle a general term for any small, discrete, microscopic structure such as a red blood cell, a sensory nerve ending, an OSTEOCYTE or a GLOMERULUS of a kidney.

corpus luteum a yellow mass of fatty material swelling out the empty GRAAFIAN FOLLICLE in the ovary after the egg (ovum) has been discharged. The cells of the corpus luteum secrete both oestrogens and progesterone and these hormones cause the lining of the womb to thicken and form a suitable bed for the fertilized ovum. If pregnancy does not occur the corpus luteum degenerates in less than two weeks.

corpus striatum a gray and white striped collection of nerve cell bodies and nerve fibres in the lower and outer part of each cerebral hemisphere. The corpus striatum is the largest subdivision of the BASAL GANGLIA and consists of the caudate and lentiform nuclei. It is concerned largely with control of movement.

corpuscle an old-fashioned term for a free-floating blood cell, such as a red or white blood cell. The term derives from the Latin *corpusculum*, the diminutive of the term for 'body'.

correlation the degree to which changes in variables reflect, or fail to reflect one another. Correlations are said to be positive when the variables change in the same direction and negative when they move in opposite directions. A common fault in statistics is to assume that correlations are significant when they are not, that is, to assume unjustifiably that changes in

variables are causally related.

Corrigan's pulse a forceful bounding pulse with a sudden, collapsing quality that is a feature of incompetence of the aortic valve at the outlet of the left ventricle of the heart. Also called a 'water-hammer' pulse. (Sir Dominic John Corrigan, 1802–80, Irish physician).

corrosive poisoning poisoning with strong acids or alkalis capable of causing rapid tissue destruction and shrinkage. Survivors often suffer severe narrowing (strictures) or obstruction of the gullet. Milk by mouth is the best readily available first aid treatment. Liver and kidney damage is common.

Cortate a trade name for CORTISONE.

Cortef a brand name for HYDROCORTISONE.

cortex the outer distinguishable zone of any solid organ. The cerebral cortex, for instance, is the outer layer of grey matter of the brain consisting of nerve cell bodies. The adrenal cortex is quite different in function from the inner part.

cortical pertaining to, or consisting of, a CORTEX.

corticoid an informal term for any steroid produced by the adrenal cortex. A corticosteroid.

corticospinal connecting the cerebral cortex and the spinal cord or pertaining to both. The corticospinal tracts are large bundles of nerve fibres largely concerned with voluntary movement.

corticosteroid drugs drugs identical to, or that simulate the actions of, the natural steroid hormones of the outer zone (cortex) of the adrenal glands. Modern synthetic steroids are often many times more powerful than the natural hormones hydrocortisone and corticosterone. They include prednisolone, methylprednisolone, triamcinolone, dexamethasone, betamethasone, deoxycortone and fludrocortisone.

corticosteroid hormones natural steroid hormones secreted by the cortex of the adrenal glands. These are cortisol, corticosterone, aldosterone and androsterone.

corticotrophin corticotropin, adrenocorticotrophic hormone (ACTH), a hormone produced by the PITUITARY GLAND which stimulates the adrenal cortex to secrete steroids in response to stress.

cortisol a hormone produced by the adrenal

cortex. Also called hydrocortisone.

cortisone the first corticosteroid produced for treatment purposes. It is converted to hydrocortisone in the liver. It was used to treat rheumatoid arthritis, severe allergies, adrenal failure and other conditions but has been largely replaced by more powerful synthetic steroids. A brand name is Cortisyl.

Corynebacterium any species of the genus *Corynebacterium*. These are GRAM POSITIVE rod-shaped bacteria and include the organism that causes diphtheria, *Corynebacterium diphtheriae*.

coryza the medical term for the common cold. See COLD.

cosmesis consideration or concern for appearance.

cosmetic surgery a branch of plastic surgery devoted to the improvement or alteration of the human appearance. Cosmetic operations include those on the nose (rhinoplasty), the ears (otoplasty), the chin (mentoplasty) and the breasts (augmentation or reduction mammoplasty). See also PLASTIC SURGERY.

costa a rib.

costal cartilages the flexible cartilagesby which the front ends of most of the ribs are connected to the breast bone (STERNUM).

costalgia pain in a rib.

costive suffering from, or causing, constipation.

costochondral pertaining to a rib and its cartilage.

cot death see SUDDEN INFANT DEATH SYNDROME.

cothymia the simultaneous association of anxiety and depression in the same person. Contast with dysthymia: a form of chronic low-grade depression, and with psychiatric comorbidity: the presence of apparently distinct psychiatric diagnoses in the same person. See also NOSOLOGY.

co-trimoxazole a combination of the sulphonamide SULPHAMETHOXAZOLE and TRIMETHOPRIM. The drug is useful in acute BRONCHITIS, urinary infections, SALMONELLA infections and in the treatment of TYPHOID carriers. Brand names are Septrin and Chemotrim.

cotyloid cavity see ACETABULUM.

cough a protective reflex by which a sudden blast of compressed air is released along the bronchial tubes and windpipe (trachea) and through the voice box (larynx). Coughing expels irritating and potentially infective or obstructive material. It is a sign of most respiratory infections and many respiratory disorders. Persistent (chronic) chest disorders feature regular coughing because of the production of excessive bronchial secretions. The quality of the cough may be diagnostic, as in WHOOPING COUGH (pertussis), partial obstruction of the larynx or paralysis of the nerves to the larynx, but is usually non-specific. It is often early in lung cancer and late in TUBERCULOSIS. Sputum may be scanty or, as in BRONCHIECTASIS, voluminous. It may contain blood (HAEMOPTYSIS).

coughing blood v. an important sign which should never be ignored. The medical term is 'haemoptysis'. Blood-streaked sputum is common in BRONCHITIS. Coughing of pure blood is almost always serious and can be a sign of lung cancer, lung abscess, TUBERCULOSIS, HEART FAILURE, PULMONARY EMBOLUS or blood clotting disorders.

cough, smoker's see SMOKER'S COUGH.

Coulter counter an electronic device for automatic blood cell count and analysis. The demands on haematological laboratories are so great nowadays, that manual methods are impracticable and automation is essential.

Coumadin a brand name for WARFARIN.

Councilman bodies red-staining dead liver cells found in YELLOW FEVER, HEPATITIS and other serious liver disorders. (William Thomas Councilman, 1854–1933, American pathologist).

counterirritant anything applied to the skin to provoke a mild inflammation and relieve deeper pain either by improving the blood supply or by interfering with the passage of sensory nerve impulses.

countertraction a pull in one direction so as to allow the full effect of a simultaneous pull in the opposite direction. Countertraction is often applied to a fractured limb undergoing surgical straightening (reduction of fracture) or sustained TRACTION for purposes of immobilization.

Coversyl a brand name for PERINDOPRIL.

cover test a test for squint (STRABISMUS). When the subject is looking at a small near object and the non-squinting eye is covered, the other eye will move to continue viewing. This repeatable observed movement indicates that a genuine strabismus is present.

Cowper's glands a pair of pea-sized, yellow, multilobed glands lying in the SPHINCTER of the male urethra and discharging into it. Under the influence of sexual interest they secrete a clear mucinous lubricant to facilitate intercourse. They are also called the bulbo-urethral glands and are the male equivalent of THE BARTHOLIN'S GLANDS. (William Cowper, 1666–1709, English surgeon).

cowpox a mild disease of cows' udders and teats that can be transmitted to people, doing manual milking. It causes skin blisters and confers immunity against SMALLPOX – a somewhat academic consideration now that this disease has been eradicated. Jenner's observations on cowpox led to vaccination and the science of immunology. (Edward Jenner, 1749–1823, English physician).

COX see CYCLO-OXYGENASE.

COX-2 inhibitors a group of drugs that block the action of the enzymes, CYCLO-OXYGENASES, which change linear fatty acids into the ring (cyclical) structures of the PROSTAGLANDINS. There are two groups, COX-1 and COX-2. Cox-2 enzymes are produced at the site of inflammation especially in joints, so inhibitors are useful in the treatment of various forms of arthritis. The group includes CELECOXIB and ROFECOXIB.

coxa the hip or hip joint.

coxalgia pain in the hip.

Coxiella a genus of micro-organisms closely related to the *Rickettsiae*.

coxitis inflammation of the hip joint.

Coxsackie viruses a large group of PICORNAVIRUS ENTEROVIRUSES of a type similar to the poliomyelitis virus. They cause HERPANGINA, BORNHOLM DISEASE (epidemic pleurodynia), MYOCARDITIS, PERICARDITIS and MENINGITIS. The group is named after Coxsackie, New York.

Cozaar a brand name for the ANGIOTENSIN II ANTAGONIST drug LOSARTAN.

Cozaar-Comp a brand name for the ANGIOTENSIN II ANTAGONIST drug LOSARTAN formulated with HYDROCHLOROTHIAZIDE.

CPH *abbrev. for* Certificate in Public Health.

CPPD *abbrev. for* calcium pysophosphate dihydrate, the crystalline substance deposited in cartilage and causing PSEUDOGOUT.

CPR *abbrev. for* cardiopulmonary resuscitation.

crab louse the human ectoparasite *Pediculus pubis* (*Phthirus pubis*), which is usually confined to the genital area, especially in the pubic hair, and is transmitted during sexual intercourse.

crack a highly purified form of COCAINE which produces an intense reaction of rapid onset. Crack is inherently more dangerous than less concentrated forms and deaths have resulted from its use.

cradle cap a type of seborrhoeic dermatitis occurring in infants and consisting of thick, yellow, greasy, crusted scales on the scalp. It is easily treated.

CRAMC *abbrev. for* Commander Royal Army Medical Corps.

cramp powerful, sustained and painful contraction of a muscle or a group of muscles. The pain persists until the contraction eases off. Cramp may be caused by salt deficiency. The cause of the common night cramps is obscure. See also WRITER'S CRAMP.

cranial nerves the 12 pairs of nerves which spring directly from the brain and brain stem. They include the nerves for smell, sight, eye movement, facial movement and sensation, hearing, taste and head movement.

cranio- *combining form denoting* the bones that enclose the brain (the CRANIUM).

cranioclast a powerful type of forceps sometimes used to crush the head of a dead baby impacted in the pelvis, so as to allow delivery.

craniofacial pertaining to the cranium and the face.

craniopharyngioma a brain tumour affecting mainly children and arising from persistent primitive cells in the region of the pituitary gland. It causes headaches, visual field loss and delayed physical and mental development. Treatment is by surgical removal.

cranioplasty surgical coverage of a bony defect in the skull, usually by means of an implant of plastic, metal or bone.

craniostenosis premature closure of the FONTANELLES and fusion of the cranial sutures so that the skull remains small and underdeveloped.

craniosynostosis premature fusion of the suture joints of the skull, usually occurring before birth and leading to a severe skull deformity. The condition can be caused by a mutation of the gene for a fibroblast growth factor receptor.

craniotomy surgical opening of the skull,

usually for the purpose of operation on the brain or to relieve dangerous pressure within the skull cavity.

cranium the skeleton of the head without the jaw bone.

CRCP *abbrev. for* Certificant of the Royal College of Physicians.

CRCS *abbrev. for* Certificant of the Royal College of Surgeons.

C-reactive proteins a group of proteins that increase rapidly in amount in the blood during infections. They promote the binding of COMPLEMENT, a process known as opsonization (From Latin, *opsonare*, to lay in provisions for the table). Human C-reactive protein consists of five identical POLYPEPTIDE units arranged in a cyclical pattern. The protein has the power of binding to micro-organisms that have phorphorylcholine in their cell membranes. The complex then activates complement and in this way encourage the destruction and removal of invaders by phagocyte cells (PHAGOCYTOSIS).

creatine a nitrogenous substance present in all muscle cells.

creatine kinases (CKs) enzymes that catalyze the bond between creatine and ATP to form creatine phosphate and ADP with the storage of energy in the phosphate bond. Creatine phosphate occurs mainly in muscle and contributes energy required for muscle contraction. CKs are released into the blood from damaged heart and other muscle cells. Creatine kinase estimations are important in the diagnosis and quantification of heart muscle damage or death after CORONARY THROMBOSIS. CK blood levels rise after strenuous exercise or intramuscular injections.

creatinine a breakdown product of the important nitrogenous metabolic substance CREATINE. Creatinine is a normal metabolic waste substance and is found in muscle and blood and excreted in the urine.

creatinine clearance test a test of the rate at which the kidneys are removing CREATININE from the blood. This is an index of the rate of filtration of the blood by the kidneys and thus of their health and efficiency.

creatinuria excess of the nitrogenous compound creatine in the urine. This occurs in conditions in which muscle is being broken down at an abnormal rate, as in acute fevers, severe DIABETES and starvation.

creationism the belief that the account of the creation of the world contained in the first chapter of the book of Genesis is literally true. The implication, often expressed, is that the scientific account, including the geological evidence, is false. Creationism denies Darwinian evolution, but a belief in, and knowledge of, evolution has become an essential component in the mental armamentarium of the medical scientist. (See EVOLUTIONARY MEDICINE.)

Credé's manoeuvre external pressure on the lower abdomen, after delivery of a baby, so as to expel the PLACENTA. (Karl Sigmund Franz Credé, 1819–1892, German gynaecologist).

creeping eruption a skin disease caused by the migration in the skin of the larvae of hookworms and certain roundworms, especially *Toxocara canis*. There is itching and eruptions in the form of wandering red lines. Also called cutaneous larva migrans.

cremaster a thin layer of muscle looping over the SPERMATIC CORD and continuous with the internal oblique muscle of the abdominal wall. Its action is to draw up the testicle.

cremation disposal of bodies by burning. Nowadays, the great majority of people dying in Britain are cremated. In most historic traditions, cremation was considered more honourable than burial.

Creon a brand name for PANCREATIN.

crepitation a fine crackling sound heard with a STETHOSCOPE when listening over lungs containing more than the normal amount of fluid secretions.

crepitus 1 the grinding or crackling sound heard when the broken ends of a fractured bone rub together. This is one of the signs of fracture. **2** the grating sensation felt when a joint affected by arthritis is moved and dry or damaged joint surfaces rub together.

CREST syndrome *acronym for* a connective tissue disorder, related to progressive systemic sclerosis, but limited to CALCINOSIS, RAYNAUD'S PHENOMENON, oesophageal involvement, hardness of the fingers (Sclerodactyly) and dilated skin blood vessels (TELANGIECTASIA). The word forming the third letter of the acronym is spelt 'esophageal' in the USA.

Crestor a brand name for ROSUVASTATIN. See STATINS.

cretinism a condition caused by thyroid

underaction from severe iodine deficiency early in life. It features dwarfism, mental retardation, dry skin, a large tongue and a puffy face. Cretinism occurs mainly in regions remote from the sea. Iodization of table salt and early screening of babies has largely eliminated the condition from such regions.

Creutzfeldt-Jakob disease (CJD) a rapidly-progressive transmissible disease of the nervous system with a long incubation period. CJD mainly affects middle-aged and elderly people as a sporadic disease causing death within a few months of onset. It is a SPONGIFORM ENCEPHALOPATHY, similar, or possibly identical, to bovine spongiform encephalopathy (BSE), KURU and scrapie in sheep and is associated with an abnormal protein called a PRION. Up to 60 cases are estimated to occur each year in Britain. There is no effective treatment. A new variant of CJD with a shorter incubation period (vCJD) appeared in 1995 and by January 2003 a total of 121 cases of new variant CJD had been confirmed in Britain. There is clear evidence that this form is caused by the same strain of prion as BOVINE SPONGIFORM ENCEPHALOPATHY. In the period 1990 –2002 the total for all types of CJD was 822. In late 2003 a patient with vCJD was treated with brain injections of pentosan polysulphate and this seemed to halt the progression of the disease. (Hans Gerhard Creutzfeldt, 1885–1964, German psychiatrist; and Alfons Maria Jakob, 1884–1931, German neurologist).

CRIB *abbrev. for* Clinical Risk Index for Babies. This is a scoring tool for assessing the initial neonatal risk of babies and for comparing the performance of neonatal intensive care units.

cribriform perforated like a sieve. The cribriform plate of the ethmoid bone allows the tiny nerve fibres of the nerve of smell (olfactory nerve) to pass though from the cranial cavity into the upper part of the nose.

cricoid 1 ring-shaped.
2 a ring-shaped cartilage in the voice-box (larynx).

cri du chat syndrome a genetic disorder caused by the absence of the short arm on chromosome number five. Affected babies have small brains (microcephaly), severe mental retardation and a peculiar, high-pitched, mewing cry, like that of a kitten. Most die before reaching adult life.

Crigler-Najjar syndrome Type I is a rare autosomal recessive disorder causing absence of an enzyme (glucuronyl transferase) essential for normal liver function. Affected new-born babies have high levels of BILIRUBIN in the blood with bilirubin staining of the basal ganglia of the brain. Mortality is high. Type II is a rare autosomal dominant, and much milder form 7of the disorder in which there is only a partial deficiency of the enzyme. Most survive. (John F. Crigler, American paediatrician, b. 1919 and Lebanese-born American molecular biologist and paediatrician Victor Assar Najjar, b. 1914).

criminal abortion illegal termination of pregnancy by any means.

Crinone a brand name for PROGESTERONE.

crisis the peak or turning-point of a disease, especially an infection like LOBAR PNEUMONIA, after which one generally knew whether the patient was going to live or die. Nowadays, patients seldom reach a crisis, because infections are rapidly brought under control with antibiotics.

crista a crest or ridge.

Crixivan a brand name for INDINAVIR.

Crohn's disease a persistent inflammatory disease affecting a segment towards the end of the small intestine (the ileum) or the beginning of the large intestine (colon), or both. The cause is unknown. Also called regional ileitis. Dietary treatment providing nitrogen in the form of free amino acids or short chain peptides have been found in some cases to compare well with corticosteroid treatment. (Burrill Bernard Crohn, 1884–1983, American gastroenterologist)

cromoglycate a drug used in allergies. It stabilizes the membrane of the mast cells that otherwise release HISTAMINE and other irritating substances when antibodies (IgE) and ALLERGENS (such as pollen grains) react on their surfaces. Brand names are Aerocrom, Cromogen, Hay-crom, Nalcrom, Opticrom, Intal Synchroner, Rynacrom and Rynacrom Spray.

Cromogen a brand name for CROMOGLYCATE.

Crosby capsule a spring-loaded device on the end of a fine tube that is swallowed and then triggered to obtain a sample of the lining of the JEJUNUM for microscopic examination for the diagnosis of malabsorption disorders. (William Holmes Crosby, American physician, b. 1914).

cross-eye the popular term for STRABISMUS or squint. This should never be ignored in young children as it almost always results in defective vision in the squinting eye. See also AMBLYOPIA.

cross-matching a test of the compatibility of blood intended to be transfused. Serum from the donor's blood is mixed with red cells from the recipient's blood. If the bloods are incompatible, the red cells will clump together (agglutination). See also BLOOD TRANSFUSION.

crossing-over the exchange of short lengths of CHROMATIDS between homologous pairs of chromosomes during one of the stages of division (meiosis) that occurs when the eggs (ova) and sperms are being formed. Crossing-over is one of the ways in which a random redistribution of genes occurs and ensures that the combinations of genes in each sperm or egg differs from the combinations in the cells of the parents.

cross-reaction the association of an ANTIBODY with an ANTIGEN that differs from the antigen that first stimulated the production of the antibody. Cross reaction is unlikely unless there is close chemical similarity between the two antigens. Some diseases are believed to result because of antigenic similarities between certain body tissues and parts of infecting organisms, such as STREPTOCOCCI.

crotamiton a drug that relieves itching. An ANTIPRURITIC drug. A brand name is Eurax.

croup inflammation and swelling of the main air tubes to the lungs (laryngotracheobronchitis) affecting young children and causing difficult, harsh, noisy and painful breathing and a typical 'barking' cough.

crown the visible part of a tooth. The part covered by enamel.

cruciate cross-shaped.

crus any leg-like structure.

crush syndrome a dangerous condition that may follow a severe crushing injury, especially if large muscles are involved. Much muscle haemoglobin is released into the blood and this seriously damages the kidneys leading to kidney failure. There is also SHOCK from fluid and blood loss.

crutch a portable support, usually in the form of a tubular light metal rod with hand grips and plastic loops for the forearms. Crutches are adjustable for height and allow mobility if one leg is severely weakened or the joints of both legs unable to bend.

crying the uttering of inarticulate sobbing or wailing sounds, associated with the secretion of tears and often with facial contortion, that expresses the emotion, usually of grief or sadness but sometimes of joy. Crying in babies and infants is prompted by minor distressful stimuli and has value in exercising the respiratory muscles, but may, if excessive, cause severe parental stress.

cryo- *combining form denoting* cold.

cryobiology the study of the effects of low temperatures on cells, tissues and organisms, including methods of using cold so as virtually to halt the processes of ageing and deterioration in living structures without causing serious damage. See also CRYOPRESERVATION.

cryonics freezing and storing the human body soon after death to preserve it indefinitely, in the hope that future scientific advances will allow correction of the process that caused the death, so that life can be restored.

cryoglobulins GLOBULINS that precipitate from solution and become visible on cooling

cryoprecipitates substances isolated or purified from a solution by lowering the temperature or by freezing and then thawing. Cryoglobulin is demonstrated, and the antihaemophilic factor, Factor VIII, is obtained, in this way from blood plasma.

cryotherapy the use of low temperatures in medical treatment. Temperatures of about −20 °C or below are useful in surgery, especially for destroying unwanted tissue such as warts, ACTINIC KERATOSIS and skin nodules (dermatofibromas). See also CRYOSURGERY.

cryopreservation the prevention of destructive bacterial action and biochemical change by maintaining biological material, such as tissue for grafting, human embryos, semen, etc., at a low temperature.

cryoprobe a surgical instrument used to apply extreme cold to tissues during CRYOSURGERY.

cryosurgery controlled tissue destruction by low temperatures, usually by means of cryoprobes by which cold can be applied with precision. The method is used in the treatment of PARKINSON'S DISEASE, cancer of the PROSTATE and other organs, RETINAL DETACHMENT and CATARACT removal.

crypt any small recess, pit or cavity in the body.

crypto- *combining form denoting* hidden.

cryptococcosis an infection with the fungus *Cryptococcus neoformans* that occurs in tropical areas and in the Southern States of the USA. It affects the lungs first and then spreads to the nervous system and to any part of the body. There are widespread nodules, filled with gelatinous material, in the tissues. A cryptococcal MENINGITIS is a common feature.

cryptogenic fibrosing alveolitis
a progressive lung disease involving thickening and fibrosis of the walls of the ALVEOLI and large mononuclear cells in the alveolar spaces. As the name implies, the cause is unknown but the condition is believed to be the end stage of a disorder brought about by one of a range of possible factors including exposure to various occupational dusts or volatile solvents, virus infections or genetic influences.

cryptorchidism cryptorchism, undescended testicle. The testicles develop in the abdomen and a testicle that fails to descend before puberty remains permanently sterile. Such a testicle is also liable to develop cancer.

Cryptosporidiosis an infection with the protozoal organism *Cryptosporidium parvum* first described in humans in 1976. It is now known to be a common cause of self-limiting acute gastroenteritis occurring in otherwise healthy people, especially children. It is a common cause of travellers' diarrhoea. In those with AIDS or other causes of immune deficiency, however, it may be a life-threatening infection with a mortality of 50%. Infection is direct or indirect via drinking water, from humans or animals. Cryptosporidium is one of the more common bowel pathogens. When treatment is necessary this may involve fluid infusion for dehydration and the use of drugs such as paromomycin (Humatin), somatostatin, azidothymidine, diloxanide furoate, furazolidone, amprolium, and the macrolide antibiotics. Unfortunately, none of the current antimicrobial dugs are reliably effective.

Crystacide a brand name for HYDROGEN PEROXIDE.

crystalline lens the internal, fine-focusing, lens of the eye, which lies immediately behind the iris diaphragm and is suspended by a delicate ligament from the CILIARY BODY. In youth the lens is elastic and changes shape easily. Elasticity, and range of focusing power, fall off almost linearly with age.

crystal violet one of the many dyes used as a

tissue and micro-organism stain for microscopic examination.

CS an irritant crystalline solid dispersed from a pressurized cannister for purposes of police control of violent persons. CS is o-chloro-benzylidene malononitrile dissolved in methylisobutylketone in a strength of 1% (USA) or 5% (UK). It causes intense burning discomfort in the eyes and on the skin, profuse watering of the eyes and nose, barely controllable spasm of the eyelids, coughing, retching and a sense of constriction in the chest. The effects may last for as long as 24 hours. Corneal damage has been claimed but it is not clear whether this is due to the active ingredient or the vehicle.

CSF *abbrev. for* cerebrospinal fluid.

CSM *abbrev. for* COMMITTEE ON SAFETY OF MEDICINES.

CSP *abbrev. for* Chartered Society of Physiotherapists.

CSSD *abbrev. for* central sterile supply department. This is a unit dedicated to bulk cleaning, packing and sterilization of all re-sterilizable material needed for surgical and medical purposes.

CTCM&H *abbrev. for* Certificate in Tropical Community Medicine & Hygiene.

CTLA4-Ig a fusion protein specific for the B7 surface receptor on T cells that has been shown to be capable of persuading T cells to recognize severely mismatched allogeneic transplanted organs as 'self' even in the absence of immuno-suppressive drugs. T cell activation requires two signals – a T cell-receptor-mediated signal and a co-stimulatory signal. Co-stimulation involves the B7 receptor. This fusion protein blocks co-stimulation and prevents T cells from mounting a rejection attack.

CT scanning computer-assisted tomography. An important method of internal X-ray scanning in which an image is built up by a computer from the data derived by analyzing and correlating the output from thousands of separate, serial, low-intensity readings, taken in successive thin planes. The radiation source is mounted on an arm that moves, between exposures, in a helix, and the radiation detector maintains a constant relationship to the source. Images can be reconstructed from the stored readings so as to appear in any desired plane or orientation. A recent development is spiral scanning that greatly speeds up the process and allows a complete chest scan within a single breath-hold. Also known as CAT scanning.

cuboid one of the bones of the foot. It lies on the outer side immediately in front of the large heel bone, the CALCANEUS, and behind the fourth and fifth metatarsal bones.

cubitus the elbow, especially the soft tissues of the elbow in front of the joint.

cubitus valgus an elbow deformity in which the forearm is tilted outward to an abnormal degree when the arms are by the sides. Some degree of such tilt, known as the 'carrying angle', is normal in women.

culdocentesis passing a needle through the upper back FORNIX of the vagina into the POUCH OF DOUGLAS so as to obtain a sample of blood, pus or other fluid for examination.

culdoscope an examining instrument used to inspect the female pelvic organs. It is passed through the vagina and then through a perforation in the cul-de-sac (FORNIX) behind the CERVIX into the pouch behind the womb. Pelvic endoscopy is now more commonly performed through the abdominal wall (LAPAROSCOPY).

cultural competence possession of the knowledge and skills required to manage cross-cultural relationships effectively. Cultural incompetence in doctors and other medical staff can seriously prejudice clinical management.

culture see BACTERIAL CULTURE, TISSUE CULTURE.

cultured arteries the artificial production of arterial tissue having no potential for rejection, by a complex process of *in vitro* cell culturing in three layers of cells taken from the proposed recipient. The technology is still experimental but shows great promise.

cuneiform 1 wedge-shaped.
2 one of the three wedge-shaped bones in the foot.

cunnilingus oral or lingual stimulation of the CLITORIS or VULVA.

cunnus the VULVA.

curare one of a group of resinous extracts from various South American trees of the genera *Chondodendron* and *Strychnos*. It was used as an arrow poison called 'woorara paste'. Curare acts at the junction between nerves and muscles and produces complete paralysis of all voluntary movement without having any effect on

consciousness. See also CURARINE.

curarine a poisonous alkaloid obtained from curare and used as a muscle relaxant or paralysant in general anaesthesia. It acts by competing with acetylcholine at the point at which motor nerves stimulate muscle fibres. The form used in anaesthesia is called tubocurarine. See also CURARE.

curarize to use a curare drug to paralyse muscles for medical purposes.

Curatoderm a brand name for TACALCITOL.

cure 1 complete resolution of a disease.
2 the failure to find any indications of a disease, especially cancer, for an arbitrary period, often five years.

curettage scraping or spooning out unwanted tissue or tissue required for examination. The instrument used is called a CURETTE.

curette a spoon-shaped instrument for performing CURETTAGE. The curette may vary in size from a tiny 2 mm spoon for scooping out meibomian cysts in eyelids, to a 2 cm instrument for general surgical use.

Cushingoid the appearance of people taking large doses of corticosteroids or suffering from CUSHING'S SYNDROME.

Cushing's syndrome the bodily changes caused by excessive secretion of corticosteroid hormones often as a result of a pituitary or adrenal tumour. A person with Cushing's syndrome is over-weight and has fat deposits on the back of the neck and shoulders. The face is 'moon-shaped' and there are often purplish streaks (striae) on the abdomen. Women often show male-pattern hairiness or baldness. There is weakness from wasted muscles, high blood pressure (HYPERTENSION), OSTEOPOROSIS, and often mental disturbances. (Harvey Williams Cushing, 1869–1939, American neurosurgeon).

cusp a projecting point.

cuspid a tooth with only one point on the crown. A canine tooth.

cutaneous pertaining to the skin.

cutaneous leishmaniasis infection of the skin with organisms of the *Leishmania* genus, such as *Leishmania tropica*. These are usually spread by the sandfly. The condition features deep crusting ulcers which may take years to heal. Also known as oriental sore. See also LEISHMANIASIS.

cuticle 1 the epidermis or outer layer of the skin.
2 the narrow strip of thickened epidermis at the

base of a fingernail or toenail.

3 the sheath of a hair follicle.

cutis the skin as a whole. The CORIUM.

cutis verticis gyrata a state of the skin of the forehead in which, as a result of hypertrophy, it is thrown into deep vertical folds so as to resemble the surface of the brain. The condition is a feature of ACROMEGALY, local inflammation and acute myeloid LEUKAEMIA. A rare primary form of the condition, which affects males only, is associated with severe learning difficulty, seizures, cerebral palsy and eye abnormalities.

CVA *abbrev. for* CEREBROVASCULAR ACCIDENT.

CVS *abbrev. for* the cardiovascular system. This consists of the heart and the blood vessels.

cyanide poisoning poisoning with a salt of hydrocyanic acid such as potassium cyanide or sodium cyanide or with hydrogen cyanide or its solution, prussic acid. Cyanide interferes with vital enzyme systems. Poisoning causes a rapid pulse, headache, convulsions and coma and may be rapidly fatal.

cyanoacrylate a powerful adhesive, popularly known as Superglue that is occasionally used in surgery as a substitute for stitches. In many cases the results are better than with sutures. The adhesive is marketed for surgical use under the generic name enbucrilate and the brand name Histoacryl.

cyanocobalamin vitamin B_{12}. This vitamin is necessary for the normal metabolism of carbohydrates, fats and proteins, for blood cell formation and for nerve function. It is used in the treatment of PERNICIOUS ANAEMIA and SPRUE. Brand names are Cytacon and Cytamen.

cyanosis blueness of the skin from insufficient oxygen in the blood. Fully oxygenated blood is bright red and imparts a healthy pinkness to the skin. Blood low in oxygen is dark reddish-blue and, through the skin, looks a dusky blue. Cyanosis may be due to lung disease, HEART FAILURE or disorders, especially congenital heart disease, in which, blood is shunted away from the lungs. 'Blue babies' have cyanosis.

cybernetics the study of the control and communication systems common to machines and animals, including the human being. The study of the analogies between complex feedback control systems and human physiology has been fruitful to both disciplines.

cyclamate an artificial sweetener 30 times sweeter than sucrose, but with no calorific value. The sodium salt of cyclohexylsulphamic acid. Cyclamate was banned in the UK and USA in 1969 after rats fed the additive throughout their lives developed bladder tumours. In 1995, however, a European panel of experts agreed that the sweetener might safely be used in limited dosage and set a daily intake threshold. Also known as Sucaryl.

cyclical vomiting periodic attacks of vomiting in children with no discernible cause.

cyclic AMP a modified form of adenosine monophosphate in which a PHOSPHODIESTER BOND links the 5'- and 3'-carbons of the sugar within the molecule. Cyclic AMP is chemical messenger within the cell which, when external hormones reach the cell membrane, conveys information to the interior to initiate an appropriate response. It is sometimes called a 'second messenger'. It plays a key role in controlling biological processes.It activates protein kinases and controls GLYCOGEN synthesis and breakdown.

Cyclimorph a brand name for MORPHINE and CYCLIZINE.

cyclins regulatory subunits of the kinases involved in the eukaryotic cell cycle. Cyclins are proteins whose concentration in the cells increases and decreases in phase with the cell cycle. Passage through the cycle is controlled by cyclin-dependent kynase complexes which are inactive unless associated with a cyclin.

cyclizine an ANTIHISTAMINE drug effective in controlling nausea and vomiting. A brand name is Valoid. Brand names of preparations containing it are Diconal, Cyclimorph and Migril.

cyclo- *combining form denoting* circular, cyclical, or the CILIARY BODY of the eye.

cyclodialysis surgical separation of the ciliary body of the eye from the sclera so as to reduce its efficiency in secreting aqueous humour and lower the pressure within the eye in GLAUCOMA.

Cyclogest a brand name for PROGESTERONE.

Cyclokapron a brand name for TRANEXAMIC ACID.

cyclo-oxygenase prostaglandin synthase, the enzyme that converts arachidonic acid to prostaglandins which are commonly mediators of pain. Inhibitors of this enzyme include aspirin and many of the large group of NSAID drugs.

cyclo-oxygenase-2 inhibitor one of a range

of drugs similar in action to NON-STEROIDAL ANTI-INFLAMMATORY drugs.

cyclopenthiazide a thiazide diuretic drug. A brand name is Navidrex.

cyclopentolate a drug used to dilate the pupils of the eyes for purposes of examination of the RETINA and other internal parts. A brand name is Mydrilate.

cyclophosphamide a drug that substitutes an open chain hydrocarbon radical for a hydrogen atom in a cyclic organic compound. It is an alkylating agent and is used as an anticancer drug for its alkylating action on the guanine molecule in DNA. The margin between the effective dose and the dangerous dose is narrow. Side effects include loss of hair, sterility, sickness and vomiting and depression of blood formation by the bone marrow. The drug is on the WHO official list. A brand name is Endoxana.

cyclopia a congenital deformity featuring fusion of the eye sockets and the eyes, so that there appears to be only a single median eye.

cycloplegia paralysis of the focusing muscle of the eye, usually caused by atropine or other similar eye drops, but occasionally a permanent state as a result of blunt injury to the eye. Cycloplegia makes it impossible to focus on near objects without spectacles.

cyclopropane a powerful, non-irritating anaesthetic gas. It has the disadvantages of being explosive and of causing heart irregularity in the presence of adrenaline.

cycloserine a drug used to treat TUBERCULOSIS caused by organisms resistant to treatment by standard drugs such as rifampicin, isoniazid, ethambutol and streptomycin. The drug is on the WHO official list.

Cyclospasmol a brand name for cyclandelate, a drug that helps to improve blood supply to any part of the body by relaxing the arteries.

cyclosporin ciclosporin, an important immunosuppressant drug that has greatly reduced the rate of rejection of grafted organs such as kidneys and hearts. It acts by interfering with the multiplication of immunocompetent T lymphocytes. Brand names are Neoral and Sandimunn.

cyclothymia a mood disorder featuring swings from elation to depression. Severe cyclothymia is sometimes known as a manic-depressive psychosis. Many normal people have cyclothymic personalities.

cyesis pregnancy.

Cyklokapron a brand name for TRANEXAMIC ACID.

cylindrical lens a lens that is plane (plano) in one meridian and has its full convex or concave curvature in the meridian at right angles. Cylindrical lenses are used to correct ASTIGMATISM. The axis is the meridian without converging or diverging power and, when used to correct an ocular refractive error, must be set at the correct orientation.

cylindromatosis a rare familial disorder featuring a 'turban' of numerous benign skin tumours affecting mainly the forehead and scalp. Cylindromas are caused by a mutation of the CYLD gene and is a condition with variable penetrance. The CYLD gene codes for an enzyme that remove ubiquitin from proteins. The loss of CYLD increases the level of a transcription factor that inhibits APOPTOSIS, thus promoting tumour formation.

cyproheptadine an antihistamine and serotonin antagonist drug used to allergies, itching disorders and migraine. A brand name is Periactin.

Cyprostat a brand name for CYPROTERONE ACETATE.

cyproterone acetate a male sex hormone antagonist drug used to treat hypersexuality and prostate gland enlargement. Brand names are Androcur and Cyprostat.

cyst an abnormal, usually spherical, walled cavity filled with secreted fluid or semi-solid matter derived from the cyst itself. Most cysts are benign but a few are malignant. Retention cysts may form when the outlet of normal glands become blocked. Sebaceous cysts and eyelid MEIBOMIAN CYSTS are of this type.

cystadenoma a non-malignant CYST-like growth of glandular tissue.

cysteamine mercaptamine, a drug used to treat NEPHROPATHIC CYSTINOSIS and prescribable only by urological specialists. A brand name is Cystagon.

cystectomy surgical removal of the urinary bladder, usually for cancer. After cystectomy, the ureters, which carry urine down from the kidneys, have to be implanted into the colon or into an artificial bladder made from an isolated length of bowel which drains out through the skin.

cysteine an AMINO ACID present in most body proteins.

cystic *adj* 1 pertaining to, or containing, a CYST or bladder.

2 contained within a cyst of bladder.

cysticercosis infestation with the larval form of the tapeworm of the genus *Taenia* acquired by eating tapeworm eggs, usually in contaminated food. When these hatch in the intestine, the larvae burrow through the bowel wall into the bloodstream and are carried all over the body to be deposited in many tissues including the muscles and the brain. These cause weakness and pain, epileptic fits, sometimes mental disorder and paralysis.

cysticercus the larval stage of many tapeworms. It consists of a head segment with attaching hooks or suckers (scolex) enclosed in a fluid-filled sac. Tapeworm in man is normally acquired by eating undercooked pork or beef containing cysticerci.

cystic fibrosis a recessive genetic disease caused by any of over 1000 mutations in a large gene on chromosome 7 known as the cystic fibrosis transmembrane conductance regulator gene (CFTR). The protein product of the gene is a chloride channel in epithelial cell membranes. Mutations result in a defect in chloride transport affecting glandular tissue throughout the body. The salivary glands, the glands of the intestine, the pancreas, the gall bladder, the lungs and the skin produce thick, sticky mucinous secretion which clogs them or tends to obstruct the passages into which they normally discharge. Children with cystic fibrosis suffer growth retardation, delay in the onset of puberty and are unable to participate normally in games and sport because of their respiratory inefficiency. There are many complications. Genetic testing of prospective parents can readily be done.

cystinosis a disease caused by failure of normal transport of cystine in lysosomes. In the infantile form, which may show itself as early as age two months, there is growth retardation, characteristic deposits in the corneas and fair hair and skin. The adult form involves the corneal changes and may affect vision to the extent that corneal grafting is necessary. Various other ocular defects may develop.

cystinuria an autosomal recessive disorder featuring abnormal amounts in the urine of the amino acids cystine, lysine, ornithine and arginine. The defect is in the kidney tubules which contain transporters for the amino acids that reabsorb them from the filtrate back into the blood. There is a second subtype of the disease in which reabsorption of cystine is normal but in which that of the other three amino acids is defective. The main disadvantage is the formation of hard cystine urinary stones. The mutated cystinuria gene codes for the amino acid transporters in the kidney tubules.

cystitis inflammation of the urinary bladder caused by infection. There is undue frequency of urination, burning or 'scalding' pain on passing urine, and sometimes incontinence. Treatment with antibiotics is usually effective.

cysto- *combining form denoting* a bladder, sac or cyst.

cystocoele a protrusion of the urinary bladder into the front wall of the vagina.

cystoid cyst-like.

cystolithiasis stones (calculi) in the urinary bladder.

cystoplasty any structural surgical procedure performed on the urinary bladder. Clam augmentation cystoplasty is a complex surgical procedure used to treat the condition of unstable or irritable (hyper-reflexive) bladder. The organ is split into two and then reconstituted using a patch of gut taken from the small intestine. This greatly weakens bladder function and prevents full voiding but is effective in controlling involuntary urination.

cystoscope a straight tubular instrument which allows illumination of the inside of the urinary bladder so that direct examination, and various forms of treatment, are possible.

cystoscopy examination of the inside the bladder with an optical instrument called a cystoscope, passed along the urethra. This requires general anaesthesia in the male but can be done under local anaesthesia in the female. Cystoscopy facilitates the diagnosis of conditions such as infections, polyps, cancers and stones in the bladder, and allows biopsies to be taken and local treatment by cautery, laser and other means to be given. It also makes it possible to pass fine catheters up the tubes leading to the kidneys (the ureters) through which a substance opaque to X-rays can be injected for X-ray studies (retrograde pyelography).

cystostomy cutting into a bladder.

cystogram see MICTURATING CYSTOGRAM.

Cystrin a brand name for OXYBUTYNIN.

Cytacon a brand name for CYANOCOBALAMIN.

Cytadren a brand name for AMINOGLUTETHIMIDE.

Cytamen a brand name for CYANCOBALAMIN.

cytarabine an antimetabolite drug used in the treatment of acute LEUKAEMIA. It is a purine antagonist (see PURINES) and acts by depriving cells of essential metabolic substances. It causes sickness and vomiting, peptic ulcers and depression of bone marrow blood formation. The drug is on the WHO official list. A brand name is Cytosar.

cytochemistry 1 the chemistry of cells.
2 an analysis of the chemical composition of cell components by staining properties and other means.

cytochrome P450 a family of enzymes responsible for the detoxification and elimination of foreign substances including many drugs by hydroxylation and increasing their solubility. The group has been intensively studied because mutations of the cytochrome P450 gene have been found to be associated with a number of diseases including Addison's disease, liver cancer and Parkinson's disease. Cytochrome P450 can also interfere with drug treatment. Selective inhibitors of aromatase-specific cytochrome P450 have been developed to assist in the treatment of breast cancer.

cytokines a general term for a range of proteins of low molecular weight that exert a stimulating or inhibiting influence on the proliferation, differentiation and function of cells of the immune system. Cytokines include INTERLEUKINS and INTERFERONS.

cytology 1 the study of cells.
2 an abbreviation of the phrase 'exfoliative cytology' the examination of isolated cells, obtained from cervical smears, sputum or elsewhere, to determine whether or not they are cancerous.

cytomegalic characterized by enlarged cells.

cytomegalovirus infection an infection caused by a virus of the herpes group which causes enlargement of the cells which it invades. In infants the infection causes liver enlargement, jaundice and blood disorders, and is sometimes fatal. Cytomegalovirus infection is a common feature of AIDS.

cytometer a laboratory instrument for counting cells, especially blood cells. Originally, a glass slide engraved in tiny squares, on which cells had to be counted one by one by human microscopists, the modern version performs the task using lasers, digital electronics and graphics imaging technology. Flow cytometry is a powerful tool in modern medicine. Its applications have expanded from cell counting and sorting, to measurement of cell surface and intracellular antigens, and the analysis of DNA. Moderns cytometers can measure several parameters on many thousands of individual cells in a very short period of time.

cytopathic pertaining to abnormal (pathological) changes in cells.

cytoplasm the part of a cell outside the nucleus and inside the cell membrane.

cytoplasmic inheritance the genetic effects of DNA situated in MITOCHONDRIA.

cytoprotectants drugs used to protect mucosal surfaces, especially of the gastointestinal tract, from ulceration, or to protect cells generally from the malign effects of cancer chemotherapy such as the combined use of cyclophosphamide and cisplatin.

Cytosar a brand name for CYTARABINE.

cytosine a pyrimidine base, one of those forming the genetic code of DNA and RNA.

cytoskeleton a complex network of ACTIN filaments within the nucleated cell. Unlike the bony skeleton in vertebrates, this skeleton has contractile properties and can alter the shape, size and even movement, of the cell. The cytoskeleton is also concerned with the adhesion of adjacent cells.

cytosol the cell contents situated between the cell membrane and the nucleus, less the endoplasmic reticulum, the mitochondria and the other structured organelles.

cytotoxic antibiotics antibiotic drugs used to treat cancer. These drugs are, in general, unsuitable for treating bacterial infections. Examples are doxorubicin (Caelyx), daunorubicin (Cerubidin), dactinomycin (Cosmegen Lyovax), epirubicin (Pharmorubicin) and idarubicin (Zavedos).

cytotoxic drugs drugs capable of damaging or killing cells. These can be used in the treatment of cancer because their effect is greatest on cells which are reproducing most rapidly. The cytotoxic drugs include alkylating agents, such as cyclophosphamide, melphalan and chlorambucil, that interfere with cell growth differentiation and function; cytotoxic antibiotics, such as dactinomycin, daunorubicin and doxorubicin, that bind to DNA blocking its transcription; antimetabolites, such as fluoruracil, cytarabine and mercaptopurine, that interfere with the action of folates; vinca alkaloids, such as vinblastine, vincristine and taxol, that block mitosis; and the TOPOISOMERASE 1 inhibitors, such as etoposide, anthracyclines and anthrapyrazoles, that interfere with nuclear enzymes required for DNA replication and the separation of daughter chromosomes.

cytotoxic immunosuppressants drugs used to modify the action of the immune system so as to help to treat autoimmune diseases and to prevent rejection of transplanted organs. An example is azathioprine (Imuran).

cytotoxicity the property of being able to cause damage to, or death of, cells.

cytotoxic T cells T lymphocytes (usually CD8 cells) that kill target cells when they identify foreign MHC molecules on their cell membranes.

d

DA *abbrev. for* Diploma in Anaesthetics.

dacarbazine an alkylating cytotoxic anti-cancer drug. The drug is on the WHO official list. A brand name is DTIC-Dome.

Da Costa syndrome a neurotic conviction that one is suffering from heart disease. The SYNDROME features PALPITATIONS, chest pain, a rapid pulse and fatigue and is essentially an ANXIETY STATE centred on the heart. Also known as neurocirculatory asthenia. (Jacob Mendes da Costa, 1833–1900, American surgeon).

dacryo- *combining form denoting* tears or the lacrimal system.

dacryoadenitis inflammation of a LACRIMAL GLAND. This sometimes occurs as a complication of MUMPS.

dacryoblennorrhoea inflammation of the LACRIMAL SAC with discharge of PUS and mucus back along the CANALICULI to appear between the lids.

dacryocystectomy surgical removal of the LACRIMAL SAC.

dacryocystitis inflammation of the tear sac (lacrimal sac) which lies in the eye socket (ORBIT), between the inner corner of the eye and the nose. Inflammation causes permanent obstruction of tear drainage and a watering eye but this can be corrected by surgery.

dacryocystography X-ray examination of the lacrimal drainage system using a radio-opaque fluid to delineate the interior.

dacryocystorhinostomy an operation to provide a new passage from the LACRIMAL SAC, through the lacrimal bone, to the inside of the nose so as to re-establish tear drainage when the nasolacrimal duct is blocked. Formerly done by cutting bone through an incision near the bridge of the nose, the procedure is now being performed using a laser probe via the nostril and a light source via a tear duct. This is called endonasal laser-assisted dacryocystorhinostomy.

dactinomycin a cytotoxic drug used to treat cancers mainly of children. Dactinomycin is an antibiotic derived from *Streptomyces pavullus* which causes breaks in DNA. This side effect renders it unsuitable as an antibacterial drug, but makes it useful as an anti-cancer drug. A brand name is Cosmegen Lyovac. There are other actinomycins in the group produced by *Streptomyces chrysomallas*.

dactyl a finger or toe. A digit.

dactylitis inflammation of the fingers and toes causing spindle-like (fusiform) swelling. This is a feature of SICKLE-CELL ANAEMIA in infants and is caused by blockage of the small arteries by clumped sickled red blood cells.

DADH *abbrev. for* Deputy Assistant Director of Health.

DADMS *abbrev. for* Deputy Assistant Director of Medical Services.

D and C see DILATATION AND CURETTAGE.

Daktacort a brand name for MICONAZOLE with HYDROCORTISONE.

Daktarin a brand name for MICONAZOLE.

Dalacin C a brand name for CLINDAMYCIN.

Dalacin T a brand name for CLINDAMYCIN.

Dalmane a brand name for FLURAZEPAM.

dalteparin sodium a low molecular weight HEPARIN used to treat acute deep vein thrombosis. The drug is given by subcutaneous injection to adults only in a single daily dose calculated on the basis of body weight. A brand name is Fragmin.

danazole a synthetic PROGESTOGEN drug that inhibits secretion by the PITUITARY gland of the sex-gland stimulating hormone gonadotrophin. It is used to treat precocious puberty, breast enlargement in the male (gynaecomastia), excessive menstruation (menorrhagia) and ENDOMETRIOSIS. A brand name is Danol.

dancing eyes see OPSOCLONUS.

dander small scales of animal skin, hair or feathers. Dander commonly cause allergic effects, especially ASTHMA.

dandruff a popular term for pityriasis capitis. The condition features scaliness of the scalp from flakes of dead skin. Some loss of surface skin cells is normal, but excessive scaliness may be due to infection with the fungus *Malassezia furfur* that causes PITYRIASIS VERSICOLOR. Dandruff responds well to medicated shampoos, especially those containing selenium and lithium. Also known as pityriasis furfuracea.

Danocrine a brand name for DANAZOLE.

Danol a brand name for DANAZOLE.

D-antigens the rhesus (Rh) ANTIGEN present in the red blood cells of 85% of people, who are said to be rhesus positive. This antigen is inherited as an AUTOSOMAL dominant. See also RHESUS FACTOR.

danthron dantron, a stimulant laxative. A brand name is Capsuvac.

dantolene a drug used to relieve muscle spasm. A brand name is Dantrium.

Dantrium a brand name for DANTROLENE.

Daonil a brand name for GLIBENCLAMIDE.

DAP&E *abbrev. for* Diploma in Applied Parasitology and Entomology.

dapsone diaminodiphenyl sulfone. For many years this has been the standard drug to treat leprosy, but irregular use has led to the development of drug resistance. Dapsone is also used in the treatment of DERMATITIS HERPETIFORMIS which may be associated with COELIAC DISEASE.

Daraprim a brand name for PYRIMETHAMINE.

Darier's disease keratosis follicularis, a rare autosomal dominant skin disease caused by mutations on chromosome 12. It features warty, foul-smelling plaques formed of coalesced greasy plaques of seborrhoeic dermatitis with severe itching and sometimes pain. The disease is chronic and may worsen with age. Treatment is with oral retinoids. Prenatal diagnosis by DNA analysis of cells obtained by CHORIONIC VILLUS sampling is possible.

dark adaptation the gradual acquisition of the ability to see in dim light that normally occurs in conditions of poor illumination. Dark adaptation becomes defective (night blindness) in vitamin A deficiency because this vitamin is necessary for the production of retinal VISUAL PURPLE. Poor dark adaptation is also a feature of RETINITIS PIGMENTOSA (tapetoretinal degeneration).

dartos muscle a thin layer of muscle lying immediately under the skin of the SCROTUM. The dartos tightens in the cold causing the skin to wrinkle and the testicles to rise.

daunorubicin an antibiotic drug used in the consolidation phase of the treatment of acute leukaemia. The drug is on the WHO official list. Brand names are Cerubidin and Daunoxome.

Daunoxome a brand name for DAUNORUBICIN.

DavMed *abbrev. for* Diploma in Aviation Medicine.

dawn phenomenon a sharp rise in the blood sugar level in the early morning in insulin-dependent diabetics. The rise is thought to be caused by nocturnal growth hormone secretion.

DBO *abbrev. for* Diploma of the British Orthoptic Council.

DCCH *abbrev. for* Diploma in Child & Community Health.

DCD *abbrev. for* Diploma in Chest Diseases.

DCDH *abbrev. for* Diploma in Community Dental Health.

Dch *abbrev. for* Doctor of Surgery.

DCH *abbrev. for* Diploma in Child Health.

DChD *abbrev. for* Doctor of Dental Surgery.

DCHT *abbrev. for* Diploma in Community Health in the Tropics.

DCM *abbrev. for* Diploma in Community medicine.

DCMT *abbrev. for* Diploma in Clinical Medicine of Tropics.

DCOphth *abbrev. for* Diploma of the College of Ophthalmologists.

DCP *abbrev. for* Diploma in Clinical Pathology.

DCPath *abbrev. for* Diploma of the College of Pathologists.

DCR *abbrev. for* Diploma of the College of Radiographers or DACRYOCYSTOR-HINOSTOMY.

DDA *abbrev. for* Dangerous Drugs Act.

DDAVP des-amino-D-arginine vasopressin or DESMOPRESSIN. A brand name for DESMOPRESSIN.

Dderm *abbrev. for* Diploma in Dermatology.

DDM *abbrev. for* Diploma in Dermatological Medicine.

DDMS *abbrev. for* Deputy Director of Medical Services.

DDO *abbrev. for* Diploma in Dental Orthopaedics.

DDR *abbrev. for* Diploma in Diagnostic Radiology.

DDS *abbrev. for* Doctor of Dental Surgery.

DDSC *abbrev. for* Doctor of Dental Science.

DDT dichloro-diphenyl-trichloroethane. This highly effective insecticide kills flies, mosquitos, lice, butterflies, moths and beetles. The use of DDT has saved millions of human lives that would otherwise have been lost from MALARIA, YELLOW FEVER, TYPHUS, PLAGUE, river blindness (ONCHOCERCIASIS), DYSENTERY, SLEEPING SICKNESS and FILARIASIS. For ecological reasons it has now been largely replaced by organophosphorous insecticides such as Malathion, Parathion and Paraquat.

deadly nightshade the source of the drug BELLADONNA.

deafness partial or complete loss of hearing. Deafness may be conductive or sensorineural. Conductive deafness results from disorders of the external ear, eardrum, middle ear and acoustical link to the inner ear; sensorineural (nerve deafness) results form disorders in the inner ear – the cochlea or acoustic nerve.

deafness gene a gene which, when mutated, leads to deafness. A mutated gene for CONNEXIN-26, for instance, can cause sensorineural deafness, as can a gene mutation leading to a defect in early development of the parts of the embryo (the branchial arches) that include the ears. Such mutations give rise to various craniofacial defects, of which the Treacher Collins Syndrome is one of the best known, that may lead to conductive hearing loss.

deaminase an ENZYME that brings about the breakdown of amino compounds.

deamination removal of the amino group from a molecule. When an NH_2 group is replaced by an oxygen atom a ketone is formed and the process is described as oxidative deamination. If the amino group is terminal, the process should, strictly, be called deamidation.

death the cessation of the processes of living. This may occur at cellular level, at tissue level (GANGRENE) or at the level of the entire organism (somatic death). Death of the whole organism results from failure of the supply of essential fuels, especially oxygen and sugar, or from inability of the tissues to use them, because of poisoning or other damage.

death cap the very poisonous mushroom, Amanita phalloides, which resembles edible mushrooms but has a prominent whitish bulb at its base. Sometimes called death cup.

death rate the ratio of the number of deaths to the total of the population concerned.

death rattle a gurgling or rattling sound caused by the passage of air through accumulated mucus and saliva in the throat of a dying person, too weak to cough or clear the throat.

death tourist a seriously ill person who seeks to terminate his or her own life by travelling to a country where medically assisted suicide is not illegal.

death wish Freud's 'thanatos', which, like so many of his concepts, was derived from classical mythology. This idea, conceived late in his career, proposed that responses such as denial and rejection of pleasure or the repeated seeking of extreme danger indicated a general wish or instinct for death.

debility lack of strength. Debility is due to loss of muscle bulk and reduction in the efficiency of the heart and respiratory system from disease or disuse. Debility is often the result of negligible demands on the body and, in this case, is remediable.

debridement the radical surgical removal of all contaminated tissue, such as the damaged edges of wounds and, especially, of all muscle suspected of being dead. After effective debridement, healing and recovery are usually rapid.

Decadron a brand name for DEXAMETHASONE.

Deca-Durabolin a brand name for NANDROLONE DECANOATE.

decalcification loss of calcium and other mineral salts from the normally mineralized tissues, bone and teeth. This occurs in OSTEOMALACIA and in OSTEOPOSOSIS.

Decapeptyl SR a brand name for TRIPTORELIN.

decarboxylases enzymes that promote the freeing of COO from –COOH. These enzymes are involved in the synthesis of amine regulators and neurotransmitters such as serotonin and dopamine.

decerebellate lacking the CEREBELLUM, or suffering the effects of loss of cerebellar function.

decerebrate suffering from the effects of loss of cerebral activity, such as thought, consciousness, sensation and the power of voluntary movement.

decerebrate rigidity the marked increase in tension (tone) that occurs in the antigravity muscles when the brain is no longer exercising control.

decibel a logarithmic unit of comparison between a standard power level and an observed level. The decibel is not a unit of sound intensity but is widely used to compare a noise level with a very low standard reference level near the limit of audibility, and to compare electrical power levels. A tenth of a bel.

decidua the thick lining of the womb (endometrium) during pregnancy with its associated membranes that are cast off with the PLACENTA after the birth of the baby.

deciduous shed or falling at a particular time or stage of growth. Sometimes applied to the primary teeth.

decomposition separation into chemical constituents or simpler compounds often as a result of bacterial enzymatic action.

decompression removal of pressure on a part. Decompression of the brain when bleeding is occurring within the skull is a life-saving procedure.

decompression sickness see BENDS, CAISSON DISEASE.

decompression, spinal see SPINAL DECOMPRESSION.

decongestant a drug or treatment that reduces the blood flow through, and swelling of, mucous membranes, especially those lining the nose and sinuses.

decortication removal of the outer covering (CORTEX) of an organ.

Decortisyl a brand name for PREDNISOLONE.

Decrin a brand name for a mixture of ASPIRIN and CODEINE.

decubitus the reclining position.

decubitus ulcers bedsores. ULCERS caused by unduly sustained skin pressure. These affect especially the buttocks, the heels, the elbows and the back of the head of people with loss of sensation from neurological damage or who are paralysed or too debilitated to move much. Bedsores may progress to complete local loss of skin with exposure of the underlying tendons or bone.

decussation a crossing so as to form an X, especially of tracts of nerve fibres.

Deep Relief a brand name for IBUPROFEN in a preparation for external use.

DEET diethyl(meta)toluamide. An insect repellent.

defecation, defaecation voluntary or involuntary emptying of the RECTUM so as to relieve oneself of accumulated faeces. Stretching of the wall of the rectum causes a conscious desire to defaecate, but if this is prevented by voluntary decision the rectal wall relaxes and the desire fades until the next movement of faeces from the colon. Deliberate inhibition is a common cause of CONSTIPATION.

defence mechanisms methods of coping with anxiety caused by conflict between desires and socially approved behaviour. The mechanisms include exclusion from consciousness (repression), denial, explaining away (rationalization), making exceptional efforts (compensation) and transfer of unacceptable qualities to others (projection). Strife commonly arises from unwise attempts to point out and demolish one another's defence mechanisms. See also DISSOCIATIVE DISORDERS.

defensive medicine medical practice in which actions, or the avoidance of actions, are importantly determined by fear of litigation. The term is relative and ranges from a decision to perform a few more tests than might strictly be necessary to a form of practice in which the first concern of the doctor is to provide his or her patients with no possible grounds for legal action. Defensive medicine is damaging both to doctors and to patients and is only partly due to the actions of ambulance-chasing lawyers who actively encourage law suites against doctors. It is also a product of public perception of the actions of a minority of practitioners for whom financial reward is the primary motive.

deferoxamine a chelating agent used to treat iron compound poisoning. The drug is on the WHO official list.

defervescence the period during which a fever is returning to normal.

defibrillation the restoration of the normal beat rhythm in a heart which is in a state of rapid, ineffectual twitching – one kind of CARDIAC ARREST. A strong pulse of electric energy (about 300 joules) is passed across the heart from two metal electrodes pressed to the chest.

defibrillator an electrical device for applying sudden high-energy shocks to the heart in the attempt to convert VENTRICULAR FIBRILLATION into normal heart rhythm. See also DEFIBRILLATION.

defibrillator, implantable a small, implantable device that detects the onset of the rapidly fatal condition VENTRICULAR FIBRILLATION and immediately applies an electrical pulse to the heart to depolarize the muscle and restore normal rhythm. Alternatively the device can stop the fibrillation by providing a pacing pulse. The device is implanted under the skin of the chest or under a pectoral muscle.

defibrination the removal of fibrin. Defibrination of blood can be achieved by stirring it with a solid rod. This is done to prevent coagulation.

deficiency diseases the large range of conditions resulting from the lack of any of the essential nutritional elements, such as protein, vitamins or minerals, or from the body's inability to digest, absorb or utilize these. See SCURVY, RICKETS, BERI-BERI, PELLAGRA, KWASHIORKOR, KERATOMALACIA.

defined daily doses published guidelines by various regulatory authorities for dosage of drugs in which precision of dosage is important.

deflazcort a CORTICOSTEROID drug. A brand name is Calcort.

deformity the state of being misshapen or distorted in body.

degeneracy in the genetic code this is a reference to the redundancy of codons arising from the fact that four bases, taken three at a time, offer 64 possibilities, while it is necessary to code for only 20 amino acids and three stop signals. The effect is that in many cases a change in the third base of a codon will not change the amino acid selected.

degeneration structural regression of body tissue or organs, from disease, ageing or misuse, which leads to functional impairment, usually progressive.

degenerative disease disease featuring DEGENERATION.

deglutition swallowing.

deglutition syncope a condition of sympathetic inhibition from vagus nerve activation due to stimulation of the oesophagus in swallowing, especially when cold beverages are taken. In a severe case there may be marked slowing of the heart, widening of peripheral blood vessels and a drop in blood pressure. This may result in dangerous dizziness, confusion and syncope.

dehiscence splitting open or separating. Often used of an operation wound which has failed to heal normally and which breaks down under internal pressure.

dehydration a reduction in the normal water content of the body. This is usually due to excessive fluid loss by sweating, vomiting or diarrhoea which is not balanced by an appropriate increase in intake.

dehydroepiandrosterone quantitatively the principal male sex hormone (ANDROGEN), of the adrenal cortex. Output declines with age, a decline thought by some to be causally related to ageing and to the development of various diseases. It is thought likely that, given to elderly people in dosage that would restore the blood levels to those of young adults, the hormone would improve physical and psychological well-being. The hormone has also been claimed to be effective in treating depression and osteoporosis.

dehydrogenases a large number of enzymes that activate oxidation-reduction reactions by the removal of a pair of hydrogen atoms from a molecule.

déjà vu the sudden mistaken conviction that a current experience has happened before. There is a compelling sense of familiarity and often a persuasion, almost always immediately disappointed, that one knows what is round the next corner.

de la Tourette syndrome see GILLES DE LA TOURETTE SYNDROME.

delayed hypersensitivity an allergic reaction occurring two to three days after the antigen contact and mediated by CYTOKINE release from sensitized T cells (T LYMPHOCYTES).

delayed speech failure of development of speech by the end of the second year of life. This may be caused by deafness, emotional disturbance or severe or prolonged childhood illness.

deletion in genetics, the removal of a segment of DNA with joining up of the cut ends. as in the loss of a segment of a chromosome. Deletion of a single BASE PAIR is one of the kinds of point mutation. Deletion of a base pair triplet (CODON) will result in a protein with a missing amino acid.

Delhi belly an old-fashioned informal term for the common intestinal infection suffered by travellers unaccustomed to the local bacterial contamination (usually faecal) of food or drink. The condition is by no means confined to the Indian subcontinent.

Delhi boil a form of LEISHMANIASIS affecting the skin. Also called oriental sore.

deliquescent having the property of taking up water from the atmosphere in sufficient quantity to dissolve itself.

delinquency, juvenile see JUVENILE DELINQUENCY.

delirium a mental disturbance from disorder of brain function caused by high fever, head injury, drug intoxication, drug overdosage or drug withdrawal. There is confusion, disorientation, restlessness, trembling, fearfulness, DELUSION and disorder of sensation (HALLUCINATION). Occasionally there is maniacal excitement.

delirium tremens a dramatic condition sometimes affecting people on withdrawal from heavy alcohol indulgence. There are purposeless body movements, shakiness, tremor, incessant and sometimes incoherent talk and a sense of threat. Vivid, unpleasant hallucinations occur. The affected person may see terrifying sights, smell horrifying smells, feel distressing touchings or hear threatening or frightening sounds or speech. Often a major seizure occurs.

delivery the process of being delivered of a child in childbirth.

delta cells cells in the pancreas or intestine that secrete SOMATOSTATINS.

Deltacortril a brand name for PREDNISOLONE.

delta hepatitis an acute, often severe, form of HEPATITIS caused by an RNA virus which is dependent on the hepatitis B virus for its replication. It is acquired along with the hepatitis B virus or it can infect hepatitis B carriers, in both cases by close personal contact or needle sharing.

Deltasolone a brand name for PREDNISOLONE.

Deltastab a brand name for PREDNISOLONE.

delta wave a low-frequency brain wave, recordable on the ELECTROENCEPHALO-GRAM, that originates in the frontal part of the brain during deep sleep in normal adults.

deltoid triangular. Shaped like the triangular Greek letter 'D'.

deltoid muscle the large, triangular 'shoulder-pad' muscle which raises the arm sideways.

deltoid ligament the strong triangular ligament, on the inner side of the ankle, which helps to bind the foot to the leg. A torn deltoid ligament may leave an unstable ankle that 'goes over' easily.

delusion a fixed belief, unassailable by reason, in something manifestly absurd or untrue. Psychotic delusions include delusions of persecution, of grandeur, of disease, of abnormality of body shape, of unworthiness, of unreality and of being malignly influenced by others.

demarcation forming a plane of separation between living and dead tissue, as in dry GANGRENE.

demeclocycline a tetracycline antibiotic used to treat ACNE and general infections. A brand name is Ledermycin.

Demerol a brand name for PETHIDINE (meperidine).

dementia a syndrome of failing memory and progressive loss of intellectual power due to continuing degenerative disease of the brain. About half are believed to be due to ALZHEIMER'S DISEASE and about one third to small repeated STROKES. A small proportion are due to PRION DISEASE (spongiform encephalopathy). It has been shown that participation in leisure activities such as playing music, games and reading, are associated with a significantly lower risk of dementia, but it is not clear whether such activities reduce the risk.

dementia praecox an outdated and inaccurate term for SCHIZOPHRENIA.

demise death.

demulcent 1 soothing.
2 an oily substance used to relieve pain or discomfort in inflamed, irritated or abraded skin or mucous membranes.

demyelination loss of the insulating fatty sheath (myelin) of nerve fibres. This usually occurs in a patchy manner. Local areas of demyelination, in the form of 'plaques' which extend across large numbers of nerve fibre bundles, is the hallmark of MULTIPLE SCLEROSIS. Also known as demyelinization.

demyelinating diseases diseases that feature loss of the myelin sheath of nerve fibres in the white matter of the central nervous system. The most important of the demyelinating diseases is MULTIPLE SCLEROSIS. Others include acute demyelinating encephalomyelitis, which may follow measles or chickenpox, and neuromyelitis optica, in which both optic nerves are affected as well as the spinal cord.

denaturation 1 alteration in the folding pattern of a protein by heat or chemical reaction from its physiological conformation to an inactive shape.

2 in the case of DNA or RNA the conversion from a double-stranded structure to a single stranded structure, usually by heating. This is an essential stage in the POLYMERASE CHAIN REACTION.

dendrite one of the usually numerous branches of a nerve cell that carry impulses toward the cell body. Dendrites allow the most complex interconnection between nerve cells, as in the brain, so that elaborate control arrangements over the passage of nerve impulses are made possible. Recent research suggests that sections of some dendrites can function independently.

dendritic cell see LANGERHANS CELL.

dendritic ulcer a branching ulcer of the CORNEA of the eye, caused by infection with the Herpes simplex virus. It may be acquired by kissing or by unknowingly rubbing the virus into the eye. See also CORNEAL ULCER.

dendron see DENDRITE.

denervation loss of the nerve supply to a part of the body, by deliberate surgical act or by a disease process.

dengue a tropical disease caused by a virus, probably of monkeys, and transmitted to humans by the mosquito Aedes aegypti. It is an acute disease with high fever, prostration, severe headache, aches in the bones, joints and muscles, and enlargement of lymph nodes. A second stage occurs with fever and a skin rash covering most of the body. The victim feels weak and unwell for weeks. Also known as breakbone fever.

Denis Browne splints splints used to correct club foot (TALIPES equinovarus) in infants. (Denis John Wolko Browne, 1892–1967, Australian-born British paediatrician).

dent- *combining form denoting* tooth or DENTAL.

dental pertaining to the teeth or to dentistry.

dental calculus a crust of chalky material from deposition of calcium and phosphorous from the saliva in the unbrushed collection of food

debris and bacteria around the teeth (plaque). Calculus leads to TOOTH DECAY and gum disease.

dental caries see TOOTH DECAY.

dental floss strong, often waxed, thread used to remove PLAQUE from around the necks of the teeth and discourage dental caries. Regular effective brushing and flossing gives excellent protection against the formation of the acids that damage the enamel.

dental hygienist a person who assists a dentist at the chair-side and who provides preventive dental care, such as scaling and cleaning.

dental technician a person who makes dental appliances, such as dentures, bridges and orthodontic devices.

dentifrice see TOOTHPASTE.

dentine the hard, calcified tissue that makes up the greater thickness of the tooth. It is denser and harder than bone, but softer than the outer enamel coating and contains tubules of cells which connect the inner pulp of the tooth to the surface.

dentinoma a benign tumour of tooth DENTINE.

dentist a person qualified to practise DENTISTRY.

dentistry the art and science of the teeth and the associated bone and soft tissue and their disorders. Dentistry is concerned with prevention, diagnosis, and management of diseases of the teeth, gums and sockets and with the supply and fitting of artificial teeth. The list that follows highlights the key entries related to medical dentistry in the dictionary: calculus (dental), canine tooth, crown, dental, dental caries, dental floss, dental hygienist, dental technician, dentine, dentist, dentistry, dentition, dentulous, dentures, edentulous, enamel, eye tooth, interdental, labiodental, osseointegrated dental implant, pulp, pulpectomy, pulpotomy, rubber dam, tooth, toothpaste, wisdom tooth.

dentition pertaining to the teeth. The primary dentition consists of 20 teeth, the secondary, or permanent, dentition, usually 32.

dentulous possessing teeth. The opposite is edentulous.

dentures artificial (prosthetic) replacements for missing teeth. Dentures are of cosmetic and functional importance, assist in the maintenance of good nutrition and allow clear speech.

deodorants preparations of aluminium or zinc

salts that act mainly by reducing the production of sweat secretion from the glands in the armpits and groins (apocrine sweat). Apocrine sweat contains ingredients that are broken down by skin bacteria to produce unpleasant-smelling compounds.

deoxy- prefix denoting removal of an oxygen atom from a molecule.

deoxygenation removal of oxygen.

deoxyribonuclease an enzyme that cuts DNA strands by breaking PHOSPHODIESTER BONDS.

deoxyribonucleic acid see DNA.

deoxyribose a sugar, part of the 'backbone' of the DNA double helix, deoxyribonucleic acid. In RNA, the equivalent sugar is ribose.

depersonalization loss of the sense of one's own reality. A dream-like feeling of being detached from one's own body or a feeling that one's body is unreal or strange. This may be a normal phenomenon.

depigmentation loss of normal pigmentation.

depilatory a preparation or procedure for removing hair or destroying the hair-forming skin tubes (follicles). Depilatories include chemical substances to soften and dissolve hair, electrolysis or waxes to grip hairs and facilitate mass removal.

Depixol a brand name for FLUPENTHIXOL (flupentixol).

depolarizing capable of bringing about depolarization. Drugs that act at the junction between a nerve fibre and a muscle fibre to cause paralysis of the muscle (neuromuscular blocking agents) may be depolarizing or non-depolarizing. Depolarizing agents so affect the electrical charges at the interface that the nerve impulse can to be passed to the muscle fibre, but because the depolarization is maintained, the muscle, after the initial contraction, cannot continue to contract. Non-depolarizing agents such as curare act by combining with and blocking the nicotinic cholinergic receptors at the post-junctional membrane.

depolarising muscle relaxants drugs used by anaesthetists to cause total relaxation of voluntary muscles by DEPOLARIZING the motor endplate and maintaining the depolarization. They include atracurium (Tracrium), rocuronium (Esmeron), gallamine (Flaxedil), mivacurium (Mivacron), cisatracurium (Nimbex), vecuronium (Norcuron) and suxamethonium (Atectine).

depolarization the immediate cause of the formation of a nerve impulse. Nerve fibres normally carry a positive charge of some 70 millivolts on the outside of the fibre, which is balanced by an equal negative charge on the inside. When movement of potassium ions causes a local reversal of this polarization, the fibre is said to be depolarized. A zone of depolarization then passes along the fibre. This is the nerve impulse.

Depo-Medrone, Depo-Medrol brand names for METHYLPREDNISOLONE used as a DEPOT INJECTION.

Deponit a brand name for GLYCERYL TRINITRATE.

Depo-Provera a contraceptive, given by DEPOT INJECTION, containing MEDROXYPROGESTERONE. See also CONTRACEPTION.

depot injection a drug formulation that allows gradual absorption, over a long period, from a quantity deposited by injection under the skin or in a muscle. Many drugs and hormones can be given in this way.

depressed fracture a bone break, commonly of the skull, in which a part of the bone is forced down below the normal level.

depression sadness or unhappiness, usually persistent. This may be a normal reaction to unpleasant events or environment or may be the result of a genuine depressive illness. Pathological depression features a sense of hopeless-ness, dejection and fear out of all proportion to any external cause. There is slowing down of body and mind, poor concentration, confusion, self-reproach, self-accusation and loss of self-esteem. Suicide is an ever-present risk.

deprivation failure to obtain or to be provided with a sufficiency of the material, intellectual or spiritual requirements for normal development and happiness.

deprivation syndrome a state of developmental retardation, both physical and emotional, and sometimes intellectual, resulting from early parental rejection. The effect is lifelong and may involve grave psychosocial disadvantage.

depth psychology 1 any school of psychology that emphasizes unconscious motivation, as distinct from the psychology of conscious behaviour.

2 PSYCHOANALYSIS.

Dequacaine a brand name for BENZOCAINE and dequalinium in lozenge form.

Dequadin a brand name for dequalinium in lozenge form.

dequalinium an antibacterial and antifungal drug used as an ingredient in medicated lozenges. A brand name is Labosept.

de Quervain's thyroiditis a condition featuring painful enlargement of the thyroid gland with suppression of thyroid hormone production. It is probably due to a virus infection and spontaneous recovery is usual. It ia also called subacute thyroiditis. (Fritz de Quervain, 1868–1940, Swiss surgeon).

Derbac-M a brand name for a preparation containing MALATHION for external use.

derealization see DEPERSONALIZATION.

derepressed the state of a gene that is turned on. Also described as induced. See also REPRESSED.

derma- *combining form denoting* skin.

dermabrasion a procedure in cosmetic plastic surgery in which rough or pitted skin is smoothed down, and its appearance improved, by sand-papering or by the use of other abrasive methods.

Dermacort a brand name for a HYDROCORTISONE skin preparation.

dermatitis inflammation of the skin from any cause. Dermatitis is not a specific disease, but any one of a large range of inflammatory disorders featuring redness, blister formation, swelling, weeping, crusting and itching.

dermatitis artefacta self-inflicted injury to the skin, usually from deliberate and prolonged scratching, but sometimes by the use of irritating substances or even sharp instruments. There is usually an underlying emotional problem but the motive may be to avoid work or obtain industrial compensation. The condition is commoner in females than in males. When the cause has been detected and removed, recovery is usually rapid but, later, other disorders may be simulated. There is a high incidence of suicide in such cases.

dermatitis herpetiformis an uncommon skin disease causing intensely itchy blistering red spots, occurring symmetrically on the elbows, shoulder-blades, buttocks and the backs of the thighs. It is thought to be due to allergy to wheat protein (gluten) and the formation of IMMUNE COMPLEXES. It may occur in COELIAC DISEASE.

dermatoglyphics the study of the patterns of the skin ridges on the fingers, palms, toes and soles of the feet. Each individual has a unique pattern and this offers a reliable means of identification.

dermatographia skin writing. A state of skin hypersensitivity in which striking white or red-edged elevated whealsoccur when the skin is firmly stroked. In this condition it is readily possible to write visibly on the skin with a blunt point, hence the name.

dermatology the study of the skin and its disorders and their relationship to medical conditions in general. The list that follows highlights the key entries related to dermatology in the dictionary: acne, acne rosacea, allergic dermatitis, alopecia, blister, cellulitis, chilblains, contact dermatitis, dermatitis, eczema, fungal infections, herpes simplex, ichthyosis, impetigo, infantile eczema, leprosy, lice, lichen planus, malignant melanoma, mole, naevus, neurofibromatosis, pityriasis, psoriasis, purpura, rodent ulcer, scabies, squamous epithelioma, striae, tinea, urticaria, varicose ulcer, verruca, warts.

dermatologist a doctor who practices DERMATOLOGY.

dermatome 1 a broad knife for taking very thin skin slices of less than full thickness (split skin) for grafting. **2** the area of skin receiving sensation from a nerve entering a single nerve root of the spinal cord.

dermatomyositis a disorder affecting both skin and muscle. There is inflammation and degeneration of connective tissue causing a rash and progressive muscle weakness. The condition is thought to be an AUTOIMMUNE disorder possibly induced by a virus.

dermatophytosis a general term for fungus infection of the skin, often called TINEA or 'ringworm'.

dermatopathology the branch of pathology concerned with disease of the skin.

dermatosis any skin disease.

Dermazole a brand name for ECONAZOLE.

dermis the true skin (cutis vera) or corium. The dermis lies under the EPIDERMIS.

dermoid cyst a benign growth caused by the abnormal infolding, during embryonic development, of a small quantity of surface tissue (ectoderm). Dermoid cysts occur mainly in the skin and ovary and often contain hair, bones or teeth. Dermoids of the ovary occasionally contain a cancer.

dermojet a device for injecting fluid without a needle, using high pressure and a very fine spurt.

Dermovate a brand name for CLOBETASOL.

Dermovate-NN a brand name for NEOMYCIN with CLOBETASOL, for external use.

DES see DIETHYLSTILBOESTROL.

desensitization 1 a method of treating allergy by injecting very small, but gradually increasing, doses of the substance to which the affected person is allergic.

2 a form of BEHAVIOUR THERAPY.

Deseril a brand name for METHYSERGIDE.

Desferal a brand name for DESFERRIOXAMINE.

desferrioxamine an iron CHELATING AGENT used in iron overload conditions or iron poisoning. A brand name is Desferal.

designer baby a baby derived from an embryo selected for a particular purpose or from one whose genome has been modified for a particular purpose.

designer drugs modifications of existing psychoactive drugs so as to produce seemingly new drugs not covered by prohibitive legislation. Designer drugs are produced in secret laboratories for profit and without regard to their dangers.

desloratadine a long-acting, low-sedation, ANTIHISTAMINE drug that does not block cardiac potassium channels and is less likely than some second generation antihistamines to have undesirable cardiac effects. It is also less prone to enter the nervous system and produce sedation. A brand name is Neoclarityn.

desmoid tumours slow-growing fibroid growths that, although not encapsulated and not capable of remote spread (METASTASIS), are locally-invasive. Their chromosomes do not suggest malignancy. They carry oestrogen receptors and affect women four times as often as men and often arise at the site of previous surgery. They are common in GARDNER'S SYNDROME.

desmoplasia the formation and proliferation of fibrous tissue, especially in tissues surrounding a CARCINOMA.

desmopressin a drug used in the treatment of

DIABETES INSIPIDUS. Desmopressin, or DDAVP, is a long-acting analogue of the natural pituitary hormone vasopressin, which is deficient in this condition. The drug is given in a nasal spray or in the form of nose drops. The drug is on the WHO official list. Brand names are DDAVP, Desmospray and Desmotabs.

desmosomes linking cross-bridges or contact sites between adjacent cells, especially epithelial cells.

Desmospray a brand name for DESMOPRESSIN.

Desmotabs a brand name for DESMOPRESSIN.

desogestrel a PROGESTOGEN hormonal ingredient in oestrogen/PROGESTOGEN oral contraceptives. Brand names of preparations containing this drug are Marvelon and Mercilon.

desoxymethasone desoxymetasone, a corticosteroid drug. Brand names for preparations containing this steroid for external use are Stiedex lotion and Stiedex LP.

desquamation shedding, peeling or scaling of skin.

detachment of the retina a separation of the neural layer of the RETINA from the underlying pigment layer as a result of a collection of fluid between the two. This is usually preceded by the development of retinal holes or tears, but detachment may be associated with traction by contracting strands of VITREOUS HUMOUR. Detachment tends to be progressive and separation of the MACULA LUTEA usually results in loss of visual acuity even if the retina is replaced.

Deteclo a brand name for TETRACYCLINE.

detoxification 1 the alteration of a substance in the body to a non-poisonous form, either as a spontaneous biochemical reaction or as a result of medical treatment with an antidote.

2 the process of treating a person for an addiction to a drug such as alcohol or heroin. This usage is largely metaphorical; in practice the process involves prohibition rather than removal of a toxic substance.

detoxification under anaesthesia a rapid and humane method of detoxifying people with heroin and other opioid addiction. The method is based on the use of opioid antagonist drugs while the patient is kept under general anaesthesia with tracheal intubation and bladder catheterization. Autonomic responses to the opiod withdrawal are monitored and

sedative drugs added to control them.
Continuous surveillance by anaesthetists
is necessary. The whole process takes about
24 hours.

detrusor 1 any entity that pushes down.
2 the muscle of the bladder.

detrusor instability involuntary contractions
of the bladder muscle causing an undesired
escape of urine. This is one of the most
important causes of incontinence, being, in
women, second only to incompetence of the
urethral sphincter. The condition is often
associated with excessive thickness of the
muscular bladder wall.

detumescence a return to normal, from a
swollen state, of an organ or part, especially
the penis.

deuteranomaly partial DEUTERANOPIA.

deuteranopia a form of colour blindness
(colour perception defect) causing a tendency
to confuse blues and greens, and greens and
reds and with a reduced sensitivity to green.

deviant behaviour behaviour that contravenes
accepted standards or rules in a society. Much
deviant behaviour is criminal.

deviation see SEXUAL DEVIATION.

dexamethasone a synthetic CORTICOSTEROID
drug used for its anti-inflammatory action and
for its value in reducing OEDEMA of the brain.
It is also used to treat severe inflammatory and
allergic disorders, shock, congenital adrenal
hyperplasia, vomiting caused by chemotherapy,
and for the diagnosis of Cushing's disease. The
drug is on the WHO official list. Brand names are
Decadron and Dexsol. The drug is also used in
various combinations.

dexamphetamine dexamfetamine, the
DEXTROROTATORY form of amphetamine
(amfetamine) sulphate, a drug sometimes used
to treat NARCOLEPSY, hyperactivity in children
and as an ANALEPTIC in hypnotic poisoning.
It is widely abused. A brand name is Dexedrine.

Dexa-Rhinaspray a brand name for
TRAMAZOLINE with DEXAMETHASONE and
NEOMYCIN.

Dexedrine a brand name for DEXAMPHETAMINE
(dexamfetamine).

dextran 70 a high molecular weight glucose
polymer used intravenously as a plasma
substitute to increase blood volume temporarily
in shock following severe blood loss, and for the
prevention of post-operative thromboembolism.

The drug is on the WHO official list.

dextrocardia the congenital anomaly in which
the apex of the heart points to the right instead
of the left. Dextrocardia is often associated with
a similar mirror-image reversal of the
abdominal organs.

dextromethorphan an opioid drug, with little
useful pain-killing action, used to control
persistent and unproductive cough. The drug
is on the WHO official list.

dextromoramide a powerful painkilling drug
used to treat intractable pain.

dextropropoxyphene a painkilling drug
similar to METHADONE. It is also dispensed in
combination with paracetamol, as Distalgesic.
Overdosage is one of the commonest causes of
death by poisoning, as absorption is rapid and
breathing is quickly paralysed. It is not much
more effective than CODEINE and some
poisoning experts think it should be
withdrawn. A brand name is Doloxene.

dextrorotary a substance which, in solution,
causes a plane beam of polarized light to rotate
to the right.

dextrose glucose. A DEXTROROTARY sugar.

dextrostix an enzyme-impregnated strip
used with a small portable electronic colour-
measuring device for convenient estimation
of the blood sugar levels by diabetics. The
dextrostix is touched to a drop of blood and
then inserted into the meter which gives a
digital reading of the blood sugar in mmol/l.

DF118 a brand name for DIHYDROCODEINE
tartrate.

DFHom *abbrev. for* Diploma of the Faculty of
Homoeopathy.

DFM *abbrev. for* Diploma in Forensic Medicine.

DGAMS *abbrev. for* Director-General of the
Army Medical Services.

DGM *abbrev. for* Diploma in Geriatric Medicine.

DGMS *abbrev. for* Director-General of Medical
Services.

DGO *abbrev. for* Diploma in Gynaecology and
Obstetrics.

DHA *abbrev. for* District Health Authority.

DHC Continus a brand name for
DIHYDROCODEINE.

DHEA *abbrev. for* DEHYDROEPIANDRO-STERONE.

DHMSA *abbrev. for* Diploma in History of
Medicine of the Society of Apothecaries.

Dhyg *abbrev. for* Doctor of Hygiene.

dhobi itch a slang term for TINEA of the groin

region (tinea crurus). It is a little unfair to blame the dhobie wallah as the trouble is more likely to be due to inadequate washing of the person, rather than the clothes.

DHyg *abbrev. for* Diploma in Hygiene.

dia- *prefix denoting* through.

diabetes see DIABETES MELLITUS.

diabetes, bronzed see HAEMOCHROMATOSIS.

diabetes insipidus a rare disease caused by inadequate production of the antidiuretic hormone (vasopressin) of the PITUITARY. Excessive quantities of dilute urine are produced and there is great thirst. Diabetes insipidus can also occur if the kidneys are abnormally insensitive to the anti-diuretic hormone. The condition should not be confused with ordinary DIABETES MELLITUS.

diabetes mellitus, Type I a disease, commonly starting in adolescence, in which the supply of INSULIN is insufficient for the body's needs. Type I diabetes results from destruction of the insulin-producing cells in the PANCREAS by an AUTOIMMUNE DISEASE process probably triggered by a virus infection.

Insulin stimulates the passage of glucose from the blood through cell membranes into the cells to be utilized as fuel. In the absence of insulin the muscles are deprived of fuel, and sugar accumulates in the blood and is excreted into the urine, taking much water with it. There is excessive urination, DEHYDRATION and great thirst. Protein and fats are consumed as fuel. The muscles waste and dangerous acidic compounds called ketone bodies are formed. These can cause diabetic coma and death. Diabetes has many serious complications, especially bleeding within the eyes from RETINOPATHY, kidney degeneration and obstruction to large blood vessels. Type I diabetes is always treated with insulin. See also ISLET TRANSPLANTATION.

diabetes mellitus, Type II also known as maturity-onset diabetes, this is due to a relative insufficiency of insulin along with impaired sensitivity to the actions of insulin. Obesity, which necessitates larger quantities of insulin, insulin resistance, abnormal beta cell function and excessively raised intracellular triglycerides are important factors. The rise in the prevalence of obesity in recent years has been accompanied by an alarming rise in the prevalence of Type II diabetes. The complications are those of Type I

diabetes and the disease may be treated by weight reduction, diet, insulin, or the use of drugs which prompt the pancreas to produce more insulin.

diabetic acidosis acidification of the blood occurring in untreated DIABETES MELLITUS as a result of the formation of excess acidic KETONE BODIES.

diabetic gangrene GANGRENE occurring in people with DIABETES MELLITUS as a result of large artery obliterative disease characteristic of the condition. Such gangrene often follows a minor injury.

diabetic retinopathy a disease of small retinal blood vessels that causes blood leakage (haemorrhages) which may be confined to the RETINA, or which may extend forward into the VITREOUS BODY with serious effects on vision. Fronds of new and fragile blood vessels may develop on the surface of the retina. Treatment is by laser destruction of much of the un-needed periphery of the retina. This is followed by disappearance of new blood vessels.

Diabex a brand name for METFORMIN.

Diabinese a brand name for CHLORPROPAMIDE.

diacetylmorphine heroin. See DIAMORPHINE.

Diaformin a brand name for METFORMIN.

diagnosis the art and science of identifying the disease causing a particular set of clinical signs and symptoms. Differential diagnosis is the selection of one from a list of diseases that present in a similar way. From the Greek *dia*, through, and *gnoskein*, to perceive.

diagnostic pertaining to DIAGNOSIS.

diakinesis one of the stages in the process of division of eggs and sperms which ensures that the number of CHROMOSOMES is halved (meiosis). In diakinesis the chromosomes shorten and thicken and the spindle fibres form, ready for the separation of the chromosomes.

dialysis separation of substances in solution by using membranes through which only molecules below a particular size can pass. Dialysis is the basis of artificial kidney machines.

Dialume a brand name for ALUMINIUM HYDROXIDE.

Diamicron a brand name for GLICLAZIDE.

diaminopyrimidines drugs used to treat or prevent MALARIA. Examples are pyrimethamine (Daraprim) and sulphadoxine with pyrimethamine (Fansidar).

diamorphine HEROIN. A semisynthetic

morphine derivative 3,6-O-diacetyl-morphine hydrochloride monohydrate. Its effects are the same as those of morphine, to which it is converted in the body, but it is much more soluble and is rapidly absorbed when taken by mouth. This is helpful when it is used in the control of severe terminal pain. The manufacture of diamorphine, even for medical use, is illegal in almost all countries. It is still used medically in Britain.

Diamox a brand name for acetazolamide, a drug used in the treatment of GLAUCOMA and sometimes in the treatment of EPILEPSY and periodic paralysis.

diapedesis the passing of blood cells through the intact CAPILLARY wall into the tissue spaces. Diapedesis is a feature of INFLAMMATION.

diaphoresis heavy perspiration, especially when medically induced.

diaphragm 1 the dome-shaped muscular and tendinous partition that separates the cavity of the chest from the cavity of the abdomen. When the muscle contracts the dome flattens, thereby increasing the volume of the chest.
2 any partitioning structure, such as the iris diaphragm of the eye.

diaphragm contraceptive a dome-shaped rubber or plastic barrier with a springy wire rim that is inserted in the vagina to cover the opening into the womb and prevent the passage of spermatozoa. Diaphragms are used in conjunction with spermicide creams or gels. See CONTRACEPTION.

diaphragmatic hernia protrusion of any abdominal organ or part or an organ through the DIAPHRAGM into the chest (thoracic) cavity.

diaphysis the shaft of a long bone. Distinguish from EPIPHYSIS, the growth zone at the ends of a long bone.

diarrhoea the result of unduly rapid transit of the bowel contents so that there is insufficient time for reabsorption of water to firm up the faeces. In consequence, the stools are loose and liquid and are passed more frequently than normal. The commonest causes are irritation from a bowel infection and psychological factors, as in the IRRITABLE BOWEL SYNDROME.

diarthrosis a freely movable joint with a SYNOVIAL MEMBRANE.

diastase an ENZYME capable of breaking down starch. An amylase.

diastasis separation of normally adjacent bones without fracture.

diastole the period in the heart cycle when the main pumping chambers (the ventricles) are relaxed and filling with blood from the upper chambers (the atria).

diastolic pertaining to DIASTOLE. The diastolic blood pressure is the pressure during diastole and is the lower of the two figures measured. The peak pressure is called the SYSTOLIC pressure.

diastolic heart failure heart failure in which systolic function is preserved – the left ventricular ejection fraction is normal. During diastole there is abnormal left ventricle relaxation with increased stiffness of the chamber. Doppler echocardiography is usually necessary to establish the diagnosis.

diathermy the use of high-frequency alternating current to heat or burn tissues. Diathermy can be used to produce a diffuse warming effect or an intense local cutting or coagulating effect for bloodless surgery.

diathesis an inherited predisposition to a disease or condition.

Diazemuls a brand name for DIAZEPAM.

diazepam a sedative and tranquillizing BENZODIAZEPINE drug. The drug is on the WHO official list. Brand names are Diazemuls, Diazepam Rectubes, Stesolid and Valclair.

Diazepam Rectubes a brand name for DIAZEPAM.

diazoxide a vasodilator drug used to treat severe high blood pressure (HYPERTENSION) and HYPOGLYCAEMIA. A brand name is Eudemine.

Dibenyline a brand name for PHENOXYBENZAMINE.

dibenzazepines drugs used to treat EPILEPSY, trigeminal neuralgia and bipolar disorders. An example is carbamazepine (Tegretol, Teril Retard.).

dibenzodiazepines drugs used to treat SCHIZOPHRENIA. An example is clozapine (Clozaril).

dibenzothiazepines drugs used to treat SCHIZOPHRENIA. An example is quetiapine (Seroquel).

dibenzoxazepines

dibromomanitol a drug used in the treatment of chronic LEUKAEMIA.

dibromopropamidine dibrompropamidine, an antibacterial and fungistatic agent used externally to treat burns, abrasions and minor skin infections. A brand name is Brulidine.

dicephaly two-headed. A gross monstrous congenital anomaly.

dichloralphenazone a hypnotic drug used for short periods for the management of insomnia and sometimes to control DELIRIUM. A brand name is Welldorm.

dichlorphenamide a DIURETIC drug with a short duration of action. It is also used in the treatment of GLAUCOMA. A brand name is Daranide.

Dick test a test of susceptibility to SCARLET FEVER. A small injection of streptococcal toxin is given. An area of inflammation indicates lack of immunity. (George Dick, 1881–1967, and Gladys Henry Dick, 1881–1963, American physicians).

diclofenac a non-steroidal anti-inflammatory drug (NSAID) used in the treatment of RHEUMATOID ARTHRITIS and other painful conditions. Brand names are Dicloflex, Diclomax, Motifene, Volraman, Volsaid Retard and Voltarol.

Dicloflex a brand name for DICLOFENAC.

Diclomax a brand name for DICLOFENAC.

Diconal a brand name for DIPIPANONE.

dicrotic having two waves, especially of a pulse.

dichromatism partial color blindness in which only two of the primary colours can be perceived.

dicoumarol an oral anticoagulant drug now mainly used as a rat poison. Other more readily controllable coumarins, such as WARFARIN, are now used.

dicyclomine hydrochloride dicycloverine, an antacid and antiflatulence drug. A brand name is Merbentyl. It is also formulated with CODEINE as Diarrest, and with DIMETHICONE (dimeticone) as Kolanticon.

Dicynene a brand name for ETHAMSYLATE (etamsylate).

didanosine a nucleoside analogue drug used in the treatment of AIDS. The drug is on the WHO official list. A brand name is Videx.

Didronel a brand name for ETIDRONATE.

Didronel PMO a brand name for EDITRONATE DISODIUM.

diencephalon the central, lower part of the brain that contains the BASAL GANGLIA, THE THALAMUS, the HYPOTHALAMUS, the PITUITARY gland.

dietary fibre a group of complex carbohydrates that includes plant cellulose, lignin, pectins and gums. These polysaccharides resist digestion and thus cannot be absorbed, but remain in the intestine until excreted, providing a useful sense of fullness or satiety. Fibre and is of value in the management of OBESITY. It bulks out the stool and is useful in the treatment of CONSTIPATION and DIVERTICULITIS. Dietary fibre reduces the risk of colorectal cancer possibly by removing carcinogens. Some soluble fibres bind bile cholesterol and prevent it from being reabsorbed. This can lower blood cholesterol. High fibre foods include vegetables and fruits, bran, beans, peas and nuts.

dietetic pertaining to diet.

dietetics the science of the principles of nutrition and their application in the pursuit of health. Dietetics includes the scientific selection of meals for people with digestive, metabolic and malnutritional disorders.

diethylcarbamazine a drug used to treat the parasitic worm diseases FILARIASIS and ONCHOCERCIASIS. The drug kills both the microfilaria and the adult worms but may provoke severe reactions when the worms die. The drug is on the WHO official list but is not available on the UK market. A brand name is Banocide.

diethylstilboestrol diethylstilbestrol, DES. A synthetic female sex hormone. This is now restricted in use to the treatment of certain cancers of the PROSTATE and the breast. If given to pregnant women it can cause cancer in the female offspring. See also STILBOESTROL.

diethyltoluamide (DEET) an insect repellant formulated as a lotion, spray or roll-on preparation that can be applied to the skin to repel mosquitos and reduce the risk of malaria. The drug is on the WHO official list.

dietician a person trained in DIETETICS.

Dietl's crisis recurrent attacks of severe pain in the loin, with nausea and vomiting, caused by partial twisting of the kidney on its vessels and kinking or obstruction of the URETER. (Jozef Dietl, 1804–78, Polish physician).

differential blood count an assessment of the percentage numbers of the various types of white cells present in the blood – the neutrophil polymorphs (40–75%), lymphocytes (20–45%), monocytes (2–10%), eosinophils (up to 6%) and basophils (up to 1%). Changes in the normal percentages are usually significant.

differentiation 1 the process by which stem cells acquire the special characteristics of the tissues into which they are developing.

2 the degree to which the cells of a tumour resemble, or fail to resemble, those of the tissue from which it arises. A high degree of differentiation implies low malignancy and *vice versa*.

3 the distinguishing of one disease from another.

differential diagnosis see DIAGNOSIS.

Differin a brand name for ADAPALENE.

Diflucan a brand name for FLUCONAZOLE.

diflucortolone valerate a powerful steroid drug used externally. A brand name is Nerisone.

diflunisal a non-steroidal pain-killing and anti-inflammatory drug (NSAID). It is a derivative of SALICYLIC ACID and is used to control symptoms in OSTEOARTHRITIS and other painful conditions. A brand name is Dolobid.

digastric 1 of a muscle having two bellies connected by a thinner tendinous part.

2 a muscle that acts to open the mouth by moving the jaw bone (mandible) down.

Di George syndrome a genetic disorder featuring many abnormalities including heart defects, facial anomalies, and congenital absence of the PARATHYROID GLANDS and the THYMUS, presenting as muscle spasms (TETANY) in a new-born baby. The associated T cell immune deficiency can be reversed by a fetal thymus transplant. The condition is due to a developmental anomaly involving the primitive structure in the neck from which both the parathyroid glands and the thymus develop. Some cases of the syndrome have recently been shown to be due to a mutation of the gene TBX1 on the chromosome. See T-box gene family. (Angelo Mario Di George, American paediatrician, b. 1921).

digestion the conversion of food into a form suitable for absorption and use by the body. This involves both mechanical reduction to a finer consistency and chemical breakdown to simpler substances.

digestive system the PHARYNX, OESOPHAGUS, STOMACH and intestines and the associated glands that secrete digestive ENZYMES (see Fig. 9).

digitalis a drug used in the treatment of HEART FAILURE. It increases the force of contraction and produces a slower, more regular pulse.

The drug is derived from the purple foxglove *Digitalis purpurea* and is usually given in the form of DIGOXIN.

digitalization dosing with a DIGITALIS preparation until the desired effect on the heart is achieved and maintained.

digital radiography a method of acquisition of an X-ray image in a form that can be stored as a computer file and reproduced as required. A phosphorescent plate is exposed in a standard X-ray cassette and the latent image on it is then scanned with a laser beam to produce a succession of light pulses that are picked up by a photomultiplier tube to produce a bit-mapped image file. This can be printed or displayed on a monitor. The phosphorescent plate can be exposed to light and reused an indefinite number of times. Images are available almost immediately and can be processed to improve contrast and detail. Reduced X-ray dosage to patients and economy in storage are further advantages.

digital subtraction angiography a method of imaging blood vessels that eliminates unwanted detail. Two digitized images are made, before and after injecting a radio-opaque dye. A negative image of one is then combined with the other, so that only differences between the two show up – in this case the dye in the vessels.

digoxin a valuable heart drug derived from the white foxglove *Digitalis lanata*. It is the most widely used of the DIGITALIS heart drugs and is a member of the group of cardiac glycosides. The drug is on the WHO official list. A brand name is Lanoxin.

DIH *abbrev. for* Diploma in Industrial Health.

dihydrocodeine a painkilling drug. Brand names are DF 118, DHC Continus and, in conjunction with PARACETAMOL, Remedeine.

dihydrofolate reductase an enzyme necessary for the synthesis of the purines of DNA.

dihydrofolate reductase inhibitors drugs that block the action of DIHYDROFOLATE REDUCTASE. Some of the drugs that inhibit this enzyme can, as in the case of METHOTREXATE, be used as anticancer drugs. Some of them have little effect on the human enzyme but a strong effect on the dihydrofolate reductases of bacterial and other parasites. Trimetrexate (Neutrexin) is a case in point; it is active against *Pneumocystis carinii*.

dihydrotachysterol a vitamin D analogue drug used to treat low blood calcium. A brand name is A.T. 10.

Dilantin a brand name for PHENYTOIN.

dilatation widening. This may be a normal process or may imply stretching beyond normal dimensions, either as part of a disease process or as a deliberate surgical act.

dilatation and curettage a common gynaecological operation that has not been entirely replaced by more recent methods such as low pressure suction curettage (SEE PIPELLE) or endoscopy. The opening into the womb is temporarily widened and a long, spoon-shaped instrument (a curette) is used to scrape the inside. This is done to treat abnormal bleeding, to remove unwanted tissue or to obtain a specimen for examination. Commonly referred to as D and C.

dilator any instrument used to widen or enlarge an opening, orifice or passage. Dilators are extensively used in surgery.

dildo a surrogate phallus. An object used as a substitute for an erect penis.

diloxanide an amoebocide drug used to treat asymptomatic patients with the cysts of *Entamoeba histolytica* (the cause of amoebic dysentery) in the stools. The drug is on the WHO official list. A brand name is Furamide.

diltiazem a calcium channel blocker drug used in the treatment of ANGINA PECTORIS and high blood pressure (HYPERTENSION). Brand names are Adizem SR, Adizem-XL, Angitil SR, Angitil XL, Dilzem SR, Dilzem XL, Slozem, Tildiem, Tildiem LA, Viazem XL, Zemtard and Zildil SR.

Dilzem a brand name for DILTIAZEM.

Dimelor a brand name for ACETOHEXAMIDE.

dimercaprol British Anti-Lewisite (BAL). A drug that takes up toxic metal ions from the body and can be life-saving in poisoning with lead, arsenic, gold, mercury, antimony, bismuth and thallium. The drug is on the WHO official list. It was developed during World War I in the course of a search for antidotes to poison war gases, particularly the arsenical Lewisite.

dimethicone dimeticone, simethicone, a drug that reduces surface tension on gas bubbles in the intestine so that they can coalesce and the gas can be more readily expelled. The drug is widely used in preparations for babies for the relief of colic.

dimethyl sulfoxide dimethyl sulfoxide, DMSO.

A colourless liquid of exceptional solvent properties that readily penetrates the surface of the skin and is used as a solvent for various drugs. Under the brand name of Rimso-50 it is used as a sterile 50% solution to wash out the bladder in certain cases of cystitis.

Dimetriose a brand name for GESTRINONE.

Dimotane a brand name for BROMPHENIRAMINE.

Dindevan a brand name for PHENINDIONE.

dinoprostone a PROSTAGLANDIN drug used by injection into the uterus to induce labour. Brand names are Prepidil, Propess-RS and Prostin E2.

Dioctyl a brand name for DOCUSATE SODIUM.

Dioderm a brand name for HYDROCORTISONE.

dioptre a measure of lens power. The reciprocal of the focal length in metres. A lens of 1 m focal length has a power of 1 dioptre. A lens of 50 cm focal length has a power of 2 dioptres. One of 33.3 cm focal length has a power of 3 dioptres. Dioptres are used by opticians in preference to focal lengths because they can immediately be added together or subtracted during vision testing.

Diovan a brand name for VALSARTAN.

Diovol a brand name for a preparation containing MAGNESIUM HYDROXIDE, DIMETHICONE and ALUMINIUM HYDROXIDE.

dioxins contaminant byproducts of the manufacture of chlorinated phenols used in herbicides, wood preservatives, dyes and other products. Dioxins are highly toxic and can cause cancer and fetal malformations. See also AGENT ORANGE.

DipBMS *abbrev. for* Diploma in Basic Medical Sciences.

DipCD *abbrev. for* Diploma in Child Development.

DipCOT *abbrev. for* Diploma of the College of Occupational Therapists.

Dipentum a brand name for OLSALAZINE.

Dip GU Med *abbrev. for* Diploma in Genitourinary Medicine.

diphenylbutylpiperidines drugs used to treat SCHIZOPHRENIA and other psychotic states. An example is Pimozide (Orap).

diphenhydramine an ANTIHISTAMINE drug with useful sedative and anti-itching properties. It is a constituent in many over-the counter cough and decongestant remedies with brand names such as Benylin Chesty Cough, Benylin

Children's Night Coughs, Benylin with Codeine, Benylin Cough and Congestion, Benylin Dry Cough, Boots Night Time Cough Syrup, Benylin Expectorant, Contac 400, Conovia Night Time Formula, Nirolex for Night Time Coughs, Nytol and so on.

Dip IMC RCS Ed *abbrev. for* Diploma in Immediate Medical Care of the Royal College of Surgeons, Edinburgh.

dipipanone an antiemetic drug formulated with CYCLIZINE under the brand name of Diconal.

DipPharmMed *abbrev. for* Diploma in Pharmaceutical Medicine.

diphenoxylate a drug related to PETHIDINE and with a codeine-like action on the bowel. It is used to treat diarrhoea. It is sold, mixed with a little ATROPINE, under the brand name of Lomotil.

diphosphonates a group of drugs that interfere with crystal formation and are used to relieve the symptoms of PAGET'S DISEASE of bone.

diphtheria a serious, and highly infectious, disease caused by the toxin of an organism *Corynebacterium diphtheriae*. This normally attacks the throat causing a membrane-like exudate of clotted serum, white cells, bacteria and dead surface tissue cells to form. This may obstruct the upper air passages, necessitating an emergency artificial opening into the windpipe (a tracheostomy) to save life. The bacterial toxin can also affect the heart.

diphtheria antitoxin a preparation of horse antibodies to diphtheria used exclusively to treat suspected cases of diphtheria in which the risk of the disease exceeds the risk of the injection. The drug is not used as a diphtheria preventive because of the severe risk of hypersensitivity. The drug is on the WHO official list.

diphtheritic myocarditis inflammation of the heart muscle caused by diphtherial toxin. There is a very fast pulse with irregularity and sometimes HEART FAILURE. Long periods of bed rest may be necessary. The condition may be fatal.

Diphyllobothrium latum a tapeworm having intermediate hosts in the freshwater crustacean *Cyclops* and then in fish. The worm is acquired by humans through eating fish. Infestation is fairly common in Finland and Scandinavia.

dipivefrin a SYMPATHOMIMETIC drug used to treat open angle GLAUCOMA. A brand name is Propine.

dipl-, diplo- *combining form denoting* double.

diplacusis a sensation of hearing two sounds of different pitch on exposure to a single sound. The condition is caused by a disorder of the COCHLEA.

diplegia paralysis of corresponding parts on both sides of the body.

diploblastic formed from two of the germ layers of the embryo.

diplococcus any one of the various cocci that occur in pairs, as does *Neisseria gonorrhoeae* that causes gonorrhoea.

diploe the spongy layer of bone between the hard outer and inner layers of the vault of the skull (cranium).

diploid having an identical (homologous) pair of chromosomes for each characteristic except sex. This is the normal state of most body cells. Eggs and sperms, however, have only a single set of half the number of chromosomes, and are said to be haploid. Red blood cells have no chromosomes.

diplopia double vision. The perception of two images of a single object. This occurs in squint (strabismus) when both eyes are not aligned on the object of interest. Diplopia with one eye is rare but possible.

Dip Pract Derm *abbrev. for* Diploma of Practical Dermatology.

DipRG *abbrev. for* Diploma in Remedial Gymnastics.

Diprivan a brand name for PROPOFOL.

diprophylline a drug similar to AMINOPHYLLINE used to relax bronchial muscle spasm in asthma and to improve the action of the heart.

Diprosone a brand name for BETAMETHASONE in a preparation for external use.

dipsogenic causing thirst.

dipsomania an uncontrollable, often episodic, craving for, and abuse of, alcohol. Between episodes the affected person may avoid alcohol altogether.

dipstix a convenient method of testing urine for protein, sugar, ketone bodies, PHENYLALANINE and other abnormal constituents. A narrow plastic or paper strip is impregnated with chemicals that change colour in the presence of the abnormal substance. See also CLINISTIX, ALBUSTIX and KETOSTIX.

-dipsia *combining form denoting* thirst or drinking.

dipterous two-winged. Belonging to the Diptera, a large order of insects which includes the flies and the mosquitoes.

Dipylidium caninum a short tapeworm of dogs and cats with the flea or louse as intermediate host. Children are occasionally infected when they swallow dog or cat fleas. Segments of the worm are seen in the stools.

dipyridamole a drug used to reduce platelet stickiness and thus the risk of STROKE in people having TRANSIENT ISCHAEMIC ATTACKS. Aspirin is more effective, but sometimes cannot be safely taken. A brand name is Persantin.

dirt eating repeated ingestion of non-nutritious and usually objectionable substances such as soil, coal, clay and paper. Medically known as pica, the practice is rare in adults except in the severely mentally retarded and sometimes in pregnant women. It is common and seldom particularly harmful in young children.

disaccharide one of the class of common sugars, including milk sugar (lactose) and cane sugar (sucrose), that can be broken down by hydrolysis, under the action of enzymes, to yield two monosaccharides.

dis- *prefix denoting* not, un-, away, apart, scattered, reverse.

disarticulation a separation at a joint.

discharge an abnormal outflow of body fluid, most commonly of pus mixed with normal secretions, or of normal secretions in abnormal amount. Discharge may occur from any body orifice or from a wound.

discectomy surgical removal of the central pulpy nucleus (nucleus pulposus) of an intervertebral disc.

disc, intervertebral see INTERVERTEBRAL DISC.

discission an outmoded operation in which the len capsule of a child's CRYSTALLINE LENS is cut with a sharp-edged needle and the lens matter allowed to disperse into the aqueous humour.

discitis inflammation of the intervertebral disc space, usually from infection and often with an associated OSTEOMYELITIS of the vertebral body or bodies. Sometimes known as infective sponmdylodiscitis.

disclosing agents stains that reveal PLAQUE on the teeth to encourage regular toothbrushing and flossing.

discontinuous gene a gene in which the coding information is split up between two or more strand lengths called EXONS, which are separated from each other by non-coding sections called INTRONS. Many genes are discontinuous.

discontinuous replication the synthesis of DNA in short lengths that later join up to form a continuous sequence.

discordance difference of phenotype in two individuals of identical, or near-identical, genotype.

disease 1 any abnormal condition of the body or part of it, arising from any cause.
2 a specific disorder that features a recognizable complex of physical signs, symptoms and effects. All diseases can be attributed to causes, known or unknown, that include heredity, environment, infection, new growth (neoplasia) or diet.

disease carrier see CARRIER.

disimpaction separation by traction of the broken ends of a bone that have been driven into each other in a position of poor alignment.

disinfection to use chemical substances to kill bacteria and other infecting agents outside the body or on the skin. Such substances include hexachlorophene, benzalkonium, cetrimide, phenol, merthiolate and various alcohols.

disinfestation the removal or destruction of ectoparasites such as lice.

disintegrins a family of snake venom anticoagulants that bind to INTEGRINS on the surface of platelets and cells, preventing their interaction with the extracellular matrix and with other cells. They inhibit tumour growth and angiogenesis and may have value in the treatment of cancer.

Disipal a brand name for ORPHENADRINE.

disjunction the separation movement of members of pairs of chromosomes to opposite poles of a cell in the process of cell division.

dislocation separation, especially the disarticulation of the bearing surfaces of a joint with damage to the capsule and to the ligaments that hold the joint together.

disodium cromoglycate disodium cromoglicate, see CROMOGLYCATE (cromoglicate).

disopyramide a drug used to prevent or control disturbances of heart rhythm. Brand names are Dirythmin SA and Rythmodan.

disorientation bewilderment or confusion about the current state of the real world and of

the affected person's relationship to it.
Awareness of time, place and person are usually
lost in that order.

dispensary a department of a hospital or clinic
supplying drugs and other medical supplies on
demand.

displacement activity one of the psychological
DEFENCE MECHANISMS. Frustrated emotions
aroused by a person, idea or object are
transferred to another person, idea or object.
Thus an aggrieved employee might take out his
resentment on a punch-bag.

Disprin a brand name for ASPIRIN.

Disprol a brand name for PARACETAMOL.

dissection 1 separation of tissues by cutting,
teasing or blunt division.
2 the act of dissecting.
3 an anatomical preparation that has been
dissected.

dissecting aneurysm of the aorta a splitting
of the wall of the largest artery in the body, into
which blood can pass under pressure. The split
tends to extend and the artery may rupture
causing immediate death. The condition may
occur in people with severe ATHEROSCLEROSIS
and high blood pressure (HYPERTENSION) or
with MARFAN'S SYNDROME.

**disseminated intravascular coagulation
(DIC)** a serious disorder of the blood clotting
mechanism in which extensive clotting occurs
within the blood vessels from the sustained and
excessive generation of thrombin, followed by a
strong activation of the clot fibrin breakdown
system (fibrinolysis) leading to a severe bleeding
tendency. DIC can be caused by severe sepsis,
extensive trauma, mismatched blood
transfusion, brain injury, extensive burns, snake
bite and liver disease. Current best treatment in
sepsis cases involves the use of a recombinant
form of human activated protein C.

disseminated sclerosis see MULTIPLE SCLEROSIS.

dissociative disorders a group of extreme
DEFENCE MECHANISMS which include loss of
memory for important personal details
(amnesia), wandering away from home and the
assumption of a new identity (fugue), splitting
of the personality into two distinct personalities
and trance-like states with severely reduced
response to external stimuli.

Distaclor a brand name for cephaclor, the
CEPHALOSPORIN antibiotic cefaclor.

distal situated at a point beyond, or away from,

any reference point such as the centre of the
body. Thus, the hand is distal to the elbow.
Compare PROXIMAL.

Distalgesic a brand name for a mixture of
PARACETAMOL and DEXTROPROPOXYPHENE.

Distamine a brand name for PENICILLAMINE.

distoclusion an improper relationship of the
teeth of the upper jaw to those of the lower, in
which those of the lower teeth are placed
further forward than (more DISTAL to) the
corresponding upper teeth.

distention an expansion or swelling from an
increase in internal pressure.

distichiasis the presence of an extra row of
eyelashes, on the inner margin of the eyelid,
that often causes severe discomfort from
contact with the eye.

distigmine an ANTICHOLINESTERASE drug used
to treat urinary retention, partial paralysis of
the intestine and MYASTHENIA GRAVIS. A brand
name is Ubretid.

distraction a pulling apart.

disulfiram a drug that interferes with the
normal metabolism of alcohol so that a toxic
substance, acetaldehyde, accumulates. This
causes flushing, sweating, nausea, vomiting,
faintness, headache, chest pain and sometimes
convulsions and collapse. It is sometimes used
to discourage drinking, but is not without
danger. A brand name is Antabuse.

dithranol a drug used in the treatment of
PSORIASIS. It is an ANTIMITOTIC agent and acts
to discourage overgrowth of epidermal cells.
The drug is on the WHO official list. Brand
names are Dithrocream, Micanol, Psorin
ointment and Psorin scalp gel.

ditiocarb the sodium salt of
diethyldithiocarbamate, a powerful
ANTIOXIDANT and CHELATING drug that has
been used to treat immune deficiency
conditions, such as AIDS. It appears to be
effective in reducing the incidence of
opportunistic infections and cancers in HIV
positive people.

Ditropan a brand name for OXYBUTYNIN.

Diuresal a brand name for FRUSEMIDE
(furosemide).

diuresis an unusually or abnormally large
output of urine.

diuretic 1 a drug or other agency that causes an
increased output of urine. Diuretics are used to
rid the body of OEDEMA fluid in conditions such

as HEART FAILURE and kidney disease.

2 causing a DIURESIS. See also LOOP DIURETICS.

Diurexan a brand name for XIPAMIDE, a thiazide diuretic drug.

diurnal pertaining to a day. Occurring daily or in a day.

divarication 1 a divergence at a wide angle.

2 the point at which divergence occurs.

divergence 1 the act or state of moving off in different directions from a point.

2 the departure from each other of two processes, modes of action or courses of evolution.

3 in genetics, the degree, usually expressed as a percentage, to which two related DNA lengths differ in nucleotide sequences, or two similar proteins differ in AMINO ACID sequence.

divergent transcription transcription started by two PROMOTERs acting in opposite directions so that transcription proceeds simultaneously in both directions from a point.

diverticulitis inflammation of abnormal outward protrusions (diverticula) of the inner lining of the large intestine (colon) through the muscular wall. Inflamed diverticula may perforate, causing the serious condition of PERITONITIS.

diverticulosis a condition in which many sac-like protrusions (diverticula) occur in the large intestine (colon).

diverticulum an out-pouching from, or sac formation on, a hollow organ or structure, such as the bowel. See also DIVERTICULOSIS.

Dixarit a brand name for CLONIDINE.

dizygotic derived from two separately fertilized eggs (ova). The term is used especially to refer to non-identical twins. Distinguished from monozygotic twins, who are derived from a single fertilized ovum and are identical.

DLO *abbrev. for* Diploma in Laryngology and Otology.

DLX *abbrev. for* Diploma in Laryngology & Otology.

DM *abbrev. for* Doctor of Medicine.

DMC *abbrev. for* District Medical Committee.

DMD *abbrev. for* Diploma in Dental Medicine.

DMHS *abbrev. for* Director Medical & Health Services.

DmedRehab *abbrev. for* Diploma in Medical Rehabilitation.

DMJ *abbrev. for* Diploma in Medical Jurisprudence.

DMARDs disease-modifying anti-rheumatic drugs, drugs used mainly in the treatment of RHEUMATOID ARTHRITIS. They act in various ways to relieve the severity of the condition.

DMO *abbrev. for* District Medical Officer.

DMR *abbrev. for* Diploma in Medical Radiology.

DMRD *abbrev. for* Diploma in Medical Radiodiagnosis.

DMRE *abbrev. for* Diploma in Medical Radiology and Electrology.

DMRT *abbrev. for* Diploma in Medical Radiotherapy.

DMS *abbrev. for* Director of Medical Services.

DMSA *abbrev. for* Diploma in Medical Services Administration.

DMSS *abbrev. for* Director Medical & Sanitary Services.

DMV *abbrev. for* Doctor of Veterinary Medicine.

DN *abbrev. for* Diploma in Nursing or District Nurse.

DNA *abbrev. for* deoxyribonucleic acid.

The very long molecule that winds up to form a CHROMOSOME and that contains the complete code for the automatic construction of the body. The molecule has a double helix skeleton of alternating sugars (deoxyribose) and phosphates. Between the two helices, lying like rungs in a ladder, are a succession of linked pairs of the four bases adenine, thymine, guanine and cytosine. The molecules of adenine and guanine are larger than thymine and cytosine and so, to keep the rungs of equal length, adenine links only with thymine and guanine only with cytosine. This arrangement allows automatic replication of the molecule. The sequence of bases along the molecule, taken in groups of three (codons), is the genetic code. Each CODON specifies a particular amino acid to be selected, and the sequence of these, in the polypeptides formed, determines the nature of the protein (usually an ENZYME) synthesized. Polypeptide formation occurs indirectly by way of MESSENGER RNA and TRANSFER RNA.

Periodicity of DNA is defined as the number of base pairs per turn of the double helix.

DNA fingerprinting the recording of a pattern of bands on transparent film, corresponding to the unique sequence of regions in the DNA (core sequences) of an individual. DNA fragments, obtained from a DNA sample by cutting it with restriction enzymes, are separated on a sheet of gel by ELECTROPHORESIS. The fragments are then denatured into single strands and the gel is blotted onto a membrane of nylon or nitrocellulose which fixes the fragments in place. Radioactive probes, complementary to the core sequences, are then added. These bind to any fragment containing the core sequence. The membrane is laid on a sheet of photographic film and a pattern of bands is produced by the action of the radiation. The arrangement of the banding pattern is unique to each unrelated person but parents and their offspring have common features. Patterns from different individuals, or from different samples from the same individual can be compared. The method can be used as a means of positive identification or of paternity testing. Only a tiny sample of blood, semen or of any body tissue is needed to provide the DNA.

DNA helicases enzymes that bring about the unwinding of DNA strands prior to replication.

DNA hybridization the use of radioactive known segments of DNA to determine the presence of complementary strands in a sample so as to determine identity, or to assess the degree of similarity between two individuals.

DNA library a collection of cloned DNA fragments that can be used as probes.

DNA ligases enzymes that reconstitutes the double strand in a DNA molecule that has a discontinuity in one strand. DNA ligases join up the broken strand by catalyzing a PHOSPHODIESTER BOND at this point. From the Latin *ligare*, to bind.

DNA methylation the addition of a methyl group to the cytosine ring that occurs in DNA when it is replicated in a dividing cell. The process forms methyl cytosine and is catalysed by enzymes called DNA methyltransferases. In humans, the change occurs only to those cytosines that preceded guanines in the DNA sequence. Methyl cytosine has a strong tendency to deaminate to form thymidine, and if this mutation is not repaired it remains. It is the commonest kind of genetic variation (polymorphism) in human populations.

DNA microarray a collection of tens of thousands of DNA single-strand molecular probes capable of detecting specific genes or measuring gene expression in a sample of tissue. A gene is expressed when it is transcribed into messenger RNA (mRNA) and forms a protein. Currently, DNA microarrays are mainly used as research tools but they have great potential as diagnostic devices and as a reliable means of predicting a patients' susceptibility to various diseases.

DNA polymerases enzymes that bring about the synthesis of a daughter strand of DNA on the basis of a complementary DNA template. They are involved in DNA replication and repair, and act by adding deoxynucleotide triphosphates to the 3'-OH group of the new DNA strand. These enzymes not only synthesize new DNA but proof-read the new strand and remove incorrect nucleotides and replace them with the correct ones.

DNA polymerase inhibitor a drug that acts against viruses by interfering with the action of the enzymes viruses use to build up their own DNA. Examples of this class of drugs are acyclovir (Soothelip, Zovirax), ganciclovir (Cymevene, Virgan), valganciclovir (Valtrex) and foscarnet (Foscavir).

DNA probe a DNA sequence labelled with a radioactive element used to identify the position of a segment with the complementary sequence by binding to it. DNA probes can also be used to identify the presence of complementary sequences in a mix of fragments.

DNA replicase an enzyme specific to DNA replication.

DNA replication the formation of new and, hopefully, identical copies of complete genomes. DNA replication occurs every time a cell divides to form two daughter cells. Under the influence of enzymes, DNA unwinds and the two strands separate over short lengths to form numerous replication forks, each of which is called a replicon. The separated strands are temporarily sealed with protein to prevent re-attachment. A short RNA sequence called a primer is formed for each strand at the fork. These primers provide a free 3'-OH end on which the new complementary sequence can be formed along the strand. The LEADING STRAND is synthesized continuously in the 5' to 3' direction, working towards the fork direction with removal of the RNA primers as the parental duplex is unwound. The LAGGING STRAND is synthesized discontinuously in the opposite direction as short fragments called Okazaki fragments. Lagging strand synthesis requires extension of the primer, then removal of the primers and gap filling. At least 20 different enzymes and factors, including DNA HELICASES, DNA POLYMERASES, RNA PRIMASES, DNA TOPOISOMERASES and DNA LIGASES are involved in the complex process of DNA replication.

DNAse *or* **Dnase** an enzyme that breaks down (hydrolyzes) bonds in DNA, releasing component nucleotides.

DNA sequencing the determination of the sequence of base pairs in a length of DNA.

DNE *abbrev. for* Diploma in Nursing Education.

DNR *abbrev. for* do not resuscitate. An instruction to refrain from energetic measures to restore the heart beat and the breathing in those people with terminal, irreversible illness in which death is expected, who suffer cardiac arrest. This has been the unwritten rule of many doctors and was enacted in American legislation in 1988.

DNS *abbrev. for* Director of Nursing Services.

DO *abbrev. for* Diploma in Ophthalmology.

Dobst *abbrev. for* Diploma in Obstetrics.

DobstRCOG *abbrev. for* Diploma in Obstetrics of the Royal College of Obstetricians and Gynaecologists.

dobutamine a drug used to assist in the management of HEART FAILURE. It increases the force of the contraction (inotropic agent) of the muscle of the ventricles and improves the heart output. It may be given by continuous intravenous drip. Brand names are Dobutrex and Posiject.

docetaxel an anticancer drug related to the natural substance taxol. A brand name is Taxotere.

doctor-assisted suicide the cooperation of a medical practitioner in bringing about the voluntary death of a patient suffering from painful or distressing terminal illness. Polls of doctors have shown that at least half agree that doctor-assisted suicide should be legalized for carefully-selected cases.

Doctor of Medicine in Britain, a person who, having obtained a basic, registrable medical qualification (Bachelor of Medicine), proceeds to further studies, research, thesis production and examination for the diploma of MD. This is equivalent to the PhD in other disciplines. In USA the basic qualification is Doctor of Medicine (MD), equivalent to Bachelor of Medicine in Britain.

doctorate the degree or status of a doctor as conferred by a university. A higher postgraduate qualification. See also DOCTOR OF MEDICINE.

docusate sodium a faecal softening drug used to treat constipation. Brand names are Dioctyl, Docusol, Fletcher's Emenette, Molcer, Norgalax and Waxsol.

Docusol a brand name for DOCUSATE SODIUM.

Doderlein's bacillus a GRAM POSITIVE bacillus, a normal inhabitant of the vagina that produces the lactic acid necessary for vaginal health. (Albert Seigmund Gustav Doderlein, 1860–1941, German gynaecologist).

dolicho- *prefix denoting* elongated.

dolichocephalic having a skull longer than it is broad.

Dolmatil a brand name for SULPIRIDE, a drug used to treat psychotic disorders.

dolor pain. One of the cardinal signs of inflammation, the other three being redness (rubor), heat (calor) and swelling (tumor).

Doloxene a brand name for DEXTROPROPOXYPHENE.

domain 1 of a protein, a discrete length of the amino acid sequence that is known to be associated with a specific function. **2** of a chromosome, a region in which supercoiling occurs independently of other domains; or a region that includes a gene of raised sensitivity to degradation by DNASE I.

dominance the power of a gene to exert its influence whether the other member of the gene pair is identical or dissimilar. GENES occur in pairs at corresponding positions (loci) on each of the paired CHROMOSOMES. A gene that has its effect only if paired with an ALLELE of the same kind is said to be RECESSIVE. The effect of a dominant gene paired with a recessive gene will be the same as if both genes had been identical to the dominant gene, but every cell in the affected person's body, including those producing sperms and eggs, contains the recessive gene. Such a person is said to be HETEROZYGOUS for that gene. When the sperms and eggs are produced, only one of the pair of chromosomes is included, so there is a 50/50 chance that this will be the one with the recessive gene. Should a sperm with the recessive gene fertilize an egg which also has the recessive gene, the recessive characteristic will be expressed because there is no other genetic material for the characteristic.

dominant see DOMINANCE.

dominant hemisphere the left half of the brain in almost all right-handed people and 85% of left-handed people. This is the hemisphere concerned with language and logical thought and containing the motor areas for voluntary use of the right side of the body. In 15% of left-handed people, the right hemisphere is dominant and subserves speech.

domiphen bromide a quaternary ammonium disinfectant drug used in lozenges. A brand name in a preparation compounded with a local anaesthetic, is Bradosol Plus lozenges.

domperidone a drug used to control nausea and vomiting. An antiemetic drug. It acts to close the muscle ring at the upper opening of the stomach (the cardia) and to relax the ring at the lower opening (the pylorus). A brand name is Motilium.

DOMS *abbrev. for* Diploma in Ophthalmic Medicine and Surgery.

donepezil an ACETYLCHOLINESTERASE inhibitor drug used in Alzheimer's disease and other forms of dementia to increase the amount of ACETYLCHOLINE available for nerve transmission. A brand name is Aricept.

donor a person, or cadaver, from whom blood, tissue or an organ is taken for transfusion or transplantation into another.

Donovan bodies the microscopic appearance caused in cell scrapings from the genital region in the tropical sexually transmitted disease GRANULOMA INGUINALE. The Donovan bodies are seen in stained mononuclear cells and are caused by the infecting agent *Donovania granulomatis*. (Lt Col. Charles Donovan, 1863–1951, Irish physican).

Donnalix a brand name for a mixture of ATROPINE, HYOSCINE and HYOSCYAMINE.

dopa decarboxylase inhibitors drugs used to treat PARKINSONISM. Examples are levodopa with benserazide (Madopar) and levodopa with carbidopa (Sinemet).

Dopacard a brand name for DOPEXAMINE.

Dopamet a brand name for METHYLDOPA.

dopamine a monoamine NEUROTRANSMITTER and hormone with an adrenaline-like action. Dopamine is the principal neurotransmitter in the extrapyramidal system. It is formed in the brain from the amino acid tyrosine via dopa and the latter, in the form of levodopa is used to treat PARKINSON'S DISEASE. Dopamine is the precursor of noradrenaline. It is also concerned with mood, memory and food intake. Excess is associated with psychiatric disorders. Dopamine is converted into at least 30 other substances some of which are hallucinogenic. The drug is on the WHO official list.

dopamine agonists drugs that have the effect of some of the actions of DOPAMINE, and are used to treat PARKINSONISM, infertility, growth hormone disorders, breast disorders and erectile dysfunction. Examples are bromocriptine, cabergoline (Cabaser), pramipexole dihydrochloride monohydrate (Mirapexin), quinagolide (Norprolac), ropinirole (Requip), lysuride, and apomorphine (Apo-go, Uprima).

dopamine receptors nerve cell membrane binding sites that are activated by dopamine molecules. Some are excitatory and some inhibitory, but both classes contain many subtypes. Some of these receptors mediate behavioural effects.

dopamine-regulating drugs drugs used to treat movement disorders caused by neurological disease or by the effects of antipsychotic drugs. An example is tetrabenazine (Xenazine).

dope a slang expression for any narcotic or addictive drug.

dopexamine a CATECHOLAMINE drug that improves the action of the heart. A brand name is Dopacard.

Doppler brain examination see TRANSCRANIAL DOPPLER ULTRASONOGRAPHY.

Doppler effect a change in the frequency of waves, such as sound or light, received by an observer, when the source is moving relative to the observer. The frequency increases when the source is approaching and decreases when it is retreating. The Doppler effect is used in a number of medical applications including measurement of blood flow and investigation of dynamic heart function. (Christian Johann Doppler, 1803–53, Austrian physicist).

Doppler ultrasound scanning a range of screening methods using the DOPPLER EFFECT to obtain information about rate of blood flow in arteries and through the heart.

Dopram a brand name for DOXAPRAM.

Doralese a brand name for INDORAMIN.

Dormonoct a brand name for loprazolam, a BENZODIAZEPINE hypnotic drug.

dornase alfa a drug used to remove sticky and tenacious secretions from the air passages of people suffering from CYSTIC FIBROSIS. A brand name is Pulmozyme.

dorsal relating to the back or towards the back. Compare VENTRAL.

dorsal root ganglia collections of the bodies of sensory spinal nerve cells lying outside but alongside the spinal cord, one for each spinal segment. The sensory spinal nerves contain the long dendrites of these cells; the axons pass into rear part of the spinal cord. Also known as posterior root ganglia.

dorsiflexion a bending backwards of any part.

DOrth *abbrev. for* Diploma in Orthodontics.

dorzolamide a CARBONIC ANHYDRASE inhibitor drug used in the form of eyedrops to treat open angle GLAUCOMA. A brand name is Trusopt.

dose 1 a stipulated quantity of a drug to be taken once or at stated intervals.
2 the amount of radiation received or administered.

dosimeter one of various devices that measure and indicate the total dose of radiation received. A dose rate meter is an instrument that measures the intensity of radiation at a particular site.

dothiepin dosulepin, a TRICYCLIC antidepressant drug. A brand name is Prothiaden.

DOTS *acronym for* Directly Observed Treatment, Short course. This is a multi-facetted American scheme of control of tuberculosis involving accurate diagnosis, an adequate supply of drugs, standardized effective treatment and systematic review of progress. In China, between 1991 and 2000, the DOTS strategy significantly reduced the prevalence of tuberculosis in certain areas.

double-blind trial a test of the real effect of a new medical treatment, in which neither the patient nor the persons conducting the trial know which of two identical-seeming treatments is genuine and which is not. Trials not conducted in this way cannot be relied on to provide reliable evidence of the efficacy of a treatment because of the power of the placebo effect and of psychological suggestion.

double jointed an informal term referring to a person with an unusual range of movement at one or more joints.

double vision see DIPLOPIA.

douche a washing out of a body cavity or opening by a stream of water or other fluid. Vaginal douching is much used by women with vaginal discharge.

doula a person, such as a woman who has experienced normal childbirth who provides emotional, physical, and informational support to a woman during and after labour.

Dovobet a brand name for CALCIPOTRIOL with BETAMETHASONE.

Dovonex a brand name for CALCIPOTRIOL.

Down's syndrome a major genetic disorder caused by the presence of an extra chromosome 21 (trisomy 21). People with Down's syndrome have oval, down-sloping eyelid openings, a large, protruding tongue and small ears. There is always some degree of learning difficulty, but this need not be severe and many people with Down's syndrome are able to engage in simple employment.

Antenatal screening for Down's syndrome has been improved since the end of the 20th century. A quadruple-test screening algorithm for all pregnant women, that includes maternal serum alphafetoprotein, human chorionic gonadotropin, unconjugated oestriol (estriol) and inhibin A is now in use to determine whether pregnant women need be offered AMNIOCENTESIS or CHORIONIC VILLUS SAMPLING. Other factors such as maternal age and ultrasound identification of fetal abnormalities are also important. (John Langdon Haydon Down, 1828–96, English physician).

downstream in genetics, at a stage in the sequence of processes in the expression of a gene that is nearer the final protein product than any stage in the direction of the DNA. The term is also used to mean in the direction of the 3'-end of a chain of bases in DNA (see PHOSPHODIESTER BOND). In both cases the opposite sense is called 'upstream'.

doxapram a drug that stimulates breathing and consciousness. An ANALEPTIC drug similar in its action to NIKETHAMIDE. A brand name is Dopram.

doxazosin a selective alpha-blocker drug used to treat urinary outflow difficulty. A brand name is Cardura.

doxepin a TRICYCLIC ANTIDEPRESSANT DRUG. A brand name is Sinequan.

doxorubicin an antibiotic, also known as Adriamycin, that interferes with the synthesis of DNA and is thus useful an anticancer agent.

It has many side effects including loss of hair, sickness and vomiting, interference with blood production and heart damage. The drug is on the WHO official list. A brand name is Caelyx.

doxycycline a tetracycline antibiotic drug, deoxytetracycline, that is well absorbed when taken by mouth, even after food. Doxycycline is also used for the prophylaxis of MALARIA. The drug is on the WHO official list. Brand names are Periostat and Vibramycin.

Doxylin a brand name for DOXYCYCLINE.

Dozic a brand name for HALOPERIDOL.

DPA *abbrev. for* Diploma in Public Administration.

Dpath *abbrev. for* Diploma in Pathology.

DPD *abbrev. for* Diploma in Public Dentistry.

DPH *abbrev. for* Diploma in Public Health.

DphilMed *abbrev. for* Diploma in Philosophy of Medicine.

DPhysMed *abbrev. for* Diploma in Physical Medicine.

DPM *abbrev. for* Diploma in Psychological Medicine.

DPMSA *abbrev. for* Diploma in Philosophical Medicine of the Society of Apothecaries.

DR *abbrev. for* Diploma in Radiology.

DrAc *abbrev. for* Doctor of Acupuncture.

DRACOG *abbrev. for* Diploma of the Royal Australian College of Obstetrics & Gynaecology.

dracontiasis infection with the GUINEA WORM *Dracunculus medinensis*.

DRACR *abbrev. for* Diploma of the Royal Australasian College of Radiologists.

drain a tube or narrow sheet inserted into a wound or cavity, or put in place during surgery, to allow free discharge of fluid, and prevent its accumulation, while healing is taking place.

drainage, surgical SEE SURGICAL DRAINAGE.

Drapolene an antiseptic skin cream containing CETRIMIDE and benzalkonium chloride.

DRCOG *abbrev. for* Diploma of the Royal College of Obstetricians and Gynaecologists.

DRCPath *abbrev. for* Diploma of the Royal College of Pathologists.

dream analysis a process purporting to derive information about the state of the unconscious mind by an interpretation of the symbolic significance of the dream content.

dreaming the subjective experience of partial consciousness during sleep. Dreaming occurs during periods of apparently light sleep, when the eyes move rapidly beneath the lids. This is called REM (rapid eye movement) sleep.

Dressler's syndrome persistent fever with inflammation of the heart sac (PERICARDITIS) and of the lung coverings (PLEURISY) during the weeks following a heart attack (MYOCARDIAL INFARCTION). It is probably an AUTOIMMUNE effect of dead heart muscle. (William Dressler, 1890–1969, American cardiologist).

DRM *abbrev. for* Diploma in Radiation Medicine.

Drogenil a brand name for FLUTAMIDE.

drop attack a tendency to fall suddenly, without warning, and without loss of consciousness. Drop attacks may be due to a temporary shortage of blood to the brain and should be investigated.

droperidol a butyrophenone antipsychotic drug that causes emotional quietening and a state of mental detachment. It is sometimes used as a premedication before surgery.

drop foot SEE FOOT DROP.

droplet infection infection acquired by contact with, or inhalation of, tiny airborne drops of water and mucus containing infective organisms, that are released from the nose or mouth during coughing or sneezing. Access is often via the CONJUNCTIVA of the eye.

dropsy an old-fashioned term for a collection of fluid in the tissues (OEDEMA).

drosophila a small fly of the genus *Drosophila*, especially the fruit fly *Drosophila melanogaster* which has been used for many years in genetic research mainly because of its four conspicuous chromosomes and relatively few and obvious characteristics.

drospirenone a progestogen drug used in combination with ETHINYLOESTRADIOL (ethinylestradiol) as a combined oral contraceptive under the brand name Yasmin.

drotrecogin alfa an anticoagulant drug used in patients with severe multiple organ failure as an adjunct to standard treatment. A brand name is Xigris.

drowning death from suffocation as a result of exclusion of air from the lungs by fluid, usually water. This may result from fluid produced within the lungs themselves (pulmonary oedema).

drug 1 any substance used as medication or for the diagnosis of disease.
2 a popular term for any narcotic or addictive substance.

drug abuse the use of any drug, for recreational or pleasure purposes, which is currently disapproved of by the majority of the members of a society. 'Hard' drugs are those liable to cause major emotional and physical dependency and an alteration in the social functioning of the user. See also COCAINE, DRUG DEPENDENCE, ECSTASY, HEROIN, MARIJUANA.

drug body packers people who smuggle drugs of abuse within the intestine or concealed in the rectum or vagina. Condoms, aluminium foil and latex material are used for packaging. The activity carries a high risk of death from poisoning.

drug dependence a syndrome featuring persistent usage of the drug, difficulty in stopping and withdrawal symptoms. Drug dependent people will go to great lengths to maintain access to the drug, often resorting to crime. Drug dependence is not limited to dependence on illegal drugs.

drug idiosyncrasy an abnormal individual response to a drug causing an effect quite different from that expected. Idiosyncracy is inherent in the person concerned and is usually due to a genetic anomaly. It may take the form of hypersensitivity so that the normal effect is produced by a dose which is a small fraction of the standard dose.

drug tolerance a progressive reduction in the effect of a drug, following repeated exposure to it, so that it no longer has the desired effect in the original dose.

drug-transporter gene one of a range of genes that code for transport proteins to which various drug molecules can attach. An example of the product of such a gene is the ABCB1 transporter (also known as MDR1) which is known to transport at least four anti-epileptic drugs. Mutations in this gene can cause multi-drug-resistant epilepsy. ABCB1 (MDR1) contributes to drug resistance in a number of diseases including several cancers, RHEUMATOID ARTHRITIS and inflammatory bowel disease.

dry gangrene GANGRENE developing as a result of loss of blood supply from arterial obstruction in which infection has not occurred. The tissues shrivel, mummify and the gangrenous extremity may drop off.

Dryptal a brand name for FRUSEMIDE (furosemide).

dry socket inflammation of the soft tissues of a tooth socket, occurring two or three days after extraction of a tooth, usually a lower molar. The condition is painful and may persist for days or weeks. The attention of a dentist is required.

DS *abbrev. for* Doctor of Surgery.

DSc *abbrev. for* Doctor of Science.

DSM *abbrev. for* Diploma in Social Medicine.

DSM IV *abbrev. for Diagnostic and Statistical Manual of Mental Disorders*, Fourth edition of May 1994. An attempt by the American Psychiatric Association to formalize and regularize psychiatric terminology and to provide clear descriptions of the various psychiatric entities. The bible of American psychiatrists, occasionally also consulted by the British. Studies are currently under way for the preparation of DSM-V.

DSS *abbrev. for* Department of Social Security.

DSSc *abbrev. for* Diploma in Sanitary Science.

DTCD *abbrev. for* Diploma in Tuberculosis and Chest Diseases.

DTCH *abbrev. for* Diploma in Tropical Child Health.

DTD *abbrev. for* Diploma in Tuberculous Diseases.

DTH *abbrev. for* Diploma in Tropical Hygiene.

DTIC-Dome a brand name for DACARBAZINE.

DTM *abbrev. for* Diploma in Tropical Medicine.

DTM&H *abbrev. for* Diploma in Tropical Medicine and Hygiene.

DTPH *abbrev. for* Diploma in Tropical Public Health.

Dubin-Johnson syndrome a rare AUTOSOMAL RECESSIVE condition featuring a failure of BILIRUBIN transport in the liver and increased levels of bilirubin in the blood. There is sickness and mild JAUNDICE but the outlook is excellent. (Isadore Nathan Dubin, Canadian pathologist, b. 1913, and Frank Bacchus Johnson, American pathologist, b. 1919).

Duchenne muscular dystrophy a hereditary, X-linked RECESSIVE muscle disorder affecting males almost exclusively. It begins in the first three years of life and first affects the legs and buttocks. Usually, the muscles appear larger than normal (pseudo-hypertrophy) but are in fact very weak. The condition spreads to affect other muscles and death is usual between the age of 20 and 30. See also DYSTROPHIN. (Guillaume Benjamin Amand Duchenne, 1805–75, French neurologist).

duck-bill speculum a hinged, two-bladed

instrument that is inserted closed into the vagina and the blades then separated. This allows for examination of the neck (cervix) of the womb (uterus) and of the vaginal walls. Also known as a Simm's speculum.

duct a tube or passage, especially one leading from a gland, through which a fluid or semisolid substance is conveyed.

ductus arteriosus a short shunting artery lying between the main artery to the lungs (pulmonary artery) and the main artery to the body (aorta). During fetal life blood need not pass through the lungs and this vessel acts as a bypass. It normally closes soon after birth. If it fails to do so (patent ductus arteriosus) the blood is insufficiently oxygenated and there may be interference with growth and development and additional strain on the heart.

dumping syndrome a feeling of drowsiness, with weakness, dizziness, nausea, sometimes vomiting, sweating and palpitations experienced after a meal by people who have had surgical removal of the stomach (gastrectomy).

duodenal ulcer a crater in the lining of the first part of the small intestine (the DUODENUM) usually caused by the action of strong acid and digestive enzymes coming from the stomach. Duodenal ulcer is also related to the presence of an organism *Helicobacter pylori*. Destruction of this organism with antibiotics, together with the use of proton pump inhibitor drugs such as OMEPRAZOLE (Losec), has been shown to cure many ulcers and to prevent recurrence. See also PEPTIC ULCER.

duodenum the C-shaped first part of the small intestine into which the stomach empties. The ducts from the GALL BLADDER and PANCREAS enter the duodenum. The duodenum is said to be 12 finger-breadths long – hence the name.

duodenitis inflammation of the lining of the first part of the duodenum. This can be seen on DUODENOSCOPY and is a condition likely to progress to DUODENAL ULCER.

duodenoscopy direct examination of the interior of the DUODENUM by means of a fibreoptic, steerable ENDOSCOPE. This is valuable in the diagnosis of DUODENAL ULCER and of cancer affecting the head of the PANCREAS or the region of the entrance of the bile and pancreatic ducts (the ampulla of Vater).

duodenostomy a surgical connection made between the duodenum and another hollow organ such as the stomach or gall bladder.

Duogastrone a brand name for CARBENOXOLONE.

Duovent a brand name for FENOTEROL with ipatropium.

Duphalac a brand name for LACTULOSE.

Duphaston a brand name for DYDROGESTERONE.

duplex a double stranded length of nucleic acid. The term is commonly used to refer to DNA in its double helical form, as distinct from a single strand of DNA.

duplex DNA normal, double-stranded DNA.

Dupuytren's contracture shortening of some of the tendons on the palm of the hand, as a result of inflammation, so that one or more fingers are pulled into a permanently bent position. The ring finger is usually the first to be affected. Treatment is by careful surgical removal of the thickened, contracted tissue. The condition is unrelated to manual labour. It is believed to be mediated by free radicals and is commoner in people with AIDS than in the general population. (Baron Guillaume Dupuytren, 1777–1835, French surgeon).

Durabolin Decadurabolin, brand names for NANDROLONE, an ANABOLIC STEROID.

dura mater a tough fibrous membrane, the outer of the three layers of the MENINGES that cover the brain and the spinal cord. The dura mater lies over the ARACHNOID and the PIA MATER.

Durogesic a brand name for FENTANYL.

dust diseases see PNEUMOCONIOSIS.

dutasteride a drug that reduces production of dihydrotestosterone by inhibiting both types of the enzyme 5-alpha-reductase and is used to control benign prostatic hyperplasia and reduce the risk of acute urinary retention. Dutasteride is said to be more effective in this role than FINASTERIDE (Proscar). Like all testosterone antagonists this drug can cause reduced sexual interest, impotence, ejaculation problems, breast tenderness and breast enlargement (gynecomastia). A brand name is Avodart.

DV&D *abbrev. for* Diploma in Venereology and Dermatology.

dwarfism abnormal shortness of stature. This may be of genetic origin as in ACHONDROPLASIA, DOWN'S SYNDROME, Trisomy 18, TURNER'S

SYNDROME and Bloom's syndrome or it may result from glandular defects such as pituitary growth hormone deficiency, primary thyroid deficiency (CRETINISM), precocious puberty or adrenal gland insufficiency. It also results from various metabolic disorders such as HURLER'S SYNDROME, TAY-SACH'S DISEASE, NIEMANN-PICK DISEASE and GAUCHER'S DISEASE.

DXA scanning dual X-ray absorptiometry scanning, a technology of bone densitometry used to measure bone mineral density as a means of assessing the degree of OSTEOPOROSIS and the risk of trouble form it. Modern DXA equipment can perform the scan in a few seconds.

dydrogesterone a PROGESTOGEN drug used to treat menstrual and premenstrual disorders, ENDOMETRIOSIS, infertility and other conditions. A brand name is Duphaston.

Dymadon a brand name for a PARACETAMOL preparation.

Dynastat a brand name for PARECOXIB.

dys- *prefix denoting* disordered, defective, difficult, bad or abnormal.

dysarthria inability to speak normally because of loss of functional control over the muscles of the tongue, lips, cheeks or larynx. This usually results from neurological disorder such as STROKE.

dysarthrosis 1 deformity, dislocation or disease of a joint.
2 development of a false joint following non-union of a bone break.

dyscalculia loss of arithmetical ability. This may occur as a specific feature of brain damage in STROKE.

dyschezia difficult or painful defaecation, usually from severe constipation and hard stools.

dyschondroplasia a rare progressive disease of the growing parts of bone (epiphyses), affecting children and causing growth retardation. The bones of the limbs are abnormally short, often unequal, and show nodular swellings.

dyscrasia a vague term meaning any abnormal condition of the body.

dysdiadokokinesis the inability to perform rapidly alternating movements involving the cessation of one movement immediately followed by the opposite movement. This is usually tested by asking the subject to oscillate the hands as rapidly as possible in a rotary manner. Dysdiadokokinesis is a sign of a disorder of the CEREBELLUM.

dysentery bowel inflammation from infection either with shigella organisms (bacillary dysentery or SHIGELLOSIS) or with the amoeba *Entamoeba histolytica* (AMOEBIC DYSENTERY). Dysentery features frequent passage of stools containing blood and mucus, abdominal pain, fever and general upset. Shigella dysentery may be more acute than amoebic dysentery but is more easily treated and the long-term implications are usually less serious. Shigellosis is treated, when necessary, with antibiotics or sulphonamides. Amoebic dysentery is treated with METRONIDAZOLE.

dysfunction any disorder or abnormality of operation or performance especially of any part of the body.

dysgenesis any abnormality of development.

dyshidrosis any anomaly of sweat production or release.

dyshormonogenesis a defect in the synthesis of the thyroid hormone thyroxine due to an enzyme failure. The low levels of thyroxine in the blood cause a large output of thyroid stimulating hormone (TSH) from the PITUITARY gland and the result is an enlargement of the thyroid gland (goitre).

dyskaryosis a visible abnormality in the nuclei of cells that appear otherwise normal. Dyskaryosis is a minimal change seen, for instance, in cells scraped from the surface of the cervix in a PAP SMEAR test and does not necessarily imply any worrying abnormality.

dyskeratosis abnormal, excessive or imperfect KERATINIZATION of cells of the EPIDERMIS. DYSPLASIA of a squamous epithelium.

dyskinesia involuntary jerky or slow writhing movements, often of a fixed pattern. The dyskinesias include the TICS, MYOCLONUS, CHOREA and ATHETOSIS.

dyslexia abnormal difficulty in reading or in comprehension of what is read, in a person of normal intelligence and emotional stability and who has had normal educational and cultural opportunities. The condition is familial and heritable and there is evidence of differences in areas of the brain that are also affected in acquired alexia. The basic difficulty appears to be in processing the sounds of speech and in the awareness that words can be broken down into smaller units of sound. Many dyslexic children respond well to remedial help especially if provided early.

dyslipidaemia any disorder of lipid metabolism reflected in abnormal levels in the blood of cholesterol or triglycerides (fats).

dysmelia deficiency or abnormality of the development of the limbs.

dysmenorrhoea painful MENSTRUATION. Around the beginning of the period, there is cramping, rhythmical pain in the lower abdomen and back, lasting usually for a few hours, but sometimes for a day or even longer.

dysmetria an inability to adjust movements accurately, without visual assistance, so as to achieve their object. Dysmetria is a sign of malfunction of the CEREBELLUM.

dysmorphogenesis severe abnormality of body development caused by influences operating at an early stage of fetal growth. Monstrous maldevelopment (TERATOGENESIS).

dysmorphophobia a conviction that other people are aware of a physical defect in the sufferer which is, in fact, non-existent. Dysmorphophobia may be a presenting symptom of schizophrenia or a neurotic disorder. Dysmorphophobia by proxy has been described in a woman who, in three consecutive pregnancies became convinced that the unborn child would suffer some physical defect. As a result she sought termination on all three occasions.

dysorexia any abnormality of the appetite.

dysostosis defective bone formation.

Dyspamet a brand name for CIMETIDINE.

dyspareunia painful sexual intercourse experienced by the woman. This may be caused by a thick, persistent HYMEN, VULVITIS, VAGINITIS, BARTHOLINITIS, URETHRITIS, episiotomy scars, vaginal dryness or atrophy of the vagina. It is often caused by tight vaginal spasm (vaginismus), a psychological problem.

dyspepsia indigestion. Any symptoms of disorder of, or abuse of, the digestive system or any symptoms attributed to digestive upset. The symptoms include discomfort in the upper abdomen, heartburn, a tendency to belching, nausea or a sense of bloated fullness (flatulence). See also PEPTIC ULCER.

dysphagia difficulty in swallowing. See also PHARYNGEAL POUCH, ACHALASIA and GLOBUS HYSTERICUS.

dysphasia impairment of speech or of the production or comprehension of spoken or written language. Dysphasia is due mainly to damage to the temporoparietal and prerolandic parts of the brain, usually from STROKE. Seven major sub-types of aphasia, including motor, sensory, conduction and ANOMIC DYSPHASIA, have been described but it is a complex disorder which cannot readily be divided into neat categories. Much can often be done to help by intensive devoted therapy. See also APHASIA.

dysphonia impairment of normal voice production, from any cause, such as LARYNGITIS, singer's nodes, 'CLERGYMAN'S THROAT', paralysis of one of the nerves to the larynx (recurrent laryngeal nerve).

dysphoria a state of unhappiness, anxiety and restlessness. The opposite of euphoria.

dysplasia an abnormal alteration in a tissue due to abnormality in the function of the component cells, but excluding cancer. There may be absence of growth, abnormal increase in growth or abnormalities in cell structure. Dysplasia in an epithelium commonly progresses to cancer.

dysplastic naevus syndrome the presence of 100 or more naevi with at least one of 8 mm or more in diameter and at least one that shows atypical features. The term is sometimes applied to patients with only one atypical naevus. People with atypical naevi are about 15 times more likely to develop malignant melanoma than those in the general population.

dyspnoea difficult, laboured or obstructed breathing. The sense of 'not getting enough air'. This is a feature of ASTHMA, partial obstruction or narrowing of the airway, lung disease, severe ANAEMIA, MOUNTAIN SICKNESS or hysterical HYPERVENTILATION. Refractory dyspnoea that has failed to respond to standard treatments has been treated effectively with sustained release morphine – a controversial measure in view of the well-known respiratory depressive effect of this drug.

dyspraxia a disturbance of voluntary movement

dysrhythmia any irregularity or disturbance of a normal body rhythm. The term is most commonly applied to the heart beat or the ELECTROENCEPHALOGRAM (EEG).

dyssynergia puppet-like movement resulting from the inability to coordinate simultaneous movement at the various joints in a limb.

Movement is broken up into its separate components. This is a sign of disorder of the CEREBELLUM.

dystaxia moderate lack of control over voluntary movement not amounting to ATAXIA.

dysthymia a degree of depression not amounting to a severe psychosis.

dystocia abnormal labour from failure of the expulsive power of the womb, from obstruction to the birth passage or from abnormalities in the size, shape or presentation of the baby.

dystonia a group of muscle disorders featuring muscle spasms, abnormal posture or muscle contraction, or interference with normal movement. The dystonias include wry-neck (TORTICOLLIS), WRITER'S CRAMP, spasmodic closure of the eyelids (BLEPHAROSPASM) and involuntary grimacing and chewing movements (Meige syndrome).

dystrophy a vague term applied to conditions in which tissues fail to grow normally, or to maintain their normal, healthy, functioning state. See CORNEAL DYSTROPHY and MUSCULAR DYSTROPHY.

dystrophia myotonica a hereditary AUTOSOMAL DOMINANT condition which presents in early adult life with wasting of the muscles of the face, neck and shoulders and spreads to the arms and legs. The muscles relax very slowly after contracting. The condition also features drooping eyelids (PTOSIS) and CATARACT.

dystrophin a large, rod-shaped structural protein situated in the sub-sarcolemmal region of the muscle fibre membrane. A mutation of the dystrophin gene that eliminates dystrophin production causes DUCHENNE MUSCULAR DYSTROPHY; a mutation that codes for a smaller amount of dystrophin or a modified molecule causes Becker dystrophy. See also MUSCULAR DYSTROPHY.

dysuria pain on passing urine. This is most commonly due to a urinary infection and is usually associated with undue frequency in the desire to urinate.

Dytac a brand name for TRIAMTERENE, a DIURETIC drug that does not lead to loss of potassium from the body.

Dytide a brand name for TRIAMTERENE in combination with another diuretic drug.

e

Eales' disease an inflammatory disorder of the retinal veins, giving rise to recurrent bleeding into the vitreous humour of the eye with severe visual disturbances. (Henry Eales, English ophthalmologist, 1852–1913).

earache pain arising from the external ear passage, the ear drum, the space between the drum and the inner ear (the middle ear) or the inner ear apparatus lying within the temporal bone of the skull. The common cause is infection, usually OTITIS EXTERNA or OTITIS MEDIA. Earache can also occur from BAROTRAUMA.

earball an acupressure device. A small ball kept in position in the ear and pressed, hopefully as a means of relieving stress.

ear, cauliflower see CAULIFLOWER EAR.

eardrum the tympanic membrane that separates the inner end of the external auditory canal (the meatus) from the middle ear. The outer side of the drum is covered with thin skin and to the inner side is attached the malleus, first of the three tiny bones, the auditory ossicles.

eardrum, perforated SEE PERFORATED EARDRUM.

ear lobe the soft, pendulous fleshy tissue at the lowest point of the external ear (pinna).

early antigens antigens on the surface of cells that are coded for by viral genes and appear very soon after cell invasion and before synthesis of viral nucleic acid starts.

ear piercing the formation of a permanent, skin-lined perforation through the earlobe, from which a decorative ring or pendant can be suspended.

ear wax the secretion of the ceruminous glands in the skin of the outer ear canal. Wax is a deterrent to small insects and traps dust. Over-production can lead to blockage of the canal and deafness which is easily corrected by wax removal.

earwig the insect *Foricula auricularia*, of the order *Dermaptera*, whose popular name derives from the widely held idea that it can burrow its way into the head after entering the ear and cause untold damage to the brain. Earwigs do occasionally enter the external auditory canal but are prevented by the eardrum from proceeding further. They can easily be floated out by instilling a little oil.

Eaton agent pneumonia lung inflammation (pneumonitis) caused by the organism *Mycoplasma pneumoniae*, a very small bacterium once thought to be a virus. Also known as primary atypical pneumonia. Outbreaks occur in institutions, mostly in children and young adults. The condition responds to tetracycline. (Monroe Davis Eaton, American bacteriologist, b. 1904).

Ebixa a brand name for MEMANTINE.

EBV *abbrev. for* for EPSTEIN-BARR VIRUS.

Ebola virus disease a severe infectious disease first described among laboratory workers in Marburg, West Germany and occurring later in the Sudan and Zaire. There is fever, muscle aching, diarrhoea, sore throat, an extensive rash, bleeding into the bowel and involvement of the brain and kidneys. The mortality may be over 90% in untreated cases and 25% in those given good supportive treatment.

ebullism the formation of water vapour bubbles in the blood as a result of an acute drop in atmospheric pressure or in the pressure to which a diver is exposed, as from too sudden a rise to the surface.

eburnation 1 the loss or thinning of the bearing cartilage of a joint, that occurs in degenerative disease such as OSTEOARTHRITIS, so that the underlying bone is exposed and becomes dense and polished by friction.
2 the burnishing or hardening of the exposed DENTINE of a tooth that results from the calcification of the soft material in the tubules.

EBV *abbrev. for* EPSTEIN-BARR VIRUS.

ecbolic causing the pregnant womb to contract and expel its contents. Oxytocic.

eccentric located away from, or deviating from, the centre or from the usual position.

ecchondroma a bony outgrowth capped with cartilage. An exostosis. Also known as osteochondroma.

ecchymosis bleeding (haemorrhage) or bruising in the skin or a mucous membrane, in the form of small, round spots or purplish discoloration.

eccrine exocrine, secreting externally, especially on to the surface of the skin, as in the case of a sweat gland.

ecdysis the shedding of the outer layer of the skin. The term is usually applied to the common process occurring during the development of various insects, such as Ophidia and many of the Arthropoda, but is sometimes used as a synonym for EXFOLIATION in humans.

ECFMG *abbrev. for* Education Council for Foreign Medical Graduates.

ECG *abbrev. for* ELECTROCARDIOGRAM.

echinate prickly or covered with spines.

echino- *combining form* denoting spiny or prickly.

echinocandins a class of lipopeptide antifungal drugs that act by inhibiting glucan synthesis, thereby damaging fungal cell walls. They are effective against *Candida* and *Aspergillus* species. Examples are caspofungin (Cancidas) and micafungin.

echinococcus one of several tapeworms of the genus *Echinococcus*, the larvae of which form large, spherical cysts in the tissues, including the brain, causing serious or fatal disease.

echinococcosis infestation by larvae of the tapeworm *Echinococcus* that results from the ingestion of faecally-carried eggs or proglottids. Also known as hydatid disease. The main causes are *E. granulosus* and *E. multilocularis* which respectively cause cystic and alveolar echinococcosis, both being serious diseases.

The definitive hosts of *E. granulosus* are dogs and wolves; those of *E. multilocularis* are red and arctic foxes. Humans are the intermediate hosts. Hydatid cysts develop mainly in the liver and lungs but may occur almost anywhere in the body. Small cysts may be symptomless, but cysts grow and may rupture causing serious complications.

echinocyte a red blood cell with a crenated or spiky surface.

echocardiography a form of ULTRASOUND imaging used to investigate heart disorders. The method can display the movement and action of the heart valves, abnormal masses in the heart and the details of congenital heart disease.

echoencephalography ULTRASOUND imaging of the brain. This is now largely superseded by CT SCANNING and magnetic resonance imaging (MRI).

echographia a form of APHASIA in which the affected person, although unable to express thoughts in writing, is able accurately to copy written or printed material.

echolalia the involuntary, parrot-like repetition of words or phrases, spoken by another person. Echolalia may occur as a feature of schizophrenia or as part of a severe tic disorder.

echopraxia an abnormal, compulsive or involuntary mimicking of the actions of another person.

ECHO virus enteric cytopathogenic human orphan virus, an enterovirus that can cause aseptic MENINGITIS and can be recovered from the cerebrospinal fluid.

eclampsia a serious complication of pregnancy in which dangerous seizures occur with a high mortality. Eclampsia is always preceded by the warning state of pre-eclampsia. This consists of raised blood pressure, OEDEMA, and protein (albumin and sometimes globulin) in the urine. The risk of eclampsia ceases soon, but not immediately, after the baby is born. It has recently been discovered that a rise in the levels of circulating angiogenic factors can predict the development of pre-eclampsia.

ecmnesia loss of short-term memory with retention of memory for earlier events.

E. coli SEE ESCHERICHIA COLI.

econazole a broad-spectrum antifungal drug used in local (topical) application. Brand names are Ecostatin, Pevaryl, Pevaryl TC and Gyno-Pevaryl.

Ecostatin a brand name for ECONAZOLE.

ecothiopate a powerful CHOLINERGIC drug of the organophosphate anticholinesterase group, used in the form of eye drops to cause prolonged contriction of the pupil. The drug is useful in the treatment of some cases of GLAUCOMA and STRABISMUS. A brand name is Phospholine iodide.

Ecotrin a brand name for ASPIRIN.

ecstasy a popular name for the drug 3,4-methylene dioxymethamphetamine (MDMA), a hallucinogenic AMPHETAMINE with effects that are a combination of those of LSD and amphetamine (amfetamine). Ecstasy is widely used to promote an appropriate state of mind at a 'rave', all-night dance sessions, but the combination of strenuous physical exercise and the direct toxic effect of the drug has led to a number of deaths in young people. Such death result from an uncontrolled rise in body temperature (hyperthermia), kidney failure, muscle breakdown (rhabdomyolysis) and sometimes liver failure. Urgent measures to reduce body core temperature can save life. The drug can also precipitate a persistent paranoid PSYCHOSIS. Claims that ecstasy can damage the dopamine system of the brain and cause Parkinson's disease have been discredited.

ECT see ELECTROCONVULSIVE THERAPY.

ectasia permanent widening, distension or ballooning of any tubular organ or part. 'Broken veins' are small ectatic skin blood vessels.

ecthyma a pus-forming, ulcerating and crusting inflammatory skin disease, similar to IMPETIGO, often affecting the forearms and legs of malnourished people.

ecto- *prefix denoting* outside or external.

ectocardia a developmental malpositioning of the heart, especially when exteriorized.

ectoderm the outermost of the three primary germ layers of an embryo, the others being the MESODERM and the ENDODERM. The ectoderm develops into the skin, the nervous system, and the sense organs.

ectogenesis having origin and undergoing early growth outside the body, as in the case of IN VITRO FERTILIZATION.

ectomorph one of the arbitrarily classified body types (SOMATOTYPES). Ectomorphic people are lean and moderately muscled.

ectoparasite any organism living on the outside of another organism and depending on it for nutrition. Lice, ticks and mites may be human ectoparasites.

ectopia malposition of an organ or structure.

ectopic situated in a place remote from the usual location. An ECTOPIC PREGNANCY is one occurring outside the womb, often in the FALLOPIAN TUBE. Ectopic foci of womb lining tissue occur on the ovaries or in various parts of the abdomen in the condition of ENDOMETRIOSIS.

ectopic expression the expression of a gene in a tissue in which it is not normally expressed. This occurs only in artificial situations such as in transgenic animals.

ectopic heart beat a contraction of the heart VENTRICLES occurring prematurely so as to disturb the regular rhythm. This usually results in a compensatory pause, experienced by the subject as a 'palpitation'.

ectopic hormone secretion hormone production at body sites not normally capable of hormone synthesis. In most cases ectopic hormone production occurs in tumours, many of which produce hormones.

ectopic pregnancy a dangerous complication of pregnancy in which the fertilized egg (ovum) becomes implanted in an abnormal site, such as the FALLOPIAN TUBE or in the pelvis or abdomen, instead of in the womb lining. The great danger is severe, and sometimes life-threatening, bleeding (haemorrhage). Treatment is by urgent operation to remove the growing embryo. This is now mainly done by laparoscopic surgery.

ectropion an out-turning of an eyelid, usually the lower, so that the wet, inner, conjunctival surface is exposed to view. Ectropion is commonest in the elderly, in whom weak and lax eyelid muscles allow the lower lid to fall away from the eye. It can also be caused by paralysis of the flat muscle surrounding the eye, as in BELL'S PALSY or by scarring and shortening (contracture) of the lid skin (cicatricial ectropion).

eculizumab an antibody against terminal protein C5. The drug has been found useful in paroxysmal nocturnal haemoglobinuria. It is well tolerated and safe and reduces haemolysis, haemoglobinuria and the need for transfusion.

eczema the effect of a number of different causes and a feature of many different kinds of skin inflammation (dermatitis). It features itching, scaly red patches and small fluid-filled blisters which burst, releasing serum, so that the skin becomes moist, 'weeping' and crusty.

edema US spelling of OEDEMA.

edentulous toothless.

edetate calcium disodium a chelating agent capable of reducing poisonous levels of heavy metals, such as lead, manganese and iron, in the body. It has the advantage over edetate sodium in that it has a lower affinity for calcium than for these heavier metals. It does not, however, remove mercury.

editronate disodium a BISPHOSPHONATE drug used to treat and prevent OSTEOPOROSIS by inhibiting osteoclastic resorption of bone. A brand name of a preparation marketed with calcium in a cyclical therapy kit is Didronel PMO.

edrophonium a drug that inactivates the enzyme CHOLINESTERASE that breaks down ACETYLCHOLINE. It is used as a test for MYASTHENIA GRAVIS, a disease in which the action of acetyl choline is impaired. The brand name is Tensilon.

EDTA *abbrev. for* ethylene-diamine-tetraacetic acid. A CHELATING AGENT, sometimes called Edetate, used in the treatment of lead poisoning or to remove excess calcium.

Edwards' syndrome a condition caused by an additional chromosome no 18 (trisomy 18). There is mental and physical retardation, rocker flat feet and deformities of the heart, kidneys and fingers. Affected babies seldom survive the first 6 months. (John Hilton Edwards, British geneticist, b. 1928)

EEG *abbrev. for* ELECTROENCEPHALOGRAM.

efavirenz a non-nucleoside reverse transcriptase inhibitor used, in combination with other antiretroviral drugs, to treat HIV infections. The drug is on the WHO official list. A brand name is Sustiva

Efcortelan a skin ointment containing HYDROCORTISONE.

Efcortesol a brand name for HYDRO-CORTISONE formulated for external use.

Efexor a brand name for VENLAFAXINE.

efferent 1 directed away from a central organ or part.

2 nerve impulses travelling away from the central nervous system to a peripheral effector.

effort syndrome see DA COSTA SYNDROME.

effusion 1 movement of fluid from its usual situation, to form a collection elsewhere.

2 the collection of fluid in an abnormal site, as in a pleural effusion, a pericardial effusion or a joint effusion.

eflornithine an antiprotozoal drug used to treat *Pneumocystis carinii* pneumonia and African TRYPANOSOMIASIS. The drug is on the WHO official list.

eformoterol formoterol, a selective beta-2 agonist drug used to treat ASTHMA. A beta-2 agonist is a drug that stimulates a certain group of adrenaline receptors in the muscle cells of the air tubes of the lungs, causing the tubes to widen. As a group, these drugs are also known as bronchodilators. The term is commonly abbreviated to beta-agonist. Eformeterol is formulated in powder form in a capsule and is administered by inhaler. Brand names are Foradil, Oxis Turbohaler.

Efudix a brand name for a preparation of FLUOROURACIL for external application.

egestion defaecation.

egg the OVUM or female reproductive cell (GAMETE). The egg contains half the chromosomes required by the new individual, and the other half are supplied by the sperm at the moment of fertilization. The egg is a very large cell, about one tenth of a millimetre in diameter, and much larger than a sperm. This is because it contains nutritive material (yolk) to supply the embryo in its earliest stages before it can establish a supply from the mother via the placenta. If more than one egg is produced and fertilized, a multiple pregnancy results, but the offspring are not identical since half the chromosomes in each come from different sperms, with different genetic material. If a fertilized ovum divides, and each of the two halves forms a new individual, these will be identical twins, with identical chromosomes.

ego 1 the Latin word for 'I'.

2 a person's consciousness of self.

3 in Freudian terms, a kind of rational internal person largely at the mercy of the 'id' (German for 'it') with its wicked and mainly sexual drives, but sometimes saved from disaster by the virtuous 'super-ego'. Freud changed his definition of the ego several times. See also FREUDIAN THEORY.

egomania a pathological degree of preoccupation with self. An abnormal degree of self-esteem.

eggshell skull doctrine a forensic principle

based on a largely imaginary possibility. If someone suffers an injury that might be expected to cause moderate but not serious damage, but that person has a pre-existing weakness so that the effects of the injury are severe, the full liability still rests with the defendant. Skulls are frequently much thicker than average, but the eggshell skull is virtually unknown.

Ehlers-Danlos syndrome a genetic disorder in which the skin is abnormally elastic so that it may be greatly stretched. It is, however, unduly fragile and gapes widely when wounded. Joints are also unusually extensible. The condition is due to a widespread defect of polymerization of the protein collagen – one of the basic constructional materials of the body. (Edvard Ehlers, German dermatologist 1863–1937 and Henri Alexandre Danlos, French dermatologist, 1844–1932).

Ehrlichiosis a rare human infection with *Ehrlichia* organisms such as *E. canis* that normally infect animals. The first known human infection was described in Japan in 1954. The illness is usually acquired by a tick bite and resembles glandular fever (infective mononucleosis). A new species, *E. chaffeensis*, was isolated in 1991 and a third in 1994. The disease is largely confined to the Southeast and mid-Atlantic states of the USA.

eicosapentaenoic acid a polyunsaturated fatty acid found in fish oils which is able to reduce the tendency to blood clotting. It is believed to be protective against CORONARY THROMBOSIS. It appears to act by antagonizing the formation of THROMBOXANE A2, one of the factors in THROMBUS formation. Brand names are Maxepa and Omacor.

eidetic strikingly vivid, detailed and accurate, allowing an extraordinarily lifelike imaging, or sometimes rehearing, of past experience.

Eisenmenger complex the structural abnormalities in the heart and the lungs that underlie the EISENMENGER SYNDROME.

Eisenmenger syndrome a congenital heart anomaly featuring a 'hole in the heart' (septal defect) or an unclosed DUCTUS ARTERIOSUS associated with serious changes in the lung blood vessels causing increased resistance to the passage of blood. Early surgical treatment of heart holes or patent ductus arteriosus may prevent the secondary lung changes from

developing. (Victor Eisenmenger, 1864–1932, German physician).

ejaculation the forceful emission of seminal fluid, caused by muscular contraction, at the time of the male ORGASM. Premature ejaculation is a common disorder. See also RETROGRADE EJACULATION.

Ekbom's syndrome see RESTLESS LEGS SYNDROME.

Elantan a brand name for ISOSORBIDE MONONITRATE.

elastic stockings supportive hosiery worn usually to assist in the control of the symptoms of VARICOSE VEINS. The external pressure applied by such stockings must be even and any local 'tourniquet' effect avoided. The compression should be greater at the ankle than at the thigh and should be graded along the leg. This requirement is now acknowledged by manufacturers and incorporated into the design of their products.

elastins extracellular scleroproteins capable of two-way stretch and rapid recoil. The amount of stretch is limited by the tethering effect of interwoven inelastic collagen fibrils. Elastins are present in quantity in the lungs, large arteries, the ligaments of the spine and in the skin.

elastosis 1 increase in elastin in a tissue. 2 degeneration and breakup of the elastic fibres of connective tissue. The condition often affects the skin as a result of ultraviolet irradiation.

Eldepryl a brand name for SELEGILINE.

Eldisine a brand name for VINDESINE.

elective a term usually used of treatment. Undertaken to achieve advantage for the patient, but not essential to life or health. Most cosmetic surgical operations can be considered elective.

Electra complex the Freudian concept, complementary to the Oedipus complex, featuring the sexual attraction of a female child for her father.

electrical injury burns caused by electrical arcs, the effects of heating from the passage of an electric current through the tissues or interference with the function of the nervous system and heart from electric currents in the body.

electric shock treatment see ELECTROCONVULSIVE THERAPY.

electro- *combining form denoting* electricity or electric.

electrocardiogram (ECG) the tracing on paper, representing the electrical events associated with the heartbeats, produced by the ELECTROCARDIOGRAPH.

electrocardiograph an instrument consisting of a series of electrical cables (leads) with a lead-switching device, a high-gain, low-noise, balanced differential amplifier and a moving coil rotary transducer that converts the amplified signal into a varying trace on a calibrated strip of moving paper. The leads are connected to low-resistance contacts on the chest of the subject and the input to the device is derived from the minute electrical currents that flow towards and away from them as a result of the heart's contractions and relaxations.

electrocardiography recording of the rapidly varying electric currents which can be detected as varying voltage differences between different points on the surface of the body, as a result of heart muscle contraction. The electrocardiograph (ECG) tracings show patterns highly indicative of a wide variety of heart disorders. Modern ECG machines usually carry out an automatic analysis of the waveform and suggest a diagnosis.

electrocautery the use of an electric current to destroy or coagulate tissue. High-frequency electrical heating (diathermy) is a convenient way of stopping bleeding during a surgical operation and is often used as a quick alternative to tying off small bleeding vessels.

electrocoagulation see ELECTROCAUTERY.

electroconvulsive therapy (ECT) a means of inducing an epileptic fit by applying a short pulse of electric current to the brain. ECT is used to treat various psychiatric conditions and is usually performed under light general anaesthesia supplemented by a short-acting muscle relaxant drug. It is most useful in cases of serious DEPRESSION and in some forms of acute SCHIZOPHRENIA. A systematic review and meta-analysis of many published reports of trials of ECT appeared in the *Lancet* in March 2003. This showed that ECT was an effective short-term treatment for depression and that it was probably more effective than drug treatment.

electrocution death from the passage of an electric current. Judicial electrocution employs a current of several amperes passing between the head and one leg by means of a high voltage and moistened electrodes to give low contact resistance.

electrodiagnosis the general term for a wide range of diagnostic methods involving the pickup, amplification, recording and display of any of the electrical events of the body. It includes ELECTROCARDIOGRAPHY, ELECTROENCEPHALOGRAPHY, ELECTROMYOGRAPHY and ELECTRONYSTAGMOGRAPHY.

electroencephalogram the multichannel tracing on paper of the output of the electroencephalograph, representing the electrical activity of the brain as occurring between pairs of electrodes in contact with the scalp and representing the algebraic sum of an immense amount of underlying electrical activity.

electroencephalography the process of making a multiple tracing, by voltmeter-operated pens, of the electrical activity of the brain. The multiple readings are of the constantly varying voltage differences occurring between pairs of points on the scalp of the subject. The electroencephalograph (EEG) is affected by sleep, HYPERVENTILATION, drugs, concussion, brain injury, brain tumours, bleeding within the brain (cerebral haemorrhage), brain inflammation (ENCEPHALITIS), EPILEPSY and various psychiatric conditions. It also assists in the determination of brain death.

electrolysis the decomposition of a solution by the passage of an electric current to separate charged particles (ions). Water can be separated into the gases hydrogen and oxygen by this means. The term is used for electrical destruction of unwanted hair follicles, but the main destructive effect is one of heating.

electrolyte balance the critical balance between the concentration in the cells and that in the tissue fluid surrounding the cells of the various inorganic IONS. The electrolytes mainly in the cells are potassium, magnesium, sulphate and phosphate. Those in the surrounding fluid are mainly sodium, chloride and bicarbonate. This balance is essential to life and is maintained by the active pumping action of the cell membranes.

electromagnetic spectrum the continuum of radiation, varying in frequency, and, correspondingly, wavelength, that includes, in order of decreasing frequency, cosmic ray photons, gamma rays, X rays, ultraviolet radiation, visible light, infrared radiation, microwaves, radio waves and heat.

electromyography a diagnostic method in which the electrical events associated with muscle contraction are amplified and recorded for analysis. The signals may be picked up by surface electrodes or a needle consisting of two insulated, coaxial conductors may be pushed into the muscle. The method allows distinction to be made between various nerve disorders, disorders affecting the junction between the nerve and the muscle and various muscle disorders.

electron carrier a compound, such as a coenzyme, capable of taking up electrons from a molecule and transferring them to another, thereby undergoing reversible reduction and oxidation.

electron microscopy a method of producing a greatly enlarged image of very small objects by using a beam of accelerated electrons instead of light. Modern instruments enable objects smaller than 1nm (one millionth of a millimetre) to be seen. This is almost down to atomic level. Focusing is done by means of magnetic fields obtained from charged plates or current-carrying coils. These fields act as lenses. Electron microscopes are essential tools in medical research and diagnosis.

electronic smart health cards an important innovation in the automation of health care administration and in the preservation and accessibility of personal health data that was adopted in France in April, 1998. Smart cards are EPROMs (erasable programmable read-only memories) that contain administrative information and details such as blood group and allergies. When inserted, along with the doctor's or pharmacist's card, into a computerized card reader, a claim form for the cost of treatment is automatically generated and the details are sent to the patient's insurer. Future versions may contain full medical records.

electronystagmography graphical recording of the small electric currents generated by eye movements. These can be picked up by metal electrodes placed near the corners of the eyes, amplified and used to deflect recording pens so

as to produce a permanent record of the eye movements. The method may be used to analyse abnormal rhythmical eye movement (NYSTAGMUS), or to record the response to CALORIC TESTS of the function of the inner ear balancing mechanism.

electrophoresis separation of charged particles in a solution (ions) by the application of an electric current. This can be done in a thin layer of solution on paper or in a gel. Ions of low weight move more quickly than those of high weight, so separation occurs and can be demonstrated by staining. The method is widely used in medicine to identify and measure the proteins present in the blood including the ANTIBODIES (IMMUNOGLOBULINS). It is used to identify the various abnormal haemoglobins causing SICKLE CELL ANAEMIA and other similar conditions. It is extensively used in genetic work such as DNA fingerprinting. Electrophoresis is remarkably sensitive. Pieces of DNA, for instance, that differ in length from each other by only one base pair can be separated into discrete bands by this method.

electroretinogram a recording of the summation of the electric changes occurring in the retina under different conditions, such as exposure to flashes of bright light. The ERG is of value in the diagnosis of some uncommon conditions affecting the RODS or the CONES.

electrospray ionization mass spectrometry a method of mass spectrometry used to obtain the chemical analysis and weight of large molecules, especially proteins and peptides using a very small sample. The electrospray provides a charge on the molecules which are then injected into a mass spectrometer to determine the ratio of charge to molecular mass.

electrovalent bond the chemical bond between an ANION and a CATION. Compounds formed by electrovalent bonds ionize when dissolved in water, with dissociation of the cations and anions.

elephantiasis the condition of enormous enlargement of a limb, the scrotum or the female external genitalia caused by obstruction to the lymph drainage channels by masses of parasitic microfilaria worms, mainly *Wuchereria bancrofti* or, in the condition of lymphogranuloma venereum, by the *Chlamydia trachomatis* organism.

eletripan a selective SEROTONIN receptor agonist used to treat MIGRAINE. A brand name is Relpax.

Elidel a brand name for PIMECROLIMUS.

ELISA test the enzyme-linked immunosorbent assay test. This is a widely used test for the presence of particular antibodies in the blood. It is a common screening test for AIDS but can be used to detect any known ANTIBODY for which the corresponding ANTIGEN is held. ELISA kits are available to test for a wide range of infections.

Elleste Solo a brand name for OESTRADIOL (estradiol) intended for the treatment of menopausal disorders.

elliptocytosis oval-shaped red blood cells. A small proportion of oval cells occurs in MEGALOBLASTIC ANAEMIA and HYPOCHROMIC ANAEMIA. A high proportion suggests an unimportant dominant hereditary disorder.

Eltroxin a brand name for THYROXINE (levothyroxine).

elution the washing out of a substance from a material into a fluid in which the material is immersed. A coronary artery stent may, for instance, be designed to elute drugs into the bloodstream.

Elwes syndrome a compulsive disorder featuring the necessity to hoard wealth and to live in poverty and self-denial in order to increase the hoard. The syndrome, which is often gravely damaging to the quality of life of the sufferer and to the affection of his associates, involves love of money to a pathological degree while denying the miser the satisfactions normally associated with the expenditure of money. There is often distorted judgement amounting almost to delusional thinking. The cause remains obscure. The syndrome is named after the notorious miser John Elwes (1714-89).

Elyzol a brand name for METRONIDAZOLE.

emaciation the state of extreme thinness from absence of body fat and muscle wasting usually resulting from malnutrition, widespread cancer or other debilitating disease.

EMAS *abbrev. for* Employment Medical Advisory Service.

embalming a method of preserving a dead body by removing the blood and replacing it with fluids, such as formaldehyde, which discourage the growth of the organisms responsible for putrefaction.

embolectomy surgical removal from a blood vessel, usually an artery, of a blood clot, or other obstruction, which has been carried to the site in the bloodstream from elsewhere in the circulation (EMBOLUS).

embolism sudden blocking of an artery by solid, semisolid or gaseous material brought to the site of the obstruction in the bloodstream. The object, or material, causing the embolism is called an EMBOLUS. See also PULMONARY EMBOLISM.

embolus any material carried in the bloodstream to a point where it causes obstruction to the blood flow. Emboli are commonly blood clots but may consist of crystals of CHOLESTEROL from plaques of ATHEROMA in larger arteries, clumps of infected material, air or nitrogen, bone marrow, fat or tumour cells.

embrocation any lotion or medicated liquid applied to the outside of the body in the hope of relieving muscle, joint or tendon pain. Embrocations have little direct effect.

embryo an organism in its earliest stages of development, especially before it has reached a stage at which it can be distinguished from other species. The human embryo is so called up to the eighth week after fertilization. After that it is called a fetus.

embryology the branch of science concerned with the process of physical development of the body, from the time of fertilization of the egg (ovum) to the time of birth.

embryopathy any developmental or biochemical disorder of an EMBRYO.

embryo research the use of early human embryos for studies into the early detection and possible correction of genetic defects and the relief of human infertility. Cloning experiments, the alteration of the genetic pattern and attempts at hybridization are prohibited. Early embryos of two weeks gestational age have no organs or nervous system and are incapable of any perception or consciousness.

embryotomy reduction of the head of an impacted dead fetus within the womb in order to aid removal.

embryonic pertaining to, or to the state of being, an EMBRYO.

embryonic reduction a method of selective

termination to avoid multiple pregnancies with three or more fetuses. This usually occurs in women who have been treated for infertility. Injections of strong salt solution may be used.

Emend a brand name for the drug APREPITANT.

Emeside a brand name for ETHOSUXIMIDE.

emergency any sudden crisis, calling for urgent intervention to avoid a serious outcome.

emergency contraception see POSTCOITAL CONTRACEPTION.

emeritus retired from an academic appointment but retaining, as an honorary title, that held before retirement. Used especially of professor.

emesis vomiting.

emetic any substance that causes vomiting.

emetine an alkaloid derived from ipecacuanha sometimes used in the treatment of AMOEBIASIS. It has now been largely replaced by the safer METRONIDAZOLE.

Emflex a brand name for ACEMETACIN.

EMG *abbrev. for* electromyogram. See also ELECTROMYOGRAPHY.

EMI scanning the same as CT or CAT (computer-assisted tomography) SCANNING. This important advance in medical imaging technology was developed in the early 1970s at the EMI laboratories by Geoffrey Hounsfield (1919–), an EMI engineer, working almost single-handed.

emission a discharge of something. A nocturnal emission is an involuntary EJACULATION of semen, usually with orgasm, during sleep.

Emla cream a brand name for a mixture of LIGNOCAINE (lidocaine) and PRILOCAINE formulated as a cream for local application to allow many diagnostic and therapeutic procedures to be carried out with minimal pain or discomfort. The name is an acronym for 'Eutetic Mixture of Local Anaesthetics'.

emmetropia the state of the normal eye, with relaxed ACCOMMODATION, in which light rays from a distance (parallel rays) focus accurately on the retina giving perfect vision.

emollient soothing. Any agent, such as a cream or ointment, that soothes or softens the skin.

emotion any state of arousal in response to external events or memories of such events that affect, or threaten to affect, personal advantage. Emotion is never purely mental but is always associated with bodily changes such as the secretion of ADRENALINE and cortisol

and their effects. The limbic system and the hypothalamus of the brain are the mediators of emotional expression and feeling. The external expression of emotional content is known as 'affect'. Repressed emotions are associated with psychosomatic disease. The most important, in this context, are anger, a sense of dependency, and fear.

emotional disorders DEPRESSION, MANIA and the 'bipolar' or 'cyclothymic' condition (MANIC-DEPRESSIVE PSYCHOSIS) in which the mood swings from an extreme of excitement to one of depression.

empathy the state said to exist between two people when one is able to experience the same emotion as the other as a result of identical responses to an event and the adoption of an identical outlook.

emphysema a lung disease in which the small air sacs (alveoli) break down so that larger air spaces are formed and the surface area available for gas exchange is reduced. There is diminished oxygen supply to the vital organs. Emphysema is commonly associated with BRONCHITIS. The chest becomes barrel-shaped and there is wheezing and shortness of breath.

emphysema, surgical see SURGICAL EMPHYSEMA.

empirical treatment treatment given without knowledge of the cause or nature of the disorder and based on experience rather than logic. Sometimes urgency dictates empirical treatment, as when a dangerous infection by an unknown organism is treated with a broad-spectrum antibiotic while the results of bacterial culture and other tests are awaited.

empty sella syndrome the radiological appearance suggesting that the hollow on top of the SPHENOID bone, the sella turcica (Turkish saddle), which normally contains the PITUITARY GLAND, is enlarged and empty. The appearance is often associated with complete normality but may indicate a pituitary tumour, atrophy of the pituitary gland, harmless herniation of the arachnoid layer of the meninges into the sella, or BENIGN INTRACRANIAL HYPERTENSION.

empyema a collection of pus in the space between the lungs and the chest wall (the pleural cavity). This usually results from PNEUMONIA, TUBERCULOSIS or cancer of the underlying lung. Empyema causes lung collapse and interferes with breathing and the pus must be removed. Also known as empyema thoracis. From Greek *empuema*, a gathering or suppuration.

EMS *abbrev. for* Emergency Medical Service.

emtricitabine a synthetic analogue of cytosine that acts as an inhibitor of HIV reverse transcriptase. The drug is taken once a day in combination with other antiretroviral drugs to treat HIV infection. It is also active against the hepatitis B virus.

Emtriva brand name for EMTRICITABINE.

Eskamel a brand name for a preparation for external use containing RESORCINOL.

ESMI *abbrev. for* Elderly Subnormal Mentally Infirm.

en- *prefix denoting* in or into.

enalapril an ANGIOTENSIN CONVERTING ENZYME (ACE) INHIBITOR drug with useful action over 24 hours. A brand name is Innovace. It is also formulated in conjunction with the diuretic drug hydrochlorothiazide as Innozide.

enamel the hard outer covering of the crown of a tooth.

enatiomers molecules that are identical to each other except that they are mirror images of each other. See also CHIRALITY and STEREOISOMERISM.

Enbrel a brand name for ETANERCEPT.

enbucrilate a CYANOACRYLIC tissue adhesive used as an alternative to stitches for minor wounds. A brand name is Histoacryl.

encapsulated enclosed in a protective, or strengthening, membrane or coating.

enceinte pregnant.

encephalins see ENDORPHINS.

encephalitis inflammation of the brain, most commonly from infection, usually by viruses. These include herpes simplex, herpes zoster, ARBOVIRUSES, polioviruses, echoviruses or Coxsackie viruses. Secondary encephalitis may follow mumps, measles, rubella, and chickenpox. Encephalitis causes severe headache, fever, vomiting, sickness, stiff neck and seizures, and may progress to mental confusion, coma and death.

encephalitis lethargica a disease of unknown cause that occurred world-wide in the 1920s affecting millions of people, especially in Europe. There was paralysis of the eye muscles and a striking tendency to sleepiness. A high proportion of those who survived developed Parkinsonism within months or years. It was also known as 'sleeping sickness' or 'von Economo's disease'.

encephalo- *combining form denoting* the brain.

encephalocoele protrusion (herniation) of the brain and MENINGES through a developmental opening in the skull, and sometimes also through the scalp.

encephalography any X ray examination of the brain. In air encephalography, the cerebrospinal fluid in the brain ventricles is replaced by air. CT SCANNING and MRI have rendered this very unpleasant procedure obsolete.

encephalomalacia softening of an area of the brain, usually as a result of loss of its blood supply (infarction).

encephalomyelitis inflammation of the brain (ENCEPHALITIS) and spinal cord (MYELITIS). Acute demyelinating encephalomyelitis may follow minor infectious diseases or vaccination and cause widespread loss of the myelin sheath of nerve fibres with paralysis, seizures and coma. The condition known as 'ME' (myalgic encephalomyelitis) is not a brain inflammation.

encephalon the brain.

encephalopathy any degenerative or other non-inflammatory disorder affecting the brain in a widespread manner.

enchondroma a benign cartilaginous tumour occurring in the ends of long bones especially those of the hands and feet.

encopresis faecal incontinence or soiling not due to organic disease or involuntary loss of control, but resulting from deliberate intent or psychiatric disorder. Encopresis occurs in toddlers resisting toilet training, in the demented and in some psychotic people.

encounter group therapy a form of group psychotherapy in which the participants concentrate on the nature and open expression of their innermost feelings, so as to increase self-awareness and improve personal communication.

endarterectomy an operation to restore full blood flow in an artery narrowed or blocked by ATHEROSCLEROSIS, by removing the diseased inner lining and any associated blood clot (thrombus). The affected segment of the artery is clamped during the operation.

endarteritis inflammation of the inner lining (intima) of an artery.

endarteritis obliterans ENDARTERITIS, mainly

affecting small arteries, and leading to occlusion of the blood vessels from overgrowth (proliferation) of the lining cells.

endemic occurring continuously in a particular population. Literally, 'among the people'. See also EPIDEMIC and PANDEMIC.

Endep a brand name for AMITRIPTYLINE.

endermic within or through the skin.

end labelling the linking of a radioactively-labelled sequence to the end of a DNA strand.

endo- *prefix denoting* within or inside.

endocarditis inflammation of the inner lining of the heart and of the heart valves, from infection, immune system disturbances or the effect of the death of overlying muscle from CORONARY THROMBOSIS. Heart valve damage from previous RHEUMATIC FEVER, congenital heart disease, the presence of artificial heart valves or damage from cardiac catheters all predispose to the condition. Intravenous drug abusers are also extremely prone to develop infective endocarditis. Without effective treatment infective endocarditis is usually progressive and the condition is rapidly fatal.

endocardium the heart lining that also covers the heart valves.

endochondral ossification bone formation occurring within cartilage, in which cartilage is replaced by bone. This is the main process of bone formation and extension during fetal life and childhood.

endocrine system the group of hormone-producing glands, controlled by the HYPOTHALAMUS and the PITUITARY gland, and consisting of the pituitary, the PINEAL GLAND, the THYROID GLAND, the PARATHYROID GLANDS, the islet tissue in the PANCREAS, the ADRENAL GLANDS, the sex hormone-producing tissue in the testicles and the ovaries, and the placenta during pregnancy. All of these release highly active chemical substances into the blood that circulate to affect cells, tissues, organs or the entire organism, as part of a complex involuntary control system, integrated with, but largely independent of, the nervous system (see Fig. 12).

endocrinologist a doctor or physiological scientist specializing in the function and disorders of the hormonal ENDOCRINE SYSTEM of the body.

endocytosis a method by which a large molecule, such as a protein, can enter a cell.

The plasma membrane of the cell is invaginated by the molecule so that an internal vesicle is formed containing the molecule. This then breaks off from the surface membrane and moves into the interior of the cell. Such vesicles are coated with a protein called clathrin.

endoderm the innermost of the three primary germ layers of an EMBRYO. The endoderm develops into the INTESTINAL TRACT and its associated structures and glands, the respiratory and urinary tracts and most of the endocrine glands. See also MESODERM and ECTODERM.

endogenous occurring without an obvious cause external to the body, and believed to result from an internal cause. A person depressed by a succession of calamities is said to have exogenous depression. In the absence of external causes, depression is said to be endogenous.

endolymph the fluid within the LABYRINTH of the inner ear.

endometrial ablation a surgical treatment for severe menstrual bleeding or fibroids situated near the inner surface of the womb, that involves destruction of the womb lining. This may be done by laser energy, by a heated wire loop, by microwave heating, or by hot fluid in a balloon. The treatment is an alternative to HYSTERECTOMY and has largely superseded D and C (dilatation and curettage).

endometrial resection see ENDOMETRIAL ABLATION.

endometrioma a tumour of abnormally placed ENDOMETRIUM. Also known as a chocolate cyst. See ENDOMETRIOSIS.

endometriosis location at abnormal sites of the glandular and blood-vessel-containing (vascularized) lining tissue of the womb (the ENDOMETRIUM). Endometrial tissue may occur in the Fallopian (uterine) tubes, on the ovaries, within the muscle wall of the womb, anywhere in the pelvis, or even at remoter sites. All endometrial tissue is subject to the hormones that control the menstrual cycle and follows the same sequence of changes that affects the womb lining. Blood produced at these abnormal sites cannot usually escape and there is local pressure and pain with each menstrual period. A large cyst can form in an ovary.

endometritis inflammation of the ENDOMETRIUM, the inner lining of the womb (uterus). This is the result of infection, the most severe form being puerperal endometritis (puerperal sepsis) which sometimes occurs following childbirth. This was once a common cause of death after delivery.

endometrium the inner mucous membrane lining of the womb (uterus) that undergoes changes in structure and thickness at different stages of the menstrual cycle, and much of which is shed at menstruation.

endomorph one of the arbitrary body types (Sheldon's SOMATOTYPES). Endomorphic people are short and stout with prominent abdomens.

endomyocardial fibrosis replacement of heart muscle by fibrous tissue, leading to severe loss of pumping action and HEART FAILURE. This is commonest in the tropics in malnourished people with heavy worm infestation. There is often EOSINOPHILIA in the heart. Fibrosis of the heart muscle is also a feature of repeated small heart attacks (MYOCARDIAL INFARCTIONS). See also CARDIOMYOPATHY.

endoneurium the CONNECTIVE TISSUE surrounding individual nerve fibres.

endonucleases enzymes that can split DNA or RNA at any point along the molecule by cutting PHOSPHODIESTER BONDS.

endophthalmitis inflammation, usually from infection, within the eyeball. Endophthalmitis, unless vigorously and effectively treated at an early stage with antibiotics, usually leads to blindness.

endophytic of a tumour that grows inwards from a surface, implying malignancy. Contrast with EXOPHYTIC.

endoplasmic reticulum a highly convoluted membrane system within cells to which RIBOSOMES attach themselves for protein synthesis. The endoplasmic reticulum is also the site of many other cell metabolic reactions.

endorphins a number of morphine-like peptide substances naturally produced in the body and for which morphine receptors exist in the brain. Many of these active substances have been found, all with the same opioid core of five amino acids. They are neurotransmitters and have a wide range of functions. They help to regulate heart action, general hormone function, the mechanisms of shock from blood loss and the perception of pain, and are probably involved in controlling mood, emotion and motivation. They are thought to be produced under various circumstances in which acute relief of pain or mental distress is required. At least some of the endorphins are produced by the PITUITARY gland as part of the precursor of the ACTH molecule. Endorphins are fragments cleaved from the beta-lipotropin component of proopiomelanocortin (POMC). The term derives from the phrase 'endogenous morphines'.

endoscopy direct visual examination of any part of the interior of the body by means of an optical viewing instrument (ENDOSCOPE) introduced through a natural orifice or through a small surgical incision. Endoscopy is much used by gastroenterologists for stomach and colon examination, by gynaecologists for LAPAROSCOPY especially for sterilization of women by tying off the FALLOPIAN TUBES (tubal ligation) and by obstetricians for examining the fetus in the womb (fetoscopy). See also ENDOSCOPE.

endoscope an internal viewing instrument. Modern endoscopes are steerable, flexible, cylindrical instruments with fibre optics for illumination and viewing and channels to allow washing of the area under view, suction, gas inflation to ease viewing, the taking of BIOPSY specimen and the use of various small operating instruments, including LASERS.

endoscopic retrograde cholangiopancreatography (ERCP) a method of X-ray examination of the bile and pancreatic ducts. Using steerable fibreoptic endoscopy, a fine CATHETER is introduced into the common opening, in the duodenum, of the two duct systems and a radio-opaque dye injected. X rays are then taken. The method is valuable in the diagnosis of GALLSTONES, bile duct disorders, PANCREATITIS and cancer of the pancreas.

endoscopic sinus surgery surgery to the sinuses surrounding the nose performed by a minimally-invasive technique using a direct-vision endoscopic approach via a nostril. Local or general anaesthesia can be used and various operations to enlarge the drainage outlets of the sinuses and remove diseases tissue.

endoscopic ultrasonography a refined form of ultrasound imaging in which the transducer is inserted into the body by way of an endoscopic port so that it may be brought closer to the point of interest. The method has been found especially useful in dealing with stones in the bile ducts or in other situations in which direct endoscopic vision is difficult.

endostatin a substance that interferes with the development of the lining of blood vessels (endothelium). Since cancers require blood vessels to grow and tumour endothelium divides up to 50 times faster than normal endothelium, this substance offers promise as an anticancer drug. Trials in mice have been remarkably promising and human trials are under way. See also ANGIOSTATIN.

endothelial dysfunction failure of the lining of blood vessels and body cavities to carry out normally any of their complex functions including the production of NITRIC OXIDE and ENDOTHELIN-1. Endothelial dysfunction reduces flow-dependent widening of arteries (vasodilatation).

endothelins a range of peptide substances, containing 21 amino acids, and believed to be the most powerful known constrictors of arteries. Very tiny amounts will raise the blood pressure. One of them, ENDOTHELIN-1, derived from the ENDOTHELIUM of blood vessels, also causes constriction of BRONCHI, inhibits the release of RENIN from the kidneys and increases the strength of the heart beat. Endothelins are formed continuously in the larger arteries. Increased output can be caused by oxidized low-density lipoproteins. Endothelin receptors are ubiquitous

endothelin-1 a peptide of 21 amino acids produced by the endothelial cells of arteries that has a powerful arterial tightening (vasoconstrictor) function. It also induces MITOSIS in cells. It has a short half-life of 1–2 minutes and its production is inhibited by endothelial-derived relaxing factor and stimulated by ANGIOTENSIN II, vasopressin, and thrombin.

endothelin-receptor antagonist any drug that blocks the receptors for the artery-narrowing hormone ENDOTHELIN-1 and that can thus be used as a treatment for high blood pressure (HYPERTENSION). An example in BOSENTAN.

endothelioid resembling ENDOTHELIUM.

endothelioma any tumour arising from blood vessel ENDOTHELIUM.

endothelium the single layer of flattened cells that lines the blood vessels, the heart and some of the cavities of the body. Endothelium is no longer regarded as simply a non-stick lining. It is now known to be a physiologically and biochemically dynamic structure that exerts a regulatory control on the tone of blood vessels and on the blood flow, mainly by the release of the hormone NITRIC OXIDE. It regulates the growth and repair of blood vessels; modulated the contraction and relaxation of the heart; protects blood cells from damage; helps to control the inflammatory process; prevents blood clotting within vessels; and offers a selectively permeable barrier to the passage through it of molecules.

endothelium-derived relaxing factor a substance produced by the lining cells of arteries that acts on the circularly placed smooth muscle in the walls of arteries to relax it and so promote widening (vasodilatation). Its action lasts for only a few seconds.

endotoxin a poisonous lipopolysaccharide formed in the cell wall of a GRAM-NEGATIVE bacterium by means of which the organism causes its damage to the host. Compare exotoxin.

endotoxin-binding proteins blood proteins that bind to the dangerous endotoxin produced by GRAM-NEGATIVE bacteria. Lipopolysaccharide binding protein (LBP) binds to a lipid component of bacterial endotoxin and delivers it to CD14 receptors on macrophages resulting in the release of inflammatory CYTOKINES. Another protein, the neutrophil granular protein bactericidal/permeability-increasing protein (BPI) competes with LBP for toxin binding at the same site, blocks endotoxin delivery to macrophages and reduces the inflammatory response and the overall toxic effect.

endotracheal within the windpipe (TRACHEA).

endotracheal tube a curved plastic tube, some 20–25 cm long, inserted through the mouth into the upper part of the windpipe (trachea), by way of the voice-box (larynx) so as to maintain a reliable AIRWAY in an anaesthetized or otherwise unconscious person. Most endotracheal tubes are cuffed with a small balloon that can be inflated to form a seal and prevent inhalation of secretions or vomit.

endourology closed diagnostic and manipulative procedures carried out within the urogenital tract.

Endoxana a brand name for CYCLOPHOSPHAMIDE.

endplate the expanded termination of a motor nerve AXON that forms a SYNAPSE with a muscle fibre.

enema the introduction of various fluids, solutions or suspensions into the rectum to treat CONSTIPATION, to assist in X-ray or endoscopic examination, or to administer drugs or nutrients.

energy the capacity of a body to do work. Energy occurs in several forms – potential as in a compressed spring or a mass in a high position, kinetic as in motion, chemical as in petroleum and nuclear as in the binding forces of the atomic nucleus. Its effect, when manifested, is to bring about a change of some kind. The term is also used metaphorically to refer to human vitality and appetite for exertion or work.

enfuvirtide the first of a new class of anti-HIV drugs. Enfuvirtide (Fuzeon) interferes with the mechanism by which the membranes of HIV and of the target T cell fuse together so as to allow insertion of the viral genome. The drug is currently unique in that it attacks the virus before the T cell is infected. It does so by binding to a region of the envelope and blocking the conformational change necessary for fusion. Unfortunately, the drug, which requires twice-daily injections, is extremely expensive. A brand name is Fuzeon.

EN(G) *abbrev. for* Enrolled Nurse (General).

EN(M) *abbrev. for* Enrolled Nurse (Mental).

EN(MH) *abbrev. for* Enrolled Nurse (Mental Handicap).

enkephalins SEE ENDORPHINS.

enolic acids the group of non-steroidal anti-inflammatory drugs (NSAIDs) that includes the pyrazolones phenylbutazone and azapropazone and the oxicam piroxicam.

enophthalmos a sinking backwards of the eyeball into its bony socket so that the lid margins cannot easily be held the normal distance apart and there is an obvious narrowing of the lid aperture. Enophthalmos is the opposite of EXOPHTHALMOS. Enophthalmos results from loss of fat within the eye socket. See also BLOWOUT FRACTURE.

enoxaparin a drug used to prevent blood clots forming in the veins after surgery or to treat formed clots. A brand name is Clexane.

enoximone a PHOSPHIDIESTERASE INHIBITOR drug used to improve the heart's action in

HEART FAILURE. A brand name is Perfan.

ensiform shaped like a broad sword blade or leaf.

ENT *abbrev. for* ear, nose and throat. Otorhinolaryngology.

enter-, entero- *combining form denoting* the intestines.

enteral within the gut (gastrointestinal tract).

enteralgia pain in the intestines.

enterectomy surgical removal of part of the intestine.

enteric pertaining to the small intestine.

enteric fever SEE TYPHOID.

enteric nervous system a collection of neurons in the intestine that can function independently of the central nervous system and has been described as the 'brain of the gut'. This system is responsible for intestinal motility including PERISTALSIS, the secretory function of the intestine, the control of blood flow in the intestinal wall and the regulation of intestinal immune and inflammatory reactions.

enteritis inflammation of any part of the intestine from any cause. The enteritides include CROHN'S DISEASE, APPENDICITIS, ULCERATIVE COLITIS, bacillary dysentery (SHIGELLOSIS), AMOEBIC DYSENTERY and diverticulitis. See also GASTROENTERITIS.

enterobiasis see THREADWORMS.

Enterobius vermicularis a threadworm. A small nematode worm commonly found in the large intestine, especially in children.

enterococcus a STREPTOCOCCUS inhabiting the intestine.

enterocolitis inflammation of both small and large intestines as a result of infection of organisms such as *Yersinia enterocolitica*, a common cause of enteritis in Europe.

enterokinase a pancreatic protein-digesting enzyme that converts trypsinogen into active trypsin. Also known as enteropeptidase.

enterolithiasis stones (calculi) in the bowel.

enteron the intestine.

enteropathy any disease of the intestinal tract.

enterorrhagia bleeding into the intestines.

enterostomy an artificial opening, usually made through the wall of the abdomen, to allow part of the intestine to discharge to the exterior. Examples are COLOSTOMY and ILEOSTOMY.

enterotomy a surgical incision into the bowel.

enterotoxin any bacterial toxin that damages intestinal tissue and causes diarrhoea and vomiting, the signs of food poisoning.

enteroviruses picornaviruses (pico RNA viruses) of the *Enterovirus* genus, that include polioviruses, Coxsackie viruses and echoviruses. Enterovirus infections are spread by faecal contamination, especially by food handlers.

enthesopathy inflammation at the sites of insertion of ligaments into bone. This is a feature of ANKYLOSING SPONDYLITIS and leads to new bone formation and fusion of the vertebra of the spine.

entrapment neuropathy disorders of nerves due to mechanical compression when they pass through narrow apertures in the body. This is a common cause of peripheral nerve disorder. See CARPAL TUNNEL SYNDROME and CERVICAL RIB.

entropion inward curling of the margin of an eyelids so that the lashes tend to rub against the eye. In severe entropion there may be complete inversion of the lid, so that the lashes are hidden. Entropion can lead to ulceration of the CORNEA.

entry inhibitors a new class of drugs that are designed to block entry of viruses into cells. Viral receptors to which viruses bind have a critical role in entry. They mediate fusion between the viral and the cell membranes. Some inhibitors bind to these receptors. Others bind to the viruses and prevent interaction with the receptors. A third class inhibit the conformational changes necessary for cell and virus membrane fusion.

enucleation removal from an enveloping capsule, sac or cover. The term is often used for the operation to remove an eyeball.

enuresis bedwetting. The involuntary passage of urine, especially during sleep.

enzootic affecting, or peculiar to, particular animals in a specific area. Used especially of a disease.

enzyme a biochemical catalyst that enormously accelerates a chemical reaction. Enzymes are complex protein molecules highly specific to particular reactions. Almost everything that happens in the body, at a chemical level, is mediated by one or more of the many thousands of different enzymes in the cells, and much of the length of each DNA molecule consists of codes for enzymes.

enzyme-linked immunosorbent assay see ELISA TEST.

enzyme replacement therapy treatment of genetic diseases in which the disorder is the result of biochemical dysfunction resulting from the absence of a particular enzyme. Enzymes can now be made by recombinant DNA technology and have to be given by intravenous injection. The method has been used successfully to treat Gaucher's disease, a sphingolipidosis caused by the absence of the lysosomal enzyme glucocerebrosidase.

enzymology the branch of biochemistry concerned with the structure and function of enzymes and coenzymes.

eosin a red dye commonly used to stain bacteria or tissue slices, for microscopic examination.

eosinophil a kind of white blood cell (leukocyte) containing granules of toxic proteins that readily stain with EOSIN. As in the cases of other classes of white cell (e.g. basophil, neutrophil) this is an adjective that has become a noun.

eosinophilia an increase in the number of EOSINOPHIL cells in the blood or in the lungs (pulmonary eosinophilia). Eosinophilia is characteristic of worm infestation, reactions to certain drugs and allergic conditions.

eosinophilia-myalgia syndrome a disorder featuring severe and persistent pain in the muscles, muscle weakness, loss of weight, fever, 'pins and needles' sensation (paraesthesia) and an exceptionally high level of EOSINOPHIL white cells in the blood. The cause is unknown but there is a strong association with ingestion of L-tryptophan.

eosinophilic enteritis an acute condition featuring severe abdominal pain, loss of weight and blood in the stools, associated with, or closely followed by a sharp rise in the levels of EOSINOPHIL white cells in the blood. The condition is probably caused by infestation with the dog hookworm Ancylostoma caninum.

Epanutin a brand name for PHENYTOIN.

ependymoma a tumour of the supporting (glial) tissue of the brain. See also GLIOMA.

ephedrine a drug with a similar action to ADRENALINE but with a more stimulant effect on the nervous system, causing tremor, anxiety, insomnia and undue alertness. It is used to treat allergic conditions and ASTHMA. Ephedrine nasal drops decongest a swollen nose lining. The drug is on the WHO official list. A brand name is CAM. Ephedrine is also formulated with other drugs under the brand names of Franol,

Franol Plus and Haymine.

epi- *prefix denoting* upon, over, outside, next to, near or beside.

epicanthus a condition in which the margin of the upper eyelid curves round and downwards on the inner side so as to conceal the inner corner of the eye. Epicanthus is common in babies and may cause an illusory appearance of in-turning of the eye (convergent STRABISMUS).

epicardium the inner layer of the bag surrounding the heart (the PERICARDIUM).

epicondylitis see TENNIS ELBOW.

epicritic pertaining to fine degrees of discrimination, as in delicate touch sensation.

epidemic the occurrence of a large number of cases of a particular disease in a given population within a period of a few weeks. Epidemics occur when a population contains many susceptible people. This is why epidemics often occur at intervals of several years.

epidemic myalgia see BORNHOLM DISEASE.

epidemiology the study of the occurrence, in populations, of the whole range of conditions that affect health. It includes the study of the attack rate of the various diseases (incidence) and the number of people suffering from each condition at any one time (prevalence). Industrial and environmental health problems are also an important aspect of epidemiology.

epidermis the structurally simple outermost layer of the skin, containing no nerves, blood vessels, or hair follicles, and acting as a rapidly replaceable surface. The deepest layer of the epidermis is the basal cell layer. Above this is the 'prickle cell' layer. The epidermis is 'stratified', the layers of cells becoming flatter towards the surface. The outermost cells of the epidermis are dead and are continuously shed.

epidermoid having the characteristics of, or pertaining to, the EPIDERMIS.

epidermoid cyst a cyst lined with epidermal cells and differing from a DERMOID CYST by the absence of other skin glands and elements.

epidermolysis separation of the outer layer of the skin from the underlying CORIUM, usually with the formation of a blister. Epidermolysis is a feature of many skin disorders.

epidermolysis bullosa one of a group of genetic disorders causing blistering of the skin and mucous membranes. In simple cases the blistering is induced by injury, but in serious cases it occurs spontaneously

epidermolytic hyperkeratosis one of a range of genetic skin-blistering diseases caused by mutations in the genes for the protein keratin expressed mainly in the basal cells of the epidermis. Children are affected most severely. There is redness, blistering and scaling of the skin at the sites of pressure or trauma especially the elbows and knees. The blistering is worsened by heat but the blisters heal without scarring and become less frequent as the child gets older. The scaling, however, persists.

epidermophytosis skin infection with any of the skin fungi including *Epidermophyton* species. Athlete's foot and tinea cruris are examples of epidermophytosis. The term literally means 'outer skin plants' and is a historic commentary on the fact that fungi were once classified as plants.

epididymis the long, elaborately coiled tube that lies behind the testicle and connects it to the VAS DEFERENS. Spermatozoa mature during their long journey through this tube and the vas deferens. They also receive stabilizing glycoproteins from the epididymal fluid.

epididymitis inflammation of the EPIDIDYMIS from infection, usually following URETHRITIS. Epididymitis may be caused by GONORRHOEA and this may lead to sterility, but most cases are caused by other infections.

epididymo-orchitis inflammation of the EPIDIDYMIS and the TESTICLE.

epidural external to the DURA MATER, the outer of the three MENINGES covering the brain and spinal cord.

epidural anaesthesia a form of local anaesthesia in which an anaesthetic drug is passed by way of a fine plastic tube into the space between the DURA MATER and the bony canal of the spine. This tube is passed in through a needle inserted between two of the lower bones of the spine. The method is popular for childbirth because it has no effect on the contractions of the womb (uterus) or on the respiratory centre of the baby.

epigallocatechin gallate (EGCG) an antioxidant substance found in green tea that is claimed to be protective against a range of common cancers. EGCG markedly reduces phosphorylation of the receptor for VASCULAR ENDOTHELIAL GROWTH FACTOR, thus disrupting the autocrine pathway that protects the cell from APOPTOSIS.

epigastrium the central upper region of the abdomen. Epigastric pain is a feature of duodenitis or duodenal ulcer.

epigenetic relating to inheritable changes in the pattern of gene expression caused by factors other than changes in the nucleotide sequence of genes. It is now recognized that cancer is caused both by genetic and epigenetic changes and that these two factors are intimately interrelated in the development of tumours.

epiglottis a leaf-like cartilaginous structure, down behind the back of the tongue, which act as a kind of lid to cover the entrance to the voice-box (larynx) and prevent food or liquid entering it during the act of swallowing.

epiglottitis inflammation of the EPIGLOTTIS. If severe, and associated with swelling, there is a risk of death from obstruction of the airway and suffocation, and it may be necessary to make an emergency opening into the windpipe (tracheostomy).

epilation removal of the hair by the roots by any means, such as plucking, waxing, chemical destruction or electrolysis.

epilepsy a physical indication of an abnormal electrical discharge in the brain. Epilepsy takes various forms. These include generalized epilepsy, or 'grand mal' which is a major fit affecting all the muscles of the body with a massive contraction (tonic stage) followed by a succession of jerky contractions (clonic stage); partial seizures, which may affect only a few muscles (simple partial seizures) or may also involve almost any of the functions of the brain and cause elaborate hallucinations (complex partial seizures); and absence attack, or 'petit mal' in which the affected person, usually a child, is momentarily inaccessible but does not fall or appear to lose consciousness.

Epilim a brand name for SODIUM VALPROATE.

epiloia a rare genetic congenital disorder, also called tuberous sclerosis or BOURNEVILLE DISEASE, in which the brain, the skin and other organs become studded with knobbly tumours derived from an abnormal overgrowth of primitive cell tissue. Epiloia occurs either as a result of a dominant gene or as a mutation, and affects about 1 baby in 20,000.

epimysium the fibrous sheath that encloses a muscle.

epinastine hydrochloride a highly-selective antihistamine drug effective topically in relieving the symptoms of conjunctival allergy arising from contact with grass and tree pollen grains, animal dander and other contact allergens. A brand name is Relestat.

epinephrine ADRENALINE. Epinephrine is the favoured medical usage in the USA, but the term 'adrenaline' is in popular use. The drug is on the WHO official list. The terms *ad* and *renal* are Latin for 'on' and 'kidney'. The corresponding terms in Greek are *epi* and *nephron*.

epineurium the connective tissue sheath of a nerve.

epiphenomenalism the belief that mental events are solely a consequence of physical events, specifically neural activity, and never the causes of them. Once considered heretical, the view is now widely held by scientists.

epiphora running over of tears as a result of failure of the normal tear drainage into the nose. This may be due to blockage of the tear duct or to ECTROPION, in which the opening of the tear drain no longer rests in the tear film.

epiphysiolysis separation of an EPIPHYSIS from the shaft of a bone.

epiphysis the growing sector at the end of a long bone. During the period of growth, the epiphysis is separated by a plate of CARTILAGE from the shaft of the bone. The edge of this plate nearest the shaft becomes progressively converted into bone, while the other edge develops new cartilage. In this way, the bone lengthens.

epiphysis, slipped see SLIPPED EPIPHYSIS.

epiphysitis inflammation of an EPIPHYSIS.

epiploon the GREATER OMENTUM.

epirubicin a CYTOTOXIC anti-cancer drug. A brand name is Pharmorubicin.

episcleritis a localized inflammation of the white of the eye (sclera). This is an uncommon cause of redness of the eye. The affected area is small, usually oval, and appears slightly raised and reddish-purple in colour. There is a dull, aching pain, worse at night, and intolerance to bright light (photophobia). The condition is treated with steroid eye drops.

episiotomy a deliberate cut made during childbirth in the margin of the vaginal opening so as to enlarge it, facilitate delivery of the baby and prevent tearing of the tissues backwards towards the anus.

epispadias a congenital abnormality of the penis, in which the urine tube (URETHRA) opens on the upper surface. Sometimes the opening is right back near the root, causing difficulties with urination and infertility. Surgical reconstruction is possible.

epistaxis nose bleed.

epithelialization the process of covering of a raw surface with EPITHELIUM. The final stage in healing.

epithelioid 1 resembling EPITHELIUM.
2 of particular cell types derived from macrophages which are a feature of granulomas.

epithelioma a cancer derived from EPITHELIUM. A carcinoma.

epithelium the non-stick coating cell layer for all surfaces of the body except the insides of blood and lymph vessels. Epithelium may be single-layered, or 'stratified' and in several layers, with the cells becoming flatter and more scaly towards the surface, as in the skin. It may be covered with fine wafting hair-like structures (cilia), as in the respiratory tract, and it may contain mucus-secreting 'goblet' cells. See also ENDOTHELIUM and EPIDERMIS.

epitope an immunologically active discrete site on an ANTIGEN to which an ANTIBODY or a B or T cell receptor actually binds. See also LINEAR EPITOPE and CONFORMATIONAL EPITOPE.

Epivir a brand name for LAMIVUDINE.

epizootic affecting a large number of animals within a short period, especially of a disease.

Epley manoeuvre an effective treatment for BENIGN PAROXYSMAL POSITIONAL VERTIGO.

epoetin human erythropoetin made by genetic engineering for use as a drug to treat severe anaemia Brand names are Eprex and Neorecormon.

eponym a name of a disease, syndrome, anatomical part, surgical instrument, etc derived from the name of the person who discovered, invented or first successfully promulgated it.

epoprostenol prostacyclin. A powerful inhibitor of clumping of blood platelets and thus of blood clotting. It is used with heart-lung (cardiopulmonary bypass) machines and artificial kidneys (dialysis machines) to preserve the platelets in the blood being pumped through them. Epoprostenol also widens (dilates) arteries. A brand name is Flotan.

Epsom salts see MAGNESIUM SULPHATE.

Epstein-Barr virus a member of the herpes family of viruses and the cause of GLANDULAR FEVER (infective mononucleosis). It is also associated with cancer of the back of the nose (nasopharyngeal carcinoma) in Chinese people and with BURKITT'S LYMPHOMA. (Michael Anthony Epstein, English pathologist, b. 1921 and Yvonne M. Barr, English virologist, b. 1932).

eptacog alfa human Factor VIIa made by genetic engineering and used to treat severe bleeding in people with Factor VIII or Factor IX deficiency (HAEMOPHILIA) A brand name is Novoseven.

epulis a localized, usually inflammatory, swelling of the gum (gingiva). Epulis may, rarely, be due to a tumour of the gingiva.

Equanil a brand name for MEPROBAMATE.

equine encephalitis one of a range of diseases of horses and humans, featuring inflammation of the brain, and caused by various strains of ARBOVIRUSES, occurring in the Americas as several types, especially Eastern, Western, Californian and Venezuelan. Epidemics of encephalitis are often preceded by death of horses. Most cases are acquired by mosquito bites. There is no specific treatment and cases often end fatally or with severe permanent brain damage.

Erb's palsy paralysis of the shoulder and arm muscles from an injury to the nerve roots emerging from the fifth and sixth spinal segments in the neck. The arm hangs down with the hand turned backwards in the 'waiter's tip' position. Erb's palsy usually results from a birth injury. (Wilhelm Heinrich Erb, German neurologist, 1840–1921).

ERCP *abbrev. for* ENDOSCOPIC RETROGRADE CHOLANGIOPANCREATOGRAPHY.

erectile capable of becoming erect. Pertaining to tissue containing many blood vessels or blood spaces that can fill with blood and become rigid. The corpus spongiosum and corpora cavernosa of the penis are the most conspicuous examples of erectile tissue.

erection a temporary state of enlargement and rigidity of the penis, due to engorgement with blood under pressure (tumescence), which, given adequate lubrication, makes insertion into the vagina possible.

ERG *abbrev. for* ELECTRORETINOGRAM.

ergocalciferol vitamin D_2. This is produced in the body by the action of ultraviolet light on ergosterol. Vitamin D is necessary for the normal mineralization of bone. Deficiency leads to RICKETS in growing children and bone softening (OSTEOMALACIA) in adults. The drug is on the WHO official list.

ergometrine an ERGOT derivative drug used to promote contractions of the muscle of the womb (uterus). This can be valuable, after the baby is born, to close off the site of separation of the after-birth (placenta) and prevent POSTPARTUM HAEMORRHAGE. It is sometimes given when delivery of the baby is almost accomplished. The drug is on the WHO official list. A brand name is Syntometrine.

ergonomics the scientific study of humans in relation to their working environment and the application of science to improve working conditions. The increasing application of complex technology has resulted in increasing human discomfort, difficulties and dangers. Ergonomics seeks to solve such problems.

ergosterol a sterol found in fungal cell membranes which, when exposed to ultraviolet light, is converted into vitamin D_2 (ergocalciferol) and to other, toxic, substances.

ergot one of various fungi of the genus *Claviceps*, that can grow on rye and other cereal plants and cause the serious condition of ERGOTISM by virtue of its alpha-adrenoceptor stimulating action. Ergot is the source of various valuable drugs such as ERGOTAMINE and ERGOMETRINE. It is also the source of lysergic acid.

ergotamine tartrate a drug that causes widened (dilated) arteries to narrow. It is thus useful in the treatment of MIGRAINE. Overdosage is dangerous. The drug is on the WHO official list. Brand names are Lingraine, Medihaler-ergotamine, and, formulated with other drugs, Cafergot and Migril.

ergotism poisoning by the ERGOT fungus. This can cause abortion, burning pain in the limbs and closure of major arteries by sustained spasm so that the blood flow is obstructed and GANGRENE may follow.

Ergotrate a brand name for ERGOMETRINE.

erogenous zones parts of the body which, when stimulated by touch in a suitable context, are especially liable to arouse sexual interest or desire.

eroticism 1 the elements in thought, pictorial imagery or literature which tend to arouse

sexual excitement or desire.
2 actual sexual arousal.
3 a greater than average disposition for sex and all its manifestations.
4 sexual interest or excitement prompted by contemplation, or stimulation, of areas of the body not normally associated with sexuality. The terms anal and oral eroticism are used in two senses – in reference to adult physical sexual activity and in a theoretical Freudian psychoanalytic sense.

ERPC *abbrev. for* evacuation of retained products of conception. An operation consisting of DILATATION AND CURETTAGE, usually performed following a missed ABORTION.

ertapenem a carbapenem broad-spectrum antibiotic active against both GRAM POSITIVE and GRAM NEGATIVE bacteria. It is used mainly to treat intra-abdominal and pelvic infections, and has the advantage over others in its class of allowing once-daily dosage. A brand name is Invanz.

eructation belching.

eruption 1 a skin rash.
2 the emergence of a tooth through the gum.

Erymax a brand name for ERYTHROMYCIN.

Erymin a brand name for ERYTHROMYCIN.

erysipelas a form of CELLULITIS from infection of the skin with streptococcal organisms. There are large, raised inflamed areas, high fever and severe illness from toxicity. The lymph nodes in the area are enlarged and tender. Treatment is with antibiotics.

erysipeloid 1 resembling ERYSIPELAS.
2 an infection caused by the bacterium *Erysipelothrix rhuscopathiae* and acquired especially by way of abrasions or cuts on the hands of people processing meat or fish.

eryth-, erythro- *combining form denoting* red or red blood cell (ERYTHROCYTE).

erythema redness of the skin from widening (dilatation) of the small skin blood vessels. This may result from one of a very large number of causes such as blushing, ROSACEA, ECTASIA of blood vessels, INFLAMMATION and rashes (exanthemata).

erythema ab igne a net-like pattern of redness on the skin, usually of the legs, caused by excessive exposure to radiant heat. The condition was common in the days of open domestic fires.

erythema migrans borreliosis the characteristic multiple ring skin eruptions of early LYME DISEASE. Early recognition and treatment with antibiotics are important if serious complications are to be avoided.

erythema multiforme a hypersensitivity disorder featuring red, raised skin eruptions of various sizes and shapes ('multiforme') occurring symmetrically on the face, neck, forearms, backs of the hands, and legs. It is associated with drug and other allergies, many infections and pregnancy.

erythema nodosum inflammation of small blood vessels (vasculitis) causing red, raised, tender nodules under the skin of both shins and sometimes elsewhere on the body. These disappear after some days or weeks. There may be fever, aches and pains and sickness. Erythema nodosum is an immunological disorder associated with a variety of conditions including TUBERCULOSIS, SARCOIDOSIS, streptococcal infections, drug allergies and LEPROSY.

erythraemic myelosis a disorder of red blood cell production similar in effect to acute myeloid LEUKAEMIA.

erythro- *combining form denoting* red.

erythroblast a primitive, nucleated red blood cell. A stage in the development of the normal non-nucleated red cell (ERYTHROCYTE) found in the circulating blood.

erythroblastosis fetalis the type of severe anaemia with JAUNDICE caused in babies by RHESUS FACTOR incompatibility when the mother is rhesus negative and the baby rhesus positive. The risk to the baby increases with successive pregnancies because of the ever rising levels of antibodies in the mother's blood.

Erythrocin a brand name for ERYTHROMYCIN.

erythrocyte a red blood cell. 'Erythro' means 'red', and 'cyte' means 'cell'. Erythrocytes are flattened discs, slightly hollowed on each side (biconcave) and about 7 thousandths of a millimetre in diameter. They contain HAEMOGLOBIN and their main function is to transport OXYGEN from the lungs to the tissues.

erythrocyte sedimentation rate see BLOOD SEDIMENTATION RATE.

erythrocytosis an increase in the number of red blood cells in a unit volume of blood. This occurs essentially as a response to an inadequate supply of oxygen to the tissues. It occurs at high altitudes, in smokers, in heart or lung disease and in the presence of certain tumours that produce substances that stimulate red cell production. Erythrocytosis also occurs in the condition of primary POLYCYTHAEMIA.

erythrodermia widespread, often permanent, redness of the skin, usually associated with flakiness (exfoliation). The redness is due to widened skin blood vessels.

erythromelalgia mottled redness and a painful burning sensation in the extremities, usually the feet, with a local rise in skin temperature.

erythromycin an antibiotic of the macrolide class with an action similar to that of the tetracyclines. It binds to the RIBOSOMES in bacterial cells and interferes with the synthesis of protein. Oral erythromycin extends cardiac repolarization. It is metabolized by cytochrome P-450 3A isoenzymes and drugs such as nitroimidazole antifungals, verapamil, diltiazen and troleandomycin that inhibit CTP3A can increase the risk of ventricular arrhythmias and sudden death. Erythromycin is on the WHO official list. Brand names are Arpimicin, Erymax, Erymin, Erythrocin, Erythroped, Tiloryth, and, formulated with other drugs for external use only, Benzamycin, Isotrexin and Zineryl.

Erythroped A a brand name for ERYTHROMYCIN.

erythropoiesis red cell production.

erythropoietic drugs drugs used to treat anaemia associated with kidney failure, mainly in people on dialysis. Examples are darbepoetin alfa (Aranesp), epoetin alfa (Eprex) and epoetin beta (Neorecormon).

erythropoietic protoporphyria a dominant genetic disease caused by a deficiency of the enzyme ferrochelatase that leads to the accumulation of protoporphyrin in the red blood cells. This causes skin hypersensitivity to light with tissue damage from oxygen free radicals causing a red crusted rash. About one sufferer in 20 develops liver failure for which the only resource is transplant. Although the condition is dominant, penetrance is incomplete and the inheritance more closely resembles that of a recessive trait.

erythropoietins hormones, produced mainly in the kidneys, that stimulates red blood cell production (eythropoiesis) in the bone marrow. The amount of hormone produced is based on monitoring of the blood flowing through the kidneys for oxygen concentration.

erythropoietin therapy the use of the hormone ERYTHROPOIETIN to promote new blood formation as an alternative to blood transfusion. This is feasible only in cases in which the patient's condition allows sufficient time for blood cell production. Erythropoietin therapy is also appropriate as a treatment for ANAEMIA caused by kidney failure, cancer or AIDS.

erythropsia red vision. A visual disorder in which all objects appear red.

eschar an area of dead, separated tissue (SLOUGH) produced by skin damage by a caustic substance or a burn.

Escherichia coli a motile, GRAM NEGATIVE, rod bacillus found in countless millions in the large intestine, and also known as coliforms. The presence of *E. coli* is presumptive evidence of faecal contamination. A strain if this organism known as O 157 was first recognized as a human pathogen in 1982 and, in 1996, it caused 600 cases of food poisoning in the USA, 490 cases in Scotland and nearly 10,000 cases in Japan. In old and frail people the mortality may reach 50%. *E. coli* have been much exploited by genetic engineers.

escitalopram a highly selective SEROTONIN reuptake inhibitor used to treat major depression and panic disorders. A brand name is Cipralex.

eserine an ANTICHOLINESTERASE drug sometimes used to constrict the pupil and treat GLAUCOMA.

Esidrex a brand name for HYDROCHLOROTHIAZIDE.

Esidrex-K a brand name for HYDROCHLOROTHIAZIDE with potassium.

Esmarch's bandage a flat, wide, rubber bandage wound progressively and tightly round a limb, from the extremity, so as to force most of the blood back into the circulation and provide a relatively blood-free field for surgery. It is commonly used in operations for varicose veins. (Johann Friedrich August von Esmarch, German surgeon, (1823–1908).

esophoria a latent tendency for the eyes to turn involuntarily inwards. When a person with esophoria has one eye covered, that eye will turn inwards. As soon as the cover is removed, the eye straightens and single binocular vision is restored. Compare EXOPHORIA.

esotropia convergent squint, or STRABISMUS. Only one eye looks directly at the object of regard, the other being turned inwards. Esotropia in children calls for urgent treatment to avoid amblyopia. Compare EXOTROPIA.

ESP *abbrev. for* EXTRASENSORY PERCEPTION.

espundia American LEISHMANIASIS. This disease is caused by the single-celled parasite Leishmania braziliensis and is spread by sandfly bites. It occurs in south Mexico, Brazil, Paraguay and Peru, causing disfiguring skin ulcers of the face and tissue destruction that extends into the cavities of the nose and mouth. It often persists for years and, if neglected, may lead to death from overwhelming secondary infection.

ESR *abbrev. for* erythrocyte sedimentation rate. See BLOOD SEDIMENTATION RATE.

essential 1 absolutely required.
2 of unknown cause.
3 (of amino acids) necessary for normal growth but not synthesized in the body.
4 extracted from, or related to an extract from, a plant (as in essential oil). Of the essence of.

essential amino acids those AMINO ACIDS that cannot be synthesized in the body and must be included in the diet. They include histidine, isoleucine, leucine, lysine, methionine, phenylalanine, threonine, tryptophan and valine.

essential fatty acid deficiency a very rare condition thought to occur only in people fed intravenously for long periods on glucose and amino acids, but without fats. The effect of deficiency is a form of scaly DERMATITIS. See ESSENTIAL FATTY ACIDS.

essential fatty acids fatty acids that cannot be synthesized in the body and that must be present in the diet for health. They are LINOLEIC acid, linolenic acid and arachidonic acid, and have at least two conjugated double bonds. These fatty acids are precursors of eicosanoids and other regulatory substances.

essential-familial tremor a genetic disorder featuring exaggerated shakiness of the hands when they are held out straight. The condition is harmless and is usually relieved by taking a small dose of alcohol.

essential hypertension high blood pressure of unknown cause. Also known as primary hypertension. In this context, the term 'essential' reflects the original view that the condition was thought to be constitutional – 'of the essence'.

essential thrombocythaemia a rare blood disorder featuring an excess of blood platelets with the increased risk of clotting of blood within the blood vessels (thrombosis). The cause is unknown.

essential tremor involuntary shaking of the hands, head, neck or voice often of genetic origin with an autosomal dominant pattern of inheritance with variable penetrance.

Estigyn a brand name for ETHINYLOESTRADIOL (ethinylestradiol).

Estracyt a brand name for ESTRAMUSTINE.

Estraderm MX a brand name for OESTRADIOL (estradiol) in a transdermal patch.

estramustine an alkylating anti-cancer drug. A brand name is Estracyt.

Estring a brand name for OESTRADIOL (estradiol) in a vaginal ring to treat post-menopausal vaginitis.

estropipate an oestrogen drug used for post-menopausal HORMONE REPLACEMENT THERAPY. A brand name is Harmogen.

etamsylate ethamsylate, a haemostatic drug used to prevent dangerous brain haemorrhage in low birth weight babies and excessive menstrual bleeding in adults. A brand name is Dicynene.

etanercept a fusion protein for the human tumour necrosis factor (TNA) receptor produced by recombinant DNA technology and engineered to block the action of TNA. It is used to treat RHEUMATOID ARTHRITIS. A brand name is Enbrel.

ethacrynic acid etacrynic acid, a LOOP DIURETIC drug. A drug that acts on the tubules in the kidneys to interfere with the reabsorption of water and thus greatly increase the output of urine. A brand name is Edecrin.

ethambutol a drug used, ideally in combination with other drugs, in the treatment of TUBERCULOSIS. Ethambutol can cause damage to the optic nerves and if persisted with after vision is affected can cause blindness. Also known under the generic name of myambutol. The drug is on the WHO official list.

ethamsylate etamsylate, a drug that reduces bleeding from small blood vessels and is used to treat excessive menstruation (menorrhagia). A brand name is Dicynene.

ethanol the chemical name for ethyl alcohol, the main constituent of alcoholic drinks. The drug is on the WHO official list.

ether a volatile and highly inflammable liquid once widely used as a safe and effective drug for the induction and continuance of general anaesthesia. Induction is slow and unpleasant and deep anaesthesia is needed for muscle relaxation. Postoperative nausea is common. Because of these disadvantages and the danger of explosion, ether is now seldom used. The drug is, however, on the WHO official list.

etherize to induce anaesthesia with ETHER.

ethics, medical see MEDICAL ETHICS.

ethinyloestradiol ethinylestradiol, a powerful synthetic oestrogen drug that can be taken by mouth and is widely used as a component of oral contraceptives and as an anti-androgen to treat female acne and hirsutism. The drug is on the WHO official list. Brand names are Dianette, Femodene, Femodette and Loestrin. The drug is also commonly formulated with a PROGESTOGEN and sold under such brand names as Binovum, Brevinor, Cilest, Eugynon 30, Femodene, Femodene ED, Loestrin 20, Logynon, Logynon ED, Marvelon, Mercilon, Microgynon 30, Microgynon 30 ED, Minulet, Norimin, Norinyl-1, Ortho-Novin 1/50, Ovran, Ovranette, Ovysmen, Schering PC4, Synphase, Tri-Minulet, Triadene, Trinordiol and Trinovum.

ethionamide a drug used in the treatment of LEPROSY or in cases of TUBERCULOSIS resistant to other drugs. The drug is on the WHO official list.

ethisterone a PROGESTOGEN drug used to treat premenstrual tension (PMT) and menstrual disorders. As norethisterone, it is also a component of oral contraceptives. A brand name is Micronor.

ethmoid bone the delicate, T-shaped, spongy bone forming the roof and upper sides of the nose and the inner walls of the eye sockets (orbits). The upper part of the ethmoid is perforated (cribriform plate) to allow passage of the fibres of the olfactory nerve, and has a central downward extension forming the upper part of the partition (septum) of the nose. The bone contains numerous air cells (ethmoidal sinuses).

ethoheptazine citrate a pain-killing drug. It is formulated with a muscle relaxant drug and with aspirin and sold under the brand name of Equagesic.

ethosuximide an antiepileptic drug used in the management of absence attacks (PETIT MAL). It has no effect against major EPILEPSY and may cause nausea and drowsiness. The drug is on the WHO official list. Brand names are Emeside and Zarontin.

ethyl alcohol see ALCOHOL.

ethyl chloride a volatile liquid sometimes used as a spray to achieve local anaesthesia of the skin by freezing. It has also been used an a general anaesthetic, by inhalation, but is dangerously potent.

ethylene glycol a compound used mainly as an antifreeze additive. If ingested it may cause severe nervous system depression that may be fatal. Metabolism may lead to severe acidosis.

ethynodiol diacetate etynodiol diacetate, a PROGESTOGEN drug used, without oestrogen, as an oral contraceptive. A brand name is Femulen.

Ethyol a brand name for AMIFOSTINE.

etidronate a drug used to treat OSTEOPOROSIS and PAGET'S DISEASE of bone. A brand name is Didronel.

etodolac a NON-STEROIDAL ANTI-INFLAMMATORY DRUG (NSAID) used to treat RHEUMATOID ARTHRITIS. A brand name is Lodine.

etomidate a general anaesthetic drug. A brand name is Hypnomidate.

etoposide an anticancer drug derived from a plant poison epipodophyllotoxin. It is used chiefly in the maintenance treatment of acute leukaemia after remission has been achieved and the bone marrow has recovered. It has been given by mouth to treat lung cancer. The drug is on the WHO official list. A brand name is Vepeside.

etoricoxib a highly selective cyclo-oxygenase-2 (COX-2) inhibitor used to treat RHEUMATOID ARTHRITIS, GOUT and chronic musculo-skeletal pain. A brand name is Arcoxia.

eu- *prefix denoting* good, well, normal.

EUA *abbrev. for* 1 examination under anaesthesia.

2 evacuation under anaesthesia. This usage refers to the removal, by suction or dilatation and curettage (D AND C), of a dead fetus and its membranes from the womb (uterus). Also known as ERPC – evacuation of retained products of conception.

Eudemine a brand name for DIAZOXIDE.

eugenics the study or practice of trying to improve the human race by encouraging the breeding of those with desired characteristics (positive eugenics) or by discouraging the breeding of those whose characteristics are deemed undesirable (negative eugenics). The concept implies that there exists some person or institution capable of making such decisions. It also implies possible grave interference with human rights. For these reasons, the principles, which have long been successfully applied to domestic animals, have never been adopted for humans except by despots such as Adolf Hitler.

eugeria the state of a high quality of life in old age. Eugeria should be the normal condition of old people, but is often precluded by physical illness or injury, psychological deficit or disturbance, and respect for defective cultural stereotypes. The term is derived from the Greek *eus-* good, and *geras* old age.

euglobulins globular proteins that are insoluble in water but soluble in saline solutions. Most of the body's globulins are euglobulins.

Euglucon a brand name for GLIBENCLAMIDE.

Eugynon, Eugynon 30 a brand name for an oral contraceptive containing ETHINYLOESTRADIOL (ethinylestradiol) and LEVONORGESTREL. See also CONTRACEPTION.

Euhypnos a brand name for TEMAZEPAM.

eukaryote any organism each of whose cells contains a well defined nucleus with a nuclear membrane in which the genetic material is carried in the chromosomes. Only bacteria and blue-green algae are not eukaryotes. The word is also spelled eucaryote.

Eumovate a brand name for CLOBETASONE.

eumycetoma a class of fungi responsible for deep mass fungal infections of the soft tissues and bones, such as MADURA FOOT, in tropical underdeveloped areas. The group includes *Madurella mycetomatis, Madurella grisea* and *Petriellidium boydii*.

eunuch a man castrated before puberty. This results in the loss of the male sex hormones and the failure of development of the secondary sexual characteristics – the beard, the deeper voice from enlarged larynx, the adult-sized penis, and the characteristic male body shape.

eupepsia good digestion.

euphenics improvement of the whole person (phenotype) through planned control and manipulation by means other than EUGENICS.

euphoria a strong feeling of well-being or happiness. The term is sometimes used to mean an abnormally exaggerated feeling of elation.

euploid 1 having a number of chromosomes that is an exact multiple of the HAPLOID number.
2 having the normal number of chromosomes.

Eurax a brand name for CROTAMITON.

euryon one of the two most widely separated points in the transverse diameter of the skull.

Eustachian tube a short passage leading backwards from the back of the nose, just above the soft palate, on either side, to the cavity of the middle ear. This allows air to pass to or from the middle ear cavity to balance the pressure on either side of the eardrum. (Bartolomeo Eustachi, Italian anatomist, b. around 1520 d. 1574).

euthanasia mercy killing.

euthyroid having normal thyroid gland function. The term is used when thyroid function is restored to normal after either THYROTOXICOSIS or HYPOTHYROIDISM.

evagination a turning inside out.

evening primrose oil a drug used in the treatment of allergic skin disease (atopic eczema) and claimed to be effective, without good evidence, for many other condition.

everolimus a new immunosuppressive agent intended for use in heart transplantation. The drug has been found more effective than AZATHIOPRINE in reducing the severity of coronary artery narrowing and occlusion in the grafted organ (cardiac-allograft vasculopathy).

eversion a turning outwards.

evidence-based medicine the use of methods of medical treatment and clinical decision-making which have been rigorously tested by properly controlled research. The latter must also be exposed to peer review, publication in respected journals and free criticism before its conclusions can be adopted as a basis for practice. A journal called *Evidence-Based Medicine* is published jointly by the British Medical Association and the American College of Physicians.

evisceration a removal of intestines or of the contents of an organ such as the eyeball.

evoked responses signals on the ELECTROENCEPHALOGRAM prompted by visual or auditory sensory input and detected by special electronic averaging techniques. Evoked responses can provide direct, objective evidence that conduction is occurring along the nerve tracts connecting the sense organ with the brain.

evolution the theory that all living organisms have developed in complexity, from a simple life form. Evolution occurs by the natural selection of those who, by the fortune of spontaneous random changes (mutations), happen to be best suited to their contemporary environment, to survive and reproduce. It does not occur by the passing on to offspring of characteristics acquired during the lifetime of an individual. Characteristics are passed on by the transmission of DNA from parents to offspring and, unless mutation has occurred, this DNA is an identical copy of the DNA of preceding generations.

evolutionary medicine a paradigm for medical education and study based on the recognition that a failure to take due account of evolution when viewing human physiology, psychology, pathology and anatomy will result in a truncated, less valid and less fruitful understanding. It should , for instance, be recognized that, the biological norm for infants and children is to be exposed to many infections – a condition that my be necessary for the 'normal' development of the immune system; and that since throughout almost the whole of human evolution life expectancy has been no more than about 30 years, systems have evolved which are largely indifferent to conditions such as OSTEOPOROSIS, PRESBYOPIA and ATHEROSCLEROSIS that do not arise until well after that age. There is good reason to believe that affluence may have much more widespread malign effects than merely obesity and that these may include greatly increased susceptibility to various cancers.

Evorel a brand name for OESTRADIOL (estradiol) in a transdermal patch.

Evra a contraceptive transdermal patch containing NORELGESTROMIN and ETHINYLOESTRADIOL (ethinylestradiol).

evulsion tearing away by force.

Ewing's tumour a very malignant bone cancer affecting children up to the age of about 15. The tumour involves the inner bone tissue, usually of long bones and has a characteristic 'onion skin' appearance on X ray. There is swelling, tenderness and pain, and often fever. The outlook is seldom favourable. (James Ewing, American pathologist, 1866–1943).

exacerbation an increase in severity or a causing of increased severity.

exanthem 1 a skin rash.

2 an infectious disease such as measles, scarlet fever or chickenpox that features a rash.

exchange transfusion the treatment given urgently to all babies with severe haemolytic disease of the newborn (ERYTHROBLASTOSIS FETALIS) from rhesus incompatibility with the mother. A fine catheter is passed along the umbilical vein into the main vein of the body (the inferior vena cava) and 20 ml of blood is withdrawn and replaced by 20 ml of donor blood. This is repeated about eight times.

excimer laser an argon fluoride laser operating in the ultraviolet part of the spectrum and producing a beam that can remove layers of tissue only a few thousands of a millimetre thick.

excimer laser coronary angioplasty the use of a vaporizing EXCIMER LASER by way of an arterial catheter to cut through and remove arterial plaque in cases of ATHEROSCLEROSIS in which the blood supply to the heart, brain, other organ or limb is prejudiced by narrowing. The catheter used contains over 200 individual 50 micron optical fibres surrounding a guide wire. The method is thought likely to be applicable in cases unsuitable for balloon angioplasty.

excimer laser refractive surgery use of the EXCIMER LASER to alter the curvature of the cornea so as to change the refraction of the eye and correct moderate degrees of short sight (myopia) and other refractive errors. Also known as excimer laser refractive keratectomy.

excipient any inert substance used to bulk up or dilute a drug, or as a vehicle for a drug.

excision cutting off and removing completely.

excision enzyme an enzyme that removes short damaged segments from the deoxyribonucleic acid (DNA) molecule of a cell.

excision repair correction of DNA damage by the removal of the damaged length of single strand by one of a number of enzymes capable of recognizing damaged nucleotides, and resynthesizing the correct nucleotide sequence complementary to the normal strand. The repair is catalyzed by DNA polymerase I and DNA ligase.

excitatory amino acids aspartic acid and glutamic acid – amino acids that act on voltage-gated ion channels in the plasma membranes of cells of the nervous system to cause them to fire.

exclusion diet a diet used to determine whether a food allergy exists. Ingredients thought to be possible allergens are eliminated individually and sequentially until an allergen is found. The procedure borders on the impracticable and may have to be modified to exclude categories of foods. Food allergy is less common than media reports might suggest.

excoriation an abrasive or tearing injury to the surface of the body.

excrescence any projection of abnormal tissue from a surface, such as a wart, heart valve vegetations or a nasal polyp.

excretion removal from the body of the waste products of metabolism.

exenteration total removal of all organs and other soft tissue from a bony cavity. Exenteration is a radical and mutilating procedure, performed only in extreme cases of cancer in which the only hope of survival is to attempt to remove all affected tissue. Exenteration is performed on the pelvis and the eye socket.

exercise muscular activity undertaken for the promotion of health and for the pleasure inherent in the use of the body. Modern sedentary life involves a dangerous degree of under-exertion and much of the bodily disorder suffered today can be attributed to the use of artificial energy sources to replace the use of one's own musculature.

exfoliation shedding of cells from a surface, such as the skin. In exfoliative dermatitis, much of the surface of the skin peels off or is shed.

exfoliative cytology a method of diagnosing cell abnormalities, such as cancer, by examining cells shed, brushed or scraped from a body surface.

exhaustion delirium an acute confusional state brought on by extreme fatigue, chronic debilitating illness or long deprivation of sleep.

exhibition the administration of a drug or other method of treatment.

exhibitionism deliberate exposure of the genitals to others to obtain sexual gratification. Exhibitionism suggests sexual inadequacy and is performed to elicit surprise, fright or disgust. Masturbation may then be used to bring about an orgasm. Exhibitionists are usually males and seldom, if ever, offer any physical danger to the victim.

exoccipital of the bony masses on the occipital bone on either side of the FORAMEN MAGNUM.

exocrine glands simple glands, such as sweat, sebaceous, or mucous glands which secrete on to a surface. Endocrine glands, by contrast, secrete into the bloodstream.

exocytosis the movement of peptides or proteins out of a cell in tiny membranous vesicles that pass through the plasma membrane.

exoenzyme an enzyme that operates outside the cell in which it was formed.

exogamy breeding between organisms that are not closely related. Outbreeding, as distinct from inbreeding.

exogenous having an external origin or cause.

exomphalos a protrusion, or herniation, of some of the abdominal contents into the umbilical cord at birth.

exon the segment of deoxyribonucleic acid (DNA) in a gene that codes for some part of the messenger ribonucleic acid (RNA). Any segment that is represented in the RNA product. Segments that do not code for RNA are called introns.

exonucleases enzymes that break down DNA and RNA molecules, starting at the ends of the molecular chains. Exonucleases split off nucleotides one at a time from the end of a chain and may be specific for either end.

exopeptidase an enzyme that acts to split off AMINO ACIDS or sometimes dipeptides from the ends of a protein molecule.

exophoria a latent tendency for the eyes to turn outwards (diverge), but which is usually controlled by the binocular fusion power. If one eye is covered in exophoria it will turn outwards under the cover. Compare EXOTROPIA, ESOPHORIA.

exophthalmic goitre overactivity of the THYROID GLAND associated with protrusion of the eyes, retraction of the upper lids and weakness of the eye movements. The hyperthyroidism causes excitability, a fast pulse, sweating and loss of weight. The EXOPHTHALMOS may be so severe as to threaten sight and the pressure in the eye sockets may have to be relieved surgically. The condition is also called Graves' disease.

exophthalmos protrusion of an eyeball. This forces the eyelids apart and causes a staring appearance. Exophthalmos is caused by an increase in the bulk of the contents of the bony eye socket (ORBIT) from any cause. The commonest cause is an immunological disorder associated with the thyroid gland, but exophthalmos, or proptosis, may be caused by tumour, bleeding or a mucous cyst from a sinus (MUCOCOELE).

exophytic of a tumour that grows outward from a surface, implying low malignancy or non-malignancy.

exostosis an outgrowth from the surface of a bone, usually in response to inflammation or repeated trauma. The commonest form of exostosis is the bunion caused by abnormal local pressure from unsuitable footwear.

exotoxin a powerful protein poison, formed by some bacteria, which is released and which may cause severe damage either locally or, if carried away by the blood, at a remote distance. Diphtheria exotoxin destroys throat lining tissue, where the organism settles, but can also travel to damage the heart and the kidneys.

exotropia divergence of the lines of vision of the two eyes. Divergent squint. In exotropia one eye points at the object of regard, the other is directed outwards. In exotropia acquired in adult life there is usually double vision (diplopia). In childhood, the false image may be suppressed and long-term visual acuity may be affected in one eye. See also ESOTROPIA.

expectant characterized by the willingness to wait hopefully. The term is used especially of medical treatment.

expected date of delivery an estimate of the date on which a baby will be born. This is an arbitrary calculation based on a statistical average gestation period of 266 days, counted as 280 days from the date of the first day of the last menstrual period.

expectoration bringing up, and spitting out, sputum. An expectorant, or cough mixture, is a medicine designed to assist in the removal of sticky mucoid sputum from the bronchial tubes. From the Latin, *ex*, out of, and *pecus*, the breast.

expiration 1 breathing out.
2 death.

expressing milk removal of excess milk from tight and uncomfortable breasts by simulating with the fingers the action of the baby's gums. Expressed milk is often offered to the baby from a bottle.

expressive motor aphasia a type of APHASIA in which language is understood and sensible responses mentally formulated but in which these cannot be expressed in speech because of damage to a small area in the dominant hemisphere. The affected person can write normally and can read silently with normal understanding. The condition is nearly always transitory.

expressivity the degree of severity shown by an AUTOSOMAL dominant trait in any particular affected individual. The main feature of expressivity is its variability.

exsanguination the loss of a substantial proportion, or almost the whole volume, of the blood. The result of a severe haemorrhage.

external auditory meatus the skin-lined external passage of the ear, leading from the outside to the eardrum (tympanic membrane).

external carotid artery a major artery that springs from the common carotid artery in the neck and supplies blood to the front of the neck, face and scalp and the side of the head and the ear. The artery also supplies the DURA MATER.

external fixator a form of bone fixation increasingly used in the management of fractures. A strong steel bar, of circular or square cross-section, lying parallel to the fractured long bone, and securely fixed to it by a number of steel pins passed in through the skin and screwed into the bone above and below the fracture site. The pins are attached to the bar by adjustable brackets.

extero- *prefix denoting* outside.

exteroceptor any sense organ receiving external stimuli.

extra- *prefix denoting* outside, beyond, additional.

extra-articular outside a joint.

extracardiac outside the heart.

extracellular in the space surrounding a cell or collection of cells. The extracellular tissue fluid is the medium of transfer of nutrient materials and oxygen, and of waste products, between the cells and the blood.

extracellular matrix non-living material secreted by cells that fills spaces between the cells in a tissue, protecting them and helping to hold them together. The extracellular matrix may be semifluid or rigidly solid and hard as in bone. It is composed mainly of protein and includes collagens, elastin, reticulin, glycoproteins, proteoglycans, fibronectin, laminins and osteopontin.

extracorporeal outside the body.

extracorporeal membrane oxygenation a method of life support, used mainly for new babies with reversible lung failure, that has been developed from adult heart-lung machines. The technology is similar to that for adults and involves the use of special silastic membranes that are freely permeable to oxygen and carbon dioxide but impermeable to blood. The baby is connected to the machine by cannulas in the right atrium and the right common carotid artery.

extracranial located or occurring outside the cranium.

extradural haemorrhage bleeding between the skull and the outer layer of brain lining (the dura mater). This usually results from a skull fracture, is often slow and insidious, and is very dangerous. A person who recovers consciousness after a head injury and then lapses once again into coma, probably has an extradural haemorrhage and is likely to be in grave danger.

extra-intracranial bypass an attempt to reduce the risk of STROKE in patients at risk by trying to improve the blood supply to the brain. A scalp artery on the outside of the skull is linked to an artery inside. Results have been disappointing.

extrapyramidal system the part of the central nervous system, supplementary to the voluntary motor (pyramidal) system, and concerned with gross movement, posture and the coordination of large muscle groups. The pyramidal system contains the main motor control pathways and includes the basal ganglia, the reticular formation and descending nerve tracts outside the pyramidal system.

extrasensory perception the claimed ability to obtain information without the use of the normal channels of communication. ESP is said to include telepathy, clairvoyance, precognition and retrocognition. There is no respectable scientific evidence for extrasensory perception, but a mass of anecdotal 'proof'.

extrasystole a premature contraction of the

heart. This is usually followed by a pause longer than the normal interval between heart beats and this is often perceptible to the subject. Extrasystoles are often described as palpitations. Ventricular extrasystoles are often described as VENTRICULAR ECTOPY.

extrauterine located or occurring outside the womb (uterus), especially of a pregnancy. See also ECTOPIC PREGNANCY.

extravasation an abnormal escape into the tissues of a fluid such as blood, serum or lymph.

extravascular outside a blood vessel or the circulatory system.

extravert a person whose concerns are directed outward rather than inward, who is positive, active, optimistic, gregarious, impulsive, fond of excitement, often aggressive, and sometimes unreliable. The concept was invented by Carl Jung who also described the opposite personality type, the introvert. Also known as extrovert. See also JUNGIAN THEORY.

extrinsic extraneous to a body or system. Originating from outside.

extroversion turning inside out.

exudate 1 a protein-rich fluid, such as serum or pus, that has leaked from blood vessels or been discharged by cells or tissues.
2 the accumulation or deposition of such fluid in or on the tissues.

exudation a slow escape of clear, cellular or other fluid from cells or blood vessels, usually in the course of inflammation.

eye, artificial see ARTIFICIAL EYE.

eye bank a storage place for donated eyes, the corneas of which are to be used for transplantation. Eyes are kept in special solutions at normal refrigerator temperature and must be used within a day or two of donation. Long-term storage of corneas, for limited purposes such as partial-thickness grafting, is possible.

eye, lazy see AMBLYOPIA.

eyelid, drooping see BLEPHAROPTOSIS.

eye strain a popular term used to describe any feeling of discomfort or distress related to the eyes or to seeing. Eye strain is not a medical concept as the eyes cannot be 'strained' or adversely affected by use. Headache and aching of the muscles around the eyes commonly result from visual difficulty.

eye tooth see CANINE TOOTH.

ezetimibe a cholesterol absorption inhibitor drug that can be used alone or, more effectively, in conjunction with a statin drug (see STATINS) to reduce blood cholesterol levels in people with hypercholesterolaemia. Such people are at risk of developing ATHEROSCLEROSIS. The drug acts specifically to inhibit cholesterol absorption and does not affect the absorption of other lipids. A brand name is Ezetrol.

Ezetrol a brand name for EZETIMIBE.

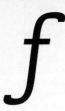

F *abbrev. for,* or symbol for, the element Fluorine.

fab the monovalent antigen-binding fragment of an antibody molecule obtained when the protein is digested with the enzyme papain. It consists of an intact light chain and the immediately-associated terminal and domains of a heavy chain.

Fabry disease see ANDERSON-FABRY DISEASE.

FACA *abbrev. for* Fellow of the American College of Anesthetists.

FACC *abbrev. for* Fellow of the American College of Cardiologists.

FACDS *abbrev. for* Fellow of the Australian College of Dental Surgeons.

face lift a cosmetic operation usually done under general anaesthesia. The skin is cut through just behind the hair line and freed from the underlying tissue by undermining. It is then pulled up tightly, the surplus removed, and the new edge stitched in place. With sublime disregard for etymological propriety, the procedure is often called rhytidectomy (literally, a cutting off of wrinkles).

facet a small flat surface on a bone or tooth or other hard body. A facet may be natural, as on the arches of the vertebrae, or the result of wear.

FACG *abbrev. for* Fellow of the American College of Gastroenterology.

facial pertaining to the face.

facial artery one of the main branches of the external carotid artery. The facial artery crosses the lower edge of the jaw bone about half way back and divides into numerous branches to supply the skin and muscles of the face and the lining of the mouth, throat and tonsil.

facial bones these are the upper jaw (maxilla), the cheek bone (zygoma), the nasal bone in the upper part of the nose, the lacrimal bone at the inner corner of the eye, the hard palate (palatine bone) and parts of the deeper ETHMOID and SPHENOID bones. The lower jaw bone is called the mandible.

facial index the ratio of the length of the face to its width multiplied by 100.

facial nerve one of the 7th of the 12 pairs of CRANIAL NERVES. Each facial nerve supplies the muscles of the face on its own side. Loss of function in a facial nerve causes partial or total paralysis of one side of the face. This is called BELL'S PALSY.

facial pain see TRIGEMINAL NEURALGIA.

facial palsy see BELL'S PALSY.

facies the facial expression or appearance characteristic of a particular medical condition or state. Typical facies are found in many conditions and may assist a doctor in diagnosis. The facies are especially characteristic in conditions such as DOWN'S SYNDROME, PAGET'S DISEASE, the TREACHER COLLIN'S SYNDROME, LEPROSY, PARKINSONISM, thyroid underactivity and ALZHEIMER'S DISEASE.

facilitation the general DEPOLARIZATION and passage of an impulse that occurs in a nerve cell when excitatory inputs at SYNAPSES exceed inhibitory inputs.

facio-scapulo-humeral dystrophy one of the forms of muscular dystrophy. This type is acquired by AUTOSOMAL DOMINANT inheritance and may appear at any age. Weakness is first noted in the facial muscles and then in the shoulders and arms. After many years the muscles of the pelvis and legs may be affected. Progress is very slow and non-continuous and the condition is compatible with normal length of life.

FACMA *abbrev. for* Fellow of the Australian

College of Medical Administrators.

FACO *abbrev. for* Fellow of the American College of Otolaryngology.

FACOG *abbrev. for* Fellow of the American College of Obstetrics & Gynecology.

FACP *abbrev. for* Fellow of the American College of Physicians.

FACR *abbrev. for* Fellow of the American College of Radiologists.

FACS *abbrev. for* Fellow of the American College of Surgeons.

FACTM *abbrev. for* Fellow of the American College of Tropical Medicine.

factor 1 any kind of biological material that causes a particular effect. 2 an effector whose function is known but which has not yet been chemically identified. 3 one of the components in the blood coagulation cascade.

Factor V Leiden mutation a mutation in the gene for the blood clotting Factor V that leads to a type of increased clotting tendency known as activated protein C resistance (APC resistance). The mutation involves a CpG dinucleotide, a common location for a mutation. APC resistance from this mutation is recognized as a cause of stroke in children but the mutation is often detected for the first time in people over 60 suffering a first episode of thrombosis. The mutation was discovered in the Thrombosis and Haemostasis Research Centre, University Hospital, Leiden, Netherlands.

Factor VIII a protein (globulin) necessary for the proper clotting of the blood. The absence of Factor VIII causes HAEMOPHILIA but it can be isolated from donated blood and given to haemophiliacs to control their bleeding tendency. The drug is on the WHO official list.

Factor IX one of the many factors necessary for blood clotting. Absence of Factor IX occurs as a result of an X-LINKED gene mutation and causes CHRISTMAS DISEASE, a form of HAEMOPHILIA almost identical to Factor VIII deficiency haemophilia. The drug is on the WHO official list. Human coagulation Factor IX is produced in freeze-dried form derived from donated blood under the brand names Mononine and Replenine.

Factor XII the factor that initiates the sequence of reactions that ends in blood clotting (coagulation). Also known as the Hageman factor.

Factor XIII an enzyme in the blood that catalyses cross-linking between molecules of fibrin so as to strengthen the forming blood clot. See also FIBRINASE. Human Factor VIII is made by genetic engineering and is sold under the brand names Kogenate and Recombinate. It is also produced in freeze-dried form from donated blood under the brand names Monoclate-P and Replenate.

facultative 1 capable of adapting in response to changing environments. Used especially of micro-organisms that can grow either in an atmosphere of oxygen (aerobic) or in the absence of oxygen (anaerobic) or of those capable of living either as parasites or non-parasites. 2 of organisms with a usual or preferred metabolic process, but which are capable, under unusual conditions, of adopting an alternative metabolic pathway.

facultative aerobe a microorganism normally reproducing without free oxygen (an anaerobe) which can sometimes grow in the presence of oxygen.

facultative anaerobe a microorganism able to flourish equally well both in the presence and absence of free oxygen.

faecalith a faece that has become so hard as to resemble a stone.

faecal softeners drugs used to treat constipation, especially in terminally ill patients. Examples are arachis oil (Fletchers), liquid paraffin, co-danthrusate (Normax), docusate sodium (Dioctyl, Norgalax) and various combinations of sodium citrate, sodium lauryl sulphoacetate and glycerol.

faeces the natural effluent from the intestinal tract. Faeces consist mainly of dead bacteria, but also contain cells cast off from the lining of the intestine, mucus secretion from the cells of the intestinal wall, bile from the liver, which colours the faeces, and a small amount of food residue, mostly cellulose.

FAGO *abbrev. for* Fellow in Australia in Obstetrics & Gynaecology.

Fahrenheit scale the temperature scale formerly used in medicine but now replaced by the CELSIUS SCALE. In the Fahrenheit scale, the melting point of ice is 32, and the boiling point of water is 212. Normal body temperature is about 98. To convert Fahrenheit to Celsius, subtract 32 and multiply by 0.555 or 5/9.

fainting temporary loss of consciousness due to brain deprivation of an adequate supply of blood and thus oxygen and glucose. This results from a reduction in blood pressure, either because the heart is pumping too slowly or less efficiently or because the arteries of the body have widened. If a fainting person is allowed to lie and the legs raised, recovery will be rapid. It is dangerous to keep a fainting person upright.

faith healing an attempt to cure disease or to improve the condition of a patient by the exercise of spiritual powers or by the influence of the personality of the healer. An important factor in determining the outcome of an illness is belief, or faith, in the probability of recovery, but 'miracles' attributed to faith healing are presumed to be due to some natural process. The psychological effect of such rituals can be powerful, and unjustified hopes for miraculous cures are commonly aroused.

falciform curved or sickle-shaped.

falciform ligament a large sickle-shaped fold of PERITONEUM extending from the front of the top of the liver to the UMBILICUS.

falciparum malaria the most dangerous form of MALARIA caused by the parasite *Plasmodium falciparum*. There is severe breakdown of red blood cells, sometimes with so much release of HAEMOGLOBIN that it appears in the urine (BLACKWATER FEVER). Falciparum malaria also features blockage of small blood vessels by parasite and toxic effects on the linings. The consequent damage to organs, including the brain, is a major danger.

fallen arches see PES PLANUS.

Fallopian tube the open-ended tube along which eggs (ova) travel from the ovaries to the womb (uterus) and in which fertilization must occur if pregnancy is to result. The open end of each Fallopian tube has finger-like processes that sweep over the surface of the ovary at the time of ovulation, wafting the egg into the tube. Also known as a uterine tube. (Gabriele Fallopio, Italian anatomist, 1523–63).

Fallot's tetralogy a common congenital heart disease consisting of four defects – narrowing of the main artery to the lungs (pulmonary artery); a hole in the wall between the two sides of the heart; defective positioning of the main artery of the body (aorta); and enlargement of the main pumping chamber on the right side of the heart (right ventricle). Affected children are breathless, tire easily and usually show bluish skin colour (cyanosis).

false rib any of the five pairs of lower ribs that are attached to cartilages rather than directly to the breastbone (sternum). See also FLOATING RIB.

false memory syndrome alleged unearthed 'memories' of childhood sexual abuse induced by psychoanalysts and other psychotherapists with more enthusiasm for Freudian theories than insight into the nature of their own activities. Cases of flagrant invitations or suggestions by therapists to their patients to 'remember' such incidents have been reported, and some of these have led to unfounded accusations and family alienation.

falx a sickle-shaped structure. The falx cerebri is the curved, vertical partition of DURA MATER that occupies the longitudinal fissure between the two cerebral hemispheres.

famciclovir an antiviral drug used to treat SHINGLES and genital HERPES. A brand name is Famvir.

familial 1 occurring in some families but not in others, as a result of genetic transmission. The term is usually applied to diseases. **2** occurring more often in a particular family than would happen by chance.

familial adenomatous polyposis an autosomal dominant genetic disorder featuring multiple ADENOMAS of the colon and rectum, desmoids, osteomas and sebaceous cysts. The condition is causes by a mutation on the adenomatous polyposis coli (APC) gene on the long arm of chromosome 5 and carries a strong risk of malignancy. About 12% of people with the gene develop a cancer of the upper intestinal tract, usually a cancer at the point where the bile and pancreatic ducts enter the small intestine (the ampulla of Vater). The APC gene is large with about 100,000 base pairs but of which only about one tenth are exons. It is a tumour suppressor gene, and the mutation allows tumours to arise. In people with familial adenomatous popyposis the normal allele of the pair is deleted.

familial atrial fibrillation a rare autosomal dominant disease caused by a mutation on chromosome 10. The features of the disease do not appear to differ from those of common ATRIAL FIBRILLATION.

familial dysautonomia an AUTOSOMAL RECESSIVE neurological disease affecting mainly

Ashkenazi Jews and featuring a marked disturbance of the function of the autonomic nervous system. This results in feeding difficulties, excessive sweating, absence of tears, indifference to pain, reduced corneal sensitivity, emotional lability and red blotching of the skin.

familial lipoprotein lipase inhibitor a substance that inhibits the fat-splitting enzyme lipase that breaks down lipoproteins. The effect of the presence of this abnormal substance in some individuals is an accumulation of very low-density lipoproteins (VLDL), chylomicrons and fats.

familial Mediterranean fever an autosomal recessive genetic disease featuring recurrent fever, PERITONITIS, ARTHRITIS, chest pain from PLEURISY and a skin rash similar to ERYSIPELAS. The disease affects families in the Mediterranean litoral especially Armenians and North African Sephardic Jews and is caused by mutation of a gene on the short arm of chromosome 16.

familial periodic paralysis a rare inherited condition featuring attacks of severe weakness lasting for hours and often following exertion or a heavy meal. In most cases the weakness is associated with a shift of potassium into the muscle cells so that blood potassium levels fall.

familial polyposis an autosomal dominant hereditary condition featuring multiple POLYPS in the small intestine and colon. There is a strong tendency to malignant change.

family balancing the wish to choose the sex of an unborn child on the basis of how many children of each sex already exist in a family. Measures to elect a gender are currently considered at least unethical and, in some countries, are illegal.

family planning a conscious decision as to the number and spacing of children born, effected by the use of CONTRACEPTION.

family therapy the treatment of behavioural and emotional problems in an individual by involvement of the whole family in the treatment process. Group interview and discussions are guided by an experienced counsellor. Many problems arise from defective interaction within the family and many are affected by the quality of family relationships. Family therapy, in which the whole family participates, can often be more effective than therapy directed only to the most seriously disturbed person.

famine oedema fluid retention in the tissues in people who are suffering from severe malnutrition in conditions such as KWASHIORKOR. In the milder cases there is puffiness around the eyes and swelling of the ankles. In severe cases the fluid retained may amount to as much as 50% of the body weight.

famotidine an H2 RECEPTOR ANTAGONIST drug used to treat peptic ulcers and reflux oesophagitis (heartburn). A brand name is Pepsid.

Famvir a brand name for FAMCICLOVIR.

Fanconi's syndrome a kidney disease in which large quantities of substances normally retained in the body are excreted in the urine. These substances include amino acids, glucose, calcium, phosphates, sodium and potassium. The result may be muscle weakness and failure to thrive and softening and distortion of the bones. There is excessive output of urine, great thirst and progressive kidney failure. Fanconi's syndrome may be of genetic origin or may be caused by out-dated tetracycline antibiotic, metal salt poisoning or vitamin D deficiency, or may occur as a complication of other conditions. (Guido Fanconi, 1892–1979, Swiss paediatrician.)

Fansidar a brand name for a mixture of PYRIMETHAMINE and SULFADOXINE.

FANZCP *abbrev. for* Fellow of the Australian & New Zealand College of Psychiatrists.

faradism the use of pulsed or alternating electric currents to stimulate muscle contraction in order to maintain the health of paralysed muscles while awaiting regeneration or recovery in damaged motor nerves.

farcy see GLANDERS.

Fareston a brand name for TOREMIFENE.

Farlutal a brand name for MEDROXYPROGESTERONE.

farmer's lung an allergic occupational lung disease caused by the repeated inhalation of dust containing the spores of fungus from mouldy straw, hay, grain or mushroom compost. There are acute attacks of fever, nausea, breathlessness and cough a few hours after exposure. Repeated attacks lead to serious lung scarring (fibrosis) and interference with oxygen transfer to the blood (respiratory failure).

fart see FLATUS.

fascia tendon-like fibrous connective tissue

arranged in sheets or layers under the skin, between the muscles and around the organs, the blood vessel and the nerves. Fascial sheaths form compartments throughout the body. Some fascia is dense and tough, some delicate. Much of it contains fat cells. The 'superficial fascia' just under the skin is one of the main fat stores of the body.

fasciculation brief, involuntary contraction of a small group of muscle fibres, causing visible twitching under the skin. In most cases fasciculation is of no importance but persistent severe fasciculation may imply nerve disease and should be reported.

fasciculus a bundle of fibres, especially nerve fibres, running together with common origins and functions.

fasciitis inflammation of FASCIA. Fasciitis is rare and is sometimes associated with conditions such as ANKYLOSING SPONDYLITIS or REITER'S SYNDROME. See also NECROTIZING FASCIITIS.

fascioliasis infection with a trematode worm or fluke of the genus *Fasciola*, especially *Fasciola hepatica*, a liver fluke parasite of sheep and cattle that can be transmitted to man on vegetation such as watercress. There is fever, loss of appetite, abdominal pain, liver tenderness, jaundice and sometimes CIRRHOSIS of the liver.

fasciolopsiasis intestinal infection with the largest human fluke parasite, *Fasciolopsis buski*, that may be up to 7.5 cm long. The condition is common in rural China and South-east Asia and is acquired by eating water plants contaminated with the larvae. Mild infections cause diarrhoea and abdominal discomfort. Heavy infections may be fatal.

fasciotomy cutting fascia, usually to relieve damaging tension in a muscle compartment or prevent compression of arteries or nerves. Fasciotomy may become necessary if the development of muscles, as in an athlete, exceeds the space available to them in their fascial compartments.

Fasigyn a brand name for TINIDAZOLE.

fastigium 1 the point of maximal severity of a disease.
2 the peak of a fever.

fasting refraining from taking food. So long as water is taken, reasonably well-nourished people can safely fast for several days. Once the fat stores are depleted, however, the voluntary muscles are consumed and soon become

severely wasted. Many people find moderate regular fasting a useful aid to health.

fatal familial insomnia a genetically-determined condition occurring between the ages of 40 and 60, involving progressively worsening insomnia, intolerance to heat, watering eyes, progressive difficulty in walking, memory deterioration, speech defect, muscle jerks, progressive physical and mental deterioration and death within 7 to 33 months of onset. The disease, which features severe loss of nerve fibres in the thalamic nuclei at the base of the brain, is one of the growing list of serious disorders caused by abnormal PRION proteins – a list that also includes Creutzfeldt-Jakob disease, new variant CJD, kuru, and Gerstmann-Strussler disease. Sporadic fatal insomnia is also a prion disease and is probably identical to fatal familial insomnia.

fat embolism the release of fat into the blood and its movement with the circulation to a point where blockage of small arteries occurs. Fat embolism usually follows fractures of long bones. Obstruction of vital arteries such as those in the brain, the lungs or in the coronary arteries of the heart is a serious complication. The acidic products of fat breakdown can also cause permanent damage to the linings of the arteries.

fatigue physical or mental tiredness. Physical fatigue is due to accumulation in the muscles of the breakdown products of fuel consumption and energy production (metabolism). Mental fatigue is usually the result of boredom, FRUSTRATION, ANXIETY, over-long concentration on a single task or dislike of a particular activity. Fatigue commonly involves both kinds.

fat mobilization increased breakdown of fats (triglycerides) with the release of fatty acids and glycerol into the blood.

fat necrosis death of body fatty tissue often as a result of exposure to pancreatic enzymes in the condition of acute PANCREATITIS.

fats also known as lipids, fats are stored as an oily liquid under the skin and in the abdomen in thin-walled cells. Fats form the body's main energy store and are converted into fuel as required. Fat stores also form an insulant against heat loss, a mechanical shock absorber and a contouring element. Body fats are triglycerides and consist of a 'backbone' of glycerol to which three fatty acids are attached.

Fats differ by virtue of different fatty acids. These may be saturated or unsaturated. Most diets contain too high a proportion of fats and especially of SATURATED FATS. Saturated fats are found in butter, milk, and other dairy products. Unsaturated fats, such as are found in vegetable and fish oils, are believed to be less harmful to health.

fat soluble able to be dissolved in fats or fat solvents. Four of the vitamins, A, D, E and K, are fat soluble.

fate map a diagram of an embryo showing the regions that will eventually form particular tissues in the adult.

fatty acids a large group of monobasic acids found in animals and plants. They are saturated or unsaturated aliphatic compounds with an even number of carbon atoms. The most abundant fatty acids are palmitic, stearic and oleic acids. Glucose and fatty acids are the two main fuel substances of the body. FATS are glyceride esters of fatty acids.

fatty degeneration an abnormal tissue state featuring the accumulation of tiny fat droplets in the CYTOPLASM of cells. This occurs in severe infections, ISCHAEMIA, and severe nutritional lack and affects especially the liver and the heart.

fauces the narrowed space at the back of the mouth and PHARYNX, under the soft palate and between the soft palatine arches (the pillars of the fauces) on either side from which the throat opens out. The term appears to be a plural of the singular word faux but is, in fact, a singular entity. From Latin, *fauces*, throat.

Faverin a brand name for FLUVOXAMINE.

favism a hereditary sensitivity to a chemical substance found in broad beans that causes severe anaemia in those so affected if they eat the beans. The condition is rare except in Iran and some parts of the Mediterranean shore. Italian, *favismo*, from Latin *favus*, a bean.

favus a persistent infection of the hair follicles, especially of the scalp (tinea capitis), caused by the fungus *Trichophyton schoenleinii*. Characteristic crusts form and in the long term there is widespread loss of hair from scarring. From Latin, *favus*, a honeycomb.

FBCO *abbrev. for* Fellow of the British College of Ophthalmic Opticians.

FBPSS *abbrev. for* Fellow of the British Psychological Society.

FBPsS *abbrev. for* Fellow of the British Psychological Society.

Fc a crystallizable, non-antigen-binding fragment of an antibody molecule obtained by brief digestion with the enzyme papain. It consists of the C-terminal part of both heavy chains, the part which binds to FC RECEPTORS.

Fc receptors cell surface receptors of a specific chemical 'shape' to bind to the Fc heavy chain terminals of the appropriate classes of immunoglobulin molecules (antibodies). IgE molecules, for instance, bind to the Fc receptors on MAST CELLS and blood eosinophil cells. IgG molecules bind to Fc receptors on phagocyte cell membranes.

FCAnaes *abbrev. for* Fellow of the College of Anaesthetists.

FCAP *abbrev. for* Fellow of the College of American Pathologists.

FCCP *abbrev. for* Fellow of the American College of Chest Physicians.

FCGP *abbrev. for* Fellow of the College of General Practitioners.

FCMS *abbrev. for* Fellow of the College of Medicine & Surgery.

FCOT *abbrev. for* Fellow of the College of Occupational Therapists.

FCP *abbrev. for* Fellow of the College of Clinical Pharmacology or Fellow of the College of Physicians.

FCPath *abbrev. for* Fellow of the College of Pathologists.

FCPS *abbrev. for* Fellow of the College of Physicians & Surgeons.

FCRA *abbrev. for* Fellow of the College of Radiologists of Australia.

FDS *abbrev. for* Fellow in Dental Surgery.

fear the response to a real or imagined perception of danger. An abnormal degree of fear, or a fear inappropriate to its cause is called a phobia. Fear is accompanied by physical symptoms such as rapid heart action, muscle tension especially in the abdomen, dryness of the throat and sweating. These symptoms are mainly caused by ADRENALINE. It is believed that separate nuclei in the amygdala mediate different aspects of fear-conditioned behaviour.

febrifuge anything that reduces a fever. From Latin *febris*, fever and *fugare*, to drive away.

febrile pertaining to, or featuring, a fever. From Latin *febris*, fever.

febrile convulsion a seizure or fit caused by a

sudden rise in temperature. Febrile convulsions are common in young children and most of these children are not epileptic. Such convulsions can, however, cause brain damage and lead to severe epilepsy. They should be avoided, if possible, by controlling high fever in children.

fecundation fertilization. Impregnation.

feedback a feature of biological and other control systems in which some of the information from the output is returned to the input to exert either a potentiating effect (positive feedback) or a dampening and regularizing effect (negative feedback). Too much positive feedback produces a runaway effect often with oscillation.

Fefol a brand name for a mixture of FOLIC ACID and IRON ('Ferrous and folic').

Fehling's solution a solution of copper sulphate, sodium hydroxide and sodium potassium tartrate once widely used to test urine for the presence of sugar. Nowadays, urine is usually tested with colour change dip sticks. (Hermann Christian von Fehling, 1812–85, German chemist).

felbinac a NON-STEROIDAL ANTI-INFLAMMATORY DRUG (NSAID) formulated in a gel for external use. A brand name is Traxam.

Feldene a brand name for PIROXICAM.

fellatio oral stimulation of the penis. From the Latin *fellatus*, to suck.

felo de se the act of committing SUICIDE.

felodipine a calcium channel blocker drug used to treat ANGINA PECTORIS and high blood pressure (HYPERTENSION). A brand name is Plendil.

Felty's syndrome RHEUMATOID ARTHRITIS associated with enlargement of the SPLEEN and a reduction in the number of white cells in the blood. There is also often anaemia, loss of weight, enlarged lymph nodes and an increased susceptibility to infection. (Augustus Roi Felty, 1885–1963, American physician).

female symbol ♀ the universally-used symbol for the female.

Femapak a brand name for OESTRADIOL (estradiol) and dydrogesterone in a transdermal patch.

Femara a brand name for LETROZOLE.

Fematrix a brand name for OESTRADIOL (estradiol) in a transdermal patch.

feminization 1 the effects of the sex hormones,

oestradiol (estradiol) and oestrone (estrone), from the ovary, bringing about the normal female secondary sexual characteristics.
2 the development of female secondary sexual characteristics in the male, as when a tumour of an adrenal gland causes the production of mainly female sex hormones (oestrogens). In testicular feminization, the male sex hormone does not bind properly to the tissue receptors. In the absence of male sex hormones before puberty, as in men castrated early, feminization occurs.

Femodene, Femodene ED an oral contraceptive containing ETHINYLOESTRADIOL (ethinylestradiol) and GESTODENE. See also CONTRACEPTION.

femoral pertaining to the thigh or the thigh bone (FEMUR). From Latin *femor*, thigh.

femoral artery the main artery of the leg in the area between the groin and the back of the knee, where it divides into two and passes down to supply the lower leg. The femoral artery supplies all the muscles and other structures of the thigh with blood.

femoral hernia the escape of a small knuckle or loop of intestine into the femoral canal – the route in the groin for the passage of the large arteries and veins from the abdomen into the legs. See also HERNIA.

femoral nerve one of the main nerves of the leg. It branches widely to run into the group of large muscles on the front of the thigh and to carry back sensation from the skin on the front and inner aspects.

femoral ring the abdominal opening of the femoral canal.

femoral vein the large vein draining the whole of the leg that lies alongside the FEMORAL ARTERY.

Femseven a brand name OESTRADIOL (estradiol) for in a transdermal patch.

Femulen a brand name for ETHYNODIOL (etynodol) DIACETATE.

femur the thigh bone. The upper end of the femur forms a ball and socket joint with the side of the pelvis. The lower end widens to provide the upper bearing surface of the knee joint.

femur fracture see FRACTURED FEMUR.

Fenbid Gel a brand name for IBUPROFEN in a preparation for external use.

Fenbid Spansule a brand name for IBUPROFEN.

fenbufen a NON-STEROIDAL ANTI-

INFLAMMATORY DRUG (NSAID). A brand name is
Lederfen.

fenestra an opening or window between two
chambers or body spaces, or an opening made
in a plaster cast or dressing to allow
examination or drainage.

fenestrated having windows or windowl-ike
openings.

fenestration 1 the surgical establishment of an
opening or the formation of a window.
2 an operation on the inner ear, to relieve the
deafness caused by OTOSCLEROSIS in which the
inner of the three tiny bones of the middle ear
becomes fused in its seating. Fenestration
creates a new window in the wall of the inner
ear to allow freer vibration of the fluid within.
It has now been largely superseded by better
procedures such as stapedectomy.

fenfluramine a drug used in the management
of obesity. It is thought to work by producing a
sense of having eaten enough (satiety) rather
than by suppressing appetite. There is evidence
that fenfluramine may be associated with heart
valve disease and PULMONARY HYPERTENSION
and it is now rarely used.

fenofibrate a fibrate anticholesterol drug used
to treat high blood cholesterol levels that fail to
respond to diet modification. A brand name is
Lipantil Micro.

fenoprofen a NON-STEROIDAL ANTI-
INFLAMMATORY DRUG (NSAID). A brand name is
Fenopron.

Fenopron a brand name for FENOPROFEN.

fenoterol a beta2-agonist, adrenaline-like drug
that is valuable in the management of asthma
while having comparatively little effect on the
heart. Its action is similar to that of
SALBUTAMOL. It is produced in combination
with the anticholinergic drug ipratropium
bromide under the brand name Duovent.

Fenox a brand name for nasal drops containing
PHENYLEPHRINE.

fentanyl a powerful, short-acting narcotic pain
killer (analgesic). Brand names are Actiq and
Sublimaze and, in trans-dermal patch form,
Durogesic.

Fentazin a brand name for PERPHENAZINE.

Feospan a brand name for an IRON preparation.

Ferfolic SV a brand name for FERROUS
FUMARATE in conjunction with FOLIC ACID and
vitamin C.

Fergon a brand name for an IRON preparation.

ferritin the principal IRON-binding protein of
the body. Ferritin acts as an iron store in the
liver and other tissues. Each ferritin molecule
can hold up to 4500 iron atoms and the amount
of iron in ferritin molecules accurately reflects
the total iron stores of the body. Ferritin also
protects against the toxic effects of excess iron.

Ferrocap F a brand name for FOLIC ACID and
IRON.

ferrochelatase a MITOCHONDRIAL enzyme
that catalyzes the process by which iron is
incorporated into the PROTOPORPHYRIN
molecule in the process of forming
HAEMOGLOBIN.

Ferrograd a brand name for FERROUS SULPHATE.

Ferrograd Folic a brand name for FERROUS
SULPHATE in conjunction with FOLIC ACID.

ferrous fumarate an iron salt used to treat
iron-deficiency anaemia. Brand names are
Fersamal and Galfer. The drug is also
formulated in conjunction with folic acid under
the brand names Galfer F.A. and Pregaday.

ferrous gluconate an iron compound used in
the treatment of iron deficiency ANAEMIA. A
brand name of a formulation with FOLIC ACID
and vitamin C is Ferfolic SV.

ferrous glycine sulphate an iron compound
used totreat iron-deficiency anaemia. A brand
name is Plesmet.

ferrous sulphate a bitter, greenish crystalline
compound of iron used in the treatment of iron
deficiency ANAEMIA. Brand names are Ferrograd
and Slow-Fe. The drug is also formulated in
conjunction with FOLIC ACID under the brand
names Ferrograd Folic, Fefol and Slow-Fe Folic.

Fersaday a brand name for FERROUS FUMARATE.

Fersamal a brand name for FERROUS FUMARATE,
an IRON preparation used to treat ANAEMIA.

fertility the power to reproduce and the
possession of such power. See also INFERTILITY.

fertility drugs drugs used to treat INFERTILITY,
usually by the induction of ovulation. The
drugs clomiphene (clomifene), tamoxifen and
cyclofenil are used to treat infertility due to
failure to produce ova. These and other similar
fertility drugs often result in multiple ovulation
and multiple pregnancies may result.

fertilization the union of the spermatozoon
with the egg (ovum) so that the full
complement of chromosomes is made up and
the process of cell division, to form a new
individual, started.

fetal pertaining to a FETUS. (See note there about spelling).

fetal alcohol syndrome the group of damaging effects caused to the growing fetus by sustained high levels of alcohol in the mother's blood during pregnancy. They include low birth weight, a small head (microcephaly) with protruding jaws and receding upper teeth, congenital heart disease, mental retardation and a high fetal death rate.

fetal anticonvulsant syndrome congenital defects caused, or thought to have been caused, by the necessary maternal intake of anticonvulsant drugs during early pregnancy.

fetal asphyxia the serious condition of deprivation of oxygen to the fetus from interference with its blood supply. This may occur from compression of the umbilical cord, as from looping round the neck of the fetus, a reduction in the blood flow to the PLACENTA or separation of the placenta from its bed. See also FETAL DISTRESS.

fetal distress observable changes in the fetus during pregnancy or, more often, labour, caused mainly by an insufficient oxygen supply via the placenta. The signs are a sustained rise in the heart rate to above 160/min, slowing of the fetal heart rate after each contraction of the womb, persistent slowness below 120/min, heart irregularity and contraction of the fetal bowel with the passage into the uterine fluid of greenish stools (meconium). These signs do not necessarily indicate lack of oxygen and fetal distress is difficult to evaluate. Fetal blood sampling, through an ENDOSCOPE, may be more useful.

fetal haemoglobin the form of HAEMOGLOBIN normally present in the red blood cells of the fetus. The haemoglobin alpha chains are identical to those of the adult, but the gamma chains are slightly different.

fetal position a position, resembling that of the fetus in the womb, sometimes adopted by a child or adult in a state of distress or withdrawal. The position is one in which the body is drawn into itself. The head is bent forward, the spine is curved, the arms are crossed over the chest and the hips and knees are fully bent (flexed).

fetation the state of pregnancy or the development of a fetus.

fetishism sexual interest aroused by an object, such as an article of clothing, or by a part of the body not normally considered sexually significant. Fetishism is essentially a male disorder and, if severe, the affected person will prefer contact with the object to contact with the owner and will often use the object to assist in masturbation.

fetor hepaticus a musty, sweet odour in the breath occurring in liver failure.

fetor oris bad breath. Halitosis.

fetoscopy visual examination of the fetus within the womb (uterus), by means of a fine fibre-optic viewing and illumination system passed into the amniotic fluid, through the wall of the uterus. Fetoscopy allows confirmation of physical abnormalities. There is a small risk of causing abortion.

fetus the developing individual from about the eighth or tenth week of life in the womb until the time of birth. The fetus has all the recognizable external characteristics of a human being. At 10 weeks, the fetus measures about 2.5 cm from the crown of the head to the rump. The face is formed but the eyelids are fused together. The brain is in a primitive state, incapable of any meaningful form of consciousness. By 3 months, the fetus is about 5 cm long (crown to rump) and by 4 months it is about 10 cm long. In the 6th month, the fetus is up to 20 cm long and weighs up to 800 g. Survival outside the womb at this stage is unlikely. Most fetuses over 2 000 grams do well if properly managed in an INCUBATOR. From the Latin *fetus*, an offspring. The common spelling 'foetus' is incorrect and is used only by journalists who should know better.

Feulgen reaction an aniline DNA-specific staining reaction. NUCLEIC ACID turns a reddish-purple colour when in contact with the Feulgen reagent which contains fuchsin and sulphuric acid. (Robert Feulgen, 1884–1955, German physiologist and chemist).

FEV FORCED EXPIRATORY VOLUME.

fever elevation of body temperature above about 37 °C, taken in the mouth. Fever is due to a resetting of the body's thermostat at a higher level so that heat production, mainly by shivering, is induced. The resetting is caused by the CYTOKINE interleukin-1 produced by white cells under the influence of bacteria, cancer, CORONARY THROMBOSIS, STROKE, crushing injury and other conditions. Fever inhibits the growth of bacteria and causes an increase in antibody production. The recognition of these advantages has led to a general abandonment of the former practice of routinely trying to reduce moderate fever.

fever blister a COLD SORE.

fexofenadine an ANTIHISTAMINE drug used to treat hay fever. A brand name is Telfast.

FFA *abbrev. for* Fellow of the Faculty of Anaesthetists.

FFCM abbrev. for Fellow of the Faculty of Community Medicine.

FFCMI *abbrev. for* Fellow of the Faculty of Community Medicine in Ireland.

FFD *abbrev. for* Fellow of the Faculty of Dental Surgeons

FFHom *abbrev. for* Fellow of the Faculty of Homoeopathy.

FFOM *abbrev. for* Fellow of the Faculty of Occupational Medicine.

FFPath *abbrev. for* Fellow of the Faculty of Pathology.

FFPHM *abbrev. for* Fellow of the Faculty of Public Health Medicine.

FFPM RCP (UK) *abbrev. for* Fellow of the Faculty of Pharmaceutical Medicine Royal College of Physicians UK.

FFR *abbrev. for* Fellow of the Faculty of Radiologists.

FIBiol *abbrev. for* Fellow of the Institute of Biology.

fibrate one of a class of drugs capable of lowering the levels in the body of lipids (fats) including cholesterol. Fibrates can reduce low-density lipoproteins and raise high density lipoproteins. Some act by interfering with cholesterol synthesis in the liver others by promoting the more rapid breakdown of lipoproteins.

fibre, dietary see DIETARY FIBRE.

fibre optics the science and technology of the transmission of light, including coherent laser light, along optical fibres and its applications. This has become important in medicine and surgery as it provides a method of internal illumination and examination through a natural orifice or through a very small artificial opening (endoscopy). Optical fibres can guide light around corners by virtue of the principle of total internal reflection. Bundles of fibres are used.

fibril a fine, slender fibre.

fibrillation uncontrolled, rapid and irregular contraction of muscle, especially heart muscle. Fibrillation most commonly affects the upper chambers of the heart (atrial fibrillation) causing an irregular pulse. Fibrillation of the main pumping chambers (ventricular fibrillation) prevents pumping and is rapidly fatal unless normal beating can be restored by electrical defibrillation.

fibrin an insoluble protein that forms as a fibrous network when the blood protein fibrinogen interacts with THROMBIN. Fibrin is the basis of a blood clot and the end product of a complex cascade of reactions set in motion by injury to a blood vessel.

fibrinase Factor XIII, an enzyme in the blood coagulation cascade that catalyzes the formation of side links between fibrin molecules so as to create a mesh of polymerized FIBRIN that stabilizes the blood clot. Fibrinase is also known as the fibrin-stabilizing factor. See also Factor VIII, IX, XII.

fibrinogen a protein in the blood that is converted to FIBRIN by the action of THROMBIN in the presence of ionized calcium, thereby bringing about coagulation of blood.

fibrinogenopenia a congenital deficiency of FIBRINOGEN in the plasma.

fibrinoid 1 resembling fibrin.
2 a homogeneous, refractile, non-cellular material resembling FIBRIN that is found in the walls of blood vessels and elsewhere in certain disease processes. Fibrinoid is also found as a layer between the PLACENTA and the womb.

fibrinolysin an enzyme that can break down FIBRIN.

fibrinolysis the use of drugs to dissolve blood clots in the circulation. Enzymes such as streptokinase or urokinase, which break down FIBRIN, are used. A combination of fibrinolysis and aspirin, given soon after a coronary attack, greatly improves the chances of survival.

fibrinous 1 rich in FIBRIN.
2 having the nature of fibrin.

fibrinous pericarditis inflammation of the PERICARDIUM with deposition of FIBRIN and white cells between the layers causing adhesions to form that may interfere with the free action of the heart. The condition occurs in rheumatic carditis and as a complication of some acute infectious diseases.

fibroadenoma a benign (non-malignant)

tumour of glandular and fibrous tissue. Most breast lumps in young women are fibroadenomas and are harmless but, unfortunately, cannot reliably be distinguished from cancers and should always be removed for examination.

fibroblast a cell that generates the protein COLLAGEN, a major component of connective tissue and the main structural material of the body. Fibroblasts are important in wound healing. They can readily be cultured artificially.

fibroblast growth factors a family of peptide regulators produced by virtually all cells. Their range of actions is wide. Only some are stimulators of the collagen-producing cells, the fibroblasts. Other effects include strong stimulation of vascular endothelial cell proliferation. Some are produced in relatively large quantities by brain tumours. Hope for people paralysed by spinal cord injuries has been raised by the discovery that a measure of rejoining in severed spinal cord tracts in rats can be achieved using a fibrin 'glue' containing a fibroblast growth factor. A mutation in the gene for a fibroblast growth factor receptor can cause CRANIOSYOSTOSIS.

fibrocartilage a tough form of CARTILAGE containing many thick bundles of COLLAGEN fibres.

fibrochondritis inflammation of FIBROCARTILAGE.

fibrocystic 1 containing fibrous tissue and cysts. 2 pertaining to a tumour of fibrous tissue, such as a FIBROMA, which has undergone degeneration with the formation of fluid-filled spaces. 3 pertaining to CYSTIC FIBROSIS.

fibroid a common, benign (non-malignant), tumour of fibrous and muscular tissue growing in the wall of the womb (uterus) usually in women over 30. A leiomyoma. Fibroids are often multiple and may become very large and cause INFERTILITY. They often cause pain and heavy menstrual periods. They may be removed surgically if causing trouble.

fibrolase an enzyme found in the venom of the American copperhead snake that degrades fibrin and fibrinogen directly and is being studied as a possible treatment for occlusive arterial disease or venous thrombosis.

fibroma a non-malignant tumour of fibrous tissue.

fibromatosis the simultaneous occurrence of a number of tumour-like collections of fibrous tissue that actively spread to cause damage, such as KELOID formation in the skin, nodules and contractures in the palms of the hands and feet, scarring in the COLON and distortion of the penis on erection.

fibromyalgia syndrome a condition featuring long-persisting general aches and pains, stiffness, fatigue and a considerable number of different points on the body that are tender to pressure. The condition affects women far more often than men. The cause is unknown and extensive investigations show no definite objective abnormality. Some experts believe that this is a psychiatric condition but the psychological problems it features are not typical of any such disorder.

fibromyoma see LEIOMYOMA.

fibronectins a family of glycoproteins occurring on cell surfaces, in most basement membranes and in blood and other body fluids. They are binding molecules that link to specific receptors on and within cells. They are involved in platelet aggregation and in the determination of cell shape and the formation of tissues. Fibronectin inhibitor drugs have been developed.

fibroplasia the formation and spread of fibrous tissue, as occurs in wound healing. See also RETROLENTAL FIBROPLASIA.

fibrosarcoma an uncommon malignant tumour of the cells that form fibrous tissue (fibroblasts). These cells are found in all parts of the body, and the tumour may affect almost any tissue, including bone, but is commonest in the leg or buttock. Radical surgery is necessary.

fibrosing alveolitis a serious lung disorder involving extensive fine scarring of, and numerous cells within, the air sacs (alveoli) of the lungs. The condition can be caused by exposure to asbestos dust, mineral dusts, fungal spores and powdered bird droppings; rheumatic disorders such as RHEUMATOID ARTHRITIS, SJÖGREN'S SYNDROME and systemic sclerosis; some of the anticancer drugs such as bleomycin and cyclophosphamide; and the heart drug amiodarone. The condition may require lung transplantation.

fibrosis scarring and thickening of any tissue or organ by the replacement of the original structure by simple collagenous FIBROUS TISSUE.

This usually follows injury or inflammation. Fibrosis is the body's main healing process and the scar tissue formed is usually strong.

fibrositis an imaginary disease that provides doctors with a plausible explanation for symptoms they cannot account for. Most cases are stress-induced muscle or tendon pain without organic abnormality. Such symptoms can sometimes be abolished by an injection of sterile water into the affected areas.

fibrous dysplasia see FIBROMATOSIS.

fibrous protein a class of insoluble proteins in the form of collagen fibrils that constitute the main structural elements of the body, especially as bone matrix, tendons, ligaments and other connective tissue. See also FIBROUS TISSUE.

fibrous tissue a simple, strong structural or repair tissue consisting of twisted stands of COLLAGEN and laid down by cells known as fibroblasts. These are among the commonest cells in the body and occur everywhere. Tissue damaged beyond recovery by disease processes is replaced by fibrous tissue (scar tissue).

fibrovascular pertaining to fibrous tissue with a good blood supply.

Fibro-vein a brand name for SODIUM TETRADECYL SULPHATE.

fibula the slender bone on the outer side of the main bone of the lower leg (tibia). The fibula is fixed to the tibia by ligaments and helps to form the ankle joint, below, but plays little part in weight-bearing.

FICS *abbrev. for* Fellow of the International College of Surgeons.

fievre boutonneuse a mild, tick-borne fever caused by the organism *Rickettsia conorii* and featuring a button-like black spot at the site of the bite, swollen lymph nodes, muscle pain, headache and a widespread skin rash. Also known as boutonneuse fever or Marseilles fever.

fight *or* **flight response** the general activation of the sympathetic nervous system in response to stress.

FIHA *abbrev. for* Fellow of the Institute of Hospital Administrators.

filamentous bacteria bacteria that take the form of branching filaments resembling the hyphae of fungi. The most important group is that of the *Actinomycetales*, which cause ACTINOMYCOSIS.

filariasis a group of parasitic worm diseases transmitted by mosquitos and other biting flies in tropical Africa, South-east Asia, the South Pacific and parts of South America. The insect vector injects large numbers of microscopic worms (microfilariae) into the blood and these settle in the tissues and grow into adult worms of from 2 to 50 cm in length. These breed thousands of new microfilariae which enter the blood and are taken up by insects and carried to other people. The filarial diseases include river blindness (ONCHOCERCIASIS), LOA-LOA and CALABAR SWELLINGS. Repeated infection with worms that inhabit the lymphatics causes blockage and ELEPHANTIASIS.

filaricide a drug that kills filarial worms. See FILARIASIS.

filgrastim human GRANULOCYTE-STIMULATING FACTOR produced by genetic engineering and used to treat severe deficiencies of some of the white cells of the blood and the immune system. A brand name is Neupogen.

filiform thread-like, as in the case of the filiform PAPILLAE of the tongue or filiform warts.

film badge a small light-tight container for a piece of photographic film which is carried, pinned to the clothing, by all staff in X-ray and radiotherapy departments. The films are regularly developed and a fogged film indicates that accidental exposure to radiation has occurred. The matter is then investigated.

filmless radiography see DIGITAL RADIOGRAPHY.

filterable virus a term with an interesting history. Originally, the term 'virus' simply meant a poison or 'morbid principle'. When it was discovered that an agent capable of causing disease could pass in a liquid through a very fine filter that would hold back bacteria, the agent was called a 'filterable virus'. In fact, the agent was what we now call a virus – a term derived by the inevitable abbreviation of popular usage.

filtrate the portion of material placed in a filter that passes through.

fimbriated fringed with finger-like processes, as at the open end of the FALLOPIAN TUBE.

finasteride an anti-androgen drug used to reduce prostate enlargement in benign prostatic hypertrophy by inhibiting the enzyme 5-alpha reductase which is concerned in the conversion of TESTOSTERONE to dihydrotestosterone, the main prostate androgen. Like all testosterone antagonists this drug can cause reduced sexual interest, impotence, ejaculation problems, breast tenderness and breast enlargement (gynecomastia). In a trial involving nearly 19,000 men the drug was found to reduce the incidence of prostate cancer by a quarter. A brand name is Proscar.

finger clubbing swelling of the ends of the fingers so that the normal depression just behind the root of the nail is replaced by a convexity. The nails can be rocked slightly on their abnormally spongy beds. Finger clubbing occurs in various disorders such as lung cancer, BRONCHIECTASIS, CONGENITAL HEART DISEASE and CIRRHOSIS of the liver. It is associated with conditions in which the supply of oxygen to the tissues is poor and often accompanies CYANOSIS. Clubbing also affects the toes.

fingerprint 1 the unique pattern printed by the ridges of epidermis on the pulpy surfaces of the ends of the fingers and thumbs.
2 of a protein, the pattern of fragments exposed by electrophoresis after splitting with a proteolytic enzyme such as trypsin.
3 of DNA, a pattern of varying-length (polymorphic) restriction fragments that differs from one individual to another and that can be used as a means of unique identification.
4 of a protein, the pattern of fragments produced on a plane surface when a protein is digested by a protein-splitting enzyme. See also DNA FINGERPRINTING.

first aid measures taken by those at the scene of an accident, or those present when a medical emergency occurs, to minimize the risk to the victim before the arrival of a medically qualified person. The essentials are to ensure free breathing (secure the airway), to prevent unnecessary loss of blood, to avoid unnecessary displacement of blood from the heart and brain (treat shock), to splint fractures and to reduce the risk of infection.

first degree burn a mild, fully recoverable degree of burning causing only redness of the skin.

first messenger a HORMONE or NEUROTRANSMITTER operating outside a cell and interacting with a cell membrane receptor. The second messenger operates within the cell.

FISH *abbrev. for* fluorescence *in situ* hybridization. This is a technique for detecting and locating gene mutations and chromosome abnormalities.

fish oils oils containing the long-chain n-3

polyunsaturated fatty acids eicosapentaenoic acid and docosahexaenoic acid. When these are incorporated into the blood platelets instead of the usual arachidonic acid, it reduces their effect in promoting blood clotting in diseased arteries and thus protects against heart disease. A 29% reduction in total mortality has been reported in people eating at least two portions of fatty fish per week. These fatty acids are also believed to modulate potassium and calcium channels and have been found effective in controlling cardiac arrhythmias.

fishskin disease see ICHTHYOSIS.

fission splitting into parts. 1 the asexual reproductive process by which a single-celled organism or a single cell in a multicellular organism splits into two daughter cells.
2 an atomic event in which the nucleus of an atom splits into fragments, with the loss of a small quantity of matter and the evolution of radiational energy of at least 100 million electron volts (MV).

fissure a deep groove or furrow that divides an organ, such as the brain, into lobes.

fistula an abnormal communication between any part of the interior of the body and the surface of the skin, or between two internal organs. Fistulas may be present at birth (congenital) or may arise as a result of disease processes such as abscesses or cancer.

fit a sudden acute attack of any disorder, especially an epileptic seizure.

fitness the ability to undertake sustained physical exertion without undue breathlessness. Fitness is associated with a sense of physical and mental well being. The achievement of fitness is possible only by making regular demands on the body to perform physical tasks. As fitness improves the bulk and strength of the voluntary muscles and the force and pumping efficiency of the heart muscle increase. The respiratory muscles perform more effectively. The subject is able to perform more work within the limits of the rate at which oxygen is supplied by the lungs and circulation (aerobic exercise). Recovery from fatigue is more rapid, a higher degree of muscle tension can be attained, the muscles are able to utilize glucose and fatty acids in the presence of less insulin, and the liver is better able to maintain the supply of glucose to the blood, and hence to the muscles, during strenuous exercise. The energy-producing elements in the muscle cells (the mitochondria) increase in size and number.

fitting suffering a sudden attack or convulsion, such as an epileptic seizure.

fixation 1 any method of holding something in a fixed position, especially holding the broken fragments of a bone in proper alignment so that they will heal together in the correct positional relationship.
2 the accurate alignment of one or both eyes on a small object.
3 a psychoanalytic term meaning an excessively close attachment to an object or person, of a kind appropriate to an earlier, immature, stage of development. See also EXTERNAL FIXATOR.

fixator 1 a muscle being used to hold a body part in a certain position or to restrict its movement, usually so that other muscles may operate effectively.
2 a device, such as an EXTERNAL FIXATOR, used to maintain parts in alignment.

flaccid flabby, limp or soft. Lacking firmness vigour or energy.

flagellant a person who whips himself, or who is whipped by another, especially for purposes of sexual arousal and gratification.

flagellar pertaining to a whip-like structure (flagellum).

flagellation 1 the act or practice of whipping.
2 the arrangement of whip-like structures (flagellae) on an organism.

flagellum a long, whip-like, filamentary process used for locomotion and present on a number of PROTOZOA and other organism, especially the class *Mastigophora* that includes *Trichomonas vaginalis*, a common cause of vaginal discharge, and *Trypanosma* species that cause TRYPANOSOMIASIS.

Flagyl a brand name for METRONIDAZOLE.

Flagyl Compak a brand name for METRONIDAZOLE formulated with the antifungal drug nystatin.

flail chest a state of abnormal mobility of the chest wall due to rib fractures.

Flamazine a brand name for SILVER SULPHADIAZINE.

flap a partially detached segment of skin and underlying tissue, having an adequate blood supply, so that it can be extended or rotated to fill an adjacent tissue deficit. Flaps are still extensively used in plastic surgery.

flash burn an injury resulting from exposure to brief periods of high-intensity radiant heat.

flash pasteurization a method of ensuring the bacteriological safety of milk and other liquid foodstuffs by subjecting it briefly to temperatures of 110 °C.

flat foot the condition in which the normal longitudinal arch of the foot has collapsed. This is mainly due to weakness of the muscles that support the arch and this may result from prolonged standing leading to muscle fatigue, or from illness. The foot turns out and the condition tends to be painful while it is developing and painless thereafter. Treatment involves strengthening the weak muscles by exercises and support of the foot so that the arch is restored.

flatline an informal term for the state of a person whose medical monitoring equipment shows a flat line rather than the normal peaks and troughs. Such a person has recently died or is very near to death.

flat pelvis a pelvis with a reduced front-to-back brim diameter. A flat pelvis sometimes causes difficulty in delivery of the baby, especially if the mother is small. A platypelloid pelvis.

flatulence a sense of fullness and discomfort in the upper abdomen associated with a desire to belch, and usually caused by air swallowing. See also AEROPHAGY.

flatus gas discharged by way of the anus. The gas is a mixture of odourless nitrogen, carbon dioxide, hydrogen and methane, and a varying quantity of hydrogen sulphide, which is said to smell like rotten eggs. Hydrogen and methane are both inflammable, but the risk to non-smokers is small. The average person farts about 20 times a day.

flavin one of a range of water soluble yellow pigments that includes the vitamin RIBOFLAVIN. Flavins occur in the tissues as coenzymes of FLAVOPROTEINS.

flavivirus a member of the *Flavivirus* genus of the Flaviviridae family. Flaviviruses are arthropod-borne (arbor) viruses and can cause encephalitic or meningitic diseases including Japanese encephalitis, West Nile virus encephalitis, St. Louis encephalitis and Murray Valley encephalitis.

flavonoids a range of many thousands of lipid-soluble polyphenols of low molecular weight, ubiquitous in the plant kingdom. *In vitro* assays have shown flavonoids to possess antimicrobial, anti-allergic, anti-inflammatory, antithrombotic and anti-neoplastic power. They can modify the actions of numerous enzymes. Some are oestrogenic, some anti-thyroidal. The principal current interest in flavonoids relates to their antioxidant and free radical-scavenging properties which is believed to be the basis of the research findings that these compounds can reduce the risk of atherosclerosis and hence heart attacks and strokes by inhibiting low density lipoprotein oxidation, reducing platelet aggregation, or reducing damage from reperfusion after ischaemia. See also FRENCH PARADOX.

flavoproteins one of the subclasses in the class of proteins known as the chromoproteins because they are combined with a coloured group. In this case the coloured group is RIBOFLAVINE (riboflavin). The flavoproteins act as enzymes concerned with tissue respiration.

Flaxedil a brand name for GALLAMINE TRIETHIODIDE.

FLCO abbrev. for Fellow of the London College of Osteopathy.

FLCOM abbrev. for Fellow of the London College of Osteopathic Medicine.

fleas small, wingless insects of the order Siphonaptera, which feed on warm-blooded animals, including man. They have powerfully muscular hindlegs and have a remarkable jumping performance. The Oriental rat flea, Xenopsylla cheopis transmits bubonic PLAGUE from rats to humans. Rat fleas also transmit mouse typhus to humans. CHIGOES penetrate the feet and toes of people walking barefoot in certain tropical regions causing pain, swelling and infection. Most fleas are no more than a nuisance.

flecainide acetate a drug used to treat severe heart irregularities. A brand name is Tambocor.

flesh fly any one of the various flies in the genus Sarcophaga. These flies lay their eggs in wounds or sores. In some cases, such as the grey flesh flies, Wohlfahrtia, the larvae will even invade the unbroken skin causing severe damage to underlying tissues.

flexibilitas cerea a now rare manifestation of catatonic SCHIZOPHRENIA in which the affected persons limbs show a wax-like resistance to bending but are said to retain the position in which they are placed for many hours. Such

accounts are probably apocryphal.

Flexin Continus a brand name for INDOMETHACIN (indometacin).

flexion the act of bending of a joint or other part or the state of being bent. A bent part.

flexion reflex a sudden automatic withdrawal movement occurring in response to a painful stimulus and effected by the contraction of the flexor muscles of all the joints on the same side.

FLEXLic(USA) abbrev. for Federation Licensing Examination (USA).

flexor a muscle that bends (flexes) a joint. A muscle that straightens (extends) a joint is called an extensor.

flexure a bend, curve, angle or fold. The hepatic flexure in the large intestine (colon) is the angle near the liver between the vertical ascending colon and the roughly horizontal transverse colon.

flies insects with one pair of wings of the order Diptera. They include the MOSQUITOES, biting midges, biting blackflies, SANDFLIES, gadflies, blowflies, botflies, the Tse-tse fly and the common house fly Musca domestica.

flight of ideas a rapid succession of thoughts manifested by continuous and constantly shifting verbalization or loosely linked play on words. The ideas are generally connected. Flight of ideas is a feature of manic mood disorders.

floaters semitransparent, shadowy bodies seen in the field of vision, usually remote from the point of observation, and moving rapidly with eye movement. For centuries, floaters have been called 'muscae volitantes' because of their resemblance to flitting flies. Most floaters are shadows of developmental remnants in the jelly-like VITREOUS HUMOUR of the eye and are harmless. Sudden onset of very conspicuous dark floaters, especially if accompanied by flashes of light (phosphenes) suggest an incipient RETINAL DETACHMENT.

floating kidney an abnormally mobile kidney.

floating rib one of the two lowest pairs of short ribs that have no attachment at the front to the breastbone or the COSTAL CARTILAGES but end among the abdominal muscles.

flocculent having a fluffy, woolly or cloudy appearance, especially of a precipitate or suspension in a fluid.

flocculus a small projecting lobe of the CEREBELLUM lying on each side of its front surface on either side of the brainstem.

Flolan a brand name for EPOPROSTENOL.

Flomax MR a brand name for TAMSULOSIN.

Flopen a brand name for FLUCLOXACILLIN.

floppy infant syndrome a state of poor muscle tension (hypotonia) in a baby so that when it is supported face down, with a hand under the chest, it droops over the hand like an inverted 'U' instead of holding its head up and keeping its back straight. Hypotonia is an indication of one of many conditions including any serious illness or birth brain injury, DOWN'S SYNDROME, TURNER'S SYNDROME or MUSCULAR DYSTROPHY. Many floppy infants do not have any of these disorders, but the condition should always be investigated.

flora 1 the entire plant life of a region. 2 in medicine, the term is used to refer to the entire bacterial life of a region of the body, as in 'intestinal flora', 'oral flora', 'skin flora' or 'normal flora' (COMMENSALS). Although often free-moving, micro-organisms were not classified under fauna. This convenient usage originated at a time when all living things were either flora or fauna. It no longer complies with current biological classification; the bacteria and the cyanobacteria now have a kingdom of their own (Monera).

florid flushed, of ruddy complexion, rosy.

Florinef a brand name for FLUDROCORTISONE.

floss see DENTAL FLOSS.

flow cytometry a medical laboratory technique used in machines that automate the analysis of cells or cell nuclei that have been labelled with fluorescent dyes specific for certain substances. The cells are suspended in a fluid, move in a flow stream, and are illuminated by a laser beam of known wavelength. The emitted light from the fluorescent markers are detected by photomultiplier tubes. Up to six variables can be measured simultaneously.

flowmeter an instrument for measuring the rate of flow of a gas or liquid. Flowmeters are important in anaesthetic practice.

Floxapen a brand name for FLUCLOXACILLIN.

FLS *abbrev. for* Fellow of the Linnean Society.

flu see INFLUENZA.

Fluanxol a brand name for FLUPENTHIXOL (flupentixol).

flucloxacillin a semisynthetic PENICILLIN antibiotic, readily absorbed when taken by mouth and effective against organisms that produce penicillin-destroying enzymes (beta-lactamases). A brand name is Floxapen. Formulated with ampicillin it is marketed as Magnapen.

fluconazole a triazole antifungal drug that can be taken by mouth and used to treat generalized fungus infections. Vaginal thrush can be cleared with a single dose. The drug is well tolerated, has few side effects and is highly effective but injudicious use may lead to the development of drug resistance. The drug is on the WHO official list. A brand name is Diflucan.

flucytosine a drug used to treat fungus infections within the body. It can be taken by mouth and is effective against CRYPTOCOCCOSIS, chromomycosis and thrush (CANDIDIASIS). Side effects are minor.

fluctuant the property of yielding to alternate pressure by palpating fingers so as to suggest that the area being felt contains fluid. Fluctuation is often exhibited by a swelling. When an abscess, for instance, has fully developed, it tends to become fluctuant.

Fludara a brand name for FLUDARABINE.

fludarabine a CYTOTOXIC anti-cancer drug. A brand name is Fludara.

fludrocortisone a steroid drug with a minor anti-inflammatory action but with a powerful sodium-retaining effect, similar to that of ALDOSTERONE. It is thus useful in the treatment of ADDISON'S DISEASE, to replace aldosterone. The drug is on the WHO official list. A brand name is Florinef.

fluent aphasia a disorder of brain function in which articulation of speech and grammatical organization are preserved but comprehension and choice of words are defective. The condition is common after STROKE.

fluid mosaic model a widely accepted account of the structure of the cell membrane, as consisting of a two-molecule layer of phospholipid with proteins embedded in it. The phospholipid layer has the physical properties of a fluid.

flukes TREMATODE flatworms or platyhelminthes. Flukes are parasitic and some, such as Chlonorchis sinensis, the liver fluke, parasitize humans causing disease.

flumazenil a drug that opposes the action of BENZODIAZEPINE drugs and can be used to reverse their sedating effect. A brand name is Anexate.

flumethasone flumetasone, a CORTICOSTEROID

drug. A brand name of a preparation in which it is combined with an antibacterial drug is Locorten-Vioform.

flunisolide a CORTICOSTEROID drug used in the form of a spray to treat hay fever. A brand name is Syntaris.

flunitrazepam a BENZODIAZEPINE drug of moderate length of action used for short periods to treat insomnia. A brand name is ROHYPNOL. The drug has acquired notoriety because of the frequency with which it has been added illegally to alcoholic drinks as an aid to rape.

fluocinolone a powerful CORTICOSTEROID drug used for external applications. A brand name is Synalar. It is marketed with other ingredients as Synalar C and Synalar N.

fluocinonide a powerful CORTICOSTEROID drug used externally to treat severe inflammatory disorders of the skin. A brand name is Metosyn.

fluocortolone a CORTICOSTEROID drug used externally. Brand names are Ultralanum and, with the local anaesthetic CINCHOCAINE to relieve symptoms of haemorrhoids, Ultraproct.

fluorescein a green dye that fluoresces bright yellow in blue or ultraviolet light. It is used to tag (label) and thus show up ANTIBODIES in tissues. It is also much used by eye specialists (ophthalmologists) to show up ulcers on the cornea and to delineate for photography the blood vessels of the retina. For the latter purpose, the dye is injected rapidly into the bloodstream (fluorescein angiography). The drug is on the WHO official list. Brand names are fluorescein, Minims fluorescein, Minims lignocaine (lidocaine, a local anaesthetic) and fluorescein, and Minims proxymetacaine (a local anaesthetic) and fluorescein.

Fluorescein a brand name for FLUORESCEIN.

fluorescein isothiocyanate (FITC) a fluorescing dye used to label antibodies in immunofluorescence tests and research techniques.

fluorescence emission of electromagnetic radiation, especially coloured visible light, during the period of absorption of radiation, which is often of a different frequency from the emitted radiation. Some substances, for instance, fluoresce visibly under ambient invisible ultraviolet light.

fluorescent antibody an antibody to which a small quantity of a fluorescent dye, especially fluorescein isothiocyanate (FITC), has been attached (conjugated).

fluorescent antibody test a laboratory test for the identification of a wide range of infective and other agents for which specific antibodies, linked to fluorescein, are held. The observation of fluorescence demonstrates that the antibody has attached to the corresponding substance (ANTIGEN), which must therefore be present.

fluoridation deliberate addition of fluorine compounds to drinking water supplies in areas in which the water is low in fluoride. The presence of about one part of fluoride per million parts of water promotes stronger and healthier teeth with reduced tendency to tooth decay. Fluoridation is a valuable public health measure.

Fluorigard a brand name for FLUORIDE intended for use as a fluorine supplement.

fluorine-18 a radioactive isotope of the element fluorine with a short half-life. Fluorine-18 is used as a tracer.

fluorine poisoning see FLUOROSIS.

fluorocarbons various organic compounds in which fluorine replaces hydrogen. The fluorocarbons are widely used as aerosol propellants, refrigerants and solvents and their release into the atmosphere is believed to offer a grave threat to the ecology of the planet because of their catalytic effect on the ozone layer. See also CHLOROFLUOROCARBONS.

fluorometholone a corticosteroid drug in the form of eye drops used to treat inflammatory external eye disorders. A brand name is FML.

fluoroscope an X-ray viewing fluorescent screen allowing continuous viewing of internal structure of the body in conditions of low illumination. Fluoroscopy has been largely replaced by IMAGE INTENSIFIER methods.

fluorosis poisoning with repeated large doses of the element fluorine. This may affect aluminium ore (bauxite) miners and workers involved in insecticide and phosphate fertilizer manufacture. The calcium in the bones is gradually replaced by fluorine and the bones become soft and crumbly. Abnormal bone protrusions occur and these may cause trouble, especially in the spine, where they may press on the spinal cord or nerve roots.

fluorouracil a pyrimidine anticancer drug. The drug is on the WHO official list.

fluoxetine an antidepressant drug that acts by

prolonging the action of the NEUROTRANSMITTER 5-hydroxytryptamine (5HT or serotonin). It is a SELECTIVE SEROTONIN RE-UPTAKE INHIBITOR. It is taken by mouth. This drug is currently being taken by some 10 million people, mainly in the USA, and is said to be the most popular psychoactive drug in the history of pharmacology. It has attracted a great deal of attention as a 'mood brightener' and enhancer of optimism. It is claimed to be capable of altering personality for the better. Possible side effects include nausea, vomiting, diarrhoea, insomnia, anxiety, outbursts of violence, fever, skin rash and convulsions. This drug can interact dangerously, even fatally, with MAOIs. A brand name is Prozac.

flupenthixol flupentixol, a phenothiazine-like (thioxanthene) antipsychotic drug used to treat schizophrenia and other psychotic disorders. Brand names are Depixol and Fluanxol.

fluphenazine a PHENOTHIAZINE derivative drug used in the treatment of psychotic conditions. It can be given by injection for long-term effect. The drug is on the WHO official list. Brand names are Modecate and Moditen. The drug is also formulated with other psychoactive substances and produced under the brand names of Modecate, Moditen and, with nortriptylene, Motival.

flurandrenolone fludroxycortide, a moderately powerful CORTICOSTEROID drug used externally to treat inflammatory skin disorders. A brand name is Haelan.

flurazepam a long-acting BENZODIAZEPINE drug. A brand name is Dalmane.

flurbiprofen a NON-STEROIDAL ANTI-INFLAMMATORY DRUG (NSAID). Brand names are Froben, Froben SR, Ocufen, Strefen and Streflam.

flutamide a drug that opposes male sex hormones (androgens) and is used to treat advances cancer of the prostate gland. Brand names are Chimax and Drogenil.

fluticasone a CORTICOSTEROID drug used as an inhalant to treat ASTHMA and hay fever. Extensive studies have shown that fluticasone is safe and effective and, in the recommended dosage, does not affect growth in childhood. Brand names are Flixonase (nasal spray), Flixotide (inhaler) and, for external use only, Cutivate. With SALMETEROL it is marketed as Seretide.

fluvastatin a statin drug (see STATINS) that blocks the synthesis of cholesterol in the body and can be used to lower unduly high blood cholesterol levels. A brand name is Lescol.

fluvoxamine a SELECTIVE SEROTONIN RE-UPTAKE INHIBITOR drug. An anti-depressant drug that acts by prolonging the action of the NEUROTRANSMITTER 5-hydroxytryptamine (5HT). A brand name is Faverin.

fly agaric a poisonous mushroom, *Amanita muscaria*. It usually has a red or orange cap with white spots.

FMC *abbrev. for* Fellow of the Medical Council.

FMCGP(Nigeria) *abbrev. for* Fellow of the Medical Council of General Practitioners (Nigeria).

FML a brand name for FLUOROMETHOLONE.

FML-NEO a brand name for FLUOROMETHOLONE formulated with neomycin.

foam contraceptive a vaginal preparation of a SPERMICIDE substance, usually dispensed in a pressurized container that produces a foam. Substances used include benzethonium and nonoxinol-9. Foams are unreliable alone and should be used only in conjunction with a BARRIER CONTRACEPTIVE method. See also CONTRACEPTION.

focal localized and circumscribed.

focal sepsis infection present, or assumed to be present, in a limited area of the body, such as the teeth, tonsils or sinuses. In the past, all sorts of disorders were said to be due to focal sepsis, but as medical knowledge has grown, such attribution has become rare.

foetus the widely-used but incorrect spelling of FETUS.

Fogarty catheter a CATHETER with a small inflatable balloon at the tip, used to remove a THROMBUS or an EMBOLUS from an artery. The uninflated balloon is pushed past the obstruction, inflated, and the catheter is then withdrawn, bringing the obstruction with it. (Thomas J. Fogarty, American thoracic surgeon, b. 1934).

folates see FOLIC ACID.

folic acid a vitamin of the B group originally derived from spinach leaves, hence the name (Latin *folium*, a leaf). The vitamin is necessary for the synthesis of DNA and red blood cells. Deficiency causes MEGALOBLASTIC ANAEMIA. Folic acid is plentiful in leafy vegetables and in liver but is also produced by bacteria in the bowel and then absorbed into the circulation.

Deficiency may occur after antibiotic treatment. Folic acid taken immediately before pregnancy and during the first few weeks can virtually eliminate the risk of embryonic neural tube defects and resulting SPINA BIFIDA or ANENCEPHALY in the baby. It will also reduce the risk of CLEFT PALATE. Normal dietary intake may not provide enough for this purpose. It has been reported, however, (January 2004) that women whose babies have neural tube defects have serum autoantibodies to folate receptors. The drug is on the WHO official list. The drug is available under the brand name Lexpec and, in conjunction with iron salts under the brand names Lexpec with iron, Folex-350, Meterfolic and Pregaday, Ferfolic SV, Ferrograd Folic, Galfer F.A., Meterfolic and Slow-Fe Folic.

folic acid antagonists drugs used to treat RHEUMATOID ARTHRITIS, PSORIASIS and various cancers. An example is methotrexate (Maxtrex).

folie à deux a rare delusional psychotic disorder affecting two, usually isolated, people who gain mutual advantage from the situation. It is sometimes called 'shared paranoid disorder'. The more dominant of the two has a delusional psychosis and the submissive person gains the approval of the other by accepting the delusions. At the same time, the dominant person retains some link with the real world through the medium of the partner. Cases ranging from *folie à trois* to *folie à douze* have been reported.

folinic acid a drug used to treat MEGALOBLASTIC ANAEMIA that has resulted from folic deficiency. A brand name is Refolinon.

folk medicine systems of medical treatment based on anecdotal tradition, empiricism and often magic, rather than experimental validation. Folk medicine is part of the cultural tradition of all societies and has, in the past, commanded wide support. Some folk remedies have had medical value, but most have been based on superstition and primitive associational reasoning; for instance, a plant root that resembles a pregnant woman might be deemed to be 'good for' pregnancy sickness.

follicle a sac-like depression or cavity, glandular or cystic in nature. Follicles may secrete new tissues as in the case of hair follicles, which synthesize and extrude hairs, and the Graafian follicles of the ovaries, which contain the eggs (ova) prior to ovulation.

follicle-stimulating hormone (FSH) a pituitary gland hormone that stimulates the Graafian follicles in the ovaries to produce eggs (ova), and the lining cells of the tubules in the testicles to produce sperms (spermatozoa). FSH may be used to treat infertility due to failure of ovulation (anovulatory infertility) or to low sperm counts. The secretion rate of follicle-stimulating hormone is controlled by feed-back of a polypeptide substance called inhibin, which is produced by the ovaries and the testicles.

follicular pertaining to, or resembling, a follicle.

folliculitis inflammation of hair FOLLICLES causing multiple small boils or pimples. The inflammation usually results from STAPHYLOCOCCAL INFECTIONS.

follitropin alpha a gonadotropin, a drug that promotes ovulation and is used to treat infertility resulting from absence of ovulation.

follitropin beta a drug that stimulated the ovaries into producing eggs and is used to treat infertility. More recently, the drug has been found to be useful in the treatment of male infertility due to hypogonadotrophic hypogonadism. A brand name is Puregon.

FOM *abbrev. for* Faculty of Occupational Medicine.

fomentation a warm, moist compress or poultice, or the application of warmth and moisture for medical purposes. Fomentation causes an increase in the blood supply to the underlying area and this can be helpful in treating inflammation.

fomites anything that has been in contact with a person suffering from an infectious disease, and which may transmit the infection to others. Fomites include sheets, towels, dressings, clothes, face flannels, crockery and cutlery, books and papers.

fondaparinux one of a new class of antithrombotic drugs used to prevent deep vein THROMBOSIS during major surgery. The drug is an inhibitor of activated Factor X which is a key enzyme in the coagulation cascade. It has been found effective in the management of pulmonary embolism. A brand name is Arixtra.

fontanelles the gaps between the bones of the vault of the growing skull of the baby and young infant that can be felt, as soft depressions on the top of the head, by gentle pressure with the fingers. The front (anterior) fontanelle lies at the junction of the two forehead (frontal) bones and the two side (parietal) bones. The rear (posterior) fontanelle lies between the two parietal bones and the single rear occipital bone. The fontanelles are covered by scalp and skin and allow moulding of the skull during birth. Both have usually closed by about 14 months. There are two other very small fontanelles on either side of the head.

food additives substances, numbered in thousands, added to food for purposes of preservation, appearance, flavour, texture or nutritional value. Without additives, much food would soon be spoiled and wasted. Common additives include vitamins, minerals and trace elements in bread, cereals, milk, margarine, table salt, fruit drinks and baby foods. Flavouring and colourings include sugar, salt, mustard, pepper, monosodium glutamate and tartrazine. Preservatives include salt, sugar, sodium nitrite, sodium benzoate, and the anti-oxidants BHT (butylated hydroxytoluene) and BHA (butylated hydroxyanisole).

food allergy sensitivity to one or more of the components of normal diets. Food allergy is much less common than unscientific claims might suggest and established methods of testing, including DOUBLE-BLIND TRIALS have shown that food allergy is not the basis of the many disorders commonly claimed to arise from it. PEANUT ALLERGY is becoming more common and may be dangerous. Monosodium glutamate can cause the 'CHINESE RESTAURANT SYNDROME'. Tartrazine sensitivity is established. Other additives, such as sulphur dioxide, sulphites, azo dyes and benzoate preservatives also sometimes cause genuine allergic reactions, such as asthma. Allergy to basic foodstuffs seldom occurs.

food irradiation deliberate exposure of food to strong ionizing radiation, such as gamma rays, to kill bacteria and insect pests and delay natural changes. Irradiation does not eliminate bacterial poisons (toxins) already formed or kill viruses, but irradiation of food tightly sealed in a suitable container, such as a polythene bag, will kill contained bacteria and further contamination does not occur. Food irradiation by gamma rays does not induce radioactivity; the effects are chemical only and may include changes in flavour and some loss of vitamins.

food poisoning a group of intestinal disorders caused either by living organisms present in food or by contamination of food by the toxins of organisms which have incubated outside the body, as from septic skin infection in food handlers. The commonest bacterial contamination of food is by *Salmonella typhimurium*, which may be found in meats and eggs. Food handled by the unconcerned is often contaminated by human faeces. Toxins in food, such as staphylococcal toxin from finger infections such as boils, cause symptoms within hours. Organisms in food cause symptoms within 2 or 3 three days. The effects are nausea, vomiting, loss of appetite, fever, abdominal pain and diarrhoea. Food poisoning can also be caused by poisonous fungi, such as *Amanita phalloides*, or berries eaten in error.

foot drop loss of the ability to bend the ankle so that the foot rises. This may be due to disorders of the lower spinal cord or of the nerves to the muscles that flex the ankle. Foot drop seriously interferes with walking. A foot brace may be necessary.

foot rot a slang term for TINEA (epidermophytosis) of the feet (tinea pedis).

Foradil a brand name for EFORMOTEROL (formoterol).

foramen a natural hole in a bone for the passage of a nerve, artery or a vein or other anatomical structure.

foramen magnum the large, almost circular hole in the centre of the base of the skull through which the spinal cord, the continuation of the medulla oblongata, passes.

foramen ovale a valve-like opening in the inner wall (septum) between the right and left upper chambers (atria) of the heart of the fetus. Before birth, about three quarters of the blood returning from the body to the right side of the heart is shunted through the foramen ovale to the left side. After birth, the pressure on the left side rises and the foramen valve closes. Soon it fuses shut.

forced expiratory volume (FEV) a measurement made with an instrument that measures expired air flow (a recording SPIROMETER). Forced expiratory volume is the maximum volume of air that can be breathed out in one second. The FEV is then compared with the maximum amount that can be breathed out in a single breath, however prolonged (the VITAL CAPACITY). The ratio FEV/VC should exceed 70% in healthy individuals but is much reduced in people with any condition that narrows the air tubes (obstructive airway disease), such as ASTHMA or chronic BRONCHITIS.

forced vital capacity the amount of air that can be expelled from the lungs by breathing out for as long as possible after a full inspiration. See also FORCED EXPIRATORY VOLUME.

forceps surgical instruments made in a wide variety of sizes and designs for different purposes, but all having opposing blades or surfaces, that are smooth, serrated or toothed, and that can be pressed together. Forceps are used to grasp or compress tissue, to extract objects, or to hold needles, swabs, LIGATURES or other medical items.

forceps delivery delivery of a baby assisted by traction on the head with obstetrical forceps after the neck of the womb (cervix) is fully widened (dilated). Forceps are used in the event of long delay in the stage after the cervix is fully dilated (the second stage of labour), if there is FETAL DISTRESS, if there is exhaustion of, or danger to, the mother (maternal distress), or if the fetus is very small and the head is liable to be damaged during passage through the vagina.

forensic medicine the application of medical science in the investigation of crime. Forensic scientists are familiar with disease processes (pathology), with the signs of assault, including rape, with some aspects of dentistry, with the action of poisons (toxicology), with the effects of firearms and other offensive weapons and with the principles of determining the time of death. They are concerned with human identification by DNA analysis, and with the evidential significance of skin scrapings, hair, seminal fluid, blood, natural and synthetic fibres, paint chips, dust, soil and many other materials. Forensic medicine is also known as medical jurisprudence or legal medicine.

forensic psychiatry the medical discipline concerned with such matters as criminal intent and the capacity to form it (see INSANITY); criminal evidence and the vulnerability of suspects; the investigation of possible wrongful convictions; confessions and how they are obtained; the psychopathology of sexual offenders; and the risks of schizophrenics in the community.

foreskin the prepuce or hood of thin skin that covers the bulb (glans) of the penis. Surgical

removal of the foreskin is called CIRCUMCISION and this is widely practised, usually for ritual or cultural reasons. The medical indications for circumcision are few.

forgetfulness the usual natural consequence of inattention or of overburdening a well-stocked mind with trivia. Failure to retrieve a memory becomes more likely the larger the number of similar memories that depend on the same cues. Abnormal (pathological) forgetfulness is the main feature of DEMENTIA and of AMNESIA.

forme fruste a disease at an early stage, or arrested by treatment, prior to the development of its full characteristics.

formication a strange 'crawling' sensation, as of ants on or under the skin, characteristic of the toxic effects of various drugs or of certain disorders of the nervous system. The word should be pronounced with care.

formoterol a long-acting beta-2 agonist drug that can be used in ASTHMA patients on inhaled steroids who continue to have symptoms. Brand names are Foradil, Oxis Turbohaler and, with BUDESONIDE, Symbicort.

formulary originally, a collection of formulas used in the preparation of medicines, but now used for a book of drug actions, side effects and dosage for the use of prescribing doctors. The *British National Formulary*, produced at regular intervals by the British Medical Association and the Pharmaceutical Society of Great Britain, is an attempt to encourage rational and cost-effective prescribing by doctors.

formulation the process of preparing a drug in a particular way or in a specific form, such as a tablet, capsule, linctus, ointment, or for one of the various forms of injection.

fornix an arch, especially one of the pair of arch-like bands of white fibres lying under the corpus callosum of the brain, or the space between the upper walls of the vagina and the neck of the womb.

Forsteo a brands name for TERIPARATIDE.

Fortagesic a brand name for a mixture of PARACETAMOL and PENTAZOCINE.

Fortipine LA a brand name for NIFEDIPINE.

Fortral a brand name for PENTAZOCINE.

Fortum a brand name for CEFTAZIDIME.

Fosamax a brand name for ALENDRONATE.

foscarnet a DNA POLYMERASE INHIBITOR drug used to treat severe herpes infections in immunocompromised people and cytomegalovirus internal eye infections in people with AIDS. A brand name is Foscavir.

Foscavir a brand name for FOSCARNET.

fosinopril an ANGIOTENSIN CONVERTING ENZME (ACE) inhibitor drug used to treat HEART FAILURE and high blood pressure (HYPERTENSION). A brand name is Staril.

fosphenytoin sodium a drug used to treat STATUS EPILEPTICUS and to prevent seizures following neurosurgery and head injury. A brand name is Pro-epanutin.

fossa a furrow or depression, especially in bone.

Foster Kennedy syndrome pallor and loss of nerve fibres in the optic nerve (optic atrophy) in one eye and swelling of the head of the optic nerve (papilloedema) in the other. This occurs if a tumour at the front of the brain compresses one optic nerve but, at the same time, causes a rise in the pressure inside the skull leading to oedema of the uncompressed nerve. (Robert Foster Kennedy, 1884–1952, American neurologist).

fourchette the small fold of skin joining the back ends of the LABIA MINORA. The fourchette is often torn during childbirth.

fourth ventricle the centrally placed, rearmost of the four fluid-filled spaces in the brain. This tent-shaped cavity for cerebrospinal fluid lies immediately behind the PONS of the brainstem and immediately in front of the CEREBELLUM. It communicates with the aqueduct of the midbrain, in front, and with the central canal of the spinal cord, below.

fovea any shallow cup-like depression. The fovea centralis of the RETINA is the central area of the macula lutea, of highest resolution and free of visible blood vessels.

foveal vision perception of objects whose images fall on the FOVEA centralis – the most discriminating part of the RETINA. Also known as photopic vision.

FPA *abbrev. for* Family Planning Association.

FPC *abbrev. for* Family Practitioner Committee.

FPHM *abbrev. for* Faculty of Public Health Medicine.

FPS *abbrev. for* Fellow Pharmaceutical Society.

FRACDS *abbrev. for* Fellow of the Royal Australasian College of Dental Surgery.

FRACGP *abbrev. for* Fellow of the Royal Australian College of General Practitioners.

FRACO *abbrev. for* Fellow of the Royal Australasian College of Ophthalmologists.

FRACOG *abbrev. for* Fellow of the Royal Australian College of Obstetricians & Gynaecologists.

FRACP *abbrev. for* Fellow of the Royal Australasian College of Physicians.

FRACR *abbrev. for* Fellow of the Royal Australasian College of Radiologists.

FRACS *abbrev. for* Fellow of the Royal Australasian College of Surgeons.

fracture a break, usually of a bone. This occurs when excessive force is applied to a healthy bone or when lesser force is applied to a bone generally weakened by a disease such as OSTEOPOROSIS, or locally weakened by a tumour or cyst. Such a fracture is called a pathological fracture. Fractures may be transverse, oblique or spiral, or the bone may be shattered into pieces (comminuted). Young bone, subjected to bending stress, often fractures on one side but bends on the other. This is called a 'greenstick' fracture. In simple fractures the overlying soft tissue is intact. In compound fractures, the fractured bone is exposed and infected. In complicated fractures there is also injury to other nearby structures such as major blood vessels and nerves. Fracture-dislocations pass across a joint and the normal relationship of the joint surfaces to one another is altered.

fractured femur a break in any part of the thigh bone, most commonly of the short neck between the top of the bone and the near-spherical head, in elderly people with OSTEOPOROSIS. Fracture of the shaft of the femur usually results from severe violence and there is often major loss of blood into the tissues causing surgical SHOCK.

fragile X syndrome a major genetic disorder caused by a constriction near the end of the long arm of an X CHROMOSOME that leads to breakage or deletion. The fragile X syndrome is second only to DOWN'S SYNDROME as a cause of mental defect. Affected men have unusually high foreheads, unbalanced faces, large jaws, long protruding ears and large testicles. They have an IQ below 50 and are prone to violent outbursts. Folic acid helps to control their behaviour. About one-third of the females with this mutation on one of their two X chromosomes are also mentally retarded. Screening for the characteristic chromosome can be done by AMNIOCENTESIS or CHORIONIC VILLUS SAMPLING.

fragilitas ossium a congenital brittle bone disease associated with blueness of the whites of the eyes due to unusual thinning of the SCLERA. Also known as OSTEOGENESIS IMPERFECTA.

Fragmin a brand name for DALTEPARIN SODIUM.

framboesia see YAWS.

frame-shift mutation a genetic mutation caused by the addition or deletion of a number of NUCLEOTIDES other than three. Because the genetic code consists of codons (groups of three nucleotides), such a change shifts the reading frame for translation so all adjacent codons are changed and a completely new set is read into the messenger ribonucleic acid (mRNA).

framycetin an antibiotic drug used externally for skin infections or as eye or ear drops. Brand names are Sofradex and Soframycin.

frangula a drug for constipation. Formulated with the bulking agent sterculia it is produced under the brand name Normacol Plus.

Franol, Franol Plus brand names for EPHEDRINE formulated with other drugs.

Frantz' tumour a cystic tumour of the pancreas of low malignancy that appears to be largely confined to young women, especially those of African origin. The tumour presents as an abdominal mass and is usually well-localized and susceptible to surgery. (First described in 1959 by the American pathologist V.K. Frantz).

fraternal twins non-identical twins produced by the simultaneous fertilization of two different eggs by different sperms (dizygotic twins). In spite of the etymology, fraternal twins need not be male or even of the same sex.

FRANZCP *abbrev. for* Fellow of the Royal Australian & New Zealand College of Psychiatrists.

FRCD *abbrev. for* Fellow of the Royal College of Dentists.

FRCGP *abbrev. for* Fellow of the Royal College of General Practitioners.

FRCN *abbrev. for* Fellow of the Royal College of Nursing.

FRCOG *abbrev. for* Fellow of the Royal College of Obstetricians and Gynaecologists.

FRCOphth *abbrev. for* Fellow of the Royal College of Ophthalmology.

FRCP *abbrev. for* Fellow of the Royal College of Physicians.

FRCPA *abbrev. for* Fellow of the Royal College of Pathologists Australasia.

FRCPath *abbrev. for* Fellow of the Royal College of Pathologists.

FRCPC *abbrev. for* Fellow of the Royal College of Physicians of Canada.

FRCPE *abbrev. for* Fellow of the Royal College of Physicians, Edinburgh.

FRCPI *abbrev. for* Fellow of the Royal College of Physicians, Ireland.

FRCPS *abbrev. for* Fellow of the Royal College of Physicians & Surgeons.

FRCPsych *abbrev. for* Fellow of the Royal College of Psychiatrists.

FRCR *abbrev. for* Fellow of the Royal College of Radiologists.

FRCRA *abbrev. for* Fellow of the Royal College of Radiologists of Australasia.

FRCS *abbrev. for* Fellow of the Royal College of Surgeons.

FRCSE *abbrev. for* Fellow of the Royal College of Surgeons, Edinburgh.

FRCSI *abbrev. for* Fellow of the Royal College of Surgeons, Ireland.

freckle a small brownish or yellowish skin blemish due to local aggregation of cells containing melanin, the normal skin pigment. Melanin-containing cells enlarge under the influence of sunlight, especially in the fair-skinned and this is usually permanent.

free association a method used in psychoanalysis to derive data from the unconscious content of the mind. The subject articulates his or her spontaneous, and deliberately unrestricted, association of mental images.

free-floating anxiety a generalized anxiety disorder. A persistent and pervasive fear not produced by any conscious cause or associated with any particular idea. There is excessive or unrealistic worry about everything. Free-floating anxiety usually lasts for at least 6 months. It is thought to be due to a disturbance of the function of NEUROTRANSMITTERS such as adrenaline or GABA, in the frontal lobes or the limbic system of the brain.

free radicals highly chemically active atoms or group of atoms capable of free existence, under special conditions, for very short periods, each having at least one unpaired electron in the outer shell. Oxygen free radicals can be very damaging to DNA and proteins and to the fat in cell membranes where a free radical chain reaction can be set up. They are normally mopped up by ANTIOXIDANTS and associated substances such as vitamins E and C, FLAVONOIDS, selenium, copper, zinc, and manganese. Produced in excess, or insufficiently opposed, free radicals are believed to be implicated in the production of ATHEROSCLEROSIS, cancer, RHEUMATOID ARTHRITIS, radiation sickness and many other conditions. They are thought to be responsible for much of the damage to the heart during the reperfusion that follows a coronary thrombosis. They are said to be promoted by many agents including radiation, atmospheric pollutants and smoking. The body's natural antioxidants include superoxide dismutase and vitamins C and E. See also NANOPARTICLES.

Frei test a skin test for LYMPHOGRANULOMA VENEREUM, now of historic interest only. (Wilhelm Siegmund Frei, 1886–1943, German dermatologist).

fremitus vibration that can be felt by a hand placed on the chest during coughing or speaking. Fremitus is increased if the lung is solidified by PNEUMONIA or if there is a large cavity near the surface. It is diminished if the associated air tubes (bronchi) are blocked and absent if the lung is separated from the chest wall by fluid in the pleural space (pleural effusion).

French paradox an informal term for the unexplained fact that, in spite of a national diet characterized by a high fat and cholesterol intake, the French enjoy almost the lowest incidence of coronary heart disease in Europe. Possible explanations include the antioxidant effect of FLAVONOID substances in red wine and the protective effect of olive oil.

frenotomy cutting of a FRENUM.

frenulum any small fold of mucous membrane.

frenum a membranous fold or sheet, such as the fold of mucous membrane under the tongue, that restrains movement or provides support.

Freon a brand name for the CHLOROFLUOROCARBONS (CFCs) used in refrigeration and as aerosol propellants.

frequency an informal term referring to the condition in which urine is passed more often than normal (frequency of urination). Frequency may be due to excessive fluid intake, bladder infection, pregnancy, the use of DIURETIC drugs, or, in men, to an enlarged prostate gland obstructing the urinary outflow so that the bladder can only be partially emptied. Frequency is occasionally of psychological origin.

frequency coding a means by which the central nervous system, limited by the all-or-none properties of nerve impulse conduction, is able to convey information about varying intensity of signals. It does this by employing frequency modulation (FM). The frequency of impulses varies with the strength of the stimulus.

frequency distribution a table or histogram showing the number of times each value of a particular variable occurs in a sample.

Freudian slip a popular term for any minor error, or muddle, in speech or writing that appears to reveal an unconscious wish or preoccupation. Such slips are inevitable in the operation of any system as complex as that of the human mind, and while there are numerous obvious instances in which errors may display opinions and prejudices we are trying to conceal, there is no reason to accept Freud's claim that they are always significant. Freud used the term parapraxis. See also FREUDIAN THEORY. (Sigmund Freud, 1856–1939, Austrian neurologist and psychiatrist).

Freudian theory a set of propositions about human personality and behaviour derived from observations of patients engaged in FREE ASSOCIATION at a time in social history when the expression of sexuality was normally repressed. Such expression, often in symbolic form, convinced Freud that sex was at the basis of most psychopathology. He asserted that the uncovering of repressed unpleasant early experiences would disperse the psychopathology which he claimed they had caused. He proposed arbitrary divisions of the mind into SUPEREGO, EGO and ID. He asserted that infants pass though three stages – oral (birth to 18 months), anal (2–5 years) and phallic (5 years onward), and that the personality could be fixed at any of these stages with serious consequences, curable only by psychoanalysis. He proposed the OEDIPUS COMPLEX and the castration complex. Freud's ideas and discoveries continue to have wide influence, but are not now generally believed to have any scientific basis. There is little convincing evidence that the application of his theories in psychoanalysis has any specific value in the treatment of psychological disturbance.

Freund's adjuvant an emulsion of killed bacteria in oil that induces antibody formation. (Jules Thomas Freund, 1890–1960, Hungarian-born American bacteriologist).

FRFPS *abbrev. for* Fellow of the Royal Faculty of Physicians & Surgeons.

friable crumbly or brittle.

Friedlander's bacillus a bacterial organism, now know as *Klebsiella pneumoniae*, that causes pneumonia. (Karl Friedlander, 1847–1887, German bacteriologist).

Friedreich's ataxia an inherited disorder of the cerebellum and spinal cord causing unsteady gait (ataxia), defective movement of the upper limbs, defective speech, and loss of sensation. The spine becomes bent sideways (scoliosis), the feet become arched (pes cavus) and the heart muscle is damaged. The condition appears first in childhood or adolescence and cases vary greatly in severity. There is no effective treatment. (Nikolas Friedreich, 1826–82, German physician).

frigidity an informal term meaning loss, in a woman, of sexual desire or of the ability to be sexually aroused, or to achieve an orgasm. The term, the usage of which is almost confined to disappointed men, is now considered pejorative and sexist. The condition may be a reflection of lack of affection, or the expression of it, by the partner, or may be due to recent childbirth, pain on intercourse (DYSPAREUNIA), fatigue, depression, fear of pregnancy or psychological trauma following rape. Some drugs, especially those given for high blood pressure (HYPERTENSION), for depression and for insomnia, reduce libido.

FRIPHH *abbrev. for* Fellow of the Royal Institute of Public Health and Hygiene.

Frisium a brand name for CLOBAZAM.

Froben SR a brand name for FLURBIPROFEN.

Frohlich's syndrome the combination of obesity and under-development of the GONADS in children associated with a tumour affecting the PITUITARY GLAND. (Alfred Frolich, 1871–1953, Austrian pharmacologist and neurologist).

Froin's syndrome changes that occur in the cerebrospinal fluid (CSF) following a complete block in its circulation. The CSF below the block is of a yellow colour (xanthochromic), has a very high protein content and often clots on standing. (Georges Froin, 1874–1932, French neurologist).

frontal pertaining to the forehead or to the FRONTAL BONE.

frontal bone the skull bone that forms the forehead and the roofs of the eye sockets (orbits). The frontal bone contains the frontal sinuses.

frontal lobe the large, foremost part of the brain. This part constitutes about one-third of the brain and is much more fully developed than in any other primate. Damage to the frontal lobe causes general disturbance of thinking, impairment of initiative and spontaneity, loss of strength of personality, and, if the rear part of the lobe is affected, paralysis.

frontal nerve a sensory nerve that emerges from the eye socket, as a branch of the OPHTHALMIC NERVE, and curls up over the upper edge of the bone to supply the skin of the upper eyelid, the forehead, and the front of the scalp.

frontal sinus one of a pair of mucous membrane-lined air spaces of variable size lying behind and above the level of the eyebrows.

frostbite freezing of bodily tissues, especially the tips of the extremities. Expanding ice crystals damage the tissues and the local blood supply is cut off. The result is local tissue death (GANGRENE).

frottage a male activity in which the unexposed genitals are rubbed against the buttocks or thighs of another person, usually a female stranger, for purposes of sexual gratification. Frottage is engaged in in densely packed crowds, as in rush hour trains. Most frotteurs are sexually or socially inadequate people who cannot achieve a more satisfactory outlet for their desires.

frovatriptan a long-acting SEROTONIN agonist drug (see TRIPTANS) used to treat MIGRAINE. A brand name is Migard.

frozen section a method of obtaining a while-you-wait opinion on a BIOPSY specimen. The tissue block is frozen solid with dry ice so that thin slices can be cut, mounted on slides, stained and immediately examined under the microscope. Frozen sections are often called for in the course of an operation for suspected cancer. The result may radically alter the surgical procedure performed.

frozen shoulder painful, persistent stiffness of the shoulder joint that restricts normal movement. The condition affects middle-aged people and usually follows injury or over-enthusiastic exercising. It may also complicate a heart attack (MYOCARDIAL INFARCTION) or STROKE, or may occur for no known reason. It is due to inflammation of the capsule of the joint, leading to thickening, and usually settles spontaneously within 2 years.

FRS *abbrev. for* Fellow of the Royal Society.

FRSE *abbrev. for* Fellow of the Royal Society of Edinburgh.

FRSH *abbrev. for* Fellow of the Royal Society of Health.

FRSM *abbrev. for* Fellow of the Royal Society of Medicine.

FRS(R) *abbrev. for* Fellow of the Royal Society of Radiographers (Radiography).

FRS(T) *abbrev. for* Fellow of the Royal Society of Radiographers (Radiotherapy).

fructose one of the simplest forms of sugar (a monosaccharide) and derived from fruit, sugar cane, honey and sugar beet. Fructose, linked to another monosaccharide, glucose, form the disaccharide sucrose which is the common domestic sugar. Fructose is sweeter than glucose, but has the same energy value. It is readily absorbed. Fructose provides direct energy for spermatozoa and is found in seminal fluid.

fructosuria a rare genetic disorder in which the metabolism of the fruit sugar fructose is abnormal, leading to appearance of the sugar in the urine.

frusemide furosemide, a drug that causes an increased output of urine (a diuretic) so as to relieve the body of unwanted retained water (oedema). Furosemide is a loop diuretic. It acts on the kidney tubules where it interferes with chloride and sodium reabsorption from the dilute filtered urine. This prevents reabsorption of water into the blood and the result is a large volume of dilute urine. The drug is on the WHO official list. Brand names are Froop, Frusol, Frusix and Lasix. The drug is one of the ingredients in a range of diuretic preparations such as Diumide-K Continus, Fru-Co, Frumil, Frusene, Lasikal, Lasilatone and Lasoride.

Frusene a brand name for TRIAMTERENE in combination with another diuretic drug FRUSEMIDE (furosemide).

frustration the emotion resulting when aims or intentions are blocked. Frustration is inevitable but some people aim for goals inherently beyond their capacity and suffer a much higher level of frustration than others. Others aim for mutually incompatible, or equally attractive but mutually exclusive, goals. Frustration breeds anger which may lead to aggression and this is often displaced and directed against an inappropriate target. Displaced anger is a common cause of marital discord.

FSH *abbrev. for* FOLLICLE-STIMULATING HORMONE.

FTA-ABS test the fluorescent treponemal antibody-absorbed test. This is a sensitive test for SYPHILIS which it can demonstrate even if the disease is latent.

Fucidin a brand name for FUSIDIC ACID.

Fucithalmic a brand name for SODIUM FUSIDATE intended for the treatment of ocular infections.

fugue a rare psychological reaction to an intolerable situation in which the affected person wanders away from the old environment, apparently in a state of AMNESIA, and takes on a new identity, occupation and life. The loss of memory is selective and does not preclude use of the previous education. If there is recovery from the fugue, amnesia for the period of the fugue occurs.

Fulcin a brand name for GRISEOFULVIN.

fulguration destruction of tissue by DIATHERMY.

fulminating sudden, severe and following an intense rapid course. Fulminant.

fumigation a method formerly used to decontaminate sick rooms after infectious disease, but not now considered of much value. In other contexts, toxic gases, vapours or volatile solids are used to kill bacteria, insect pests or rodents in buildings and food stores. Poisons used include chlorine gas, organophosphorous agents and arsenic and cyanide compounds.

functional disorders see CONVERSION DISORDER.

functional dysphonia hoarseness of the voice caused by factors other than organic changes to the larynx, vocal cords or their nerve supply. Women are affected more often than men and most patients are young or middle aged introverted adults with a history of stressful events. The condition will usually respond to skilled speech therapy.

functional electrical stimulation the

application of pulsed or alternating electric current in order to cause natural contractions and maintain their health in expectation of recovery of spontaneous function.

fundus the inner surface of an organ furthest from the opening. The fundus of the eye is the inner area covered with the RETINA. The fundus of the uterus is the inner surface of the dome of the womb.

fungating forming an elevated, irregular growth mass. Commonly implying malignancy.

fungi a large group of spore-bearing organisms that derive their nourishment by decomposing non-living organic matter and absorbing nutrients through their surface (saprophytic activity). Many fungi can infect the body but, in people with healthy immune systems, infection tends to be limited to the epidermis of the skin and the mucous membranes of the genital tract. Malnourishment and poor living conditions predispose to deeper fungus infections following penetrating injuries to the feet and other parts. Immune deficiency allows widespread opportunistic fungus infections of all parts of the body.

fungiform papilla one of the broad, flat, slightly raised, nipple-shaped protuberances scattered over the top and sides of the tongue.

Fungilin a brand name for AMPHOTERICIN.

Fungizone a brand name for AMPHOTERICIN.

fungus infections infection of any part of the body with any fungal organism. Fungus infections of the skin (EPIDERMOPHYTOSES), the mouth and vagina are common, but those of the interior of the body are rare except in people with IMMUNE DEFICIENCY. Skin fungus infections include various forms of 'ringworm' (TINEA) from infection with fungi of the genus *Trichophyton*. THRUSH (candidiasis) is infection with the fungus *Candida albicans*, a yeast fungus which favours the mouth and the vagina. 'Opportunistic' fungi are those attacking very debilitated people, people with AIDS, those on immunosuppressive treatment or people with widespread cancer, severe diabetes or long-term (chronic) infections such as tuberculosis.

fungicidal capable of killing fungi. The term is used both for drugs that can do this without, at the same time, damaging the infected person, and for agencies that can destroy fungi and their spores outside the body.

funiculitis inflammation of the SPERMATIC CORD. Also known as corditis.

funiculus any cord-like structure.

funnel chest a condition in which the breastbone is hollowed backwards, especially at its lower end. This greatly reduces the front-to-back dimension of the chest and the heart is displaced to the left and may be compressed. There is restricted chest expansion and reduced VITAL CAPACITY.

funny bone a popular term for the part of the back of the elbow containing a groove in which the ulnar nerve runs near the surface and is easily accessible to trauma. The severe pain experienced if the nerve is struck will evoke a conspicuous physical response that may seem funny to an unsympathetic observer. The victim is unlikely to be amused.

Furadantin a brand name for NITROFURANTOIN.

Furamide a brand name for DILOXANIDE.

furuncle a boil.

furunculosis widespread or repeated boils.

fusafungine an anti-inflammatory and antibiotic spray preparation for throat infections. A brand name is Locabiotal.

fusidic acid a steroid antibiotic used in the form of sodium fusidate against penicillin-resistant (beta-lactamase-producing) staphylococci. It has no value against streptococci and is usually given in conjunction with another antibiotic such as FLUCLOXACILLIN. Brand names are Fucidin and Fucithalmic.

fusiform spindle-shaped. Tapering to a point at each end.

fusiform bacillus a spindle-shaped micro-organism such as the GRAM NEGATIVE *Fusobacterium fusiforme*, the cause of Vincent's angina.

fusion inhibitors a new class of antiviral drugs that function by preventing the fusion of the VIRUS with the cell membrane of the host cell. These drugs can reduce plasma levels of HIV in patients in whom standard combinations of antiretroviral drugs are no longer effective. See ENFUVIRTIDE.

Fuzeon a brand name for the HIV fusion inhibitor drug ENFUVIRTIDE.

FVC abbrev. for FORCED VITAL CAPACITY.

Fybogel a brand name for ISPAGHULA.

Fybogel Mebeverine a brand name for MEBEVERINE formulated with ISPAGHULA.

g

G1 the period in the cell cycle between the last MITOSIS and the start of DNA replication.

G2 the period between the end of DNA replication and the start of the next MITOSIS.

GABA gamma-aminobutyric acid. GABA is a NEUROTRANSMITTER substance derived from glutamic acid that performs important dampening (inhibitory) functions in the brain. BENZODIAZEPINE drugs enhance the action of GABA. In PARKINSON'S DISEASE there is a considerable reduction in the number of GABA binding sites in the SUBSTANTIA NIGRA of the brain.

GABA analogues drugs used to treat partial seizure epilepsy, myoclonus, neuritic pain and drug and alcohol dependency. Examples are acamprosate (Campral EC), gabapentin (neurontin), piracetam (Nootropil) and vigabatrin (Sabril).

gabapentin an analogue of the natural NEURO-TRANSMITTER GABA used in the management of certain types or epilepsy. A brand name is Neurontin.

GABA derivative muscle relaxants drugs used to treat muscle spasm. An example is baclofen (Lioresal).

GABA uptake inhibitors drugs used as an adjunct to the treatment of EPILEPSY. An example is tiagabine (Gabitril).

gag 1 a viral gene necessary for viral replication. 2 a device used by dental and other surgeons to keep the mouth wide open and allow oral treatment.

gait the particular way in which a person walks. From the Middle English gate, a way or passage.

galact-, galacto- *combining form denoting* milk or milky.

galactagogue any agent that promotes the flow of milk.

galactocoele a cystic, milk-filled swelling in a milk duct of the breast caused by obstruction.

galactopoiesis milk formation by the cells of the glandular structure of the breast. Also known as lactogenesis.

galactorrhoea excessive flow of breast milk or spontaneous milk production at times other than after pregnancy. Galactorrhoea can occur in men as well as women, if the milk-stimulating hormone prolactin is present, as from a tumour of the PITUITARY gland. Babies' breasts can produce milk from the hormone in the mother's blood. From the Greek *gala*, milk and *rhein*, to flow. See also WITCHES' MILK.

galactosaemia a genetic disorder due to the absence of an enzyme necessary for the breakdown of milk sugar (galactose) to glucose. The accumulating galactose may cause diarrhoea, vomiting, cataracts, mental retardation, liver damage with jaundice and malnutrition. Infants fed on a galactose-free diet can grow up entirely normal.

galactose a monosaccharide sugar that is a constituent of LACTOSE, the main sugar of milk. Also known as cerebrose.

galactosuria the presence of GALACTOSE in the urine.

galantamine an ACETYLCHOLINESTERASE inhibitor drug used in Alzheimer's disease to increase the amount of ACETYLCHOLINE available for nerve transmission. A brand name is REMINYL.

Galenamet a brand name for CIMETIDINE.

Galenamox a brand name for AMOXICILLIN.

Galenism medical theory and practices as taught by the Greek physician Claudius Galen ca. 130–200. Galen brought some science into medicine but was mistaken in many of his ideas.

His influence was so great that for 15 centuries it was considered heretical to question his dicta. Many important advances, such as the concept of the circulation of the blood and the appreciation of the dangers of blood-letting, were thereby delayed.

Galenphol a brand name for PHOLCODINE.

Galfer a brand name for FERROUS FUMARATE.

gall the old term for BILE, but still preserved in the word GALL BLADDER and GALLSTONES.

gallamine triethiodide a synthetic, short-acting muscle relaxant used by anaesthetists to allow passage of an ENDOTRACHEAL tube at the beginning of anaesthesia. A brand name is Flaxedil.

gall bladder the small, fig-shaped bag, lying on the under side of the liver, into which bile secreted by the liver passes to be stored and concentrated. When fatty food enters the beginning of the small intestine (the DUODENUM), the gall bladder empties into it, by way of the common bile duct.

gall bladder cancer a rare form of cancer, almost unknown in the absence of GALLSTONES. It is much commoner in women than in men and is usually found to be inoperable at the time of diagnosis.

Gallie's operation the use of strips of FASCIA lata taken from the side of the thigh to repair a defect in a hernial ring. (William Edward Gallie, 1882–1959, Canadian surgeon).

gallipot a small well-glazed earthenware container for medical solutions. The modern gallipot is made of tin-foil or polypropylene. From the Dutch *gleipot*, meaning pottery brought in galleys from abroad.

gallium scan a method of demonstrating tumours and inflammation in the liver and elsewhere. Gallium is an element that concentrates in tumour and inflammatory cells to a greater extent than in normal liver cells. The radioactive isotope, gallium-67, which is chemically identical, can therefore be used in conjunction with a GAMMA CAMERA to reveal liver cancers or areas of inflammation.

gallop rhythm a characteristic pattern of heart sounds sometimes heard with a stethoscope when the heart rate is rapid and the third and fourth heart sounds coincide. Third and fourth heart sounds may indicate heart abnormality such as HEART FAILURE or undue stiffness of the muscle walls.

gallows traction a method of treating fractures of the thigh bone (femur) in young children. Skin traction is applied to both legs and the child is suspended from a beam so that the buttocks are just clear of the bed. Also known as Bryant's gallows traction.

gallstones round, oval or faceted masses of cholesterol, chalk (calcium carbonate), calcium bilirubinate, or a mixture of these. Gallstones vary in size, from less than a millimetre to several centimetres, and are often present but unsuspected. They are commoner in women than in men and are more likely if the composition of the bile is abnormal or there is infection or blockage of outflow of bile. They tend to cause inflammation of the gall bladder (cholecystitis) and can be fragmented by LITHOTRIPSY.

Galpseud a brand name for PSEUDOEPHEDRINE.

galvanic pertaining to direct current electricity, or to the shock produced by a direct current. See also FARADIC. (Luigi Galvani, 1737–98, Italian scientist).

gam-, gamo- *combining form denoting* joined, especially sexually united.

Gamanil a brand name for LOFEPRAMINE.

gamete a cell, such as a sperm or ovum, possessing half the normal number of chromosomes (haploid) and capable of fusing with another gamete in the process of fertilization, so that the full (diploid) number of chromosomes is made up. From the Greek *gamos*, marriage.

gamete intrafallopian transfer (GIFT) direct placement of up to three harvested and incubated human eggs, together with a quantity of spermatozoa, into a fallopian tube via a fine catheter. GIFT, which implies *in vivo* fertilization, is a method of achieving pregnancy that in some cases offers a better alternative to *in vitro* fertilization (IVF).

gametocyte a cell from which a GAMETE is developed by division. In the ovary, a gametocyte is an oocyte; in the testicle it is a spermatocyte.

gametogenesis the production of gametes. See GAMETE.

gamma the third letter of the Greek alphabet. Often used in medicine to denote a particular class.

gamma-aminobutyric acid see GABA.

gamma camera a device consisting of a large

crystal of a material that produces a tiny point of light where it is struck by a gamma ray. Between the crystal and the subject is interposed a thick lead plate drilled with numerous parallel holes (a collimator) that ensures that only parallel rays strike the crystal. In this way an image is formed on the crystal corresponding to the pattern of gamma rays given off by the subject. The gamma camera is used in conjunction with selective radionuclides that concentrate in certain parts of the body, such as the bones, the thyroid gland or a tumour. See also RADIONUCLIDE SCANNING.

gamma globulin a group of soluble proteins, present in the blood, most of which are IMMUNOGLUBULINS (antibodies), and which show the greatest mobility towards the cathode during ELECTROPHORESIS. Gamma globulin provides the body's main antibody defence against infection. For this reason it is produced commercially from human plasma and used for passive protection against many infections, especially HEPATITIS, MEASLES and POLIOMYELITIS.

gamma-glutamyl transferase an enzyme widely distributed in body tissues and released into the blood when tissue, especially liver tissue, is damaged. Increased levels occur in liver damage from any cause. Measurements can be used as an index of alcohol abuse. Increased blood levels may sometimes occur without liver cell damage.

gamma radiation electromagnetic radiation of energy greater than several hundred thousand electron volts. With the development of very high voltage X-ray equipment there is now a technological overlap between X-ray and gamma radiation. Formerly, gamma was obtained only from decay of radioactive elements. Gamma radiation is highly penetrative and is valuable in RADIOTHERAPY.

gammopathy any abnormality, in quality or quantity, of the IMMUNOGLOBULINS present in the blood. Benign monoclonal gammopathy is an abnormal production of a single clone of an immunoglobulin. Gammopathies are associated with MULTIPLE MYELOMA.

ganciclovir a DNA POLYMERASE INHIBITOR drug used to treat CYTOMEGALOVIRUS infections in people with AIDS. Brand names are Cymevene and Virgan.

ganglion 1 any large, discrete collection of nerve cell bodies, from which bundles of nerve fibres emerge.
2 a rubbery, compressible, cystic swelling arising from the fibrous sheath of a tendon or the capsule of a joint, commonly on or around the wrist.

ganglionectomy surgical removal of a GANGLION.

ganglioneuroma a benign tumour composed of sympathetic ganglion cells and neural fibrous tissue.

ganglionitis inflammation of a ganglion.

ganglioside a compound of fat and carbohydrate (glycolipid) that is an important component in cell membranes.

gangliosidosis a disorder of GANGLIOSIDE metabolism resulting in accumulation of gangliosides in nerve tissue, especially in the lysosomes. Gangliosidoses are usually due to gene mutation causing an enzyme defect or deficiency. An example is TAY-SACH'S DISEASE.

gangosa the grotesque facial mutilation sometimes caused by untreated late YAWS, in which the nose and upper lip are destroyed so that the mouth and nasal orifice become a single open cavity.

gangrene death of tissue, usually as a result of loss of an adequate blood supply. Gangrene is most commonly caused by disease of arteries that cause narrowing and obstruction, but may result from any other cause of arterial obstruction. If uninfected, this is called dry gangrene. The extremities are most commonly affected. Infection in gangrenous tissue causes putrefaction, producing wet gangrene. Gas gangrene is the result of deep infection, especially of muscle, with ANAEROBIC organisms, such as Clostridium welchii. This organism produces gas within the tissues.

ganja a form of MARIJUANA resin derived from the flowering tops and leaves of specially selected plants.

Ganser's syndrome a pattern of fraudulent and exaggerated simulation of psychiatric behaviour, usually detectable by the expert as revealing the subject's notion of madness rather than any recognized psychiatric pattern. It is common among prisoners awaiting trial especially when they believe they are being watched. Recovery is sudden when no further advantage is perceived. (Sigbert Joseph Maria Ganser, 1853–1931, German psychiatrist).

Garamycin a brand name for GENTAMICIN.

Gardnerella vaginalis an organism commonly infecting the vagina and giving rise to an irritating vaginal inflammation with a thin discharge having a fishy odour when in contact with alkali ('whiff test'). The organism is transmitted sexually and the condition is treated with metronidazole.

Gardner's syndrome an autosomal dominant hereditary disorder featuring multiple benign bony tumours (osteomas), EPIDERMOID CYSTS, soft tissue tumours including DESMOID TUMOURS, POLYPS in the intestine, and a 95% chance of developing cancer of the colon. (Eldon John Gardner, American geneticist, b. 1909).

gargoylism the effect of one of a number of X-linked or autosomal recessive disorders of MUCOPOLYSACCHARIDE metabolism that cause coarsening of the features, excessive hairiness and often mental retardation.

gas and oxygen nitrous oxide and oxygen. This is a common general anaesthetic combination but being only mildly anaesthetic, is often used as a vehicle for other, more potent, gases, such as vaporized HALOTHANE, or is supplemented by other drugs. Nitrous oxide usefully reduces pain sensation and gas and oxygen is sometimes used alone to relieve labour pains.

gas embolism see AIR EMBOLISM.

gas gangrene the effect of deep muscle infection with the dangerous anaerobic, gas-producing organism *Clostridium welchii* or *Clostridium oedematiens*. There is extensive tissue death, gas production and severe general upset. Energetic surgery may be necessary to preserve life.

Gasserian ganglion a large collection of nerve cells forming the sensory root of the 5th cranial (trigeminal) nerve. Also known as the semilunar ganglion. (Johan Ludwig Gasser, 1723–65, Austrian anatomist).

gastr-, gastro- *combining form denoting* the stomach, belly or abdomen.

gastrectomy surgical removal of the stomach. Partial gastrectomy is commoner than total gastrectomy and is performed for the treatment stomach and duodenal ulcers that cannot be controlled medically, and for cancer of the lower part of the stomach. Surgery for peptic ulceration is usually combined with an operation to cut the nerves responsible for stimulating acid production in the stomach (VAGOTOMY). Since the development of drugs such as CIMETIDINE and RANITIDINE (Zantac), gastrectomy has been performed less often.

gastric pertaining to the stomach. The word derives from the Greek *gaster*, the belly.

gastric erosion minor damage to the stomach lining causing areas with many fine, superficial bleeding points. Gastric erosion is the first stage in the development of a stomach ulcer. It is caused by local irritants such as alcohol and aspirin, but is also a feature of severe stress, blood infection (SEPTICAEMIA) and large burns.

gastric juice the watery mixture of hydrochloric acid, pepsin and mucin secreted by the glands in the lining of the stomach. Gastric juice has a powerful digestive action on protein and is also protective against many infective organisms.

gastric lavage stomach washout. This is done to remove or dilute drugs or non-corrosive poisons taken in suicide attempts. Lavage is avoided if corrosive poisons have been taken. A wide-bore soft plastic or rubber tube is pushed down the gullet (oesophagus) into the stomach, the end held high, and water run in through a funnel. The end of the tube is then lowered so that the washings drain out. This process is repeated until the returning water is clear.

gastric ulcer a local defect in the mucous membrane lining of the stomach as a result of the loss of mucus and other protection against the action of acid and digestive enzymes. Stomach ulcers are treated with ANTACIDS and H$_2$ receptor antagonist drugs such as CIMETIDINE.

gastrin a peptide hormone secreted by the stomach on the stimulus of the sight, smell or contemplation of food. The hormone is released into the blood. The entry of protein into the stomach stimulates even more gastrin production and this hormone returns to the stomach to stimulate the production of acid and pepsin (GASTRIC JUICE) from the cells of the stomach lining (gastric mucosa).

gastritis inflammation of the stomach from any cause. See also GASTRIC EROSION.

Gastrobid Continus a brand name for METOCLOPRAMIDE.

Gastrobrom a brand name for a mixture of MAGNESIUM TRISILICATE, MAGNESIUM HYDROXIDE, MAGNESIUM CARBONATE and chalk (calcium carbonate).

gastrocnemius the main muscle forming the bulge of the calf. The gastrocnemius arises by two heads from the back of the lower end of the thigh bone (femur) and is inserted, with the SOLEUS muscle, by way of the ACHILLES TENDON into the back of the heel bone (CALCANEUS). Its action is to extend the ankle joint in walking and standing on tiptoe.

gastrocolic pertaining to the stomach and the colon. A gastrocolic fistula is an abnormal connection between the inside of the stomach and the inside of the colon.

gastrocolic reflex the reason so many of us visit the toilet after breakfast. The intake of food causes PERISTALSIS in the colon which culminates in the desire to defaecate.

gastroduodenal pertaining to the stomach and the DUODENUM.

gastroduodenitis inflammation of the stomach and duodenum.

gastroduodenostomy a surgical junction made between the stomach and the duodenum so that the contents can flow readily from one to the other.

gastroenteritis inflammation of the lining of the stomach and the small intestine from infection with organisms, such as *Salmonella*, various viruses and *Escherichia coli*. There is fever, abdominal pain, diarrhoea and vomiting. Gastroenteritis kills millions of children each year in Third World countries, mostly from dehydration and malnutrition.

gastroenterologist a doctor specializing in the digestive system and its disorders. Gastroenterologists are concerned not only with the OESOPHAGUS, stomach and intestines, but also with the major associated glands – the LIVER and the PANCREAS.

gastroenterology the medical specialty concerned with the stomach, the intestines and the associated structures, including the liver. The list that follows highlights the key entries related to gastroenterology in the dictionary: atrophic gastritis, colorectal, colon cancer, colostomy, duodenal ulcer, duodenum, duodenoscopy, fissure, fistula, gastrectomy, gastric, gastric erosion, gastric juice, gastric lavage, gastric ulcer, gastrin, gastritis, gastrocolic, gastroduodenal, gastroenteritis, gastroenterologist, gastroenterology, gastroenterostomy, gastrointestinal, gastrojejunostomy, gastro-oesophageal, gastroplication, gastroptosis, gastroscope, gastroscopy, gavage, haemorrhoids, hourglass stomach, intestine, intestinal obstruction, large intestine, nasogastric tube, pentagastrin test, rectal cancer, rectal examination, rectal prolapse, stomach cancer, stomach disorders, stomach pump, stomach ulcer, stomach washout.

gastroenterostomy a surgical operation for DUODENAL ULCER in which the normal outlet of the stomach into the DUODENUM is closed off and a side-to-side junction (anastomosis) made between the stomach and the beginning of the small intestine. This effectively bypasses the duodenum, keeping stomach acid away from it and allowing the ulcer to heal.

gastroepiploic artery one of a pair of arteries that runs round the greater curvature of the stomach.

gastrointestinal pertaining to the stomach and intestines.

gastrojejunostomy see GASTRO-ENTEROSTOMY.

gastro-oesophageal pertaining to the stomach and the OESOPHAGUS.

gastroplication a surgical operation to correct severe ballooning (dilation) of the stomach. Redundant tissue is folded over and stitched in place.

gastroptosis a sagging or downward displacement of the stomach.

gastroscope an illuminating and viewing instrument for examining the inside of the stomach. An ENDOSCOPE used for the stomach. See also GASTROSCOPY.

gastroscopy direct visual examination of the inside of the stomach. This is done when barium X-ray reveals an ulcer, so that malignancy can be excluded by BIOPSY. The healing of ulcers can also be confirmed by gastroscopy. Various treatments can also be performed by gastroscopy. These include the injection of adrenaline around a bleeding ulcer to constrict the blood vessels.

gastrosplenic ligament a fold of PERITONEUM running from the stomach to the spleen. Also known as the gastrosplenic OMENTUM.

gastrostomy a surgical opening made into the stomach with the formation of a temporary or permanent passage from the outer surface of the abdomen, for purposes of feeding or drainage.

gastrotomy an incision into the stomach.

gastrula the stage in the development of an EMBRYO following the BLASTULA stage when the ECTODERM, ENDODERM and primitive GUT have developed.

Gaucher's disease a rare hereditary metabolic disease due to an enzyme defect that interferes with the proper function of cell LYSOSOMES. The condition features massive accumulation of materials called glucocerebrosides in the lysosomes. There is great enlargement of the liver and spleen, bone marrow displacement, bleeding tendency, bronzing of the skin, and anaemia. Also known as cerebroside lipidosis. (Philip Charles Ernst Gaucher, 1854–1918, French physician).

Gaussian distribution normal distribution. The distribution of characteristics found in large populations subject to many causes of variability. The graph of the Gaussian distribution of any characteristic (such as body height) is a symmetrical bell shape, centred on the mean. (Johann Karl Friedrich Gauss, 1777–1855, German mathematician).

gavage 1 forced feeding through a tube passed down into the stomach through the mouth. 2 the use of a high calorie, large volume diet to improve nutrition (superalimentation).

Gaviscon a brand name for a range of antacid preparations containing various ingredients such as sodium alginate, MAGNESIUM TRISILICATE, ALUMINIUM HYDROXIDE and SODIUM BICARBONATE.

Gaviscon Infant a brand name for a preparation containing sodium alginate and MAGNESIUM ALGINATE.

gay an informal term for homosexual, usually male.

gay bowel syndrome the damaging effects on the lower bowel caused by male homosexual practices resulting in injury to, and infection of, the margin of the anus and the rectum from finger or hand insertion (fisting) or from the insertion of other objects. Other features include ANAL FISSURES, and ANAL FISTULAS, haemorrhoids and ulcers.

G banding a method of identifying the different members of a haploid set of metaphase chromosomes by means of staining that reveals their individual pattern of stripes.

gel a largely liquid colloid, retained in a semisolid state by molecular chains, usually cross-linked.

gelatin film a thin sheet of sterile processed gelatin used in surgery to repair defects in membranes. The film absorbs within six months.

gelatin sponge a surgical sponge of sterile water-insoluble gelatin used to control capillary bleeding. The sponge is left in place and will absorb within about six weeks.

Geltears a brand name for CARBOMER.

Gelusil a brand name for a mixture of ALUMINIUM HYDROXIDE, MAGNESIUM HYDROXIDE and the foam-dispersing agent simethicone.

gemcitabine a CYTOTOXIC anticancer drug. A brand name is Gemzar.

gemfibrozil a FIBRATE cholesterol-lowering drug. A brand name is Lopid.

Gemzar a brand name for GEMCITABINE.

-gen *combining form denoting* something that produces or creates, as in PATHOGEN.

gender a classification of organisms based on their sex. From the Latin *genus*, a kind.

gender identity the inherent sense that one belongs to a particular sex. In almost all cases that sex corresponds to the anatomical sex, but for a small minority, the gender identity is for the opposite anatomical sex. See also GENDER REASSIGNMENT.

gender reassignment acknowledgement of the true mental and emotional sex (gender identity) of an individual when this does not correspond to the apparent anatomical sex. Gender reassignment is a necessary, and serious, preliminary to any serious consideration of sex-change surgery.

gender role all behaviour that conveys to others, consciously or otherwise, a person's GENDER IDENTITY as male or female.

gene the physical unit of heredity, represented as a continuous sequence of bases, arranged in a code, in groups of three (codons), along the length of a DNA molecule (nucleic acid). The gene is the transcription code for a sequence of AMINO ACIDS linked to form a single POLYPEPTIDE chain and includes lengths on either side of the coding region known as the leader and the trailer, and non-coding sequences (INTRONS) that intervene between the coding segments. The latter are called EXONS. Exons tend to be conserved throughout a long evolutionary period; introns may vary considerably in length. The length of a gene is largely determined by the introns. The function of genes can be altered by changes (MUTATIONS) in the base sequences and their operation is regulated by adjacent, or even remote, parts of the DNA molecule. All genes are present in all nucleated cells, but only genes relevant to the particular cell are 'switched on' as required.

gene action the operation of genes in determining the whole body constitution (phenotype) of an individual.

gene cloning the identification and isolation of a gene and the production of a number of identical copies of it.

gene family a group of genes whose exons are related, having been derived from an ancestral gene.

gene frequency the number of occurrences of a particular gene in a population.

gene library a collection of cloned deoxyribonucleic acid (DNA) fragments together with information about the gene function. See also GENETIC MAPPING.

General Medical Council the governing and registering body of doctors in the United Kingdom. For many years the qualification for full medical practice in the UK was inclusion in the Medical Register. But in 2004 a new system was introduced. Under this, the Register was strengthened by a specific licence to practice supported by periodic REVALIDATION. This change was made to ensure that doctors remained up-to-date in their knowledge, and fit, throughout their careers, to provide adequate, safe and effective medical care for their patients. Registered and validated doctors are expected to make the care of their patients their first concern. They must respect patients' views, dignity and privacy; provide information in a form patients can understand; respect the rights of patients to be involved in decisions about themselves; recognize the limits of their professional competence; behave honestly and be trustworthy; avoid allowing personal beliefs to prejudice patient care; cooperate with colleagues; and act quickly to protect patients if they have good reason to believe that they, or another doctor may not be fit to practice.

gene silencing the inhibition of transcription of a gene. DNA METHYLATION is an important cause of gene silencing and when this affects tumour-suppressor genes may be a cause of cancer.

gene therapy medical treatment in which genes are deliberately introduced into general body cells. The method has been in use since 1989. Genes may be delivered directly to target cells by viruses from which viral genes have been removed and replaced by therapeutic genes. In addition, genes may be carried into cells by nutrient substances such as fats proteins or a mineral such as calcium phosphate. Alternatively, some of a person's cells may be removed, genetically modified outside the body, and then reintroduced. The conditions currently most commonly treated by gene therapy are CANCER, AIDS and CYSTIC FIBROSIS. The method is in its early infancy but promises great things. Modification of the human germ line so as to change the heritable state is currently forbidden.

genera the plural of GENUS.

general anaesthesia a state of unconsciousness and immobility, brought about by drugs, so as to allow surgical operations or other physical procedures to be performed without pain or awareness. Deep levels of unconsciousness, formerly necessary to achieve the required degree of muscle relaxation, are no longer used. Light anaesthesia, associated with the use of drugs to relax muscles and prevent pain, shock and autonomic disturbance, is now standard. The action of general anaesthetic drugs is now better understood. Pain responses are suppressed primarily at spinal cord level; hypnosis and amnesia are mediated by the brain. These drugs are now believed to operate on ion channels in nerve cells by binding directly to the protein sites. Different anaesthetic drugs bind specifically to different ion channels.

general anaesthetics drugs used to induce and maintain GENERAL ANAESTHESIA. Examples are thiopentone (Thiopental) for induction; etomidate (Hypnomidate) for induction; nitrous oxide, halothane, isoflurane, desflurane and sevoflurane for maintenance; propofol for induction and maintenance; and ketamine (Ketalar) for production of a trance-like dissociative anaesthesia for minor surgical procedures.

generalized anxiety disorder see FREE FLOATING ANXIETY.

general paralysis of the insane (GPI) a now rare form of dementia from SYPHILIS of the nervous system. GPI was a feature of the third (tertiary) stage of untreated syphilis and occurred 10–20 years after infection in a small proportion of cases. The condition is characterized by delusions of grandeur, mania and sometimes delusions of persecution.

general paresis see GENERAL PARALYSIS OF THE INSANE.

general practitioner a doctor who does not specialize in any particular branch of medicine but who treats a wide variety of relatively minor medical conditions and is able to discern those conditions requiring specialist attention.

generation 1 a single stage of reproductive descent in the history of an organism.
2 the average or normal time between the birth of parents and the birth of their offspring. In humans, this may be taken to be 25 years.

generative pertaining to reproduction.

gene redundancy the presence of many copies of the same gene within a cell.

generic drug a drug sold under the official medical name of the basic active substance. The generic name is chosen by the Nomenclature Committee of the British Pharmacopoeia Commission and is used in publications such a the *British National Formulary*. Doctors are encouraged to prescribe generic drugs as these are generally cheaper than the same drug under a trade or brand name.

genesis origins, beginnings or the process of being formed.

gene splicing the process in GENETIC ENGINEERING in which a short length of DNA from one organism is inserted into the DNA of another.

gene suppression the situation in which a normal PHENOTYPE develops in an individual or cell with a mutant gene due to a second mutation either in the same gene or in a different gene.

genetic carrier see CARRIER.

genetic code the sequence of the bases, adenine, guanine, cytosine and thymine, lying along the nucleic acid (DNA) molecules, the chromosomes. The bases occur in groups of three, each group being called a codon and each codon contains any three of the four in any order. This gives 64 different combinations, allowing some redundancy. A particular codon selects a particular one of the 20 amino acids or an instruction such as 'gene starts here' or 'end of gene'. The sequence of codons ensures that a number of particular amino acids are linked together in a particular order so as to form a protein molecule – usually an ENZYME that promotes some biochemical process.

genetic counselling the process of trying to determine, for the purpose of advising prospective parents, the probability that a future child will suffer from a particular genetic disorder known to occur in the family. Genetic counsellors must have a detailed knowledge of the principles of genetics and of the nature of the conditions caused by gene defect. They must be skilled in constructing family pedigrees and in interpreting them. Counselling is best done in specialized centres where the necessary expertise can be obtained.

genetic dogma the idea, proposed by Francis Crick and James Watson, that genetic information is invariably transferred in the direction DNA to RNA to protein. The discovery of reverse transcription organisms, such as HIV, in which information passes from RNA to DNA, knocked this theory on the head.

genetic engineering the deliberate alteration, for practical purposes, of the GENOME of a cell so as to change its hereditable characteristics. This is done mainly by recombinant DNA techniques using gene copies obtained by the POLYMERASE CHAIN REACTION. Enzymes (restriction enzymes) are used to cut the nucleic acid molecule at determinable positions and short lengths of DNA from another organism are inserted. The second cell will now contain genes for the property or characteristic borrowed from the first cell. The genes might, for instance, code for the production of a useful protein such as insulin or some food material. Bacteria, yeasts and other organisms are used as the hosts for the new gene sequences and these organisms can be cloned in enormous numbers to produce the desired effects, or substances, for which the new genes code. Well over 100 valuable drugs and vaccines have been produced in this way, including human insulin, growth hormone, interferons, hepatitis vaccine, digoxin monoclonal antibody, orthoclonal OK3, somatotropin, TISSUE PLASMINOGEN ACTIVATOR

(TPA), erythropoietin, granulocyte MACROPHAGE colony-stimulating factor (GM-CSF), granulocyte colony stimulating factor (G-CSF) and Factor VIII. Cloned copies of the genes for many genetic diseases have been made available for use as probes for the identification of the disease by AMNIOCENTESIS, before birth. The possibility also arises of correcting genetic defects in early embryos. Genetic engineering offers almost unlimited possibilities for the advancement of medicine, science and technology, but strict control is also necessary if the many manifest dangers are to be avoided.

genetic fingerprinting see DNA FINGERPRINTING.

genetic immunodeficiency disorders inherited disorders that affect the function of the immune system. Also known as primary immunodeficiencies. X-linked immunodeficiency disorders include some forms of the severe combined immunodeficiencies (SCID); Wiskott-Aldrich syndrome; X-linked hypogammaglobulinaemia; X-linked agammaglobulinaemia; chronic granulomatous disease; and the X-linked lymphoproliferative syndrome. Autosomal recessive immunodeficiency disorders include other forms of SCID; Di George syndrome; bare lymphocyte syndrome (MHC deficiency); ataxia telangiectasia; and selective immunoglobulin G deficiency.

genetic load the totality of abnormalities caused in each generation by defective genetic material carried in the human gene pool.

genetic mapping 1 the process of determining the location of the genes for various characteristics and diseases in the chromosomes. 2 the determination of the sequence of bases in the chromosomes corresponding to the genes. The human GENOME mapping project is now under way and is hoped to be completed by the beginning of the 21st Century.

genetic marker a gene or DNA sequence that indicates the presence of a disease or a probable risk of developing it.

genetics the branch of biology concerned with the structure, location, abnormalities and effects of the genes. Medical genetics is mainly concerned with the expression of abnormal genes or gene combinations in the production of disease. Knowledge of such matters allows useful genetic counselling. William Bateson,

(1861–1926) was the English physiologist whose studies and publications led to his being known as the 'father of genetics'. Curiously, Bateson persistently opposed the chromosome theory of heredity. The list that follows highlights the key entries related to genetics in the dictionary: ABC genes, ABCA3 gene, adenovirus early region genes, alpha-2-macroglobulin gene (A2M gene), ancestral genes, androgen receptor gene, BRCA genes, complementary genes, contiguous gene syndrome, deafness gene, discontinuous gene, discontinuous replication, drug-transporter gene, epigenetic, gametogenesis, gene, gene action, gene cloning, gene family, gene frequency, gene library, gene silencing, gene therapy, gene splicing, gene suppression, genetic carrier, genetic code, genetic counselling, genetic dogma, genetic engineering, genetic fingerprinting, genetic mapping, genetic marker, genetics, genetic screening, homeobox genes, homologous genes, housekeeping genes, immune response genes, jumping genes, karyogenesis, leaky mutant gene, major immunogene complex, molecular genetics, mosaic gene, multigene family, mutation, ob gene, oncogenes, operator gene, orphan genes, parthenogenesis, preimplantation genetic diagnosis, proto-oncogene, regulator gene, repressor gene, stress genes, structural gene, suppressor gene, T-box gene family, V gene.

genetic screening the use of AMNIOCENTESIS or CHORIONIC VILLUS SAMPLING before birth to obtain fetal cells or a small portion of fetal tissue on which chromosomal, and to some extent gene, studies can be made. A number of serious genetic disorders can, in this way, be diagnosed at a very early stage after conception so that the option of terminating the pregnancy can be considered.

-genic *combining form denoting* producing or creating, as in TERATOGENIC.

geniculate 1 bent at an angle, like a knee. 2 capable of bending at an angle. The term comes from the Latin *geniculatus* meaning with bended knee.

geniculate body one of the four small oval prominences on the base of the brain lying in relation to the optic pathways and the THALAMUS. The lateral geniculate bodies contain important links (synapses) in the route of visual information from the eyes to the visual cortex at the back of the brain.

genioglossus one of the small extrinsic muscle of the tongue. It arises from centre of the back of the jaw bone (mandible).

genital pertaining to the GENITALIA.

genital herpes infection with the Herpes simplex virus, Type II, usually acquired during sexual intercourse. The blisters that form on the GENITALIA, in crops, resemble cold sores but are typically more widespread and severe than those occurring around the mouth and nose. The drug Acyclovir can reduce the frequency and severity of attacks but is not curative.

genitalia a term usually implying the external organs of generation – the labia majora and minora and the clitoris in the female and the penis, scrotum and testicles of the male. Strictly, the genitalia also include all the other parts concerned with reproduction – the vagina, uterus, fallopian tubes and ovaries in the female; and the spermatic cords, vasa deferentes, seminal vesicles and prostate gland in the male.

genital stage the last and most mature of the stages of psychosexual development as described by Sigmund Freud. This stage is said to be reached in late adolescence or early adult life.

genital warts warts occurring on the external genitalia. These are caused by the same papillomaviruses, of the *papovavirus* family, as any other warts but are sexually transmitted and, because of their situation are often more extensive and exuberant than other warts. They are often called condylomata acuminata and are commonly associated with cancer of the cervix of the uterus.

genito-urinary medicine the current term for the speciality formerly described as venereology. Genito-urinary medicine has acquired a new status, prominence and importance since the appearance of AIDS.

genome the complete set of CHROMOSOMES, together with the MITOCHONDRIAL DNA, containing the entire genetic material of the cell.

genomic pertaining to the GENOME.

genomic imprinting the concept, derived from an increasing body of compelling evidence, that the expression of some of the genes depends on whether they have been derived from the father or from the mother. It has been shown, for instance, that chromosomal deletion in chromosomes of paternal origin may differ in their effect from the same deletion in the homologous chromosome of maternal origin. Many cancers are associated with loss of a particular chromosome derived from a particular parent – usually the mother. The DNA of some genes is modified during the formation of gametes so as to have altered expression and be activated or inactivated.

genomics the study of the GENOME.

Genotropin a brand name for SOMATOTROPIN.

genotype 1 the total genetic information contained in a cell.

2 the genetic constitution of an individual organism. Compare PHENOTYPE.

gentamicin an aminoglycoside antibiotic used mainly for the treatment of serious GRAM NEGATIVE infections. Otherwise, gentamicin is used topically for external infections, such as those of the eye or ear. In large dosage it can cause TINNITUS, deafness and kidney damage. Recently, gentamycin has been shown to be capable of bypassing a STOP MUTATION and has been shown to be helpful in controlling CYSTIC FIBROSIS and other genetic disorders caused by stop mutations. The drug is on the WHO official list. Brand names are Cidomycin, Garamycin, Genticin and Minims gentamicin. See also PTC124.

gentian violet a solution of methyl-rosanilinium chloride, a pigment once widely used as a conspicuous skin application in cases of IMPETIGO but now considered politically incorrect in the Western world and has been replaced by more effective remedies. The drug is on the WHO official list.

Genticin a brand name for GENTAMICIN.

genu a knee or any knee-like or bent anatomical structure.

genus the taxonomic category above species and below family. The generic name, in the Linnaean classification, is always written with a capital letter, the specific name in lower case. Thus, in *Homo sapiens*, *Homo* is the genus and *sapiens* the specific name.

genu valgum knock knee. Some degree of genu valgum occurs normally in about one infant in five but this has usually corrected itself spontaneously by the age of seven. It may also be caused by RICKETS and is not uncommon in RHEUMATOID ARTHRITIS.

genu varum bow or bandy legs. This is common and normal in healthy toddlers and usually corrects itself by about 18 months. Severe bowing can be caused by OSTEOCHONDROSIS of the main lower leg bone (the tibia) or by rickets. In these cases the condition can be cured by early treatment with night splints.

geometric mean the average value of a set of n integers quantities, expressed as the nth root of their product. The geometric mean is used to determine the average of a skewed frequency distribution.

ger-, gero- *combining form denoting* old age or relating to the elderly.

Geref a brand name for SERMORELIN.

geriatrician a doctor specializing in the medical aspects of old age.

geriatric medicine the medicine of old age. The branch of medicine concerned with the practical application of the science of GERONTOLOGY to the improvement of the quality of life of elderly people. Modern geriatrics is a growing and positive discipline much concerned with the abolition of conventional stereotypes. The emphasis is on the encouragement of maximal activity and achievement, regardless of age, and the avoidance, and when necessary, management, of conditions such as ATHEROSCLEROSIS, STROKE, heart disease, defects of vision and hearing, OSTEOPOROSIS, DIABETES, ARTHRITIS, CANCER and DEMENTIA.

germ a popular term for any organism capable of causing disease. Germ plasm is living primitive tissue capable of developing into an organ or individual.

German measles see RUBELLA.

germ cells sexual reproductive cells. See OVA and SPERMATOZOA.

germicide an antiseptic agent that kills micro-organisms.

germ layer any one of three layers of tissue, the ectoderm, the mesoderm and the endoderm, into which the embryo differentiates.

germ line 1 the lineage of cells leading to the contemporary GERM CELLS.
2 often used loosely to refer to the cells of the ovary and testes that give rise, respectively, to the ova and spermatozoa, and to the ova and spermatozoa themselves.

geroderma the characteristic skin changes occurring in old age – atrophy, pigmentation, drying, loss of fat and loss of elasticity.

gerontology the study of the biology, psychology and sociology of ageing. Gerontology is concerned with the changes that occur in the cells, tissues and organs of the body with age, with the natural limits of cell reproduction, the causes of natural cell death, the effects of life style and physical activity on longevity and the psychological and sociological effects of ageing.

Gerstmann's syndrome a combination of agraphia, right-left disorientation, finger agnosia and acalculia caused by a parietal lobe tumour. (Josef Gerstmann, 1887-1969, Austrian neurologist.)

gestalt a physical, mental or symbolic pattern or figure so arranged that the effect of the whole differs from, or is greater than, that of the sum of its parts. A unified whole, the full nature of which cannot be grasped by analyzing its parts.

gestalt psychology a school of psychology that held that phenomena, to be understood, must be viewed as structured, organized whole entities (gestalten). Thus the gestalt of a melody remains recognizable whether it be sung, played on a flute or heavily orchestrated. Gestalt theories have had an impact on the physiology of perception, but the philosophic view that psychological phenomena are irreducible gestalts no longer commands much support.

gestation period the period from fertilization of the egg (ovum) to the birth of the child. The human gestation period is 40 weeks, plus or minus 2 weeks.

gestodene the PROGESTOGEN component of a range of combined oral contraceptives such as Femodene, Femodene ED, Minulet, TriMinulet and Triadene.

Gestone a brand name for a PROGESTERONE drug used to treat excessive menstrual bleeding.

gestrinone a testosterone-like drug that interferes with the release of GONADOTROPHIC HORMONES and can be used in women to treat ENDOMETRIOSIS. A brand name is Dimetriose.

GH *abbrev. for* GROWTH HORMONE.

Ghon complex the association of a small focus of TUBERCULOSIS just under the lung covering (pleura) with tuberculosis in the corresponding lymph nodes at the root (hilum) of the lung. (Anton Ghon, 1866–1936, Czech pathologist).

GHRF *abbrev. for* GROWTH HORMONE releasing factor.

GHRIH *abbrev. for* GROWTH HORMONE release inhibiting hormone (SOMATOSTATIN).

giant cell a large multinucleate cell formed from the fusion of many MACROPHAGES. Giant cells are often a feature of granulomas.

giant cell arteritis see TEMPORAL ARTERITIS.

giant cell tumours these bone tumours usually affect young adults, causing swelling and pain in a long bone near a joint. The X ray shows a typical 'soap bubble' appearance. They may be BENIGN or MALIGNANT but the outlook after reasonably early surgery is usually good.

giardiasis intestinal infection with the single-celled protozoan organism *Giardia lamblia*. This is usually acquired in contaminated drinking water but may be transmitted sexually. Giardiasis causes DIARRHOEA with cramping abdominal pain, flatulence and bulky malodourous stools. Medical treatment is effective. (Vitem Dusan Lambl, 1824–95, Czechoslovakian paediatrician).

giddiness see VERTIGO.

gigantism excessive body growth. This is usually the result of an abnormal production of growth hormone by the pituitary gland in childhood, before the growing ends of the bones (the epiphyses) have fused. The excess hormone production is almost always due to a benign tumour – a pituitary adenoma. The height may exceed 2.4 m. Excess growth hormone after fusion of the epiphyses causes ACROMEGALY.

Gilbert's syndrome a form of mild JAUNDICE affecting about 5% of the population, most commonly adolescents and young adults, and often brought on by fasting. Fasting produces ketone bodies that displace BILIRUBIN from its link with the blood protein albumin. The jaundice is due to the excess of bilirubin in the blood. There is yellowing of the skin. Many people affected have no symptoms but there may be loss of appetite, a feeling of sickness and pain in the upper abdomen. The liver function tests are normal but there is a deficiency of a liver enzyme, glucuronyl transferase. The syndrome is sometimes a result of a dominant genetic defect and is also known as benign familial non-haemolytic hyperbilirubinaemia. (Nicolas Augustin Gilbert, French physician, 1858–1927).

Gilles de la Tourette's syndrome a major TIC featuring involuntary body movements such as grimaces, shrugs, twitches and jerks, and the uncontrollable emission of cough-like sounds, barks or grunts and sometimes compulsive utterances, usually of an obscene nature (coprolalia). Effective treatment with drugs is possible. It seems probable that Dr Samuel Johnson, subject of Boswell's great biography, suffered from this syndrome. (George Edouard Albert Brutus Gilles de la Tourette, 1855–1909, French neurologist).

gingiva the gum.

gingival pertaining to the gums.

gingivectomy a dental operation to remove part of the gum.

gingivitis inflammation of the gums. Gingivitis almost always implies neglect of dental hygiene with accumulation of PLAQUE around the necks of the teeth and the development of dental CALCULUS. There is inflammation and bleeding and, if the condition is neglected, damage to the PERIODONTAL MEMBRANE that secures the teeth in place. Gingivitis is also a feature of SCURVY.

gingivostomatitis inflammation of the gums and the mucous membrane lining of the mouth.

ginko biloba a plant extract containing FLAVONOIDS, terpenoids and organic acids that is claimed to be effective in peripheral vascular disease and in slowing the progress of dementia.

ginseng the root of two perennial Chinese and Korean herbs of the genus *Panax* – *P. quinquefolium* or *P. schinseng*. Ginseng is credited with the power to cure many diseases including cancer, rheumatism and diabetes, and to have powerful aphrodisiac properties. There is no evidence that the herb has any medical or other value.

girdle the ring of bones at either the shoulder (shoulder girdle) or the pelvis (pelvic girdle) that, respectively, support the arms and the legs.

glabella the normally hairless area between the inner ends of the eyebrows immediately above the nose. From the Latin *glabellus*, hairless.

glabrous smooth. The term is applied to a hairless surface.

gland a cell or organized collection of cells capable of abstracting substances from the blood, synthesizing new substances, and secreting or excreting them into the blood (endocrine glands), into other bodily structures or on to surfaces, including the skin (exocrine glands). The simplest glands are single mucus-secreting goblet cells. Glands also produce digestive enzymes, hormones, tears, sweat, milk and sebum. LYMPH NODES are often miscalled 'glands'.

glanders an infectious disease of horses occasionally transmitted to humans. It is caused by the organism *Pseudomonas mallei* and features chest infection with high fever and prostration or many abscesses throughout the body, especially in the skin.

glandular 1 pertaining to, functioning as or resembling a gland or the secretion of a gland. 2 possessing glands.

glandular fever infectious mononucleosis. An infection caused by the Epstein-Barr virus of the herpes family. It is spread by close contact, especially kissing, and is commonest in young adults. The disease appears after an incubation period of 4–7 weeks. There is fever, weakness, headache, sore throat, and enlargement of lymph nodes and the spleen. Spontaneous recovery, within a month, is usual. Sometimes there is prolonged fatigue and recurrences of fever.

glans the acorn-shaped bulb at the end of the penis or the small piece of erectile tissue at the tip of the CLITORIS. From the Latin word *glans*, an acorn.

glass eye an ARTIFICIAL EYE worn for cosmetic purposes. An ocular prosthesis. Artificial eyes are made of acrylic plastic, never of glass.

Glasgow coma scale a numerical method of evaluating the level of coma by assigning numbers to the response to three groups of responses to stimulation – eye opening, best obtainable verbal response, and best obtainable movement (motor) response. The scores are added and a deteriorating total suggests the need for a change in management.

glatiramer a mixture of synthetic polypeptides that act on the immune system and are claimed to reduce substantially the frequency of relapses in people with relapsing MULTIPLE SCLEROSIS. Its use is restricted to those who have suffered a relapse in the previous two years. The drug is unsuitable for patients who are severely affected and unable to get about unaided. A brand name is Copaxone.

glaucoma a rise in the pressure in the fluids within the eye of sufficient degree to cause internal damage and affect vision. There are several kinds of glaucoma, the commonest,

chronic simple glaucoma, being almost symptomless but causing insidious and gradual narrowing of the fields of vision. Acute congestive glaucoma causes exquisite pain and sudden blinding. Subacute glaucoma causes eye-ache, misting of vision and the perception of rainbow coloured rings around lights. Glaucoma can be CONGENITAL. See also GONIOSCOPE.

Gleason score a method of grading malignancy of prostate cancers, based on the pattern of glandular differentiation. Both the dominant and secondary patterns of differentiation are scored on a scale of 1 to 5, and the Gleason score, is the sum of the two scores.

gleet a discharge of mucus and pus from the URETHRA as in GONORRHOEA.

glenoid 1 of any smooth, shallow depression, especially in a bone, as in the glenoid cavity of the shoulder blade (scapula) with which the head of the upper arm bone (humerus) articulates.

2 the cavity of the scapula on the outer aspect.

gliadin one of the two main components of wheat protein and the one that contains the factor responsible for damaging the intestinal lining and causing COELIAC DISEASE.

glial tissue binding or connective tissue, especially in the nervous system. The glial cells of the brain, long believed to have only a supporting, nutritional and antipathogenic role, are now known to communicate with neurons and with one another, to have a function in the formation of synapses, and can determine which neural connections become stronger or weaker over time. It thus appears that glial cells are as important in thinking, learning and in the emotions as are neurons. Almost all intrinsic brain tumours are neoplasms of glial cells.

glibenclamide a SULPHONYLUREA drug, similar in action and effect to CHLORPROPAMIDE, and used to treat maturity onset (Type II) DIABETES. The drug is on the WHO official list. Brand names are Daonil, Euglucon, and Semi-daonil.

Glibenese a brand name for GLIPIZIDE.

gliclazide a SULPHONYLUREA drug used to treat maturity onset (Type II) DIABETES. A brand name is Diamicron.

glimepiride a SULPHONYLUREA drug used to treat maturity onset (Type II) DIABETES.

A brand name is Amaryl.

glio- *combining form denoting* glue-like; relating to GLIAL TISSUE.

glioma a tumour of the binding (glial) tissue of the brain – the neurological connective tissue. Gliomas are the commonest kind of brain tumour. They vary widely in malignancy and rate of growth. Depending on the type of glial tissue involved, or on their structural characteristics, gliomas may be called astrocytomas, glioblastomas, oligodendrogliomas, ependymomas and medulloblastomas.

GLP-1 a glucagon-like neuropeptide claimed to be an obesity mediator. Starved rats given the drug behave as if satiated and this state is reversed if given a GLP-1 antagonist.

gliosis propagation (proliferation) of nerve connective tissue (neuroglia) in the brain or spinal cord. This may occur as a repair process or as a response to inflammation.

gliotoxin a poisonous substance produced by the fungus Aspergillus fumigatus that has been found to interfere with the 'stickiness' of MACROPHAGES and to inhibit the process by which the immune system recognizes transplanted tissue, infecting organisms and cancer cells as 'foreign'.

glipizide a SULPHONYLUREA drug used to treat maturity onset (Type II) DIABETES. Brand names are Glibenese and Minodiab.

gliquidone a SULPHONYLUREA drug used to treat maturity onset (Type II) DIABETES. A brand name is Glurenorm.

glitazones thiazolidinedione derivative drugs used to treat type II (non-insulin-dependent) diabetes mellitus. Glitazones act by altering fatty acid metabolism by way of peroxisome proliferator-activated receptors which, in effect, increase cell sensitivity to insulin.

Glivec a brand name for IMATINIB.

globular protein any protein readily soluble in a weak salt solution. GLOBULINS are globular proteins. Also known as eublobulins.

globulins a group of blood proteins that include the family of IMMUNOGLOBULINS (Ig) or antibodies, comprising IgG, IgM, IgE, IgA, and IgD; FACTOR VIII, the antihaemophilia globulin; antilymphocytic globulin; thyroxine-binding globulin; fibrinogen; prothrombin; vitamin D-binding globulin; and many others. Gamma globulins are the most strongly positively

charged of the blood globulins and most of them are immunoglobulins.

globus hystericus the sensation of having a 'lump in the throat' which cannot be swallowed. This is due to an abnormal constriction of the muscles surrounding the lower part of the throat (pharynx) and is a feature of acute anxiety, depression or mental conflict.

glomerulonephritis acute or chronic inflammation of the GLOMERULI of the kidneys. The condition is mainly caused by immune complexes. These are bacteria, such as streptococci, to which are linked quantities of antibody insufficient to destroy them. Glomerulonephritis commonly affects children causing fever, headache, loss of appetite, vomiting and puffiness of the face and body (oedema). The urine contains blood and protein and the kidneys may, briefly, cease to function. Recovery is usual but there may be persistent abnormality of kidney function.

glomerulosclerosis a kidney disease in which many glomeruli (see GLOMERULUS), previously damaged by inadequate blood supply or GLOMERULONEPHRITIS, become replaced by a non-functioning glassy (hyaline) material. It sometimes occurs without prior damage. The effects resemble those of the NEPHROTIC SYNDROME and kidney function gradually deteriorates. Kidney failure is a common outcome.

glomerulus a microscopic, spherical tuft of blood capillaries, especially that within the BOWMAN'S CAPSULES of the kidney, through which urine is filtered. From the Latin *glomus*, a ball of thread.

glossal pertaining to the tongue. From the Greek *glossa*, a tongue.

glossalgia pain in the tongue.

glossectomy surgical removal of the tongue. This mutilating procedure may be the only safe option in cancer of the tongue.

glossitis inflammation of the tongue, usually from nutritional deficiency, especially of iron and vitamin B. It also occurs in iron-deficiency ANAEMIA, in SYPHILIS, ERYTHEMA MULTIFORME, PEMPHIGUS, BEHÇET'S SYNDROME, LICHEN PLANUS and may be caused by any persistent irritant, such as tobacco smoke, roughened teeth, badly fitting dentures or over-use of mouth-washes.

glossolalia 'speaking in tongues'. The

production of a stream of usually meaningless sounds resembling words. Glossolalia is a skill acquired by some people who enjoy a high state of religious excitement and is often accorded respect by like-minded observers.

glossopharyngeal nerves the 9th of the 12 pairs of cranial nerves arising directly from the brain and providing taste sensation to the back of the tongue and sensation in the lining of the throat. They also supply the CAROTID BODY and the CAROTID SINUS and a pair of muscles that assist in swallowing.

glottal pertaining to the GLOTTIS.

glottal stop a speech characteristic in which there is sudden interruption of the voice sound from a momentary complete closure of the vocal cords (GLOTTIS).

glottis the narrow, slit-like opening between the vocal cords and between the false vocal cords and the space between them. The vocal apparatus of the larynx.

glove-and-stocking anaesthesia loss of sensation in the areas of skin covered by gloves and stockings. This occurs in certain peripheral nerve disorders from B vitamin deficiency and other causes, from SYPHILIS and sometimes as part of a neurotic conversion disorder.

Glucagen a brand name for GLUCAGON.

glucagon one of the four hormones produced by the Islet cells of the PANCREAS, the others being insulin, somatostatin and a polypeptide of unknown function. The action of glucagon opposes that of insulin. It causes liver glycogen, a polysaccharide, to break down to glucose, thereby increasing the amount of sugar in the bloodstream. It can also mobilize fatty acids for energy purposes. Glucagon is a 20-amino acid peptide secreted by the alpha Islet cells. A brand name is Glucagen.

Glucobay a brand name for ACARBOSE.

glucocorticoids CORTISOL and other similar hormones produced by the outer zone (cortex) of the adrenal gland. The glucocorticoids suppress inflammation and convert AMINO ACIDS from protein breakdown into glucose, thus raising the blood sugar levels. Their effect is thus antagonistic to that of INSULIN.

glucogenesis the formation of glucose from GLYCOGEN.

gluconeogenesis the formation of glucose from non-carbohydrate sources, especially from AMINO ACIDS from protein. GLUCOCORTICOID hormones stimulate gluconeogenesis.

Glucophage a brand name for METFORMIN.

glucose grape or corn sugar. Glucose is a simple monosaccharide sugar present in the blood as the basic fuel of the body. Glucose is essential for life; a severe drop in the blood levels rapidly leads to coma and death. It is stored in the liver and the muscles in a polymerized form called GLYCOGEN. It is derived from carbohydrates in the diet, but in conditions of shortage can be synthesized from fats or proteins. The sugar is on the WHO official drug list.

glucose-6-phosphate dehydrogenase deficiency an X-linked recessive disorder, common among black African people, that can cause red blood cells to break down (haemolyse) if certain drugs are taken. Glucose 6PD is necessary for a biochemical pathway by which red cells obtain their energy. In its absence red cells are easily injured. The drugs that can precipitate HAEMOLYSIS include sulphonamides, antimalarial drugs, antibiotics and aspirin. Large doses are usually necessary to produce the effect.

glucose tolerance test a test of the body's response to a dose of glucose after a period of fasting. The blood sugar levels are measured at various intervals after the sugar is taken and the results plotted on a graph. A characteristic shape of the curve occurs in DIABETES because the blood sugar levels rise to an abnormal height and take longer than usual to return to normal. A urine test also shows sugar, in diabetes.

glucosidase inhibitors drugs, such as acarbose (Glucobay), that interfere with the absorption of carbohydrates and are used as aids to weight loss. Acarbose is used to treat Type 2 diabetes that is inadequately controlled by diet and oral hypoglycaemics.

glucuronic acid a substance formed from glucose that combines with many body waste products to form glycosides that are excreted in the urine.

glue ear secretory OTITIS MEDIA. A condition affecting the middle ears of children in which the free movement of the chain of bones linking the eardrum to the inner ear is impeded by sticky mucus. This causes deafness which is often unsuspected as the child does not complain. Early treatment is essential if the education, and possibly intellectual development, are not to suffer.

glue sniffing see SOLVENT ABUSE.

glutamate a negatively-charged ion derived from GLUTAMIC ACID and an important excitatory neurotransmitter in the central nervous system. Glutamate can be used as a marker of progression in stroke; concentrations of glutamate are higher in the blood and cerebrospinal fluid of patients with progressive stroke than in those with stable cerebral infarcts. Glutamate, which is produced by neurons deprived of oxygen, prompts the production of highly reactive free radicals that can kill brain cells. There is some evidence that cannabinoids from marijuana can protect against this damage by donating electrons in the manner of the antioxidant vitamins C and E.

glutamic acid glutamate, an AMINO ACID present in most proteins. One of its salts, MONOSODIUM GLUTAMATE, is widely used as a seasoning and flavouring agent and has been suspected as the cause of the CHINESE RESTAURANT SYNDROME.

glutamic acid decarboxylase autoantibodies autoantibodies that can be predictors DIABETES and that also occur in the STIFF MAN SYNDROME. Glutamic acid decarboxylase is the enzyme that catalyzes the decarboxylation of the amino acid glutamic acid, the product being 4-aminobutyrate. The immunological link between diabetes and the stiff man syndrome remains obscure.

glutamic pyruvic transaminase an enzyme released from damaged heart and liver cells and which provides quantitative evidence of disease of these organs.

Glutarol a brand name for a preparation of GLUTARALDEHYDE.

glutaraldehyde an antiviral drug used in solution for external application to treat warts on the sole of the foot (plantar warts) and elsewhere. A brand name is Glutarol.

glutathione a tripeptide amino acid derivative that protects red cells from oxidative damage and, in the form of the enzyme glutathione peroxidase, plays an important role in detoxifying hydrogen peroxide and organic peroxides produced in the body. Glutathione also participates in the transport of amino acids from one cell to another.

glutathione synthetase one of the enzymes

concerned in the synthesis of GLUTATHIONE from glutamate.

glutathione synthetase deficiency a rare autosomal recessive inborn error of metabolism dur to a mutation in the gene for glutathione synthetase. There are low levels of GLUTATHIONE, raised blood acidity, a tendency to red cell breakdown (haemolysis) and excretion of large quantities of 5-oxoproline in the urine. 5-oxoproline is a stage in the gamma-glutamyl cycle by which amino acids are transported. The antioxidant vitamin E has been used to treat cases.

gluteal pertaining to the buttock region.

gluten the insoluble, glue-like protein constituent of wheat that causes stickiness in dough. Gluten consists of two proteins – gliadin and glutenin. Some people are sensitive to gluten and in these it causes the intestinal malabsorption disorder COELIAC DISEASE which is treated by a strict gluten-free diet. Gluten is found in wheat, oats, barley, rye and similar grain cereals.

gluten-induced enteropathy see COELIAC DISEASE.

gluteus maximus the largest of the three flat buttock or rump muscles. The gluteal muscles arise from the back of the pelvis and are inserted into the back of the upper part of the thigh bone (femur). They straighten (extend) the hip joint in rising from a stooping position and in running, climbing and going upstairs.

gluteus medius the buttock muscle lying between the GLUTEUS MAXIMUS and GLUTEUS MINIMUS.

gluteus minimus the smallest, thinnest and deepest of the three buttock muscles.

glycaemia the presence of glucose in the blood. This is essential for life but the amounts must remain within strict limits. See also HYPERGLYCAEMIA and HYPOGLYCAEMIA.

glycaemic index a measure of the effect a given food has on blood sugar levels, expressed in terms of a comparison with glucose, which has a value of 100. Fast-releasing foods that raise blood sugar levels quickly are high on the index, while slow-releasing foods, at the bottom of the index give a slow but sustained release of sugar.

glycyrrhiza licorice. The drug is derived from the roots of *Glycyrrhiza glabra* and is of little medical importance other than as a flavourant.

glyceryl trinitrate nitroglycerine, a drug

highly effective in controlling the pain of ANGINA PECTORIS. The oral preparation may be taken in a tablet that is allowed to dissolve under the tongue and the pain is usually relieved in two to three minutes. The drug is also available in patches to be applied to the skin (transdermal patches). Nitrates have a powerful action in widening (dilating) arteries, including the coronary arteries, thus improving the blood supply to the heart muscle. SILDENAFIL (Viagra) should not be taken by people using glyceryl trinitrate. Nitroglycerine is a well-know explosive but is formulated for medical purposes in safe dilution. The drug is on the WHO official list. Brand names are Coronitro, Deponit, Glytrin, Minitran, Nitro-Dur, Nitrocine, Nitrolingual, Nitromin, Nitronal, Percutol, Suscard Buccal, Sustac and Transiderm-Nitro.

glyco- *combining form denoting* sugar or glycine.

glycobiology the study of the role of carbohydrates in biological events and their association with disease processes and mechanisms. Major advances in the understanding of the roles of glycoproteins and glycolipids has, in recent years, elevated glycobiology into a discipline in its own right.

glycogen a polysaccharide formed from many molecules of the monosaccharide glucose and found in the liver and in the muscles. It is the primary energy store of the body as it breaks down readily to release molecules of glucose. Glycogen has been called 'animal starch'.

glycogenesis the formation of the polymer GLYCOGEN from many GLUCOSE molecules.

glycogenolysis the process of breakdown of GLYCOGEN to release molecules of GLUCOSE.

glycogen storage diseases a group of about a dozen rare conditions due to absence or defect in one of the many enzymes involved in the process of storage of glucose as GLYCOGEN. Type I, for instance, is due to deficiency of the enzyme glucose-6-phosphatase and causes the infant to be obese and doll-like with poor muscles and soft bones. Some survive to adult life but are liable to suffer from gout and to have dangerous attacks of HYPOGLYCAEMIA. Also known as the glycogenoses.

glycolysis the breakdown of glucose or other sugars under the influence of enzymes, with the formation of lactic acid or pyruvic acid and the release of energy in the form of adenosine triphosphate (ATP). The complex biochemical sequence by which glucose-6-phosphate is converted to pyruvate and ATP.

glycoprotein any member of a class of proteins linked to carbohydrate units. They are called conjugated proteins and are of comparatively small molecular weight. Some, such as follicle stimulating hormone, luteinizing hormone and chorionic gonadotropin, lose their function if the sugar part is removed; others can continue to function even if deglycosylated. Some glycoproteins are cell adhesion molecules.

glycopyrronium bromide an ANTICHOLINERGIC drug used by anaesthetists to dry up secretions during general anaesthesia. Brand names are Robinul and Robinul neostigmine.

glycosuria sugar in the urine. This is one of the cardinal signs of DIABETES.

glycosaminoglycans mucopolysaccharides, a range of polysaccharides containing amino sugars or monosaccharides in which the –OH group is replaced by an NH_2 group. Heparin is a glycosaminoglycan. All six classes contain substantial amounts of D-glucosamine and D-galactosamine.

glycosylated haemoglobin a normal chemical linkage between haemoglobin and glucose. The amount of glucose linked in this way is proportional to the average levels of glucose in the blood. This provides an independent check of the quality of blood sugar control in DIABETES and is a useful monitoring aid.

glymidine a sulphonurea drug used in the treatment of non-insulin dependent DIABETES. Like the other sulphonureas, such as TOLBUTAMIDE and CHLORPROPAMIDE it is taken by mouth and reduces the blood sugar (oral hypoglycaemic drug).

Glypressin a brand name for TERLIPRESSIN.

Glytrin a brand name for GLYCERYL TRINITRATE.

GMC *abbrev. for* General Medical Council.

gnath-, gnatho- *combining form denoting* the jaw.

gnathalgia jaw pain.

gnathoplasty cosmetic or plastic surgery to correct a protruding jaw (PROGNATHISM) or a receding chin (retrognathism).

gnathostomiasis infestation with the dog and cat parasitic worm *Gnathostoma spinigerum* that is common in the Far East. The intermediate hosts are fish and the tiny crustacean water flea Cyclops and the worm is acquired by eating undercooked fish or drinking water containing the flea. The adult worm settles in the tissues and can damage the lungs, kidneys, brain or eyes. The worm may settle visibly under the skin; otherwise the diagnosis is by antibody tests. Treatment is difficult.

GnRH *abbrev. for* GONADOTROPHIN-releasing hormone.

GOBI a UNICEF mnemonic for four essential measures for the maintenance of child health in developing areas. The letters stand for Growth monitoring, Oral rehydration, Breast-feeding and Immunization. It is believed that effective attention to these four factors in such children could halve the present death rate.

goitre enlargement of the THYROID GLAND from any cause. This may be due to overactivity of the gland in THYROTOXICOSIS, to HASHIMOTO'S THYROIDITIS, to infective thyroiditis, to DYSHORMONOGENESIS, to cancer of the gland or to iodine deficiency.

Golden Eye a brand name for eye drops containing PROPAMIDINE.

Goldenhar's syndrome oculo-auriculo-vertebral dysplasia, a congenital disorder in which one side of the face is malformed, often with an enlargement of one side of the mouth. There may also be hearing loss, curvature of the spine, and mild retardation.

gold treatment the use of gold salts, such as sodium aurothiomalate (Myocrisin), to treat RHEUMATOID ARTHRITIS. These are effective in slowing progress of the disease, especially in early cases, but side effects, such as mouth and tongue inflammation, itching, liver and kidney damage and blood disorders, are common.

golfer's elbow inflammation of the tendon attachment at the bony prominence on the inner side of the lower end of the upper arm bone (humerus). A number of forearm muscles are inserted at this point and overuse, as in inept golf causes partial tearing or strain. 'Tennis elbow' is the same condition. Rest is essential.

Golgi apparatus a collection of stacked, flattened, cup-shaped sacs situated in the CYTOPLASM of cells near the nucleus and concerned with the movement of materials within the cell. The Golgi apparatus receives protein-containing vesicles from the endoplasmic reticulum, glycosylates them, sorts them into groups for different locations and transports them to other parts of the cell or to the cell membrane for export. (Camillo Golgi, 1843–1926, Italian microscopic anatomist).

gomphosis a non-moving joint, such as those between the bones of the CRANIUM.

gonadal agenesis failure of development of the GONADS.

gonadomimetic drugs drugs used to treat postmenopausal symptoms. An example is tibolone (Livial).

gonadotrophic hormones PITUITARY GLAND hormones that stimulate the testicles and the ovaries to produce sperms (spermatozoa), eggs (ova) and sex hormones. Follicle stimulating hormone promotes the growth and development of the eggs ova and sperms, and luteinizing hormone prompts the production of sex hormones. Gonadotrophic hormones are used as drugs to treat infertility, delayed puberty and underdevelopment of the gonads.

gonadotrophin, chorionic see CHORIONIC GONADOTROPHIN.

gonadotrophin release inhibitors drugs used to treat ENDOMETRIOSIS, MENORRHAGIA, gynaecomastia and benign breast cysts. Examples are danazol (Danol) and gestrinone (Dimetiose).

gonads the sex glands. The gonads are the ovaries in the female, that produce eggs (ova) and the testicles in the male, that produce sperms (spermatozoa). Both also produce sex hormones.

gonioscope an optical device consisting of a thick contact lens incorporating an angled mirror that allows examination of the otherwise visibly inaccessible angle between the back of the CORNEA and the front of the IRIS. This angle is important as the site of drainage of the aqueous humour from the eye, and may be blocked in some forms of GLAUCOMA.

goniotomy an operation to open up the abnormal internal drainage angle in congenital GLAUCOMA.

gonococcal arthritis joint inflammation occurring as a consequence of an infection with Neisseria gonorrhoeae.

gonococcal epididymitis inflammation of the EPIDIDYMIS due to a gonorrhoeal infection.

gonococcus the GRAM NEGATIVE bacterium, Neisseria gonorrhoeae, that causes GONORRHEA and is often found, in pairs (diplococcus) within white cells.

gonorrhoea a sexually transmitted disease once very prevalent among the sexually promiscuous but now, because of its ease of treatment with antibiotics, overtaken by CHLAMYDIAL infections and AIDS. As a result of antibiotic resistance, gonorrhoea may be due for a come-back. It causes a discharge of pus and mucus (mucopurulent discharge) and can lead to SALPINGITIS in women and narrowing of the urine tube (urethra) and ORCHITIS in men. From the Greek words *gonos*, semen and *rhoia*, a flow.

good cholesterol an informal term for cholesterol carried in high density LIPOPROTEINS (HDL).

Good Medical Practice a booklet, published by the General Medical Council (GMC) for the attention of all doctors. It lays down the principles of high quality practise and the standards of competence, care and conduct they are expected to maintain in their professional work. From 2005 registration with the GMC will no longer be a sufficient qualification for British doctors. All will require a licence to practise for which they must be revalidated. The purpose of REVALIDATION is to establish that a doctor complies with the standards laid down in this pamphlet. *Good Medical Practice* requires that every doctor must be professionally competent, honest and trustworthy; must perform consistently well; practise ethically; do patients no harm; avoid allowing personal beliefs to prejudice patient care; be an effective team player; and take action if poor practise by a colleague places patients at unnecessary risk. Patients' welfare must be their first concern; they must treat patients politely and considerately; respect their dignity, privacy and right to be involved in decisions concerning them; listen to them and respect their views; and explain medical matters clearly in terms they can understand.

Goodpasture's syndrome a severe disorder featuring glomerular inflammation (glomerulonephritis), leading to kidney failure and sometimes dangerous bleeding in the lungs. The syndrome is due to defects in basement membrane Type IV collagen caused by autoantibodies (auto-immune disease) and urgent treatment with immunosuppressive drugs and plasma exchange transfusion may be necessary to save life. (Ernest William Goodpasture, 1886–1960, American pathologist).

goose flesh skin in which the tiny erector pili muscles have contracted, causing the hairs to stand upright and the skin around each hair to form a small papilla. These muscles contract in response to cold or fear.

goose pimples see GOOSE FLESH.

Gopten a brand name for TRANDOLAPRIL.

GORD, *acronym for* gastro-oesophageal reflux disease. (See REFLUX OESOPHAGITIS).

Gorlin syndrome a rare autosomal dominant genetic disorder featuring a strong predisposition to various tumours, especially multiple BASAL CELL CARCINOMAS; brain tumours; ovarian FIBROIDS; multiple cysts in the jawbone (mandible); MILIA; and skull and rib abnormalities. Thousands of skin tumours may be present. The condition is believed to be due to a mutation on chromosome 9 affecting tumour suppressor genes. (American oral pathologist Robert J. Gorlin, b. 1923).

goserelin a gonadotrophin-releasing hormone used as a drug to treat ENDOMETRIOSIS, uterine FIBROIDS, MENORRHAGIA and cancer. A brand name is Zoladex.

GOT *abbrev. for* the enzyme glutamate oxaloacetate transaminase. This enzyme is released when heart and liver cells are damaged. Its detection and measurement provide helpful diagnostic information.

gout an acute inflammatory joint disorder (ARTHRITIS) caused by deposition of monosodium urate monohydrate crystals around joints, tendons and other tissues, especially the near joint of the big toe. This occurs when there is excess uric acid in the body, probably as a result of a genetic abnormality. There is excruciating pain and inflammation. Treatment is by non-steroidal anti-inflammatory drugs (NSAIDS), such as indomethacin (indometacin) or naproxen, used early and throughout the attack. Colchicine is also effective. Gout can be prevented by the use of allopurinol which lowers the levels of uric acid in the blood. See also GOUTY TOPHI.

gouty tophi chalky crystalline nodules of a urate salt which may accumulate in the ear cartilage in gout and break through the skin to appear externally.

GP *abbrev. for* GENERAL PRACTITIONER.

GP IIb/IIIa inhibitors drugs that block the glycoprotein receptor sites on activated PLATELETS thereby preventing the binding of fibrinogen and other ligands to these sites. The result is an inhibition of platelet aggregation and the reduced tendency to form clots. These drugs are used to prevent heart attacks in patients with unstable ANGINA and to reduce the risk of blockage of coronary artery stents. Examples are abciximab (Reopro), eptifibatide (Integrilin) and tirofiban (Aggrastat).

GPI *abbrev. for* GENERAL PARALYSIS OF THE INSANE.

G proteins cell messengers that relay signals from over 1000 different cell membrane receptors to many different intracellular effectors such as enzymes and ion channels. G proteins have three subunits, alpha, beta, and gamma, each coded for by a different gene, selected from a total of 34 genes. G protein function is switched on and off by the binding and hydrolysis of guanosine triphosphate to the alpha subunit which is loosely attached to the others. Binding causes the beta and gamma fragments to separate as a dimer and to activate downstream effectors.

G protein diseases a group of diseases caused by abnormalities in G PROTEINS so that hormonal stimulation is reduced or is abnormally persistent. They include essential HYPERTENSION, CHOLERA, ACROMEGALY, night blindness, pseudohypoparathyroisism, and adenomas of the thyroid, adrenal and ovary.

Graafian follicle a nest of cells in the ovary that develops into a fluid-filled cyst containing a maturing egg (ovum). One or more of these develops in each menstrual cycle, releasing one or more ova into the FALLOPIAN TUBE and leaving behind the CORPUS LUTEUM. (Regnier de Graaf, 1641–73, Dutch anatomist).

gracilis a long slender muscle lying on the inner side of the thigh.

grade the degree of malignancy of a tumour as determined by its microscopic characteristics. Grade should not be confused with STAGE.

graft a tissue or organ, taken from another part of the body or from another donor person, and surgically implanted to make up a deficit or to replace a defective part. To be successfully retained, a graft must quickly establish an adequate blood supply and must be able to resist immunological rejection responses.

graft-versus-host disease a complication usually appearing two to three weeks after a bone marrow transplantation and caused by cytotoxic T cells in the donated marrow graft. These attack the host tissues causing liver inflammation (hepatitis) with obstruction to bile flow, diarrhoea and a severe scaling skin disease called exfoliative dermatitis. Drugs such as CYCLOSPORIN (ciclosporin) and high dose steroids must be used as the condition, once fully established, has a mortality of about 30%.

gramicidin an antibiotic used externally in ointments and creams, often in conjunction with the antibiotics NEOMYCIN and FRAMYCETIN and with CORTICOSTEROIDS. It is too toxic for internal use. Brand names of various combinations with other drugs are Adcortyl, Graneodin, Neosporin, Sofradex, Soframycin and Tri-Adcortyl.

Gram negative used of a micro-organism that when stained by Gram's method does not retain the purplish dye, methyl violet, but only the red counter-stain carbol fuchsin. Stained Gram negative organisms appear red. The whole class of medically important bacteria can be divided into a large GRAM POSITIVE group and a smaller Gram negative group. This division is an important step in identification. (Hans Christian Joachim Gram, 1853–1938, Danish physician).

Gram positive used of a micro-organism that when stained by Gram's method resists decolorization with acetone and retains the methyl violet dye, thus appearing blue, purple or black. The reaction to Gram's stain depends on the structure of the cell wall of the organism. Most infective organisms, such as staphylococci and streptococci are Gram positive.

grand mal a major epileptic seizure. The fit may include a prodromal stage, an AURA, a tonic stage with sudden contraction of all muscles, a clonic stage in which the muscles undergo a succession of convulsive jerky contractions, and a period of unconsciousness or sleep.

Graneodin a brand name for an ointment containing GRAMICIDIN and NEOMYCIN.

granins a family of acidic, soluble secretory proteins that include various chromogranins and secretogranins. The granins occur in vesicles in neurons and neuroendocrine cells. They are prohormones and give rise to bioactive peptides and can be used as markers of sympathoadrenal activity and of secretion from normal and neoplastic neuroendocrine cells into the bloodstream. Some granins are sensitive markers. Raised levels of chromogranin A, for instance, may allow confident diagnosis of PHAEOCHROMOCYTOMA, VON HIPPEL-LINDAU DISEASE or NEUROFIBROMATOSIS.

Granisetron a serotonin antagonist drug that blocks the nausea receptors in the small intestine and is used to control sickness and vomiting after surgery and in patients on anticancer chemotherapy. It can be used in children. A brand name is Kytril.

Granocyte a brand name for LENOGRASTIM.

granulation tissue the tissue that forms on a raw surface or open wound in the process of healing. It consists of rapidly budding new blood capillaries surrounded by newly generated COLLAGEN fibrils secreted by cells called FIBROBLASTS, and many embedded inflammatory cells.

granulocyte a white blood cell (LEUKOCYTE) containing granules. Granulocytes include NEUTROPHILS, BASOPHILS, EOSINOPHILS and their precursors. MAST CELLS are also granulocytes. These cells are components of the immune system.

granulocyte colony stimulating factor a circulating hormonal substance that controls the growth of some of the white cells of the blood. The human gene for this factor has been sequenced and the factor is produced by recombinant DNA techniques (genetic engineering) and sold under brand names such as Granocyte and Neupogen.

granulocytic leukaemia a kind of cancer of white blood cells in which neoplastic change occurs in GRANULOCYTES, especially the NEUTROPHILS. Also known as myelogenous or myeloid leukaemia.

granulocytopenia deficiency of GRANULOCYTES in the blood.

granulocytosis an increase in the number of GRANULOCYTES in the blood. Compare AGRANULOCYTOSIS.

granuloma 1 a localized mass of GRANULATION TISSUE forming a nodule. Granulomas are often a response to the presence of foreign material within the tissues, and are commonly associated with persistent infection and inflammation. **2** an aggregate of EPITHELIOID macrophages often including multinucleated giant cells, plasma cells and eosinophils.

granuloma annulare a skin condition commonly affecting the back of the feet or hands of children and young adults. It appears as an incomplete ring of confluent, slightly raised bumps, usually of skin colour but sometimes red or red-blue. The cause is unknown and recovery is spontaneous.

granuloma inguinale a sexually transmitted disease, caused by an organism *Donovania granulomatis*, and almost confined to coloured people in the tropics. It starts as a small papule on the genitals which enlarges to form an extensive, velvety ulcer covering the genital area, the upper thighs and the buttock cleft. Streptomycin and oxytetracycline are effective.

granulomatosis any disease featuring multiple granulomas.

granulosa cells epithelial cells that surround the oocyte in developing ovarian follicles.

Graves' ophthalmopathy a severe eye disorder associated with thyroid gland dysfunction affecting mainly women in their 30s and 40s. It is an autoimmune disorder involving a massive cellular and fluid infiltration of the soft tissues of the bony orbit so that the upper eyelids are retracted, the eyeballs protuberant, eye movement limited and parts of the corneas often exposed and liable to drying. Optic nerve compression may lead to visual loss. Surgical decompression of the orbit may be necessary. See also EXOPHTHALMOS and THYROTOXICOSIS.

gravid pregnant. The term may be applied either to a woman or to a womb (uterus). From the Latin *gravid*, heavy or burdensome. See also PRIMIGRAVIDA.

gray a unit of absorbed dose of radiation equal to an energy absorption of 1 Joule per kilogram of irradiated material. 1 Gy is equivalent to 100 RADS. In radiotherapy, radiation is commonly applied to the area of the tumour in a dosage of around 2 Gy a day, five days a week for periods of 3–6 weeks.

greater omentum a large double fold of PERITONEUM attached to the greater curvature of the stomach and hanging down like an apron over the intestines. It contains many fat cells and is translucent and partially fragmented.

greenstick fracture a type of long bone break common in children in which the fracture is incomplete, the bone being bent on one side and splintered on the other.

grey baby syndrome a dangerous condition of acute failure of the blood circulation caused by the antibiotic CHLORAMPHENICOL. In premature and young babies the liver cannot adequately render the drug safe by linking with other substances (conjugation) and high levels occur in the blood. For this reason chloramphenicol is never given to premature babies.

grey matter that part of the CENTRAL NERVOUS SYSTEM consisting mainly of nerve cell bodies. The grey matter of the brain includes the outer layer (the cortex) and a number of centrally placed masses called nuclei. In the spinal cord, the grey matter occupies the central axis. The white matter consists of nerve fibres – axons of the nerve cells.

grey platelet syndrome a genetic disorder of platelet granule secretion in which the platelets, which are reduced in number, show a distinctive grey appearance with Romanowsky stains and have few or no granules. The condition features a mild bleeding tendency. This is one of the range of inherited throbocytopenias.

greenhouse effect the progressive earth-heating effect resulting from the transparency of the atmosphere to sun (solar) radiation at high frequencies and its relative opacity to energy re-radiated by the earth at a lower, less penetrative, frequency. Water vapour and carbon dioxide are the main elements concerned, and any increase in these, mainly from the burning of fossil fuels, enhances the heating effect. A rise in surface temperature could melt polar ice and cause widespread flooding.

green monkeys any of several African monkeys of the genus *Cercopithecus*. Simian immunodeficiency viruses (SIV) are the closest known relatives of the human immuno-deficiency virus (HIV) and these have been isolated from green monkeys and other primates. 20% to 50% of green monkeys in their native habitat harbour the virus, but it is by no means established that this was the origin of AIDS. An SIV with an even closer genetic sequence has been found in a chimpanzee.

grief the mental and physical responses to major loss of whatever kind, especially loss of a loved person. The mental aspects include unhappiness, anguish and pain, guilt, anger and resentment. The physical aspects are caused by overaction of the sympathetic part of the autonomic nervous system. This causes rapid breathing and heart rate, loss of appetite, a sense of a lump in the throat (GLOBUS HYSTERICUS), a fluttering sensation in the upper abdomen and sometimes severe restlessness. Grief follows a pattern of recognizable stages, some of which are: a sense of being stunned; refusal to accept the event; denial; a feeling of alarm; anger; a sense of guilt; and, eventually, consolation, adjustment and forgetting.

grinding-in a method of obtaining improved relationship of the opposing (occlusal) surfaces of teeth by inserting abrasive paste and moving the jaws relative to one another.

grippe a popular term for INFLUENZA.

gristle see CARTILAGE.

griseofulvin an antifungal drug derived from a *Penicillium* mould that concentrates in the outer layers of the skin and in the nails and is thus useful in the treatment of 'ringworm' (TINEA) infections. Skin infections settle quickly, but tinea of the nails requires treatment for months. Brand names are Fulcin and grisovin.

Griseostatin a brand name for GRISEOFULVIN.

Grisovin a brand name for GRISEOFULVIN.

groin the area between the upper part of the thigh and the lower part of the abdomen. The groins slope outwards and upwards from the central pubic region and includes an obvious crease when the hip is flexed. The term is sometimes confused with loin, which is on the back between the lowest ribs and the back of the pelvis.

groin strain any minor stretching of the tendinous attachments of the several muscles that are inserted into the central ligament of the groin and the adjacent bones of the pelvis.

grommet a tube, shaped so as to be retained in a hole, being narrower in the centre than at the ends. Tiny plastic grommets are used to secure and maintain drainage of the middle ear, through the eardrum, in cases of 'glue ear' (secretory OTITIS MEDIA).

gross anatomy body structure visible with the naked eye, as distinct from HISTOLOGY which is the structure visible on microscopy.

group therapy a method of psychotherapy

used especially to treat emotional disorders featuring defective relationships. Selected groups of 4 to 12 patients are guided in discussion by a therapist. The method provides a forum in which each member can demonstrate, for the critical perusal of the others, his or her particular aberration in human interaction. Different schools of therapy, including behaviourist, transactional analysis, family therapy and 'psychodrama', have adopted the method. A notable example of group therapy use is Alcoholics Anonymous.

growing pains a popular medical fiction. Growth is never painful. Possible causes of pains so described are hairline traumatic fractures, muscle and tendon strain from overuse, ligament strain and partial dislocation (subluxation) of joints.

growth hormone (GH) the hormone, somatotropin, produced by the pituitary gland, that controls protein synthesis and hence the process of growth. Excess growth hormone during the normal childhood growth period causes gigantism. Deficiency causes dwarfism. In adult life, excess causes ACROMEGALY. GH is secreted during periods of exercise and stress and for an hour or two after falling asleep. Growth hormone is also produced by breast tissue and in excess by breast cancers. GH encourages cancer cells to metastasize. Somatotropin is available as a commercial product under brand names such as Genotropin, Humatrope, Norditropin, Saizen and Zomacton.

growth hormone releasing factor (GHRF) a hormone used as a drug to test the function of pituitary growth hormone. A brand name is sermorelin (Geref).

gryphosis see ONYCHOGRYPHOSIS.

gryposis curvature or hooking.

guaiacum resin a resinous extract from the heart wood (lignum vitae) of the *Guiacum officinale* tree of India. The resin was used in the 16th century as an alternative to mercury for the treatment of syphilis. Since then it has been used to treat rheumatic disorders but this use is abandoned. Today guaiac is used in a test for the presence of inapparent traces of blood (occult blood) in the stools.

guanethidine sulphate an adrenergic receptor blocker drug used in the treatment of high blood pressure (HYPERTENSION) and

GLAUCOMA. A brand name is Ismelin.

guanine one of the two purine bases of double-ring structure (the other being ADENINE) which, with the PYRIMIDINE bases form the 'rungs of the ladder', and the genetic code, in the double helix deoxyribonucleic acid (DNA) molecule. Guanine is also one of the ribonucleic acid (RNA) bases.

guanine analogues drugs that closely resemble GUANINE and that are taken up by viruses or neoplastic cells to their disadvantage. Examples are famciclovir (Famvir) used to treat herpes zoster and tioguanine (Lanvis) used to treat acute leukaemias.

guarding reflex tightening of the muscles of the abdominal wall when pressed upon by the examining hand in the presence of underlying tenderness from inflammation. Guarding makes examination difficult but is, in itself, of diagnostic significance.

guar gum an edible natural material with the property of binding carbohydrates in the intestine and reducing the rate of absorption so as to prevent a sudden increase in blood sugar. This is helpful in DIABETES.

gubernaculum any guiding structure such as the fibrous cord that extends from the fetal testicle in the abdomen down to the scrotum and forms a mould for the canal down which the testicle moves into the scrotum around the time of birth.

guidelines in a medical context, guidelines are a series of suggestions, issued by official bodies, such as the Department of Health or by independent experts, for the conduct of medical practice. They include advice on the treatment of particular disorders or on effective ways of dealing with any clinical or human-relational problem. Guidelines are not prescriptive or directive, but doctors who fail to follow widely-recognized guidelines risk criticism and may even, in the event of poor outcomes be at risk of legal action. The practice of publishing guidelines, and of amending and updating them regularly, has grown steadily in recent years.

Guillain–Barré syndrome a serious immunological disorder affecting nerves in which damage occurs to the insulating fatty sheaths (myelin). The condition almost always follows a virus or bacterial infection. Cytomegalovirus, Epstein-Barr virus, *Campylobacter jejuni* and *Mycoplasma* *pneumoniae* have been implicated. Spinal roots are infiltrated with T cells and macrophages and the latter invade and strip off the myelin sheaths. In mild cases axons remain unaffected and remyelinization occurs; in severe cases axon degeneration also occurs. There is backache, tingling and numbness extending from the hands and feet to other parts of the body and progressive muscle weakness, sometimes amounting to complete paralysis. So long as the breathing is maintained, by artificial means if necessary, even these serious cases usually recover completely within two months. (Georges Guillain, French neurologist, 1876-1961 and Jean Alexandre Barré, French neurologist, 1880-1967).

guilt a state of distress usually caused by the belief that one has contravened accepted moral, ethical, religious or legal standards of behaviour. Early conditioning in such matters remains powerful throughout life and guilt may be experienced even when early precepts have been long-since been abandoned as illogical. A deep, and seemingly inappropriate, sense of guilt is often a feature of psychiatric disorder.

Guinea worm the parasitic worm *Dracunculus medinensis*. This occurs in many areas of tropical Africa and America. The worm is acquired by drinking water containing Cyclops water fleas that have ingested the worm larvae. The adult female worm, about 1 m long, settles under the skin and breaks through to release larvae, especially when the skin is in contact with water. She can be removed by winding her carefully out on a twig.

guillotine a sharp-edged instrument sometimes used in the operation of tonsillectomy.

gular pertaining to the gula or upper part of he throat (GULLET).

Gulf War syndrome a disorder, or group of disorders as yet unproven to be related to service in the Persian Gulf War against Iraq of early 1991. About 1500 UK troops and many more Americans are convinced that they, and even, in some cases, their subsequently-born children, suffered, or suffer, one or other of a wide variety of disorders as a result of this military service. Most believe these to be caused by the large range of vaccines and drugs given to them as protection against possible biological and chemical warfare, or by exposure to organophosphate agents. The matter has been the subject of long study in the United States by a Presidential Advisory Committee which submitted its final report in September 1997. No single cause had been found and the Committee suggested that stress was the most likely explanation for post-Gulf War symptoms experienced by miliary personnel. This opinion is hotly challenged by many.

gullet the common term for the OESOPHAGUS.

GUM *abbrev. for* genitourinary medicine. This specialty has absorbed and replaced the former discipline known as venereology.

gumboil an abscess in the gum and the outer bone covering (periosteum) arising from a spread of infection from a decayed tooth. There is redness, swelling and tenderness, all relieved when the gumboil bursts or is drained through a small surgical incision.

gumma one of the principle features of late (tertiary) SYPHILIS. The gumma is a localized mass of GRANULATION TISSUE, with a necrotic centre of a gum-like consistency. It occurs as a result of toxic destruction of tissue and can occur anywhere in the body, including the intestines, the liver and the brain.

gustatoreceptor a TASTE BUD on the tongue.

gustatory pertaining to the sense of taste.

gustducin a protein that is released when the taste receptors in the mouth detect a bitter compound. This protein triggers a cascade of reactions that finally sends sensory messages to the brain which cause the experience of a bitter taste. Gustducin blockers have been developed in the expectation that a food additive might remove unpleasant flavours from foods. This may be expected to exacerbate the obesity pandemic in the Western world.

gut the intestine. The term is neither slang nor popular. A major gastro-enterology journal is called *Gut*. The term is also sometimes used as an abbreviation for CATGUT.

gut-associated lymphoid tissue (GALT) patches of lymphoid tissue in the intestine comprising the Peyer's patches, solitary lymphoid nodules under the gut mucous membrane, and the vermiform appendix.

gut failure a condition in which the intestinal tract cannot process enough food to maintain adequate nutrition. Permanent gut failure most commonly results from removal of too great a length of the small intestine or from Crohn's disease or local loss of blood supply. Other causes include failure of neurological control of intestinal motility and DIABETES. Life must be maintained by tube feeding (parenteral nutrition).

Guthrie test a sensitive test for PHENYLKETONURIA that can be done on the new-born baby. The test requires a few drops of blood from a heel stab and the blood is then cultured with bacteria that grow well in an environment of phenylalanine. Heavy growth indicates an abnormal concentration of the substance. (Clyde Graeme Guthrie, 1880–1931, American physician).

gutta a drop, such as an eye or ear drop.

guttate 1 in the form of drops.
2 speckled or spotted as if by drops. Drop-shaped.

gynae- 1 *combining form denoting* woman or female.
2 Informal *abbrev. for* GYNAECOLOGY.

gynaecologist a doctor specializing in the wide range of disorders of the reproductive organs and the breasts of women. Gynaecologists are also usually experts in the management of pregnancy and childbirth (obstetrics). From the Greek *gyne*, a woman. See also GYNAECOLOGY.

gynaecology the speciality concerned with abnormality and disease of the female external genitalia (vulva), the vagina, womb (uterus), Fallopian tubes, ovaries and other structures in and about the female pelvis, and with the breasts. It is concerned, in particular, with menstrual disorders, endometriosis, pelvic infection, cancer of the uterus and adjacent organs, cysts and tumours of the ovaries, infertility, contraception and complications of child-bearing including ectopic pregnancy and breast lactation disorders. The list that follows highlights the key entries related to gynaecology in the dictionary: abortion, amenorrhoea, bacterial vaginosis, carcinoma in situ, cervix,

dilatation and curettage, dysmenorrhoea, ectopic pregnancy, endometrial ablation, endometrial resection, endometrioma, endometriosis, endometritis, endometrium, extrauterine, fibroid, gynaecologist, gynaecology, infertility, menstruation, menorrhagia, menopause, oligomenorrhoea, ovarian dysmenorrhea, ovarian hyperstimulation syndrome, ovarian tumours, prolapse, sterilization, transcervical endometrial ablation, transcervical endometrial resection, uterine dystocia, uterus, uterus disorders, vaginal discharge.

gynaecomastia the occurrence in the male of breasts resembling those of the sexually mature female. Gynaecomastia is often temporary as a result of a transient hormonal upset, but it may be caused by treatment with oestrogens or steroids, by liver disease, by a tumour of the PITUITARY GLAND or the testicle, or by the use of the diuretic drug spironolactone. Persistent gynaecomastia has, traditionally, been treated by plastic surgery, but the preferred treatment now appears to be the drug TAMOXIFEN. From the Greek *gynae*, a woman and *mastos*, a woman's breast.

gynandromorph a person having both male and female external genitalia and secondary sexual characteristics. A person displaying HERMAPHRODITISM.

gynaephobia an abnormal fear of women.

gynatresia a congenital closure of any part of the female genital tract, especially the VAGINA.

Gyne-Lotremin a brand name for a vaginal preparation containing CLOTRIMAZOLE.

Gyno-Daktarin a brand name for MICONAZOLE.

Gyno-Pevaryl a brand name for ECONAZOLE.

gyrus one of the many lobe-like rounded elevations on the surface of the brain resulting from the infolding of the adjacent grooves (sulci). From the Greek *guros*, a circle.

h

H-2 receptor antagonist one of a range of drugs that block the action of HISTAMINE on RECEPTORS, mainly in the stomach, that are concerned with the secretion of acid. The most important of these drugs are CIMETIDINE (Tagamet), famotidine (Pepcid), nizatidine (Axid) and RANITIDINE (Zantac). Although these drugs are ANTIHISTAMINES, this term is normally restricted to blockers of the H-1 receptors in the blood vessels.

HAART *abbrev. for* highly active antiretroviral therapy. Life prolongation by HAART of HIV-infected people has brought new problems, such as the increasing incidence of hepatitis C, which has a route of infection in common with HIV.

habenular nucleus one of a pair of collections of nerve cells in the brain, situated on either side of the stalk of the PINEAL BODY, and having a strap-like form.

habilitation training of the disabled in needed skills.

habit a predictable sequence of reactions to common stimuli or behaviour occurring in particular contexts. Habits are conditioned, are often performed automatically and unconsciously, and avoid the need for decision-making.

habit-forming tending to lead to physiological ADDICTION.

habitual abortion a strong tendency to recurrent, spontaneous termination in successive pregnancies. See also ABORTION.

habituation the development of a tolerance or dependence by repetition or prolonged exposure. From the Latin *habituare*, to bring into a condition.

haem- *combining form denoting* blood. From the Greek *haima*, blood.

Haelan a brand name for FLURANDRENOLONE (fludroxycortide).

haemagglutination clumping together of red blood cells.

haemagglutination pregnancy test a test based on the fact that red blood cells treated with human CHORIONIC GONADOTROPHIN will clump together, but that this can be prevented by urine from a pregnant woman.

haemagglutinin an antibody that causes HAEMAGGLUTINATION of red blood cells bearing the corresponding ANTIGEN.

haemangioma a benign tumour of blood vessels occurring mostly in the skin as 'birthmarks'. Haemangiomas include STRAWBERRY NAEVI, PORT-WINE STAINS, CAVERNOUS HAEMANGIOMAS and cirsoid aneurysms (widened and twisted vein-like vessels fed directly by an artery).

haemarthrosis blood within a joint space. This can occur from injury or disease such as SCURVY or HAEMOPHILIA. There is pain, heat, swelling and muscle spasm. Such blood soon absorbs but repeated episodes cause damage and crippling deformity.

haematemesis vomiting blood. This may indicate stomach or duodenal ulcers, gastric erosions, varicose veins in the gullet (OESOPHAGEAL VARICES) or the MALLORY-WEISS SYNDROME. Stomach cancer does not commonly cause haematemesis. Vomited partially digested blood resembles coffee grounds.

haematin the iron-containing portion of HAEMOGLOBIN. A complex of PORPHYRIN, iron and hydroxide ion.

haematinic pertaining to any substance that promotes blood production.

haematocoele a collection of blood in a body cavity that forms a cyst-like or tumour-like mass.

haematochezia the passage of unaltered blood via the anus, indicating recent lower intestinal bleeding.

haematocolpos an accumulation of blood in the vagina as a result of an imperforate HYMEN.

haematocrit 1 a CENTRIFUGE used to separate the cells from the fluid part of the blood. 2 the proportion of the volume of cells to the total volume after the blood has been centrifuged.

haematogenous originating in, or carried by, the blood.

haematologist a specialist in disorders of the blood.

haematology the study of the blood and blood disorders. The main subjects of concern are the various forms of anaemia, polycythaemia, the haemoglobinopathies such as sickle-cell disease and thalassaemia, purpura, haemophilia, clotting disorders and the leukaemias. Haematology is also concerned with all aspects of blood transfusion and its complications. The list that follows highlights the key entries related to haematology in the dictionary: ABO blood groups, aleukaemic leukaemia, antiphospholipid syndrome, antiplatelet antibodies, aplastic anaemia, anaemia, autologous blood donation, blood, blood cells, blood clotting, blood count, blood culture, blood groups, blood substitute, blood clotting (coagulation), differential blood count, grey platelet syndrome, haemoglobinopathies, haemolysis, haemolytic, haemolytic anaemia, haemolytic disease of the new-born, haemolytic-uraemic syndrome (HUS), haemophilia, hairy cell leukaemia, Kell blood group system, leukaemias, myeloma, lymphocytic leukaemia, myeloid leukaemia, platelet, platelet activating factor, platelet-associated autoantibodies, platelet disorders, polycythemia, purpura, red blood cell, sickle cell anaemia, sickling crisis, thalassaemia, white blood cell.

haematoma an accumulation of free blood anywhere in the body, that has partially clotted to form a semi-solid mass. Haematomas may be caused by injury or may occur spontaneously as a result of a bleeding or clotting disorder. In some sites, as within the skull, enlarging haematomas may be very dangerous. Infected haematomas may form abscesses.

haematoma auris 'cauliflower ear' resulting from repeated bleeding into the tissues of the ear, usually caused by boxing, with the formation of much internal scar tissue and distortion.

haematophagous bloodsucking.

haematopoiesis the growth and maturation of the blood cells and other formed blood elements in the bone marrow. Haematopoiesis normally occurs in the flat bones, such as the pelvis, breastbone and shoulder-blades, but in times of extra demand may extend to other bones or even other tissues such as the liver. All haematopoiesis, including both red and white cells, develops from a single type of stem cell.

haematopoietic growth factors haemopoietins, factors including GRANULOCYTE COLONY STIMULATING FACTOR and granulocyte-macrophage stimulating factor that bring about the maturation of bone marrow stem cells to form normal blood cells.

haematosalpinx a collection of blood in a Fallopian tube.

haematospermia blood in seminal fluid.

haematoxylin a reddish or yellow dye used to stain biological material for microscopic examination.

haematuria blood in the urine. In large quantity this causes a smoky, bright red or brownish appearance, but small quantities may be unnoticed. OCCULT blood can be detected by simple tests. Haematuria may result from bleeding from any part of the urinary system, from the kidneys to the URETHRA and must always be investigated.

haemo- *combining form denoting* blood.

haemochromatosis a rare genetic disease featuring abnormal absorption and retention of iron. Total body iron may rise from the normal 4 or 5 g to as much as 60 g and the stored iron may cause CIRRHOSIS of the liver, DIABETES, IMPOTENCE, HEART FAILURE and bronzing of the skin. Treatment is by regular weekly bleeding until the levels of serum iron reach normal. The drug desferrioxamine is also useful.

haemoconcentration thickening of the blood from loss of plasma or water. This occurs in dehydration and after severe burns.

haemoculture culture of blood for the isolation of organisms.

haemocytoblast the precursor cell from which any of the formed blood elements can be derived.

haemocytometer a glass plate accurately engraved with a grid of squares on which a thin film of blood is allowed to spread so that cell counts can be done under the microscope. Also known as a counting chamber.

haemodialysis a method of removing excessive natural waste products from the blood of people whose kidneys are no longer able to perform this function. The haemodialysis apparatus is commonly described as an artificial kidney. The blood is passed through a long semi-permeable plastic tube immersed in constantly changed water and the unwanted substances diffuse out.

haemofiltration a technique similar to HAEMODIALYSIS used to remove waste products from blood in cases of kidney failure. A membrane filter is used to remove an ultra-filtrate of plasma containing undesirable small molecules in solution and this is replaced with an artificial solution containing physiological levels of the normal electrolytes. The process may be done either by continuous arteriovenous haemofiltration driven by the patient's own blood pressure, or by vein to vein haemofiltration using an extracorporeal pumping mechanism.

haemoglobin the iron-containing protein that fills red blood cells. Haemoglobin combines readily but loosely with oxygen in conditions of high oxygen concentration, as in the lungs, and releases it when in an environment low in oxygen, as in the body tissues. In health, each 100 ml of blood contains 12–18 g of haemoglobin. The various genetically induced abnormalities of haemoglobin are called HAEMOGLOBINOPATHIES.

haemoglobin A the normal form of the haemoglobin molecule, containing two alpha chains and two beta chains.

haemoglobinopathies a group of inherited diseases in which there are specific abnormalities in the HAEMOGLOBIN molecule. The group includes SICKLE-CELL DISEASE and the THALASSAEMIAS.

haemoglobinaemia a rise in the normal concentration of free HAEMOGLOBIN in the plasma.

haemoglobinuria free HAEMOGLOBIN in the urine. This rare event occurs when large quantities of haemoglobin have been released from the red cells in the blood, as in severe MALARIA, causing the complication 'blackwater fever' or other forms of HAEMOLYTIC ANAEMIA. The free haemoglobin is able to pass through the kidneys into the urine. Compare HAEMATURIA.

haemolysis destruction of red blood cells by rupture of the cell envelope and release of the contained HAEMOGLOBIN. This occurs when red cells are placed in fluids more dilute than serum or as a result of an immune-mediated process. It may result from excessive trauma to red cells as in passage through artificial heart valves. Haemolysis also occurs when there is an inherent weakness in the cell membrane as in HEREDITARY SPHEROCYTOSIS. It also occurs in many other conditions including GLUCOSE-6-PHOSPHATE DEHYDROGENASE DEFICIENCY, various HAEMOGLOBINOPATHIES, THALASSAEMIA, rhesus factor incompatibility (ERYTHROBLASTOSIS FETALIS) and vitamin K overdosage.

haemolytic pertaining to HAEMOLYSIS.

haemolytic anaemia a form of ANAEMIA arising from haemoglobin loss as a result of increased fragility of red blood cells. See also HEREDITARY SPHEROCYTOSIS.

haemolytic disease of the new-born see ERYTHROBLASTOSIS FETALIS and RHESUS FACTOR.

haemolytic-uraemic syndrome (HUS) the combination acute kidney insufficiency, haemolytic anaemia and a low platelet count (thrombocytopenia). Biopsy of kidney tissue shows a blood vessel disorder with thrombosis of the glomerular and other small vessels. In spite of the thrombocytopenia, blood clotting times are normal. The syndrome has many causes including Shiga toxin-producing *E. coli* infection in post-diarrhoea cases, other infections, pregnancy, drugs, cancers, systemic lupus erythematosus and organ transplants, but most probably relate ultimately to endothelial injury. Its effects may be very serious as almost any system of the body may be involved.

haemoperfusion a method of removing poisons from the blood. The blood is passed through a tube containing either treated charcoal or ION-EXCHANGE RESINS. Clotting is prevented by using HEPARIN.

haemopericardium blood in the space between the layers of the heart coverings (PERICARDIUM).

haemoperitoneum free blood within the PERITONEAL CAVITY.

haemophagocytic syndrome a disease in which the large scavenging cells, the MACROPHAGES or histiocytes, attack blood forming tissues in the bone marrow, causing severe anaemia and bleeding tendency. Some cases are due to infection with herpes viruses, such as the cytomegalovirus and the EPSTEIN-BARR VIRUS, and these tend to be very serious.

haemophilia an X-linked recessive blood clotting disorder causing a life-long tendency to excessive bleeding. It cannot be passed from father to son because the father transmits only the Y chromosome to his sons. All the daughters of a haemophilic man are carriers of the gene but do not suffer the disease. There is a 50% chance that each of their sons will be a haemophiliac. Females can acquire the disease only if both X chromosomes carry the gene. Haemophilia A is due to the absence of Factor VIII, one of the coagulation factors. Haemophilia B (Christmas disease) is due to deficiency of Factor IX. Both feature bleeding, either spontaneous or on minor trauma, most commonly into the joints. This causes severe pain, swelling and muscle spasm. Repeated episodes lead to damage and severe joint disability. Tooth extraction or external injury are followed by prolonged bleeding. Spontaneous bleeding may occur into the bowel. Haemophilia is treated by repeated injections of Factor VIII or IX obtained from donated blood.

haemophiliac a person suffering from HAEMOPHILIA.

Haemophilus a genus of small GRAM NEGATIVE rod-shaped micro-organisms that includes *H. influenzae* which can cause MENINGITIS, *H. haemolyticus* which is often found in the throat, and the causative organism of CHANCROID, *H. ducreyi*.

haemophobia a pathological fear of blood.

haemopneumothorax the presence of both blood and air in the space between the two layers of PLEURA, the pleural cavity.

haemopoiesis see HAEMATOPOIESIS.

haemoptysis coughing up blood. This is most often an indication of BRONCHITIS or BRONCHIECTASIS or the result of a bout of heavy coughing but may also be caused by TUBERCULOSIS or, more probably nowadays, lung cancer.

haemorrhage an abnormal escape of blood from an artery, a vein, an arteriole, a venule or a capillary network. Haemorrhage may occur into a body cavity or organ, into tissues such as muscles, or externally by way of a wound. Internal haemorrhage often causes a HAEMATOMA. Severe haemorrhage results in dangerous loss of circulating blood volume and there may be insufficient to supply the heart muscle and the brain. This is inevitably fatal unless a rapid transfusion of blood is given. Insufficient circulating fluid causes the syndrome of surgical SHOCK for which fluid replacement is urgently needed. This need not be whole blood; an infusion of salt water (saline) can save life.

haemorrhagic disorders these include the PURPURAS, hereditary haemorrhagic TELANGIECTASIA, PLATELET excess, deficiency or defect, HAEMOPHILIA, CHRISTMAS DISEASE, VON WILLEBRAND'S DISEASE and the effects of vitamin K deficiency and advanced liver disease.

haemorrhagic fevers fevers that involve internal bleeding or bleeding into the skin. These include DENGUE, Kyasanur forest disease, Marburg-Ebola fever, meningococcal septicaemia, PLAGUE, RELAPSING FEVER, ROCKY MOUNTAIN SPOTTED FEVER and YELLOW FEVER.

haemorrhoidectomy the surgical operation for the removal of large, internally placed piles (HAEMORRHOIDS). A tight string (ligature) is tied around the base of the pile to control bleeding and the pile is cut off.

haemorrhoids varicose veins in the anal canal. Haemorrhoids may involve the veins near the upper end of the canal, causing internal piles, or those at the lower end, just under the skin, causing external haemorrhoids. Both may be affected. They cause bleeding, pain and a sense of incompleteness when defaecating. Internal piles may pass out of the anus (prolapse). Treatments include direct surgical excision (haemorrhoidectomy), injection (sclerotherapy), laser coagulation, infra-red coagulation, radiofrequency coagulation, or rubber band encirclage. From the Greek *haimorrhoia*, a flow of blood.

haemosiderin one of the two forms in which iron is stored in the body. The bulk of the iron is stored as haemosiderin. See also FERRITIN.

haemosiderinuria the presence of HAEMOSIDERIN in the urine. This occurs in cases of excessive breakdown of red blood cells with release of haemoglobin. Most of this is taken up by a serum protein haptoglobin, but if all the haptoglobin is consumed free haemoglobin damages the kidney tubules and haemosiderin appears in the urine.

haemosiderosis excessive deposition of iron in the tissues. When this is severe enough to cause tissue damage it is known as HAEMOCHROMATOSIS.

haemostasis 1 deliberate arrest of bleeding by local compression or clamping of bleeding vessels, by the use of ties (ligatures) around arteries and by various forms of cautery. Haemostasis is essential during surgical procedures to prevent the field of operation becoming obscured by blood.
2 the natural processes by which bleeding stops – small damaged arteries and blood clotting (coagulation).

haemostat 1 anything that stops bleeding.
2 a pair of artery forceps.

haemothorax blood in the normally potential space between the outer covering of the lung (visceral PLEURA) and the inner lining of the chest wall (parietal pleura). Haemothorax is the result of injury or disease. Unless the blood is removed and the bleeding stopped, adhesions tend to occur between the two layers, causing restriction in the free movement of the lung.

hair the filamentary keratin secretion of follicles in the skin. The outer layer, or cuticle, of each hair is made of overlapping flat cells arranged like roofing slates. Below this is the thick cortex of horny cells and the core of softer rectangular cells. The hair colour comes from pigment cells (melanocytes) of uniform colour present in differing concentration. Very curly hair comes from curved follicles.

hair cycle the repetitive sequence of growth and rest affecting the production of the hair follicles. The growth phase is known as anagen and this varies in length in different sites. The scalp anagen may last for several years. The rest phase is called the telogen. After about three months of telogen the hair is shed and a new anagen starts. Between these is the brief catagen during which the base of the hair becomes club-shaped.

hairball see BEZOAR.

hairiness, excessive see HIRSUTISM.

hairy cell leukaemia a rare disease featuring overgrowth of B. LYMPHOCYTES usually in men between 40 and 60 years of age. The lymphocytes show prominent hair-like projections. There is a profound drop in the numbers of all blood cells and the spleen, which is the site of the bulk of the abnormal lymphocytes, is enlarged. Treatment is by spleen removal (splenectomy) and the use of drugs such as alpha-INTERFERON and deoxycoformycin.

hairy tongue overgrowth (hyperplasia) of the normal small, fir-tree-like projections (papillae) of the tongue.

Halciderm a brand name for HALCINONIDE.

halcinonide a powerful CORTICOSTEROID drug used for external application. A brand name is Halciderm.

Haldol a brand name for HALOPERIDOL.

Haliborange a brand name for a range of preparations containing vitamins A, D and C.

halitosis bad breath. Most cases result from neglect of tooth brushing and flossing, odorous foodstuffs or drinks, smoking, gum infection (GINGIVITIS) or dental decay. Less common causes include DIABETES, BRONCHIECTASIS, lung abscess, atrophy of the nose lining (atrophic rhinitis), kidney failure or liver failure.

Haldol a brand name for HALOPERIDOL.

Hallpike manoeuvre a clinical test to diagnose BENIGN PAROXYSMAL POSITIONAL VERTIGO.

hallucination a sense perception in the absence of an external cause. Hallucinations may involve sights (visual hallucinations), sounds (auditory), smells (olfactory), tastes (gustatory), touch (tactile) or size (dimensional). Hallucinations should be distinguished from delusions – which are mistaken ideas.

hallucinogenic causing HALLUCINATION.

hallucinogenic drugs drugs that cause HALLUCINATION. Most are derived from plants such as the desert peyote cactus, *Lophophora williamsii* from which mescaline is derived, the psilocybin-containing 'sacred mushrooms' and the seeds of the morning glory flower, which contains lysergic acid. These drugs can precipitate a PSYCHOSIS in predisposed people.

hallucinosis an abnormal mental state featuring hallucinations.

hallux the big toe.

hallux rigidus a painful condition in which the joint between the first long foot bone (the metatarsal) and the nearer of the two bones of the great toe is unable to bend properly. This causes severe walking disability. An operation on the tendons may be necessary or a rocker bar may be fitted to the shoe.

hallux valgus a common foot deformity in which the two bones of the big toe are angled in the direction of the little toe. There is a prominent bump on the inner edge of the foot and this is subjected to undue pressure and forms a bunion (BURSITIS). Hallux valgus is caused by unsuitably pointed footwear.

halofantrine a phenanthrene anti-malarial drug used to treat both main types of malaria, those caused by *Plasmodium falciparum* and *Plasmodium vivax*. A brand name is Halfan.

haloperidol a butyrophenone drug used in the treatment of psychiatric disorders. It is similar in its effects to the PHENOTHIAZINE derivative drugs. The drug is on the WHO official list. Brand names are Dozic, Haldol, Haloperidol and Serenace.

halothane a pungent, volatile, non-inflammable liquid anaesthetic agent. Halothane is a powerful drug that induces anaesthesia in a concentration of less than 1%. Severe liver damage occurs very occasionally, usually after a second exposure to the drug in a sensitized subject. The drug is on the WHO official list. A brand name is Fluothane.

Halsted's radical mastectomy a mutilating surgical operation for breast cancer involving total removal of the breast and the underlying muscles, the fat under the skin, the lymph nodes in the arm pit (axilla) and a wide area of skin. This kind of radical surgery is now rarely performed. (William Stewart Halsted, 1852–1922, American surgeon)

halzoun an acute swallowing and breathing difficulty occasioned by inflammation and swelling of the gullet and larynx caused by ingestion of the nymphs of *Linguatula serrata* in undercooked mutton liver and lymph nodes.

hamartoma a rare BENIGN tumour of mixed normal cells that can affect any organ and that contains tissues normal to the organ. A lung hamartoma containing bronchial lining cells, connective tissue and cartilage, may cause obstruction of a BRONCHUS. As a rule, hamartomas do little harm.

hamate 1 Hooked at the tip.
2 one of the bones of the wrist.

HAMLET *acronym for* human alpha-lactalbumin made lethal to tumour cells. See ALPHA-LACTALBUMIN.

hammer toe a toe permanently bent so that the outer bone points downward like the head of a hammer. The condition is caused by excessive tightness of the tendon that bends the toe (flexor tendon) and is often treated by cutting tight tendons and fusing the two toe bones together (ARTHRODESIS).

hamstrings the tendons of the three long, spindle-shaped muscles at the back of the thigh (the hams). These prominent tendons can be felt at the back of the knee on either side.

hamstring muscles the three large muscles on the back of the thigh – the semimembranosus, the semitendinosus and the biceps femoris. These muscles arise from the lower back part of the pelvis and are inserted, by way of the HAMSTRINGS, into the back of the bone of the lower leg (the TIBIA). Contraction of the hamstring muscles bends the knee and straightens the hip joint.

hand-arm vibration syndrome
see VIBRATION-INDUCED DISORDERS.

handedness the natural tendency to use one hand rather than the other for skilled manual tasks such as writing. Ambidexterity – the indifferent use of either hand – is rare. About 10% of people are left-handed.

hand-foot-and-mouth disease a disease caused by *Coxsackie A 16* virus affecting especially young children. It has an incubation period of 4 to 6 days and features small blisters in the mouth and on the hard palate and these also appear on the hands and feet. The blisters give way to shallow ulcers that heal in a few days. The condition settles without treatment.

handicap any physical, mental or emotional disability that limits full, normal life activity. Handicap may be CONGENITAL or acquired as a result of injury or disease especially to the nervous or musculoskeletal systems.

Hand-Schuller-Christian disease a condition of multiple destructive HISTIOCYTOSIS of bone causing skull defects, pituitary gland disturbances with DIABETES INSIPIDUS, middle ear infection and loss of teeth. (Alfred Hand, American paediatrician, 1868–1949, Artur Schuller, Austrian neurologist, 1874–1958, and Henry Asbury Christian, American physician, 1876–1951).

hanging a method of judicial execution or of committing suicide. Judicial hanging by the drop method causes separation (disarticulation) of the upper neck vertebrae and severance of the spinal cord. Suicidal hanging usually causes death by strangulation.

hangnail a narrow strip of partly separated skin at the base of the nail (the cuticle). This leaves the deeper tissue exposed to infection and the nerve endings to undue stimulation. See also PARONYCHIA.

hangover the state of general distress experienced on the morning after an evening of alcoholic over-indulgence. The symptoms include headache, depression, remorse, shakiness, nausea and VERTIGO. With the possible exception of stomach irritation, these are not caused by alcohol, most of which has already been metabolized. The breakdown products, such as acetaldehyde, and some of the other constituents (congeners) of alcoholic drinks are, however, toxic. Other factors such as smoking, dehydration, overeating, the recollection of indiscretion and the loss of sleep may contribute.

Hansen's disease leprosy. An infection of the skin and the nerves, caused by the slowly replicating organism *Mycobacterium leprae*. Infectivity is low and the incubation period of the disease is from 2–5 years. Untreated Hansen's disease may cause loss of fingers and toes due to trauma to anaesthetized parts, and severe facial disfigurement and blindness. In the lepromatous form the body's immune reaction is poor and tissue destruction is great. In the tuberculoid form there is a good immune response and the disease is milder and non-infectious. Treatment with the drug dapsone is now less effective because of bacterial resistance and this has been replaced by drugs such as rifampicin, clofazimine and ethionamide, used in combination. Thalidomide is also valuable in the treatment of Hansen's disease.

hantavirus disease a disease caused by viruses of the *Hantavirus* genus. In Britain it can affect farm, nature conservancy and sewage workers and those engaged in water sports. Many cases are mild and inapparent but severe cases feature high fever, headache, shock, nausea and vomiting and small blood spots (PETECHIAE) in the skin. The eyes are red and the face, neck and shoulders flushed. Blood pressure drops and

kidney failure may occur. In 10% of severe cases there is significant bleeding. The virus is carried by rats, field mice and bank voles and probably passed to humans by inhaling dried animal secretions.

hantavirus pulmonary syndrome acute respiratory illness featuring a brief period of fever, muscle pains, headache, nausea and cough followed by severe shock and pulmonary oedema simulating the acute adult RESPIRATORY DISTRESS SYNDROME (ARDS). The mortality without specific treatment is 50–75% but the drug ribavirin is effective. The disease is caused by a strain of hanta virus and was originally though to be acquired only from rodents. Human case-to-case infection has now been demonstrated.

haploid having half the number of chromosomes present in a normal body cell. The germ cells, the sperms and eggs (ova) are haploid, so that, on fusion, the full (DIPLOID) number is made up. From the Greek *haploeides*, single.

haploidy the state of being HAPLOID.

haplosis the process of halving of the DIPLOID number of chromosomes by reduction division (MEIOSIS).

haplotype the entire set of allelic variants that may be found at any particular genetic location.

hapten an incomplete antigen that cannot, by itself, promote antibody formation but that can do so when conjugated to a protein. Most haptens are organic substances of low molecular weight. From the Greek *haptein*, to fasten.

haptic 1 *adj* pertaining to the sense of touch. A haptic contact lens is a large lens fitting under the eyelids and covering the white of the eye as well as the cornea.
2 the part that touches. The haptic of an intraocular lens is the peripheral supporting part.

haptoglobin alpha$_2$-globulin, a plasma protein that binds free haemoglobin to form a complex too large to pass out of the kidneys into the urine.

hardening of the arteries see ARTERIOSCLEROSIS and ATHEROSCLEROSIS.

hare lip a lay term for the appearance caused by a badly repaired CLEFT LIP.

Harmogen a brand name for ESTROPIPATE.

Hartman's procedure a surgical operation,

performed mainly for cancer of the rectum and lower colon, in which the segment of the bowel containing the cancer is removed, the rectal stump is over-sewn, and the lower end of the sigmoid colon is brought out as a COLOSTOMY. (Robert Hartman, 1831–93, German surgeon).

Hartnup disease a rare genetic metabolic disease in which the amino acid tryptophan is not normally absorbed causing a PELLAGRA-like syndrome. The condition is named after Edward Hartnup who was found to suffer from the disorder.

Hashimoto's thyroiditis a common form of thyroid gland swelling (GOITRE). This form of thyroid gland inflammation affects mostly middle-aged women and is an AUTOIMMUNE disorder, due to attack by antibodies mainly to the protein thyroglobulin produced by the gland. Other antibodies are also present. The resulting inflammation causes pain and sometimes difficulty in swallowing from gland enlargement. There is reduced output of thyroid hormone (thyroxine) and replacement therapy may be needed. A short course of steroids is also effective. (Hakaru Hashimoto, 1881–1934, Japanese surgeon).

hashish see CANNABIS.

Haverhill fever an epidemic of RAT-BITE FEVER caused, not by rat bites, but by contamination of milk with the causal organism, *Streptobacillus moniliformis*. Haverhill is a township in Massachusetts where the first outbreak was recognized in 1926.

Haw river syndrome a rare genetic disorder, similar to Huntington's disease, caused by a gene mutation on chromosome 12. It was found in five generations of a family from the Haw River area of North Carolina, USA. The condition starts in adolescence or early adult life and features lack of coordination, ataxia, paranoia, delusions, hallucinations, chorea, generalised seizures, and dementia, with death occurring 15 to 20 years after onset.

Hay-Crom a brand name for CROMOGLYCATE (cromoglicate).

hay fever a term remarkable for its imprecision, the condition being neither a fever nor caused by hay. See ALLERGIC RHINITIS.

Haymine a brand name for EPHEDRINE formulated with other drugs.

HDL *abbrev. for* high density LIPOPROTEINS.

head banging 1 a dangerous form of dancing in which the head is shaken vigorously and rapidly in a flapping manner. This can cause serious brain or other internal injury from over-stressed structures and has been the cause of several deaths.
2 a generally harmless activity engaged in by babies impressed by the effect it has on parents.

head injury see BRAIN DAMAGE, EXTRADURAL HAEMORRHAGE, SKULL FRACTURE, SUBDURAL HAEMORRHAGE.

head-standing an activity popular with practitioners of Hatha yoga, gymnasts and others. It has been recommended to relieve some forms of backache. Head-standing, or body inversion is generally harmless, but is dangerous to people with glaucoma because it causes a sharp rise in the fluid pressure within the eyes and affects the field of vision, possibly permanetly.

heaf test see TUBERCULIN TEST.

healing 1 the natural processes of tissue repair or restoration following an injury.
2 a power often wrongly attributed to doctors. Healing is a homeostatic function of the body and occurs automatically unless prevented by infection, continuing injury of any kind, radiation, cancerous change, the presence of foreign material or great age.
3 a claimed paranormal ability to perform miracles.

health 1 the general state of a person or organism. This may be good or bad.
2 the state of being in excellent condition of body or mind and free from disease, abnormality or disorder.

health action zone a designated geographic area, such as a county, a large town or a borough of a large city, in which purchasers and providers of healthcare in the British National Health Service cooperate to integrate all the different aspects of medical care, reduce health inequalities and ensure the best possible value for money.

health care practitioner a proposed new additional model of medical care designed to relieve the shortage of conventionally-qualified medical staff. Drawn from nursing, occupational therapy, physiotherapy or other sources not necessarily medical, the health care practitioner would undergo a one-year training course of seven modules. On qualifying, HPCs would be capable effectively of taking medical histories and carrying out examinations, ordering tests, providing basic treatment, patient education and nursing care, identifying unusual and difficult conditions and coping with medical emergencies.

health education the inculcation of knowledge the possession of which can help to promote health and reduce the chances of disease. Health education is concerned with such matters as personal hygiene, cleanliness, exercise of body and mind, good diet, care of the skin and hair, and the avoidance of hazards such as smoking, excessive drinking and the abuse of drugs.

health food food claimed or believed to be more beneficial to health than the generality of nutriments. Numerous claims are made explicitly or implicitly for the medical benefit of various foods but many of these are of dubious authority. Some measure of control in the UK is provided by the Health Claims Initiative of the National Food Alliance and the Food and Drink Federation which produces guidelines for food manufacturers. In the USA the Food and Drug Administration (FDA) serves a similar, if more draconian function.

hearing aid any device capable of increasing sound intensity at the ear, so as to assist the deaf. Electronic hearing aids traditionally consist of a microphone, an integrated circuit amplifier and an earpiece, often combined into a single device. Many include an electro-magnetic pickup for use in buildings or with telephones equipped with electro-magnetic sound radiation devices. Latest designs are intended for ear implantation and, instead of producing amplified sound from an earphone, apply output vibrations directly to the auditory ossicles, so eliminating feedback squeal. Amplification cannot relieve all cases of deafness.

hearing loss failure of normal perception of sounds or of sounds of a particular range of frequencies. Most hearing loss involves the higher frequencies. Hearing loss may be conductive, due to mechanical defects or obstruction in the ear, or sensorineural, due to damage to the inner ear nerve mechanisms.

hearing tests see AUDIOGRAM.

heart the twin-sided, four-chambered controlled muscular pump that, by means of regular rhythmical tightening (contractions) of the chambers and the action of valves, maintains the twin circulations of blood to the lungs and to the rest of the body. The right side of the heart pumps blood through the lungs and back to the left side. The left side pumps the blood returning from the lungs through all parts of the body and back to the right side.

heart, arrest see CARDIAC ARREST.

heart, artificial see ARTIFICIAL HEART.

heart attack a serious disorder of sudden onset in which part of the heart muscle is acutely deprived of its blood supply (MYOCARDIAL INFARCTION) usually as a result of blockage by blood clot of a branch of one of the coronary arteries (CORONARY THROMBOSIS) or as a result of coronary artery spasm. The usual predisposing cause of coronary thrombosis is ATHEROSCLEROSIS. Unless the blood supply is immediately restored part of the heart muscle dies. This is not necessarily fatal; the outcome usually depends on the size of the area affected. There is severe, persistent pain or a crushing sense of pressure in the centre of the chest and a terrifying conviction of impending death, which is all too often justified. The pain may spread in all directions – to the back, neck and arms. Half of those who die do so within 3 or 4 hours. As methods of dissolving the blood clot and other effective treatments exist, no time must be lost in getting a person with a coronary thrombosis to hospital. Ambulance crews are trained in emergency management and have saved many lives. There have been repeated suggestions that infection with *Chlamydia pneumoniae* may be a causal or contributory factor. See also CORONARY SYNDROME.

heart block a functional dissociation between the contractions of the upper chambers of the heart and those of the lower, due to interruption of the specialized conducting muscle fibres in the heart that normally coordinate this relationship. Such damage is usually due to inadequate coronary blood supply to the heart muscle but may be due to other causes such as rheumatic fever, syphilis or tumour. In heart block the pulse is generally very slow, as the lower chambers can only beat at their intrinsically low rate. Heart block is one of the major indications for the implantation of an artificial PACEMAKER.

heartburn a boring or aching sensation felt behind the lower part of the breastbone (sternum) when acid from the stomach regurgitates into the gullet (oesophagus). The symptom can also be caused by spasm of the oesophagus. Heartburn is usually due to dietary indiscretion but is also a central feature of HIATUS HERNIA. It can often be prevented by eating more slowly, more wisely and more continently.

heart disease, congenital see CONGENITAL HEART DISEASE.

heart enlargement an increase in the thickness of the muscular walls of the heart, mainly of the lower chambers (ventricles), usually as a result of increased work demand. Enlargement often results from high blood pressure (HYPERTENSION), heart valve disease or increased resistance to blood flow through the lungs. It is a feature of various CARDIOMYOPATHIES and can also occur from an increase in the volume of the chambers (dilatation).

heart examination see ANGIOGRAPHY, ECHOCARDIOGRAPHY, ELECTROCARDIOGRAPHY, HEART MURMURS, HEART STRESS TEST, PULSE, STETHOSCOPE.

heart failure the condition in which the heart is no longer capable of pumping a sufficient volume of blood to meet the body's needs for oxygen and nutrition. The result is engorgement of the veins and other small blood vessels and fluid accumulation in the tissues (OEDEMA). Failure may affect either side of the heart, or both. In left heart failure most of the effects are apparent in the lungs, in right heart failure most of the effects are in the body generally. Heart failure causes swelling and pitting oedema, accumulation of fluid in the abdominal cavity, breathlessness and moist sounds in the lungs. The commonest cause of heart failure is ischaemia from coronary narrowing or blockage, leading to progressive loss or dysfunction of heart muscle cells. The condition is treated with DIURETIC drugs to get rid of accumulated fluid, INOTROPIC AGENTS to increase the power of the heart, and drugs of the ACE-INHIBITOR class to reduce the resistance against which the heart has to pump blood. The latest advance in heart failure treatment is transplantation of genetically-altered cardiac fibroblasts combined with stem-cell mobilization by granulocyte COLONY STIMULATING FACTOR. See also DIASTOLIC HEART FAILURE.

heart inflammation carditis is the general term. ENDOCARDITIS is inflammation of the inner lining (the endocardium). MYOCARDITIS is inflammation of the heart muscle. PERICARDITIS is inflammation of the PERICARDIUM, the outer fibrous covering of the heart.

heart-lung machine a bulky device that is able to carry out the functions of the heart and the lungs, during the period of a surgical operation on the heart. The machine includes atraumatic rotary pumps powerful enough to maintain the circulation through the body, blood filters for particles, bubbles and foam, a blood oxygenator and carbon dioxide extractor, a cooler and a re-heater. Blood from the patient's main veins is carried in tubes to the machine and the machine output is connected to the main body artery (the aorta). ANTICOAGULANTS are used to prevent blood clotting.

heart-lung transplant the insertion of a donated heart with its associated lungs, connected as a unit, into the chest of a patient with severe destructive heart and lung disease. The operation involves fewer major connections than a heart transplant, but immunological reactions may be greater and the connection to the windpipe (trachea) may cause problems. A common rejection reaction is a severe inflammation of the small bronchi, called obliterative bronchiolitis. Even so, the results are remarkable and about 70% of patients are alive and well 2 years after the operation.

heart massage a lay term for cardiopulmonary resuscitation in which the circulation of the blood is artificially maintained by compressing the heart between the lower part of the breast-bone and the spine. This is done about 80 times a minute, but for every 15 compressions the lungs must be inflated twice by mouth-to-mouth respiration. In the average adult subject the breast-bone should be depressed about 5 cm and the weight of the body should be applied through straight arms. The activity is very tiring.

heart murmur a sound caused by turbulent blood flow or vibration of a heart valve that may or may not indicate abnormality. Many heart murmurs are innocent.

heart output see CARDIAC OUTPUT.

heart rate the number of contractions of the pumping chambers of the heart per minute. This varies with the degree of exertion. A low resting rate is, in general, an indication of the heart's efficiency. The average rate is between 70 and 85 beats per minute, but an athletic person may have a PULSE rate as low as 40 or 50.

heart reduction a surgical technique to reduce the volume of muscle in the left ventricle of a heart that has failed as a result of dilated CARDIOMYOPATHY. A full-thickness segment is cut out of the wall of the ventricle and the edges stitched together. Increased ventricular size raises the tension disproportionately and interferes with the contractions of the ventricle. By reducing the volume of the cavity, contractility and the heart output per beat is improved. The procedure is still experimental.

heart sounds the sounds heard with a STETHOSCOPE applied over the heart. The most prominent sounds are caused by the closure of the heart valves. Heart abnormalities, especially valve disorders, cause additional sounds, called MURMURS. The timing and characteristics of these give much information about the state of the heart.

heart, stopped see CARDIAC ARREST.

heart stress test see CARDIAC STRESS TEST.

heart surgery surgical procedures performed on the heart and its blood vessels. They include heart valve stretching (valvotomy), valve replacement, coronary artery BALLOON ANGIOPLASTY, CORONARY ARTERY BYPASS operations, HEART REDUCTION, HEART VALVE REPLACEMENT, the closure of 'holes in the heart' (congenital septal defects) and PATENT DUCTUS ARTERIOSUS, the correction of other congenital abnormalities and HEART TRANSPLANTATION.

heart transplantation the replacement of a heart irremediably damaged by disease with a healthy heart from a donor. Ideal tissue matching is seldom obtained but problems with immunological rejection reactions have largely been overcome.

heart valve replacement a method of treating the effects of a leaking or narrowed heart valve by removing it and substituting a donated human valve, a pig heart valve or a mechanical prosthesis.

heat disorders bodily dysfunction resulting from exposure to excessive heat, from disorders of the heat regulating mechanisms or from the excessive production of body heat. The heat disorders include PRICKLY HEAT, heat cramps, HEAT EXHAUSTION and HEAT STROKE.

heat exhaustion a disorder usually caused by

undue exertion in a hot climate with inadequate water and salt intake. Heat exhaustion features severe weakness, headache, nausea, sweating, vertigo, collapse and failure of the peripheral circulation from loss of fluid content in the blood. Treatment involves urgent fluid and salt replacement.

heat-shock proteins a range of peptides that are well conserved throughout a wide range of organisms and are produced by the body in response to various stressors. They are found in high concentration in plaques of ATHEROSCLEROSIS and levels of heat-shock proteins in people who have suffered strokes and heart attacks, and women with breast cancer, are higher than in controls. Antibodies against bacterial HSP can cross-react with human HSP60 causing cytotoxic damage to endothelial cells stressed by FREE RADICALS or infection. Heat-shock proteins are also associated with oral ulcers and Behçet's disease. They are found in a variety of bacteria.

heatstroke the effect of environmental temperature too high to be managed with the body's heat regulating mechanisms. The body temperature rises, the skin is dry and there is headache, nausea and confusion. Untreated heatstroke is often fatal. Also known as heat hyperpyrexia.

heavy chains polypeptides forming the main part of the Y structure of an ANTIBODY, including the stalk and the inner edges of the two upper arms. Each heavy chain contains one variable region and three or four fixed domains. Attached to the outer side of the upper arm parts of the heavy chains are the two LIGHT CHAINS. The area between the free upper ends of the two pairs of chains is known as the N terminal. This is the antigen combining site and is the variable part of the antibody allowing for the enormous range of different specificities.

hebephrenia one of the patterns of SCHIZOPHRENIA. Hebephrenia features regression to inappropriately youthful speech and behaviour, foolish mannerisms, delusions of omnipotence or religiosity and hallucinations. From the Greek *hebe*, youth and *phrenia*, the mind.

Heberden's nodes bony swellings around the furthest joints of the fingers, occurring in OSTEOARTHRITIS. (William Heberden, English physician, 1710–1801)

hectic 1 characterized by wide swings of temperature or daily recurrence of fever. 2 feverish and flushed.

hedonism the philosophic and psychological proposition that pleasure, or gratification, is the only ultimate good, and that the pursuit of pleasure is the ultimate motivating force. The concept of 'pleasure' is, of course, susceptible to a variety of definitions.

Hegar's dilators graded round-ended metal sounds used to achieve progressive widening of the canal of the neck (cervix) of the womb (uterus). See also DILATATION AND CURETTAGE. (Alfred Hegar, German obstetrician and gynaecologist, 1830–1914)

Hegar's sign softening of womb (uterus) due to its increased blood supply, perceptible on gentle finger pressure on the neck (cervix). This is one of the confirmatory signs of pregnancy and is usually obvious by the 16th week.

Heimlich manoeuvre a first aid procedure used to try to relieve choking caused by an inhaled foreign body such as a bolus of food. The upper part of the abdomen is encircled from behind, the hands are clasped together in front and the fists are suddenly and firmly forced upwards into the gap between the lower ribs so as to compress the air in the chest. (Henry Jay Heimlich, American surgeon, b. 1920)

HeLa culture a vigorously growing tissue culture cell line, established more than half a century ago and apparently immortal, that is used in laboratories all over the world for research and diagnostic purposes. The original cells occurred in a cervix cancer in a woman from whose name (Henrietta Lack) the term was derived. Artificial cell cultures of cancer cells achieve immortality by virtue of the enzyme TELOMERASE.

helicase an enzyme that breaks the hydrogen bonds between the BASE PAIRS in DNA thus separating the two strands of the double helix in the process of replication. Helicase works in conjunction with single-strand binding proteins that attach to the outer side of each single strand preventing the two from rebonding so that two rows of free-ended bases are left as templates on which new complementary strands can be formed.

Helicobacter pylori an organism found in the stomach and duodenum in at least half of the world's population. Whether or not it causes disease depends on several factors including the presence or absence in the organism of the *babA2* (bacterial adhesion) gene. In people with PEPTIC ULCER *H. pylori* with this gene is more than three times as common as in people without peptic ulceration. The bacterium has also been linked with other gastrointestinal diseases including gastric cancer and gastric mucosa-associated lymphoid tissue (MALT) lymphoma. Destruction of the organisms with METRONIDAZOLE or clarithromycin used in combination with a proton pump inhibitor drug such as OMEPRAZOLE is often followed by ulcer healing and appears to prevent recurrence. Eradication of the infection can be confirmed with a urea breath test. It is not yet clear whether this organism actually causes peptic ulcer but it certainly causes a diffuse gastritis. The genome of *H. pylori* has been sequenced.

helix the folded margin of the outer ear. The form of the helix is determined by the underlying cartilage.

Heller's operation a treatment for failure of the lower end of the gullet to relax (ACHALASIA of the cardia). The tight encircling muscle is slit down to the mucous membrane lining but without perforating. (Ernst Heller, 1877–1913, German professor of surgery).

HELLP syndrome *acronym for* haemolysis, elevated liver enzymes, low platelet syndrome.

helminth a worm, especially a parasitic NEMATODE or fluke (TREMATODE). From the Greek *helmins*, a worm.

helminthemesis vomiting of worms. This occurs only in very heavy worm infestation.

helminthiasis any disease caused by worm infestation.

helper T cell a subclass of T lymphocytes which provides essential assistance to MACROPHAGES of the immune system. When organisms have been ingested by a MACROPHAGE, antigen is expressed on the macrophage surface at the site of the MAJOR HISTOCOMPATIBILITY COMPLEX (MHC) surface markers. Helper T cells bind to the combination of antigen and MHC and produce the CYTOKINE gamma-interferon. This diffuses to the MACROPHAGE and switches on the killing function so that the organism is destroyed. In the absence of helper T cell assistance the protective function of the immune system is seriously undermined. The HIV attacks and kills helper T cells thus causing acquired immune deficiency (AIDS).

helper virus a virus that supplies deficient functions in a damaged virus, so as to allow the latter to complete its invasion of a cell.

hemeralopia inability to see as well in bright light as in dim. From the Greek *hemera*, day, *alaos*, blind and *ops* an eye.

hemi- *combining form denoting* half. From the Greek *hemi*.

hemianopia loss of half of the field of vision of one or both eyes. Hemianopia usually affects corresponding halves of the visual fields of both eyes as it is usually due to damage to the optical nerve tracts behind the eyes that contain fibres from both eyes. In homonymous hemianopia there is loss of corresponding halves of the field of each eye. In bitemporal hemianopia both outer halves are lost. Hemianopia is a common symptom of STROKE or pituitary gland tumour.

hemiballismus a condition of sudden onset, usually in elderly people, featuring violent, involuntary, spasmodic movements of large amplitude on one side of the body only. The movements are constant and exhausting but cease during sleep. Hemiballismus is caused by a loss of blood supply to one of the subthalamic nuclei in the brain or its connections.

hemicolectomy surgical removal of one half of the large intestine (colon).

hemicorporectomy surgical removal of the lower half of the body, including the pelvis and its contents.

hemicranial headache pain in one half of the head, a characteristic of classical MIGRAINE, hence the name.

hemiglossectomy surgical removal of half the tongue, usually for cancer.

Heminevrin a brand name for CHLOMETHIAZOLE.

hemiparesis muscle weakness on one side of the body.

hemiplegia paralysis of the right or left half of the body. This is the result of damage to one side of the main motor nerve pathways which run down from the surface of the brain to the spinal cord. Hemiplegia is a cardinal sign of STROKE but can be caused by MULTIPLE SCLEROSIS, brain inflammation (ENCEPHALITIS), brain tumour or injury. The arm is usually more severely affected than the leg and the face

may or may not be involved.

hemipterous belonging to the Hemiptera order of bugs, a large group of insects that includes the cone-nose bugs that transmit CHAGAS' DISEASE and the bed-bugs. From the Greek *hemi*, half and *pteron*, a wing.

Henoch-Schonlein purpura a bleeding disorder, mainly affecting children and caused by an allergic (anaphylactoid) reaction. There is bleeding into the skin, the intestines and the joints, causing abdominal pain and arthritis. See also PURPURA. (Eduard Heinrich Henoch, German paediatrician, 1820–1910, and Johann Lukas Schonlein, Bavarian pathologist, 1793–1864).

heparin a complex polysaccharide organic acid found mainly in lung and liver tissue. Heparin is thought to bind to THROMBIN and antithrombin in plasma thereby assisting in their combination and interfering with the cascade of reactions that end in blood clotting (coagulation). From the Greek *hepar*, the liver. The drug is on the WHO official list. Heparin is widely used as an anticoagulant under brand names such as Calciparine, Canusal, Hepsal, Monoparin and Multiparin. See also LOW MOLECULAR WEIGHT HEPARIN.

heparin-induced thrombocytopenia a blood platelet deficiency disorder caused by a reaction to heparin. The condition is caused by antibodies, usually of the IgG class against a heparin-platelet Factor IV complex on the surface of platelets. Paradoxically, the condition features thrombosis and embolism with the risk of stroke and other serious arterial occlusion effects. This is because the immune complexes formed combine with the antibody Fc receptors of platelets causing their activation and the initiation of clotting.

hepat-, hepato-, hepatico- *combining form denoting* liver.

hepatectomy removal of part or the whole of the liver.

hepatic pertaining to the liver.

hepatic coma loss of consciousness associated with liver failure.

hepatic encephalopathy brain disorder associated with severe liver disease with loss of liver function. Neurological malfunction, with behavioral and psychological changes, occurs.

hepatitis A liver inflammation caused by the hepatitis A virus (HAV), which is excreted in the faeces and acquired by the ingestion of contaminated food. There is fever, severe loss of appetite, enlargement and tenderness of the liver, yellowing of the skin (JAUNDICE), darkening of the urine and pale, clay-like stools. There is no specific treatment but full recovery is the rule.

hepatitis B liver inflammation caused by the hepatitis B virus (HBV), which is transmitted in blood or blood products or in other body fluids and can be spread from mother to baby during, or soon after, birth. The commonest mode of spread is by shared intravenous needles. Male homosexuals are greatly at risk. The disease is similar to hepatitis A, but more severe. There is a significant death rate in the acute stage and 10% of those who recover become carriers and may develop complications, including CIRRHOSIS and cancer of the liver. Vaccination against HBV is effective.

hepatitis B vaccine a vaccine containing inactivated hepatitis B virus surface antigen produced by recombinant DNA technology and adsorbed on aluminium hydroxide. The vaccine is given to people at high risk of acquiring hepatitis B. These include close family contacts of a patient with hepatitis B, intravenous drug abusers, sexually promiscuous people, patients on haemodialysis, those receiving frequent blood transfusions and medical staff in regular contact with blood or body fluids or tissues. The drug is on the WHO official list.

hepatitis C formerly called hepatitis non-A, non-B, this liver disease is caused by a small single-stranded RNA virus, 30–38 nm in diameter known as the hepatitis C virus (HCV). The disease occurs world-wide and is spread mainly by intravenous drug abuse, tattooing, needle-stick injuries, inadequately-sterilized medical equipment and transfusion of blood or blood products. Sexual transmission occurs, but is rare. Only a minority of infected people develop symptoms and the clinical course is usually mild with jaundice in only 10%. Unfortunately the infection persists in about 80% of cases and 20 to 30% develop CIRRHOSIS OF THE LIVER within 30 years of acquiring the infection.

hepatitis, delta a liver inflammation caused by a very small virus, hepatitis delta virus (HDV) that can reproduce only in the presence of the hepatitis B virus (HBV). This superinfection

occurs in about 5% of cases and consideravly worsens the outlook. HDV infection has caused serious epidemics and is endemic in the Mediterranean area. The method of spread is not clearly understood.

hepatitis E a liver inflammation caused by a single-strand, non-enveloped RNA virus 27–34 nm in diameter, known as hepatitis virus E (HEV), that is spread, waterborne, by the faecal-oral route. The first outbreak in Delhi, spread by sewage and flooding, caused 30,000 cases of jaundice. By early 2005 the disease was endemic or epidemic throughout the whole of north Africa, the middle East, south Asia and China, parts of south-east Asia and central America. There is a mortality of up to 4 per cent, but in pregnant women the mortality may be as high as 20%.

hepatocellular pertaining to liver cells.

hepatocyte a liver cell. Hepatocytes are metabolically very active and are rich in MITOCHONDRIA, LYSOSOMES and ENDOPLASMIC RETICULUM. Each is surrounded by highly permeable capillaries.

hepatojugular reflux a visible upward movement of the jugular vein pulse in the neck on pressure on the abdomen. This is a way of distinguishing venous from arterial pulsation.

hepatolenticular degeneration see WILSON'S DISEASE.

hepatoma a primary cancer of the liver (hepatocellular carcinoma). Primary liver cancer is rare in the Western world while secondary cancer is very common. Hepatomas are common in areas in which exposure to HEPATITIS B and AFLATOXINS occur frequently. In these areas, males with CIRRHOSIS are especially prone. There are high blood levels of ALPHAFETOPROTEIN. Surgery is sometimes feasible but the outlook is poor.

hepatomegaly enlargement of the liver. Possible causes include HEPATITIS, HEART FAILURE, secondary cancer, constrictive PERICARDITIS, LYMPHOMA, LEUKAEMIA, amoebic abscess, MALARIA, KALA AZAR and SCHISTOSOMIASIS.

hepatorenal syndrome a form of kidney failure occurring in CIRRHOSIS of the liver, not because of kidney disease but probably because of greatly diminished blood flow through the kidneys because of renal vasoconstriction. The outlook is very poor unless liver transplantation is performed.

hepatosplenic pertaining to the liver and the spleen.

hepatotoxicity the state of being poisonous (toxic) to the liver, or the degree to which a substance is toxic to the liver.

Hepsera a brand name for ADEFOVIR DIPIVOXIL.

HER2 human epidermal receptor 2, a growth factor receptor that plays an essential role in cell proliferation and differentiation. The 20 to 25% of breast cancers that over-express HER2 have a high rate of recurrence in the first two or three years after surgery. The monoclonal antibody drug trastuzumab which blocks this receptor is effective in reducing the dangers of HER2-expressing breast cancers.

herbal 1 a book containing identifying descriptions of plants and an account of their alleged medicinal properties.

2 pertaining to, or containing herbs.

herbal medicine a form of medical treatment using extracts of herbs. Many orthodox and important drugs are derived from herbs, but herbalists concentrate on those not considered by pharmacologists to be of sufficient medical value to exploit. Because of the variability of the amounts of the active ingredients in herbs and because these medicines are not assayed, instances of poisoning by herbal remedies regularly appear in the medical press. There are moves to regulate this trade.

hereditary haemorrhagic telangiectasia a rare autosomal dominant genetic disorder caused by mutations of the gene for endoglin, on chromosome 9, part of the receptor complex for transforming growth factor. The result is a disorder of the smallest blood vessels (capillaries) which become widened (dilated) and have a tendency to bleed. It presents with typical featuring characteristic lesions on the lips, face, and mouth and can also extend to the gastrointestinal tract causing anaemia and to the lungs causing HAEMOPTYSIS.

hereditary spherocytosis a genetic disorder of the red blood cells which tend to be spherical rather than disc-shaped and are unduly fragile, breaking easily to release HAEMOGLOBIN. This leads to ANAEMIA, and the scavenging of the destroyed red cells causes enlargement of the spleen (splenomegaly).

hereditary tyrosinaemia a metabolic disorder due to an inherited deficiency of the enzyme fumarylacetoacetate hydrolase. There is progressive liver and kidney damage, low blood phosphate, RICKETS and sometimes severe neurological complications and muscle weakness. Tyrosine is excreted in the urine. In acute cases death occurs in the first year of life. Most cases are fatal unless treated. A diet low in tyrosine and phenylalanine is given.

heredity the transmission from parent to child of any of the characteristics coded for in the molecular sequences on DNA known as the GENES. Heredity is mediated by way of the CHROMOSOMES which, essentially, consist of DNA. Of the 46 chromosomes in each body cell, 23 come from the mother and 23 from the father. The pattern of genes on the chromosomes is called the genotype; the resulting physical structure with all its characteristics is called the phenotype.

Hering—Breuer reflex a feedback system for controlling breathing. The stimulation of stretch receptors in the bronchi and lungs, occasioned by breathing in, eventually causes the DIAPHRAGM and the muscles between the ribs (intercostal muscles) to cease contracting. (Heinrich Ewald Hering, 1866–1918, German physiologist; and Josef Breuer, 1843–1925, Austrian physician)

hermaphroditism the rare bodily condition in which both male and female reproductive organs are present, often in an ambiguous form. Some hermaphrodites are said to be capable of sexual intercourse with either sex. Most hermaphrodites are raised as males but about half of them menstruate and most develop female breasts. The term derives from the mythical Hermaphroditos, who so inflamed the passions of a young woman called Salmacis that she prayed for total union with him. Her wish was granted and the two were fused into one body.

hernia abnormal protrusion of an organ or tissue through a natural or abnormal opening. Hernias commonly involve a loop of bowel and occur at weak points in the walls of body cavities, especially the abdomen. They are common in the groin region INGUINAL HERNIA and FEMORAL HERNIA, at the umbilicus (UMBILICAL HERNIA) and at the opening in the diaphragm for the gullet (oesophagus). Herniation of the stomach up through the diaphragm is called a HIATUS HERNIA. Hernias that cannot be returned to their normal position are said to be incarcerated and if the blood supply is cut off by swelling they are said to be strangulated. Hernias should be corrected by surgery. External supports (trusses) are not generally satisfactory. Although the great majority of hernias involve displaced bowel, many other structures or tissues can herniate from their normal position. These include part of the brain through the large opening for the spinal cord or through a defect in the skull; muscle tissue through its compartment wall; synovial membrane of a joint through the joint capsule; and the pulpy centre of an intervertebral disc (nucleus pulposus).

hernial sac a bag of PERITONEUM pushed through a hernial orifice and containing the loop of bowel or other body part that has herniated.

herniated intervertebral disc an inaccurate term used to describe the squeezing out of part of the pulpy centre (nucleus pulposus) of one of the discs between two adjacent bones of the spine (vertebrae).

herniorrhaphy an operation for repair of a HERNIA and the closure and strengthening of the orifice through which it has passed by means of natural tissue, such as strips of FASCIA, or artificial material.

heroin see DIAMORPHINE.

heroin babies babies who have received a regular morphine dosage via the placenta before birth and who show withdrawal signs after birth. These include diarrhoea, vomiting, sweating, sneezing, shakiness, hyperactivity, breathing difficulties and convulsions and persist for 1–3 weeks.

herpangina a virus infection mainly affecting children under 7 and featuring fever, severe sore throat, loss of appetite (anorexia), and greyish-white blister-like spots on and around the tonsils. Herpangina is caused by a coxsackie virus and is similar to HAND, FOOT AND MOUTH DISEASE.

herpes viruses a group of eight different viruses that includes the herpes simplex virus, types I and II, causing, respectively, 'cold sores' and venereal herpes, herpes zoster virus, that causes CHICKEN POX and SHINGLES, the Epstein Barr virus, that causes GLANDULAR FEVER (infective mononucleosis), the cytomegalovirus that affects people with immunodeficiency disorders, and human herpes virus 8 that causes

KAPOSI'S SARCOMA. From the Greek *herpein*, to creep.

herpes gestationis an uncommon skin disease affecting pregnant women and causing red-based blisters anywhere on the body but usually symmetrically on the elbows, shoulder blades, buttocks and backs of the thighs. The condition resolves as soon as the baby is born but recurs in subsequent pregnancies or even on taking oral contraceptives.

herpes zoster see HERPES VIRUSES and SHINGLES.

herpetiform herpes-like.

Herpid a brand name for IDOXURIDINE.

Herceptin a brand name for TRASTUZUMAB.

Herxheimer reaction see JARISCH-HERXHEIMER REACTION.

Hess test a test for PURPURA in which a SPHYGMOMANOMETER cuff is left inflated for 5 min and the skin then inspected for PETECHIAL HAEMORRHAGES. (Alfred Fabian Hess, 1875–1933, American physician)

hetero- *combining form denoting* different. From the Greek *heteros*, meaning other.

heterochromatin a length of chromatin in the genome that is permanently highly condensed and whose DNA is not transcribed.

heterocyclic of organic compounds with one or more closed rings consisting of carbon atoms and atoms of other elements such as nitrogen, oxygen or sulphur.

heterograft a transplant of tissue taken from one species and grafted into another.

heterologous 1 derived from a different source. 2 of a transfusion or transplant from a different species.
3 of tissue not normally present at a particular site.
4 of parts of different organisms that differ in structure.

heteroploid having an abnormal number of chromosomes.

heterosexuality the common state of sexual orientation directed towards a person of opposite anatomical sex.

heterotopic occurring in an abnormal location, especially of normal tissue, as, for instance in ENDOMETRIOSIS.

heterotopic ossification the development of mature lamellar bone in soft tissue that does not normally contain bone. The condition is usually associated with trauma in or around a joint or following severe head or spinal cord injuries. Heterotopic ossification is also found in the rare autosomal dominant condition of MYOSITIS OSSIFICANS.

heterozygous of a person carrying different genes at the same gene locus in corresponding chromosomes. The ALLELES are different. A single DOMINANT gene can manifest itself in a heterozygous person. Recessive genes are only manifest if both are present (HOMOZYGOUS).

heterozygosity the state of possessing two different ALLELES for one or more genes. Loss of heterozygosity from all the abnormal cells in a lesion indicates monoconal proliferation and is a molecular marker of neoplasia.

hexachlorophane hexachlorophene, a bactericidal agent used in soaps and for skin cleansing. A chlorinated phenol. Brand names are Ster-Zac Powder and, formulated with other ingredients, Dermalex.

hexamine hippurate methenamine hippurate, an antibacterial drug used to assist controlling urinary tract infections. A brand name is Hiprex.

hexetidine an antiseptic used in a weak solution as a mouthwash or gargle to treat oral ulcers, sore throat, gum inflammation (gingivitis) and bad breath. A brand name is Oraldene.

Hexopal a brand name for INOSITOL.

HFEA *abbrev. for* Human Fertilisation and Embryology Authority.

Hg the symbol for the element mercury. Blood pressure is measured in terms of the weight of a column of mercury measured in millimetres, as in 140/80 mm Hg (Systolic/Diastolic).

HGPRT deficiency deficiency of hypoxanthine-guanine-phosphor-ibosyl transferase. The absence of this enzyme occurs as the result of a rare X-linked recessive inheritance and leads to severe over-production of uric acid, spastic paralysis, ATHETOSIS, mental deficiency and a strong tendency to self-mutilation. Also known as LESCH-NYHAN SYNDROME.

hiatus a gap or abnormal space.

hiatus hernia abnormal mobility of the stomach allowing the junction with the gullet (oesophagus) to pass up through the opening in the DIAPHRAGM into the chest cavity. As a result, the mechanism normally preventing regurgitation of stomach contents into the

oesophagus fails, and acid moves up into the oesophagus, damaging the lining (reflux oesophagitis) and causing burning pain. Treatment is with drugs such as RANITIDINE (Zantac), OMEPRAZOLE (Losec) or surgery.

Hibitane a brand name for CHLORHEXIDINE.

HIB vaccine a vaccine against *Haemophilus influenzae*, type B. This vaccine was introduced in October, 1992 following which there was a rapid reduction in the number of reported cases of this infection especially in children under 5.

hiccup repetitive involuntary spasms of the diaphragm causing inspirations, each followed by sudden closure of the vocal cords. In most cases the cause is unknown and it can be stopped by re-breathing into a small bag. Pathological hiccup is a feature of various conditions including kidney failure with URAEMIA, pleurisy, pneumonia and intestinal disorders. It can be dangerously exhausting but can often be controlled with the muscle relaxant drug baclofen (Lioresal). In some cases it may have to be treated by temporarily paralysing the nerve to the diaphragm. Also called 'hiccough'.

hidr-, hidro- *combining form denoting* sweat or sweat gland.

hidradenitis inflammation of sweat glands.

hidradenoma a benign tumour of a sweat gland.

hidrosis sweating. Excessive sweating is caller HYPERHIDROSIS.

high density lipoproteins SEE LIPOPROTEINS.

hilum a small gap or opening in an organ through which connecting structures such as arteries, veins, nerves or ducts enter or leave.

hindbrain the part of the embryonic brain from which the CEREBELLUM and the brainstem, with the nuclei of most of the cranial nerves, develop. Technically known as the rhombencephalon.

hindbrain hernia headache one of the rarer forms of headache. In this condition part of the CEREBELLUM passes into the large opening for the spinal cord at the base of the skull (the foramen magnum). This may occur during straining, coughing, sneezing or laughing. It can be relieved by enlarging the foramen magnum.

hinge region the part of the immunoglobulin (antibody) molecule between the Fab and Fc regions that allows flexibility.

Hioxyl a brand name for HYDROGEN PEROXIDE.

hip-clicking test a method of detecting

CONGENITAL DISLOCATION OF THE HIP in babies, a condition often missed, because unsuspected.

hip, congenital dislocation of see CONGENITAL DISLOCATION OF THE HIP.

hippocampus an infolded ridge of the surface of the brain (cerebral cortex) on either side. Each hippocampus forms a ridge on the floor of the LATERAL VENTRICLE. Disease or injury to the hippocampus causes memory defects. PET scanning in young subjects shows that the act of memorization is associated with a 5% increase in blood flow to the hippocampus. From the Greek *hippos*, a horse, and *kampos*, a sea monster.

Hippocratic oath an ethical code for doctors that has been observed, to varying degrees, since the times of ancient Greece. Contrary to popular belief doctors are not required to take the oath as part of their graduation ceremony. A modern version was drawn up by the World Medical Association in Geneva in 1948, the general terms of which are that the doctor pledges to serve humanity without consideration of race, religion or social standing, to respect his or her teachers, to practise conscientiously, to put the welfare of the patient before every other consideration, to keep patients' secrets and to maintain the best traditions of the profession. (Hippocrates of Cos, Greek physician, 460–367 BC).

hip replacement an operation in which the upper end of the thigh bone (femur) is sawn off, a short, angled metal shaft with a smooth metal or ceramic ball on its upper end is forced down into the hollow of the bone, and a plastic cup to fit the ball is fitted to the natural hollow on the side of the pelvis (the ACETABULUM). Advances reported late in 2003 include the use of two short incisions rather than one long incision and access via the separation of muscle planes rather than by cutting muscle. These technical improvements have made it possible for patients to return home the day after their operation.

Hiprex a brand name for HEXAMINE HIPPURATE (methenamine hippurate).

Hirschprung's disease a congenital failure of development of the nerve supply to the lower part of the large intestine. This causes failure of PERISTALSIS and effective obstruction of the bowel. Treatment is by surgical removal of the affected segment. (Harald Hirschprung,

1830–1916, Danish paediatrician).

hirsutism excessive hairiness. Hirsutism in women may, rarely, be due to an excess of male sex hormone from an ovarian or adrenal gland tumour but is usually hereditary, ethnic or just unfortunate. Certain drugs such as STEROIDS, PHENYTOIN and STREPTOMYCIN can cause hirsutism.

hirudin a substance secreted by the salivary glands of leeches to prevent blood coagulation so that they can continue to feed on blood. The leeches are, of course, unaware that their hirudin acts by blockade of the glycoprotein IIb/IIIa receptors on blood platelets. Hirudin has been found capable of preventing restenosis after coronary angioplasty.

hist-, histio-, histo *combining form denoting* tissue.

histamine a powerful hormone synthesized and stored in MAST CELLS and basophil cells from which it is released when antibodies attached to the cells are contacted by ALLERGENS such as pollens. Free histamine acts on H_1 receptors to cause small blood vessels to widen (dilate) and become more permeable to protein, resulting in the effects known an allergic reactions. It causes smooth muscle cells to contract. Histamine also acts on receptors in the stomach (H_2 receptors) to promote the secretion of acid. H_2 receptor blockers, such as cimetidine and ranitidine (Zantac) are widely used to control acid secretion.

histamine analogues drugs used to treat the symptoms of MÉNIÈRE'S DISEASE. An example is betahistine (Serc).

histidine an essential amino acid and precursor of HISTAMINE.

histiocyte a fixed scavenging cell (phagocyte) found in connective tissue. Histiocytes are also known as reticuloendothelial cells and reticulum cells. A macrophage that does not migrate.

histiocytosis one of several disorders in which HISTIOCYTES occur in abnormal numbers, in localized areas, without any of the usual causes, such as infection. Histiocytosis LESIONS may be single or multiple. The condition is also known as histiocytosis X.

Histoacryl a brand name for ENBUCRILATE.

histochemistry the biochemistry of cells and tissues.

histocompatibility sufficient affinity between

the genetic composition (genotypes) of donor and host to allow successful tissue or organ grafting.

histocompatibility antigens genetically determined glycoprotein groups situated on the outer membrane of all body cells to provide an identifying code unique for each person (except identical twins). These groups act as ANTIGENS and, in a foreign environment, provoke the production of ANTIBODIES against them. This is the basis of graft rejection. They are also called HLA antigens because they were first found on human white blood cells (LEUKOCYTES). There are three classes: class 1 proteins are found on the surface of most cells, even on red blood cells; class 2 proteins are found on the surface of B cells, antigen-presenting cells and some endothelial cells; class 3 proteins are components of the complement system. See also MAJOR HISTOCOMPATIBILITY COMPLEX (MHC).

histology the study of the microscopic structure of the body. All healthy tissues are identifiable microscopically and a knowledge of normal histology is an essential basis for the recognition of the specific microscopic changes occurring in disease. The microscopic study of diseased tissue and the identification of diseases by this means is called histopathology.

histolysis breakdown of the structure of body tissue.

histones strongly alkaline proteins commonly associated with DNA. Histones may be released into the blood and appear in the urine when tissue breaks down in wasting illnesses.

histopathology the microscopic study of disease processes in tissues.

histoplasmosis a lung infection caused by the fungus *Histoplasma capsulatum*. The condition is usually mild and self-limiting, except in immunodeficient people who may develop a severe and sometimes fatal tuberculosis-like disease. Histoplasmosis is largely confined to limited areas of the United States of America, such as the Ohio basin.

history a medical history is the record of everything that is relevant to a person's health. A full history includes an account of the previous medical conditions, the social and family record and the details of the present complaint. Taking a good medical history is a fine art.

histrionic personality disorder a type of hysterical personality disorder manifested by ostentatious, flamboyant dress, exaggerated speech and manner, and theatrical, attention-seeking, behaviour. The conduct appears calculated to impress or shock. There is often inability to maintain deep relationships and psychosexual disorder is common.

HIV the human immunodeficiency virus and the cause of AIDS. HIV binds avidly to CD4 cell surface receptors so its greatest affinity is for helper T cells. It will, however, also infect MACROPHAGES and the microglial cells of the brain, which also have CD4 receptors. HIV is an RNA retrovirus and uses the enzyme reverse transcriptase to convert its RNA into DNA which is then incorporated into the genome of the host cell where it can remain latent for years. The host DNA produces more HIV RNA by transcription and the cell then releases large numbers of new HI viruses which infect other cells. The virus was identified in 1983 by Dr Francoise Barré-Sinoussi (1950–) working at the Pasteur Institute in Paris. Two years later she proved that it was the cause of AIDS. She is now Head of the Retrovirus Biology Unit at the Institute and was awarded one of the French Republic's highest honours – the Chevalier de l'Ordre National de Merité.

hives see URTICARIA.

HIV lipoatrophy a subset of lipodystrophy that is liable to complicate prolonged multidrug antiretroviral therapy for HIV infection. There is peripheral breakdown of subcutaneous fat and central fat accumulation associated with type 2 diabetes. The effect is thought to be due to the use of nucleoside-analogue reverse-transcriptase inhibitors and HIV-PROTEASE INHIBITORS.

HIV-protease inhibitor one of a range of drugs that interfere with the enzyme produced by the human immunodeficiency virus (HIV) that allows it to replicate itself in human cells. Recent guidelines for the early treatment of HIV infection recommend that all such patients should be given HIV-protease inhibitor drugs. Currently, these drugs are indinavir (Crixivan), nelfinavir (Viracept), ritonavir (Norvir) and saquinavir (Invirase). A further drug, amprenavir, is under investigation. These drugs, used in combination with other antiretroviral drugs cause a sustained reduction in HIV replication and reduce morbidity and prolong life. Their side effects include excess weight gain from fat deposition.

HLA human leukocyte antigen; the MAJOR HISTOCOMPATIBILITY COMPLEX.

HLA antigens see HISTOCOMPATIBILITY ANTIGENS and MAJOR HISTOCOMPATIBILITY COMPLEX.

HMG-CoA reductase inhibitors
see HYDROXYMETHYL GLUTARYL COENZYME A REDUCTASE INHIBITORS.

hoarseness the result of thickening of the vocal cords usually from inflammation (LARYNGITIS) but also from nodules on the cords (SINGERS' NODES) or by partial paralysis of the muscles that tighten the cords from involvement of a laryngeal nerve by neck cancer or trauma.

Hodgkin's lymphoma a form of cancer of lymphatic tissue especially lymph nodes. There is widespread, painless lymph node enlargement and, later, spleen and liver enlargement, fever and anaemia. Sometimes the bone marrow is involved, usually at a late stage of the disease. Treatment is with radiotherapy and, if necessary, with drugs such as cyclophosphamide, chlorambucil and vincristine. In general, the outlook for this once invariably fatal disease, is now good. (Thomas Hodgkin, 1798–1866, English physician)

hole in the heart SEE INTERATRIAL SEPTAL DEFECT and INTERVENTRICULAR SEPTAL DEFECT.

hol- or **holo-** *combining form denoting* wholly, entire. From the Greek *holos*.

holistic medicine a medical philosophy in which the patient is regarded, not simply as the site of a diagnostic and therapeutic problem, but as a whole person in his or her cultural and environmental context, with feelings, attitudes, fears and prejudices. The best medical practice is invariably holistic.

holmium laser prostate resection
an advance in the use of lasers for the closed internal (endourological) treatment of enlargement of the prostate gland (prostate hyperplasia). The holmium laser appears to have significant advantages over earlier types of YAG laser used for this purpose.

holoblastic cleavage cleavage of a fertilized egg into two parts (blastomeres), each of which can form an entirely separate individual.

holocrine pertaining to a gland whose secretion is a breakdown product of the gland's own lining cells. A sebaceous gland is a holocrine gland.

holoenzyme a complete enzyme that includes its prosthetic coenzyme. An enzyme without its coenzyme is called an apoenzyme.

Holter monitoring continuous recording of the ELECTROCARDIOGRAPH (ECG) using a small, portable cassette recorder. The method is valuable for detecting transient abnormalities that are likely to be missed during the short period of a normal ECG examination.

Homans' sign the eliciting of a sharp pain in the calf and behind the knee by passively forcing the foot backwards (dorsiflexion). This is an indication of deep vein THROMBOSIS in the calf. The test is now regarded as dangerous as it may dislodge an EMBOLUS. (John Homans, 1877–1954, American surgeon)

homatropine a drug used in the form of eyedrops to widen the pupils for ophthalmic examination and temporarily to paralyze the muscles of the iris to assist in the treatment of iris inflammation (anterior UVEITIS).

homeo- *combining form denoting* similar. From the Greek *homoios*, of the same kind.

homeobox genes a highly CONSERVED family of genes, found in a large range of different species, including insects. Homeobox genes are expressed early in embryonic development and are the determinants of body shape. These genes divide the early embryo into fields of cells each with the potentiality to develop into a particular part such as an arm, leg, tissue or organ. This is the key to the long-unexplained problem of how bodily configuration is determined by genetics. Mutations in homeobox genes cause severe bodily defects such as PHOCOMELIA.

homeopathy, homoeopathy a system of medical practice based on two questionable, not to say absurd, premises – that diseases can be cured by giving substances that cause the same symptoms and that the more thoroughly these substances are diluted, the more powerful is their effect. The method is claimed to work even if successive dilution has eliminated the last molecule of the original substance. Compare ALLOPATHY. See also ALTERNATIVE MEDICINE.

homeostasis the principle of self-regulating information feedback by which constant conditions are maintained in a biological system such as the human body. Homeostasis is essential to life and applies to thousands of bodily parameters. Some of the more obvious examples are temperature regulation, blood acidity control, blood pressure control, heart rate, blood sugar levels and hormone secretion.

hom-, homo- *combining form denoting* same, like. From the Greek *homos*.

homocystinuria the abnormal presence of homocystine in the urine. This may be caused by vitamin B12 deficiency, a B12 metabolic defect, drugs or urinary infection but is usually due to an autosomal recessive enzyme-defect disorder. The hereditary form features sparse blond hair, OSTEOPOROSIS with overgrowth of long bones, a hollowed chest, dislocation of the lenses of the eyes and mental retardation.

homograft a graft taken from a member of the same species as the recipient. Compare HETEROGRAFT.

homolateral situated on the same side. Ipsilateral. Compare CONTRALATERAL.

homologous 1 of corresponding structure, position, function or value.
2 having the same consecutive sequence of genes as another chromosome.
3 belonging to a series of organic compounds of which the successive members differ by constant chemical increments.
4 of transplantation in which the donor and recipients are of the same species.

homologous chromosomes chromosomes with the same genetic loci that occur in pairs, one derived from the mother and one from the father.

homologous genes genes from organisms of different species that code for the same enzyme or other product. Homologous genes need not have the same base sequences.

homonymous corresponding to the same side, as in HOMONYMOUS HEMIANOPIA.

homonymous hemianopia loss of half of the field of vision of each eye, the loss being either of both right halves or both left halves.

homophobia a slang term meaning fear of homosexuality.

homosexuality sexual preference for a person of the same anatomical sex. The term derives from the Greek *homos*, the same (not from the Latin *homo*, a man) and is applicable correctly to women as well as to men. In 1991, differences in the size of a hypothalamic nucleus between heterosexual and homosexual men were reported; and in 1993 it was reported that a region of the long arm of the X chromosome

was associated with male homosexuality. It is still not universally accepted, however, that homosexuality is genetically induced.

homozygous having identical gene pairs (ALLELES) at corresponding positions (loci) on the chromosome pairs. People who are homozygous for a quality or condition will always manifest it.

honeycomb lung an X-ray appearance found in some cases of INTERSTITIAL PULMONARY FIBROSIS and in some rare conditions such as HISTIOCYTOSIS and TUBEROUS SCLEROSIS.

hookworm infestation parasitization by one of the roundworms (nematodes) *Ancylostoma duodenale* or *Necator americanus*. Hookworm infestation (ancylostomiasis) occurs worldwide in areas where people go barefoot. The mouth parts of the worms are equipped with securing hooks. Large infestations cause abdominal pain, diarrhoea, severe anaemia and debility. There are effective ANTHELMINTIC drugs to remove the worms.

hordeolum a STYE. A small staphylococcal infection of the root of an eyelash.

hormones chemical substances produced by the ENDOCRINE and other glands or cells and released into the bloodstream to act upon specific receptor sites in other parts of the body, so as to bring about various effects. Hormones are part of the control and feedback system of the body by which HOMEOSTASIS is achieved. The pituitary hormones are adrenocorticotropin, to prompt cortisone release from the adrenal cortex; follicle-stimulating and luteinizing hormones to produce sperm and egg maturation in the testis and ovary; prolactin for milk secretion in the breast; thyroid stimulating hormone for the thyroid; growth hormone for the bones and muscles; melanotropin for the pigment cells (melanocytes); and antidiuretic hormone for water reabsorption in the kidneys. Under these influences, each of the endocrine glands produces its own hormones.

hormone replacement therapy HRT, the long-term prescription of synthetic or natural hormones to people whose endocrine glands have had to be removed or, for other reasons, no longer secrete adequate quantities of the natural hormones. The term is often applied to the treatment of postmenopausal women with oral, trans-dermal (patch) or depot OESTROGEN or combined oestrogen and progestogen preparations, to alleviate menopausal symptoms and to try to prevent rapid progression of OSTEOPOROSIS. Commonly abbreviated to HRT. After years of general medical approval, HRT has recently come in for criticism on the grounds that it does not, as was formerly believed, protect post-menopausal women against coronary heart disease, and that it slightly increases the risk of breast cancer and venous thromboembolism. In spite of its obvious advantages in reducing the risk of bone fracture and other complications of osteoporosis, it is no longer recommended indiscriminately for all post-menopausal women. Women who stop taking HRT and who have enjoyed an increase in bone-mineral density will lose most of this gain in the two years following cessation. A report of the experience of over 1 million women between 1996 and 2001, published in August 2003, concerned itself with the increased risk of breast cancer and showed that five years of HRT would produce 5 to 6 additional cases of breast cancer in every 1000 women. Other research has shown that HRT also produces 6 additional cases of coronary heart disease per 100,000 women.

Hormonin a brand name for OESTRADIOL (estradiol).

horn a rare, age-related local overgrowth of the horny layer of the skin so that a short, cylindrical, horn-like protrusion occurs. Cutaneous horns are easily removed but the base may be found to be cancerous.

Horner's syndrome the association, on one side, of a drooping upper eyelid, an apparently slightly sunken eyeball, a pupil reduced in size compared with the other, and absence of sweating on the same side of the face. This syndrome is an indication that certain nerves in the neck have been damaged, possibly by cancer. (Johann Friedrich Horner, 1831–1886, Swiss ophthalmologist)

horseshoe kidney a congenital kidney anomaly in which the two organs are fused at the upper or lower ends so as to form a single organ lying across the midline of the body. The condition is not necessarily harmful but is associated with an increased incidence of HYDRONEPHROSIS, kidney stones and infection.

hosiery, supportive SEE ELASTIC STOCKINGS.

hospice a hospital specializing in the care of the terminally ill. Hospices are dedicated to providing the physical, emotional and psychological support and expert pain management needed to help the dying to accept the reality of death and to die in dignity and peace of mind.

host 1 an organism that provides a residence and nourishment for a parasite.
2 a person receiving a graft of a donated organ or tissue.

hot-dog headache headache induced by sodium nitrite preservative in certain foods. See also ICE CREAM HEADACHE.

hot flushes waves of sudden widespread relaxation of the muscle walls of skin blood vessels so that they dilate and cause the skin to become reddened and warm. Hot flushes are common around the time of the MENOPAUSE and can be controlled by HORMONE REPLACEMENT THERAPY. Women in the USA experience hot flashes rather than flushes

hourglass stomach a stomach with a central narrowing, usually due to contracted scar tissue around an ulcer.

house fly *Musca domestica* the common fly. This insect finds faeces attractive and is one of the vehicles of spread of diseases such as TYPHOID, SHIGELLOSIS (dysentery), POLIOMYELITIS, and AMOEBIC DYSENTERY.

housekeeping genes constitutive genes, genes that provide the basic routine functions required by all cells for their sustenance.

housemaid's knee see CLERGYMAN'S KNEE.

house officer a doctor in training, the most junior member of the medical staff of a hospital, usually resident in the hospital.

HRT *abbrev. for* HORMONE REPLACEMENT THERAPY.

HTLV–I human T lymphotropic virus, type I, a virus associated with adult T cell LEUKAEMIA or T cell lymphomas and other conditions, such as tropical spastic paraparesis and POLYMYOSITIS. See also HTLV–III.

HTLV–III the earlier, and now outdated, term for the AIDS virus, now known as the HIV. HTLV–III was an abbreviation of 'human T cell lymphotropic virus, type III'.

Hughes' syndrome an autoimmune condition caused by an antibody to phospholipid, a major constituent of cell plasma membranes, or an antibody to cardiolipin. It features recurrent thromboses causing strokes, heart attacks and other arterial obstruction effects, or recurrent fetal loss during pregnancy, and is commonly secondary to systemic lupus erythematosus or a lupus-like disease. Antiphospholipid antibodies are believed to accelerate atheroma by interacting with low-density lipoproteins (LDLs). They can also occur as drug reactions or in certain infectious diseases. There is commonly an abnormally low level of blood platelets (thrombocytopenia). Also known as the antiphospholipid syndrome. (Graham Hughes, who described the syndrome in 1983)

Humalog a brand name for INSULIN LISPRO.

Human Actrapid a brand name for a preparation of neutral INSULIN.

human chorionic gonadotrophin see CHORIONIC GONADOTROPHIN.

human cloning the production of a person genetically identical to another person by the insertion of a genome from a somatic cell into an ovum from which the DNA has been removed (somatic cell nuclear transfer). Human cloning is currently almost universally proscribed. At the present time it is also scientifically unfeasible. Because nuclear cloning bypasses the normal processes of gametogenesis and fertilization, it prevents the reprogramming of the clone's genome necessary for the development of an embryo into a normal human being. There is evidence that surviving cloned animals have serious abnormalities of gene expression.

Human Fertilization and Embryology Authority an organization set up by act of Parliament in 1990 to control research involving embryos. The HFEA regulates and inspects all UK clinics providing IVF, donor insemination or the storage of eggs, sperm or embryos. It maintains a register of persons whose gametes are used for assisted conception and licenses and monitors all human embryo research being conducted in the UK.

human genome the entire gene map of all the chromosomes that contains all the information needed to make a human being. The genome contains about 6000 million chemical bases forming about 30,000 genes. The completion of the sequencing of these bases, along the length of each chromosome, in the massive research programme known as the human genome project, was formally announced on 14 April 2003, but well before that date the information obtained had already had a major impact on medicine. As an index of the speed of progress in genomic medicine, this announcement was made only a few days prior to the 50th anniversary of the publication of the structure of DNA by Watson and Crick.

human givens a term that is becoming popular with psychotherapists, psychologists, educationists and others concerned with the nature and pathology of the mind. It refers to a body of organizing but tentative ideas that are being developed from scientific advances in understanding of brain function and of the rich inheritance of innate knowledge patterns with which we are all born and which manifest themselves as emotional and physical needs.

human herpesvirus 1 the HERPES SIMPLEX virus mainly responsible for causing cold sores at the skin/mucous membrane junction of the mouth or nose.

human herpesvirus 2 the herpes simplex virus mainly responsible for causing sexually-transmitted herpes.

human herpesvirus 3 the varicella-zoster virus causing CHICKENPOX and SHINGLES.

human herpesvirus 4 the Epstein-Barr virus that is shed in the saliva of most adults and causes infectious mononucleosis (glandular fever).

human herpesvirus 5 the CYTOMEGALOVIRUS.

human herpesvirus 6 the herpes virus that causes the childhood disease roseola infantum (exanthema subitum).

human herpesvirus 7 a virus found in association with human T lymphocytes and is present in the saliva of most adults. It is not currently known to cause disease.

human herpesvirus 8 a herpes virus that causes KAPOSI'S SARCOMA in people with immune deficiency, especially AIDS. The virus is also associated with several otherwise rare forms of lymphoma that occur in AIDS patients.

Human Insulatard a brand name for ISOPHANE INSULIN.

human leukocyte antigen (HLA) the human MAJOR HISTOCOMPATIBILITY COMPLEX.

human metapneumovirus a recently-discovered respiratory virus that is a major cause of acute lower respiratory infections especially in the first ten years of life. Infections feature bronchiolitis, croup, pneumonia and exacerbation of asthma. It is related to, and roughly equal in importance to, the respiratory syncytial virus.

Human Mixtard a brand name for human INSULIN.

Human Monotard a brand name for human zinc INSULIN.

Human Ultratard a brand name for human zinc suspension INSULIN.

Human Velosulin a brand name for human neutral INSULIN.

humanistic psychology a school of psychology that views people as individuals responsible for, and in control of, their destinies and that emphasizes experience as the source of knowledge. It suggests that we can acquire insight into the inner life of another person by trying to see things from that person's own point of view.

Humatrope a brand name for SOMATOTROPIN.

Humegon a brand name for MENOTROPHIN.

humeral pertaining to, or the region of, the HUMERUS.

humerus the long upper arm bone that articulates at its upper end with a shallow cup in a side process of the shoulder blade (scapula) and, at its lower end with the RADIUS and ULNA bones of the lower arm.

humira a brand name for ADALIMUMAB.

humoral 1 pertaining to extracellular fluid such as the blood plasma or lymph.
2 pertaining to B cell, antibody-mediated immunity.
3 pertaining to the aqueous and vitreous humours of the eye.
4 an obsolete term referring to the ancient medical theory, propagated mainly by Galen (see GALENISM), that the body contains four humours (blood, phlegm, yellow bile and black bile) and that health results from their correct balance.

humour the possession of, or the capacity to perceive, those things which excite laughter or the desire to laugh. Humour is one of the more mysterious characteristics of the human being and its nature has been endlessly argued. We laugh when we are painlessly surprised; when we perceive foolishness or qualities to which we consider ourselves superior; when we see the pompous deflated, the powerful threatened or the consciously superior mocked. Theories abound, none of them entirely convincing. Humour is, however, a valuable human

attribute and its absence is a personality defect.

Humulin I a brand name for human ISOPHANE INSULIN produced by recombinant DNA technology.

Humulin Lente a brand name for human zinc INSULIN produced by recombinant DNA technology.

Humulin S a brand name for neutral INSULIN produced by recombinant DNA technology.

Humulin Zn a brand name for zinc suspension INSULIN produced by recombinant DNA technology.

hunch back extreme curvature or angulation of the spine. This may be caused by congenital malformation, postural defect, crush fracture of a vertebra, spontaneous collapse of a vertebra from disease such as tuberculosis (POTT'S DISEASE) or exaggeration of the natural curve by OSTEOPOROSIS.

hunger the symptoms of abdominal discomfort, pain, contractions of the stomach and craving for food induced by a drop in the level of sugar in the blood passing through the HYPOTHALAMUS of the brain.

hungry bones syndrome a condition that sometimes follows removal of a tumour that has been causing excessive output of parathyroid hormone (HYPERPARATHYROIDISM). Calcium is withdrawn so rapidly from the blood that lowered blood levels occur, causing TETANY.

Hunter's syndrome an X-LINKED RECESSIVE genetic disorder similar to, but less severe than, Hurler's syndrome. It is a MUCOPOLYSACCHARIDOSIS causing GARGOYLISM and some degree of mental retardation. (Charles H. Hunter, 1872–1955, Canadian physician)

Huntington's disease a rare, dominant, genetic brain disorder caused by a defective gene on chromosome number 4 that has complete penetrance. The disease appears most often in middle-aged adults and leads to loss of nerve cells and a buildup of the neurotransmitter dopamine. This causes involuntary twitching or jerking movements of the face and body (chorea), alternating excitement and depression, and progressive DEMENTIA. The chorea can be controlled by drugs but there is no treatment for the central problem. When the disease starts in childhood the inheritance is four times as likely to be from the father than from the mother. The mechanism of the disease is unknown but it is thought that neural toxicity results from the accumulation of amino-terminal fragments containing an expanded polyglutamine region. (George Huntington, 1850–1916, American General Practitioner)

Hurler's syndrome one of the mucopolysaccharidoses, a group of inherited disorders. Hurler's syndrome is due to the absence of the enzyme alpha-iduronidase. There is dwarfism, many skeletal deformities, corneal opacity, heart abnormalities, mental retardation and early death. The condition was once known as 'gargoylism'. (Gertrude Hurler, Austrian paediatrician, who described the condition in 1920)

Hutchinson's teeth notching of the biting edge of the permanent incisor teeth due to congenital SYPHILIS. The phenomenon is now rare. (Jonathan Hutchinson, 1828–1930, English surgeon)

Hyalase a brand name for HYALURONIDASE.

hyaline translucent or glassy, as in hyaline cartilage. Of amorphous texture.

hyalitis see ASTEROID HYALITIS.

hyaloid HYALINE.

hyaluronans drugs analogous to HYALURONIC ACID used as protectives, lubricants or synovial fluid substitute, to treat interstitial CYSTITIS, osteoarthritis, and to maintain the anterior chamber of the eye in ophthalmic surgery. Examples are sodium hyaluronate (Cystistat, Orthovisc, Ophthalon, Ostenil), polyvinylpyrrolidone (Gelclair) and Hylan G-F 20 (Synvisk).

hyaluronic acid hyaluronate, a long polymer glycosaminoglycan, consisting of repeating disaccharide units, found in basement membranes, mature oocytes, skin, cartilage, the vitreous body of the eye and the synovial fluid of joints.

hyaluronidase an enzyme that breaks down proteins holding tissue planes together. Its use assists in the dispersal of tissue fluids or injected drugs. A brand name is Hyalase.

hybernating myocardium areas of the heart muscle that show failure of contraction (asynergy) as a result of coronary artery disease but that are capable of returning to function if an adequate blood supply is restored as by bypass grafting. All such areas were formerly thought to have suffered irreversible change.

hybridization probing the use of a radioactively-labelled single-strand sequence of DNA to form a hybrid complementary pairing with an RNA strand and thus identify it; or the use of a labelled RNA strand to pair with and identify a DNA strand.

hybridoma a cell line (CLONE) formed by the fusion of two or more different types of cells, such as a B LYMPHOCYTE and a lymphoid tumour cell (myeloma). Malignant tumours can be immortal so a hybridoma, suitably nourished, can continue permanently exercising the function of the B lymphocyte to produce specific antibodies (MONOCLONAL ANTIBODIES).

Hycamtin a brand name for TOPOTECAN.

hydantoins drugs used to treat epilepsy and spasticty of voluntary muscle. Examples are phenytoin (Epanutin), dantrolene (Dantrium) and fosphenytoin (Pro-epanutin).

hydatid disease a disorder caused by ingesting tapeworm eggs so that the part of the worm life-cycle that normally occurs in dogs or pigs affects a human person. The worm embryos enter the bloodstream from the intestines and are carried to the liver, lungs, muscles and brain where they form cysts that gradually increase in size, causing variable damage. Brain cysts can cause EPILEPSY. Surgical removal of dangerous cysts may be necessary.

hydatidiform mole a tumour arising from the part of the embryo that normally forms the PLACENTA. A normal pregnancy is assumed but, instead of containing a fetus, the womb fills with a mass of grape-like cystic bodies of various size. Often, all the chromosomal material comes from the father. There is usually vaginal bleeding and the woman is often ill. Early diagnosis and removal is important as some hydatidiform moles change into the highly malignant CHORION EPITHELIOMA.

Hydopa a brand name for METHYLDOPA.

hydr, hydro- *prefix denoting* water. From the Greek *hydro*, water.

hydraemia excessive water in the blood.

hydralazine a drug that causes arteries to widen (vasodilatation) and can be used as an adjunct to the treatment of high blood pressure (HYPERTENSION) and moderate degrees of HEART FAILURE. It is seldom used alone. The drug is on the WHO official list. A brand name is Apresoline.

hydramnios an excess of AMNIOTIC fluid in the pregnant womb (uterus). This is one of the common complications of pregnancy.

hydrarthrosis an abnormal accumulation of fluid in a joint.

Hydrea a brand name for HYDROXYUREA (hydroxycarbamide).

hydrocephalus 'water on the brain' – an abnormal accumulation of cerebrospinal fluid within, and around, the brain. This occurs if the fluid, which is continuously secreted, cannot be normally reabsorbed, usually because of obstruction of the passages to the site of reabsorption, by a congenital abnormality or later acquired disease. In babies, the head becomes greatly enlarged, and if the cause cannot be removed, an artificial shunt, or bypass, must be inserted to carry the fluid down to the heart or the abdominal cavity. Unrelieved hydrocephalus causes brain damage by compression.

hydrochloric acid a strong acid, produced by the lining of the stomach, that breaks down connective tissue and cell membranes in the food, so that it can more easily be acted on by digestive enzymes. Hydrochloric acid also kills most of the bacteria ingested with the food.

hydrochlorothiazide a drug used to increase the output of urine so as to relieve the body of surplus water. A thiazide DIURETIC drug. The drug is on the WHO official list. A brand name is Hydrosaluric. Hydrochlorothiazide is formulated in conjunction with a variety of drugs. It is available with potassium under the brand name Amil-Co; with another diuretic as Dyazide, Moduret 25, Moduretic, Triam-Co; with ANGIOTENSIN CONVERTING ENZYME inhibitor drugs as Accuretic, Acezide, Capozide, Carace 10 Plus, Innozide and Zestoretic 20; with BETA BLOCKER drugs as Co-Betaloc, Kalten, Moducren and Monozide 10; and with an angiotensin II antagonist drug as Cozaar-Comp.

hydrocoele a painless collection of fluid around the testicle. The condition is usually BENIGN, but may be secondary to testicular cancer. It is usual to draw off some of the fluid for examination.

hydrocortisone a natural steroid hormone derived from the outer layer (cortex) of the adrenal gland. The drug CORTISONE is converted into hydrocortisone in the liver. Hydrocortisone has anti-inflammatory and sodium-retaining properties. It is widely used as a mild CORTICOSTEROID drug mainly for skin disorders. The drug is on the WHO official list. Brand names are Colifoam, Corlan, Dioderm, Efcortelan, Efcortesol, Hydrocortistab, Hydrocortone, Midison Lipocream. The drug is also formulated, for external use, with a variety of other drugs such as allantoin, antibiotics, azole antifungal drugs, coal tar extracts, crotamiton (anti-itch drug), hydrating agents, local anaesthetics, zinc oxide, etc. At least 40 preparations containing hydrocortisone are available on the UK drug market.

Hydrocortistab a brand name for HYDROCORTISONE.

Hydrocortisyl a brand name for HYDROCORTISONE.

Hydrocortone a brand name for HYDROCORTISONE.

hydroflumethiazide a thiazide diuretic drug. A brand name is Aldactide.

hydrogen bond a bond in which a hydrogen atom is shared by two other atoms. The hydrogen is more firmly attached to one of these (which is called the hydrogen donor) than to the other (which is called the hydrogen acceptor). The acceptor has a relative negative charge, and, as unlike charges attract each other, a bond is formed to the hydrogen atom. Hydrogen bonds are weak and easily broken but occur extensively in biomolecules. The link between the bases in the two chains of DNA are hydrogen bonds. Adenine links to thymine by two hydrogen bonds, and guanine links to cytosine by three hydrogen bonds.

hydrogen ion concentration the number of free hydrogen ions in a given quantity of fluid, such as blood. Hydrogen ion concentration (pH) determines acidity. In the blood it must be kept within the narrow limits of pH 7.37–7.45 or a fatal condition occurs.

hydrogen peroxide a powerful oxidizing and antibacterial agent. It is formulated as a cream for external use on skin infections, ulcers and pressure sores. Brand names are Crystacide and Hioxyl.

hydrolases enzymes that promote the splitting of large molecules by attaching –OH from water to one moiety and –H from water to the other.

hydrolysis splitting of a compound into two parts by the addition of water (H_2O), the hydrogen atom (H) joining to one part and the hydroxyl group (OH) joining to the other. Hydrolysis is usually effected by a hydrolytic ENZYME.

Hydromet a brand name for a mixture of HYDROCHLOROTHIAZIDE and METHYLDOPA.

hydromorphone a powerful narcotic pain-killer drug used to relieve severe cancer pain. A brand name is Palladone.

hydronephrosis ballooning out of the urine collecting system of the kidney, as a result of obstruction to the free outflow of urine at any point below the kidney. This may be due to simple or malignant prostate enlargement, external pressure on, or a stone or blood clot in, a URETER, tumour of the bladder, inflammatory narrowing of the URETHRA or even a very tight foreskin (phimosis). There is pain in the loin, and infection leads to fever and sometimes blood in the urine. Unrelieved hydronephrosis often proceeds to kidney failure.

hydropathy a form of ALTERNATIVE MEDICINE in which water with alleged medicinal properties is used either externally or internally to try to cure disease or improve health.

hydropericardium an accumulation of fluid in the membranous bag (pericardial sac) that surrounds the heart. See also PERICARDITIS.

hydroperitoneum excess fluid in the PERITONEAL CAVITY.

hydrophobia violent and painful spasms of the throat muscles occurring as one of the principal symptoms of RABIES. Literally, fear of water.

hydropneumothorax the presence of both air and fluid EXUDATE in the space between the layers of the PLEURA.

hydrops fetalis the most severe form of HAEMOLYTIC DISEASE OF THE NEWBORN. The fetus dies in the womb from the overwhelming toxic effect of the BILIRUBIN released during excessive breakdown of red blood cells. See also RHESUS FACTOR.

hydroquinine a drug that has been used to treat muscle cramps. The drug may be dangerous in people with kidney inadequacy because of accumulation in the body.

Hydrosaluric a brand name for HYDROCHLOROTHIAZIDE.

hydrotalcite an antacid drug used to treat flatulence and dyspepsia. Brand names of preparations containing this drug are Altacite and Altacite Plus.

hydrotherapy the use of water as a form of medical treatment, as in spa baths and the drinking of spa water. Small swimming pools are routinely used by physiotherapists to facilitate the return of function in very weak muscles unable to operate unsupported.

hydroxocobalamin vitamin B_{12}. This is the specific treatment for PERNICIOUS ANAEMIA and is highly effective unless neurological damage has already occurred. The drug is on the WHO official list. Brand names are Cobalin-H and Neo-Cytamen.

hydroxyapatite 1 a principal ingredient in tooth enamel. A paste containing the compound has been used experimentally to seal small enamel cavities without drilling.
2 a calcium and phosphorus supplement used to treat OSTEOPOROSIS, RICKETS, OSTEOMALACIA and to maintain body minerals during breast feeding. A brand name is Ossopan.

hydroxychloroquine a drug used to reduce the activity of RHEUMATOID ARTHRITIS. A brand name is Plaquenil.

hydroxymethyl glutaryl coenzyme A reductase inhibitors also known as statins (see STATINS), these are drugs that block the liver's production of cholesterol by competitive inhibition of the enzyme that catalyzes the rate-limiting step of cholesterol synthesis. These drugs can lower the levels of low-density lipoproteins (LDLs) by 25–45% and a number of major trials have shown their benefits in preventing heart attacks and other effects of ATHEROSCLEROSIS. Up to 30% of patients, however, have genetic variations that prevent them from responding to these drugs. The HMG Co-A reductase inhibitors include atorvastatin, cerivastatin, fluvastatin, pravastatin, rosuvastatin and simvastatin.

hydroxyprogesterone hexanoate a progestogen drug used by depot injection during early pregnancy to prevent spontaneous abortion. A brand name is Proluton.

5-hydroxytryptamine see SEROTONIN.

hydroxyurea hydroxycarbamide, a CYTOTOXIC drug used in the chemotherapy of cancer. The drug is also capable of effecting a substantial reduction in the frequency and severity of crisis in SICKLE CELL ANAEMIA. A brand name is Hydrea.

hydroxyzine an antihistamine drug used as a sedative for anxiety and to control itching (pruritus). Probably the only English word containing 'xyz' in sequence. Brand names are Atarax and Ucerax.

hygiene the study of the promotion of health. Hygiene includes rules for personal conduct and cleanliness and Public Health measures such as preventive medicine. From the name of *Hygieia*, daughter of Aesculapius, the Greek God of medicine. Her sister, *Panacea*, sometimes called *Therapia*, provided healing.

hygroma a lymph vessel tumour (LYMPHANGIOMA) featuring a fluid-filled cystic cavity.

Hygroton a brand name for CHLORTHALIDONE.

hymen the thin, fringe-like ring of skin that partly occludes the lower end of the vagina in the virgin. Hymens vary considerably in thickness and extent and may even be imperforate, requiring a minor operation to allow menstruation. The hymen is usually torn during the first sexual intercourse and this may cause some bleeding. From the Greek *Humen*, the God of marriage.

hymen reconstruction a surgical procedure often forced on women who are the victims of a male-dominated culture which insists on proof of virginity – such as the display of a bloody bed sheet at the time of marriage. The procedure has been criticised on various grounds one of which is that it involves the collusion of the surgeon concerned in a deceitful act.

Hymenolepsis nana a dwarf tapeworm that commonly infests children living in poor conditions in tropical areas. Children are infected directly by ingesting the eggs and no intermediate host is involved. Heavy infestations can cause ENTERITIS.

hymenotomy surgical cutting of a rigid or imperforate HYMEN.

hyoid bone the delicate U-shaped bone suspended from muscles in the upper part of the front of the neck, like a spar in rigging. It provides a base for the movements of the tongue and is usually fractured in manual strangulation. From the Greek letter *upsilon*, 'U' and *eides*, like.

hyoscine scopolamine. A drug structurally related to ATROPINE and having similar properties. It is used to treat painful menstruation and bowel colic. A brand name is Buscopan.

hyoscyamine an ATROPINE-like drug used to

relax smooth muscle spasm, as in colic, and for its sedative effect.

hyper- *prefix denoting* above, beyond, over, excessive. Hyper- is one of the most widely-used prefixes in medicine and covers a range of senses all of which imply an excess over the normal. It may refer to growth of a body part, for instance, indicating an abnormal increase in size, as in hypertrophy or hyperplasia. It may qualify over-production of the secretion of a gland, as in hyperhidrosis, or the excessive effect of excessive glandular secretion, as in hyper-thyroidism. It may refer to over-sensitivity of a sense organ, as in hyperacusis, or overactivity of a part or of the whole organism, as in hyper-activity. It can mean an abnormal range of movement, as in hyperextension of a joint, or an abnormally high pressure, as in hypertension. It is commonly used to indicate an abnormally high level of a substance in the body or in the blood, as in hypercholesterolaemia. In almost all these senses and usages the antonym HYPO can also be applied. From the Greek *huper*.

hyperacidity 1 the secretion of more than the normal amount of acid in the stomach.
2 any condition featuring a higher than normal degree of acidity or quantity of acid.

hyperacusis undue sensitivity to sound which is perceived as uncomfortably loud. The perception of sounds of normal intensity as unusually loud is known as recruitment. These are features of various conditions including many cases of SENSORINEURAL DEAFNESS and of BELL'S PALSY. Hyperacusis should be distinguished from phonophobia (fear of sound) and misophonia (dislike of sound).

hyperactivity an unduly high level of restlessness and aggression with a low level of concentration and a low threshold of frustration, especially as resulting from minimal brain dysfunction. The term is usually applied to children and is sometimes called the 'hyperkinetic syndrome'.

hyperaemia an increase in the amount of blood in a part, organ or tissue as a result of widening (dilatation) of the supplying arteries.

hyperaesthesia increased or exaggerated sensitivity to any sensory modality, especially touch.

hyperaldosteronism the effect of excessive output of ALDOSTERONE from the outer layer (cortex) of the adrenal gland. There is muscle weakness from potassium deficiency, excessive urine output and consequent great thirst, and high blood pressure (HYPERTENSION). When the condition is due to a tumour of the aldosterone-secreting cells it is called Conn's syndrome.

hyperalimentation 1 nutritional intake in excess of normal.
2 total feeding by intravenous means (parenteral nutrition).

hyperbaric oxygen treatment treatment by exposure of the whole body to oxygen at pressures up to three times that of the atmosphere. This can be valuable in conditions, such as heart and lung disorders in which the oxygen supply to the tissues is inadequate, DECOMPRESSION SICKNESS (the 'bends'), carbon monoxide and cyanide poisoning, NECROTIZING FASCIITIS, crush injury, COMPARTMENT SYNDROME, severe burns and GAS GANGRENE. The patient is placed in a pressure chamber.

hyperbilirubinaemia an excess of BILIRUBIN in the blood. This may cause JAUNDICE.

hypercalcaemia an excess of calcium in the blood. This may be due to excessive intake of calcium in the diet, prolonged immobilization, over-production of PARATHYROID hormone causing undue release of calcium from bones, malignant disease of bone and various non-bony cancers that produce a parathyroid hormone-like polypeptide.

hypercalcuria an excess of calcium in the urine. This may be due to HYPERCALCAEMIA or to reduced reabsorption of filtered calcium in the tubules of the kidneys. Hypercalcuria can cause stones (calculi) to form in the kidney, ureters or bladder.

hypercapnia a higher than normal level of carbon dioxide in the blood. This suggests that ventilation in the air sacs of the lungs (alveoli) is inadequate possibly because the sensitivity of the respiratory centre to raised CO_2 levels has been affected. In health, hypercapnia always causes an increased rate and depth of breathing.

hypercatabolism unduly rapid breakdown of body tissues. This may occur in fevers.

hyperchlorhydria excessive acid (hydrochloric acid) in the stomach.

hypercholesterolaemia abnormally high levels of CHOLESTEROL in the blood. This may be dietary or may, rarely, be due to an inherited defect. See also HYPERLIPIDAEMIA.

hyperchromatic of increased density of histological staining.

hypercoagulable states conditions in which the tendency for the blood to clot is greater than normal so that coagulation may occur within the blood vessels. Hypercoagulabilty occurs in people with excessive numbers of blood platelets, in the Budd-Chiari syndrome, in women on the oral contraceptive pill and in people with cancer.

hyperemesis gravidarum a condition of excessively severe and protracted sickness and vomiting occurring as one of the complications of pregnancy. Hyperemesis can be dangerous, but admission to hospital, without treatment, is often sufficient to relieve it.

hyperextension 'over-straightening' of a joint beyond its normal limits.

hyperflexion bending beyond the normal limits.

hypergammaglobulinaemia an excess of the immune protein gamma globulin in the blood. This occurs in chronic liver disease and indicates increased activity of the B lymphocytes of the immune system.

hyperglycaemia excessive levels of glucose in the blood. This is a feature of untreated or undertreated DIABETES MELLITUS.

hyperhidrosis excessive sweating. This is not usually the result of disease but may be caused by fever, overactivity of the thyroid gland and occasionally nervous system disorders. It is commonly the result of a stress reaction or other psychological upset.

hyperkalaemia excessive levels of potassium in the blood. This may be due to abnormally high intake of potassium supplements, kidney failure, circulatory failure, severe untreated DIABETES or other conditions. Excess potassium causes muscle weakness and paralysis, irregular heart action and CARDIAC ARREST.

hyperkeratosis undue thickening of the outer layer of the skin so that a dense horny layer, such as a corn or callosity, results. This is a normal and essentially protective response to local pressure. Hyperkeratosis may also occur as an inherited disorder of the palms and the soles, or as ICHTHYOSIS.

hyperkinesis excessive movement or activity. Hyperactivity.

hyperlipidaemia an abnormal increase in the levels of fats (lipids), including cholesterol, in the blood. This may be of dietary origin or may be due to PANCREATITIS or bile system disorder or may be a dangerous familial disorder of dominant inheritance. Most people with familial hyperlipidaemia develop serious coronary artery disease before the age of 50.

hyperlipoproteinaemia an increase in blood levels of LIPOPROTEINS. These are the tiny particles in which lipids (fats and CHOLESTEROL) are conveyed in the blood.

hypermetropia an inherent, dimensional eye defect in which neither distant nor near objects can be seen clearly when the eye in a state of relaxed focus. Vision can be clarified by ACCOMMODATION and this is easy for the young, who are often unaware of hypermetropia. As the power of accommodation falls off with age, however, hypermetropia inevitably becomes manifest and convex spectacles will be needed.

hypermobility syndrome a condition of abnormally lax ligaments and joints that affects up to 10% of all people. The result is an undue tendency to dislocations, recurrent sprains and joint pain.

hypernatraemia excessive sodium in the blood.

hypernephroma a malignant kidney tumour that often remains clinically silent until a late stage. Treatment is by surgical removal of the affected kidney. The term arises from a mistaken belief that the tumour arose from tissue of the adrenal gland situated above (hyper) the kidney.

hyperostosis abnormal thickening or growth (HYPERTROPHY) of bone, either generally or, more commonly, locally.

hyperparathyroidism the result of excessive output of hormone from the PARATHYROID GLANDS that control deposition of calcium and phosphorus in the bones. The over-production is usually due to a tumour of the hormone-producing cells. There is OSTEOPOROSIS and excessive deposition of calcium in the soft tissues of the body such as the joint cartilages, tendons and muscles.

hyperperistalsis excessive activity of the bowel in passing along its contents.

hyperphagia overeating.

hyperphosphataemia excessive levels of phosphates in the blood.

hyperpigmentation abnormally increased numbers of pigment cells (melanocytes) in a particular area of the body.

hyperpituitarism an abnormal excess of production of PITUITARY hormones, especially growth hormone.

hyperplasia an increase in the number of cells in a tissue or organ causing an increase in the size of the part. Hyperplasia is not a cancerous process. It is often a normal response to increased demand and ceases when the stimulus is removed. To be distinguished from HYPERTROPHY.

hyperpnoea abnormally rapid and deep breathing.

hyperprolactinaemia excessive levels in the blood of the pituitary hormone PROLACTIN. Very high levels suggest a pituitary tumour, but abnormal levels may be caused by oestrogens, kidney failure and various drugs.

hyperpyrexia body temperature above 41.1 °C (106 °F). Hyperpyrexia calls for urgent treatment to lower the temperature, if permanent brain damage is to be avoided.

hypersensitivity an allergic state in which more severe tissue reactions occur on a second or subsequent exposure to an ANTIGEN than on the first exposure. A particular group of antibodies (IgE) is involved in many hypersensitivity reactions.

hypersomnia abnormally prolonged sleep from which the affected person can be aroused only with difficulty and for brief periods.

hypersplenism a condition in which an enlarged spleen is associated with a reduction in the levels of white cells and platelets in the blood. It is thought that the deficiency of these elements in the blood is due to their concentrating in the spleen.

hypertelorism an abnormal increase in the distance between bodily parts, usually referring to an abnormal separation of the eye sockets (orbits) due to a much widened and enlarged SPHENOID bone. Such hypertelorism is a congenital condition and is sometimes associated with other developmental abnormalities and with mental retardation.

hypertension abnormally high blood pressure. A pressure of 135/85 or less is considered normal. A sustained pressure of 159/99 or over that fails to respond to weight loss, salt reduction, dietary adjustment and smoking and stress avoidance, requires drug treatment. Hypertension seldom causes symptoms until an advanced stage is reached in which secondary complications affecting the arteries, kidneys, brain or eyes develop. The condition is, however, potentially dangerous as it can induce a vicious circle of arterial damage resulting in higher blood pressure. Hypertension is a principal cause of STROKE and cardiovascular disease and of DIABETES. Everyone should have regular routine checks of blood pressure. See also KOROTKOFF SOUNDS.

hypertensive retinopathy damage to the RETINA as a result of bleeding from small retinal blood vessels and an inadequate retinal blood supply from arterial disease. There are widespread haemorrhages and signs of local retinal death with sometimes severe visual loss. Hypertensive retinopathy is a sign of dangerously high blood pressure calling for urgent treatment. Untreated, the mortality is high.

hyperthermia see HYPERPYREXIA, MALIGNANT HYPERTHERMIA.

hyperthyroidism overactivity of the thyroid gland. See THYROTOXICOSIS.

hypertonia increased muscle tension (tone).

hypertrichosis see HIRSUTISM.

hypertrophy an increase in the size of a tissue or organ caused by enlargement of the individual cells. Hypertrophy is usually a normal response to an increased demand as in the case of the increase in muscle bulk due to sustained hard exercise. Compare HYPERPLASIA.

hyperuricaemia an abnormal level of uric acid in the blood. This results in the deposition of crystals of monosodium urate monohydrate in joints and tendons, causing GOUT. Hyperuricaemia is most commonly due to a genetically determined defect in the excretion of urates by the kidneys.

hypervariable regions the parts within the antibody and T cell receptor variable regions which show the greatest variability.

hyperventilation unusually or abnormally deep or rapid breathing. This is most commonly the result of strenuous exercise but the term is more often applied to a rate and depth of breathing inappropriate to the needs of the body. This results in excessive loss of carbon dioxide from the blood and sometimes a consequent spasm of the muscles of the forearms and calves. Hyperventilation can, rarely, be a feature of BRAIN DAMAGE, poisoning, fever or THYROTOXICOSIS.

hyperventilation syndrome a state in which the affected person, most often a woman, will, from time to time, begin to breathe at an abnormally rapid rate and abnormally deeply. The effect is to increase the rate at which carbon dioxide is lost from the blood causing a rise in the pH. This brings on a temporary physiological upset with tingling sensation in the skin, cramping or spasm of the fingers and toes and a feeling of faintness or actual fainting. These effects can be relieved by rebreathing into a small plastic bag. The syndrome mainly affects people with generalised anxiety disorder or sometimes chronic fatigue syndrome. It is also known as psychogenic hyperventilation.

hypervitaminosis one of a number of disorders that can result from excessive intake of certain vitamins, especially vitamins A and D. Overdosage with vitamin D can cause deposition of calcium in arteries and other tissues and kidney failure.

hypervolaemia an abnormal increase in the blood volume.

hyphaema a layer of blood in the front chamber of the eye between the back of the CORNEA and the front of the IRIS. This usually results from blunt injury and in most cases the blood reabsorbs without complication and vision is restored. In some cases a serious secondary bleed occurs 3–5 days after the injury.

hypnagogic 1 causing sleep.
2 pertaining to the period during which a person is falling asleep. Of images, dreams or hallucinations occurring during this period.

hypno- *combining form denoting* sleep.

Hypnomidate a brand name for ETOMIDATE.

hypnopompic pertaining to the period during which a person is waking up from sleep. Of images, dreams or hallucinations occurring during this period.

hypnosis a state of abnormal suggestibility and responsiveness, but decreased general awareness often brought about by concentration on a repetitive stimulus. In the hypnotic state, the instructions of the hypnotist are usually obeyed, opinions apparently modified and hallucinations experienced. Many widely-believed myths are associated with hypnotism. It does not involve any kind of sleep; it is impossible without the full cooperation of the subject; and a hypnotized person will not perform actions that would normally be unacceptable. There is, however, inevitably some loss of personal will. Long-forgotten memories of obscure detail are not uncovered by hypnotism.

hypnotherapy treatment by HYPNOSIS.

hypnotic any drug or agent that induces sleep. There are various classes of hypnotic drugs. These include acylic ureides; alcohols; amides; barbiturates; BENZODIAZEPINES; carbamates; CHLORAL derivatives; quinazolone derivatives; piperidineduines; and certain ANTIHISTAMINES.

Hypnovel a brand name for MIDAZOLAM.

hyp, hypo- *prefix denoting* below, beneath, less than. Hypo- is the exact opposite of HYPER-. Reference to that entry will indicate the range of uses. Almost all the hyper-entities mentioned there have their hypo-counterparts. There is, however, one usage in which hypo- is commoner than hyper-. This is when it is used to refer to position in the body, as in hypochondrium or hypogastric. In this sense, the body is to be understood as standing upright, so hypo-indicates that the entity is nearer the soles of the feet than the part it qualifies. Hypo- is, however, also used in the sense of 'deep to' as in hypodermic. From the Greek *hupo*. Compare HYPER-.

hypoaesthesia less than normal sensitivity to any sensory modality.

hypoalbuminaemic malnutrition a condition in which there is increased breakdown of body protein, as after major trauma or burns, but the protein intake is so low that normal levels of blood albumin cannot be maintained. The condition is sometimes called adult QWASHIORKOR.

hypocalcaemia inadequate blood levels of calcium. This may be caused by inadequate intake or absorption, low output of hormone by the parathyroid glands (HYPOPARATHYROIDISM) or PANCREATITIS. The result may be TETANY. The proportion of blood calcium in the ionized form is reduced in ALKALOSIS and this, too may cause tetany.

hypocapnia reduced amounts of carbon dioxide in the blood, as after HYPERVENTILATION.

hypochlorhydria reduced amounts of acid in the stomach.

hypochondriac a person manifesting HYPOCHONDRIASIS.

hypochondriasis, hypochondria a state of constant unjustified conviction of usually serious illness such as heart disease or cancer. The hypochondriac often experiences symptoms that are taken to be manifestations of the feared disease, but still has full insight and is not deluded. The basis of hypochondriasis is unknown. It does not respond to antidepressive treatment. It may be no more than a defect of personality featuring a low fear threshold and an unusually high awareness of the normal functions of the body. Trials conducted between 1997 and 2001 showed that short-term individualized cognitive behaviour therapy can have a long-term beneficial effect in reducing hypochondriacal symptoms.

hypochondrium the region of the abdomen immediately below the cartilages that join the lower ribs on either side to the breastbone. The term, literally, means 'below the cartilages'.

hypochromia a condition of the red blood cells in which they contain less than the normal amount of HAEMOGLOBIN. On microscopic examination the red cells appear pale in the centre. Hypochromia is a feature of iron deficiency ANAEMIA.

hypochromic anaemia ANAEMIA featuring HYPOCHROMIA.

hypodermic under the skin, as in a hypodermic injection or injection needle.

hypodermic syringe a SYRINGE for giving HYPODERMIC injections.

hypogammaglobulinaemia abnormally low levels of the immunoglobulin gammaglobulin in the blood. This is a feature of some kinds of immunodeficiency and can be corrected by monthly injections of gamma globulin.

hypogastrium the lowest of the 3 central regions of the ABDOMEN. The central area below the navel.

hypoglossal nerves the 12th and last of the pairs of nerves which arise directly from the brain (cranial nerves). They supply the muscles of the tongue and are necessary for talking and swallowing.

hypoglycaemia abnormally low levels of sugar (glucose) in the blood. Hypoglycaemia is dangerous as the brain is critically dependent on glucose and is rapidly damaged if this fuel is absent. Hypoglycaemia causes trembling, faintness, sweating, palpitations, mental confusion, slurred speech, headache, loss of memory, double vision, fits, coma and death.

Behaviour is often irrational and disorderly and may simulate drunkenness. The commonest cause is an overdose of insulin in a diabetic. Diabetics are advised always to carry sugar lumps or glucose sweets for use as an emergency treatment of hypoglycaemia.

hypoglycaemic drugs drugs used in the treatment of Type II (maturity-onset) DIABETES. The term is not normally applied to INSULIN.

hypogonadism failure of the normal production, by the testicles or ovaries, of sex hormones, or failure of production of sperms (spermatozoa) or eggs (ova).

hypogonadotropic hypogonadism a usually congenital condition in which there is a severe deficiency of the gonadotropin-releasing hormone (GnRH) of the pituitary gland. As a rule the penis remains infantile and the testes do not descend into the scrotum (cryptorchidism). No sexual development occurs at puberty. In rare cases the condition may develop in men who had previous normal secondary sexual development and a normal puberty. This leads to loss of libido, impotence and infertility. In these cases, treatment with gonadotropin-releasing hormone can reverse all the features of the disorder.

hypokalaemia abnormally low levels of potassium in the blood. This is usually due to excessive loss in the urine or from the bowel. Hypokalaemia causes muscle weakness, paralysis, heart irregularities, mental confusion and disorientation, and cardiac arrest.

hypomania a sustained, but mild or moderate, degree of abnormal elation and hyperactivity.

hyponatraemia abnormally low levels of sodium in the blood. This may be due to excessive salt loss in sweat, overtreatment with DIURETICS, ADDISON'S DISEASE, chronic diarrhoea, or to heart, liver or kidney diseases featuring severe OEDEMA. There is low blood pressure, a fast pulse, a reduction in blood volume, reduced secretion of urine (OLIGURIA), muscle cramps and cold, pale skin.

hypoparathyroidism reduced production of parathyroid gland hormone. This is rare except when two or more of the four glands have been accidentally removed in the course of a THYROIDECTOMY operation. There is a reduction in the level of calcium in the blood causing spontaneous production of nerve impulses and TETANY.

hypophoria a latent tendency to vertical squint in which a covered eye becomes oriented downwards but resumes straight binocular FIXATION when uncovered.

hypophosphataemia a reduction in the levels of phosphate in the blood.

hypophysectomy surgical removal or destruction of the pituitary gland. This may be necessary to remove a pituitary tumour or to prevent the secretion of pituitary hormones which encourage certain cancers of the breast, testicle or ovary.

hypophysis the PITUITARY gland. From the Greek *hupophusis*, an attachment underneath.

hypopigmentation a lower than normal concentration of pigment cells (melanocytes).

hypopituitarism abnormal under-production of pituitary hormones. This is usually due to damage by a tumour known as a chromophobe adenoma, but may be due to an acute loss of blood supply (infarction) occurring as a sequel to POSTPARTUM HAEMORRHAGE.

hypoplasia underdevelopment of a tissue or organ as a result of a failure of production of a sufficient number of cells. Compare HYPERPLASIA.

hypopnoea abnormally slow and shallow breathing. Compare HYPERPNOEA.

hypoprothrombinaemia a deficiency of the protein PROTHROMBIN or prothrombin activity in the blood. Prothrombin is necessary for normal blood clotting.

hypopyon a layer of pus cells in the aqueous humour at the bottom of the front chamber of the eye, immediately behind the CORNEA. Hypopyon does not necessarily signify intraocular infection (ENDOPHTHALMITIS) but is often the result of sterile inflammation as in UVEITIS.

hyposmia a reduced sense of smell.

hypospadias a congenital abnormality of the penis in which the urine tube (URETHRA) opens on the underside of the organ, either at the neck of the bulb (glans) or further back. The prevalence of the condition has doubled in the last 30 years. Hypospadias causes inconvenience in urination and possible infertility, but surgical correction is possible. Tissue culture can be used to provide sheets of artificially grown natural material to line the extended portion of the urethra.

hypotension low blood pressure. This may be a feature of various serious conditions such as surgical SHOCK from massive fluid loss, or HEART FAILURE, but British and American medicine does not recognize the existence of a state of low blood pressure compatible with normal life activities. In Germany and other countries such hypotension is widely accepted. Postural hypotension is a drop in blood pressure occurring on standing up. This causes faintness or dizziness.

hypothalamus the region of the under-surface of the brain immediately above the pituitary gland. The hypothalamus is the area in which the nervous and hormonal systems of the body interact. It receives information relating to hormone levels, physical and mental stress, the emotions and the need for physical activity, and responds by prompting the pituitary appropriately. Nuclei in the lower region of the hypothalamus contain neurons that secrete growth hormone releasing hormone, gonadotropin releasing hormone, somatostatin and other regulating substances.

hypothenar eminence the minor muscle bulk on the palm of the hand on the little finger side opposite the ball of the thumb (the THENAR eminence).

hypothermia below-normal body temperature. This may occur, especially in the elderly, as a result of prolonged exposure to low temperatures or may be brought about deliberately to reduce tissue oxygen requirements during surgery, especially HEART SURGERY.

hypothesis a tentative proposition used as a basis for reasoning or experimental research, by means of which it may be rejected or incorporated into accepted knowledge. See NULL HYPOTHESIS.

hypothesis test a statistical procedure to determine the probability (p) that the observed result of a test or trial could have been obtained if the NULL HYPOTHESIS were true.

hypothyroidism underactivity of the THYROID GLAND. See MYXOEDEMA.

hypotonia a condition in which the muscles offer reduced resistance to passive movement. Hypotonia may be a result of damage to, or malfunction of, the CEREBELLUM. See also FLOPPY INFANT SYNDROME.

Hypovase a brand name for PRAZOCIN.

hypoventilation reduced depth and rate of breathing.

hypovitaminosis any disorder due to vitamin deficiency.

hypovolaemia an abnormal reduction in the circulating blood volume from any cause.

hypoxaemia deficiency of oxygen in the blood. This is usually due to relative failure of the passage of oxygen from the atmosphere to the blood because of lung disease, or inadequate or inappropriate movement of blood through the lungs because of heart disease, either congenital or acquired. Hypoxaemia often causes CYANOSIS.

hypoxia deficiency of oxygen in the tissues. Local hypoxia can lead to GANGRENE; general hypoxia to the death of the individual. Hypoxia occurs mainly as a result of obstructive artery disease, especially ATHEROSCLEROSIS. It may also occur from respiratory disease that prevents access of oxygen to the blood, ANAEMIA, certain forms of poisoning and suffocation.

hypromellose a preparation of METHYL CELLULOSE used as a vehicle in eye drops and as an ingredient in artificial tears.

Hypurin Bovine Lente a brand name for bovine zinc suspension INSULIN.

Hypurin Bovine Isophane a brand name for bovine ISOPHANE INSULIN.

Hypurin Bovine Neutral a brand name for neutral bovine INSULIN.

hysterectomy surgical removal of the womb (uterus). This may be done through the vagina (vaginal hysterectomy) or through an incision in the abdominal wall (abdominal hysterectomy). The operation is performed to treat extensive FIBROIDS, cancer of the womb, ENDOMETRIOSIS, excessive menstruation (MENORRHAGIA), for purposes of sterilization or out of fear of possible later womb cancer. In some affluent countries hysterectomy is grossly over-performed. In California, for instance, almost half of all women undergo hysterectomy.

hysteria a disturbance of body function not caused by organic disease but resulting from psychological upset or need. The affected person is apparently unaware of the psychological origin of the disorder. The term 'hysteria' has become politically incorrect and is now usually referred to as a CONVERSION DISORDER.

hysterosalpingectomy surgical removal of the womb (uterus) and one or both Fallopian tubes.

hysterosalpingostomy a surgical

reimplantation of a Fallopian tube into the side of the womb so as to re-establish continuity in the passage for the ovum and, hopefully, restore fertility.

hysteroscopy direct visual examination of the inside of the womb using an illuminating optical device. Hysteroscopy, which can be done under local anaesthesia, is a valuable diagnostic technique that allows biopsy specimens of the womb lining (endometrium) to be taken from suspicious areas. It has largely replaced D AND C (dilatation and curettage).

hysterotomy an opening into the womb for surgical purposes or to procure an abortion.

Hytrin a brand name for TERAZOSIN.

Hytrin BPH a brand name for TERAZOSIN.

Hz *abbrev. for* Hertz, the unit of frequency equal to one cycle per second. (Heinrich Rudolph Hertz, 1857–94, German physicist).

i

-ia *suffix denoting* a disease or pathological condition.

IAMC *abbrev. for* Indian Army Medical Corps.

IARC *abbrev. for* International Agency for Research on Cancer.

-iasis *suffix denoting* a pathological condition produced by a specified cause, as in CANDIDIASIS, or relating to or resembling, as in ELEPHANTIASIS.

-iatric *suffix denoting* a specified form of medical treatment or care, as in psychiatric.

-iatrics *suffix denoting* a class of medical treatment or study, as in PAEDIATRICS.

iatrogenic pertaining to disease or disorder caused by doctors. The disorders may be unforeseeable and accidental, may be the result of unpredictable or unusual reactions, may be an inescapable consequence of necessary treatment, or may be due to medical incompetence or carelessness. *Iatros* is the Greek word for a doctor.

iatrocognition a thinking style characteristic of many doctors, featuring linear and reductionist logic, intolerance of ambiguity, and an unduly critical and pessimistic outlook. This thinking style is a severe impediment to effective leadership.

-iatry *combining form denoting* medical treatment, as in PSYCHIATRY.

ibandronic acid a biphosphonate drug that act directly on bone to inhibit osteoclastic activity. The drug is used to treat high levels of blood calcium caused by malignant tumours whether or not bone secondaries are present. It is also used to prevent pathological fractures. A brand name is Bondronate.

Ibugel a brand name for IBUPROFEN in a preparation for external use.

ibuprofen a painkilling (analgesic) drug with anti-inflammatory properties, useful in mild rheumatic and muscular disorders and in the relief of menstrual pain. The drug is on the WHO official list. Brand names are Brufen, Fenbid Spansule and Motrin. Brand names of preparations for external use include Deep Relief, Fenbid Gel, Ibugel, Ibuspray and Proflex.

Ibuspray a brand name for IBUPROFEN in a preparation for external use.

IC *abbrev. for* Intensive Care.

-ic *suffix denoting* pertaining to, or characterized by, as in RHEUMATIC.

ICD *abbrev. for* 1 Intrauterine contraceptive device.

2 Implantable cardioverter-defibrillator.

ice cream headache one of the commonest causes of headache, experienced by at least one third of ice cream afficionados when ingestion is rapid and mouthfuls large. The pain is induced by narrowing of arteries following cooling of the back part of the hard palate. It is felt in the forehead or temporal region, starts soon after the first mouthful, and reaches a climax within a minute. Occasionally it persists for as long as five minutes. There is no reason to suppose that this form of referred pain is harmful, but it can be avoided by a more restrained habit of consumption.

ichor a watery, SEROUS, or blood-tinged discharge from an ulcer or wound.

ichthyo- *combining form denoting* fish.

ichthyism a general term for food poisoning caused by eating infected or decomposing fish.

ichthyosis a fishscale-like disorder of the skin, usually genetically determined and present from birth. The skin is unable to retain water and tends to dry out. Protective and waterproof barrier creams are used.

ICRF *abbrev. for* Imperial Cancer Research Fund.

icthyosis bullosa of Siemens an autosomal dominant disorder with blistering and over-thickening of the horny surface layer of the epidermis (hyperkeratosis). The condition features an unusually heavy shedding (moulting) of the surface layers of the skin and a grey, lichenoid appearance.

-ician *suffix denoting* someone who practices or is a specialist in, as in physician.

icterogenic causing JAUNDICE.

icterus an alternative term for JAUNDICE. The Roman author Pliny, the Elder, believed that jaundice could be cured by gazing on the small yellow bird, the oriole. *Icteros* is the Greek word for a yellow bird.

icterus gravis neonatorum
see ERYTHROBLASTOSIS FETALIS, HAEMOLYTIC DISEASE OF THE NEW-BORN.

ictus a sudden attack of disease such as a STROKE.

ICU *abbrev. for* Intensive Care Unit.

id a Freudian term for that primitive part of our nature concerned with the pursuit of mainly physical and sexual gratification and unmoved by considerations of reason, logic or humanity. The id manifests the forces of the libido and the death wish, but is said to be the source of much of our psychic energy. Freud's choice of the term may have been a little prudish in its lack of specificity; *id* is a Latin rendering of the Greek *es* meaning it. See also FREUDIAN THEORY.

idarubicin a CYTOTOXIC anti-cancer drug. A brand name is Zavedos.

IDDM *abbrev. for* insulin dependent diabetes mellitus (Type I DIABETES).

ideation the formation of ideas, thought, the use of the intellect.

ideational apraxia the inability to carry out normal motor functions, such as using objects properly, because of mental confusion resulting from organic brain disease.

idée fixe a fixed idea or obsession, often delusional, and having a marked effect on behaviour.

identical twins twins derived from the same egg (ovum) which, after the first division, has separated into two individuals. Identical twins thus have the same genetics.

ideogram a graphics representation of the G BANDING pattern of a CHROMOSOME.

ideomotor mental processes that immediately result in movement.

idio- *combining form denoting* personal, individual, originating within oneself, without external cause.

idiocy the state of a person with a mental age of less than three. The term is little used in medicine.

idiopathic of unknown cause.

idiosyncrasy 1 a physiological or mental peculiarity.
2 a tendency to react abnormally to a drug, often in a manner characteristic of the response to a much larger dose than that taken. An individual hypersensitivity to a drug, not of an allergic nature.

idiot a person of severe mental deficit, incapable of coherent speech or of normal response to danger.

idiot savant a person, severely backward in most mental respects, who shows great precocity and ability in one particular direction, such as mental arithmetical calculation or data recall. The idiot savant often has an IQ of less than 50 and the particular skill is seldom of practical use.

idiotypes the molecular structure of the variable region of an IMMUNOGLOBULIN molecule that confers its antigenic specificity.

idoxuridine a drug effective against HERPES SIMPLEX viruses. Idoxuridine is chemically very similar to thymine, which it replaces in the viral DNA thereby preventing replication. The drug is on the WHO official list. A brand name for a preparation for external use is Herpid.

ifosfamide an ALKYLATING AGENT used as an anticancer drug. A brand name is Mitoxana.

Ig *abbrev. for* IMMUNOGLOBULIN.

IgA immunoglobulin class A, an antibody class concerned with protection against virus and other infections in the mucous membranes of the body, especially in the respiratory and digestive systems.

IgA nephropathy a form of GLOMERULO-NEPHRITIS associated with deposition of the immunoglobulin IgA in the glomeruli of the kidneys. There is occasional blood and protein in the urine and kidney failure may occur. The cause is unknown and there is no effective treatment.

IgD immunoglobulin class D, an antibody class probably concerned with the regulation of B LYMPHOCYTES. IgD is found almost exclusively on the surface of B lymphocytes.

IgE immunoglobulin class E, an antibody class concerned with immediate hypersensitivity reactions, such as hay fever (ALLERGIC RHINITIS). IgE has an affinity for cell surfaces and is commonly found on MAST CELLS.

IgG immunoglobulin class G. This antibody accounts for three quarters of the immunoglobulins in the blood of healthy people. It is widely distributed in the tissues and is the only immunoglobulin class that passes through the placenta to the fetus. It is concerned with protection against a wide range of infecting organisms. Note that the term gamma globulin refers to the whole class of immunoglobulins, not simply to IgG.

IgM immunoglobulin class M, an antibody class concerned especially with the breakdown of foreign cells and with preparing foreign material for PHAGOCYTOSIS.

ileal conduit the use of part of the small intestine (ileum) as a disposal route for urine by implanting the URETERS into it after surgical removal of the bladder.

ileitis see REGIONAL ILEITIS.

ileocaecal pertaining to the ILEUM and the CAECUM. The ileocaecal valve is an internal fold of lining mucous membrane that prevents reflux of bowel contents from the caecum into the ileum.

ileocolic intussusception an abnormal INVAGINATION of the ILEUM through the ILEOCECAL valve into the COLON.

ileocolitis inflammation of both ILEUM and COLON.

ileocolostomy a surgical connection between the ILEUM and the COLON usually to bypass an obstruction or a disease process in the CAECUM or ascending colon.

ileostomy a surgical operation in which the lower part of the small intestine (the ileum) is cut and the upper end brought out through the front wall of the abdomen so that the bowel contents can discharge externally into a bag. Ileostomy is necessary when there is bowel obstruction, or when the lower bowel requires to be rested to recover from disease, injury or surgical operation.

ileum the third part of the small intestine lying between the JEJUNUM and the start of the large intestine, the CAECUM. The contents of the ileum are of the consistency of a watery mud

and almost all nutrients have been absorbed by about the middle of the ileum.

ileus failure, usually temporary, of the process of PERISTALSIS by which the bowel contents are moved onwards. More correctly known as adynamic ileus, or sometimes paralytic ileus, the condition is caused by injury, severe infection, loss of blood, shock, or deficiency of potassium, calcium or magnesium. There is persistent vomiting and abdominal distention. Treatment is to keep the bowel as empty as possible by use of a suction tube and to deal with the original cause.

iliac arteries the two large arteries into which the abdominal AORTA divides in the lower abdomen, and which supply blood to the pelvic region and the legs.

iliacus the part of the ILIOPSOAS muscle arising from the inside of the back wall of the pelvis (the iliac fossa and sacrum) and being inserted into the top of the front of the FEMUR. The iliacus helps to flex the hip joint in walking.

iliac veins the three large veins on each side of the body that drain the pelvis and legs and accompany the ILIAC ARTERIES.

iliofemoral ligament a strong fibrous band running from the front of the pelvis to the top of the thigh bone (femur).

ilioinguinal pertaining to the iliac region and the groin.

iliopsoas a large muscle group arising from the inside of the back wall of the pelvis and lower abdomen and consisting of the ILIACUS and PSOAS major and minor muscles. These muscles are inserted into the front of the top of the thigh bone (femur) and act to bend the hip joint or to flex the trunk on the thigh as in sitting up from lying.

iliotibial tract a thickening in the sheet of tough fibrous tissue (fascia lata) that covers the outer side of the thigh. The iliotibial tract extends upwards from the prominence on the upper part of the main lower leg bone (tibia) (the lateral condyle) to the crest of the pelvis (the iliac crest).

ilium the uppermost of three bones into which the INNOMINATE bone of the pelvis is arbitrarily divided. Its most conspicuous feature is the iliac crest forming the upper brim of the pelvis on either side.

illusion a false sense perception from misinterpretation of stimuli. Most illusions are normal and harmless, but some are features of psychiatric conditions, especially depression. Compare DELUSION and HALLUCINATION.

iloprost trometamol a synthetic prostacycline analogue formulated as an aerosol spray for inhalation. It is used in the treatment of primary pulmonary hypertension to improve exercise capacity. Iloprost inhibits platelet aggregation and adhesion and dilates small blood vessels, resulting in an improvement in cardiac output and blood oxygen saturation.

Ilotycin a brand name for ERYTHROMYCIN.

IMA *abbrev. for* Irish Medical Association.

image intensifier a device used in radiology by means of which weak X-ray images obtained by low dosage radiation may be converted into television images and improved in brightness and contrast by purely electronic means. This allows continuous X-ray sceening for various procedures, such as the insertion of arterial catheters, without exposing the patient to unaceptably large doses of radiation.

imaging techniques any of the various methods of visual screening display of internal features of the body. They include X-ray, CT SCANNING, MAGNETIC RESONANCE IMAGING (MRI), ULTRASOUND SCANNING, ANGIOGRAPHY, DIGITAL SUBTRACTION ANGIOGRAPHY and fibreoptic closed circuit television.

imatinib an anticancer drug of the protein-tyrosine kinase inhibitor class used to treat some cases of chronic myeloid leukaemia. Imatinib is used in cases of adult leukaemia with the Philadelphia chromosome which causes the production of an abnormal protein tyrosine kinase. The drug is indicated if interferon-alpha treatment fails or if the disease is in a highly active phase. Brand name: Glivec.

imbecile an obsolete term for a mentally retarded person or, nowadays, a person with severe learning difficulty.

imbibition the taking up of fluid as by absorption into a gel.

imbrication an overlapping of the free edges of a tissue as in the surgical correction of a tissue defect or of a weakened area.

Imdur a brand name for ISOSORBIDE MONONITRATE.

imidazoles a class of antifungal and antibacterial drugs effective against a wide range of bacteria and fungi. The group includes METRONIDAZOLE (Flagyl), MEBENDAZOLE, THIABENDAZOLE (tiabendazole), CLOTRIMAZOLE (Canesten), ketoconazole and miconazole.

imidazopyridine hypnotics drugs used for the short-term treatment of insomnia. An example is zolpidem (Stilnoct).

Imigran a brand name for SUMATRIPAN.

imipenem an ANTIBIOTIC enzyme inhibitor resistant to breakdown by most beta-lactamases. It is active against a wide range of bacteria. The drug is on the WHO official list. A brand name with cilastatin is Primaxin.

imipramine a widely used tricyclic anti-depressant drug. A brand name is Tofranil.

immersion foot a form of cold injury resulting from prolonged immersion in cold water. Long-term constriction of the blood vessels results in tissue damage from deprivation of oxygen and nutrition. Permanent loss of sensation and abnormal sensitivity to cold result. In the most severe cases GANGRENE occurs. Also known as trench foot.

immobilization the avoidance of movement of an injured or diseased part, especially a bone fracture, so that healing may take place. Effective fracture immobilization demands that the joint above and below the fracture should be unable to flex. Immobilization is achieved by means of slings, splints, plaster of Paris casts, cold-setting plastic casts and external steel bar fixators of variable design.

immortalization a change in a eukaryotic cell line that confers the ability to go on dividing and reproducing indefinitely. Immortalization implies the ability to continue to reform TELOMERES.

Immukin a brand name for INTERFERON GAMMA-1b.

immune complexes combinations of ANTIGEN and ANTIBODY and sometimes COMPLEMENT proteins. These complexes may be deposited in the walls of small blood vessels where they react with complement, MAST CELLS, other white cells or PLATELETS to trigger local inflammation. Immune complexes are involved in long-term infections such as ENDOCARDITIS, various kinds of ARTHRITIS, allergic ALVEOLITIS (Farmer's lung, bird-fancier's lung), and a range of kidney, arterial and skin diseases.

immune response genes genes, including all those within the MAJOR HISTOCOMPATIBILITY COMPLEX (MHC) that determine the total response to a given antigen.

immune surveillance a body mechanism by which early cancers are detected as being foreign and are attacked and usually destroyed. Immune surveillance is a T cell-mediated process without which cancer would be much commoner. See also CTLA4-IG.

immunity the relative ability to resist infection or the effects of any toxic or dangerous substance. Immunity may be inherent or acquired as a result of prior infection or immunization. Active immunity involves the production of ANTIBODIES. Passive immunity is that conferred by antibodies derived from another person or animal and injected or received across the placenta or in the breast milk. Passive immunity is much less persistent than active immunity.

immunization the process of conferring a degree of protection or IMMUNITY against infection or the effects of infection. The terms 'immunization' and 'vaccination' are interchangeable. See also INOCULATION.

immuno- *combining form denoting* immune or immunity.

immunoassay a method of testing for, and measuring the concentration of, various antibodies. Various methods, including RADIOIMMUNOASSAY, enzyme linked immunosorbent assay (ELISA) and immunoelectrophoresis may be used.

immunochemistry the science of the chemical processes underlying the antigen-antibody reaction and of the other chemical reactions involved in the operation of the immune system.

immunocompromized in a condition of diminished ability to resist infection, to reject foreign material gaining access to the body, and to react aggressively at a cellular level to early cancerous change. People may become immunocompromized by heavy and prolonged antibiotic treatment, by exposure to large doses of CORTICOSTEROIDS or other IMMUNO-SUPPRESSANT DRUGS, or by disorders affecting the immune system such as AIDS.

immunodeficiency disorders any one of a number of congenital or acquired conditions in which the body's immunological system of defence against infection, foreign material and some forms of cancer, is defective. Immunodeficiency may be of genetic origin, may be IATROGENIC or may be caused by infection with the human immunodeficiency virus (HIV) that has led to the development of AIDS. See also GENETIC IMMUNODEFICIENCY DISORDERS.

immunofluorescence the detection and identification of antigenic material by observing, under the microscope, the fluorescence of known, specific, fluorescein-linked (conjugated) antibodies that have become attached to it.

immunogen any substance that can elicit an immune response. An antigen.

immunoglobulins ANTIBODIES, protective proteins produced by cloned B lymphocyte-derived plasma cells. There are five classes of immunoglobulins, the most prevalent being immunoglobulin G (IgG), or gammaglobulin which provides the body's main defence against bacteria, viruses and toxins. Immunoglobulins are Y-shaped protein molecules consisting of two inner heavy POLYPEPTIDE chains, forming a Y, and, attached to the outer side of the short arms of the Y, two light polypeptide chains. The heavy chains are held together and the light chains held to the arms, by disulphide bonds. The short arms of the Y, with the light chains, are called the Fab (fragment antigen binding) section of the antibody. The antigen combining site lies between the open ends of the light and heavy chains. See also IgA, IgD, IgE, IgG and IgM. Some immunoglobulins are prepared as drugs for the management of RHESUS incompatibility and antibody deficiency; for the prophylaxis of MEASLES and hepatitis A; to minimize fetal damage when a pregnant woman is exposed to RUBELLA; and to assist in the treatment of TETANUS and RABIES. They are marketed under such brand names as Flebogamma, Gammabulin, Gammagard, Octagam, Rhophylac, Sandoglobulin, Vigam liquid and Winrho SDF.

immunology the science and study of the many complex cellular and biochemical interactions involved in the functioning of the immune defences of the body and of the mechanisms that allow the body to distinguish 'self' from 'non-self'. The list that follows highlights the key entries related to immunology in the dictionary: AIDS, allergy, allograft, anaphylaxis, antibody, antigen, atopy, autoimmunity, basophil, B cell, BCG, complement, eosinophil, HLA, mast cell, immune complex, immunity, immunodeficiency, immunoglobulins, interferon, killer cell, lymphocyte, lymphoma, major histocompatibility complex (MHC), major histocompatibility locus, phagocyte, plasma cell, polymorph, T cell, transplantation, thymus.

immunopathology the study of the role of immunological processes in the production of disease and in its diagnosis and treatment.

immunomodulators drugs that can act on the immune system in a therapeutically helpful manner. They include INTERFERONS and glatiramer acetate (Copaxone) for multiple sclerosis; tacrolimus (Protopic) and pimecrolimus (Elidel) for severe atopic eczema; and inosine pranobex (Imunovir) for herpes simplex infections.

immunoprophylaxis prevention of disease by the use of vaccines.

immunosuppressant drugs drugs that act on any part of the immune system of the body so as to interfere with the normal reactions to the presence of any ANTIGEN. Such drugs are used to prevent graft rejection and to treat conditions caused by immune phenomena, such as immune complex disorders or autoimmune disease. They include AZATHIOPRINE, corticosteroid drugs, CYCLOSPORIN (ciclosporin), mycophenolate motefil (Cellcept), etanercept (Enbrel), anakinra (Kineret), tacrolimus (Prograf), sirolimus (Rapamune), infliximab (Remicade), daclizumab (Zenapak) and the anti-lymphocyte monoclonal antibody OKT3. See also CTLA4-IG.

immunotherapy 1 passive immunization by means of serum containing immunoglobulins. 2 mainly experimental cancer treatment based on attempts to stimulate the immune system into a more vigorous attack on cancer cells. Methods employed have included the use of BCG, antisera from cancer patients, INTERFERONS and the injection of modified cancer cells. 3 treatment of allergic conditions by repeated injections of the ALLERGENS responsible, so as to build up tolerance. Also known as desensitization.

Imunovir a brand name for INOSINE PRANOBEX.

Imodium a brand name for LOPERAMIDE.

impaction 1 the condition of being forced into and retained in any part of the body. 2 the situation in which the ends of a fractured

bone are firmly driven into each other so that movement at the fracture site does not occur. 3 retention of an unerupted tooth in the jaw by obstruction by another tooth, especially a molar, so that its normal appearance is prevented.

impalpable unable to be felt.

imperforate having no opening. Used of a structure normally having an opening, as of an imperforate hymen or anus.

impetigo a common, highly infectious, skin disease caused by STAPHYLOCOCCUS infection. Impetigo is commonest in children, and in hot, moist climates. In temperate areas, widespread impetigo can be an indication of inadequate standards of personal hygiene. It feature rapidly spreading small blisters which soon turn to golden-green crusts. Treatment is by thorough skin cleaning and the use of antibiotic ointment.

implantable defibrillator see DEFIBRILLATOR, IMPLANTABLE.

implantation 1 partial penetration of, and attachment to, the lining of the womb by the fertilized egg. 2 the introduction into the body of a donated or transferred tissue or organ or a prosthetic part, such as an intraocular lens.

implant defibrillator an experimental device that senses VENTRICULAR FIBRILLATION in patients liable to recurrent episodes of this form of heart stoppage (cardiac arrest) and automatically applies electric shocks to the heart to reverse the condition.

impotence the inability to achieve or sustain a sufficiently firm penile erection (tumescence) to allow normal vaginal sexual intercourse. The great majority of cases are not caused by organic disease and most men experience occasional periods of impotence. It is often related to anxiety about performance and is usually readily corrected by simple counselling methods which prescribe sensual massage but forbid coitus. Organic impotence may be caused by DIABETES, MULTIPLE SCLEROSIS, spinal cord disorders and heart disease. Many cases can be helped by the drug SILDENAFIL (Viagra).

impregnation the act or process of making pregnant, fertilizing or inseminating.

impression in dentistry, a negative mould of the teeth or other mouth structures, made in plastic, which is later filled with Plaster of Paris to provide a perfect copy of the anatomy.

imprinting 1 the rapid early development in young animals of the ability to recognize and to be attracted to others of their own species or to similar surrogates.
2 in genetics, changes that occur in a gene in passing through the egg or the sperm so that maternal and paternal alleles differ at the start of embryonic life.

IMS *abbrev. for* Indian Medical Service.

Imunovir a brand name for INOSINE PRANOBEX.

Imuran a brand name for AZOTHIAPRINE.

in- *prefix denoting* not or in, into, within.

inactivated viruses commercially-prepared vaccines against various viral infections. Vaccines include those against HEPATITIS A, (marketed as Avamix, Epaxal, Havrix Monodose and Vaqta Paediatric); hepatitis A and B (Twinrix); hepatitis A and TYPHOID (Hepatyrix and Viatim); and RABIES (Rabipur).

Inadine a brand name for POVIDONE-IODINE.

inanition a state of exhaustion or a bodily disorder arising from lack of any of the nutritional elements such as calories, protein, vitamins, minerals or water.

in articulo mortis at the exact moment of death.

inborn of qualities or characteristics that are genetically determined rather than being acquired after conception.

inborn errors of metabolism genetic defects that interfere with the normal biochemical processes of the body. The term was coined in 1908 Sir Archibald Garrod (1857–1936) to describe the inherited diseases ALKAPTONURIA, ALBINISM, CYSTINURIA, and PENTOSURIA. Many other such conditions are now known and their genetic mechanism understood. All metabolic processes are mediated by enzymes and these are coded for by genes. When a gene mutation results in the absence or defect of one or more of these enzymes, inborn errors of metabolism result.

inbreeding mating of the closely related. Inbreeding tends to promote similarities and to deny access to new genes. It increases the chances of offspring being HOMOZYGOUS for RECESSIVE genes and thus manifesting the effect but, in itself, has no inherent tendency to produce bad characteristics. Its reputation so to do arises from the observation of the undesirable effects of inbreeding in the genetically disfavoured.

incarcerated hernia a hernia in which the loop of bowel that has prolapsed has become permanently trapped in the hernial sac and cannot be reduced.

incest sexual intercourse between close blood relatives, especially between brothers and sisters, fathers and daughters, or mothers and sons. The 'prohibited degrees' vary in extent in different legal systems. There is a strong social taboo against incest now thought to be based on social and psychological, rather than genetic, factors.

incestuous pertaining to INCEST.

incidence the number of cases of an event, such as a disease, occurring in a particular population during a given period. Incidence is usually expressed as so many cases per 1000, or per 100,000, per year. Compare PREVALENCE.

incision a surgical cut made to achieve access or to allow discharge of unwanted material such as pus. The placement of surgical incisions is often a matter for judgement involving considerations of subsequent wound strength as well as good access.

incisional hernia the separation of the edges of an operative INCISION by the protrusion through it of an internal structure such as a loop of bowel. An incisional hernia may also occur through an accidental wound.

incisor one of the four central teeth of each jaw, with cutting edges for biting pieces off food. The incisors are situated immediately in front of the canine teeth.

incisura an indentation or notch in a structure.

inclusion bodies microscopically visible masses of virus material, or areas of altered staining behaviour, seen within cells in a number of virus infections such as RABIES, herpes infections, papovavirus infections and adenovirus infections.

inclusion conjunctivitis an acute inflammation of the CONJUNCTIVA caused by Chlamydia trachomatis and featuring discharge of mucus and pus. Virus masses (inclusion bodies) may be demonstrated in conjunctival cells. The condition is usually acquired as a sexually transmitted disease and responds to treatment with TETRACYCLINE. Also known as inclusion blennorrhoea.

inclusion cyst an encapsulated, usually spherical, buried body formed in tissue by implantation of a surface layer of cells (epithelium) which continues to produce its normal secretions.

incompetent cervix a laxity or undue wideness of the inner mouth (internal os) of the outlet of the womb that commonly leads to repeated, painless miscarriages after the 16th week of pregnancy. The condition is treated by the insertion of a purse-string stitch of non-absorbable material which is removed shortly before term.

incompetent heart valve a valve that has been damaged by disease or congenital defect so that its cusps do not close completely and blood is able to pass in a direction contrary to the normal. This causes regurgitation and flow turbulence and imposes an abnormal load on the heart muscle of the affected chamber.

incompetent vein valve a valve, defective either by constitution or by stretching, that fails to support a column of blood and promotes stagnation, increased pressure on the vein wall and varicosity.

incomplete abortion loss of part of the products of conception, usually the embryo or fetus, with retention in the womb of the placenta or some of the membranes. Se also ABORTION.

incomplete dominance failure of one or other of two ALLELES to exert a dominant effect with the result that the PHENOTYPE has a form somewhere in between those of the two phenotypes that would be produced were either gene homozygous.

incontinence loss of voluntary control of one or both of the excretory functions. Faecal incontinence is the inability to control the evacuation of the rectum. Urinary incontinence is loss of complete control over the voiding of urine. Stress incontinence features the escape of small quantities of urine on coughing, laughing or otherwise sharply increasing the pressure within the abdomen.

incoordination the inability accurately to time and phase the various components of movement so that these tend to be effected separately causing clumsiness and lack of smoothness in MOTOR activity.

incubation period the interval between the time of infection and the first appearance of symptoms of the resulting disease. Incubation periods vary widely, from as little as a few hours in the case of CHOLERA to many weeks in some cases of RABIES.

incubator an equipment providing a closed controllable environment in which optimum conditions may be established for the nutrition, growth and preservation of organisms, whether bacterial or human. Incubators are used to culture bacteria and to promote the survival of premature babies.

incubatory carrier a person harbouring an infectious disease which is still in its INCUBATION PERIOD.

incurable not able to be remedied by currently available medical means. The progress of medical science in the 20th century repeatedly showed that what is incurable today is often remediable tomorrow.

incus the middle of the three tiny bones (auditory ossicles) that form a chain across the middle ear linking the eardrum to the inner ear. The incus is anvil shaped.

indapamide a diuretic drug used to treat high blood pressure (HYPERTENSION). Brand names are Natramid and Natrilix.

Inderal a brand name for PROPRANOLOL.

index finger the finger adjacent to the thumb.

index of refraction a measure of the optical density of a transparent material such as glass or the cornea. It is the ratio of the speed of light through the material to its speed in a vacuum.

indicator a substance that undergoes an observable change, usually a change of colour, when a chemical alteration occurs in its environment. Indicators may demonstrate changes in acidity, the presence of various substances, such as sugar or protein in body fluids, or alterations in the concentrations of substances. Indicators are widely used in chemistry and in clinical medicine.

indigestion see DYSPEPSIA.

indirect-acting sympathomimetics beta agonist drugs that act indirectly and are used to treat bronchospasm, nasal congestion and some allergic disorders. Examples are ephedrine hydrochloride (Cam); ephedrine with theophylline (Franol); and ephedreine with chlorpheniramine (chlorphenamine) (Haymine).

indium-111 a radionuclide that emits gamma rays and can be used as a tracer for localizing tumours.

indinavir a PROTEASE INHIBITOR drug used in combination with antiviral drugs to treat AIDS. The drug is on the WHO official list. A brand name is Crixivan.

Indocid a brand name for INDOMETHACIN (indometacin) .

Indocid PDA a brand name for INDOMETHACIN (indometacin).

Indolar a brand name for INDOMETHACIN (indometacin).

indole 2,3-benzopyrrole, an unpleasant-smelling product of protein breakdown that contributes to the odour of the faeces. In high dilution, indole has a pleasant smell and has been used in the perfumery industry. See also SKATOLE.

indolent of slow progression or taking a long time to heal. Causing little or no pain. Often used of skin ulcers.

indomethacin indometacin, a non-steroidal painkilling (analgesic) and anti-inflammatory drug (NSAID) of the indole acetic acid group. Brand names are Flexin Continus, Indocid, Indocid PDA and Indomod.

Indomod a brand name for INDOMETHACIN (indometacin).

Indoramin a selective adrenergic alpha-blocker drug used to treat high blood pressure (HYPERTENSION). Brand names are Baratol and Doralese.

inducer a molecule that causes a gene to be expressed by binding to a repressor protein so as to prevent it from acting to prevent expression.

induction of labour the artificial initiation of the processes of birth, usually at a late stage in the pregnancy, before this has occurred spontaneously. This is done in cases in which the continuation of the pregnancy would be dangerous either to the mother or baby by reason of such conditions as PRE-ECLAMPSIA, POSTMATURITY, ANTEPARTUM HAEMORRHAGE, DIABETES or HAEMOLTYIC DISEASE (rhesus incompatibility). Induction may also be done if the fetus has died or is severely abnormal.

induration 1 abnormal hardness of tissue as a result of a disease process or injury.
2 hardening of tissue.

industrial diseases diseases specifically caused by the effects of work processes or working conditions on health or by exposure to substances involved in work processes.

indwelling of a CATHETER or draining tube that is left in situ for a length of time.

inebriety drunkenness.

inevitable abortion a separation of the placental attachment to the wall of the womb that has proceeded to such an extent that the death of the embryo or fetus cannot be prevented. See also ABORTION.

in extremis *adv.* near to death, in extreme danger of dying.

Infacol a brand name for DIMETHICONE (dimeticone).

infanticide killing of an infant.

infantile spasms an epilepsy-like syndrome affecting babies in the first year of life. The baby suddenly flexes the neck and trunk as if bowing (salaam attacks), the arms are thrown out and the legs are either extended sharply or drawn up. The spasm last for only a second or so but may be frequent. Possible causes include a congenital brain defect, brain injury at birth, prenatal infection, the effects of earlier meningitis or untreated PHENYLKETONURIA. In many cases no such cause is found. The outlook is often poor.

infantilism persistence of child-like characteristics of body and mind into adult life. Arrested development in an adult.

infant mortality the number of infants per 1000 live births who die before reaching the age of 1 year. Infant mortality is a sensitive index of the standards of public health in a society. The rate in Britain was about 150 in 1900. Today, in the best regions, it is as low as 8.

infarct a volume of dead tissue lying within living tissue, the death being caused by local loss of blood supply. Infarcted tissue swells and becomes firm, and blood vessels around an infarct widen. Plasma and blood may pass into the infarct, increasing the swelling. Later the infarct becomes pale and shrinks and soon it is replaced by fibrous tissue and is converted into a scar which is usually at least as strong as the original tissue. Function is, of course, lost.

infarction the deprivation of a part of a tissue or organ of its blood supply so that a wedge-shaped area of dead tissue (an infarct) forms. Infarction of part of the heart muscle is the process underlying a heart attack.

infection 1 the process by which organisms capable of causing disease gain entry to the body and establish colonies.
2 the state of injury or damage to part of the body resulting from this process.

infectious diseases diseases caused by organisms that can spread directly from person to person. Diseases requiring a transmission agent (vector) such as malaria, yellow fever and leishmaniasis, are usually excluded from this group. Common infectious diseases are CHICKENPOX, DIPHTHERIA, FOOD POISONING, GASTROENTERITIS, GLANDULAR FEVER, HEPATITIS, INFLUENZA, MEASLES, MENINGITIS, MUMPS, RUBELLA, TUBERCULOSIS and the SEXUALLY TRANSMITTED DISEASES.

infectious mononucleosis see GLANDULAR FEVER.

infective capable of causing INFECTION.

infecundity infertility. Inability to bear children.

inferior situated below. An anatomical term referring to relationships in the upright body. The heart is inferior to the head, but no value judgement is implied. From the Latin *inferus*, below.

inferiority complex a concept of the Austrian psychiatrist Alfred Adler (1870–1937) indicating a general sense of unworthiness resulting from repressed perception of one's bodily defects. In popular usage the term simply implies a generally self-critical attitude or a boastful, self-exalting manner that compensates for feelings of inferiority.

infero- *combining form denoting* anatomically INFERIOR.

infertility the apparent inability of a particular couple to reproduce. The problem may rest either with the female or with the male or, rarely, with both. Male causes are largely confined to a low sperm count or abnormal sperms and cigarette smoking. So the first step in investigation is to investigate this by examination of a sample of seminal fluid. Female causes are more numerous and include failure of ovulation, blockage of the fallopian tubes, uterine fibroids, adhesions within the womb, sperm-hostile mucus in the cervix, thyroid disorders, DIABETES, obesity, and excessive physical exercise. Joint causes include cigarette smoking, excessive caffeine intake, use of recreational drugs and ignorance of basic reproductive processes.

infestation the condition of being invaded or inhabited by ectoparasites such as lice, mites or ticks. The term is also sometimes applied to large internal parasites such as intestinal worms, but this is more usually referred to as INFECTION.

infibulation female CIRCUMCISION with stitching together of the LABIA MAJORA so as to prevent sexual intercourse.

infiltration the movement into, or accumulation within, a tissue or organ, of cells or material not normally found therein. Cellular infiltration, as with LYMPHOCYTES, is often part of an immunological response.

inflammation the response of living tissue to injury, featuring widening of blood vessels, with redness, heat, swelling and pain – the cardinal signs 'rubor', 'calor', 'tumor' and 'dolor' of the first century physician Celsus. Inflammation also involves loss of function and is the commonest of all the disease processes. It is expressed by the ending '-itis'. Inflammation involves release of PROSTAGLANDINS which strongly stimulate pain nerve endings. It is, in general, protective and assists the immune system to restore normality, but persistent (chronic) inflammation may lead to the formation of undesirable scar tissue.

infliximab a monoclonal antibody used to treat severe cases of CROHN'S DISEASE which have failed to respond to treatment with corticosteroids or immunosuppressant therapy. The drug is also used to treat rheumatoid arthritis. Brand name: Remicade.

influenza a respiratory infection caused by a virus of the *Orthomyxoviridae* family and spread mainly by the aerosol of droplets coughed and sneezed by sufferers. It is highly infectious to the susceptible, spreads rapidly, and tends to occur in epidemics in the winter time. There are three main types – A, B and C – distinguishable by antibody tests. Type B is the main cause. Influenza features fever, sore throat, running nose, dry cough, headache, backache, muscle pains, loss of appetite, insomnia and prostration. In most cases the acute stage lasts for only a few days and the symptoms then gradually resolve. Complications include HYPERPYREXIA, BRONCHITIS, PNEUMONIA and REYE'S SYNDROME. There is a significant mortality rate, especially in old people. Vaccines are available and are especially important for the elderly.

informed consent the formal agreement to a surgical or medical procedure by a patient who has been adequately briefed on what is proposed and who is fully aware of all reasonably possible side effects or complications.

infra- *prefix denoting* below, beneath, INFERIOR to.

infraclavicular under the collar-bone.

infraocclusion failure of a tooth to erupt fully so that the biting or grinding surface is unable to contact that of its fellow in the other jaw. Also known as infraclusion.

inframandibular below the lower jaw.

infraorbital lying below the ORBIT.

infrapatellar below the knee cap.

infra-red pertaining to electromagnetic radiation of wavelengths between 780 nanometers (nm) and 1 mm, being greater than those of visible light but shorter than those of microwaves. Heat radiation.

infrascapular below the shoulder blade.

infraspinatus muscle a muscle that runs from the back surface of the shoulder blade (SCAPULA) to the back of the upper part of the upper arm bone (HUMERUS). Its action is to rotate the arm outwards.

infraspinous situated below any spine or spinous process.

infrasplenic below the SPLEEN.

infrasternal below or deep to the breastbone.

infratemporal below the temporal region of the skull. Below the TEMPORAL FOSSA.

infratrochlear situated below the pulley for the tendon of the superior oblique eye-moving muscle.

infraumbilical below the navel.

infundibulum any funnel shaped bodily passages or structure, such as the stalk of the PITUITARY GLAND.

infusion 1 the administration of a fluid other than blood into a vein. Blood infusion is called TRANSFUSION. Fluids given by intravenous infusion include saline (sodium chloride) solutions, DEXTRAN solution, DEXTROSE solution, lactic acid solution, bicarbonate solution and a variety of special mixtures, such as Ringer's and Hartmann's solution. 2 the soaking of a solid substance in a solvent, such as water, for the purpose of extracting an active ingredient.

ingestion the process of taking food or other material into the stomach. Ingestion is followed by DIGESTION, ABSORPTION and, finally, ASSIMILATION.

ingrown toenail an inaccurate lay term for inflammation and swelling of infected soft tissues surrounding the nail. The swollen tissue overlaps the edge of the nail causing an appearance as if the nail had grown into the tissue. The growth of the nail is normal.

inguinal pertaining to the groin.

inguinal hernia a HERNIA in which, under the influence of intra-abdominal pressure, a sac of PERITONEUM is forced down the inguinal canal, followed by a loop of bowel. In men the inguinal hernia descends alongside the spermatic cord into the scrotum which, in time, may become greatly enlarged by the bulk of its abnormal contents.

inguinal ligament a slightly downward-sloping and downward-curving ligament that runs from a bony spine on the upper and outer front edge of the pelvis (anterior superior iliac spine) to the PUBIS. The ligament forms part of the tendinous attachment (aponeurosis) of one of the main abdominal muscles, the external oblique muscle. Also known as Poupart's ligament. (Francois Poupart, 1661–1709, French surgeon and naturalist).

inhalers devices for delivering medication in aerosol, vapour or powder form to the bronchial tubes and lungs, especially for the treatment of ASTHMA. Propulsion of the drug may be by gas under pressure or by an inhaled current of air. Drugs commonly taken in this way include BRONCHODILATORS and CORTICOSTEROIDS.

inherent of a quality or part, existing naturally or intrinsically.

inheritance 1 the acquisition of a particular set of genes (GENOME) from the entire series of a person's forebears, by way of an equal number of genes from each parent. 2 the characteristics transmitted in this way.

inhibition arrest or limitation of a function or activity.

Initard a brand name for a slow acting INSULIN.

injection the introduction of any substance, especially medication or nutritional substances, into the body, usually by means of a hollow needle and a syringe. Injections may be given into the skin (intradermally), under the skin (subcutaneously), into a muscle (intramuscularly), into a vein (intravenously), into an artery (intra-arterially), into the SUBARACHNOID SPACE or into a sheath (intrathecally), or into an organ. The term is also sometimes used to refer to the introduction of substances into a body orifice such as the URETHRA, the vagina or the rectum.

injury any permanent or semi-permanent disturbance of structure or function of any part of the body caused by an external agency. Such agency may be mechanical, thermal, chemical, electrical or radiational. The term may also be applied to damage caused by infecting organisms or to psychological trauma.

ink blot test any of several psychological tests, such as the Rorschach test, in which the subject indicates his or her perception of a random-shape pattern produced by folding a sheet of paper over a large ink-blot. It is doubtful whether the method has any real objective analytic value independently of the qualities of the analyst.

inlay dental restorative material that is cemented into a prepared cavity in a tooth.

innervation 1 the supply or distribution of nerve fibres to any part of the body.
2 the provision of nerve stimuli to a muscle, gland or other nerve.

innocent INNOCUOUS, non-malignant, BENIGN.

innocuous having no ill effect, harmless.

Innohep a brand name for TINZAPARIN.

innominate artery a major, unpaired, artery that arises from the arch of the aorta, towards the right side of the body, and immediately divides into the right subclavian and right carotid arteries.

innominate bone the bone that forms each side of the pelvis. Each innominate bone is attached, behind, to the sides of the SACRUM and, in front, to the other innominate at the pubic junction (symphysis pubis). The innominate is nominally divided, for convenience, into the ilium, above, the ischium, below, and the pubis, in front. Bones were commonly named because of their resemblance to other things. The innominate bone bears little resemblance to any other shape, hence the term which means nameless.

innominate vein one of a pair of veins which drain the head and upper chest by way of the JUGULAR and SUBCLAVIAN veins. The two innominate veins join to form the SUPERIOR VENA CAVA.

Innovace a brand name for ENALAPRIL.

Innozide a brand name for ENALAPRIL in conjunction with HYDROCHLOROTHIAZIDE.

inoculation immunization or vaccination. The procedure by which the immune system is stimulated into producing protective antibodies (IMMUNOGLOBULINS) to specific infective agents, such as viruses and bacteria by the introduction into the body of safe forms of the organism or of its ANTIGENIC elements.

inoperable referring to the stage in a disease, normally treated by surgery, beyond which surgery is not feasible or useful. The term is commonly applied to cancer that has spread widely. Many conditions once universally considered inoperable are now treated by surgery.

inorganic of chemical compounds, not having the structure of, or derived from, compounds found in living organisms. Not containing carbon.

inosculate to join by small openings.

inosine pranobex isoprinosine. An antiviral drug used to treat oral and genital herpes and genital warts. The drug also enhances the efficiency of the immune system by increasing the number of T cells and enhancing the activity of natural killer cells. A brand name is Imunovir.

inositol nicotinate a nicotinic acid derivative that is used to treat disorders such as RAYNAUD'S DISEASE that involve arterial spasm. A brand name is Hexopal.

inotropic influencing the force or speed of muscular contractility. Inotropic agents, such as dobutamine and dopamine are used to improve the output of the heart in the treatment of HEART FAILURE and sometimes in acute circulatory failure (SHOCK).

inotropic agents generally, any measure used to change the force of a muscle. In practice the term is used for drugs that increase the force of contraction of the heart and whose use is usually limited to cases of low-output HEART FAILURE. They include ADRENALINE and NORADRENALINE, isoprenaline, PHOSPHODIESTERASE INHIBITORS, DIGITALIS, DOPAMINE derivatives, dopexamine (Dopacard) and dobutamine (Dobutrex, Posiject). Their use calls for great skill and knowledge and is generally confined to cardiologists. From the Greek *inos*, a muscle and *tropos*, a turning.

inpatient a person staying in a hospital, at least overnight, for treatment.

inquest a judicial inquiry usually into the cause of a death. Inquests are presided over by coroners who are either barristers, solicitors or medical practitioners. Inquests are held in cases of violent or unnatural death, deaths in prison, deaths from industrial disease or poisoning and in other cases of death in which the coroner has discretion as whether or not to hold an inquest. A jury may or may not be called.

INR *abbrev. for* International Normalized Ratio. This is a measure of a patient's prothrombin time based on what it would be if measured using the WHO international reference reagent. The INR is used as a standard for monitoring the effects of anticoagulant treatment with WARFARIN.

insanitary unhygienic.

insanity a legal rather than a medical term, implying a disorder of the mind of such degree as to interfere with a person's ability to be legally responsible for his or her actions. The term is little used in medicine but might equate to PSYCHOSIS. A defence of insanity, in law, is governed by the McNaughten Rules. These state, in part, 'The jurors ought to be told in all cases that every man is presumed to be sane and to possess a sufficient degree of reason to be responsible for his crimes, until the contrary be proved to their satisfaction: and that to establish a defence on the grounds of insanity, it must be clearly proved that, at the time of the committing of the act, the party accused was labouring under such a defect of reason, from disease of the mind, as not to know the nature and quality of the act he was doing or, if he did know it, that he did not know he was doing what was wrong.'

insecurity the sense of concern and anxiety caused by uncertainty over any aspect of living, whether physical, social, spiritual or financial. Insecurity is believed by some psychiatrists to be a major cause of neurotic disorder, but feelings of insecurity are also often responsible for valuable creative achievement.

inseminate v. to introduce semen into the genital passage of a female whether by coitus or otherwise. Potentially to impregnate.

insensate lacking sensation, feeling or sensibility.

insensible lacking the power of feeling. Unconscious.

insertion mutation a mutation caused by the insertion into a DNA sequence of one or more nucleotides.

insidious of disease, occurring or progressing in an imperceptible manner so as to reach a harmful stage before being suspected.

insight 1 ability to appreciate the real nature of a situation.
2 awareness of the nature of one's own psychiatric symptoms with some appreciation of the possible causes or precipitating factors.

People suffering from neurotic illnesses usually have considerable insight; those with psychotic disorders are often, by definition, deemed to be lacking in insight.

in situ in a normal position. The term is used also of cancer that remains at the site of origin and has not yet spread locally or remotely.

insomnia difficulty in falling asleep or in remaining asleep for an acceptable period. Insomnia is very common and is often caused by worry, tension, depression, pain or old age. Sleep requirements vary widely from person to person and those who sleep for apparently short periods seldom, if ever, suffer any harmful effects.

insomniac a person habitually suffering INSOMNIA.

inspiration the process of breathing in. Inhaling.

inspissated thickened or condensed, as by absorption of water, boiling or evaporation.

instincts complex, unlearned, inherited fixed action patterns or stereotyped behaviour shown by all members of a species. Instinctive responses are essential for survival and the physical basis for these patterns is 'hard-wired' into the brain. Much of social activity consists in the complex interplay of instinctive responses and education.

instrument 1 a means by which something is done. An agency used to accomplish some purpose.
2 a surgical instrument.
3 a displaying or recording device.

insufflate 1 to blow into or upon.
2 to treat by blowing a drug in powder, gaseous, or vaporous form into a body cavity.

Insulatard a brand name for a slow acting INSULIN.

insulin a peptide HORMONE produced in the beta cells of the Islets of Langerhans in the PANCREAS. Insulin facilitates and accelerates the movement of glucose and amino acids across cell membranes. It also controls the activity of certain enzymes within the cells concerned with carbohydrate, fat and protein metabolism. Insulin production is regulated by constant monitoring of the blood glucose levels by the beta cells. Deficiency of insulin causes DIABETES. Insulin preparations may be in the 'soluble' form for immediate action or in a 'retard' form for prolonged action or as mixtures of these.

Most insulins for medical use are now produced by RECOMBINANT DNA methods (GENETIC ENGINEERING) and are identical to human insulin. Bovine and porcine insulins are still used. Brand names include: Neutral Insulin injections: Humalog, Actrapid, Velosulin, Humulin S, Hypurin Bovine Neutral, Hypurin Porcine Neutral, Insuman Rapid, NovoRapid and Pork Actrapid. Biphasic Insulin injections: Humalog Mix25 and Mix50, Mixtard, Humulin, Hypurin Porcine, Insuman Comb, NovoMix 30 and Pork Mixtard 30. Isophane Insulin injections: Insulatard, Humulin, Hypurin Bovine Isophane, Isuman Basal and Pork Insulatard. Insulin Zinc Suspension (Mixed): Monotard, Humulin Lente and Hypurin Bovine Lente. Insulin Zinc Suspension (Crystalline): Ultratard and Humulin Zn. Protamine Zinc Insulin injection: Hypurin Bovine PZI. Long-acting Insulin Analogue: Lantus. The prefix 'Human' was deleted from insulin products in mid-2003.

insulin glargine a basal human insulin analogue modified so as to produce peakless release and a duration of effective action in DIABETES of as long as 24 hours. A brand name is Lantus.

insulin lispro very rapidly-acting INSULIN. A brand name is Humalog.

insulinoma a rare tumour of the INSULIN-producing cells of the PANCREAS. Insulinomas can produce large quantities of insulin and lead to the dangerous condition of HYPOGLYCAEMIA.

insulin pumps automated devices that deliver an appropriate amount of insulin directly into the bloodstream or via the peritoneal cavity after monitoring the blood sugar levels. Insulin pumps can be implanted and require a battery change at intervals of 3–5 years. Various complications may arise but patients using insulin pumps enjoy better control of blood sugar, fewer hypoglycaemic episodes and do not have to give themselves injections. Most report a better quality of life. It is hoped that insulin pumps will reduce the incidence of major diabetic complications.

insulin resistance a state in which normal levels of insulin in the blood fail to produce the normal biological response. A feedback mechanism results in higher than normal levels of insulin and the blood sugar levels may be normal or raised. Insulin resistance is commonly associated with type II DIABETES (non-insulin dependent diabetes mellitus), obesity and essential HYPERTENSION. It may be exacerbated by various drugs including corticosteroids, beta blockers, and high dosage of thiazide diuretics.

insulin shock 1 HYPOGLYCAEMIA resulting from excessive insulin in the blood. 2 an outmoded treatment for psychiatric disorders in which hypoglycaemia is deliberately induced and then terminated with intravenous glucose.

insult any injury, trauma, poisoning or irritation to the body.

Intal a brand name for CHROMOGLYCATE.

Intal Synchroner a brand name for an inhaler containing CROMOGLYCATE (cromoglicate).

integrins a family of linked polypeptide chains, alpha and beta, that mediate adhesions and other interactions between cells and the extracellular matrix and between cells and other cells. Integrins are expressed on endothelial cells, leukocytes, other cells and platelets, and act as receptors for fibrinogen, fibronectin, thrombospondin, von Willebrand factor, and vitronectin. See also DISINTEGRINS.

integument any outer covering, such as the skin or the outer membrane layer of an organ or the capsule of an organism or spore. When the term is used without qualification, the skin is implied.

intellection the act or process of performing a mental act.

intellectualization a DEFENCE MECHANISM in which a personal problem is analysed in purely intellectual terms, the emotional aspects being deliberately excluded.

intelligence a group of separate, but correlated, abilities, such as memory, speed of perception of relationships, verbal skills, numerical skills and visuo-spatial perception, each of which is present to a varying degree. There is no single entity which may be described as raw, undifferentiated intelligence. The IQ (INTELLIGENCE QUOTIENT), which attempts to quantify these abilities, generally equates well with scholastic performance and with subsequent success in business or professional life, but a severe deficiency in motivation may nullify a high IQ.

intelligence quotient (IQ) a figure obtained by dividing the mental age, as assessed by various tests such as the Stanford-Binet test, by the chronological age, and multiplying the result by 100. Versions of the Stanford-Binet test include sections for every age level, from 2 to 20. These tests involve such activities as making copies of simple pictures, putting shapes in appropriate holes, stringing beads, answering questions, identifying absurdities in pictures, selecting words that have something in common, pairing off abstract shapes, predicting future terms in an arithmetical or graphical series, and so on. The IQ increases with age up to about 18 and then remains fairly static during most of adult life. People of IQ over 130 are exceptionally intelligent, and people below 70 are retarded in their ability to learn.

intemperance lack of restraint in personal indulgence in any activity, such as alcoholic consumption, likely to be harmful in excess.

intensive care the application of close and continuous monitoring of the condition of patients in a critical or unstable condition who are liable to die suddenly unless certain danger signs are detected early and appropriate action taken.

intention tremor a physical sign of disease of the CEREBELLUM or associated neural pathways, in which shakiness occurs on performing a voluntary action often of increasing excursion as the action proceeds. The tremor ceases on rest.

inter- *prefix denoting* between, among, shared or mutual.

interarticular situated between articulating joint surfaces.

interatrial between the upper chambers of the heart.

interatrial septal defect a congenital abnormal opening in the wall (septum) between the two upper chambers (atria) of the heart. One of the forms of 'hole in the heart' defect.

intercalary occurring, or interposed, between parts.

intercellular among or between cells.

interclavicular between the collar bones.

intercondylar situated between two CONDYLES.

intercostal lying between adjacent ribs, as in the case of the respiratory INTERCOSTAL MUSCLES and the intercostal arteries, veins and nerves.

intercostal muscles voluntary muscles, situated between each pair of adjacent ribs, which, on contracting, raise the rib cage upwards and outwards so as to increase the

volume of the chest and cause air to be forced in by atmospheric pressure.

intercourse 1 any form of human communication.
2 a popular term for SEXUAL INTERCOURSE, COITION or COPULATION.

intercristal between two crests.

intercurrent pertaining to any disease, especially an infectious disease, affecting a person already suffering from another disease.

interdental *adj* 1 between the teeth.
2 a consonant pronounced with the tip of the tongue between the teeth, as 'th-'.

interdigital between the fingers or the toes.

interdigitation arranged in the manner of clasped fingers.

interface a surface forming a common barrier or boundary between two objects.

interferons a considerable range of antiviral protein substances produced by cells that have been invaded by viruses. Interferons are released by such cells and provide protection to other cells liable to be invaded, not only by the original virus, but also by any other infecting organism. They also modify various cell-regulating mechanisms and slow down the growth of cancers. Alpha-interferons are derived from various white cells of the immune system; interferon beta from fibroblasts; and interferon gamma from T LYMPHOCYTES (T cells). Interferons can be produced in quantity by GENETIC ENGINEERING methods and are effective in the treatment of a variety of virus-associated conditions including Kaposi's sarcoma, the common cold, herpes simplex infections, genital warts and an uncommon form of leukaemia, hairy cell leukaemia.

interferon alfa an INTERFERON class containing at least 15 functional proteins some of which are used as drugs to treat metastatic kidney cancers, chronic myeloid leukaemia, hairy cell leukaemia, hepatitis B and C, genital warts and AIDS-related KAPOSI'S SARCOMA. Brand names are Intron A, Roferon-A, Viraferon and Wellferon.

interferon beta a INTERFERON used as a drug to reduce the severity, and frequency of relapses, of MULTIPLE SCLEROSIS. Unfortunately, there is little clear evidence that this interferon can affect the long-term outcome. In addition, it may cause an influenza-like effect for several months after starting treatment. Brand names are Avonex and Betaferon.

interferon gamma an INTERFERON used as an antiviral drug. A brand name is Immukin.

interictal pertaining to the interval between seizures in EPILEPSY.

interleukins a range of CYTOKINES secreted by white cells of the immune system. Effector cells have surface receptors for the various interleukins.

interleukin-1 a powerful polypeptide hormone produced by MACROPHAGES and fibroblasts that acts on LYMPHOCYTES to increase their ability to respond to ANTIGENS. Interleukin-1 is also responsible for resetting the temperature regulating mechanism at a higher level and thus causing fever, for the induction of the release of ACUTE PHASE PROTEINS, and for promoting the absorption of bone by OSTEOCLASTS.

interleukin-2 a peptide chemical mediator released by helper T LYMPHOCYTES that stimulates clonal T cell and B cell division and proliferation. It is known as the T cell growth factor and is responsible for the activation on natural killer T cells.

Interleukin-2 receptor antagonists IMMUNOSUPPRESSANT DRUGS used to help to prevent organ rejection after transplant. An example is daclizumab (Zenapax).

interleukin-3 a CYTOKINE produced by T cells amd MAST CELLS that promotes the growth and differentiation of blood forming cells and thegrowth of mast cells.

interleukin-4 a CYTOKINE produced by HELPER T CELLS, MAST CELLS and bone marrow that has a wide range of actions. It promotes the proliferation of B cells, T cells, MAST CELLS and blood forming cells; it induces the formation of MAJOR HISTOCOMPATIBILITY COMPLEXES on B cells; and it is believed to promote class switching in B cells from one class of antibodies to another.

interleukin-5 a CYTOKINE produced by HELPER T CELLS and MAST CELLS that assists in the proliferation of activated B cells and eosinophil cells and in the production of IgM and IgA.

interleukin-6 a CYTOKINE produced by HELPER T CELLS, MACROPHAGES, fibroblasts and MAST CELLS that promotes the growth and differentiation of B cells, T cells and blood stem cells and the induction of ACUTE PHASE PROTEINS.

interleukin-7 a CYTOKINE produced by the bone marrow stromal cells responsible for the proliferation of B cell precursors, helper and cytotoxic T cells and activated mature T cells.

interleukin-8 a CYTOKINE produced by MONOCYTES that is the substance causing CHEMOTAXIS of T cells and NEUTROPHIL polymorph phagocytes.

interleukin-9 a CYTOKINE produced by T LYMPHOCYTES (T cells) that promotes the growth and proliferation of T cells.

interleukin-10 a CYTOKINE produced by helper T cells, B cells, MACROPHAGES, and the placenta that inhibits gamma-interferon secretion and mononuclear cell inflammation.

interleukin-11 a CYTOKINE produced by bone marrow stromal cells that promotes the induction of ACUTE PHASE PROTEINS.

interleukin-12 a CYTOKINE produced by T LYMPHOCYTES that inactivates natural killer cells.

interleukin-13 a CYTOKINE produced by T LYMPHOCYTES that inhibits mononuclear cell inflammation.

interlobar situated between lobes.

intermediate-filament proteins protein elements in the cytoskeleton of diameters intermediate between those of microfilaments and microtubules. They include keratins, vimetin, desmin, peripherin, syncoilin, alpha-internexin, nestin and synemin. The gene family has at least 65 members and more than 30 diseases are related to mutations of these genes.

intermenstrual 1 occurring between menstrual periods.
2 pertaining to the interval between menstrual periods.

intermittent catheterization see CATHETERIZATION, INTERMITTENT.

intermittent claudication sudden crippling pain in the leg muscles, occurring after walking for a certain, usually relatively constant, distance. Claudication is caused by inadequacy of blood supply to the muscles usually from arterial disease such as ATHEROSCLEROSIS. From the Latin verb *claudicare*, to be lame or limping and is associated with the limping, grimacing Claudius, Emperor of Rome.

intermuscular between muscles or muscle groups. Compare INTRAMUSCULAR.

intermuscular septa fibrous connective-tissue sheets that partition muscle groups in the limbs.

intern (USA) a recent medical graduate undergoing practical training under supervision.

internal capsule a corridor within the brain

for bundles of nerve fibres, especially the motor PYRAMIDAL TRACTS descending from the motor cortex. Each internal capsule lies on the outer side of the THALAMUS and CAUDATE NUCLEUS and on the inner side of the LENTICULAR NUCLEUS. Bleeding within an internal capsule is a common cause of paralytic STROKE.

internal carotid artery one of the two main divisions of the common CAROTID ARTERY. The internal carotid supplies blood to the main part of the brain (CEREBRUM) and associated structures, including the eye.

internal fistula an abnormal passageway connecting two or more internal parts of the body. A fistula not opening on to the surface of the skin.

internal secretion any secretion absorbed directly into the blood rather than passed out on to an internal surface or to the exterior.

international medical agencies bodies concerned with the sharing of medical knowledge and cooperation in research and treatment. Among the many such agencies are the International Agency for Research on Cancer; International Bone Marrow Transplant Registry; International Commission on Radiological Protection; International Committee for the Advancement of Neuroscience and Psychiatry; International Committee of the Red Cross; International Cooperative Biodiversity Groups Program; International Fertility Research Program; International Society for Pharmacoepidemiology; International Technology Transfer; Medical Emergency Relief International; and International Union against Tuberculosis.

interneuron a nerve that connects other nerves. An internuncial neuron.

internist (USA) a physician who specializes in the study and treatment of non-surgical diseases in adults. A specialist in internal medicine.

internuncial linking two neurons.

interorbital lying between the eye sockets (ORBITS).

interphalangeal between the bones of a finger, especially the finger joints.

interphase the resting stage between mitotic cell division when chromosomes are loosely coiled and cannot be seen by light microscopy. The interphase is divided into periods designated G1, S and G2.

interpupillary between the pupils of the eyes. Situated or occurring between the pupils. The interpupillary distance must be measured when glasses are being prescribed so that the lens centring will be correct.

intersegmental reflex a spinal REFLEX arc in which the input (sensory) and output (motor) nerves are connected by tracts running within the spinal cord between different segments of the cord.

intersex a person with bodily or psychological characteristics of both man and woman. A person of ambiguous sex. See also HERMAPHRODITISM.

interspinous situated between, or joining, spinous processes of the spinal column or elsewhere.

interstices small spaces or gaps between parts of an organ or between cellular structural elements of tissues.

interstitial pertaining to, or existing in, INTERSTICES.

interstitial keratitis a corneal disorder affecting people suffering from CONGENITAL SYPHILIS or TUBERCULOSIS, in which the deep layers of the cornea are invaded by tiny blood vessels growing in from the periphery. Severe haziness, with loss of vision, results. Treatment is with antibiotics and steroids.

interstitial pulmonary fibrosis a lung disorder involving widespread deposition of fine scar tissue fibrosis. This interferes with oxygenation of the blood and with the release of carbon dioxide. The condition may be caused by long-term irritation by chemical fumes or industrial dusts, but is usually of presumed AUTOIMMUNE origin. There is breathlessness, cough, chest pain and FINGER CLUBBING and progressive deterioration. There is no specific treatment for the established condition, short of lung transplantation.

interstitial radiotherapy radiation therapy applied by implanting a radioactive source within or near the diseased tissues. Also known as brachytherapy. Compare INTRACAVITARY THERAPY.

intertrigo a DERMATITIS occurring in areas where skin surfaces come into contact with, and chafe, each other. It is a feature of obesity and occurs under the breasts, between the buttocks and between the thighs. The condition responds to loss of weight and attention to washing and to the care of the skin in the intertriginous areas.

intertrochanteric between the bony protuberances (greater and lesser trochanters) at the top of the thigh bone (femur).

interventricular foramen one of two holes (foramina) that connect the THIRD VENTRICLE of the brain to each LATERAL VENTRICLE. Also known as the foramen of Monro.

interventricular septal defect an abnormal congenital opening in the wall (septum) between the two lower chambers (ventricles) of the heart. One of the 'hole in the heart' disorders.

intervertebral situated between adjacent vertebrae, as in the case of an INTERVERTEBRAL DISC.

intervertebral disc a disc-shaped, fibrocartilage, shock-absorbing structure lying between the bodies of adjoining vertebrae in the spinal column. Each disc consists of an outer fibrous ring called the annulus fibrosus and an inner soft core called the nucleus pulposus.

intestine the part of the digestive system lying between the outlet of the stomach (the PYLORUS) and the ANUS. It consists, sequentially, of the DUODENUM, the JEJUNUM, the ILEUM, the wide, pouch-like caecum, that carries the APPENDIX, the large intestine, or COLON, the S-shaped SIGMOID colon, the RECTUM and anus.

intestinal obstruction blockage of the inner bore of the INTESTINE so that forward movement of the contents is prevented. This may occur as a congenital condition, as a result of twisting of the bowel (VOLVULUS), from STRANGULATION by swelling in a HERNIA, by a sleeve-like 'telescoping' into itself (INTUSSUSCEPTION), by impaction of hard faeces, by an internal or encircling tumour, or by a failure of the normal mechanism of PERISTALSIS by which the contents are moved along. See also ILEUS. Obstruction causes severe colicky abdominal pain, distention, constipation and often vomiting. Treatment is urgent.

intestinal tract the INTESTINE. The whole of the tubular structure of the digestive system stretching from the outlet of the stomach to the anus. Also known as the intestinal canal.

intestinal transplantation surgical insertion and connection of a donated length of small intestine as a treatment for short gut syndrome or other forms of intestinal failure or extensive intestinal tumour. The procedure is a radical alternative to intravenous feeding (total

parenteral nutrition). In most cases the liver is transplanted along with the intestine. Currently, less than half the patients who have this major procedure survive for three years but the operation is still in its infancy and improved results are to be expected with time and experience.

intima the innermost layer of a blood vessel or hollow organ.

intolerance a tendency to react adversely to stimuli of any kind or to drugs or foodstuffs.

intoxication 1 the action of a poison of any kind on an organism.
2 drunkenness or alcoholic poisoning. From the Latin *intoxicare*, meaning to smear with poison.

intra- *prefix denoting* within, inside.

intra-abdominal lying or occurring within the cavity of the ABDOMEN.

intra-arterial within an artery.

intra-articular within a joint.

intracapsular within its capsule. In an intracapsular cataract operation the whole affected CRYSTALLINE LENS, including its capsule, is removed. This method is now almost obsolete.

intracardiac within one of the chambers of the heart.

intracavernous aneurysm a local swelling (dilatation) in the part of the INTERNAL CAROTID artery that lies within the CAVERNOUS SINUS.

intracavitary therapy a form of treatment in which radioactive material or anticancer medication is placed within a cavity of the body so as to affect a tumour within the cavity, or nearby.

intracellular within a cell.

intracerebral within the brain.

intracerebral haemorrhage bleeding inside the brain, usually from a small artery predisposed by ATHEROSCLEROSIS, but sometimes from rupture of a pre-existing small ANEURYSM. Intracerebral haemorrhage causes STROKE.

intracranial within the skull.

intractable resistant to cure.

intracutaneous within the skin. Intradermal.

intracytoplasmic sperm injection a method of in vitro fertilization (IVF) in which a single SPERMATOZOON is injected directly into an ovum which is then implanted into the womb. The method, which was introduced in 1993, allows women to become pregnant by partners who may be totally sterile as a result of low sperm counts, poor sperm mobility or even AZOOSPERMIA. Anxieties that the method may result in an unacceptably high number of defective babies seem to have been exaggerated. There are indications, however, that there is an increased risk of mild delays in development at 1 year in babies produced by this method of fertilization.

intradermal within the thickness of the skin.

intraepidermal epithelioma a skin cancer confined to the EPIDERMIS of the skin, as in the case of an early SQUAMOUS CELL or BASAL CELL CARCINOMA. Carcinoma in situ.

intraepithelial within the epithelium.

intrahepatic within the liver.

intraluminal within any tubular structure. Within the lumen.

intramedullary 1 within the innermost tissue (medulla) of any organ.
2 within the bone marrow.
3 within the MEDULLA OBLONGATA.

intramural 1 within the walls of an organ.
2 within the substance of a wall.

intramuscular within a muscle. In an intramuscular injection the needle is passed deeply into the substance of a muscle before the fluid is injected.

intranasal within the nose.

intraocular within the eyeball.

intraocular lenses rigid, or flexible and folding, plastic optical lenses that are placed in the lens capsular bag after the cataractous and opaque contents have been removed either by emulsification or extrusion, and washout. Loss of the natural lens defocuses the eye markedly and additional optical power averaging 15 dioptres is required. This can readily be provided by an intraocular lens. Foldable lenses allow the whole cataract operation to be performed through a very short incision that may require no sutures.

intraocular pressure the hydrostatic pressure within the otherwise collapsible eyeball necessary to maintain its shape and allow normal optical functioning. Intraocular pressure must be adequate but not excessive as this may compress blood vessels within the eye and deprive important structures of blood. Damagingly raised pressure is called GLAUCOMA. Intraocular pressure is measured with a TONOMETER.

intraoral within the mouth.

intraorbital within an ORBIT.

intraosseous infusion the process of supplying urgently needed fluid into the marrow cavity of a bone in a life-threatening condition in which normal access to the circulation is difficult, and delaying, or impossible.

intraparietal 1 INTRAMURAL.
2 within the parietal lobe of the brain.

intrapartum occurring during childbirth (parturition).

intraperitoneal within the cavity of the PERITONEUM.

intraperitoneal dialysis solution a solution run into the peritoneal cavity, left for a time and then withdrawn. While the solution is in situ, metabolic waste products diffuse into it and can thus be removed from the body. The drug is on the WHO official list.

intraspinal block a form of regional anaesthesia in which an anaesthetic drug is injected into the spinal canal.

intrapulmonary within the substance of a lung.

intrarenal within a kidney.

intrathecal 1 within a sheath.
2 within the SUBARACHNOID SPACE.

intrathoracic within the chest (thoracic) cavity.

intratracheal within the TRACHEA.

intrauterine within the womb (uterus).

intrauterine contraceptive device (IUCD, IUD) a loop, ring, coil, T-shaped or 7-shaped body made of plastic or other material and inserted into the body of the womb in order to prevent pregnancy usually by interfering with the implantation of fertilized eggs. Each device has a fine nylon tail that protrudes through the canal of the cervix so that its presence can be confirmed and so that it can easily be removed. Some IUDs release PROGESTOGENS; others are wound with fine copper wire that releases copper ions. Copper interferes with the action of enzymes concerned with implantation. IUDs are second in effectiveness after oral contraceptives. See also CONTRACEPTION.

intravaginal 1 within the vagina.
2 within a tendon sheath.

Intraval a brand name for SODIUM THIOPENTONE (thiopental).

intravascular within a blood vessels within the lymphatics.

intravascular coagulation blood clotting abnormally within a blood vessel.

intravascular oxygenation an experimental method of raising the oxygen levels of the blood and reducing the carbon dioxide levels by means of a device, the intravenous oxygenator (IVOX), introduced into a vein. IVOC consists of a bundle of about 1000 very fine siloxane-coated polypropylene hollow fibres through which oxygen is passed. The bundle is about 50 cm long and is inserted into the largest vein in the body, the inferior vena cava.

intravascular ultrasonography the use of ultrasound imaging by means of a transducer within a blood vessel. This has become possible by the development of ultrasound probe catheters small enough to be inserted into a coronary artery and other peripheral arteries. The method produces detailed images of the interior walls of arteries and is especially useful in assessing plaque morphology and volume in cases of ATHEROSCLEROSIS. The method can also be used for STENT placement and the assessment of plaque regression during statin therapy.

intravenous 1 within a vein.
2 into a vein. Intravenous injection of a drug achieves rapid action. It also permits the giving of irritating substances because these are rapidly diluted and dispersed in the blood.

intravenous pyelography a method of X-ray visualization of the drainage systems of the kidneys and the URETERS by giving an INTRAVENOUS injection of a radio-opaque substance that is rapidly excreted in the urine. The injection is followed by a series of X rays taken at intervals. These show the shape of the internal bore of the urinary drainage channels.

intraventricular within a ventricle of the heart or brain.

intraventricular heart block an interference with the propagation of the stimulus to the heart beat occurring in the wall between the two lower chambers (ventricles) of the heart, or in the ventricular walls themselves, usually as a result of MYOCARDIAL INFARCTION.

intravesical within the urinary or other bladder.

intrinsic belonging to or situated within, the body or part of the body.

intrinsic factor a glycoprotein substance produced by the lining of the stomach (gastric mucosa) that complexes with vitamin B12 and promotes its absorption by the stomach, without itself being absorbed.

intro- *prefix denoting* into, inward or directed into.

introitus the entrance into any hollow organ or body cavity. The term is often used to refer to the entrance to the vagina.

intron a non-coding segment of a DISCONTINUOUS GENE. Introns are lengths of DNA interposed between coding segments (EXONS) in a gene and are transcribed into MESSENGER RNA but are then removed from the transcript and the exons spliced together. Introns do not contain biological information.

Intron A a brand name for INTERFERON ALFA-2b.

Intropin a brand name for DOPAMINE.

introspection examination, usually prolonged, of one's own thoughts, feelings, and sensations.

introversion 1 a physical turning in upon itself, as may occur with a hollow organ.
2 a directing of psychic energy in upon the self. See also INTROVERT.

introvert a person whose tendency of mind is to look inwards, to contemplate his or her own thoughts, feelings and emotions rather than to seek social intercourse. The introvert is often OBSESSIVE, anxious, HYPOCHONDRIACAL and solitary, more concerned with thought than with action. Compare EXTROVERT.

intubation the passage of any tube, such as a CATHETER or windpipe (tracheal) AIRWAY into any organ or tubular structure in the body. Intubation may be done to keep a passageway, such as the LARYNX, open, to withdraw a specimen for analysis, or to administer a drug.

intuition knowledge apparently acquired without either observation or reasoning. The idea, although romantically attractive, wilts in the presence of modern psychological and physiological ideas. Few experts now believe that anything can come out of the brain that has not previously gone in, in however fragmentary a form. Intuition is probably the result of the synthesis of information from partly-conscious observations.

intumescence 1 the process of swelling or becoming engorged, as in the erection of the penis.
2 the condition of being swollen.

intussusception the movement of a length of bowel into an adjacent segment in the manner of a telescope. Invagination of a bowel segment. The condition is commonest in children. Once started, intussusception rapidly progresses until the supplying blood vessels are also drawn in and become obstructed. GANGRENE may result.

Urgent surgical correction is required.

inunction the act or process of rubbing in an ointment.

in utero within the womb.

invagination a folding into or ensheathing. The process of invagination occurs in the early development of the embryo when part of the BLASTODERM folds inward so that the hollow sphere becomes cup-shaped and double-walled.

Invanz a brand name for ERTAPENEM.

invasive 1 involving entry to the body through a natural surface, usually referring to entry for diagnostic purposes.
2 having a natural tendency to spread, as of a cancer.

inversion mutation a mutation resulting from the removal of a length of DNA which is then reinserted facing in the opposite direction.

inverted nipple a breast nipple that is turned inwards, like a navel, rather than outwards. The condition, if constitutional, is inherently harmless, except that breast-feeding may be difficult, but it can often be corrected by regular pulling. A normal nipple that inverts should be investigated without delay as breast cancer may have this effect.

in vitro occurring in the laboratory rather than in the body. Literally, 'in glass'. Compare IN VIVO.

in vitro fertilization (IVF) fertilization of an egg that has been withdrawn from the body, by sperms that have been obtained by masturbation. The procedure is done by adding semen to the eggs in a glass receptacle. A successfully fertilized ovum may then be artificially implanted into the womb (uterus) so that the pregnancy may continue. Fertilization can also be achieved by intracytoplasmic sperm injection. Recently CYTOPLASM containing known mitochondrial genetic defects has been eliminated by a process in which a fertilized NUCLEUS is transferred into another ovum. Babies born from such a procedure can be said to have three parents.

in vivo occurring naturally within the body. Compare IN VITRO.

involucrum 1 a sheath or covering of a part.
2 new bone growing around a piece of dead bone (a sequestrum) usually in the condition of OSTEOMYELITIS.

involuntary muscle smooth muscle, usually within an organ or blood vessel, that contracts under the influence of unconscious processes

mediated by the AUTONOMIC nervous system rather than by the conscious will.

involution 1 decay, retrogression or shrinkage in size.
2 a return to a former state.
3 an infolding or INVAGINATION.

iodine a halogen element which, in small quantities, is an essential component of the diet. Iodine is poisonous in excess and is sometimes used in an alcoholic or aqueous potassium iodide solution as an antiseptic. The radioactive isotope, iodine 131, is extensively used for thyroid imaging and thyroid function tests. The drug is on the WHO official list.

iodo- *combining form denoting* iodine or violet.

Iodoflex a brand name for CADEXOMER IODINE.

iodoform a yellowish iodine compound, containing about 96% iodine, used as an antiseptic.

iodosorb a brand name for CADEXOMER IODINE.

iohexol a contrast medium used to assist in X-ray examination of the spinal canal, the arteries and the urinary system. The drug is on the WHO official list.

ion an electrically charged atom, group of atoms, or molecule. A positive ion is an atom that has lost an electron; a negatively charged ion is one that has gained an electron. See also IONIZATION.

ion channels protein ports in cell membranes that are specific for the passage of sodium, potassium, calcium and chloride ions in solution. Changes in the protein configuration, under the influence of various hormone molecule attachment, intracellular ion or other chemical concentration, or electrical potential, cause ion channels to open or close as required. Many diseases result from disordered function of ion channels.

ion exchange a reversible chemical reaction in which ions in a solution are replaced by others with like charge from an insoluble solid such as an ION EXCHANGE RESIN. The process is used for softening hard water, purifying sugar, separating radioactive isotopes and for other purposes.

ion exchange resins synthetic organic polymers through which fluids can be passed so as to effect ION EXCHANGE. These resins contain anionic groups neutralized by small mobile cations and it is these that are exchanged for others in the fluid. The composition of ion exchange resins is adjusted according to the particular requirement.

ionization the state of an atom or group of atoms that has become positively charged by the loss of an orbital electron, or negatively charged by gaining an electron. All body electrolytes such as sodium, potassium, calcium and magnesium become ionized in solution. Gases may be ionized by means of electrical discharges.

ionized bracelets device claimed by their manufacturers to 'balance positive and negative ions in the body' and thereby improve health. A randomized, double-blind, placebo-controlled trial on people with shoulder, neck, low back or knee pain has failed to show any difference between placebo bracelets and the genuine article.

ionizer a device that purports to alter the state of IONIZATION of the domestic atmosphere is a manner claimed to be conducive to health and well-being.

ionizing radiation radiation capable of causing ionization by breaking electron linkages in atoms and molecules. Such radiation includes alpha particles (helium nuclei), beta particles (electrons), neutrons, X-rays and gamma rays.

iontophoresis a little-used method of applying medication to the tissues in ionic form by means of electrodes to which an electric current is applied.

iopanoic acid a contrast medium used to assist in X-ray examination. A brand name is Telepaque. The drug is on the WHO official list.

Iopidine a brand name for APRACLONIDINE.

ipecacuanha a drug once widely used to promote vomiting in people known to have taken poisons. Ipecacuanha is no longer recommended. It is not believed to prevent absorption even if given early and it may increase the risk of aspiration of the poison. The drug is, however, on the WHO official list.

Ipral a brand name for TRIMETHOPRIM.

ipratropium bromide an ANTICHOLINERGIC drug used to treat asthma. The drug is on the WHO official list. Brand names are Atrovent, Ipratropium Steri-Neb, Rinatec.

Ipratropium Steri-Neb a brand name for IPRATROPIUM BROMIDE.

ipsilateral being located on, affecting or referring to, the same side of the body. HOMOLATERAL. Compare CONTRALATERAL.

IQ *abbrev. for* INTELLIGENCE QUOTIENT.

irbesartan an ANGIOTENSIN II ANTAGONIST drug used to treat high blood pressure (HYPERTENSION). Brand names are Aprovel and CoAprovel.

iridectomy surgical removal of part or all of the IRIS of the eye, for the treatment of an iris tumour or to allow free circulation of the AQUEOUS HUMOUR. The term 'peripheral iridectomy' is used to refer to the production of a small hole in the iris near the root, but this should more properly be called an iridotomy. Iridotomy is usually performed, as an outpatient procedure, with a laser.

irido- *combining form denoting* the iris of the eye.

iridocyclitis an obsolescent term for anterior UVEITIS.

iridodonesis a trembling of the iris on eye movement that occurs when it has lost the support of the crystalline lens, normally situated immediately behind it, after intracapsular cataract extraction or lens dislocation.

iridology medical diagnosis by examination of the iris of the eye and the location of 'clefts' in areas said to represent the various parts of the body. The procedure, which is roughly analogous to REFLEXOLOGY, is rejected by orthodox ophthalmologists as having no scientific or rational basis.

iridotomy a cutting into the iris.

irinotecan an anticancer drug used to treat widespread secondary cancer of the colon or rectum. A brand name is Campto.

iris the coloured diaphragm of the eye forming the real wall of the front, water-filled, chamber and lying immediately in front of the CRYSTALLINE LENS. The iris has a central opening, the pupil. It contains circular muscle fibres to constrict the pupil and radial fibres to enlarge (dilate) it.

iritis inflammation of the IRIS. See also UVEITIS.

iron an element essential for the formation of HAEMOGLOBIN. Lack of iron, or excessive loss leads to IRON-DEFICIENCY ANAEMIA. Iron is provided in a variety of chemical forms for the treatment of anaemia and is usually taken by mouth. In urgent cases, or if oral therapy fails, iron can be given by injection.

iron-deficiency anaemia ANAEMIA caused either by inadequate dietary intake of iron, poor absorption of iron or excessive loss of iron from bleeding. Most cases are due to iron losses in menstrual bleeding not being balanced by adequate intake. Often there are no symptoms, but the condition may cause tiredness, lack of energy, sore tongue, cracks at the corners of the mouth and brittle finger nails. Treatment with supplementary iron is effective.

iron dextran an iron hydroxide dextran complex given by injection to treat iron deficiency anaemia in adults who have shown intolerance to oral iron preparations. The drug is on the WHO official list.

iron lung a now obsolete device used to maintain breathing in patients with paralysis of respiration. It consisted of a coffin-like metal box in which the patient lay with only the head protruding, and with an air-tight seal around the neck. Air was pumped in and out of the box at the normal breathing rate, causing the patient's chest to expand and collapse. The iron lung has long been replaced by much more portable and less restricting positive pressure pumping equipment.

iron polysaccharide complex a form of iron used to treat iron deficiency anaemia in premature babies. A brand name is Niferex.

irradiation exposure to any form of ionizing or other radiation either for purposes of treatment, as in radiotherapy, or to sterilize medical or surgical material and instruments.

irreducible incapable of being replaced or restored to a former state, as in the case of a HERNIA or a fracture. Irreversible.

irremediable not able to be remedied or cured.

irrigation the act of flushing with water or some other solution, especially of a wound or body cavity.

irritability 1 the state of being normally excitable or able to respond to a stimulus. 2 the state of abnormal excitability featuring an exaggerated response to a small stimulus.

irritable bowel syndrome a persistent disorder of unknown cause characterized by recurrent abdominal pain, abdominal rumblings (borborygmi), excessive gas production, urgency to empty the bowels and intermittent diarrhoea often alternating with constipation. It most commonly affects women between 20 and 40 especially those of an anxious disposition. After full investigation and reassurance the symptoms will often settle on simple treatment. There is no consensus of opinion and no hard evidence as to the cause of this common disorder. Also known as spastic colon, mucous colitis, colonic spasm or nervous diarrhoea.

irritable colon see IRRITABLE BOWEL SYNDROME.

ISAAC *acronym for* International Study of Asthma and Allergies in Childhood. The study reported its findings, in over 400,000 children in 56 countries, in April, 1998.

ISABEL an advanced Internet artificial intelligence computer program for the differential diagnosis of children's disorders available for doctors to use free of charge. ISABEL is a charity at http://www.isabel.org.uk. It was founded by the stockbroker Jason Maude after his three-year-old daughter Isabel nearly died from toxic shock and necrotizing fasciitis when doctors were slow to recognize these complications of chickenpox. The charity is currently working on the extension of the scheme to adult patients.

ischaemia inadequate flow of blood to any part of the body. It is a serious disorder usually due to narrowing, from disease, of the supplying arteries. It accounts for a high proportion of serious ill-health in the Western World and is the basis of conditions such as ANGINA PECTORIS, CORONARY THROMBOSIS, STROKE and INTERMITTENT CLAUDICATION.

ischaemic necrosis local tissue death (GANGRENE) due to an inadequate blood supply.

ischaemic neuropathy a nerve disorder due to inadequate blood supply and featuring tingling, numbness and pain and sometimes loss of motor function.

ischaemic tolerance the transient protection against the grave effects of severe and sustained reduction in cerebral blood supply afforded by a period of a few minutes of local or global sublethal cerebral ISCHAEMIA.

ischium the lowest of three bones into which the innominate bone, comprising one side of the pelvis, is divided. The ischial tuberosities are the bony prominences on which we normally sit.

Isib 60XL a brand name for ISOSOBIDE MONONITRATE.

islet cell antibodies autoantibodies to the cytoplasm of the insulin-producing beta cells of the islets of Langerhans in the pancreas. Autoimmune damage to the beta cells is the main cause of DIABETES, and the presence of these antibodies and of antibodies to glutamic acid decarboxylase (which are markers of autoimmune beta cell damage) can be a predictor of diabetes.

Islets of Langerhans INSULIN secreting collections of cells lying in the INTERSTITIAL tissue of the PANCREAS. (Paul Langerhans, 1847–1888, German medical student, later anatomy professor).

islet transplantation, an alternative to pancreatic transplantation in patients whose conventional diabetic control is threateningly poor and whose risk of diabetic complications and shortening of life is considered high. A lesser degree of immunosuppression is required than pancreas transplantation and the surgery is minor. Purified ISLETS OF LANGERHANS are digested from a donor pancreas and are infused through a catheter passed through the liver into the portal vein from whence the islets pass into the sinusoids of the liver. The method is still considered experimental.

Ismo a brand name for ISOSOBIDE MONONITRATE.

iso- *combining form denoting* equal or equivalent.

Iso-Autohaler a brand name for ISOPRENALINE in an inhaler.

isocarboxazid a monoamine oxidase inhibitor (MAOI) antidepressant drug.

isochromosome an abnormal chromosome formed when, during the ANAPHASE of cell division, the CENTROMERE divides horizontally rather than longitudinally, thus producing a chromosome with two long arms and one with two short arms.

Isogel a brand name for ISPHAGULA.

isogenic pertaining to individuals who are genetically alike, such as identical twins or closely inbred animals. Isogenic individuals are ideal donors to each other of organs for transplantation.

isograft transplantation of tissue or an organ from one ISOGENIC person to another.

isoimmune of immune disease in which the ANTIBODIES are produced as a result of ANTIGENS from another person. An example is HAEMOLYTIC DISEASE OF THE NEW-BORN. Compare AUTOIMMUNE in which the antigens come from the same person.

Isoket a brand name for ISOSORBIDE DINITRATE.

isolation the state of separation from other people of a person suffering from an infectious disease, or carrying infective organisms, so as to prevent spread of infection. Isolation is also

used to protect immunocompromised people from organisms carried by healthy people (reverse barrier nursing).

isoleucine an essential AMINO ACID.

isomer a chemical compound having the same number of each type of atom (same percentage composition and molecular weight) as another compound, but having different chemical or physical properties.

isometheptene a SYMPATHOMIMETIC drug used to treat MIGRAINE. A brand name of a preparation with paracetamol is Midrid.

isometric 1 of equal dimensions or length. 2 of muscular contraction, in which an increase in tension occurs without shortening.

isometric exercises muscular exercises in which muscle groups are pitted against each other so that strong contraction occurs without movement.

isoniazid a drug used in the treatment of TUBERCULOSIS. The drug occasionally produces side effects such as skin rash and fever, and rarely nerve involvement. The drug is on the WHO official list. Brand names of preparations in combination with other drugs are Rifater, Rifinah and Rimactazid.

isonicotinic acid derivatives drugs used to treat TUBERCULOSIS. Examples are isoniazid and rifampicin. These are used in combination.

Isophane Hypurin a brand name for ISOPHANE INSULIN.

isophane insulin a form of insulin modified by adsorption on to a protein molecule protamine so as to act for up to about 12 hours with delayed onset of action. Brand names are Humulin I, Hypurin Bovine Isophane, Hypurin Porcine Isophane and Hypurin Porcine Biphasic Isophane.

isoprenaline an ADRENALINE-like drug given by injection to treat surgical SHOCK and HEART BLOCK. The drug is on the WHO official list. A brand name is Saventrine.

Isopto Carpine a brand name for PILOCARPINE eye drops in HYPROMELLOSE.

Isopto Tears a brand name for artificial tears containing HYPROMELLOSE.

isosorbide dinitrate a drug used to prevent or relieve ANGINA PECTORIS and to treat HEART FAILURE. The drug is on the WHO official list. Brand names are Angitak, Cedocard Retard, Isoket and Isotek Retard.

isosorbide mononitrate a drug used to treat

ANGINA PECTORIS and HEART FAILURE. Brand
names are Elantan, Imdur, Isib 60XL, Ismo,
MCR-50, Monit, Mono-Cedocard and
Monomax SR.

isosporiasis an infection with the protozoal
parasite *Isospora belli* usually acquired by
ingestion of egg cysts in water or food
contaminated with human faeces. The
condition most commonly affects people with
AIDS, and 15% of AIDS sufferers in Haiti are said
to be affected. Isosporiasis causes abdominal
colic, watery diarrhoea, fatty stools from
malabsorption and dehydration, and is
effectively treated with a combination of
trimethoprim and sulphamethoxazole.

Isotard XL a brand name for ISOSORBIDE
MONONITRATE.

isotonic of a fluid that exerts the same OSMOTIC
PRESSURE as another, especially as that of the
body fluids. Body cells, such as red blood cells,
can be immersed in an isotonic solution
without being caused to change shape. 'Normal'
saline is isotonic with blood.

isotope chemically identical elements whose
atomic nuclei have the same number of protons
but different numbers of neutrons. The number
of protons determines the number of orbital
electrons and hence the chemical properties.
Radioactive isotopes are called radionuclides.
From the Greek *iso-*, equal and *topos*, place.
Isotopes occupy the same place in the Periodic
table of the elements.

isotope scanning the use of radioactive
elements incorporated in molecules of
substances that can safely be introduced into
the body, or into certain blood cells, and which
tend to concentrate in particular organs, parts
or diseased areas, such as tumours. The GAMMA
CAMERA can then be used to measure the local
uptake of these substances or to identify local
concentrations.

isotretinoin a RETINOID drug used to treat
ACNE. The oral preparation is used under
strictly controlled conditions to exclude
pregnancy because of the known risks to the
fetus. Brand names are Roaccutane, and, for
external use Isotrex and Isotrexin.

Isotrex a brand name for ISOTRETINOIN
formulated for external use.

Isotrexin a brand name for ISOTRETINOIN and
ERYTHROMYCIN formulated for external use.

islet transplantation an alternative to

pancreatic transplantation in patients whose
conventional diabetic control is threateningly
poor and whose risk of diabetic complications
and shortening of life is considered high. A
lesser degree of immunosuppression is required
than panceras transplantation and the surgery
is minor. Purified ISLETS OF LANGERHANS are
digested from a donor pancreas and are infused
through a catheter passed through the liver into
the portal vein from whence the islets pass into
the sinusoids of the liver. The method is still
considered experimental.

ispaghula a mucilaginous plant that swells in
water to provide bulk in the intestine and
promote movement of the contents. Ispaghula
is used to treat constipation. Brand names are
Fybogel, Fybozest, Konsyl and Regulan.

isradipine a calcium channel blocking drug
used to treat high blood pressure
(HYPERTENSION). A brand name is Prescal.

Istin a brand name for AMLODIPINE.

itching a tickling or irritating sensation causing
a desire to rub or scratch. Itching is caused by
the stimulation of certain nerve-endings in the
skin, probably by certain enzymes called
endopeptidases. Severe itching is called
PRURITUS. See also FORMICATION.

-itis *suffix denoting* inflammation of.

ito cell one of numerous star-shaped cells lying
in the spaces between the main liver cells
(hepatocytes) and the blood channels (sinusoids)
that store vitamin A.

itraconazole a triazole antifungal drug use
to treat thrush and other fungal infections.
A brand name is Sporanox.

IUCD, IUD *abbrev. for* INTRAUTERINE
(CONTRACEPTIVE) DEVICE.

IUS abbrev. for intrauterine system. The term
refers to a hormonal contraceptive coil, such as
MIRENA, that carries a supply of progestogen,
which is released in small amounts over a
period of three to five years.

IVC *abbrev. for* inferior vena cava, the largest
vein in the body.

ivermectin a drug used to kill MICROFILARIA in
the treatment of ONCHOCERCIASIS and other
microfilarial diseases. Ivermectin has also been
used to treat severe SCABIES in elderly
institutionalized people, but an unusually high
death-rate in this group cast doubt on the safety
of the application. The drug is on the WHO
official list.

IVP *abbrev. for* intravenous PYELOGRAPHY.

IVU *abbrev. for* intravenous UROGRAPHY. This is the same as IVP.

ixodidae a family of ticks, some of which are capable of taking considerable quantities of blood and causing bite infections. Other can transmit diseases such as the allergic tick-bite fever, tick paralysis, tick-borne typhus, Q FEVER and TULARAEMIA.

j

Jaccoud's arthritis a form of arthritis secondary to long-standing SYSTEMIC LUPUS ERYTHEMATOSUS that features tendon contractures and joint deformity but without X-ray indications of joint erosion. (S. Jaccoud, 1839–1913, French professor of internal pathology).

jackscrew a dental device used to pull together or push apart teeth or jaw fragments.

Jacksonian epilepsy a type of epilepsy arising from a definite focus in the brain, usually in the MOTOR CORTEX, and showing a progressive spread of effects as the abnormal brain excitation spreads over the surface. (John Hughlings Jackson, 1835–1911, English neurologist).

Jacquemier's sign blueness of the vaginal lining due to increased blood flow, suggesting pregnancy. This is not, in itself, a reliable sign of pregnancy. (Jean Marie Jacquemier, 1806–79, French obstetrician).

jactitation 1 the extreme restlessness and tossing of delirium.
2 sudden, irregular jerking or twitching. From the Latin *jactitare*, to throw out or to make a display.

Jakob-Creutzfeldt disease see CREUTZFELDT-JAKOB DISEASE.

jamais vu a strong sense that one has never before seen what is currently being perceived, although logic contradicts it. There is also a sense of unreality and DEPERSONALIZATION. Jamais vu may be a feature of temporal lobe EPILEPSY but also sometimes occurs in severe anxiety (phobic) disorders.

Jamaica vomiting sickness see ACKEE POISONING.

Japanese B encephalitis a brain inflammation caused by an ARBOVIRUS transmitted by *culicine* mosquitoes. The disease occurs mainly in South-east Asia but is spreading into India and can cause major epidemics with a high mortality rate. There is headache, stiff neck, fever, vomiting, tremors, muscle twitching, coma and death in 15% to 40% of cases. There is no specific treatment but an effective vaccine has been developed.

jargon 1 technical or specialized language used in an inappropriate context to display status or exclusiveness.
2 the formulation of fluent but meaningless chatter by combining unrelated syllables or words. Jargon is sometimes a feature of APHASIA.

Jarisch-Herxheimer reaction a sudden acute feverish reaction, often associated with a flare-up of a skin rash, sometimes occurring within hours of beginning treatment of SYPHILIS, LEPTOSPIROSIS or RELAPSING FEVER with penicillin. The reaction is thought to be caused by allergy to some of the products of destroyed spirochaetes. (Adolf Jarisch, 1850–1902, Austrian dermatologist; and Karl Herxheimer, 1861–1944, German dermatologist).

Jarvik artificial heart a pioneering but unsuccessful mechanical heart prosthesis that failed largely because of its uncontrollable tendency to throw off blood clots that were then carried to the brain and caused STROKES. (Robert Jarvik, American biomedical engineer, b. 1946).

jaundice yellowing of the skin and of the whites of the eyes (scleras) from deposition of the natural pigment, bilirubin, that is released when HAEMOGLOBIN is broken down. Bilirubin is normally excreted in the bile but cannot do so in certain liver diseases and in obstruction to the outflow of bile into the intestine. In such cases it accumulates in the blood causing jaundice.

jaw 1 the mandible, the U-shaped bone that articulates with the base of the skull high up in front of the ears. In biting and chewing (mastication) the mandible is pulled upwards by powerful muscles running down from the base and temples (temporal bones) of the skull. **2** the MAXILLA, or upper jaw.

jaw winking an inherited condition, also known as the Marcus Gunn syndrome, in which there is a drooping eyelid (ptosis) that retracts suddenly and momentarily when the mouth is opened wide or the jaw is moved firmly to one side. In some cases, the same stimulus causes a normal eye to close tightly. The condition is caused by an abnormal distribution of twigs of the motor nerves of the facial and jaw muscles. (R. Marcus Gunn, 1850–1909, Scottish ophthalmologist).

jaw wiring the securing of the jaws in a proper relationship by means of malleable wire bound round the necks of the teeth. This is commonly done to splint single or multiple fractures of either jaw and is sometimes done to limit food intake in the treatment of severe obesity. Weight loss is rapid but old habits usually prevail when the wiring is removed.

jazz ballet bottom development of an abscess in the region of the cleft between the buttocks in people who engage in a form of jazz dancing in which the full weight is repeatedly taken on this region of the body. A collection of blood (haematoma) occurs and this becomes infected to produce an abscess.

JCC *abbrev. for* Joint Committee on Contraception.

JCHMT *abbrev. for* Joint Committee for Higher Medical Training.

JCPTGP *abbrev. for* Joint Committee on Postgraduate Training in General Practice.

jealousy in childhood syndrome emotional disturbance resulting from competition between siblings or occasioned by the arrival of a new baby. The condition features regression to more childish behaviour, temper tantrums, bedwetting or manifest anxiety and is managed by scrupulous parental fairness.

jeep disease cyst-like cavities, containing a quantity of hair, occurring in the skin of the cleft between the buttocks. These cysts have

narrow openings to the exterior. Abscess formation is common. The condition is believed to be either a form of PILONIDAL SINUS or a form of DERMOID CYST.

Jehovah's Witnesses a widespread religious group who interpret certain passages in the bible, which they take as a literal record of God's word, as a prohibition of blood transfusion. Many have died after refusing critically needed medical treatment. Most doctors respect this view except when it is applied to young children.

jejunal pertaining to the JEJUNUM.

jejunal biopsy taking a small sample of the lining of part of the small intestine for microscopic examination. This is an important investigation in cases of MALABSORPTION. The biopsy is obtained by means of a small, spring-loaded device called a Crosby capsule that is swallowed suspended from a string and triggered when in place. In some forms of malabsorption there is a characteristic atrophy or absence of the small finger-like processes (villi) through which absorption occurs.

jejunoplasty surgical repair or alteration of the first part of the small intestine (JEJUNUM).

jejunostomy a surgical procedure in which an opening is cut in the JEJUNUM and the upper end brought out through the wall of the ABDOMEN so that the bowel contents can discharge to the exterior.

jejunum the length of small intestine lying between the DUODENUM and the ILEUM and occupying the central part of the ABDOMEN. Much of the enzymatic digestion of food, and most of the absorption, takes place in the jejunum. Absorption occurs through the thin walls of millions of tiny finger-like processes on the lining, called villi.

Jekyll and Hyde disorder an uncommon schizophrenic-like illness featuring alternating periods of social conformity and strongly antisocial behaviour.

jellyfish stings injection of highly irritating substances from the stinging capsules (nematocysts) of jellyfish. Most jellyfish stings are almost harmless but certain species, such as the box jellyfish *Chironex fleckeri* of the Pacific and Indian oceans, can cause severe reactions and even paralysis of breathing. An antivenom is available.

Jelonet a proprietary dressing for wounds and

burns consisting of an open gauze mesh impregnated with a soft paraffin base. This type of dressing is also known as Vaseline gauze and some similar preparations also incorporate antibiotics.

Jennerian vaccination the original method of protection against the now non-existent disease of SMALLPOX originated by Jenner. Jenner's contribution marked the real beginning of the science of IMMUNOLOGY. (Edward Jenner, 1749–1823, English physician).

jerk 1 a sudden involuntary movement, usually of the head or a limb.
2 a reflex muscle or muscle group contraction in response to a sudden stretching by briskly tapping the tendon. A tendon reflex.

jet lag a loss of synchronization between the local time and the internal body rhythms as a result of rapid long-distance easterly or, to a lesser extent, westerly air travel. Sleep is disturbed, digestion and bowel habit affected, memory and mental efficiency impaired and there is a persistent sense of fatigue. The pineal gland hormone, melatonin, is believed to control some of the biorhythms and has been used experimentally in attempts to prevent jet lag.

JHMO *abbrev. for* Junior Hospital Medical Officer.

jigger flea see CHIGOE.

Jocasta's crime see INCEST.

jogger's heel any disorder of the heel, such as blistering, strain of the Achilles tendon, or persistent bony tenderness, that can be attributed to jogging.

jogger's nipple painful inflammation of the nipple caused by constant rubbing against a garment in the course of recreational running.

jogging slow running conducted within the limits of the subject's ability to supply oxygen to the muscles for an indefinite period. Regular jogging increases the capacity for exertion, lowers blood pressure, improves the function and performance of the heart and may diminish the progress of arterial disease. Beginners should build up distance very gradually and should be equipped with suitable footwear.

joints junctions between bones whether or not obvious movement is possible. There are three types – fibrous, cartilaginous, and synovial. Fibrous joints, such as those between the bones of the vault of the skull (CRANIUM) allow little or no movement. Cartilaginous joints, such as

those between the ribs and the breast-bone (sternum), allow limited movement. Synovial joints, such as the shoulder, elbow, hip and knee joints, are freely movable and have lubricated bearing surfaces. Synovial joints are enclosed in capsules and are reinforced by internal and external ligaments. The range of movement varies with the construction of the joint.

joint-break fever see O'NYONG-NYONG FEVER.

joule a unit of work, energy and heat. A watt-second. The joule is being used increasingly to replace the CALORIE in nutritional contexts. The calorie is equal to 4.187 J. (James Prescott Joule, 1818–89, English physicist).

jugular pertaining to the throat or neck.

jugular veins the six main veins – the right and left internal and external jugulars and the front anterior jugulars – that run down the front and side of the neck, carrying blood back to the heart from the head. The internal jugulars are very large trunks containing blood at low pressure. The external and anterior jugulars are much smaller.

jugular venous pulse the visible movement of the skin caused by movement of blood in an internal jugular vein when the subject reclines with the neck at 45. Examination of the pulse can provide information about the function of the right side of the heart. See also HEPATOJUGULAR REFLUX.

jumping genes see TRANSPOSONS.

junctional at the interface between two structures.

junctional naevus a flat or slightly raised, brown, hairless skin mole arising from pigment cells lying at the junction between the EPIDERMIS and the underlying true skin (CORIUM). Junctional naevi occur on any part of the skin. All coloured moles on the palms and soles are junctional naevi. About half of all MALIGNANT MELANOMAS arise from junctional naevi, but such malignant change is rare. Any alteration in the appearance of a pigmented mole should be reported at once.

Jungian theory a body of psychoanalytic theory offered as an alternative to Freud's with its central emphasis on sex. Carl Gustav Jung (1875–1961) defined 'libido', more widely, as a general creative life force that could find a variety of outlets. He identified EXTRAVERSION and INTROVERSION and suggested that people could be divided into four categories by their primary interests – the intellect, the emotions, intuition and the sensations. Like Freud, Jung was deeply concerned with symbols which he considered central to the understanding of human nature. He postulated the existence of a layered unconscious psyche, both personal and collective, the latter being common to all humankind. He proposed the concept of 'archetypes' – inherent tendencies to experience and symbolize universal human situations in distinctively human ways. Never very scientific, Jung later in life moved even further into the airy realms of metaphysical speculation about which no scientific comment is possible. Compare FREUDIAN THEORY.

Junifen a brand name for IBUPROFEN.

junk food a popular term for highly refined and processed, readily assimilable and palatable food with a low level of roughage. Junk food has a high calorific value but is often low in vitamins and minerals and usually has a high content of saturated fats. Junk food encourages excessive intake and commonly leads to obesity. The full extent of the dangers of an largely junk food diet has not been established but few experts deny that the dangers exist.

junkie *or* **junky** a slang term for a narcotic, especially heroin, addict.

jurisprudence the science of law. Medical jurisprudence is another term for FORENSIC MEDICINE.

jury-mast an upright bar incorporated into a Plaster of Paris jacket and used as a head support in the treatment of spinal disease.

juvenile angiofibroma a rare benign tumour occurring at the back of the nasal cavity affecting male adolescents almost exclusively. The tumour is probably a form of vascular malformation and consists of irregular vascular endothelial-lined spaces embedded in a fibrous stroma. Its blood supply is derived from the sphenopalatine artery and sometimes also from the internal carotid artery.

juvenile delinquency criminal behaviour by a young person. Juvenile delinquency has a peak incidence around fifteen or sixteen years of age and is commonly associated with peer pressures to conform, parental neglect and lack of social opportunity to direct energy into more acceptable channels. There is often a poor school record, with truancy and resentment of authority. Most delinquents eventually learn to conform to generally acceptable patterns of behaviour.

juvenile rheumatoid arthritis see STILL'S DISEASE.

juxta- *combining form denoting* near to or alongside.

juxta-articular adjacent to a joint.

juxtaglomerular situated near to a kidney GLOMERULUS.

juxtamedullary situated in the CORTEX of the kidney near to the MEDULLA.

juxtapapillary near the head of the optic nerve (the optic disc) on the RETINA.

juxtaposition in apposition or side-by-side.

K the symbol for potassium; for temperature in the absolute scale; for kilo- as applied to many other units; and for the weight of large molecules in KILODALTONS.

Kabikinase a brand name for STREPTOKINASE.

kala azar one of the forms of LEISHMANIASIS, caused by *Leishmania* organisms and spread by the bite of sandflies. Kala azar occurs mainly in the Mediterranean area and in India, but is spreading westward into Europe. There is fever, anaemia, lymph node swelling, enlargement of the spleen and liver, damage to the bone marrow, malnutrition and loss of immune capacity (immunosuppression). The condition can be diagnosed by the ELISA test and is treated with drugs containing antimony. Also known as visceral leishmaniasis.

Kallmann's syndrome absence of the sense of smell associated with a deficiency of the hormone from the HYPOTHALAMUS that prompts the PITUITARY GLAND to secrete a sex gland stimulating hormone (gonadotrophic releasing hormone). (Franz Josef Kallman, 1897–1965, German-born American geneticist and psychiatrist).

Kalspare a brand name for TRIAMTERENE in combination with another diuretic drug chlorthalidone.

Kalten a brand name for HYDROCHLOROTHIAZIDE formulated with AMILORIDE and the BETA BLOCKER drug ATENOLOL.

Kaltostat a brand name for a dressing impregnated with CALCIUM ALGINATE.

Kamillosan a brand name for CHAMOMILE.

kanamycin a broad spectrum aminoglycoside ANTIBIOTIC derived from a oil actinomycete. Kanamycin is active against GRAM NEGATIVE organisms but is now largely replaced by gentamicin. The aminoglycosides can cause deafness, TINNITUS and kidney damage. The drug is on the WHO official list. A brand name is Kannasyn.

kangaroo mother method a method of care for small babies in the first few months of life involving frequent breast feeding, maximal skin-to-skin contact of mother and baby, and early discharge from the maternity unit. The method implies careful selection after detailed examination.

Kaofort a brand name for KAOLIN and CODEINE.

kaolin a fine clay powder used as a suspension in the treatment of DIARRHOEA and sometimes as a thick paste POULTICE to apply local heat. The term is derived from the name of the Chinese province where it was first obtained.

Kaposi's sarcoma a slow-growing tumour of irregularly-shaped, round capillary, and slit-like endothelial-lined vascular spaces and spindle-shaped cells with mononuclear cell infiltrates. The lesions appears on the skin as multiple, firm, bluish-brown nodules scattered about, especially on the limbs. Before 1981 the condition was so rare as to deserve only a bare mention in medical textbooks. It is now familiar to the lay person and feared by people infected with HIV. 18% of people with AIDS develop Kaposi's sarcoma and in these cases it often spreads to affect the internal organs, especially the lymphatic and digestive systems. In spite of this, AIDS patients showing only Kaposi's sarcoma usually live longer than those presenting with OPPORTUNISTIC INFECTIONS. It is treated with anticancer drugs such as vinblastin, adriamycin, bleomycin, vincristine and dacarbazine. (Moricz Kohn Kaposi, 1837–1902, Austrian dermatologist).

kappa the tenth letter of the Greek alphabet, sometimes used to denote the tenth in a series.

Kartagener's syndrome the combination of congenital malfunction of the brush borders of the respiratory hair cells (cilia) with BRONCHIECTASIS, SINUSITIS and reversal (transposition) of the internal organs of the body. (Manes Kartagener, Swiss physician, b. 1897).

karyapsis see KARYOGAMY.

karyo- or **caryo-** *combining form denoting* a cell nucleus. From the Greek *karuon*, a nut.

karyocyte a nucleated cell.

karyogamy the coming together and fusing of the nuclei of GAMETES.

karyogenesis the formation of a cell nucleus.

karyokinesis MITOSIS.

karyolysis destruction of a cell nucleus.

karyon the cell nucleus.

karyolymph the fluid in the nucleus of a cell.

karyomegaly an increase in the size of the nuclei of the cells of a tissue.

karyoplasm the PROTOPLASM of the cell nucleus. Nucleoplasm.

karyorrhexis fragmentation of the nucleus of a cell as seen in a dead cell.

karyosome a spherical mass of aggregated CHROMATIN material in a resting (interphase) nucleus.

karyotype 1 the individual chromosomal complement of a person or species. The GENOME.

2 the CHROMOSOMES of an individual set out in a standard pattern and obtained from a photomicrograph taken in METAPHASE that has been edited with software so that the separate chromosomes are arranged in numerical order. This is done for the diagnosis of chromosomal disorders, as in prenatal detection of fetal abnormality.

katabolism see CATABOLISM.

katal a unit of enzyme activity in the SI system. 1 international unit is equal to 16.6 nanokatal.

Katayama syndrome a set of allergic phenomena associated with the penetration of the skin and invasion of the body by the larval stage (CERCARIAE) of SCHISTOSOMIASIS. The effects include local itching, URTICARIA, fever, headache, muscle aches, abdominal pain, cough, patchy pneumonia and enlargement of the SPLEEN. (Kunika Katayama, 1856–1931, Japanese physician)

Katayama fever a manifestation of acute SCHISTOSOMIASIS believed to be an immune complex response to eggs laid by maturing schistosomes. Four to six weeks after a schistosomal infection there is fever, enlarged liver and spleen, an urticarial rash and an asthma-like bronchospasm. The diagnosis is important because lack of treatment may lead to severe and permanent neurological damage.

Kawasaki disease a world-wide disease of infants and young children that causes fever, swollen lymph nodes, a measles-like rash, red eyes, inflamed tongue, dry cracking lips, peeling skin and, in just under half the cases, local widening (ANEURYSMS) in the CORONARY arteries. These are usually transient but 10% have long-term involvement of the coronaries. The disease is probably a retrovirus infection possibly spread by house-dust mites or cat fleas. Aspirin has been found useful in the treatment and appears to reduce the incidence of heart complications. Less than 1% of affected children die from the disease and most make a complete recovery. The condition was first recognized in 1967 by the Japanese paediatrician Dr Tomisaku, in the port of Kawasaki.

Kay-Cee-L a brand name for POTASSIUM (KCl).

Kayser-Fleischer ring a golden-yellow coloured ring seen near the edge of the corneas on examination with a SLIT-LAMP MICROSCOPE in WILSON'S DISEASE. The ring is due to deposition of copper. (Bernhard Kayser, 1869–1954, German ophthalmologist; and Richard Fleischer, 1848–1909, German physician).

kb *abbrev. for* kilobase (1000 base pairs of DNA or RNA). This is a convenient measure of the length of a gene or other segment of nucleic acid.

KB-141 a synthetic form of thyroid hormone that stimulates the receptors that mainly increase the metabolic rate and lower LOW-DENSITY LIPOPROTEINS without increasing the heart rate. KB-141 has been shown to be effective in substantially reducing the weight of monkeys on a fixed diet.

K cells see KILLER CELLS.

Kearns-Sayre syndrome (KSS) a syndrome caused by major rearrangements of, and often large deletions from, the MITOCHONDRIAL DNA. The condition features paralysis of the eye-moving muscles with double vision; drooping eyelids; degeneration of the retinas; defects in the conducting muscle tissue of the heart; respiratory distress; and in some cases staggering walk, deafness and DIABETES.

Kefadim a brand name for CEFTAZIDIME.

Kefadol a brand name for CEFAMANDOLE.

Keflex a brand name for CEPHALEXIN (cefalexin).

Keftid a brand name for CEFACLOR.

Kefzol a brand name for CEPHAZOLIN (cefazolin).

Kegel exercises exercises designed to strengthen and rehabilitate the pelvic-floor muscles of those suffering stress incontinence.

Kell blood group system a family of red blood cell ANTIGENS designated as the ALLOTYPES KK, Kk, kk and K-k-, believed to be on the short arm of chromosome 2. Antibodies to the K-antigen occur in about 10% of people in England and can cause red cell breakdown (haemolytic) transfusion reactions. The group system is next in importance to the ABO and rhesus systems and is named after a woman whose serum contained the antibodies.

Keller's operation a surgical treatment for HALLUX VALGUS or HALLUX RIGIDUS, in which the near (proximal) half of the nearer toe bone is removed together with any bony outgrowth (exostosis) and a false join allowed to form. (Colonel William Lordan Keller, 1874–1959, American surgeon).

keloid an abnormal healing response causing scars that are markedly overgrown, thickened and disfiguring. Keloids are commoner in black people than in white and may follow any injury or surgical incision. Surgical removal of keloids is followed by even more extensive keloid formation but they can be helped by injection of corticosteroid drugs. Untreated keloids eventually flatten.

keloid acne a persistent (chronic) inflammation of the hair follicles, especially on the back of the neck, that produces hard reddish or white KELOID-like scars.

keloidosis having multiple keloids.

Kemadrin a brand name for PROCYCLIDINE.

Kemicetin a brand name for CHLOROMYCETIN.

Kenalog a brand name for TRIAMCINOLONE.

Kennedy's syndrome see FOSTER-KENNEDY SYNDROME.

kenophobia cenophobia. Abnormal fear of large, empty spaces. This is not quite the same as AGORAPHOBIA.

kerat-, kerato- *combining form denoting* CORNEA or horny KERATOSIS. From the Greek *keras* horn.

keratectasia bulging of the CORNEA due to weakening from thinning or softening (KERATOMALACIA). In keratectasia there is a danger of rupture under the influence of the normal intraocular pressure and urgent measures are needed to avoid this. Sometimes a 'bandage' contact lens is used; more often a corneal graft is performed.

keratectomy surgical removal of part, or rarely all, of the CORNEA.

keratin a hard protein (scleroprotein) of cylindrical, helical molecular form occurring in horny tissue such as hair and nails and in the outer layers of the skin. Hair and nails consist almost wholly of keratin. Keratins are insoluble and cannot generally be split by PROTEOLYTIC enzymes.

keratinization the formation of, or conversion into, keratin. This normally occurs to a limited degree in the outer layers of the skin, but is especially prominent when skin is exposed to constant localized pressure. Corns and callosities are areas of keratinization. Also known as cornification or hornification.

keratitis inflammation of the outer lens of the eye (the CORNEA). This implies a prior invasion of the cornea with blood vessels (vascularization). Keratitis commonly follows inadequately or incorrectly treated infections with cold sore (Herpes simplex) viruses and is also a feature of TRACHOMA and congenital SYPHILIS. There is pain, watering and acute sensitivity to light. Vision is severely affected if the centre of the cornea is involved. See also KERATOCONJUNCTIVITIS.

keratoacanthoma a wart-like growth, usually occurring on the face in elderly people, that rapidly increases in size over the course of two months until it is about a centimetre in diameter, hemispherical and with a central white horny plug. If left alone for a month or two, the keratoacanthoma begins to get smaller and eventually disappears leaving a depressed scar. Doubt as to diagnosis, however, often dictates removal for examination.

keratochromatosis discoloration of the CORNEA.

keratocoele a small, blister-like bulge on the CORNEA at a point at which local weakness, as from injury or incision, allows the inner, elastic membrane, Descemet's membrane, to balloon through. Also known as a descemetocoele. (Jean Descemet, 1732–1810, French professor of anatomy and surgery).

keratoconjunctivitis a severe inflammation of the membrane covering the white of the eye (the CONJUNCTIVA), with involvement of the CORNEA, associated with a disorder of the outer lens (the cornea). This is most commonly caused by an ADENOVIRUS acquired by contact, via towels, fingers or eye drops. A week or two after onset, the cornea may develop a number of small, whitish opacities that may disturb vision. These often last for months, but will eventually disappear. There is no specific treatment. See also KERATOCONJUNCTIVITIS SICCA.

keratoconjunctivitis sicca dry eye. A state of inadequate wetting and lubrication of the cornea as a result of defective tear production. This results from damage to the tear glands by the same AUTOIMMUNE DISEASE process that causes RHEUMATOID ARTHRITIS, SJÖGREN'S SYNDROME, systemic lupus erythematosus and other related conditions. Dry eye is common in all these disorders. There is constant discomfort, foreign-body sensation and sometimes pain and the condition may progress to infection and ulceration of the cornea. Treatment is by the regular use of artificial tears.

keratoconus a growth disorder (dystrophy) of the CORNEA causing central peaking or conicity and affecting vision. The main disability is from image distortion. Keratoconus is a familial condition that usually starts in adolescence, affecting girls more than boys. Spectacles may help at first, the progressive distortion usually calls for correction with hard contact lenses. Corneal grafting is often eventually required but the results are usually good.

keratocyte 1 one of the cells of the main body of the CORNEA.
2 an abnormally-shaped red blood cell bearing horn-like projections. Keratocytes may occur in cases of poisoning or adverse drug reactions in which the red cells are damaged.

keratodermia thickening of the horny outer layer of the skin. This sometimes occurs in a patchy manner symmetrically on the palms and soles. Keratodermia may be a feature of the MENOPAUSE, or may occur in REITER'S SYNDROME. In many cases the cause is obscure.

keratoglobus a condition in which the cornea bulges abnormally causing MYOPIA and distorted vision.

keratolysis peeling off and shedding of the outer layer of the skin (the epidermis) or of the horny layer of the epidermis from the lower, still-living zone. In some cases affecting the soles of the feet, the condition is caused by the organisms *Acinomyces* or *Corynebacterium*.

keratolytic drugs drugs able to break down or soften keratinized epidermis that are used, often in combination with other ingredients, to treat ACNE, dry skin conditions, WARTS and PSORIASIS. Examples are salicylic acid, benzoyl peroxide, silver nitrate, formaldehyde solutions and podophyllum resin.

keratomalacia softening or 'melting' of the cornea usually in severely malnourished children whose body stocks of vitamin A have become exhausted. Corneal melt leads to internal infection and irremediable blindness and this is the fate of millions of children every year in economically depressed parts of the world. A small regular dose of vitamin A, as from a few fleshy green leaves, will prevent this.

keratome an obtusely angle-bladed ophthalmic knife, sharp on both edges, sometimes used to cut into the CORNEA.

keratometer an optical instrument used to measure the radius of curvature of the cornea. See also KERATOMETRY.

keratometry measurement of the curvature of the front surface of the CORNEA in various meridia. This is done to assist in the fitting of contact lenses, to determine the optical constants of the eye for the purposes of determining the required power of an intraocular lens, and to diagnose conditions such as KERATOCONUS or KERATOGLOBUS.

keratomycosis fungus infection of the CORNEA.

keratopathy any disorder of the outer lens of the eye (the CORNEA).

keratophakia a method of altering the refractive power of the CORNEA, as by introducing an artificial lens or a lens-shaped piece of donated cornea between its layers.

keratoplasty see CORNEAL GRAFT.

keratoscope an instrument from which bright concentric circles can be reflected by the CORNEA so as to reveal optical irregularities of the surface.

keratosis small white patches in the skin arising

from excessive local reproduction of the horny outer cells, so that more than the normal amount of KERATIN is formed. Solar keratosis, caused in the elderly by over-exposure to the sun, is a precancerous condition. Keratosis may also affect the hair follicles causing baldness, the outer and middle ears causing obstruction of the ear canal and CHOLESTEATOMA, and the mucous membranes of the lip and of the throat.

keratosis follicularis see DARIER'S DISEASE.

keratotomy any surgical cut (incision) into the cornea. Radial keratotomy is an operation purporting to reduce short-sight (MYOPIA) by inducing scarring to flatted the cornea. Eight or more deep radial cuts are made. The operation is of dubious propriety and is being replaced by less crude methods.

keraunophobia abnormal fear of thunder and lightning. From the Greek *keraunos*, a thunderbolt.

Kerecid a brand name for the antiviral drug idoxuridine. This drug was the first to show effective action against herpes simplex viruses but has now been largely superceded by ACYCLOVIR.

kerion a localized boggy swelling on the scalp with oozing of pus and serum from the hair follicles. Kerion is a reaction to fungus infection of the scalp (TINEA CAPITIS) and is self-curing. It is commonest in agricultural workers and is often contracted from farm animals.

kernicterus jaundice of the brain resulting from RHESUS FACTOR disease in babies in which excessive red cell breakdown results in the release of large quantities of BILIRUBIN. Death is common before, or within a week or two after, birth. Surviving infants feed poorly, suffer varying degrees of paralysis, epilepsy, spasticity of the muscles, mental retardation, deafness and blindness. Kernicterus is preventable by prenatal diagnosis and treatment.

Kernig's sign an indication of irritation of the membranes surrounding the brain and spinal cord (the meninges) as in meningitis. Attempts to bend the hip with the knee straight (straight leg raising) cause pain and are strongly opposed by irritative spasm in the hamstring muscles that extend the hip and bend the knee. (Vladimir Michailovich Kernig, 1840–1917, Russian physician).

Ketalar a brand name for KETAMINE.

ketamine a drug used to produce insensitivity

to pain, mental and emotional dissociation and lack of awareness so that surgical procedures can be carried out on a conscious patient. It is related to PHENCYCLIDINE. The drug is on the WHO official list. A brand name is Ketalar.

ketoacidosis see KETOSIS.

Ketocid a brand name for KETOPROFEN.

ketoconazole an imidazole antifungal drug. Ketoconazole is absorbed into the blood from the intestine and can be used to treat internal (systemic) fungal infections as well as skin fungal infections. It can, however, damage the liver. Brand names are Daktarin Gold and Nizoral.

ketogenesis the formation of acid KETONE BODIES, as in uncontrolled DIABETES, starvation or as a result of a diet with a very high fat content.

ketonaemia KETONES in the blood. Low levels are normal.

ketones a class of acidic organic compounds that includes acetone and aceto-acetic acid. Ketones have a carbonyl group, CO, linked to two other carbon atoms. They are formed in states of carbohydrate deficiency such as starvation or in conditions, such as DIABETES, in which carbohydrates cannot be normally utilized. Acetone, aceto-acetic acid and beta-hydroxybutyric acid are called ketone bodies. Ketones are volatile substances and confer on the breath the sickly, fruity odour of nail-varnish remover. See also KETOSIS.

ketonuria the presence of the ketone bodies acetone, aceto-acetic acid or beta-hydroxybutyric acid in the urine, usually in cases of untreated DIABETES.

ketoprofen a drug in the non-steroidal anti-inflammatory (NSAID) and pain killing (analgesic) group. Brand names are Ketocid, Orudis, Oruvail and, for external use, Oruvail gel and Powergel.

ketorolac a NON-STEROIDAL ANTI-INFLAMMATORY (NSAID) drug. Brand names are Acular and Toradol.

ketosis the presence of abnormally high levels of KETONES in the blood. These are produced when fats are used as fuel in the absence of carbohydrate or available protein as in DIABETES or starvation. Ketosis is dangerous because high levels make the blood abnormally acid and there is loss of water, sodium and potassium and a major biochemical upset with nausea, vomiting, abdominal pain, confusion, and, if the condition is not rapidly treated, coma and death. Mild ketosis also occurs in cases of excessive morning sickness in pregnancy.

ketosteroid a steroid hormone to which an oxygen molecule has been attached, especially at the 17th carbon atom (C-17). An oxosteroid. A 17-ketosteroid is a steroid with a CO (carbonyl) group at C-17. 17-ketosteroids are excreted in the urine as breakdown products of ANDROGENS and are present in excess in adrenal and gonadal overactivity.

ketostix a convenient dipstick urine test for KETONES. A paper strip impregnated with sodium nitroprusside turns a deep permanganate colour in the presence of ketones. The test is very sensitive. If the urine tests positive both for sugar and ketones the diagnosis of DIABETES is virtually certain.

ketotic pertaining to KETOSIS.

ketotifen a drug that prevents the release of HISTAMINE and other irritating substances from MAST CELLS in allergic conditions. Its action is similar to that of CROMOGLYCATE (cromoglicate) but has the disadvantage of causing drowsiness. A brand name is Zaditen.

keyhole surgery a lay term for LAPAROSCOPIC SURGERY.

keyway an undercutting made in a drilled tooth cavity so that the filling, when hardened, will be less likely to fall out.

Kiditard a brand name for QUINIDINE.

kidney one of the paired, reddish brown, bean-shaped structures lying in pads of fat on the inside of the back wall of the ABDOMEN on either side of the spine, just above the waist. The kidneys filter the blood, removing waste material and adjusting the levels of various essential chemical substances, so as to keep them within necessary limits. In so doing, they produce a sterile solution of varying concentration known as urine. This passes down the ureters to the bladder where it is stored until it can be conveniently disposed of. The kidneys are largely responsible for regulating the amount of water in the body and controlling the acidity of the blood. Most drugs or their products are eliminated through the kidney. Kidneys control fluid and chemical levels by both filtration and selective reabsorption under the control of various hormones such as ALDOSTERONE from the adrenal gland, the ANTIDIURETIC HORMONE

from the pituitary gland and PARATHYROID hormone from the parathyroid glands. Sodium, potassium, calcium, chloride, bicarbonate, phosphate, glucose, amino acids, vitamins and many other substances are returned to the blood and conserved. Proteins, fats and all the cells of the blood remain in the circulation. The kidneys produce ERYTHROPOIETIN, which stimulates the rate of formation of blood cells in the bone marrow. When blood pressure falls below normal the kidneys release the enzyme renin into the blood. This results in the formation of a further hormone, angiotensin, which rapidly causes blood vessels throughout the body to constrict and raise the blood pressure.

kidney cysts small, fluid-filled cavities in the kidneys that are common and benign and usually cause neither symptoms nor danger. But see POLYCYSTIC KIDNEY.

kidney disorders see ALPORT'S SYNDROME, GLOMERULONEPHRITIS, HORSE-SHOE KIDNEY, HYPERNEPHROMA, KIDNEY FAILURE, NEPHRITIS, NEPHROSIS, POLYCYSTIC KIDNEY, · PYELONEPHRITIS, WILM'S TUMOUR.

kidney failure the stage in kidney disease in which neither organ is capable of excreting body waste products fast enough to prevent their accumulation in the blood. Kidney failure is inevitably fatal unless the affected person is treated by DIALYSIS or has a kidney transplant.

kidney grafting see KIDNEY TRANSPLANT.

kidney, polycystic see POLYCYSTIC KIDNEY.

kidney stones crystallization out of various substances dissolved in the urine, especially during DEHYDRATION when the urine is most concentrated. Stone formation is promoted by infection or by any increase in the amount or character of substances dissolved in the urine. Some drugs can form stones, others can potentiate the formation of stones. Stones may occur in inherited disorders in which abnormal amounts of substances such as cystine and xanthine are excreted, but most kidney stones contain various combinations of calcium, magnesium, phosphorus, and oxalate. Uric acid stones tend to develop when the blood levels of this substance are abnormally high, as in gout.

kidney transplant the insertion of a donated kidney into the body and connection of its blood vessels to the host vessels and its ureter to the host bladder. The donated kidney is usually placed in the right side of the pelvis, alongside the bladder and connected to the ILIAC vessels. The results of kidney transplantation are excellent, with success in more than 80% of cases.

Kikuchi's disease a disease usually affecting young women who present with painless enlarged lymph nodes in the neck or elsewhere, fever and liver damage. The condition may be confused with malignant LYMPHOMA or HODGKIN'S DISEASE but usually settles within three months.

killer cells a subclass of large, granular LYMPHOCYTES that includes the natural killer (NK) cells and the killer (K) cells. These are important elements in the immune system and are the final effectors in the process by which damaged, infected or malignant cells are recognised and destroyed. At this stage in the process, killer cells act in conjunction with activated MACROPHAGES and cytotoxic T cells.

kilo- *prefix denoting* one thousand, as in KILOCALORIE.

kilobase a unit of measurement of the length of a DNA or RNA sequence equal to 1000 base pairs of DNA or 1000 bases of RNA.

kilocalorie the amount of heat needed to raise the temperature of a kilogram of water by 1 °C. This has been the standard nutritional unit of energy for years, but is now being replaced by the kilojoule. 1 kcal = 4.187 kJ. See JOULE.

kilodalton one thousand daltons. A dalton is the weight of a hydrogen atom. The kilodalton is the standard unit used to represent the weight of large molecules such as proteins. It is normally abbreviated to K or Kd.

kiloton 1 1000 tons.
2 a unit of 'yield' for atomic bombs, equivalent to the explosive force of 1000 tons of TNT.

Kimmelstiel-Wilson bodies rounded masses of glassy (hyaline) material found in areas of kidney damage in the nodular type of diabetic NEPHROPATHY that may occur in people who have had DIABETES for several years. The condition features protein in the urine, generalized OEDEMA and high blood pressure (HYPERTENSION). (Paul Kimmelstiel, 1900–1970, German physician; and Clifford Wilson, English physician, b. 1906)

kinaesthesia perception of bodily movement, or of the sensation of movement. Compare PROPRIOCEPTION.

kinase see TRANSFERASE.

Kineret a brand name for ANAKINRA.

kinesiology the study of muscles and their effects on movements, especially in relation to physical therapy.

King's evil the historic term for tuberculosis of the tonsillar lymph nodes in the neck (scrofula). As late as the beginning of the 18th century it was believed that scrofula could be cured by a touch from the King. The great lexicographer Dr Samuel Johnson was touched for the King's evil by the queen but, being a lifelong sceptic in such matters, enjoyed no advantage.

Kinidin Durules a brand name for QUINIDINE.

kinin one of a family of POLYPEPTIDES, released as a part of the inflammatory process, which increase the leakiness of small blood vessels and cause smooth muscle fibres to contract.

Kinsey reports the first large-scale studies of human sexual behaviour. The reports, *Sexual Behavior in the Human Male* (1948) by Alfred C. Kinsey, Wardell B. Pomeroy and Clyde E. Martin, and *Sexual Behavior in the Human Female* (1953) by the same authors and Paul H. Gebhard, had a profound effect on public and private attitudes to sex and helped to overcome repressive taboos about open discussion on the subject.

Kirschner wire a stout wire or fine metal rod passed through bone, tensioned, and secured at either end in a metal stirrup. Kirschner wire is used to apply traction. (Martin Kirschner, 1879–1942, German surgeon).

kissing the widespread human practice of pressing the lips against some part of the body of another person, especially the mouth. Kissing has social as well as sexual functions and these are usually kept apart. Some societies accept public kissing between adult males; others do not. Kissing can be dangerous, as, for instance, a means of transmission of infectious mononucleosis. It can be fatal when an adult with an oral cold sore kisses a child with eczema, producing the life-threatening Kaposi's varicelliform eruption.

kissing cancer a cancer implanted in a new site by prolonged local contact from another affected site.

kissing bug the *reduviid* bug that transmits CHAGAS' DISEASE. It is so called because its nocturnal bite is barely felt.

kissing disease see GLANDULAR FEVER.

kissing ulcer a pair of ulcers on opposite sides of a tubular structure, such as the DUODENUM.

kiss of life mouth-to-mouth or mouth-to-nose artificial respiration.

Klean-prep a brand name for POLYETHYLENE GLYCOL.

Klebsiella pneumonia inflammation of the lung (pneumonia) caused by the GRAM NEGATIVE organism *Klebsiella pneumoniae*. This is a rare but very severe disease with a high mortality. One or more lobes of the lungs become solidified and partially destroyed. Large amounts of purulent, brownish sputum are produced. The organisms is resistant to many antibiotics.

kleptomania a rare impulse disorder featuring recurrent stealing of things neither needed nor wanted. The object is the emotional relief of tension accompanying a successful theft rather than acquisition. This is often followed by strong guilt feelings. Only 1 person in 20 arrested for shop-lifting behaves in a manner consistent with the diagnosis. The cause is unknown.

Klinefelter's syndrome a male bodily disorder caused by one or more additional X (sex) chromosomes. Instead of the normal X and Y sex chromosomes, men with Klinefelter's syndrome have an XXY configuration. This has a feminizing effect. The penis and testicles are small and there may be female breast development and diminished sexual interest (libido). Homosexuality and transvestism are common. The diagnosis can easily be confirmed by chromosomal analysis. Hormonal and plastic surgical treatment can help. (Harry Fitch Kleinfelter, American physician, b. 1912).

Klumpke's paralysis loss of function and wasting of the muscles of the forearm and hand due to injury of the nerve roots emerging from the spine in the lower part of the neck. (Augusta Dejerine-Klumpke, 1859–1927, French neurologist)

knee the hinge articulation between the lower end of the thigh bone (FEMUR) and the upper end of the main lower leg shin bone (TIBIA). The knee cap (PATELLA) is a flat bone lying within the massive tendon of the thigh muscles and is not an intrinsic part of the joint.

knee disorders see BAKER'S CYST, CHONDROMALACIA PATELLAE, CLERGYMAN'S KNEE, HAEMARTHROSIS, KNEE LOCKING, LOOSE BODIES, OSTEOARTHRITIS and SYNOVITIS.

knee-locking a common effect of a tear in a semilunar (meniscus) cartilage of the knee joint or of its attachment. A fragment of cartilage may slip between the bearing surfaces of the joint and prevent either full straightening or full bending. The treatment is surgical removal of the affected cartilage (meniscectomy).

knock-knee see GENU VALGUM.

knuckle the common name for a finger joint.

Koch's postulates a set of criteria to be obeyed before it is established that a particular organism causes a particular disease. The organism must be present in every case and must be isolated, cultured and identified; it must produce the disease when a pure culture is given to susceptible animals; and it must be recoverable from the diseased animal. (Robert Koch, 1843–1910, German bacteriologist)

Kohler's disease 1 OSTEOCHONDRITIS of the SCAPHOID bone of the foot. A condition affecting children and adolescents. There is a defect in the blood supply to the bone, from compression of the foot arch, leading to central bone death (necrosis). Weight-bearing must be avoided during the active stage of the disease, but spontaneous healing occurs. 2 osteochondritis of the head of the bone in the palm articulating with the forefinger (second metatarsal bone). (Alban Kohler, 1874–1947, German radiologist).

koilo- *prefix denoting* hollow or empty.

koilocytosis the appearance of spaces (vacuoles) in cells. Cervical or dermal epithelial koilocytosis is characteristic of infection with the human PAPILLOMAVIRUS.

koilonychia thin, brittle, concave fingernails. This may result from iron deficiency ANAEMIA or injury to the nail bed. Koilonychia also occurs in the itchy skin disease LICHEN PLANUS and in the rare inherited condition dystrophic epidermolysis bullosa. From the Greek *koilos*, concave or hollow and *onyx*, a finger or toenail.

koilorachic having a backward curve in the lumbar spine.

Kolanticon a brand name for a preparation containing ALUMINIUM HYDROXIDE, MAGNESIUM OXIDE, DICYCLOMINE HYDROCHLORIDE (dicycloverine) and DIMETHICONE (dimeticone).

Konakion a brand name for vitamin K (PHYTOMENADIONE).

Koplik's spots tiny white spots, surrounded by a red base, occurring on the inside of the cheeks and the inner surface of the lower lip during the INCUBATION PERIOD of MEASLES. (Henry Koplik, 1858–1927, American paediatrician).

kopophobia an abnormal fear of fatigue.

koro a delusional disorder of males in which the sufferer becomes convinced that his penis is shrinking and that when it disappears into his body, he will die. To prevent this, he will tie his penis to a heavy stone or persuade friends to hold it, in relays. The delusion is limited to certain areas in South-east Asia and relates to the belief that ghosts have no genitals. Epidemics occur.

Korotkoff sounds the sounds heard through a stethoscope held over a compressed artery with each pulse beat as the compression is gradually released, in the process of measuring the blood pressure with a SPHYGMOMANOMETER. The first pulse sound heard as blood is able to pass through the narrowed artery is Korotkoff phase I. The sounds get louder as the cuff pressure continues to fall, but then there is a sudden muffling. This is Korotkoff phase IV; the cuff pressure at this point has, in the past, been taken as the diastolic pressure. Soon after that the sounds disappear altogether. This is Korotkoff phase V, the cuff pressure at which is now generally taken as the diastolic. (Nikolai Sergeivich Korotkov, 1874–1920, Russian physician).

Korsakoff's psychosis see WERNICKE-KORSAKOFF SYNDROME.

kosher a rabbinic term derived from the Hebrew word for proper or fit and most commonly applied to the food authorized for orthodox Jews. Kosher foods include the meat of cattle, sheep, goats, chickens and fish with scales and fins. Animals must be killed in accordance with prescribed rules and carcasses inspected for disease. Meat must be immediately broiled or salted. Such observances are of significant hygienic value.

KP *abbrev. for* keratic precipitates. Collections of inflammatory cells that are deposited on the inside of the CORNEA in UVEITIS.

kraurosis vulvae a form of VULVITIS involving drying and shrivelling of the VAGINA and VULVA with itching and pain. The condition is related to post-menopausal oestrogen deficiency. From the Greek *krauros*, dry or brittle.

Krause's corpuscles spheroidal, laminated, delicately capsuled endings to nerve fibres, found in the skin and mucous membranes. They are receptors for cold stimuli. Also known as end bulbs of Krause. (Wilhelm Johann Friedrich Krause, 1833–1910, German anatomist)

Krebs cycle a cyclical sequence of 10 biochemical reactions, brought about by mitochondrial enzymes, that involves the oxidation of a molecule of acetyl-CoA, to two molecules of carbon dioxide and water. Each turn of the cycle can result in the formation of 12 molecules of ATP per molecule of acetyl-CoA. ATP is the direct source of energy for all work performed in any cell. The Krebs cycle is one of the most important in all body biochemistry and occurs in all organisms that oxidise food totally to carbon dioxide and water. Also known as the citric acid cycle or the tricarboxylic acid cycle. (Hans Adolf Krebs, 1900–89, German-born English biochemist).

Kuntscher nail a large, strong, stainless steel nail with a clover-leaf cross-section, used to maintain alignment in fractures of the shaft of the thigh bone (FEMUR) or TIBIA. The nail is hammered into the hollow canal of the bone. (Gerhard Kuntscher, 1902–72, German surgeon)

Kupffer cells fixed MACROPHAGE cells that line the fine blood sinuses (capillaries) of the liver and act as scavengers to remove senescent red blood cells, bacteria and other foreign material. (Karl Wilhelm von Kupffer, 1829–1902, German anatomist)

kuru a slow, fatal brain infection that appeared to be limited to natives of the highlands of New Guinea among whom it was spread by the practice of eating the brains of dead relatives. The disease is thought to be caused by a subvirus particle, called a PRION, which has none of the usual properties of a virus except the ability to produce a characteristic disease process. The prion was, apparently, transmitted through skin abrasions during the preparation of the meal. This explained why kuru affected the women only. The prion is resistant to most of the normal methods of sterilization. The condition features headache, aching joints and limbs, progressive inability to walk and, later, even to sit up, inability to speak and to swallow, sometimes DEMENTIA and eventual death. See also CREUTZFELDT-JAKOB DISEASE and BOVINE SPONGIFORM ENCEPHALOPATHY.

Kveim test a test for SARCOIDOSIS involving the introduction of some tissue, prepared from a person suffering from the condition, into the skin. A typical tissue reaction occurs after a few weeks. (Morton Ansgar Kveim, Norwegian physician, b. 1892).

kwashiorkor a serious nutritional deficiency disease of young children resulting from gross dietary protein deficiency with a high intake of carbohydrate of low nutritional value. There is retarded growth and development, a protuberant abdomen, muscle wasting, tissue fluid retention (OEDEMA), red discolouration of the hair, irritability or apathy and enlargement of the liver. The protein deficiency results in inadequate antibody levels and seious infections. Children under two years of age who develop kwashiorkor and survive are likely to suffer life-long ill effects.

Kwells a brand name for HYOSCINE.

Kyasanur forest disease an ARBOVIRUS haemorrhagic fever that occurs in Mysore State, India, in the villages around the Kyasanur forest. The disease is caused by a virus of the same group as that causing JAPANESE B ENCEPHALITIS and the infection is transmitted by tick bite. There is sore throat, headache, muscle aches, abdominal pain and diarrhoea and the condition may progress to brain inflammation (ENCEPHALITIS).

kyphoscoliosis an abnormal degree of backward curvature of the dorsal spine (KYPHOSIS) combined with curvature to one side (SCOLIOSIS).

kyphosis an abnormal degree of backward curvature of the part of the spine between the neck and the lumbar regions. Backward curvature is normal in this region and kyphosis is an exaggeration of the normal curve. It is commonly the result of bad postural habits in adolescence or of OSTEOPOROSIS. From the Greek *kyphos*, meaning bowed or bent.

Kytril a brand name for GRANISETRON.

labetalol a combined alpha- and beta-blocking drug, sometimes found to be more effective in the treatment of high blood pressure (HYPERTENSION) than beta-blockers. It is also used to treat ANGINA PECTORIS. A brand name is Trandate.

labia the four lips of the female genitalia. The inner pair, the labia minora, surround the entrance to the vagina and the external opening of the urine tube (URETHRA) and join at the front to form a hood over the front of the head of the clitoris. The outer pair, the labia majora, are long, well-padded folds, containing muscle and fibro-fatty tissue, and covered with hair. They are normally closed and conceal the rest of the genitalia.

labial pertaining to the lips or labia.

labile liable to change. The term is applied to the emotions as well as to physiological change.

labiodental *adj* a sound articulated by contact between with the lip and teeth, as in the sound 'f'.

labiomental pertaining to the lower lip and the chin.

labionasal pertaining to the lips and the nose.

labium the singular of LABIA.

Labosept a brand name for DEQUALINIUM.

labour the three stage process of delivering a baby and the PLACENTA by contractions of the muscles of the womb (uterus), of the DIAPHRAGM and of the wall of the abdomen. The first stage lasts from the onset of pains to full widening (dilatation) of the CERVIX, the second to the delivery of the baby and the third to the delivery of the placenta.

labyrinth any group of communicating anatomical cavities, especially the internal ear, comprizing the vestibule, semicircular canals and the cochlea.

labyrinthectomy surgical removal of part or all of the LABYRINTH. This operation is sometimes performed for the relief of MENIERE'S DISEASE and leads to total deafness on the same side.

labyrinthitis inflammation, usually as a result of an influenza or mumps virus infection, of the part of the inner ear responsible for balance. Labyrinthitis causes VERTIGO, vomiting and a ringing or hissing in the ears (TINNITUS). Deafness may follow, but the condition usually clears up spontaneously within days or weeks.

laceration a wound made by tearing. An irregular wound of the tissues, as distinct from a clean cut (incised wound).

lachesine a drug sometimes used to widen (dilate) the pupils in people sensitive to ATROPINE.

lachrymal an arbitrary and incorrect spelling of LACRIMAL.

lacidipine a CALCIUM CHANNEL BLOCKER drug. A brand name is Motens.

lac operon a sequence of genes found in many bacteria that codes for the enzymes needed to break down lactose to glucose and galactose so that the sugars can be utilized. Studies on the lac operon have been important in genetic research. The lactose repressor protein controls the transcription of the lac operon.

lacrimal pertaining to the tears, to their production and to their disposal. Note that the spelling 'lachrymal' has neither logical nor etymological justification. The term comes from Latin *lacrima*, a tear.

lacrimal bone a small plate of bone, situated just inside the inner wall of the eye socket (orbit), with a shallow hollow to accommodate the LACRIMAL SAC.

lacrimal canaliculus one of four tiny tubes that carry tears from the inner corners of the four eyelids to the LACRIMAL SAC.

lacrimal gland the tear-secreting gland lying in the upper and outer corner of the bony eye socket (orbit) and opening by many small ducts into the upper cul-de-sac of the CONJUNCTIVA behind the upper lid. Lacrimal glands secrete during emotional weeping and when the eye is irritated. The eye is normally kept wet by tiny accessory lacrimal glands in the conjunctiva.

lacrimal sac the small bag lying under the tissues just inwards and below the inner corner of the eye. Tears drain into the lacrimal sac before being discharged down the nasolacrimal duct into the nose.

lacrimal system the tear-producing LACRIMAL GLANDS and the drainage system – the CANALICULI and the NASOLACRIMAL DUCT – that carry surplus tears down into the nose.

lacrimation secretion of tears, especially excessive production as in weeping or in the presence of a foreign body or corneal ulcer. Compare EPIPHORA.

lacrimator tear gas.

lact-, lacto- *combining form denoting* milk, milk production or lactic acid.

lactagogue any agent that promotes the secretion or flow of milk.

lactalbumin any of a group of proteins contained in milk.

lactase an enzyme that brings about the HYDROLYSIS of LACTOSE to glucose (dextrose) and galactose. Beta-galactosidase.

lactase deficiency syndrome a condition featuring excessive intestinal gas and diarrhoea on taking milk or milk products caused by a congenital or acquired deficiency of LACTASE. Lactose is not broken down and is acted on by gas-forming intestinal bacteria.

lactate dehydrogenase (LDH) one of the cell enzymes released into the blood when heart muscle cells are damaged during a heart attack (myocardial infarction). A measure of the concentration of these enzymes can indicate the severity of the attack.

lactation the secretion and production of milk in the breasts (MAMMARY GLANDS) after childbirth.

lacteal 1 pertaining to milk.
2 a lymph vessel that absorbs and carries emulsified fat from the small intestine to the

THORACIC DUCT and hence to the bloodstream.

lactic acid an acid formed when muscles are strongly contracted for long periods. Also formed from carbohydrates in the vagina by the action of DODERLEIN'S BACILLUS. Lactic acid is an ingredient in a range of drug formulations.

lactic dehydrogenase an enzyme that catalyzes the dehydrogenation of l-lactic acid to pyruvic acid. Dehydrogenation involves removing hydrogen atoms, usually two, from a molecule.

lactiferous able to produce, secrete, or convey milk.

lactobacillus any of the genus of GRAM POSITIVE bacilli that produce LACTIC ACID from carbohydrates by fermentation. Lactobacilli are normal inhabitants of the mouth, intestine and vagina. They ferment milk to yoghurt and are responsible for its acid flavour.

lactofelicine an antibiotic derived from the protein lactofeline in human milk. It is a single peptide and has been found to be selectively effective against various bacteria that cause diarrhoea and food poisoning, especially *Listeria* species and *Escherichia coli*.

lactoferrin an iron-binding protein found in milk and other body fluids and in neutrophil polymorph LEUCOCYTES in which its action helps to retard bacterial reproduction.

lactogenic promoting milk production (LACTATION).

lactoglobulin one of the proteins present in milk.

lactose the main sugar in milk. It is broken down by the digestive enzyme lactase (beta-galactosidase) to galactose and glucose.

lactose intolerance the result of an insufficiency of the lactose-splitting enzyme lactase (beta-galacosidase) in the lining of the small intestine. Lactose in milk is acted on by gas-forming intestinal bacteria, causing abdominal discomfort, colicky pain and diarrhoea. Asian and African people who have undergone a change of diet to one with a higher lactose content are often affected in this way.

lactosuria LACTOSE in the urine.

Lactugal a brand name for LACTULOSE.

lactulose a disaccharide sugar that acts as a gentle but effective LAXATIVE. It is not absorbed or broken down but remains intact until it reaches the colon where it is split by bacteria and helps to retain water, thereby softening the stools. Brand names are Duphalac, LACTUGAL and Regulose.

lacuna any empty space, missing part, cavity or depression.

lacus any small lake or collection of fluid.

Laennec's cirrhosis a form of liver CIRRHOSIS known as micronodular cirrhosis and featuring widespread nodules of regeneration of about 1 mm in diameter. This type is characteristic of the damage caused by alcohol. Also known as portal cirrhosis. (Rene-Theophile-Hyacinthe Laennec, 1781–1826, French physician, who also invented, but, one hopes, did not so name, the STETHOSCOPE.).

laetrile a substance, amygdalin, derived from the seeds of bitter almonds, apricots and other fruit, that has been claimed to be effective in treating cancer. It is said to yield a cyanide-containing compound, mandelonitrile, under the action of enzymes said to be more plentiful in cancers than in normal tissue. There is no medically acceptable evidence that laetrile has any value in the treatment of cancer.

laevocardia a reversal of the position of the abdominal organs (situs inversus) but with a normal position of the heart. Situs inversus is more commonly associated with a heart so placed that the apex points to the right instead of the left (DEXTROCARDIA).

laevulose fructose or fruit sugar, a monosaccharide found in honey and fruit. Combined with glucose, it forms the disaccharide cane sugar (sucrose).

lagging strand in DNA replication, the single strand forming a duplex in the direction away from the fork in the parental DNA. Replication on the lagging strand is discontinuous and can occur briefly in both directions.

lagophthalmos the condition in which the eyelids are unable to close, usually because of forward protrusion or enlargement of the eyeball, as in dysthyroid eye disease (Graves' ophthalmopathy) or tumour in the ORBIT. From the Greek *lagos*, a hare.

LAH *abbrev. for* Licentiate of the Apothecaries Hall, Dublin.

-lalia *suffix denoting* a disorder of speech.

laliophobia an abnormal fear of talking or stuttering.

lalo- *combining form denoting* speech.

lalopathology the study of speech disorders.

lalopathy any disorder of speech.

laloplegia paralysis of the speech muscles.

Lamarckism the discredited doctrine that species can change into new species as a result of characteristics acquired as a result of striving to overcome environmental disadvantages. It was claimed that such acquired characteristics became hereditary. (Jean Baptiste Pierre Antoine de Monet, Chevalier de Lamarck, 1744–1829, French naturalist).

lambdoid 1 resembling an inverted Y junction as in the Greek letter *lambda*.
2 pertaining to the SUTURE between the OCCIPITAL bone at the back of the skull and the PARIETAL bones on either side.

lamella any thin plate, layer or sheet, as of bone.

Lamictal a brand name for LAMOTRIGINE.

lamina any thin sheet or layer of tissue, especially the flat surfaces on the arch of a vertebra.

lamina cribrosa 1 the multiperforated plate of ethmoidal bone in the roof of the nose through which the fine fibres of the OLFACTORY NERVE pass.
2 the ring of perforations in the white of the eye, at the back of the globe, through which bundles of OPTIC NERVE fibres, and the central artery and vein of the RETINA, pass (lamina cribrosa sclerae).

laminar arranged in layers.

laminectomy an operation to relieve pressure on spinal nerve roots following PROLAPSED INTERVERTEBRAL DISC. A part of side of the arch of a VERTEBRA is removed to gain access to the site at which some of the pulpy material from the centre of an intervertebral disc is protruding. This material is removed.

Lamisil a brand name for TERBINAFINE.

lamivudine a reverse transcriptase inhibitor drug used to treat infections with retroviruses, such as HIV. The drug has also been used to treat hepatitis. The drug is on the WHO official list. A brand name is Epivir.

lamotrigine a drug used to control the type of epilepsy known as 'petit mal' or absence attacks. It is taken by mouth. Possible side effects include skin rash, a serious inflammatory condition of mucous membranes (Stevens-Johnson syndrome), headache, indigestion, double vision, blurred vision, vertigo, drowsiness, reduced white cell count and liver failure. A brand name is Lamictal.

lance to cut into or incise a part, such as an

abscess for the purposes of DRAINAGE of PUS or other fluid. In these days of disposable scalpel blades, the term is no longer used as a noun.

Lancefield's streptococcal classification a division of STREPTOCOCCI (see STREPTOCOCCUS) into four groups on the basis of the antigenic differences in the polysaccharide structure of the cell walls of the organisms. Group A, *Streptococcus pyogenes*, are the most dangerous. (Rebecca Craighill Lancefield, 1895–1981, American bacteriologist).

lancet 1 (obsolete) a small surgical knife used for making incisions for DRAINAGE. Almost all surgical cutting is now done with disposable surgical scalpels or disposable blades fitted to reusable handles.
2 (*The Lancet*) a long-established and highly-respected British journal of medicine and surgery, rivalled in status and popularity in Britain only by the *British Medical Journal*.

Landry's paralysis a disorder of sudden onset featuring paralysis of the arms and due to an AUTOIMMUNE, DEMYELINATING process affecting the spinal cord. See GUILLAIN-BARRE SYNDROME. (Jean Baptiste Octave Landry, 1826–65, French physician).

Langerhans cell an antigen-presenting dendritic cell found in the skin. These cells pick up and process antigen in the skin and then move to the nearest lymph node where the antigen is presented to T cells. In this way the immune system may become sensitized to a contact allergen. (Paul Wilhelm Langerhans 1847-88, German physician, who described these cells when he was a medical student.).

lanolin a mixture of esters of fatty acids derived from animal skin secretions on wool. Lanolin is used, in conjunction with other ingredients such as zinc oxide, to form various soothing skin ointments.

Lanoxin a brand name for DIGOXIN.

lanreotide a SOMATOSTATIN analogue drug used to treat the growth disorder acromegaly prior to surgery on the pituitary gland. Somatostatin is a hormone produced by the hypothalamus of the brain, which inhibits the release of the natural growth hormone, somatotropin as well as of other pituitary gland-stimulating hormones. Brand name: Somatuline LA.

lansoprazole a PROTON PUMP INHIBITOR drug. A brand name is Zoton.

Lantus a brand name for INSULIN GLARGINE.

lanugo the short, downy, colourless hair that covers the fetus from about the fourth month to shortly before the time of birth. Similar hair sometimes grows on people with cancer, on those taking certain drugs and on girls with ANOREXIA NERVOSA.

Lanvis a brand name for THIOGUANINE (tioguanine).

laparo- *combining form denoting* the flank, loin or abdominal wall.

laparoscopic cholecystectomy removal of the gall bladder without a large surgical incision, using LAPAROSCOPY. The postoperative recovery is more rapid and the cosmetic effect excellent, but there is a slightly higher probability of operative complications.

laparoscopic colectomy removal of the large intestine by LAPAROSCOPIC SURGERY.

laparoscopic hernia repair repair of HERNIA using LAPAROSCOPIC SURGERY.

laparoscopic sterilization closure of the Fallopian tubes in the female by means of LAPAROSCOPY so that eggs (ova) cannot be contacted by sperms. This is an established and safe procedure. The tubes may be clipped, cut and sealed with electric cautery or occluded by small circular plastic bands. The latter method allows possible reversal.

laparoscopic surgery a range of surgical techniques performed through small metal or plastic ports inserted through short incisions in the skin. The instruments are externally controlled and the operation site is internally illuminated and is commonly viewed on a computer-type monitor. Since much of post-operative morbidity relates to the use of large skin and muscle incisions, this method is popular with patients and substantially shortens recovery time. Older surgeons must master some entirely new techniques and adapt to the change in the relationship of hand and eye. The method is rapidly replacing earlier and cruder methods.

laparoscopy direct visual examination of the interior of the abdomen, through a narrow optical device (endoscope) passed through a small incision in the abdominal wall. Endoscopes use fibre optic illumination and viewing channels. Laparoscopy allows a range of operations to be performed using instruments passed in through the endoscope.

laparoscopy, three-dimensional a system

357

of LAPAROSCOPIC SURGERY that provides the operator with a three-dimensional display of the abdominal organs. The method uses a single-rod-lens endoscope with two miniaturized video cameras. Active liquid-crystal shutter spectacles must be worn. A three-dimensional view improves accuracy, dexterity, speed, and safety.

laparotomy 1 a surgical incision through the flank.

2 (colloquial) an exploratory operation performed for purposes of diagnosis.

Largactil a brand name for CHLORPROMAZINE.

large granular lymphocyte one of a range of larger-than-average lymphocytes with granules in the cytoplasm which function as natural killer and killer cells. The group also includes activated cytotoxic T cells.

large intestine the part of the intestine that extends from the end of the ILEUM to the ANUS. It starts in the lower right corner of the abdomen with the caecum, from which the APPENDIX protrudes, proceeds as the ascending COLON to the upper right corner, loops across to the upper left corner as the transverse colon then descends to the lower left corner as the descending colon. The intestine then swings down and centrally as the sigmoid colon and continues as the rectum and the anal canal. The main function of the colon is to reabsorb water from the bowel contents. The rectum is a temporary store for faeces.

Lariam a brand name for MEFLOQUINE.

Larodopa a brand name for LEVODOPA.

Laroxyl a brand name for AMITRIPTYLENE.

larval therapy the use of maggots that feed on dead and infected tissue to assist in the healing of serious wounds. Used in rare cases in which healing is hampered by the resistance of the infecting organisms to ANTIBIOTICS.

larva migrans 1 the skin irritation caused by the penetration of hookworm and other larvae (cutaneous larva migrans).

2 the allergic effects associated with the invasive stage of an infection with the worm parasite Toxocara canis (visceral larva migrans). These include ASTHMA and EOSINOPHILIA.

larvicide any agent that kills the larval form of an organism, especially a human parasite.

laryng-, laryngo- *combining form denoting* the voice-box (LARYNX).

laryngeal 1 pertaining to the larynx.

2 produced in or with the larynx, as of a sound.

laryngectomy surgical removal of the Adam's apple (LARYNX). Laryngectomy is performed for otherwise untreatable cancer of the larynx. The cut upper end of the windpipe (trachea) must be brought out through an opening in the front of the neck to allow breathing. Normal speech is impossible after laryngectomy.

laryngitis inflammation of the voice-box (LARYNX), usually as part of a common cold or other upper respiratory tract infection (URTI), but sometimes as a result of overuse of the voice. There is hoarseness, pain and difficulty in speaking. In most cases full recovery may be expected in a few days, especially if the voice is rested. See also CLERGYMAN'S THROAT and SINGERS' NODES.

laryngology the branch of medicine concerned with the study and treatment of the LARYNX and its disorders. Laryngology is usually clinically associated with the study of the ear (otology) and of the nose (rhinology). An ear, nose and throat (ENT) specialist is called an otorhinolaryngologist (ORL).

laryngopharynx the lower part of the PHARYNX adjacent to the LARYNX.

laryngoscopy examination of the LARYNX either directly by extending the recumbent subject's neck and using a rigid metal instrument, called a laryngoscope, to depress the tongue, or indirectly by way of an angled mirror held behind the back of the tongue. Direct laryngoscopy allows BIOPSY of the vocal cords and removal of polyps, nodules or foreign bodies.

laryngospasm sudden tight and sustained closure of the vocal cords caused by irritation to the LARYNX or ALLERGY. Laryngospasm prevents breathing and can be very dangerous. It is a problem commonly encountered by anaesthetists.

laryngostenosis narrowing of the space between the vocal cords (GLOTTIS).

laryngotomy a surgical opening into the LARYNX.

laryngotracheal pertaining to the LARYNX and the TRACHEA.

laryngotracheobronchitis widespread inflammation of the voice box (LARYNX), the wind-pipe (TRACHEA) and the main air passages of the lungs (the BRONCHI). Laryngotracheobronchitis commonly causes croup, especially in children.

larynx the 'Adam's apple' or voice box. The larynx is situated at the upper end of the windpipe (TRACHEA), just in front of the start of the gullet (OESOPHAGUS). At its inlet is a leaf-shaped flap of cartilage, the EPIGLOTTIS, that prevents entry of swallowed food. It has walls of cartilage and is lined with a moist mucous membrane and contains the vocal cords. These are two folds of the mucous membrane that can be tensed by tiny muscles to control their rate of vibration as air passes through them, and hence the pitch of the voice. The gap between the folds is called the glottis.

Lasegue's sign a clinical sign of pressure on nerve roots in the lumbar region in SCIATICA. With the patient lying on his or her back there is limitation of thigh bending (flexion) on the affected side, on attempts to raise the straight leg. The sign can also be elicited by attempting to flex the ankle with the straight leg raised. This causes pain. (Charles Ernest Lasegue, 1816–83, French neurologist).

laser *acronym for* Light Amplification by Stimulated Emission of Radiation. A device that produces light of a single, precisely defined wavelength, in which all the waves are in phase with each other (coherent light). This allows the beam to be intensely concentrated, with little tendency to spread out, and permits focusing into a spot of microscopic size. The properties of the various lasers make them invaluable for a variety of medical and surgical purposes, and a many laser types, including argon lasers, various YAG lasers, carbon dioxide lasers, various pumped dye lasers and high-precision excimer lasers, are being exploited for this purpose. See also LASER THERAPY.

laser in-sutu keratomileusis (LASIK) a method of correcting refractive errors of the eye that uses a laser to vaporize a thin layer of the centre of the cornea after a shallow flap of the outer surface has been raised. In correcting myopia (short sight) this procedure reduces the degree of curvature of the optical zone of the cornea so that its power as a lens is reduced and the image is formed further back in the plane of the retina.

laser photocoagulator an ophthalmic laser used to produce tiny spot burns on the RETINA. See LASER.

laser therapy any medical use of lasers for purposes designed to improve the state of patients. Laser therapy includes simple bloodless tissue cutting; destroying or sealing unwanted blood vessels; tumour destruction; unblocking obstructed FALLOPIAN TUBES to restore fertility; removal of tattoos and birthmarks; removal of atherosclerotic plaque and thrombosis inside arteries so as to restore patency; removal of prostate gland tissue causing outflow obstruction; precision corneal curvature adjustment to correct refractive errors; treatment of glaucoma by opening eye aqueous drainage channels (see LASER TRABECULOPLASTY); destroying peripheral parts of the retina so as to allow regression of dangerously fragile new blood vessels in DIABETIC RETINOPATHY; and attempting to promote healing in sprains, inflamed tendons and painful joints. See also LASER.

laser trabeculoplasty the use of an argon laser to cut multiple tiny holes in the trabecular meshwork of the eye so as to cause scars that, on contraction, widen the outflow channels of the meshwork and increase the facility of outflow. The method has proved effective in many cases of chronic simple GLAUCOMA.

laser weapon eye injuries severe dazzling, after-image formation and blinding caused by military laser rangefinders, target designators, anti-optical sensor systems and anti-personnel laser weapons. Many military lasers in current use are capable of immediate permanent destruction of vision in both eyes by photocoagulation of the foveal regions to the retinas. This effect is made more probable because of the physiological mechanism that aligns the foveas on the object of regard. Protective goggles are effective only if they also eliminate useful vision.

Lasix a brand name for FRUSEMIDE (furosemide).

Lassa fever an infectious disease caused by an arenavirus and first noted in 1969 in West Africa. The disease is maintained in the rat population and spread by rat urine. Lassa fever features a high temperature for 7 to 17 days, slow pulse, sore throat, red eyes, prostration, vomiting and pain in the chest wall and abdomen. Yellow spots and ulcers appear on the tonsils. There is a drop in the white cell count in the blood (leukopenia), internal bleeding and often liver and kidney failure. The most severely affected pass into coma and die of inadequate circulation (shock), respiratory insufficiency, or cardiac arrest. The mortality rate may be as high as 50% but many mild cases occur. Strict isolation is necessary. Treatment is with the antiviral drug RIBAVIRIN and with plasma from convalescent patients.

lassitude a disinclination to make an effort to achieve anything. Lassitude may indicate organic disease or depression, but is often due to boredom from lack of interests.

latanoprost a PROSTAGLANDIN drug used in the form of eye drops once daily to control intraocular pressure in chronic simple GLAUCOMA.

latent present but not manifest. Not yet having an effect.

lateral of, at or towards the side of the body. From the Latin military word *latus*, a flank or wing. Unilateral means occurring only on one side; bilateral means relating to both sides.

laterality 1 pertaining to one side.
2 a tendency to use or occur in one side rather than the other.
3 dominance of one hemisphere of the brain over the other.

lateral ventricles the fluid-filled cavities in each half of the brain (cerebral hemispheres) that communicate with the THIRD VENTRICLE by way of the interventricular foramen.

laterodeviation displacement to one side.

lateroflexion a bending to one side.

latex test a test for immunoglobulin M (IgM), the rheumatoid factor, in RHEUMATOID ARTHRITIS. Small polystyrene particles coated with human immunoglobulin G (IgG) are clumped in the presence of IgM. The latex test is positive in about 80% of cases of rheumatoid arthritis.

lathyrism spastic paralysis with loss of sensation in the legs caused by poisoning with vetch (Lathyrus peas). Lathyrism occurs in some parts of India.

latissimus dorsi the broadest muscle of the back. It arises from the spines of the six lower thoracic vertebrae and from the FASCIA attached to the lumbar vertebrae and back of the pelvis and sweeps up and forward to be inserted by a short, broad tendon into the back of the top of the upper arm bone (humerus). It acts to pull the body upward in climbing and assists in heavy breathing.

Latrodectus a genus of poisonous spiders. *L. mactans* is known as the black widow spider.

latus the side of the body. The plural form is latera.

Latycin a brand name for a TETRACYCLINE eye ointment.

laudanum a solution of crude opium in alcohol (tincture of opium). The alkaloids of opium are now refined and separated and prescribed as specific drugs. Laudanum was once casually recommended for a wide range of conditions.

laughing gas a popular term for the anaesthetic drug NITROUS OXIDE.

Laurence-Moon-Biedl syndrome a rare genetic disorder featuring mental retardation, extra toes or fingers, and a retinal degeneration, RETINITIS PIGMENTOSA, that may progress to blindness. There is no treatment and attempts should be made, by GENETIC COUNSELLING, to prevent further transmission of the gene. (John Zacharias Laurence, 1830–1874, English physician; Richard C. Moon, b. 1926, American pathologist; and Artur Biedl, 1869–1933, Austrian physiologist).

LAV lymphadenopathy-associated virus. This was the name first given to the human immunodeficiency virus (HIV) when it was discovered in the Pasteur Institute in Paris, by researchers Francoise Barré-Sinoussi, C. Cherman and F Rey, working under Luc Montagnier. The same virus was called HTLV–III (human T cell lymphotropic virus, Type III) by workers under Robert Gallo when it was isolated in the National Cancer Institute, Bethesda, Maryland.

lavage washing out of a hollow organ or cavity, especially by irrigation. Stomach washout.

laxative drugs drugs used to promote free emptying of the rectum, especially in the treatment of CONSTIPATION. Laxative drugs are much less used than formerly as it is recognized that constipation is better treated by a high fibre diet and regular habits.

Laxoberal a brand name for SODIUM PICOSULPHATE (sodium picosulphate).

lazy eye a lay term applied both to an abnormal inturning of the eye (convergent STRABISMUS or esotropia) and to the defect of vision often resulting from untreated squint in young children (AMBLYOPIA).

LCPS *abbrev. for* Licentiate of the College of Physicians & Surgeons.

LD see LACTATE DEHYDROGENASE.

LDL *abbrev. for* low density LIPOPROTEINS.

LD₅₀ the dose of a poison that kills half the subjects exposed to it. Used as a measure of the toxicity of drugs and other substances.

LDSC *abbrev. for* Licentiate in Dental Science.

LDS *abbrev. for* Licentiate in Dental Surgery.

leaching the washing or dissolving out of a substance by contact with a percolating fluid.

lead 1 a malleable heavy metal with poisonous salts.
2 an electrical connection or electrode by which currents are conveyed to or from the body.

lead poisoning the toxic effect of lead and lead compounds. Acute poisoning, from a large dose, causes abdominal pain, vomiting, diarrhoea, muscle weakness, convulsions, coma and death. Small amounts of lead taken in over long periods accumulate in the body and cause damage to brain function with headache, loss of physical coordination, loss of intellectual ability and memory, and abnormal behaviour.

lead encephalopathy degeneration of brain nerve cells and fluid collection in the brain (cerebral oedema), due to acute lead poisoning.

leading strand in DNA replication, the separated strand that is being converted to a duplex in the direction of the fork, or the opening of the fork, in the parent DNA. Replication is continuous along the leading strand. Compare LAGGING STRAND.

lead polyneuropathy damage to peripheral nerves, especially those supplying the hands and feet, occurring in long-term (chronic) lead poisoning. There is muscle weakness, pain, pins-and-needle sensation (paraesthesia) and numbness in the glove-and-stocking areas.

leaflet any small, leaf-like structure such as the cusps of a heart or other valve.

leaky mutant gene one of a pair of genes (ALLELE) that is less active than its normal partner. A leaky mutation produces only partial loss of a characteristic.

learning disability a well-meaning euphemism for mental retardation. Other terms include developmental reading disorder and developmental word blindness. The condition should not be confused with DYSLEXIA which is a specific disorder. Young people with learning disability experience exceptional difficulty in acquiring an average standard of education. Learning disability is always apparent by the age of seven or, in severe cases, earlier. In spite of considerable research, the causes and nature

remain obscure and controversial. There is no disagreement, however, that in mild cases the best treatment is intensive, individually-tailored, one-to-one instruction in reading and writing by an experienced remedial teacher. Behavioural and emotional problems, often secondary to the learning disability, also require appropriate skilled attention.

Leber's hereditary optic neuropathy a rare genetic disease inherited from the mother caused by a point mutation in MITOCHONDRIAL DNA. Onset is usually about the 20th year and males are affected more often than females. It features changes in the small retinal blood vessels progressing to a degree of atrophy of the optic nerves in both eyes with a severe defect in visual acuity. In most cases a visual acuity of about 6/60 – one tenth of normal – is retained. (T. von Leber, 1040–1917, German ophthalmologist and professor of ophthalmology at Heidelberg).

lecithins a group of phosphoglycerides, plentiful in egg yolk, and occurring widely in the body, especially as a major constituent of cell membranes and in nerve tissue. Lecithins are important emulsifying agents and surfactants and are concerned, for instance, in the normal expansion of the fetal lung at the time of birth. Also known as phosphatidyl cholines.

lecithinase an enzyme that breaks down lecithin.

lectins a group of proteins that bind firmly to specific small sugar (oligosaccharide) parts of glycoproteins and glycolipids. Most lectins in humans are cell membrane proteins with binding sites on the outside of the membranes, and are concerned in cell migration, tissue formation, fertilization, phagocytosis, agglutination, etc.

Ledclair a brand name for SODIUM CALCIUM EDETATE.

Ledercort a brand name for TRIAMCINOLONE.

Lederfen a brand name for FENBUFEN.

Lederspan a brand name for TRIAMCINOLONE.

leech 1 an annelid worm of the class Hirudinea, some of which are blood-suckers. Leeches were formerly much used to withdraw blood, to reduce HAEMATOMAS and to attempt to treat varicose veins.
2 a facetious term for a medical practitioner.

leflunomide a disease-modifying antirheumatic drug used to treat RHEUMATOID ARTHRITIS. The drug has numerous possible side effects and may interact adversely with several other forms of treatment. It is used only under careful medical supervision by an expert. The drug has been suspected of causing serious lung complications since October 2003; a number of Japanese patients taking the drug have, since then, died from an interstitial pneumonia. Brand name: Arava.

left ventricle volume reduction see HEART REDUCTION.

Legionella pneumophila a thin GRAM NEGATIVE rod organism that grows in a medium rich in iron and cysteine. It is the cause of LEGIONNAIRES' DISEASE.

Legionnaires' disease a type of PNEUMONIA caused by *Legionella* bacteria which can propagate in warm, moist places such as air-conditioning towers and are spread into the air in water droplets. The disease features headache, muscle aches, diarrhoea, cough, high fever, pneumonia, mental confusion, and kidney and liver damage. The lungs may suffer irremediable damage, and this is the common cause of death. The death rate is about 4%. Most deaths occur among the elderly, the infirm, heavy smokers and heavy drinkers. Treatment is by antibiotics such as ERYTHROMYCIN and RIFAMPICIN. The disease was first recognized in members of the American Legion attending a convention in a hotel in Pennsylvania in 1976.

leg lengthening an orthopaedic surgical technique used to equalize leg length in children in cases of severe leg length discrepancy or to correct short stature. An EXTERNAL FIXATOR is applied, the bone is cut through with preservation of the outer bone membrane (periosteum), and very gradual lengthening is applied via the fixator at a rate of about 1 mm per day. Once the desired length is achieved no further lengthening traction is applied but the fixator must be left in place until bone consolidation has occurred. The treatment may take months.

legumen a protein present in peas and beans.

Leiden mutation see FACTOR V LEIDEN MUTATION.

leiomyo- *combining form denoting* smooth muscle.

leiomyoma a benign tumour of smooth muscle found most commonly in the womb (uterus). Leiomyomas often contain much fibrous tissue. Also known as FIBROID, fibromyoma or leiomyofibroma.

leiomyosarcoma a rare malignant tumour of smooth muscle sometimes affecting the womb or the stomach. The leiomyosarcoma of stomach accounts for less than 1% of stomach cancers. Unlike stomach carcinomas it grows slowly and spreads late and the outlook after surgery is usually good.

Leishman-Donovan bodies the form in which *Leishmania* parasites appear in MACROPHAGE cells in LEISHMANIASIS. They appear as oval, nucleated, non-flagellated structures in the CYTOPLASM of the MACROPHAGES. Also known as *amastigotes*. (Major-General Sir William Boog Leishman, 1865–1926, English Army pathologist, and Lt Col Charles Donovan, 1863–1951, Irish physician).

Leishmania a genus of single-celled organisms equipped with a whip-like motility organ (flagellated protozoon). The genus contains many species responsible for the various forms of LEISHMANIASIS, known by such names as KALA AZAR, ESPUNDIA, forest yaws, chiclero ulcer, uta, diffuse cutaneous Leishmaniasis, oriental sore, Aleppo boil, Baghdad boil, bouton d'Orient and Delhi boil.

Leishmaniasis a group of infections, caused by single-celled microscopic parasites of the genus LEISHMANIA, and spread by sandflies. It can affect either the skin (cutaneous Leishmaniasis) or the internal organs (visceral Leishmaniasis or KALA AZAR). A seriously disfiguring form, ESPUNDIA, occurs in various parts of south America. Leishmaniasis is becoming increasingly important because of the volume of holiday traffic to areas in which it is endemic, especially the Mediterranean. See also DELHI BOIL, ORIENTAL SORE.

lemniscus a bundle of nerve fibres in the brain or spinal cord.

lemon balm extract extract of *Melissa officinalis* that is said to increase the activity of ACETYCHOLINE and improve memory both in healthy people and in those with ALZHEIMER'S DISEASE. The effect of the extract is claimed to be comparable to that of some drugs licensed for use in the disease. Lemon balm extract can also be obtained from the sagebrush *Salvia officinalis*. Interestingly, the name Salvia derives from a Latin term for good health.

Lenium a brand name for a shampoo containing SELENIUM.

lenograstim human GRANULOCYTE-STIMULATING FACTOR produced by genetic engineering and used to treat severe deficiencies of some of the white cells of the blood and the immune system. A brand name is Granocyte.

lens a regular transparent solid having convex or concave surfaces such that incident beams of light are bent so as to converge (convex lenses) or diverge (concave lenses). The CORNEA is the main light-bending lens of the eye. The internal CRYSTALLINE LENS effects fine adjustments to the focus by an alteration of curvature. Fixed lenses are used in spectacles or in contact with the corneas to correct inherent errors of eye focusing.

lens implant a tiny, plastic lens of high optical quality supported by delicate plastic loops, that is inserted into the eye at the end of a cataract operation to replace the opaque natural lens that has been removed.

Lentard MC a brand name for INSULIN.

Lente insulin a general term for slow-release INSULIN.

lenticonus a condition in which one or both surfaces of the internal crystalline lens of the eye is conical rather than spherical. This causes distortion of vision.

lenticular pertaining to, or shaped like, a lens.

lentiform 1 lens- or lentil-shaped.
2 pertaining to the lenticular nucleus of the BASAL GANGLIA of the brain.

lenticulo-striate pertaining to the lenticular nucleus and CORPUS STRIATUM of the brain and their interconnections.

lentigo a local concentration of pigment-containing cells (melanocytes) in the skin. Lentigos (often called lentigenes) resemble freckles but occur as commonly on covered as on uncovered parts and do not become less conspicuous in winter time. They are harmless.

leontiasis the lion-like appearance of the face, featuring deep furrows and ridges, that occurs in some cases of advanced leprosy (HANSEN'S DISEASE).

leper a person suffering from leprosy (HANSEN'S DISEASE).

lepra leprosy (HANSEN'S DISEASE).

leprology the study of leprosy (HANSEN'S DISEASE).

leproma the nodular skin manifestation of leprosy (HANSEN'S DISEASE).

lepromatous leprosy a severe form of HANSEN'S DISEASE in people with reduced cell-mediated immunity to the causal organism Mycobacterium leprae and widespread dissemination of the organism.

lepromin test a test for determining the type of HANSEN'S DISEASE suffered by a known leprosy patient. A suspension of dead Mycobacteria leprae is injected into the skin. A positive result – a local reaction – can be seen after 4 weeks. It is negative in LEPROMATOUS LEPROSY and positive in TUBERCULOID LEPROSY.

leprosarium an institution for the treatment of people suffering from HANSEN'S DISEASE.

leprosy see HANSEN'S DISEASE.

-lepsis *combining form denoting* a seizure.

leptin a HORMONE produced by fat cells which signals the state of repletion. The substance was discovered at the end of 1994 and showed so much promise that more than 600 papers appeared on the topic within three years. Leptin is a protein of 167 amino acids coded for by the ob gene (for 'obesity'). Its receptor is expressed in the HYPOTHALAMUS in an area known to be concerned with satiety and hunger. Leptin was at first thought to be the complete answer to appetite control but its action in humans has been found to be more complex than its action in rats. Only about one fifth of people respond to a high concentration of leptin by reducing food intake.

Leptin provides a FEEDBACK SIGNAL from fat to the nervous system, stimulates the neurons that express PROOPIOMELANOCORTIN. When this molecule is split by proteolytic enzymes the anorexogenic peptide alpha MELANOCYTE-STIMULATING HORMONE is produced.

lepto- *combining form denoting* fine, soft, delicate, slender or weak.

leptocytosis the condition in which red blood cells are thinner than normal and contain less HAEMOGLOBIN. Leptocytosis is a feature of iron deficiency ANAEMIA, THALASSAEMIA, liver disease and sometimes after SPLENECTOMY.

leptomeningeal pertaining to the two soft inner layers of membrane that surround the brain, the PIA MATER and the ARACHNOID MATER, but not the DURA MATER.

leptomeningitis inflammation of the two fine inner layers of the MENINGES, the PIA and

ARACHNOID maters.

Leptospira a genus of spiral micro-organisms of the order Spirochaetales. See also LEPTOSPIROSIS.

leptospirosis an infection caused by a fine spiral-shaped organism (SPIROCHAETE) *Leptospira icterohaemorrhagiae* or *L. canicola* and transmitted in the urine of rats or dogs to farm and veterinary workers, fish-market workers, sewer workers and miners. The organism can penetrate the intact skin and the infection may be mild. Severe cases feature headache, muscle aches and tenderness, red eyes, loss of appetite, vomiting and sometimes a skin rash. JAUNDICE, HEART FAILURE and MENINGITIS may occur and are signs of danger. The mortality in such cases may be as high as 20%. Those who recover do so completely. The organisms are sensitive to penicillin and this drug is effective, if given early. Also knows as Weil's disease. (H. Adolph Weil, German physician, 1848–1916).

lercanidipine a calcium channel blocker drug used to treat high blood pressure (HYPERTENSION). A brand name is Zanidip.

lesbianism female homosexuality. Long-term stable lesbian relationships are common, as in male homosexuality. The term comes from the Greek female poet *Sappho*, who lived on the island of Lesbos with her followers during the 7th century BC.

Lesch-Nyhan syndrome a rare X-linked recessive disease of male children in which a severe over-production of uric acid causes gout, CEREBRAL PALSY, mental retardation, CHOREA and compulsive self-mutilating biting. The disease is due to a deficiency of the enzyme hypoxanthine-guanine phosphoribosyl transferase. (Michael Lesch, American cardiologist, b. 1939, and William Leo Nyhan, American paediatrician, b. 1926).

Lescol a brand name for FLUVASTATIN.

lesion a useful and widely used medical term meaning any injury, wound, infection, or any structural or other form of abnormality anywhere in the body. Doctors would be at a loss without this term, but it is commonly wrongly regarded by lay people as implying some specific condition such as an adhesion. The word is derived from the Latin *laesio*, an attack or injury.

lethal injection an increasingly widely-used method of execution of condemned criminals. Since the method involves intravenous skills rarely available to non-medical people, doctors are commonly asked to advise or even participate – which few, if any, can contemplate without revulsion.

lethal mutation a mutation whose effect is so serious that the cell is killed. Lethal mutations will often result in the death of the organism concerned.

lethargy an abnormal state of apathy, sleepiness, drowsiness or lack of energy. Lethargy may be due to organic brain disease or to DEPRESSION. In Greek mythology the river Lethe flowed through Hades and the dead were required to drink its water so as to forget their past lives.

letrozole an AROMATASE INHIBITOR drug used to treat breast cancer in menopausal women that has resisted anti-oestrogen drugs. A brand name is Femara.

Letterer-Siwe disease a fatal disease of infants in which there is fever, generalized lymph node, liver and spleen enlargement, an eczematous skin rash and anaemia. The condition is brought about by an enormous increase in the number of antigen-presenting cells of the immune system known as Langerhans cells. These produce grossly excessive CYTOKINES resulting in great proliferation. The mortality varies but may be as high as 50%. Experts argue as to whether or not the condition is a form of cancer. The preferred name for the condition is now Langerhans cell histiocytosis. (Erich Letterer, German pathologist, b. 1895, and Sture August Siwe, Swedish paediatrician, b. 1897).

leuc-, leuco-, leuk-, leuko- *combining form denoting* white or LEUCOCYTE.

leucapheresis a method of harvesting white cells from a compatible donor for the treatment of uncontrollable infection in a patient with acute LEUKAEMIA. White cells for this purpose can be obtained from patients with chronic granulocytic leukaemia.

leucine one of the essential AMINO ACIDS.

leucoblast an immature white blood cell.

leucocyte any kind of white blood cell. The leukocytes include the neutrophil POLYMORPHONUCLEAR LEUKOCYTES ('Polymorphs'), EOSINOPHILS, BASOPHILS, LYMPHOCYTES and MACROPHAGES.

leucocytosis an increased concentration of white cells (LEUKOCYTES) in the blood other than one caused by one of the LEUKAEMIAS. Leukocytosis is an important indication that an inflammatory, usually infective process is occurring somewhere in the body.

leucoderma lack of normal skin pigmentation causing abnormally white skin, usually in patches. See ALBINISM, PIEBALDISM and VITILIGO.

leucodystrophies a group of conditions featuring degeneration of the white matter of the central nervous system with DEMYELINATION. Most are due to genetic errors of fat (lipid) metabolism. The leucodystrophies lead to widespread paralysis, muscle contracture and progressive DEMENTIA.

leucoencephalopathy a rare disorder occurring in the late stages of LYMPHOMA or other cancers. Scattered throughout the brain are areas of DEMYELINATION with changes in the supporting (glial) cells characteristic of PAPOVA VIRUS infection. The resulting damage to nerve function causes widespread effects including paralysis, speech and visual defects, DEMENTIA and convulsions and the condition is fatal within a matter of weeks.

leucoerythroblastosis a condition in which primitive blood cells of both the red and white series are present in the circulation. This indicates a major disturbance of the bone marrow blood forming function and is seen in ANAEMIA, bone marrow cancer and MYELOFIBROSIS.

leucoma a dense, white opacity of the CORNEA resulting from disease or injury. A leucoma near the centre of the cornea causes blindness, but vision can be restored by corneal grafting.

Leucomax a brand name for MOLGRAMOSTIN.

leuconychia white discoloration of, or white patches in, the fingernails.

leucopenia an abnormal reduction in the number of circulating leucocytes.

leucorrhoea any whitish VAGINAL DISCHARGE containing mucus and pus cells. Leucorrhoea is purely descriptive and is not a specific disease.

leukaemias a group of blood disorders in which white blood cells reproduce in a disorganized and uncontrolled way and progressively displace the normal constituents of the blood. The leukaemias are a form of cancer (neoplasia) and unless effectively treated are usually fatal. Death occurs from a shortage

of red blood cells (ANAEMIA), or from severe bleeding or from infection. The different types of leukaemia arise from different white cell types and have different outlooks. In most cases the cause is unknown but there are definite associations with radiation, with certain viruses, with some anticancer drugs and with some industrial chemicals such as benzene. Treatment is, at present, primarily by chemotherapy. Removal of the spleen may help. Blood transfusions and antibiotics are commonly required. Other treatments include RADIOTHERAPY, white cell transfusions, bone marrow transfusion after total body radiation, bone marrow removal, treatment to destroy malignant cells and its replacement. Some of these methods are still experimental.

Leukeran a brand name for CHLORAMBUCIL.

leukoplakia a thickened white patch occurring on a mucous membrane, especially inside the mouth, on the lips or on the female genitalia. Leukoplakia is a response to long-term irritation and is a PRECANCEROUS condition that should never be ignored.

leukorrhoea see VAGINAL DISCHARGE, LEUCORRHOEA.

leukotrienes powerful chemical agents released by MAST CELLS, basophil cells and MACROPHAGES and involved in many allergic and other immunological reactions. Leukotrienes are derived from ARACHIDONIC ACID and cause CHEMOTAXIS and increase the leakiness of small blood vessels. In asthma they cause the narrowing of the air passages and the secretion of mucus. They can be inhibited by corticosteroid drugs.

leukotriene receptor antagonists drugs that prevent the action of LEUKOTRIENES by blocking their receptors on cell membranes, such as those of smooth muscle. These drugs have a useful dual effect in relaxing the smooth muscle of the air passages (bronchi) and in combatting inflammation in the bronchial linings – both features of ASTHMA. They have also been found useful in hay fever. Examples are montelukast (Singulair) and zafirlukast (Accolate).

leuprorelin a GONADOTROPHIN-releasing hormone drug used to treat ENDOMETRIOSIS in women and PROSTATE CANCER in men. In prostate cancer, the effect of leuprorelin is said to be equivalent to that of orchiectomy, and disease progression is prevented in up to 95% of patients. A brand name is Prostap.

levallorphan a morphine-related drug that acts as a morphine antagonist and is used to treat morphine poisoning, especially when this is causing dangerous depression of respiration.

levamisole an ANTHELMINTIC drug used to remove roundworms. It has also been found to have an unexpected effect in stimulating the immune system by increasing T cell responsiveness and encouraging the activity of polymorphonuclear LEUCOCYTES and MACROPHAGES. It is effective in RHEUMATOID ARTHRITIS. Adverse side effects limit its use. The drug is on the WHO official list.

levator 1 any muscle that acts to raise a part of the body.
2 an elevator. A surgical instrument used to prize up a depressed piece of bone as after a fracture of ZYGOMA or skull.

LeVeen shunt a valved plastic tube used to drain accumulated fluid in the peritoneal cavity (ascites) directly into a main vein. (Harry LeVeen, American surgeon, b. 1914).

Levitra a brand name for VARDENAFIL.

levobunolol a beta-blocker drug used in the form of eye drops to treat chronic simple GLAUCOMA. A brand name is Betagan.

levocabastine an ANTIHISTAMINE drug formulated as eye and nasal drops for the treatment of allergic CONJUNCTIVITIS and hay fever. A brand name is Livostin.

levocarnitine a nitrogenous muscle constituent necessary for the transport of long-chain fatty acids across the inner mitochondrial membrane. It is used as a drug to correct a deficiency of carnitine in people on dialysis. A brand name is Carnitor.

levodopa L-dopa. A drug used in the treatment of PARKINSON'S DISEASE. Levodopa relieves symptoms in the majority of cases and often effects a remarkable reduction in disability. Brand names of the drug, in combination, respectively, with benserazide and carbidopa, are Madopar and Sinemet.

levodopa with carbidopa DOPAMINE precursor drugs used to treat PARKINSON'S DISEASE. The drug combination is on the WHO official list. A brand name is Sinemet.

levofloxacin an ANTIBIOTIC used to treat mild to moderately severe respiratory and urinary tract infections. The drug is on the WHO official list. A brand name is Tavanic.

Levonelle-2 a LEVONORGESTREL (progestogen-only) drug used as an emergency contraceptive. The two-tablet course must be started as soon as possible, but within 72 hours of unprotected sexual intercourse or known failure of another method of contraception. The second tablet must be taken at an interval of 12 to 16 hours.

levonorgestrel a PROGESTOGEN drug used in oral contraceptives. The drug is on the WHO official list. Brand names of the progestogen-only product are Microval, Mirena, Norgeston and Norplant. It is also formulated with ETHINYLOESTRADIOL (ethinylestradiol) as an oral contraceptive under such brand names as Eugynon 30, Eugynon 30, Microgynon 30, Microgynon 30 ED, Ovran, Ovranette, Schering PC4 and Trinordiol.

levothyroxine THYROID hormone as a sodium salt used to treat hypothyroidism. The drug is on the WHO official list. A brand name is Thyronine.

Lewy bodies abnormal intracellular proteins that occur in the nerve cells of the cerebral cortex, basal ganglia and pigmented brainstem neurons, causing PARKINSONISM. If present in large quantities they as associated with dementia (diffuse Lewy body disease). (Frederic H. Lewy 1885–1950, US neurologist of German origin).

libido sexual desire or its manifestations. In psychoanalytic theory, the term is used more generally to mean the psychic and emotional energy associated with instinctual biological drives.

Libman-Sacks endocarditis a condition in which warty growths, discernible on ECHOCARDIOGRAPHY develop on the heart lining and especially on the valves. Unlike most forms of endocarditis these growths are not associated with bacterial infection. They are a feature of SYSTEMIC LUPUS ERYTHEMATOSUS (SLE). (Emanuel Libman, American physician, 1872–1946, and Benjamin Sacks, 1896–1939, American physician).

Librium a brand name for CHLORDIAZEPOXIDE.

LicAc abbrev. for Licentiate in Acupuncture.

lice small, wingless, insect parasites of humans. There are three kinds of human lice – the head louse, *Pediculus humanus capitis*, that lives on the scalp and feeds by sucking blood, the body louse, *Pediculus humanus corporis*, that lives in the seams of clothing close to the skin and move on to the body only to feed, and the crab louse, *Phthirius pubis*, that infests the pubic hair and, occasionally, the chest hair, armpit hair or eyebrows. *Phthirius pubis* is usually transmitted by sexual contact. Body lice transmit epidemic TYPHUS and RELAPSING FEVER.

lichen any skin eruption.

lichenification hardening and thickening of the skin so as to produce the condition of LICHEN SIMPLEX.

lichen planus an uncommon skin disease featuring small, intensely itchy, slightly raised, reddish-purple patches that enlarge and run together to form flat-topped plaques up to 2 cm in diameter. They are usually found on the fronts of the wrists and forearms, the sides of the calves and ankles and the lower back. The cause is unknown. Lichen planus usually clears up within 2 years. Itching can be relieved by hydrocortisone ointment.

lichen sclerosus a form of skin atrophy affecting the vulva in women and occasionally other areas. The skin becomes white, glazed and sometimes severely shrunken and even ulcerated. Although usually painless, the condition may cause itching and sometimes pain. In about 5% of severe cases occurring after puberty, the condition progresses to vulval cancer, sometimes after it has been present for 20 years or more. Treatment is by local steroid ointment for a limited time, and sometimes surgery.

lichen simplex hardened and thickened skin epidermis caused by abnormally persistent scratching. This is usually a response to some long-term (chronic) skin condition but may be the result of mental agitation and the establishment of a scratch-itch-scratch-itch cycle. Lichenification soon disappears if scratching can be avoided.

lid lag the failure of the normal downward following movement of the upper lids on looking downward. Lid lag causes a strange staring appearance. It is a feature of undue protrusion of the eyes (EXOPHTHALMOS) and occurs in overactivity of the thyroid gland (THYROTOXICOSIS).

lidocaine LIGNOCAINE or Xylocaine. The drug is on the WHO official list.

Lidothesin LIDOCAINE or Xylocaine.

lie the position or attitude of the fetus in the womb in relation to the long axis of the mother's body. Lie may be longitudinal (normal) or transverse.

lie detector a popular terms for the polygraph – a collection of devices used to monitor and record various parameters of the body, such as the pulse rate, the blood pressure, the evenness and rate of breathing and the moistness, and hence the electrical resistance, of the skin. These vary with the state of the emotions and the results can be thought to cast light on significance to the subject of certain questions or statements. Emotional responses do not, however, necessarily indicate that the subject is lying or concealing the truth. Lie detection is a function of the interpreter, not the machine and it is the sensitivity, intelligence, imagination and experience of the operator that determines the forensic value of the procedure. This should always be challenged if lie detector evidence is used in court.

lienal pertaining to the SPLEEN.

lienorenal pertaining to the spleen and kidney.

life expectancy a statistical estimate of the number of years a person, of any particular age, is likely to live.

life support system medical equipment used to maintain respiration or the heart action, and possibly nutrition, in a person unable to survive without such support.

ligamentous 1 of the characteristics of LIGAMENTS.

2 pertaining to a ligament or ligaments.

ligaments bundles of a tough, fibrous, elastic protein called COLLAGEN that act as binding and supporting materials in the body, especially in and around JOINTS of all kinds. Ligaments are flexible but very strong and, if excessively strained, may pull off a fragment of bone at their attachment.

ligand a MOLECULE or ION that binds to a central chemical entity. A general term for any molecule that is recognized by a surface receptor.

ligase an ENZYME that promotes the linkage of chemical groups. Also known as a synthetase.

ligation the surgical process in which a string (LIGATURE) is placed tightly around a tissue and tied. This is most commonly done to tie off a blood vessel to prevent bleeding, or to close a duct. Tubal ligation is a form of female sterilization in which the Fallopian tubes are tied off.

ligator a surgical instrument used to facilitate LIGATION of inaccessible blood vessels.

ligature any thread-like surgical material tied tightly round any structure. Ligatures are commonly made of absorbable material, such as catgut or collagen, but may be non-absorbable.

light chains the short polypeptide chains that form the outer parts of the upper arms of the Y-shaped ANTIBODY molecule. The light chains of all antibodies have one length (domain) that is the same for all (the constant domain) and one terminal domain that varies in its amino acid sequence (the variable domain). A domain is a single loop of about 110 amino acids. See also HEAVY CHAINS.

lightening the sense of relief felt, during the last three or four weeks of pregnancy, with the descent of the presenting part of the fetus, usually the head, more deeply into the pelvis so that the womb occupies a smaller volume of the abdomen. This reduces abdominal distention and occasions some easing of breathing and general discomfort. Lightening is usual in first pregnancies but may not be apparent later.

lightning pains severe, shooting, stabbing pains in the legs and sometimes around the trunk occurring in the syphilitic condition of TABES DORSALIS. These are due to damage to the roots of the sensory nerves in the lower back and lumbar regions.

lignocaine LIDOCAINE, a widely used local anaesthetic drug which may be given by injection or as a topical application. It is also used by intravenous injection in the treatment or prevention of acute disorders of heart rhythm such as VENTRICULAR TACHYCARDIA and VENTRICULAR FIBRILLATION.

LIHSM *abbrev. for* Licentiate of the Institute of Health Services Management.

limbic system a centrally situated, ring-shaped structure in the brain consisting of a number of interconnected nerve cell nuclei. The limbic system represents much of what constitutes the brain in the lower mammals and is concerned with unconscious and automatic (autonomic) functions such as respiration, body temperature, hunger, thirst, wakefulness, sexual activity and their associated emotional reactions. Diseases of the limbic system cause emotional disturbances, and these can include emotional lability, forced or spasmodic laughing and crying, aggression, anger,

violence, placidity, apathy, anxiety, fear, depression and diminished sexual interest.

limbal pertaining to the LIMBUS.

limbus an edge or distinct border, especially the margin of the CORNEA.

Limclair a brand name for TRISODIUM EDETATE.

lincosamides a group of ANTIBIOTICS reserved for serious infections with ANAEROBIC and other organisms. They may have serious side effects. An example is CLINDAMYCIN (Dalactin, Dalactin C, Dalactin D and Zindaclin). Clindamycin as a cream can be used locally to treat ACNE.

linea a line.

linea alba the central strip of white FASCIA running down the front wall of the abdomen from the bottom of the breastbone (STERNUM) to the PUBIS.

linear accelerator a machine that uses high voltages to accelerate particles so that they can be used in RADIOTHERAPY.

linear epitope a section of a protein, consisting of a sequence of amino acids, to which an antibody can bind. Compare CONFORMATIONAL EPITOPE.

linear regression a statistical method of predicting the value of one variable, given the other, in a situation in which a CORRELATION is known to be significant. The equation is $y = a + bx$ in which x and y are, respectively, the independent and dependent variables and a and b are constants. This is an equation for a straight line.

lingam a symbol for the penis in Indian religion. The Hindu phallic image of the god Siva. See also YONI.

Lingraine a brand name for ERGOTAMINE TARTRATE.

lingual pertaining to, or pronounced with, the tongue.

lingual artery a branch of the external CAROTID artery that runs forward underneath the tongue to supply the tongue muscles.

lingual nerve a sensory nerve providing sensation to the inside of the jaw and tongue. It is a branch of the mandibular nerve – the lower of the three divisions of the great sensory nerve of the face, the trigeminal nerve.

lingula any tongue-shaped structure or process.

lingular tongue-shaped.

liniment an irritating fluid rubbed into the skin to promote a mild inflammatory increase in the blood supply to the underlying tissues.

Liniments are of limited therapeutic value, but usually have an impressive smell.

linitis inflammation of the layer of the stomach wall below the mucous membrane lining. Linitis plastica, or leather bottle stomach, is a spread in this area of fibrous tissue as a response to cancer of the stomach. The outlook in this condition is poor.

Lioresal a brand name for BACLOFEN.

liothyronine sodium a thyroid hormone preparation used to treat severe thyroid hormone deficiency. A brand name is Tertroxin.

linin the delicate, thread-like material in the cell nucleus to which chromatin granules appear to be attached.

linkage 1 the location of genes on the same CHROMOSOME so that the characteristics they determine tend to remain associated.
2 the tendency of genes to remain together during recombination. This is proportional to their proximity to each other. Sex linkage simply implies that the particular gene is located on an X or a Y chromosome.
3 the force that holds atoms together in a molecule.

linkage disequilibrium the occurrence of combination of genes (linkages) in a population more often, or less often, than would be expected from their distance apart in the genome.

linkage map a CHROMOSOME map showing the relative positions of known genes.

Linnaean pertaining to the system of taxonomic classification and the binomial nomenclature widely used in medicine, in which the name of the genus (generic name) is followed by the name of the species (specific name). Examples are *Staphylococcus aureus* and *Fasciola hepatica*. (Carolus Linnaeus, or Carl von Linne, 1707–78, Swedish biologist)

linoleic acid the principle fatty acid in plant seed oils. An essential polyunsaturated fatty acid, interconvertible with LINOLENIC ACID and arachidonic acid and needed for cell membranes and the synthesis of PROSTAGLANDINS. It is plentiful in vegetable fats. Essential fatty acid dietary deficiency is rare.

linolenic acid an essential fatty acid. Like LINOLEIC and arachidonic acids it is polyunsaturated and found in vegetable oils and wheat germ.

linsidomine a NITRIC OXIDE donor drug which, with a similar compound molsidomine, has

been studies as a possible treatment to improve the outlook in cases of heart attack. Regrettably there was no significant difference in effects between these drugs and a placebo.

lip-, lipo- *combining form denoting* fat or lipid.

lipaemia an increase in amount of emulsified fat in the blood, causing undue turbidity of the PLASMA.

Lipantil Micro a brand name for FENOFIBRATE.

lipase an enzyme that catalyzes the breakdown (hydrolysis) of fat molecules to glycerol and fatty acids.

lipase inhibitors drugs used to treat obesity in patients with a body mass index (BMI) of greater than 30. An example is orlistat (Xenical).

lipectomy fat removal, usually by suction. A form of cosmetic plastic surgery designed to improve body contours. Small incisions are made in the skin and a blunt-ended metal sucker is passed through and moved around under the skin to suck out fat cells. Human frailty being what it is, the effect is usually temporary.

lipidosis any disorder of fat metabolism featuring a generalized deposition of lipids in RETICULOENDOTHELIAL SYSTEM cells. Also known as lipid storage disease. See also GAUCHER'S DISEASE and NIEMANN-PICK DISEASE.

lipid profile a clinical chemistry assessment of the levels of fats in a patient's blood. The measurements include total cholesterol, total triglycerides, high- and low-density lipoproteins, and sometimes apolipoprotein E.

lipids see FATS.

Lipitor a brand name for ATORVASTATIN. See STATINS.

lipoatrophy local shrinkage and loss of the fat under the skin often caused by repeated injections of insulin into the same area in diabetics.

lipochromes natural fatty pigments, such as carotene or LIPOFUSCIN.

Lipocream a brand name for HYDROCORTISONE.

lipodystrophy a condition of disordered fat metabolism. There may be abnormal breakdown of fats with loss of weight, excessive levels of fats in the blood, raised blood sugar levels, enlargement of the liver and abnormal thyroid gland function. In some cases there is breakdown of fat from the upper part of the body and abnormal deposition around the buttocks and thighs. The condition can be caused by prolonged multiple antiretroviral therapy.

lipofuscin a golden-brown pigment that occurs in granules in muscle and nerve cells in numbers proportional to the age of the individual. Also known as age pigment.

lipogranulomatosis a rare metabolic disease in which the absence of an enzyme results in the accumulation of fatty material (ceramides and gangliosides) in nerve cells. This causes severe brain damage and death usually by the age of 2.

lipolysis lipid breakdown (HYDROLYSIS) into free fatty acids and glycerol under the influence of LIPASE. This is increased in DIABETES. Also known as adipolysis.

lipolytic pertaining to the breakdown of fat (LIPOLYSIS).

lipoma a non-malignant tumour of fatty tissue. Lipomas may occur in fat anywhere in the body and grow slowly to form soft, smooth swellings. They seldom cause problems but can be removed if disfiguring.

lipomatosis the condition of having many LIPOMAS.

lipomatous pertaining to a LIPOMA.

lipoproteins any complex of fats with protein. A conjugated protein consisting of a simple protein combined with a fat (lipid) group. The blood lipoproteins, which are the cholesterol carriers of the body, are classified by density, in accordance with the proportions of protein, as very low density (VLDL), low density (LDL) and high density (HDL). LDLs contain relatively large amounts of cholesterol. HDLs contain 50% of protein and only 20% of cholesterol. LDLs transport lipids to muscles and to fat stores and are associated with the arterial disease ATHEROSCLEROSIS and thus heart disease and STROKE. HDLs are protective against these diseases because their main role is to transport cholesterol from the periphery back to the liver. They also carry paraoxanase enzymes that limit oxidative modification of LDLs necessary before cholesterol can be laid down in arterial walls. Blood concentration of HDL cholesterol shows a strong inverse correlation with the risk of coronary heart disease.

liposarcoma a very rare malignant tumour of fatty tissue. Liposarcomas usually occur in the fat on the inside of the back wall of the abdomen or in the MEDIASTINUM of elderly people.

Liposic a brand name for CARBOMER.

Lipostat a brand name for PRAVASTATIN. See STATINS.

lipping the formation of a curled edge at the bearing joint surface of a bone in OSTEOARTHRITIS and other degenerative bone disease.

lip-print the lip analogue of the fingerprint. Lip-prints are much less reliable as means of identification because, unlike fingerprints, they change with age.

lipreading a means of communication with the deaf. English speech involves more than forty distinct sounds but less than ten visibly distinguishable mouth patterns can be reliably identified. Other facial, bodily and contextual clues are, however, provided and a skilled lipreader can often discern or infer 60% of spoken information.

Liquifilm Tears a brand name for artificial tears containing polyvinyl alcohol.

lisinopril an ANGIOTENSIN CONVERTING ENZYME inhibitor drug use to treat HEART FAILURE and high blood pressure (HYPERTENSION). Brand names are Carace and Zestril and, in conjunction with a thiazide diuretic, Carace 10 Plus and Zestoretic.

Liskonum a brand name for LITHIUM.

lisp an anomaly in the production of 'sssss' sounds (sibilants) in speech in which the tip of the tongue is protruded between the teeth instead of being placed high and close to the hard palate behind the upper front teeth. The lisp is largely under voluntary control and can be corrected by speech therapy.

listeriosis an infection with the organism, *Listeria monocytogenes*, which is found in most meats, poultry, fish, crustaceans and in soft cheeses and various precooked foods. Proper cooking will kill the organism which, however, varies considerably in its ability to cause disease (virulence). Listeriosis is commonest in babies and old people and most cases are mild and pass unremarked. Severe cases feature fever, CONJUNCTIVITIS, inflammation of the salivary glands as in mumps, sometimes skin pustules and, rarely, arthritis, bone inflammation and abscesses in the brain and spinal cord. Listeriosis responds well to PENICILLIN, ERYTHROMYCIN and TETRACYCLINE.

Litarex a brand name for LITHIUM.

-lith *suffix denoting* stone, as in FAECALITH.

lithiasis the formation of stones (calculi)

anywhere in the body, but especially in the urinary and bile secretion and storage systems.

lithium an element, the lightest known solid, used as the citrate or carbonate for the control of MANIC DEPRESSIVE states. Lithium is also used as the succinate in ointments for the treatment of seborrhoeic dermatitis and in shampoos for the control of dandruff. The drug is on the WHO official list. Brand names are Camcolit, Li-liquid, Liskonum, Litarex and Priadel. A preparation for external use is Efalith.

litho- *combining form denoting* stone.

lithopaedion lithopedion, a dead fetus, sometimes of full-term development, that has been retained in the womb, or in the abdominal cavity, and eventually calcifies. Literally, a 'stone child', lithopaedion is a very rare phenomenon. There is a recorded case of a woman of 69 who had carried her lithopaedion in her womb for 28 years.

lithotomy a now abandoned surgical operation for bladder stone. It was originally performed through the floor of the pelvis via an incision along the crease at the inside of the top of the thigh. A successful cut was rewarded by a gush of urine and blood and the appearance of the stone. The more refined modern lithotomy operations have, in turn, now largely been replaced by LITHOTRIPSY.

lithotomy position the position in which a patient is placed for gynaecological operations or for any surgical procedure on the PERINEUM. The patient lies on his or her back with the knees up and the thighs spread wide. The feet and thighs are usually supported in slings.

lithotripsy a method of fragmenting stones in the urinary system and in the gall bladder, by focused and concentrated ultrasonic shock waves. High energy ultrasound waves, generated by a high-voltage spark discharge, can be focused to a point by parabolic reflectors and aimed so that the point of focus coincides with the stone. The stone shatters and is reduced to particles small enough to be passed naturally in the urine or into the bile duct and bowel. Up to 90% of stones, which previously could have been removed only by open surgery, can now be dealt with by this method.

lithotrite a surgical instrument used to crush stones within the body so as to allow easy or spontaneous removal.

lithotrity a surgical operation involving the crushing of stones in the bladder or external urine passage (URETHRA).

litmus a powder derived from certain lichens that contains the natural dye azolitmin. This turns red in an acidic medium at pH below 4.5 and blue at an alkaline pH above 8.3. Paper strips impregnated with litmus form convenient indicators for checking urine acidity.

Little's disease a common form of spastic paralysis (CEREBRAL PALSY) (William John Little, 1810–94, English surgeon).

live attenuated vaccines vaccines containing live viruses and other organisms that have been rendered safe by chemical or other means. They include vaccines against measles, mumps and rubella (M-M-R II, Priorix), rubella alone (Erevax), yellow fever (Arilvax), chickenpox (Varilrix), tuberculosis (BCH vaccine) and poliomyelitis.

livedo reticularis an irregular, mottling of the legs in a wide-mesh, fishnet pattern which occurs in CUSHING'S SYNDROME and various collagen diseases. A similar brownish mottling, called erythema ab igne, used to be common in women who sat too close to the fireplace.

liver the largest organ of the ABDOMEN occupying the upper right corner and extending across the midline to the left side. It is wedge-shaped, with the thin edge pointing to the left, of a spongy consistency, reddish-brown in colour and moulded to fit under the domed DIAPHRAGM so that most of it lies behind the ribs. The liver receives chemical substances in the blood, especially in the nutrient-rich blood from the intestines (glucose, amino acids, fats, minerals and vitamins) and processes these according to the needs of the body. It takes up the products of old red blood cells and converts these into a pigment, bilirubin, which together with other substances, form the bile. It breaks down toxic substances into safer forms. Ammonia produced from protein breakdown is converted into urea, which is excreted in the urine. Alcohol and other drugs are altered to safer forms. To a remarkable degree, the liver is able to regenerate itself after disease, toxic damage or injury. But if this capacity is exceeded, functional liver cells form nodules and are replaced by inert fibrous tissue (CIRRHOSIS) and the whole function of the body is severely affected.

liver abscess a walled-off collection of pus in

the liver, usually from the spread of AMOEBIASIS of the large intestine, but also from spread of infection from APPENDICITIS, DIVERTICULITIS, pelvic inflammation or gall bladder disease. There is high fever, tenderness over the liver, pain in the upper right corner of the abdomen and prostration. Liver abscesses must be drained surgically and the original cause treated.

liver biopsy the taking of a small core of liver tissue by means of a special cutting needle introduced between the lower ribs on the right side, under local anaesthesia. The method allows precise diagnosis to be made, by microscopic examination, of a wide range of liver disorders such as CIRRHOSIS, the different kinds of HEPATITIS and JAUNDICE, the damage caused by drugs, and the various forms of cancer, including LYMPHOMAS.

liver cancer malignant disease, primary or secondary, affecting the liver. Secondary cancer, spread from a primary site elsewhere, is very common. Primary cancer originating in the liver is rare in Britain. In many tropical areas primary liver cancer is common. This is believed to be due to the association of chronic HEPATITIS B infections, liver CIRRHOSIS, and ingestion of food contaminated with the fungus *Aspergillus flavus*, which produces the poison AFLATOXIN.

liver, cirrhosis of see CIRRHOSIS OF THE LIVER.

liver extract a former, crude but effective, treatment for PERNICIOUS ANAEMIA, now superseded by the active principle hydroxycobalamin.

liver failure the end stage of severe liver disease in which liver function is so impaired that it cannot meet the metabolic needs of the body. There is JAUNDICE, an accumulation of toxic substances in the blood such as ammonia, fatty acids and nitrogenous compounds causing a sweet musty odour in the breath, nausea and vomiting and brain damage with restlessness, disorientation, coarse tremor of the hands, sometimes aggressive outbursts, convulsions, weakness, coma and death.

liver fluke one of several types of flatworm (trematode) which can gain access to the liver by way of the bile duct and cause a feverish illness with liver tenderness and enlargement. The common form of liver fluke, *Fasciola hepatica*, is a parasite of sheep which produces

eggs that are passed in the sheep faeces. The intermediate host is an aquatic snail from which further larvae are released to congregate on the leaves of water plants such as cress or water-chestnut. If these are eaten by humans, the infestation may be acquired. Diagnosis is by microscopic identification of the fluke eggs in the stools. ANTHELMINTIC drugs are used to kill the worms.

liver spot a popular term used to describe various skin blemishes including LENTIGENES, spots sometimes known as Pityrosporon versicolor, caused by the skin yeast fungus MALASSEZIA FURFUR, or the SPIDER NAEVUS, which is the only one with any connection with the liver.

liver transplant the introduction of a donated liver or liver segment into the body of a person suffering from liver failure. Organ rejection is prevented by triple therapy with CYCLOSPORIN (ciclosporin), prednisolone and AZATHIOPRINE and about three-quarters of patients have an acceptable outcome. Failures are mainly due to infection or multi-organ failure. The first liver transplant in Britain was performed in 1968 by Professor Sir Roy Calne one of the great pioneers of modern British surgery.

Livial a brand name for TIBOLONE.

livid black or bluish-black discoloration from accumulation of free blood in the tissues. Bruised or 'black-and-blue'. Post mortem lividity is the extensive bruising seen in the dependent areas of the body, indicating the position in the first 8–12 hours after death.

living will a document requesting and directing what should be done in the event of a person's later inability to express his or her wishes on medical management. The purpose is usually to try to ensure that exceptional measures are not taken to maintain life in the event of a terminal illness. The respecting of such a will has long been accepted in most States in the USA and has, since January 1998, also been a statutory right in Britain. The term refers to the fact that the writer's deposition may be enacted when he or she is still living. The Voluntary Euthanasia Society has recently produced a new draft that will also provide an opportunity for the patient to express the desire to be kept alive for as long as is reasonably possible.

Livostin a brand name for LEVOCABASTINE.

LLCO *abbrev. for* Licentiate of the London

College of Osteopathy.

LLCOM *abbrev. for* Licentiate of the London College of Osteopathic Medicine.

LM *abbrev. for* Licentiate in Midwifery.

LMC *abbrev. for* Local Medical Committee.

LMCC *abbrev. for* Licentiate of the Medical Council of Canada.

LMP *abbrev. for* last menstrual period.

LMS *abbrev. for* Licentiate in Medicine and Surgery.

LMSSA *abbrev. for* Licentiate in Medicine and Surgery of the Society of Apothecaries of London.

LOA *abbrev. for* left occipitoanterior, a common position of the fetus in the womb, with the head down and the back of the head pointing to the front and a little to the left.

Loa loa a filarial worm, known as the African eye worm. 2.5–6 cm long the worms are acquired by the bite of the *Chrysops* fly and may live in the tissues under the skin for over 15 years, causing Calabar swellings. Occasionally a worm can be observed passing across the white of the eye under the CONJUNCTIVA. See also LOIASIS.

lobar pneumonia an acute inflammation of one or more lobes of the lung caused by the organism Streptococcus pneumoniae. The onset is sudden with high fever, vomiting or convulsions in children; chest pain, especially on breathing; a cough, at first dry then with much rusty-coloured sputum; rapid breathing; flushed face; and often cold sores around the mouth or nose. The condition responds well to antibiotics. Also known as pneumococcal pneumonia.

lobe a well-defined subdivision of an organ. Many organs, such as the brain, the lung, the liver, the pituitary, the thyroid gland and the prostate gland, are divided into lobes.

lobectomy surgical removal of a lobe.

lobeline a mixture of alkaloids with action similar to nicotine. Lobeline is derived from plants of the *Lobelia* genus and has been used as a respiratory stimulant, but is of little medical importance.

lobotomy, prefrontal see PREFRONTAL LEUKOTOMY.

lobule a small LOBE or subdivision of a lobe.

Locabiotal a brand name for FUSAFUNGINE.

local anaesthetic an ANAESTHETIC affecting only part of the body and not affecting

consciousness. Local anaesthetics may be applied, usually by injection, directly to the part to be operated upon, or may be applied, at a distance, to the sensory nerves coming from the part (nerve block).

Loceryl a brand name for AMOROLFINE.

lochia the discharge of blood, mucus and particles of tissue from the womb, mainly coming from site of the afterbirth (PLACENTA), during the first 2 or 3 weeks after birth. The discharge is red for the first 3 or 4 days and usually disappears by about the tenth day. Offensive-smelling lochia suggests infection and is a danger sign.

locked-in syndrome a state of total paralysis, except for eye movements, in which the victim remains conscious and able to communicate by eye movement codes. This nightmarish situation usually results from a basilar artery haemorrhage or thrombosis, or other damage, affecting the ventral pons with preservation of the dorsal tegmental area. This destroys almost all motor function, but leaves the higher mental functions intact. Compare PERSISTENT VEGETATIVE STATE.

lockjaw a lay term for uncontrollable contraction (spasm) of the powerful chewing muscles that occurs in established TETANUS. The spasm clamps the teeth together so that they can barely be separated. The medical term is trismus.

Locoid a brand name for HYDROCORTISONE.

Locoid C a brand name for a preparation for external use containing HYDROCORTISONE and CHLORQUINALDOL.

locomotor pertaining to the function of voluntary movement.

locomotor ataxia see TABES DORSALIS.

Locorten-Vioform a brand name for FLUMETHASONE (flumetasone) combined with an antibacterial drug Vioform (clinoquinol).

loculated divided into small spaces, compartments or cavities.

locum tenens a person, especially a doctor, who substitutes for another for a period of days, weeks or months. The term is usually abbreviated to 'locum'. The phrase is Latin for holding a place.

locus the position on a chromosome at which the gene for a particular characteristic resides. The plural is loci. A locus can contain any of the ALLELES of the gene.

Lodine a brand name for ETODOLAC.

Iodoxamide a mast cell-stabilizing drug that prevents the release of HISTAMINE in allergic conditions, formulated as eye drops for the treatment of allergic CONJUNCTIVITIS. A brand name is Aldomide.

Loeffler's syndrome a form of patchy pneumonia featuring fever, cough, difficulty in breathing, associated with a marked rise in the numbers of EOSINOPHIL white cells in the lungs and the circulating blood. (Wilhelm Loeffler, Swiss physician, b. 1887).

Loestrin 20 a brand name for an oral contraceptive containing ETHINYLOESTRADIOL (ethinylestradiol) and NORETHISTERONE. See also CONTRACEPTION.

lofepramine a TRICYCLIC ANTIDEPRESSANT DRUG. A brand name is Gamanil.

lofexidine a drug used to control withdrawal symptoms during OPIATE detoxification. A brand name is Britloflex.

logarithmic growth phase the stage of growth in which cells are doubling in number during consecutive equal lengths of time. This rapidly leads to an enormous increase in the number of cells.

logo- *combining form denoting* word or speech.

logorrhoea an abnormal flow of words, some or all of which may be meaningless or invented (neologisms). Severe logorrhoea may amount to logomania. See also JARGON.

-logy *suffix denoting* study, science, theory, thesis or creed.

Logynon, Logynon ED brand names for oral contraceptives containing ETHINYLOESTRADIOL (ethinylestradiol) and LEVONORGESTREL.

loiasis a type of FILARIASIS caused by the microfilarial worm parasite *Loa loa*. The disease occurs in Central and West Africa and features prominent lumps under the skin (Calabar swellings) caused by inflammatory reaction to the migrating worms. The adult worm sometimes appears under the CONJUNCTIVA of the eye. Also known as eye worm.

loin the soft tissue of the back, on either side of the spine, between the lowest ribs and the pelvis. Compare GROIN.

Lomotil a brand name for a mixture of DIPHENOXYLATE and ATROPINE.

longsightedness see HYPERMETROPIA.

Loniten a brand name for MINOXIDIL.

long-QT syndrome a genetic disorder in which the interval between the Q and the T waves of the electrocardiogram is usually, but not necessarily, prolonged to 500 msec or more. The condition is due to defects of potassium ion or sodium ion channels in heart muscle and features fast heart rate, heart irregularities, fainting and sometime sudden death. Six different mutations of genes coding for the ion channels have been detected, but in about 50% of cases these mutations do not produce symptoms. Sudden death occurs only in about 4% of affected persons.

loose bodies small pieces of bone or of the CARTILAGE bearing surface of joints that have become detached and may interfere with the smooth functioning of the joint. They are a feature of OSTEOARTHRITIS.

loop diuretics drugs that lead to a large output of water in the urine by interfering with the reabsorption of sodium and chloride in the loop of Henle tubules in the kidneys. They include FRUSEMIDE (furosemide) (Fru-Co, Frumil, Frusene, Frusol, Lasikal, Lasilactone, Lasix); BUMETANIDE (Burinex, Burinex A, Burinex K); and torasemide (Torem). Frusemide is commonly formulated in combination with the thiazide diuretic AMILORIDE.

lop-eared having ears with a folded down or drooping upper border.

loperamide a synthetic narcotic analogue drug used to control mild diarrhoea. Brand names are Imodium and Norimode.

Lopid a brand name for GEMFIBROZIL.

Lopresor a brand name for METOPROLOL.

Lopurin a brand name for ALLOPURINOL.

loratadine an ANTIHISTAMINE drug used to treat hay fever and other allergic disorders.

lorazepam a benzodiazepine tranquillizer drug similar to diazepam). A brand name is Ativan.

lordosis an abnormal degree of forward curvature of the lower part of the spine, often associated with abnormal backward curvature of the upper part (KYPHOSIS). Lordosis is an exaggeration of the normal forward curve and often causes the buttocks to appear unduly prominent.

Loron a brand name for SODIUM CLODRONATE.

losartan an ANGIOTENSIN II ANTAGONIST drug used to treat high blood pressure (HYPERTENSION). In the LIFE trial of this drug, reported on in 2003, a subgroup of diabetic patients taking the drug showed a 37 percent reduction in mortality from heart attacks or strokes and a 39 percent reduction in overall mortality over people on other treatment. The drug appears to be effective in preventing sudden death from heart arrhythmias. A brand name is Cozaar. The drug is available combined with the diuretic drug HYDROCHLOROTHIAZIDE under the brand name Cozaar-Comp.

Losec a brand name for OMEPRAZOLE.

Lotremin a brand name for CLOTRIMAZOLE.

loupe a small monocular or binocular magnifying lens, usually set in an eyepiece or head frame, used for examination or operation when fine detail is involved. Operating loupes have now largely been replaced by operating microscopes.

louse see LICE.

low-density lipoproteins the complexes by which cholesterol and other fats (lipids) are transported in the blood in conjunction with protein. High levels of low-density LIPOPROTEINS are associated with the serious arterial disease of ATHEROSCLEROSIS.

low molecular weight heparins heparins that can be isolated from standard heparin by differential precipitation with ethyl alcohol or by gel filtration chromatography or other means. These heparins differ in their mode of action and pharmacological and immunological properties from normal heparin and are useful in cases in which side effects such as heparin-induced THROMBOCYTOPENIA have occurred. They have advantages over heparin in the treatment of venous thrombosis. They bind much less avidly to heparin-binding proteins than does heparin. This increases their bioavailability at low doses and makes their anticoagulant response more predictable. The group includes certoparin (Alphaparin), dalteparin sodium (Fragmin), enoxaparin (Clexane), reviparin sodium (Clivarine) and tinzaparin (Innohep).

lower motor neuron disease damage, by injury or disease, to one or more motor nerves supplying voluntary muscles. The result may be flaccid paralysis of muscle, absent or diminished reflex jerks and progressive muscle atrophy. Compare UPPER MOTOR NEURON DISEASE.

Loxapac a brand name for LOXAPINE.

loxapine a TRICYCLIC drug used to treat psychotic disorders. A brand name is Loxapac.

Loxosceles reclusus the North American brown recluse spider whose venom is more powerful than that of a rattlesnake but is received in a much smaller dose. The bite of this spider is as dangerous as that of the black widow *Latrodectus mactans*.

Lp(a) lipoprotein a low-density lipoprotein particle containing apolipoprotein B-100 linked by a single disulphide bridge to the glycoprotein apoprotein(a). This lipoprotein plays an essential part in artherothrombogenesis and its level is a reliable predictor of death from atherosclerotic pathology in elderly men.

LRCP *abbrev. for* Licentiate of the Royal College of Physicians.

LRCPE *abbrev. for* Licentiate of the Royal College of Physicians of Edinburgh.

LRCPI *abbrev. for* Licentiate of the Royal College of Physicians of Ireland.

LRCPS *abbrev. for* Licentiate of the Royal College Physicians & Surgeons.

LRCS *abbrev. for* Licentiate of the Royal College of Surgeons.

LRCSI *abbrev. for* Licentiate of the Royal College of Surgeons of Ireland.

LRFPS *abbrev. for* Licentiate of the Royal Faculty of Physicians & Surgeons.

LSA *abbrev. for* Licentiate of the Society of Apothecaries London.

LSD *abbrev. for* lysergic acid diethylamide, a hallucinogenic drug derived from lysergic acid, once used in psychiatric research and treatment but now largely confined to illicit use. The drug is a powerful SEROTONIN antagonist and can induce a psychotic state with PARANOID delusions that can last for months.

L-selectin an adhesion molecule that triggers off the interaction between leukocytes and blood vessel endothelium. It is shed from the surface membrane of haematopoietic cells and circulates in the blood as a functional receptor.

LSM *abbrev. for* Licentiate of the School of Medicine.

Ludiomil a brand name for MAPROTILINE HYDROCHLORIDE.

Ludwig's angina an acute spreading bacterial infection of the floor of the mouth, causing severe swelling and tenderness, with fever, pain and difficulty in opening the mouth and in swallowing. There is some danger that the swelling might extend to the voice box (LARYNX) and cause ASPHYXIA. The usual source of infection is grossly neglected teeth. Antibiotics are necessary. (Wilhelm Friedrich von Ludwig, 1790–1865, German surgeon).

lues an obsolete term for SYPHILIS, sometimes used by doctors as a euphemism.

Lugacin a brand name for GENTAMICIN.

lumbago severe and incapacitating pain in the LUMBAR region. Lumbago is a symptom, not a disease, and may be caused by many different conditions.

lumbar relating to the LOINS and lower back.

lumbarization fusion of the side processes of the lowest lumbar vertebra to the SACRUM.

lumbar puncture passage of a needle between two vertebrae of the spine, from behind, into the fluid-filled space lying below the termination of the spinal cord. Lumbar puncture is usually done to obtain a sample of cerebrospinal fluid for laboratory examination in the investigation of disorders of the nervous system. It also allows antibiotic drugs, anaesthetic agents and radio-opaque substances to be injected.

lumbo- *combining form denoting* the LOINS or lumbar.

lumbosacral pertaining to the region of the LUMBAR vertebrae and the curved central bone at the back of the pelvis (SACRUM).

lumbrical 1 pertaining to the LUMBRICAL MUSCLES.

2 pertaining to, or resembling, an earth worm, especially in reference to the intestinal parasite Ascaris lumbricoides.

lumbrical muscles the four small intrinsic muscles of the hand lying between the METACARPAL BONES and acting on tendons of another muscle, the flexor digitorum profundus, to straighten the fingers and bend the joints between the fingers and the palms. Similar muscles, with similar actions, occur in the feet and assist in walking.

lumen the inside of any tube, such as a blood vessel, an air passage (bronchus) or the intestine.

Lumogan a brand name for BIMATOPROST.

luminal pertaining to a LUMEN.

luminous emitting or reflecting light.

lumpectomy a minimal operation for breast cancer in which no attempt is made to remove more than the obvious lump. Supplementary treatment with radiation or chemotherapy is then given. See also MASTECTOMY.

lunacy a legal term for psychotic disorder, no longer used by doctors. The origins of the word derive from the old belief that madness was caused by the full moon. From the Latin *luna*, the moon.

lunate bone one of the bones of the wrist (carpal bones). The lunate is the middle of the three bones in the row nearest to the forearm.

Lundh test a test of the digestive enzyme function of the PANCREAS. A tube is passed into the DUODENUM and a liquid meal is given by mouth to stimulate production of pancreatic enzymes. The digestive juice is sucked out through the tube and analysed.

lung abscess a lung infection with organisms such as *Staphylococcus aureus* or *Klebsiella pneumoniae* which has proceeded to tissue destruction, suppuration and the formation of a pus-filled cavity lined with condensed inflammatory tissue. Lung abscesses commonly rupture into a bronchus so that pus is coughed up.

lungs the paired, air-filled, elastic, spongy organs occupying each side of the chest and separated by the heart and the central partition of the chest known as the mediastinum. Each lung is surrounded by a double-layered membrane called the PLEURA. The function of the lungs is continuously to replenish the oxygen content of the blood and to afford an exit path from the blood for carbon dioxide and other unwanted gases. The right lung has three lobes and the left two. An air tube (BRONCHUS) and a large artery and vein enter each lung on its inner aspect and these branch repeatedly as they pass peripherally. The smallest air passages end in grape-like clusters of air sacs, the alveoli, the walls of which are very thin and contain the terminal branches of the blood vessels. In this way the air comes into intimate contact with the blood so that interchange of gases can readily occur.

lung cancer an inaccurate term usually referring to cancer of the lining of one of the air tubes (bronchi). The medical term is bronchial carcinoma. This tumour accounts for more than half of all male deaths from cancer and the incidence in women is rising rapidly. In most cases it is caused by cigarette smoking. The first sign of lung cancer may be a change in the character of the cough with a little blood in the sputum. Collapse of a lung lobe may cause breathlessness. Pain in the chest is common, especially if the cancer has spread to the lung lining (pleura) or the chest wall. Often there are no symptoms until the cancer has spread to other parts of the body, such as the brain, the liver or the bones. Diagnosis is by X-ray examination or CT scanning or by BRONCHOSCOPY. If the tumour is localized to one lobe or one lung, surgical removal of the lobe or lung offers the best chance of survival. Even in these cases, the 5 year survival rate is only about 30%. If there has been further spread, the outlook is poor. Chemotherapy and radiotherapy may sometimes prolong life a little, but cannot cure the condition.

lung collapse see ATELECTASIS, PNEUMOTHORAX.

lung disorders see ACTINOMYCOSIS, ANTHRACOSIS, BAGGASOSIS, BIRD FANCIER'S LUNG, BRONCHIAL ASTHMA, BRONCHITIS, BRONCHO-PNEUMONIA, EMPHYSEMA, FARMERS' LUNG, HAEMOTHORAX, LARYNGOTRACHEOBRONCHITIS, LEGIONNAIRES' DISEASE, LUNG ABSCESS, LUNG CANCER, OBSTRUCTIVE AIRWAY DISEASE, PIGEON FANCIER'S LUNG, PNEUMONIA, PNEUMOTHORAX, PULMONARY EMBOLISM, PULMONARY FIBROSIS, PULMONARY HYPERTENSION, PULMONARY OEDEMA, RESPIRATORY DISTRESS SYNDROME, SARCOIDOSIS, SILICOSIS, TRACHEITIS AND TUBERCULOSIS. See also PULMONARY FUNCTION TESTS.

lung surfactant drugs substances that replace a deficiency in natural SURFACTANT in the lungs for the treatment of RESPIRATORY DISTRESS SYNDROME or HYALINE MEMBRANE DISEASE in very low-weight new-born babies. Examples are beractant (Survanta) and poractant (Curosurf).

lungworm any one of various parasitic worms that can affect the lungs in the course of their life cycles.

lupoid resembling LUPUS VULGARIS.

lupus a general and imprecise term referring to one of a variety of severe skin disorders, especially LUPUS VULGARIS.

lupus anticoagulant an antibody, or groups of antibodies, to negatively-charged phospholipids liable to be associated, paradoxically, with a tendency for blood to clot within the blood vessels. This may lead to deep vein thrombosis, arterial thrombosis with strokes and heart attacks and, in pregnant women, a strong tendency to fetal death and abortion. Some patients with LUPUS ERYTHEMATOSUS are known to have a positive result in tests for syphilis while not suffering from the disease. This effect is caused by the lupus anticoagulant. See also HUGHES' SYNDROME.

lupus erythematosus a general inflammatory disease of CONNECTIVE TISSUE caused by a disturbance of the immune mechanisms with AUTOIMMUNE processes and the formation of IMMUNE COMPLEXES. It may be induced by drugs. The disease takes two forms – chronic discoid lupus erythematosus (DLE) and the more serious, and sometimes life-threatening, form, systemic lupus erythematosus (SLE). DLE features red, raised bumps in the skin, usually on the face and scalp and often a 'butterfly' rash across the bridge of the nose and hair loss (ALOPECIA). SLE can involve the joints and tendons, causing ARTHRITIS and sometimes deformities, and the heart, lungs, kidneys, liver and nervous system may be damaged. Lupus erythematosus is treated with steroid drugs and sometimes other immunosuppressive drugs.

lupus pernio a form of SARCOIDOSIS affecting the skin and causing raised purple swellings or plaques on the nose, cheeks and ears.

lupus vulgaris a now rare tuberculous skin infection, formerly the cause of much tissue destruction and facial deformity, especially around the nose and the inside of the mouth. From the Latin *lupus*, wolf.

Lustral a brand name for SERTRALINE.

luteal pertaining to the CORPUS LUTEUM, its functions and its hormones, especially progesterone.

luteinizing hormone a hormone released by the PITUITARY GLAND that stimulates egg production (ovulation) from the ovary, in the female, and testosterone from the testicle, in the male. In men, rising blood levels of testosterone inhibit secretion of luteinizing hormone, while, in women, rising levels of oestradiol (estradiol) prompt an increased secretion of luteinizing hormone in the middle of the menstrual cycle.

luteoma a collection of multiplied CORPUS LUTEUM cells in the ovary sometimes occurring in the last 3 months of pregnancy. The luteoma occasionally secretes male sex hormones. It is not a true tumour and regresses after the baby is born.

luxation dislocation.

LVAD abbrev. for left ventricular assist device; an implanted device that, for a time, can boost the heart output, maintaining life until a heart transplant can be done. The LVAD is not an 'artificial heart'.

Lyclear a brand name for PERMETHRIN.

lycopene a carotenoid antioxidant pigment occurring in ripe fruit especially tomatoes. The colour of tomatoes is due to lycopene. Organic tomato ketchup is a fruitful source. The substance has been shown to be protective against breast, pancreatic, prostatic and colonic cancer.

Lyme borreliosis see LYME DISEASE.

lymecycline a tetracycline ANTIBIOTIC used to treat acne and general infections. A brand name is Tetralysal.

Lyme disease a disease caused by the spiral organism (spirochaete) *Borrelia burgdorferi*, and transmitted by the bite of the tick *Ixodes dammini*. A slightly itchy red spot appears, within a month at the site of the mite bite. This expands to form a ring. Up to 100 other similar spots may soon appear and there is fever, fatigue, headaches, stiff neck, muscle and joint pain and enlarged lymph nodes. The Borrelia organism can affect almost every organ of the body. Several weeks or months after onset, up to 15% of affected people develop nervous system complications such as MENINGITIS, ENCEPHALITIS, nerve paralysis, muscle weakness or shingles-like pain in the skin. Some develop mental illness and others have a profound fatigue and weakness that may last for months or years. The joints are affected in at least half the cases, usually intermittently and mildly, but sometimes severely with joint damage similar to mild RHEUMATOID ARTHRITIS. Heart involvement occurs in about 8%, usually HEART BLOCK but also heart enlargement and inflammation of the heart capsule (PERICARDITIS). Lyme disease can be passed from a mother to her unborn baby, and *Borrelia* have been found in children with severe congenital defects. If the early skin pattern is recognized and treatment with antibiotics given, all these complications are avoided. Lyme disease was first reported among the inhabitants of Old Lyme, Connecticut, in 1975, but is now occurring in Britain and in many other parts of the world.

lymph tissue fluids drained by the lymph vessels and returned to the large veins. Lymph varies in character in different parts of the body. Lymph from the tissues contains large numbers of white cells, mainly LYMPHOCYTES, and is usually clear. Lymph from the intestines is milky, especially after a meal, because of the large number of fat globules which it contains. Fat-laden lymph is called CHYLE.

lymph-, lympho- *combining form denoting* LYMPH or lymphatic tissue.

lymphadenectomy surgical removal of LYMPH NODES.

lymphadenitis inflammation of LYMPH NODES, usually secondary to infection in the area draining to the affected nodes. Thus an infection in the leg may cause lymphadenitis in the groin.

lymphadenomatosis see LYMPHOMA.

lymphadenopathy any disease process affecting a LYMPH NODE. Also known as lymphadenosis.

lymphangiectasis local widening (dilation) of the wall of a LYMPH vessel.

lymphangiectomy surgical removal of LYMPH vessels.

lymphangioendothelioma a tumour of the cells lining a lymph vessel.

lymphangioma a benign tumour of lymph vessels, often congenital. Cystic lymphangiomas are called hygromas.

lymphangitis inflammation of lymphatic vessels, usually caused by virulent organisms, often STREPTOCOCCI (see STREPTOCOCCUS). Lymphangitis causes conspicuous red streaks under the skin with fever and general upset. The condition indicates a potentially dangerous infection and calls for urgent antibiotic treatment.

lymph gland the incorrect term for a LYMPH NODE. These are not glands, although commonly so described, even by doctors.

lymph nodes small oval or bean-shaped bodies, up to 2 cm in length, situated in groups along the course of the LYMPH drainage vessels. The nodes have fibrous capsules and are packed with lymphocytes. The main groups of lymph nodes are in the groins, the armpits, the neck, around the main blood vessels in the abdomen, in the MESENTERY and in the central partition of the chest (the MEDIASTINUM). Lymph nodes offer defence against the spread of infection by producing ANTIBODIES, and become involved in the spread of cancer. They can become cancerous, forming LYMPHOMAS.

lymphoblast an immature LYMPHOCYTE.

lymphoblastoma a LYMPHOMA consisting of cells mainly of the lymphocyte precursor type.

lymphoblastosis an excessive number of primitive lymphocytes (lymphoblasts) in the blood and, occasionally, in the tissues, as in acute lymphoblastic LEUKAEMIA.

lymphocytes specialized white cells concerned in the body's immune system. Several different types can be distinguished. B lymphocytes produce antibodies (IMMUNOGLOBULINS) and are divided into the plasma cells that secrete the immunoglobulins and memory cells that act when the event that stimulated antibody selection recurs. T lymphocytes help to protect against virus infections and cancer and are divided into helper cells, suppressor cells, cytotoxic cells, memory cells and mediators of delayed hypersensitivity. There are also large granular lymphocytes. These are the KILLER CELLS (K cells) and the natural killer cells (NK cells).

lymphocytic choriomeningitis an acute viral MENINGITIS caused by an arenavirus, the lymphocytic choriomeningitis virus, spread by house mice. There is fever, aches and pains, a brief recovery, then a second stage with recurrenceof fever, headache and sometimes meningeal symptoms such as stiff neck. The condition is usually mild with complete recovery.

lymphocytic leukaemia a LEUKAEMIA in which the cells undergoing uncontrolled increase (proliferation) are LYMPHOCYTES. Chronic lymphocytic leukaemia is a variable disease: some patients require no treatment; others have a poor outcome. ZAP-70 estimations provide a guide to the prognosis.

lymphocytosis a abnormal increase in the number of LYMPHOCYTES circulating in the blood. A form of LEUKOCYTOSIS.

lymphoedema persistent swelling of the tissues as a result of inadequate drainage from blockage or absence of the LYMPH channels. Absence may be congenital or the result of cancer surgery. Obstruction may be by cancer cells or by filarial parasitic worms. The latter causes ELEPHANTIASIS.

lymphogranuloma venereum a sexually transmitted disease caused by *Chlamydia trachomatis* organisms causing transient genital ulcers, enlargement and matting of the groin lymph nodes, fever, weight loss, enlargement of the liver and spleen, and later complications such as narrowing of the urine passage (URETHRAL STRICTURE), abscesses and stricture of the rectum and the formation of drainage SINUSES. The condition responds to TETRACYCLINE antibiotics but corrective surgery may be necessary.

lymphoid pertaining to LYMPH or lymphatic tissue.

lymphokine-activated killer cells cells artificially produced by incubating lymphocytes from cancer patients with INTERLEUKIN-2 (IL-2). The result is a class of natural-killer cells whose targets are not restricted to cells carrying particular antigens. They offer potential as treatment modalities.

lymphokines CYTOKINES produced by lymphocytes. Lymphokines attract MACROPHAGES to the site of foreign material and activate them to kill organisms, cause other T cells to clone and provide other cells with protection against virus invasion. They include INTERFERONS, CHEMOTACTIC factor, transfer factor and INTERLEUKIN-2.

lymphomas a group of cancers of lymphoid tissue, especially the lymph nodes and the spleen. There are two kinds. If certain large, irregular, multinucleated cells, called Reed-Sternberg cells, are present, the disease is called HODGKIN'S LYMPHOMA. If not, it is called a non-Hodgkin's lymphoma. 90% of non-Hodgkin's lymphomas are of clonal masses of B cells, 10% of T cell origin. They vary considerably in their degree of malignancy and have many features in common with certain leukaemias. There is tiredness, loss of weight and sometimes fever. At a certain stage there may be pressure on various structures of the body. This may cause paralysis by compression of the spinal cord, difficulty in swallowing from pressure on the oesophagus, difficulty in breathing, obstruction of the bowel causing vomiting, and obstruction of the lymph vessels causing lymphoedema. Treatment depends on the cell type and on the extent of spread. In some cases, no treatment is needed and often patients are watched for years without intervention. But when treatment is required, radiotherapy is often best and may be curative. See also BURKITT'S LYMPHOMA.

lymphopoiesis the production of LYMPHOCYTES.

lymphosarcoma the term formerly used for non-Hodgkin's LYMPHOMA.

lyo-, lyso- *combining form denoting* loosened or dispersed.

Lyon hypothesis see X-INACTIVATION.

Lyonization see X-INACTIVATION.

lyophilic 1 readily dissolving.
2 of a colloid, quickly dispersing because of an affinity between the dispersed particles and the dispersing medium.

lyophilized freeze dried.

lysergic acid an ergot alkaloid, one of the components of ERGOTAMINE.

lysergic acid diethylamide see LSD.

lysin any substance capable of causing LYSIS, especially a specific antibody that brings about a COMPLEMENT FIXATION reaction.

lysis the destruction of a living cell by disruption of its membrane. Haemolysis is lysis of red blood cells. This will occur if the cells are placed in plain water.

lyso- *combining form denoting* LYSIS or decomposition.

lysosomal storage diseases genetic diseases in which defects in lysosomal enzymes result in the accumulation in the LYSOSOMES of unsplit large molecules, such as glycosaminoglycans (mucopolysaccharides) and glycogen, engorging them and distorting other cell contents, affecting their function. These diseases include cystinosis, sialic acid storage disease and glycogen storage disease. They affect many parts of the body.

lysosome one of the types of ORGANELLE found in cell cytoplasm. Lysosomes contain various hydrolytic enzymes capable of digesting large molecules (macromolecules), the products of which can then leave the lysosomes. Injury to lysosomes may release enzymes that can damage the cell.

lysozyme an enzyme found in tears, milk and other body fluids and capable of destroying certain bacteria by breaking down their walls by the digestion of their peptidoglycans.

lyssavirus a single strand RNA virus that causes RABIES or a potentially fatal encephalitis indistinguishable from rabies. To date, seven different lyssavirus genotypes have been identified. Apart from the rabies strain, most of the lyssaviruses are endemic in bats.

lysuride lisuride, a DOPAMINE agonist drug used to treat Parkinson's disease. A brand name is Revanil.

Maalox a brand name for a preparation containing ALUMINIUM HYDROXIDE and MAGNESIUM HYDROXIDE.

Macaca mulatta the rhesus monkey, whose red cells are agglutinated by an antibody that also agglutinates the blood cells of 83% of people (rhesus positive people). The ANTIGEN that stimulates the production of this antibody was originally found in the blood of *Macaca mulatta* and the antibody was first isolated from the serum of rabbits and guinea pigs immunized against the red cells of the monkey.

MACD *abbrev. for* Member of the Australasian College of Dermatology.

Mace a tear gas made from the lacrimatory agent chloracetophenone combined with a dispersant and an aerosol propellant.

macerated softened by prolonged contact with liquid.

MACGP *abbrev. for* Member of the Australasian College of General Practitioners.

Mackie's syndrome a corneal disorder featuring small areas of epithelial drying and disruption near the margin on the nasal and the temporal side, sometimes with the formation of a distinct depression (dellen). The condition, which is common, is the result of abnormal blinking in wearers of hard contact lenses. If neglected, it may progress to PINGUECULA and even PTERYGIUM. Also known as three and nine o'clock keratopathy. (Ian A. Mackie, b. 1927, London consultant ophthalmologist).

MACO *abbrev. for* Member of the Australian College of Ophthalmologists.

MACR *abbrev. for* Member of the American College of Radiology.

macro- *combining form denoting* large.

Macrobid a brand name for NITROFURANTOIN.

macrobiotics a non-scientific system of diet based on the yin-yang (opposing, light–dark, male–female) principle. The principles of sound nutrition are well established on demonstrable scientific grounds that do not involve this idea. Over-enthusiastic adherence to a macrobiotic dietary could lead to ill-health.

macrocephalous having an abnormally large head.

macrocheilia abnormally large lips.

macroencephaly the state of having an abnormally large brain.

macrocrania having an abnormally large skull in proportion to the size of the face.

macrocytic anaemia anaemia in which the red blood cells are unusually large, as in PERNICIOUS ANAEMIA.

macrocytosis the condition in which the blood contains large numbers of enlarged red blood cells (macrocytes). This occurs when red cells are being produced more rapidly than normal to try to compensate for reduced oxygen carrying capacity.

macrodactyly abnormally large fingers or toes.

Macrodantin a brand name for NITROFURANTOIN.

macrodontia abnormally large teeth.

macrogamete 1 the mammalian ovum, which is much larger than the male sex cell, the microgamete or spermatozoon.
2 the female sex cell of the malarial parasite and other PROTOZOA.

macroglia one of the two forms of neurological connective tissue (glia).

macroglobulin see IgM.

macroglobulinaemia a rare disease featuring abnormal quantities of a monoclonal immunoglobulin-M and a tendency to develop undue thickness (hyperviscosity) of the blood. The condition progresses to immune deficiency and susceptibility to infection.

macroglossia enlargement of the tongue.

macrolide one of a range of antibiotics with a wide spectrum of action that can be used as an alternative to the penicillins to treat respiratory infections including LEGIONNAIRES' DISEASE. The group includes erythromycin, azithromycin and clarithromycin.

macrognathia an abnormally large jaw.

macromastia abnormally enlarged breasts.

macromelia abnormal enlargement of one or more limbs.

macromolecule a very large molecule, such as a protein or other long polymer. DNA is a macromolecule, as is the polysaccharide glycogen.

macronormoblast an abnormally large form of any of the precursor series of cells that lead to mature red blood cells.

macrophage an important cell in the immune system. Macrophages are scavenging cells, large PHAGOCYTES derived from blood MONOCYTES, and are found all over the body, especially in the liver, lymph nodes, spleen and bone marrow. Some are stationary within the tissues (fixed macrophages), others are free and move about, being attracted to sites of infection. Connective tissue (fixed) macrophages are called histiocytes; those in the liver are called Kupffer cells; and those in the nervous system are called microglial cells. Macrophages are AMOEBOID and ingest foreign material and bacteria, which they destroy. In order to bring about an immune response, most ANTIGENS must first be processed by macrophages so that their antigenic elements can be presented to LYMPHOCYTES on the macrophage surfaces. The term derives from the Greek *macros*, large and *phageo* to eat.

macrophage activation factor a LYMPHOKINE that prompts a MACROPHAGE into action.

macrophagic myofasciitis a recently-described apparently new disease featuring fever, muscle and joint pain, muscle and general weakness and infiltration of the tissues around the muscles by sheets of large, finely-granular MACROPHAGES. The muscle fibres, themselves are minimally affected. The microscopic appearances are unlike those of any previous muscle or fascial disorder. The condition

appears to respond to treatment with various combinations of antibiotics and steroids. It was first described by the French physicians and histopathologists Professor R.K. Gerardi, M. Coquet, F-J Authier, P. Laforêt,L. Bélec, D. Figarelle-Branger, J-M Mussini, J-F Pellissier and M. Fardeau.

macropsia abnormal perception of the size of objects so that they seem larger than they actually are.

macroscopic visible to the naked eye.

macula any small flat spot.

macula lutea the yellow spot in the centre of the RETINA on which the image of the point of greatest visual interest falls when something is observed. The macula is the most sensitive part of the retina and is devoid of blood vessels. Here, the concentration of colour-sensitive cones is maximal and the visual resolution is greatest. The full visual acuity is possible only by The use of the centre of the macula – the fovea.

macular degeneration see AGE-RELATED MACULAR DEGENERATION.

macular translocation a new technique for treating age-related MACULAR DEGENERATION. The procedure involves moving the fovea of the eye so that it lies over an area in which the underlying tissues are healthy. The most effective procedure appears to be a full translocation achieved by a peripheral 360 degree retinal incision and rotation of the free RETINA by 25 to 50 degrees so as to place the fovea over healthy tissue. The retina is then reattached with laser burns.

maculopapular pertaining to small, circumscribed, usually discoloured, slightly raised spots on the skin.

madarosis loss of the eyelashes or eyebrows or both.

Madopar a brand name for LEVODOPA in combination with BENSERAZIDE.

madura foot see MYCETOMA.

Madurella a widely distributed genus of fungi, the cause of MYCETOMA.

maggots eyeless, short-lived, worm-like larvae of flies that are devoid of appendages but are able to feed on organic matter and often help to clean septic wounds. Maggots acquired a new respectability in the year 2004 when they became prescribable on the British National Health Service under the brand name Larve.

One or two applications, each lasting for up to three days, during which the maggots are restrained by a net, have been found effective in cleaning up most wounds. See also MYIASIS.

magic the belief that thoughts or acts can influence unrelated events, or the use of ritual to attempt to summon supposed supernatural forces. Historically, there has been considerable overlap between religion, magic and science and these have been separated only with great difficulty and, even today, incompletely. The reduction, by science, of the status of magic to childish superstition has been one of the triumphs of human achievement. Magical thinking is a feature of early childhood and of the mental processes of some adults.

Magnapen a brand name for a mixture of the penicillin antibiotics AMPICILLIN and FLUCLOXACILLIN.

magnesium alginate a drug used to treat dyspepsia and heartburn. Brand names of preparations containing it are Algicon and Gaviscon Infant.

magnesium carbonate a mild antacid drug used to treat DYSPEPSIA. Brand names of preparations containing it are Algicon and Topal.

magnesium hydroxide an ANTACID and LAXATIVE drug. The drug is on the WHO official list. Brand names of preparations containing it are Diovol, Maalox, Mucaine and Mucogel.

magnesium oxide an antacid drug. Brand name of preparations containing magnesium oxide and DIMETHICONE (dimeticone) are Asilone and Kolanticon.

magnesium sulphate a drug formerly used by mouth or by ENEMA to treat CONSTIPATION and by injection to treat magnesium deficiency. Was also much used by local application in a paste or poultice to draw water from wounds. Also known as Epsom salts. The use of magnesium sulphate, especially in people with kidney disorders, can lead to severe toxicity. The drug is on the WHO official list.

magnesium trisilicate a drug used as an antacid in the treatment of DYSPEPSIA. Brand names of preparations containing it are Gastrocote, Gaviscon and Pyrogastrone.

magnetic nanoparticles particles of iron oxide coated with DEXTRAN to which specific ANTIBODIES will readily adhere. If such particles are injected into a person infected with the relevant virus they will large form clusters of nanoparticles and viruses. On MRI scanning the nanoparticles become magnetized and are detectable. Adenoviruses and herpes simplex viruses have been detected by this technique. It has also been used to demonstrate secondary spread to lymph nodes of prostate cancer.

magnetic resonance imaging (MRI) an important method of body scanning offering a degree of resolution of detail unequalled by any other method. The body is exposed to an intense magnetic field which forces spinning atomic nuclei into a standard orientation. Brief radio waves (electromagnetic signals) applied to the body cause certain atoms, especially the hydrogen in water, to take up a new alignment. In returning to the standard orientation these atoms emit small radio waves that can be picked up and their origin computed. The MRI scanner then reconstitutes images of cross-sections of the body in much the same way as does the CT scanner. The MRI scanner is capable of resolving subtle abnormalities in soft tissue such as brain and nerves. The characteristic plaques of multiple sclerosis, for instance, are clearly revealed as is an area of brain deprived of its blood supply. No ionizing radiation is involved. See also CT SCANNING.

magnetic resonance spectroscopy an advanced method of chemical analysis using a technique similar to that employed in nuclear magnetic resonance imaging. The method is based on the fact that the electrons in a molecule shield the nucleus to some extent from the strong applied external field, causing different atoms to absorb at slightly different frequencies. It is applicable to molecules in the living body or in other organisms. The method has, for instance, been used to prove that the structure of the protein capsid surrounding the genome of HIV consists of seven alpha helices, two beta-hairpins and a single exposed loop.

main accoucheur the hand attitude, similar to that of a gynaecologist making a vaginal examination, that occurs in TETANY or in some forms of MUSCULAR DYSTROPHY. The fingers are held straight but the joints between the fingers and the metacarpals are bent.

major histocompatibility complex (MHC) cell surface protein markers, coded for by a large cluster of genes on chromosome 6, that control the activities of cells of the immune system. The

MHC molecules indicates the tissue type and are important in organ donation. They have, however, wider functions in the immune system. Infected cells used their MHC sites to signal the fact to helper T cells and cytotoxic T cells so that they can be attacked. There are two classes of MHC. Class I MHC molecules are present on virtually all body cells other than red blood cells; class II MHC molecules occur on antigen-presenting cells such as MACROPHAGES and B cells. Cytotoxic T cells (CD8) bind to MHC class I, while helper T cells (CD4) bind to MHC class II. MHC variations have been used extensively in human population studies.

major histocompatibility locus a region on chromosome 6 that contains a large number of genes coding for lymphocyte cell surface ANTIGENS that determine the tissue type and immunological responses of the individual.

major immunogene complex a gene region that codes for the HISTOCOMPATIBILITY ANTIGENS, for the LYMPHOCYTE surface antigens, for the control factors of the plasma cells that produce antibodies, and for the proteins of the COMPLEMENT system.

mal- *combining form denoting* disease, bad, abnormal or defective.

malabsorption one of a number of disorders in which there is a failure of movement of some of the elements of the diet from the small intestine into the bloodstream so that MALNUTRITION may occur in spite of an adequate diet. See LACTASE DEFICIENCY SYNDROME, COELIAC DISEASE, STEATORRHOEA, RICKETS and OSTEOMALACIA.

-malacia *suffix denoting* softening.

malacoplakia a form of persistent inflammation of the urinary bladder featuring soft, pale, elevated plaques composed of MACROPHAGES and LYMPHOCYTES. The condition most commonly affects middle-aged women.

malady any disease, disorder or illness.

malaise a vague general term for feeling unwell. Although included in the list of symptoms of most diseases, the term has no diagnostic value.

malar bone see ZYGOMA.

malar relating to the cheek bone (zygoma) or to the prominence caused by the cheek bone. From the Latin *mala*, the cheek or cheekbone, and perhaps also the Latin *malum*, an apple.

malar flush a high flush over the cheek bones,

with a bluish tinge that has, in the past, been taken to be an important sign of narrowing of the MITRAL valve of the heart. Sometimes called the 'mitral facies'.

malaria one of a number of infections that cause recurrent fevers and are responsible for at least a million deaths each year throughout the world. Malaria is caused by one of several different species of single-celled parasites (protozoa) of the genus *Plasmodium*. *Plasmodium falciparum* causes a 24 hour cycle, with bouts of fever, shaking, headache and general aches and pains occurring every day. The common *Plasmodium vivax*, and the *Plasmodium ovale* have a 48 hour cycle and *Plasmodium malariae* a 72 hour cycle. Heavy infection can be very dangerous, especially with *P. falciparum* which can block the small blood vessels of the brain and cause grave illness. This parasite also often causes so much red blood cell destruction that the released haemoglobin colours the urine dark red or black, giving the name 'blackwater fever'. The disease is transmitted from person to person by certain species of *Anopheles* mosquito which breed in stagnant water. The parasites undergo breeding cycles in the blood but can also settle in the liver and undergo breeding cycles there, occasionally breaking out into the blood. Because of the liver cycle, people who have had malaria and have been inadequately treated may appear to have fully recovered, but may develop severe attacks months or years later. Treatment is with the antimalarial drugs. These include AMODIAQUINE, CHLOROQUINE, MEFLOQUINE, PROGUANIL and QUININE. From the Italian *mala*, bad and *aria*, air.

Malarone a brand name for PROGUANIL in conjunction with ATOVAQUONE.

Malassezia furfur a skin yeast fungus, previously known as *Pityrosporon* thought to be implicated in causing SEBORRHOEIC DERMATITIS and DANDRUFF. The drug LITHIUM in ointment or cream form is used to treat these conditions. Rare cases of dangerous systemic infections in newborn babies requiring central venous catheters have been reported.

malathion a poisonous organophosphate insecticide drug used in very low concentration in preparations for external use to destroy lice. Brand names are Derbac-M, Prioderm and Suleo-M.

maleruption abnormal positioning, or failure of appearance, of teeth.

male symbol ♂ the universally used biological symbol for the male. The symbol is the zodiac sign of Mars the Roman God of war, epitomizing maleness, and represents a shield and a spear rather than an erect penis.

malformation any bodily deformity or structural abnormality resulting from a defect in development or growth.

malic acid a drug used to clean external wounds and ulcers and remove dead tissue. A brand name is Aserbine.

malignant a term usually applied to cancerous tumours but also used to qualify unusually serious forms of various diseases tending to cause death unless effectively treated. The term is opposite in meaning to benign and derives from the Latin *malignus*, evil.

malignant hypertension a severe and dangerous form of high blood pressure that follows a rapid course with progressive damage to blood vessels and to the eyes and the kidneys. There is a major danger of STROKE. Unless effectively treated the condition is often fatal.

malignant hyperthermia a rare inherited muscle disorder that leads to dangerously high fever from intense muscle contraction when the affected person is given a general anaesthetic drug such as halothane, cyclopropane or ethyl ether, or a muscle relaxant drug such as succinylcholine. Emergency treatment to cool the patient, to neutralize the rapid rise in blood lactic acid from the muscles, and to reverse the abnormal muscle response, is needed to save life.

malignant melanoma a dangerous cancer of the skin or the eye. About 1% of cancers are malignant melanomas. Half of them arise from pigmented moles and this is more likely if there is much exposure to sunlight. Only about one mole in a million, however, becomes malignant. Suspicious changes include alteration in outline shape, size or protuberance from the surface, colour change, especially darkening and colour irregularity, itching or pain, softening, crumbling or the development of satellite moles around the original one. Any such change in a mole, or the appearance of a new coloured mole with these characteristics, should be reported at once. Treatment is by widespread removal. Malignant melanoma of the CHOROID of the eye is painless but causes RETINAL DETACHMENT.

malignant pustule one of the forms of ANTHRAX, occurring when the organism penetrates an abrasion in the skin. There is a boil-like LESION with a black dead centre surrounded by a hard inflamed swelling. This is the commonest manifestation of anthrax in humans and, although serious, usually responds to antibiotics.

malingering a pretence to be suffering from a disease, or the simulation of signs of disease, so as to gain some supposed advantage such as avoidance of work or of presumed danger, or to obtain money by fraudulent claims for compensation. See also MUNCHAUSEN'S SYNDROME.

malleolus either of the two bony protuberances on either side of the ankle. The inner (medial malleolus) is a process on the lower end of the TIBIA, the outer (lateral malleolus) is a process on the lower end of the FIBULA.

malleus the outermost and largest of three small bones of the middle ear, the auditory ossicles. From the Latin *malleus*, a hammer.

Mallory-Weiss syndrome a tear at the lower end of the gullet (OESOPHAGUS) caused by violent movements of the DIAPHRAGM during retching or vomiting. There is vomiting of blood. In most cases the tear heals well, often without treatment. (George Kenneth Mallory, b. 1900, American pathologist; and Konrad Weiss, 1898–1942, American physician).

malnutrition any disorder resulting from an inadequate diet or from failure to absorb or assimilate dietary elements. The term is now often used to describe the effects of an ill-chosen, even if calorifically adequate, diet or of excessive food intake. See also SPRUE, MALABSORPTION, COELIAC DISEASE, CROHN'S DISEASE, ANOREXIA NERVOSA, VITAMIN DEFICIENCY, BERI-BERI, PELLAGRA, SCURVY, XEROPHTHALMIA, RICKETS and KWASHIORKOR.

malocclusion a poor physical relationship between the biting or grinding surfaces of the teeth of the upper jaw and those of the lower. Malocclusion is readily correctable by ORTHODONTIC TREATMENT.

Malpighian corpuscle a tiny spherical body, one of millions in the kidney, consisting of a bundle of CAPILLARIES enclosed in a capsule which is attached to a tubule for the drainage of urine. (Marcello Malpighi, 1628–94, Italian anatomist).

malposition 1 abnormal location of any part of the body.

2 during pregnancy, an abnormal lie of the fetus in the womb.

malpractice professional misconduct including professional negligence. Medical malpractice includes the failure to provide proper standards of medical care, engaging recklessly in dangerous treatments, abusing professional privileges in any way, giving fraudulent certificates, procuring illegal abortions, using medical status to exert improper influence such as establishing sexual relationships with patients, betraying professional confidences, engaging in improper self-promotion and disparaging colleagues. Doctors behaving in any of these ways may be brought before the Professional Conduct Committee of the General Medical Council and, the allegations being proved, may have their names erased from the Medical Register so that they may no longer legally practise. Some forms of malpractice are also criminal offences for which a doctor may also have to answer in law.

malpresentation any position (lie) of the fetus before or during labour that would result in a part other than the vertex of the head appearing first at birth. Malpresentations include breech, face (head extended), shoulder and arm PRESENTATIONS.

Malta fever see BRUCELLOSIS.

maltase an enzyme that splits MALTOSE.

Malthusian theory the theory that populations tends to increase faster than the means of their subsistence so that starvation, poverty and misery are inevitable unless populations are controlled by disease, famine, celibacy, 'vicious practices' (contraception), infanticide or war. The theory was proposed in An Essay on the Principle of Population, 1798 (Thomas Robert Malthus, 1766–1834, English theorist).

maltose a disaccharide sugar consisting of two linked molecules of glucose. It is produced by the enzymatic splitting, during digestion, of starches and glycogen.

maltworker's lung an ALLERGIC ALVEOLITIS caused by fungal spores of Aspergillus clavatus from malting barley.

malunion healing of a bone fracture in an unsatisfactory position. This may interfere with the mechanics of adjacent joints and lead to OSTEOARTHRITIS.

mamillary bodies paired, rounded, breast-like swellings on the underside of the HYPOTHALAMUS of the brain just behind the stalk of the PITUITARY GLAND.

mammary artery grafting a method of bypass for coronary narrowing used to overcome the strong tendency of vein grafts to become arterialized and eventually blocked by athero-sclerosis and thrombosis. It has been found that grafts using one or both of the internal mammary arteries instead of a length of leg vein remain open longer and are far more resistant than veins to these dangerous disease changes.

mammary gland the BREAST. This is rudimentary in the male but developed and capable of the function of long-term milk production in the female. The word *mamma* is both Greek and Latin for breast and may derive originally from the sound made by hungry babies. See also BREAST ABSCESS, BREAST CANCER, BREAST ENLARGEMENT and BREAST-FEEDING.

mammography a method of X-ray examination of the breasts using low-radiation (soft) X-rays and specially designed apparatus to reveal density changes that might imply cancer. Mammography is used in cases of suspected breast cancer and as a screening procedure on groups of women. It cannot be relied on to exclude cancer and does not distinguish between benign and malignant tumours, but tumours that cannot be felt may be detected. Mammography has been found to be more reliable if its timing is properly phased with the menstrual cycle. Breast tissue is more dense during the luteal phase (days 15–28).

mammoplasty plastic surgery on the breasts. Surgery to increase the bulk is called augmentation mammoplasty; surgery to make breasts smaller is called reduction mammoplasty. When breasts have been removed for cancer, breast reconstruction is possible.

mancinism the condition of left-handedness.

mandelic acid an antiseptic drug used in sterile solutions for washing out the bladder, especially if a permanent catheter is in use. A brand name is Uro-Tainer.

mandible the lower jaw bone. The head of the mandible, on either side, articulates with a hollow on the underside of the temporal bone, just in front of the ear. This is called the temporo-mandibular joint. The mandible is pulled upwards by powerful masticatory muscles. In dislocation of the mandible, the heads slip forward out of the hollows in the temporal bone and the mouth remains wide open until the dislocation is reduced by downward pressure on the back teeth.

manganese poisoning an industrial disease largely confined to miners who breathe manganese ore dust and workers exposed to manganese compounds. Brain damage occurs, resulting in rigidity of the muscles with loss of facial expression, slowness of movement, speech impairment, and delusions, hallucinations and compulsive disorders.

mange a common skin disease of domestic animals sometimes transmitted to people. It is caused by any one of a range of skin mites, such as *Sarcoptes scabei* that burrow into the skin causing intense itching. See also SCABIES.

mania a state of physical and mental overactivity featuring constant compulsive and sometimes repetitive movements and unceasing loquacity. The manic phase of a MANIC DEPRESSIVE ILLNESS. From the Greek *mania*, raving madness.

-mania *suffix denoting* exaggerated feeling for, compulsion towards, or obsession with.

manic-depressive illness an emotional (affective) disorder of unknown cause featuring an association of abnormal elation (mania) and pathological depression. The depressive phase usually comes first and for 6 to 12 months there is mental and physical slowing, loss of interest and energy, sadness, pessimism, self-blame and thoughts of suicide. Five or six such episodes usually occur over a period of about 20 years. The manic phase, if it occurs, usually follows two to four depressive episodes. It features speeding up of thought and speech, inappropriate elation, disordered judgement, ever-changing flights of ideas, grandiose notions, deceitful behaviour, unrealistic plans and sometimes socially or financially ruinous behaviour. The spontaneous recovery rate in manic-depressive illness is about 90%. Treatment is with antidepressant drugs and, in the manic phase, with LITHIUM.

manipulation any operation performed with the hands, especially one purporting to restore displaced parts to a normal relationship. See also OSTEOPATHY.

mannitol a SUGAR sometimes given by injection as a concentrated solution to draw water from the brain in cases of ENCEPHALITIS or head injury. The drug is on the WHO official list.

mannosidosis an autosomal recessive lysosomal storage disease similar to Hurler's disease, caused by a deficiency of the enzyme alpha mannosidase. There are two types; Type 1 leads to an early death from severe systemic disturbances. Type II is less severe.

manometer a glass U-tube containing mercury or other liquid, and having a graduated scale, used to measure pressure in a gas. One end of the tube is left open, the other is connected by a flexible pipe to the source of pressure.

Mantoux test a skin test for resistance to TUBERCULOSIS in which a small quantity of a sterile liquid derived from a culture of tubercle bacilli (tuberculin) is injected into the skin and the local reaction noted. A negative result suggests susceptibility to tuberculosis and may prompt vaccination with BCG. The test is now performed by a rapid multiple puncture technique, similar to the Heaf test, but using disposable, multiple-tine test units. (Charles Mantoux, 1887–1947, French physician).

manubrium the shield-shaped upper part of the breastbone (STERNUM). The inner ends of the collar bones (clavicles) and of the first and second ribs articulate with the manubrium.

Manusept a brand name for TRICLOSAN.

MANZCP *abbrev. for* Member of the Australian & New Zealand College of Psychiatrists.

MAO *abbrev. for* Master of the Art of Obstetrics.

MAOI see MONOAMINE OXIDASE INHIBITOR.

maple bark disease an ALLERGIC ALVEOLITIS caused by inhalation of the saprophytic fungus *Coniosporium corticale* from the bark of maple trees.

maple syrup urine disease a hereditary defect of protein metabolism in which the breakdown of amino acids is defective because of the absence of an oxidase enzyme. The result is the presence of keto-acids with an odour of maple syrup in the urine. The condition causes serious neurological disturbances and death within a few months of birth.

mapping the process of determining the order of GENES, and their functions, on the CHROMOSOMES. The human genome project, currently under way, is designed to map the entire collection of the human chromosomes, with incalculable potential benefit to humankind, and a huge increase in responsibility for the application of the knowledge.

maprotiline hydrochloride a tetracyclic antidepressant drug. A brand name is Ludiomil.

marasmus a state of wasting or emaciation from starvation, usually in infants. There is weakness, irritability, dry skin and, unless rapidly corrected by feeding, retardation of growth and of mental development.

Marcaine the long-acting local anaesthetic drug BUPIVACAINE. The effect lasts for about 4 hours.

Marburg disease a severe infectious disease that first occurred in laboratory workers in Marburg, West Germany, handling monkey tissue from Uganda. The disease subsequently occurred in Zaire. It is caused by the Marburg/Ebola virus and features fever, severe aching in the muscles, diarrhoea, sore throat, an extensive livid rash, enlarged lymph nodes, internal bleeding, pneumonia, ENCEPHALITIS and kidney failure. There is no specific treatment and the mortality can be as high as 90% in untreated cases. With good supportive care the mortality is about 25%.

march fracture a hairline break in a long bone of the foot caused by repeated trauma as by stamping the feet in marching. The condition is also common in joggers. There is pain, tenderness in the sole of the foot and swelling. Displacement is unusual and the bone will usually heal without immobilization if the stress is removed.

Marcus Gunn phenomenon see JAW WINKING.

Marevan a brand name for the anticoagulant drug WARFARIN.

Marfan's syndrome a rare AUTOSOMAL DOMINANT genetic disorder involving weakness of the structural COLLAGEN protein fibrillin. The disease is caused by a defective gene on chromosome 15. People with Marfan's syndrome are tall with long extremities and strikingly spider-like fingers (ARACHNODACTYLY). Their joints are unusually mobile and dislocate easily and the internal lenses of the eyes commonly become displaced. The main artery of the body (the AORTA) is abnormally floppy and heart disease commonly occurs. (Antonin Bernard Jean Marfan, 1858–1942, French physician).

marijuana see CANNABIS.

marital counselling the process of analysis of relational problems between spouses and the giving of advice on how they may be relieved.

marker 1 a trait, condition, gene, or substance that indicates the presence of, or a probable increased predisposition to, a medical or psychological disorder.

2 a gene whose location on a chromosome is known so that it can be used as a point of reference for MAPPING new mutations.

marrow transplant see BONE MARROW TRANSPLANT.

Marplan a former brand name for the monoamine oxidase inhibitor ANTIDEPRESSANT drug isocarboxazid. The brand name is still in use in the USA.

marsupialization a surgical procedure for dealing with cysts when complete removal is impracticable. The CYST is widely opened and the opening maintained but gradually reduced until the cyst shrinks.

Marvelon an oral contraceptive containing ETHINYLOESTRADIOL (ethinylestradiol) and DESOGESTREL. See also CONTRACEPTION.

Marzine a brand name for the ANTIHISTAMINE and ANTIEMETIC drug CYCLIZINE. Also known as Valoid.

masculinization see VIRILIZATION.

masochism the achievement of sexual arousal or gratification by the experience of physical or mental pain or humiliation. Masochism is said to derive from a partly repressed sense of guilt which inhibits orgasm but which can be assuaged by punishment so that orgasm becomes possible. (Leopold von Sacher-Masoch, 1835–95, Austrian pornographic novelist).

massage stimulation of skin and muscle by rubbing, kneading, stroking, pummelling or hand-hammering with therapeutic intent. Massage has little physical effect but the psychological and symbolic effect of human touch can be deeply soothing and can relieve symptoms, especially those of undue muscle tension.

masseter a short, thick, paired muscle in each cheek running down from the cheekbone (zygomatic arch) to the outer corner of the jawbone (mandible). The masseters act to raise the lower jaw and compress the teeth together in the act of chewing.

mast- *combining form denoting* breast or breast-like.

mastalgia pain in the breast.

mastatrophy shrinkage of the breasts.

mast cell a connective tissue cell found in large numbers in the skin and mucous membranes and in the lymphatic system. The mast cell plays a central part in allergic reactions. It contains numerous large granules – collections of powerfully irritating chemical substances such as HISTAMINE; SEROTONIN; HEPARIN; the proteases tryptase and chymase; CYTOKINES; PROSTAGLANDINS; and LEUKOTRIENES. In people with allergies, the antibody (immunoglobulin), IgE, remains attached to specific receptors on the surface of the mast cells. When the substance causing the allergy (the ALLERGEN) contacts the IgE, the mast cell is triggered to release these substances and the result is the range of allergic symptoms and signs. CHROMOGLYCATE can stabilize the mast cell membrane and prevent the release of the contents. Mast cells closely resemble blood BASOPHIL cells, and the latter also carry receptors for IgE. The mast cell has recently emerged as an important element in the inflammatory events leading to joint damage in RHEUMATOID ARTHRITIS. See also ATOPY.

mastectomy surgical removal of the breast (mammary gland). This is done almost exclusively for the treatment of cancer. Radical mastectomy, now a relatively uncommon operation, involves the removal of all breast tissue and skin, the underlying pectoral muscles and the lymph nodes in the armpit. In simple mastectomy, only the breast tissue is removed. In lumpectomy only the obvious mass is removed through a short radial incision.

mastication chewing.

mastitis inflammation of the breast. This is commonest during LACTATION and is usually caused by infection with organisms such as Staphylococcus aureus entering through cracks or abrasions in the nipples. There is high fever, redness, hardening and tenderness. Treatment is with antibiotics but an abscess may form which may have to be drained surgically.

mastocytosis an excessive proliferation of MAST CELLS in the tissues or in the bone marrow.

mastoid bone a prominent bony process which can be felt behind the lower part of the ear. This is not a bone in its own right but a protuberance on the lower, outer aspect of the TEMPORAL BONE. The mastoid process is honeycombed with air cells and these communicate with the middle ear. Infection can spread to the air cells

from the middle ear, causing a MASTOIDITIS. The term refers to a fanciful breast-like appearance.

mastoidectomy an operation to chisel off part of the surface bone of the mastoid process behind the ear so as to release pus, allow drainage and prevent inward spread of infection in MASTOIDITIS.

mastoiditis inflammation of the mastoid air cells from infection usually spread from an OTITIS MEDIA. This is potentially dangerous as the infection may proceed through the bone into the interior of the skull and cause a brain abscess.

mastopathy any disease or disorder of the breast (mammary gland).

mastoplasia breast enlargement from an increase in the bulk of the milk-secreting tissue.

mastoptosis sagging of the breasts.

masturbation self-stimulation of the genitals, with sexual fantasizing, in order to reach orgasm. Repetitive movement of the skin of the penis or gentle massage of the clitoris is the usual method. Over 90% of males and 75% of females are believed to masturbate at one time or another. Kinsey found that the frequency varied from three or four times a week in adolescence to once or twice a week in adult life. Urologists have long been aware that male masturbation can be beneficial but have refrained from mentioning it. Recent research has, however, brought the matter out into the open by showing that frequent male masturbation between the ages of about 20 and 50 substantially reduces the risk of prostate cancer. An equal frequency of orgasm by sexual intercourse does not, apparently, provide the same advantage.

materia medica an out-dated term for PHARMACOLOGY especially in relation to the treatment of disease by drugs (therapeutics).

maternal mortality the number of women who die each year, from causes associated with pregnancy or childbirth, for every 1000 total births. Deaths during pregnancy from causes unrelated to pregnancy are excluded but causally related deaths are counted, even if they occur months or years after the pregnancy. Maternal mortality is a useful index of the standards of medical care in a community.

matrix the scaffolding or ground substance of a tissue which supports the specialized functional cells.

maturity-onset diabetes DIABETES MELLITUS developing in or after middle age and caused by a relative insufficiency of INSULIN production by the PANCREAS. The condition is of more gradual development than insulin-dependency diabetes and can often be treated by diet or oral HYPOGLYCAEMIC drugs rather than by insulin. In general, it is associated with less severe symptoms than juvenile-onset (Type I) diabetes, but complications such as eye and kidney disease are common. Also known as Type II diabetes.

MAustCOG *abbrev. for* Member of the Australian College Obstetrics & Gynaecology.

Maxepa a brand name for EICOSAPENTAENOIC ACID.

Maxidex a brand name for the steroid drug DEXAMETHASONE in the form of eyedrops.

maxilla one of a pair of joined facial bones that form the upper jaw, the hard palate, part of the wall of the cavity of the nose and part of the floor of each eye socket. The maxillae bear the upper teeth and each contains a cavity called the maxillary antrum or sinus.

maxillary sinus the mucous membrane-lined air space within each half of the maxillary bone. The maxillary sinuses drain into the nose. Also known as the maxillary antrum.

maxillofacial pertaining to the MAXILLA and the rest of the face. Maxillofacial surgery is much concerned with the treatment of facial injuries and fractures of the facial skeleton.

Maxitrol a brand name for NEOMYCIN with DEXAMETHASONE, for external use.

Maxolon a brand name for the anti-emetic and anti-nausea drug METOCLOPRAMIDE.

Maxtrex a brand name for METHOTREXATE.

MB *abbrev. for* Bachelor of Medicine.

MBACA *abbrev. for* Member of the British Acupuncture Association.

MBBS *abbrev. for* Bachelor of Medicine, Bachelor of Surgery.

MBChB *abbrev. for* Bachelor of Medicine, Bachelor of Surgery.

MC *abbrev. for* Master of Surgery.

McArdle's dissease an autosomal recessive disorder of muscle carbohydrate metabolism in which glycogen breakdown is blocked because of non-functioning of the enzyme myophosphorylase. The effect is a considerable reduction in exercise capacity. Attempts at strenuous activity cause cramps, muscle injury, RHABDOMYOLYSIS and MYOGLOBINURIA. Ingestion of sucrose before exertion can markedly improve exercise capacity.

MCB *abbrev. for* Master of Clinical Biochemistry.

McBurney's sign tenderness on gentle pressure at a point (McBurney's point) on the right side of the abdomen two-thirds of the way from the navel to the bony prominence on the front of the hip (anterior superior iliac spine). This is a fairly reliable sign of APPENDICITIS. (Charles McBurney, 1845–1913, American surgeon).

MCCM *abbrev. for* Member of the College of Community Medicine (New Zealand).

MCDH *abbrev. for* Mastership in Community Dental Health.

MCFP *abbrev. for* Member of the College of Family Practitioners.

Mch *abbrev. for* Master of Surgery.

MChir *abbrev. for* Master of Surgery.

MChD *abbrev. for* Master of Dental Surgery.

MChOrth *abbrev. for* Master of Orthopaedic Surgery.

MchOtol *abbrev. for* Master of Otology.

MCISC *abbrev. for* Master of Clinical Science.

MclinPsychol *abbrev. for* Master of Clinical Psychology.

McNaughten rules see INSANITY.

McommH *abbrev. for* Master of Community Health.

MCPA *abbrev. for* Member of the College of Pathologists of Australia.

MCPath *abbrev. for* Member of the College of Pathologists.

MCPS *abbrev. for* Member of the College of Physicians & Surgeons.

MCR-50 a brand name for ISOSOBIDE MONONITRATE.

MCRA *abbrev. for* Member of the College of Radiologists of Australia.

MD *abbrev. for* Doctor of Medicine. See DOCTOR OF MEDICINE.

MDD *abbrev. for* Doctor of Dental Medicine.

MdentSc *abbrev. for* Master of Dental Surgery.

MDR *abbrev. for* multi-drug resistant.

MDR1 multi-drug-resistant protein No 1. see DRUG-TRANSPORTER GENES.

MDS *abbrev. for* Master of Dental Surgery.

MDSC *abbrev. for* Master of Dental Science.

MDU *abbrev. for* Medical Defence Union, the world's largest legal defence membership organization run by doctors in the interests of doctors and to provide them with legal advice and assistance.

measles a highly infectious, often epidemic, disease of childhood caused by a paramyxovirus usually acquired by droplet inhalation. The incubation period is 10–14 days and just before the rash appears KOPLIK'S SPOTS may be seen in the mouth. There is fever, cough, running nose, misery, CONJUNCTIVITIS, and an irregular, red, mottled, slightly raised rash which lasts for about a week and then fades. Complications include OTITIS MEDIA, BRONCHITIS, PNEUMONIA and sometimes ENCEPHALITIS. The disease can be prevented by a vaccine which should be given to all children, aged 1–2 years, especially those who are debilitated and chronically ill and for whom there is no valid medical objection.

meat substitutes non-animal protein food products, derived from soya beans, wheat gluten, yeast or other sources, and usually flavoured and textured to resemble natural muscle protein. These products are a reasonably effective substitute for animal protein but may not contain all the essential AMINO ACIDS.

meatus any passage or opening in the body.

mebanazine a monoamine oxidase inhibitor (MAOI) drug used in the treatment of severe depression.

mebendazole an ANTHELMINTIC drug used to get rid of roundworms, hookworms, threadworms and whipworms. The drug is on the WHO official list. A brand name is Vermox.

mebeverine an antispasmodic drug used to treat bowel colic. Brand names are Colofac and Fybogel Meberverine.

Meckel's diverticulum a small pouch-like sac that protrudes from the interior of part of the small intestine (ILEUM) in about 2% of people. Normally harmless, it sometimes becomes infected and causes a condition indistinguishable from APPENDICITIS. Meckel's diverticulum may also lead to twisting (VOLVULUS) or infolding (INTUSSUSCEPTION) of the bowel. (Johann Friedrich Meckel II, 1781–1833, German anatomist).

meclozine an anticholinergic drug that has an inhibitory action on the vomiting centre of the brain and is used to prevent motion sickness. A brand name is Sea-legs.

meconium the thick, greenish-black, sticky stools passed by a baby during the first day or two of life, or before birth if the fetus is deprived of an adequate oxygen supply (fetal distress). Meconium consists of cells from the lining of the fetal bowel, bowel mucus and bile from the liver. Once feeding is established meconium is replaced by normal stools.

meconium ileus obstruction of the intestine in a new-born baby with CYSTIC FIBROSIS due to failure of digestion of the MECONIUM which becomes very firm and packs the lower ILEUM with a putty-like material. There is vomiting and distention. Surgery may be needed to remove the obstructed section of the bowel.

media the middle wall of an artery or vein. The media is composed of smooth muscle and elastic fibres and is the thickest of the three layers. Also known as the tunica media.

medial situated toward the midline of the body. Compare LATERAL.

median 1 situated in or towards the MEDIAN PLANE of the body.
2 in statistics, the middle value when observations are ranked in order of magnitude.

median plane the vertical plane that divides the body into right and left halves.

median nerve one of the two major nerves of the arm, supplying most of the muscles and providing sensation in the two-thirds of the hand on the thumb side.

mediastinitis inflammation of the MEDIASTINUM.

mediastinoscopy direct examination by fibreoptic ENDOSCOPY of the internal structures of the central compartment of the chest (the MEDIASTINUM). The endoscope is passed through an opening in the base of the neck under general anaesthesia. The procedure is relatively easy on the right side but is more difficult and dangerous on the left and other methods are often preferred.

mediastinum the central compartment of the chest, flanked on either side by the lungs, and containing the heart, the origins of the great blood vessels, the TRACHEA and the main BRONCHI, the OESOPHAGUS and many lymph nodes.

medical 1 pertaining to the whole discipline of healing, exercised by whatever means.
2 pertaining to those disorders that are treated by drugs and advice rather than by surgical methods.

medical bacteriology the branch of BACTERIOLOGY concerned with the micro-organisms that cause disease or otherwise affect health.

medical computing the application of computers to clinical and administrative medicine. Software expert systems have been written that enable a computer to take a more detailed and accurate medical history than is possible with the time available to the average doctor. It has been found that patients will often communicate more freely with a computer than with a doctor. Computer programs now make a better job of interpreting electrocardiograms than most doctors. Expert diagnostic systems that learn by experience are beginning to rival the best doctors in accuracy. They also provide considerable help in selecting appropriate drugs and dosage. Computers have a major role to play in a wide range of medical administrative tasks. The list that follows highlights the key entries related to medical computing in the dictionary: ADAM software, BIS monitor, computerized axial tomography, computers in medicine, medical computing, digital radiography, digital subtraction angiography, Holter monitoring, ophthalmic digital imaging systems, personal digital assistant, PET scanning, robotics, robotic surgery, spiral computed tomography, telemedicine.

medical education the provision of instruction and information in the sciences basic to medicine and in clinical practice, ideally in such a manner as to inculcate in the recipient the desire to continue the process, spontaneously, throughout life. Literally, a 'drawing out'. The importance of medical education is highlighted by the recent decision of the General Medical Council to issue licences to practice only to doctors whose knowledge and skills have been validated and shown to conform to the standards laid down in the GMC pamphlet GOOD MEDICAL PRACTICE. This applies to all doctors from 2005. John Locke insisted that the aims of education, in order of importance, were virtue, wisdom, breeding and learning. There is much to be said for this view.

medical entomology the science concerned with the identification and study of insects that affect health, especially those that act as transmitters (vectors) of disease-producing organisms.

medical ethics a code of practice by which doctors govern their professional behaviour. As well as the avoidance of MALPRACTICE, medical ethics is concerned with the many moral questions and dilemmas that have arisen in consequence of medical advances – questions such as the rightness of prolonging life by extraordinary means, choices in allocating limited resources, decisions about organ transplantation, the propriety of psychosurgery, how far research on fetuses is justified, how trials of new drugs should be conducted, whether the diagnosis of genetic defects in embryos is always justified and how far genetic engineering may ethically proceed.

medical geography the relationship between geographic factors and disease. With the growth of world travel, medical geography has assumed ever-increasing importance in the contexts of both public health and research.

medical information highway the linked network of thousands of readily accessible medical web pages on the Internet that can be used to obtain medical information updates. The principal difficulty is the *embarras de richesse*. Reliability can be assessed in much the same way as in paper publications by an assessment of the status of the institutions publishing in this way and of the professional status of the authors, and a careful and critical review of the content. The full text of nearly all major general medical journals is accessible on the Internet and most now publish regular lists of addresses of reliable medical websites. See also MEDICAL COMPUTING and TELEMEDICINE.

medical jurisprudence the study or practice of those aspects of medicine that relate in any way to the law. Also known as forensic medicine.

medicinal marijuana SEE CANNABIS.

medical microbiology the study of micro-organisms that can affect health. Medical microbiology includes the study of certain classes of VIRUSES (medical virology), BACTERIA (medical bacteriology), FUNGI (medical mycology) and PROTOZOA (medical protozoology).

Medical Officer of Health an obsolete term for the principal medical administrator in a local government area. Now known as a Community Physician.

medical parasitology the study of the relationship between man and the many life-forms that adopt his body as a habitat and source of support and nutrition. Human parasites include ectoparasites such as lice, fleas, mites and some flies and endoparasites such as the wide range of worms. Bacteria and other infective micro-organisms are also parasites.

medical rationing the allocation of scarce or inadequate medical resources to an ever-expanding and increasingly-demanding population of patients. The avoidance of rationing (in the sense of denying essential treatment to a proportion of patients) is currently a major preoccupation of the medical profession and has led to healthy expansion in the used of specialist nurses, nurse practitioners, nurse prescribing, TELEMEDICINE and the increasing of the clinical scope of paramedical personnel of all kinds.

medically-unexplained symptoms symptoms for which investigation, even if extensive, fails to reveal an organic cause. This substantial class of complaints, which is a frequent cause of patient dissatisfaction and is one of the most common reasons for attendance at general medical outpatient clinics, has been seriously neglected in the training of doctors. Routine prescription of analgesics or other drugs is of negative value, and these complaints call for acknowledgement, counselling, reassurance and appropriate follow-up.

medicated of soaps, shampoos, lotions, confections, etc., containing a drug or other medication.

medication an Americanism for prescribed medicine now coming into common usage in Britain.

medicine 1 the branch of science devoted to the prevention of disease (hygiene), the restoration of the sick to health (therapy) and the safe management of childbirth (obstetrics). Medicine is a scientific discipline but the practice of medicine involves social skills and the exercise of sympathy, understanding and identification, not normally demanded of a scientist.
2 medical practice not involving surgical operative intervention. In this sense, medicine and surgery are distinguished.
3 any drug given for therapeutic purposes.

medicochirurgical pertaining to both medicine and surgery.

medicolegal pertaining to both MEDICINE and law.

Mediterranean diet a diet featuring a high intake of vegetables, legumes, fruit, nuts, cereals and olive oil; a moderately high intake of fish; a low to moderate intake of cheese and yoghurt; a low intake of other dairy products, saturated fats, meat and poultry; and a moderate and regular intake of wine taken with meals. Research has shown that close adherence to the traditional Mediterranean diet is associated with a significant increase in longevity. The diet was found to reduce deaths both from coronary heart disease and from cancer.

Mediterranean fever see BRUCELLOSIS.

medium any substance in which micro-organisms may be cultured in an incubator. Most culture media use AGAR jelly or gelatine containing additional materials such as blood or meat broth to encourage bacterial growth. Selective media contain substances that discourage the growth of unwanted organisms or specifically foster the growth of others.

Medizip a surgical dressing and wound-closing device in the form of two multi-layered, microporous adhesive supportive strips which are applied one to each side of an incised wound or surgical incision and are then drawn together by closing a slide zip fastener attached to the two inner free edges. Medizip is a trade mark of Atrax Medical Group Ltd.

Medline a large computer database containing a substantial proportion of the papers produced in the best medical journals over a period of years. Medline contains millions of entries and is accessible free of charge to almost any doctor interested enough to wish to consult it. A search, however, requires special skill if one is not to be inundated with references.

Medrone a brand name for the steroid drug METHYLPREDNISOLONE.

medroxyprogesterone a PROGESTOGEN drug that can be taken by mouth and is used to treat excessive menstrual bleeding (MENORRHAGIA), the PREMENSTRUAL SYNDROME, ENDOMETRIOSIS, infertility and oestrogen-dependent cancers. The drug is on the WHO official list. Brand names are Adgyn Medro, Climanor, Provera, Depo-Provera, Farlutal and Premique.

It is also available formulated as an adjunct to oestrogen for menopausal HORMONE REPLACEMENT THERAPY under the brand names

Improvera, Premique, Premique Cycle and Tridesta.

medulla 1 the inner part of an organ, especially of the kidney, the adrenal and the shaft of long bones. Compare CORTEX.

2 the MYELIN layer of nerve fibres. See also MEDULLA OBLONGATA.

medulla oblongata the part of the BRAINSTEM lying below the PONS and immediately above the spinal cord, just in front of the CEREBELLUM. The medulla oblongata contains the nuclei of the lower four CRANIAL NERVES, the vital centres for respiration and control of heart-beat, and the long motor and sensory tracts running down to and up from the spinal cord. Disease or injury to the medulla is always serious, often fatal.

medullated MYELINATED.

medulloblastoma a malignant brain tumour, most commonly affecting children and usually occurring in the CEREBELLUM or in the nearby roof of the FOURTH VENTRICLE.

medulloepithelioma 1 a rare eye tumour affecting the CILIARY BODY or RETINA. May be BENIGN or MALIGNANT. Also known as dictyoma.

2 a rare malignant tumour of the nervous system.

mefenamic acid a NON-STERODIAL ANTI-INFLAMMATORY DRUG (NSAID) and painkilling (analgesic) drug used to treat arthritis, and menstrual disorders. Brand names are Meflam and Ponstan.

mefloquine a drug used to prevent and treat MALARIA. The drug is effective but has been criticized for its neuropsychological side effects which include fatigue, depression, headache, insomnia and distressing dreams. The drug is on the WHO official list. A brand name is Lariam.

mega- 1 *prefix denoting* one million.

2 *combining form denoting* large.

megabase a unit of measurement of the length of a segment of DNA equal to 1,000,000 base pairs. Usually contracted to Mb.

Megace a brand name for MEGESTROL.

megacolon enlargement (hypertrophy) and widening (dilation) of part or all of the COLON associated with severe and intractable CONSTIPATION. Megacolon may be CONGENITAL or acquired. Congenital megacolon is an AUTOSOMAL RECESSIVE condition caused by the local absence of the nerves responsible for PERISTALSIS.

megakaryocyte an unusually large bone marrow cell that releases many small fragments of its CYTOPLASM as the blood PLATELETS essential for clotting (blood coagulation).

megakariocytopoenia an abnormal deficiency of MEGAKARYOCYTES in the bone marrow.

megakaryocytosis an increase in the number of MEGAKARYOCYTES in the bone marrow.

megalo-, -megaly combining forms denoting abnormal enlargement.

megaloblastic anaemia anaemia that features large numbers of abnormally large, nucleated red blood cell precursor cells in the bone marrow and in the blood. This occurs in PERNICIOUS ANAEMIA and in other similar types of anaemia.

megalomania a delusion of power, wealth, omnipotence or grandeur.

megaureter considerable widening of the tube carrying urine down from the kidney to the bladder (the ureter). This usually results from obstruction to outflow in the lower part of the ureter or from reflux of urine upwards from the bladder.

megestrol a PROGESTOGEN drug used to assist in the treatment of breast or endometrial cancer. A brand name is Megace.

meglumine iotroxate a biliary contrast medium used in cholecystangiography. A brand name is Biliscopin. The drug is on the WHO official list.

meibomian cyst a small, pea-like swelling in an eyelid caused by accumulation of secretion in one of the lid lubricating glands (MEIBOMIAN GLANDS) that open on to the lid margin, just behind the line of the lashes. Meibomian cysts commonly become infected. Treatment is by a minor operation under local anaesthesia in which the contents are scooped out through the inner surface of the lid. Also known as a chalazion.

meibomian gland one of the 20 to 30 glands that occupy each eyelid, lying parallel to each other and perpendicular to the lid edge and opening on to the lid margin. The meibomian glands secrete an oily fluid that prevents adhesion between the lids and forms an outer layer on the tear film over the cornea and conjunctiva so as to retard drying. (Heinrich Beibom, 1638–1700, German professor of Medicine, History and Poetry).

meibomianitis inflammation of one or more of the glands of the eyelid. See also MEIBOMIAN CYST.

Meigs syndrome an accumulation of fluid in the abdomen (ASCITES) or in the space between the lungs and the chest wall (PLEURAL EFFUSION) associated with a FIBROMA or other tumour of an ovary. The condition is being treated with BOTULINUM TOXIN. (Joe Vincent Meigs, 1892–1963, American gynaecologist).

meiosis the process in the formation of the sperms (spermatozoa) and eggs (ova) in which chromosomal material undergoes recombination (meiosis I) and the chromosomes are reduced to a single set of 23 (haploid number) instead of the normal 23 pairs (meiosis II). This allows the restoration of the normal number when the spermatozoon fuses with the ovum. See also MITOSIS.

Meissner's plexus a network of nerve fibres, from the PARASYMPATHETIC NERVOUS SYSTEM, lying in the wall of the intestines between the mucous membrane lining and the muscle layer. These fibres control and coordinate the movements and changing contractions of the intestines. (Georg Meissner, 1829–1905, German anatomist).

melaena blackening of the stools by altered blood that has been released into the bowel from bleeding in the OESOPHAGUS, STOMACH, or DUODENUM. Melaena implies loss of at least 60 ml of blood and is an important warning sign that should never be ignored.

melan-, melano- *combining form denoting* black.

melancholia DEPRESSION.

melanin the body's natural colouring (pigment) found in the skin, hair, eyes, inner ears and other parts. In body cells, melanin is bound to protein. It is a complex POLYMER formed from the amino acid TYROSINE (4-hydroxphenyl-alanine) by oxidation via dopa and dopaquinone.

melanin concentrating hormones small peptides formed in the pituitary and brain that regulate skin colour by altering the concentration of melanin.

melanocortin 4 receptor (MC4R) a cell receptor that is strongly stimulated by the alpha MELANOCYTE-STIMULATING HORMONE – a peptide that produces a sense of fullness after eating. Mutations of the gene that codes for MC4R are commonly associated with severe uncontrollable overeating and pathological obesity. Such mutations can be found in nearly 6% of people with a life-long history of obesity.

melanocyte a pigment cell of the skin. A cell carrying MELANIN or capable of producing melanin.

melanocyte-stimulating hormone the PITUITARY GLAND hormone that promotes the synthesis of MELANIN in MELANOCYTES. Also known as melanotropin. Alpha melanocyte-stimulating hormone is an ANOREXOGENIC peptide produced by the enzymatic cleavage of proopiomelanocortin (POMC) that is a powerful agonist of the MELANOCORTIN 4 RECEPTOR.

melanocytoma a harmless benign tumour, mainly of melanocytes, found on the OPTIC DISC, especially in black people.

melanocytosis excessive numbers of MELANOCYTES.

melanoderma abnormal darkening of the skin from excessive numbers of MELANOCYTES.

melanoma any benign or malignant tumour of MELANOCYTES. See also MALIGNANT MELANOMA.

melanonychia blackening of the nails with MELANIN.

melanosis abnormal pigmentation of the tissues from excessive deposition of MELANIN. Melanosis coli is pigmentation of areas of the COLON due to an accumulation of MACROPHAGES containing melanin or a similar pigment.

melanotic freckles uneven, light to dark brown, blotchy areas of pigmentation containing abnormal MELANOCYTES that sometimes occur on the cheek prominences of people after middle age. Melanotic freckles are precancerous and may progress to MALIGNANT MELANOMAS. Also known as malignant lentigo.

melanuria the presence of the black pigment MELANIN in the urine of people suffering from widespread MALIGNANT MELANOMA.

melarsoprol a combination of melarsan oxide and dimercaprol used to treat TRYPANOSOMIASIS. The drug is highly effective but must be used with caution because of sometimes dangerous side effects including the JARISCH-HERXHEIMER REACTION. The drug is on the WHO official list.

MELAS syndrome the combination of Mitochondrial myopathy, Encephalopathy, Lactic Acidosis and Stroke-like attacks. The syndrome also features retinal degeneration leading to visual field defects, and sometime hemiplegia.

melatonin a hormone synthesized from serotonin in the pineal gland and elsewhere. Melatonin production has a strong circadian rhythm, being secreted mainly in the period between about 2100 hours and 0800 hours. Bright light suppresses melatonin secretion and exogenous melatonin can alter the timing of the body clock. For these reasons it has been proposed as a means of combatting jet lag. Other methods have been found more generally useful.

melioidosis a severe infection caused by *Pseudomonas pseudomallei* acquired through skin abrasions. The disease features high fever, prostration and multiple abscesses in the liver, lungs and spleen with PNEUMONIA and other severe effects. Early treatment with large doses of TETRACYCLINE antibiotics and CHLORAMPHENICOL may save life, but treatment must be continued for weeks or months.

Melleril a brand name for the PHENOTHIAZINE antipsychotic drug thioridazine.

melphalan a drug used in the treatment of POLYCYTHAEMIA VERA, chronic LEUKAEMIA and MYELOMA. A brand name is Alkeran.

memantine an inhibitor of glutamate NMDA RECEPTORS used with the expectation of delaying the progress of ALZHEIMER'S DISEASE and other forms of dementia. It has been shown to have some value even in the later stages of dementia. A brand name is Ebixa.

membrane attack complex a ring-like complex of COMPLEMENT proteins that form a pore in the membrane of target cells leading to the inflow of water and sodium ions so that the cell is often destroyed.

membrane fluidity the ability of lipid molecules to move sideways within their own single-molecule-thick layer.

membrane-protein ion channels voltage-controlled and gated cell membrane pores through which currents of sodium and potassium ions pass in water solution. The movement of these ions through the controlled channels underlie all electrical activity of the nervous system, including the brain and are thus responsible for all behaviour, thinking, and emotional activity. Voltage-gated ion channels have a central pore domain surrounded by voltage-sensor regions.

memory the persistent effect on behaviour and thought of past experience. Short-term memory stores are small and the contents are soon lost unless repeatedly refreshed. Long-term memory stores are very large but are not always readily accessible. The physical basis of long-term memory has not yet been established, but most researchers seem to favour the circulating nerve impulse hypothesis rather than the idea of bit-coding by protein molecules.

memory cells B LYMPHOCYTES that retain information about previous challenge, as by infective organisms, so that ANTIBODIES can be more rapidly produced in response to a subsequent infection with the same agent.

memory pill an informal term for a drug purporting to improve memory. Currently the main interest in the 'ampakines' – drugs that are said to amplify the signal of the neurotransmitter GLUTAMATE, which is used in neurons in the memory circuits.

menarche the onset of MENSTRUATION. Compare MENOPAUSE.

Mendelian disease a disease caused by a single mutated gene. Also known as a 'single gene disorder'. Although some 5,000 such diseases are known, nearly all of them are comparatively rate. Some of the more common are CYSTIC FIBROSIS, SICKLE CELL DISEASE, THALASSAEMIA, HAEMOPHILIA, MARFAN'S SYNDROME, PHENYLKETONURIA, one form of RETINITIS PIGMENTOSA, DUCHENNE'S MUSCULAR ATROPHY, HUNTINGTON'S DISEASE and adult POLYCYSTIC DISEASE.

menhidrosis monthly sweating, sometimes with blood in the sweat, as a form of vicarious menstruation. Also known as menidrosis.

Ménière's disease a usually progressive, episodic middle ear disease caused by an increase in the fluid pressure within the LABYRINTH and featuring a combination of dizziness (VERTIGO), nausea, variable hearing loss, a sense of fullness in the head and singing in the ears (TINNITUS). During episodes of vertigo the deafness and tinnitus temporarily increase. Treatment is mainly that of the symptoms but in some cases surgery is advised to try to control the pressure. Vertigo can also be relieved by removing the balancing mechanism on one side (LABYRINTHECTOMY) but this causes total deafness on that side. (Prosper Ménière, 1799–1862, French physician).

Ménière's syndrome see MÉNIÈRE'S DISEASE.

meninges the three layers of membrane that surround the brain and the spinal cord. The innermost, the PIA MATER, dips into the brain furrows (sulci). The intermediate ARACHNOID MATER bridges over the furrows, leaving the subarachnoid space which contains cerebrospinal fluid and many blood vessels. The outer later, the dura mater, is a tough, fibrous protective covering attached, in the skull, to the overlying bone and forming a tube to enclose the spinal cord.

meningioma a tumour of the cells of the MENINGES. Most meningiomas are fixed to the DURA MATER and are benign but, because of their location and the bony surroundings of the nervous system, may do serious damage by compression of neurological structures. Treatment is by surgical removal and this is often successful.

meningism a collection of signs and symptoms, such as headache, stiff neck and fever, suggestive of MENINGITIS but occurring in the absence of an unequivocal diagnosis of the condition.

meningitis inflammation of the MENINGES. This can be caused by many different organisms, especially the HERPES SIMPLEX virus, the VARICELLA-ZOSTER virus that causes CHICKEN POX and SHINGLES, the meningococcus, the POLIO virus, the echo virus, the COXSACKIE virus and the MUMPS virus. Meningitis may also complicate LYME DISEASE, LEPTOSPIROSIS, TYPHUS, TUBERCULOSIS and other infections. Viral meningitis may be a minor illness but can be acute, with headache, stiff neck, fever and drowsiness progressing rapidly to deep coma. There may be weakness or paralysis of the muscles, speech disturbances, double vision, loss of part of the field of vision and epileptic fits. Most patients recover completely, but some have residual nervous system damage. There is no specific treatment for most virus infections, but herpes meningitis responds to the drug ACYCLOVIR. See also MENINGOCOCCAL MENINGITIS.

meningococcal meningitis an epidemic form of MENINGITIS, sometimes called cerebrospinal fever or spotted fever, and commoner in children than in adults. The organism responsible, *Neisseria meningitidis*, is spread by coughed or sneezed droplets. There is a sore throat, fever, severe headache, marked neck stiffness and vomiting. A rash of red spots appears on the trunk and the affected person may be gravely ill within a day of onset and

quickly become confused, drowsy and comatose. Without treatment, death may occur within days or even hours but an intensive course of antibiotics is usually successful, resulting in full recovery. Vaccines are available. Contacts are sometimes given protective antibiotics.

meningocoele protrusion (herniation) of the two outer layers of the MENINGES, the dura and arachnoid maters, through a usually developmental bony defect in the skull or spine, to form a cyst filled with cerebrospinal fluid, lying under the skin. Meningocoele is most commonly found in the condition of SPINA BIFIDA.

meningoencephalitis inflammation of the brain and the surrounding membranes (MENINGES).

meningoencephalocele protrusion of part of the brain with the covering membranes (MENINGES) through a defect in the skull. An encephalocoele.

meningomyelocele an abnormal protrusion of the spinal cord and its covering membranes (MENINGES) through a congenital defect in the bone of the spine (SPINA BIFIDA). The meningomyelocele forms a swelling under the skin and the condition is usually associated with a severe neurological disturbance with loss of function in the legs and bladder. Folic acid taken just before, and during the first few weeks of, pregnancy can eliminate this disaster.

meningovascular pertaining to the MENINGES and to the blood vessels supplying the brain.

meniscectomy surgical removal of a torn or displaced semilunar cartilage from the knee joint.

Menogon a brand name for MENOTROPHIN.

menopause the end of the reproductive period in women when the ovaries have ceased to form GRAAFIAN FOLLICLES and produce eggs (OVA) and menstruation has stopped. The menopause usually occurs between the ages of 48 and 54. There is reduced production of OESTROGEN hormones by the ovaries and this may cause accelerated loss of bone bulk (OSTEOPOROSIS) and thinning and drying of the vagina (atrophy) with difficulty and discomfort in sexual intercourse. The common menopausal symptoms (hot flushes, night sweats, insomnia, headaches and general irritability) have not been proven to be due to oestrogen deficiency, but these usually settle if oestrogens are given. HORMONE REPLACEMENT THERAPY may be indicated for osteoporosis and vaginal atrophy. The term is derived from the Greek *meno*, a month, and *pausos*, cessation.

Menophase a brand name for MESTRANOL.

Menorest a brand name for OESTRADIOL (estradiol).

menorrhagia abnormally heavy and prolonged MENSTRUAL PERIODS. This is often due to an excessive buildup of the womb lining (the ENDOMETRIUM) but may be due to a spontaneous abortion or FIBROID TUMOURS. Cancer of the endometrium usually causes irregular bleeding, rather than menorrhagia. The condition can often be treated with the contraceptive pill.

menotrophin a GONADOTROPHIN drug used to treat both female and male infertility and inadequate development of the sex organs. Brand names are Humegon, Menogon and Pergonal.

menstrual disorders see AMENORRHOEA, OLIGOMENORRHOEA, DYSMENORRHEA, MENSTRUAL IRREGULARITY, MITTELSCHMERZ, MENORRHAGIA, POLYMENORRHOEA, METRORRHAGIA and PREMENSTRUAL TENSION (PMT).

menstrual irregularity an alteration in the regular timing of the MENSTRUAL PERIODS. This is normal at the beginning of the menstrual life (menarche) and before the menopause. At other times it may be due to missed periods, pregnancy followed by early miscarriage, ANOREXIA NERVOSA, excessive dieting, strenuous athletics or midcycle bleeding.

menstrual period the sequence of days, usually 3 to 7 but averaging 4 days, during each menstrual cycle when the lining of the womb (the endometrium), together with a quantity of blood, is being shed via the cervix and the vagina. The volume lost varies between 50 and 150 ml. Menstrual blood is dark in colour and does not clot.

menstruation the periodic shedding of the lining (ENDOMETRIUM) of the womb (uterus) at intervals of about 28 days causing bleeding through the vagina of 3 to 7 days duration in the non-pregnant female. The purpose of menstruation is to renew the endometrium so that it is in a suitable state to ensure implantation of a fertilized egg (ovum).

mental pertaining to the mind.

mental deficiency SEE MENTAL RETARDATION.

mental retardation intellectual ability so much below average as to preclude the performance of most forms of work or other social functions. Mentally retarded people usually require supervision and guidance if they are to avoid distress or danger. There are degrees of mental deficiency. So far as INTELLIGENCE QUOTIENTS (IQs) can be measured in the mentally retarded, the mildly defective have IQs from 70 down to about 55; the moderately defective have IQs from 54 to 40; and the severely defective have IQs below 40.

menthol a volatile oil used as a local application to relieve itching or as an embrocation. Menthol can also be used as an inhalant to relieve nasal congestion. Excessive inhalation can be dangerous and menthol can cause skin allergy. Brand names of preparations for external use containing menthol are Balmosa, Fradol, Radian B and Salonpas.

mento- *prefix denoting* the chin.

mentum the chin.

meperidine see PETHIDINE.

meprobamate a mildly tranquillizing carbamate drug with muscle-relaxant properties used in combination with painkilling drugs to treat muscle and joint pain. A brand name is Equagesic.

Meptid a brand name for the mild narcotic-like painkiller meptazinol.

meralgia paraesthetica pain and numbness over the front and side of the thigh due to entrapment of the sensory nerve to the part (lateral cutaneous nerve of thigh) by the INGUINAL LIGAMENT.

Merbentyl a brand name for DICYCLOMINE HYDROCHLORIDE (dicycloverine).

mercaptopurine a CYTOTOXIC drug used in combination with others in the treatment of acute LEUKAEMIA. The drug is on the WHO official list. A brand name is Puri-Nethol.

Mercilon a brand name for ETHINYLOESTRADIOL (ethinylestradiol) formulated with the PROGESTOGEN drug DESOGESTREL as an oral contraceptive.

mercury poisoning the toxic effect of ingestion of mercury compounds either in large doses (acute poisoning) or in small doses over a period (chronic poisoning). Acute mercury poisoning causes nausea and vomiting, pain in the abdomen and diarrhoea. Chronic poisoning, as from the inhalation of mercury vapour, causes brain damage with staggering, tunnel vision, garbled speech, severe tremor and emotional disturbances.

mercy killing EUTHANASIA.

Merkel's discs Merkel's corpuscles, small cup-shaped touch receptors in the epidermis, each consisting of a single sensory nerve fibre ending in contact with an epithelial cell. (Friedrich S. Merkel, German anatomist and physiologist, 1845–1919).

Merocets a brand name for CETYLPIRIDINIUM CHLORIDE.

Meronem a brand name for MEROPENEM.

merozoite one of the stages in the life cycle of the malarial parasite. Merozoites are small motile bodies released in large numbers after asexual division of the schizont in red blood cells. They invade further red cells or liver cells where they continue to reproduce asexually or initiate a sexual reproduction cycle by the formation of male and female sex cells.

MERLIN *abbrev. for* Medical Emergency Relief International.

meropenem a CARBAPENEM antibiotic drug. A brand name is Meronem.

mes-, meso- *prefix denoting* middle, MEDIAL, intermediate or connective.

mesalazine a salicylate drug used to treat, and prevent recurrences of, ULCERATIVE COLITIS. Brand names are Asacol, Pentasa and Salofalk.

mesencephalon the middle section of the embryonic brain.

mesentery the complex, double-layered folded curtain of PERITONEUM that encloses the bowels and by which they are suspended from the back wall of the abdomen. Blood and lymphatic vessels run to and from the intestines between the two layers of the mesentery.

mesenteric adenitis inflammation, probably from virus infection, of the lymph nodes in the MESENTERY. The condition is common in children and can be very difficult to distinguish from APPENDICITIS. Also known as mesenteric lymphadenitis.

mesna a drug used to prevent damage to the urinary tract of people being treated with the anticancer drugs cyclophosphamide or ifosfamide. A brand name is Uromitexan.

mesoappendix the small MESENTERY of the APPENDIX.

mesocolon the folded membrane of PERITONEUM by which the colon is suspended from the inside of the back wall of the abdomen.

mesoderm the intermediate of the three primary germ layers of the developing embryo, lying between the outer ECTODERM and the inner ENDODERM. Mesoderm develops into the bones and muscles, the heart and blood vessels and most of the reproductive system.

mesomorph a person of powerful musculature and large, strong bones. One of the SOMATOTYPES.

mesothelioma a slow-growing benign or malignant tumour of MESOTHELIUM. Malignant pleural mesothelioma is almost entirely the result of exposure to asbestos dust 25 to 50 years previously. In Britain today there are about 1800 deaths per year from this cause and these are expected to peak between 2011 and 2015. Mesothelioma can also occur in the abdomen and in the tunica vaginalis of the testis. Radical surgery has been advocated for malignant pleural mesothelioma. Suggestions that SV40 may have an aetiological link have been challenged.

mesothelium lining cells originating in the primitive MESODERM of the developing embryo. Mesothelium occurs in the PERITONEUM, PLEURA and PERICARDIUM as well as elsewhere in the body.

messenger 1 pertaining to ribonucleic acid (RNA) that carries the coded information for protein synthesis from the DNA to the site of protein synthesis, the RIBOSOMES.
2 a HORMONE or other effector capable of acting at a distance from its site of production. A second messenger is a hormone, produced within a cell and operating on internal structures, when another hormone acts on the outer cell membrane.

messenger RNA commonly written as mRNA, this is the molecule that reads the genetic code from DNA. Before this can happen the double helix must separate into two single strands. One of these carries the same sequence as the mRNA and is called the coding strand. The other is called the template, or antisense, strand and it is this strand that directs the synthesis of the mRNA by complementary base pairing. In RNA the base uracil replaces thymine. The messenger RNA molecule then leaves the cell nucleus and passes out through a nuclear membrane pore to the site of protein synthesis. There the appropriate amino acids are selected and placed in the right order by TRANSFER RNA which, using its anticodons, reads the code on the messenger RNA.

mesterolone a male sex hormone (androgen) drug used to treat male infertility from androgen deficiency. A brand name is Pro-Viron.

mestranol an OESTROGEN drug, used in combination with a PROGESTOGEN as an oral contraceptive or as a hormone replacement therapy for post-menopausal women. A brand name of a combination with the progestogen NORETHISTERONE is Norinyl-1.

met-, meta- *prefix denoting* beyond, after, following, with, next to, transcending, changed or transformed.

meta-analysis an attempt to improve the reliability of the findings of medical research by combining and analyzing the results of all discoverable trials on the same subject. In crude terms the advantages are obvious: trials that find against a hypothesis will cancel out the effect of those that find for it. Pooling of raw data is not, however, without statistical hazard and it has become apparent that meta-analysis can introduce its own sources of inaccuracy. The method is currently undergoing refinement.

metabolic syndrome a dangerous development in obese people that features low levels of high-density lipoprotein cholesterol, raised triglycerides, glucose intolerance with insulin resistance and raised blood pressure. The syndrome seriously increases the risk of DIABETES and CARDIOVASCULAR DISEASE. The metabolic syndrome is common in Western populations with a high prevalence of obesity. The US Centers for Disease Control and Prevention reported in 2003 that 24% of the US adult population had the metabolic syndrome. The syndrome is transmitted through the mother and there are recent indications that it is the result of a mutation in the MITOCHONDRIAL DNA.

metabolism the totality of the body's cellular chemical activity, largely under the influence of enzymes, that results in work and growth or repair. The 'building-up' aspects of metabolism are known as anabolic and the 'breaking-down' as catabolic. Metabolism involves the consumption of fuel (glucose and fatty acids), the production of heat and the utilization of many constructional and other biochemical

elements provided in the diet, such as AMINO ACIDS, fatty acids, carbohydrates, vitamins, minerals and trace elements. The basal metabolic rate is increased in certain disorders, such as hyperthyroidism, and decreases in others. Anabolism can be artificially promoted by the use of certain steroid male sex hormones (androgens or anabolic steroids).

metabolite any substance involved in METABOLISM either as a constituent, a product or a byproduct.

metacarpal bone one of the five long bones situated in the palmar part of the hand immediately beyond the CARPAL bones of the wrist and articulating with the bones of the fingers (PHALANGES).

metacarpus the five bones of the palm of the hand.

metacentric of a chromosome in which the CENTROMERE is at or near the centre.

metachromasia the variations in colour produced in different parts of a tissue when stained with a single dye.

metamorphopsia distortion or breakup of the perceived visual image either as a result of disruption of the normal relationship of the cones in the central part of the RETINA or as a result of brain damage or malfunction or the effects of HALLUCINOGENIC drugs.

metamorphosis major alterations in structure and appearance occurring in an organism, such as the human embryo, in the process of its development from egg (ovum) to baby.

metaphase stage of MITOSIS or MEIOSIS during which the chromosomes are aligned around the equator of the cell and are visible on microscopy. The stage at which the banding pattern of the chromosomes is apparent.

metaphysis the growing part of a long bone. The metaphysis lies between the growth plate (the EPIPHYSIS) and the shaft (the diaphysis).

metaplasia an abnormal change in the character or structure of a tissue as a result of changes in the constituent cells. Metaplasia often involves a change of cells to a less specialized form and may be a prelude to cancer.

metaraminol a SYMPATHOMIMETIC drug used as a heart stimulant in states of abnormally low blood pressure (hypotension) or to relieve PAROXYSMAL TACHYCARDIA caused by hypotension.

metatarsal one of the five long bones of the foot lying beyond the TARSAL bones and articulating with the bones of the toes (PHALANGES).

metatarsus the five bones of the foot.

metastasis 1 the spread or transfer of any disease, but especially cancer, from its original site to another place in the body where the disease process starts up. Metastasis usually occurs by way of the bloodstream or the lymphatic system or, in the case of lung disease by coughing and re-inhalation of particles to other parts of the lung.
2 the new focus of disease, so produced.

metatarsalgia pain in the long bones of the foot (METATARSALS).

Metatone a brand name for a mixture of THIAMINE and glycerophosphates widely popular as a 'tonic'.

metazoa all the members of the animal kingdom that consist of more than one cell. All animals more complex than the one-celled PROTOZOA.

metencephalon the part of the hindbrain of the embryo from which the CEREBELLUM and the PONS develop.

Metenix a brand name for METOLAZONE.

metenkephalin one of the several ENDOGENOUS opium-like substances having a sequence of five amino acids. See also ENDORPHINS.

meteorism tightness and distention of the abdomen as a result of internal gas under pressure in the peritoneal cavity or in the bowel. Also known as tympanites.

-meter *suffix denoting* a measuring instrument.

metformin a biguanide oral HYPOGLYCAEMIC drug used in the treatment of MATURITY ONSET DIABETES. The drug may be dangerous to those with liver or kidney disease or a high alcohol intake. The drug is on the WHO official list. A brand name is Glucophage.

methadone a synthetic narcotic painkilling (analgesic) drug with properties similar to those of MORPHINE. It is also used as a substitute for HEROIN in attempts to manage addiction, but is widely abused. A brand name is Physeptone.

methaemoglobin HAEMOGLOBIN that has been altered by oxidation of the iron fraction from the ferrous to the ferric state by drugs such as PHENACETIN, DAPSONE and related compounds or by nitrites. It is of a brown colour and does not combine reversibly with oxygen.

methaemoglobinaemia the presence of METHAEMOGLOBIN in the blood in excess of the normal 1%. This may occur as a hereditary condition or as a result of absorption of nitrites from the intestine. Methaemoglobinaemia causes CYANOSIS.

methaemoglobinuria the presence of methaemoglobin in the urine.

methimazole a drug used in the treatment of overactivity of the thyroid gland. It is effective in reducing thyroid activity but may cause AGRANULOCYTOSIS. A sore throat is a warning symptom.

methionine an antidote used to treat PARACETAMOL poisoning from overdose. A drug used in combination with paracetamol to protect the liver against the serious damage that is caused by deliberate overdosage. A brand name of the combination is Paradote.

Methoblastin a brand name for METHOTREXATE.

methocarbamol a centrally-acting muscle relaxant drug used to treat conditions of severe muscle spasm. A brand name is Robaxin.

methotrexate an ANTIMETABOLITE and IMMUNOSUPPRESSIVE drug used to treat cancer and help in the treatment of RHEUMATOID ARTHRITIS. It acts by interfering with the metabolism of FOLIC ACID. The drug is on the WHO official list. A brand name is Maxtrex.

methotrimeprazine levomepromazine, a phenothiazine derivative anti-psychotic drug. A brand name is Nozinan.

methoxamine an alpha-adrenergic agonist drug that constricts arteries and is sometimes used in emergency to raise falling or dangerously low blood pressure. A brand name is Vasoxine.

methyl cellulose an inert and non-absorbable substance that has been used to bulk out meals in the hope of achieving weight loss. It is also used as a laxative and in artificial tears. A brand name is Celevac.

methylcyanoacrylate sterilization the use of a surgical tissue adhesive for closure of the fallopian tubes as a method of female sterilization. A small balloon pump device is used to apply the material via the cervix. The method was developed as an alternative to the much-criticized but widespread practice of inserting pellets of quinacrine. Tests of toxicity have been passed.

methyldopa an alpha adrenergic agonist drug that, paradoxically, is effective in the treatment of high blood pressure (HYPERTENSION). The drug is said to act centrally on the brainstem by stimulating adrenergic receptors in such a way as to reduce the normal action of the sympathetic nervous system on arteries. This explanation is not universally accepted. The drug is on the WHO official list. A brand name is Aldomet.

methylene blue a solution of methylthioninium chloride that has been used to treat METHAEMOGLOBINAEMIA. It is also used as a bacterial stain and sometimes in surgery to demonstrate fistulas. The drug is on the WHO official list.

methylphenidate a nervous system stimulant drug that, paradoxically, has been found effective in the management of ATTENTION-DEFICIT HYPERACTIVITY DISORDER in children. A brand name is Ritalin. The current consensus of opinion on the use of this drug for this purpose is that it is grossly over-prescribed, especially in the USA.

methylprednisolone a CORTICOSTEROID drug used in a wide range of conditions to control severe inflammation, treat allergies and replace stroid deficiencies. It is commonly used in depot form for long-term action. Brand names are Medrone, Depo-Medrone and Solu-Medrone.

methyl salicylate an aromatic compound used externally as an embrocation often in combination with other ingredients. Also known as Oil of Wintergreen. Brand names of formulations containing methyl salicylate are Balmosa, Monphytol, Phytex, Radian B and Salonpas.

methyltestosterone a male sex hormone drug sometimes used to treat severe itching caused by CIRRHOSIS OF THE LIVER.

methylxanthine derivatives drugs such as THEOPHYLLINE and AMINOPHYLLINE used in the treatment of ASTHMA.

methysergide a SEROTONIN antagonist ERGOT derivative drug used to treat resistant cases of MIGRAINE and some cases of persistent diarrhoea. A brand name is Deseril.

metoclopramide an ANTI-EMETIC drug also useful in the control of severe heartburn (REFLUX OESOPHAGITIS) in HIATUS HERNIA. The drug is on the WHO official list. Brand names are

Gastrobid Continus, Gastromax and Maxolon. The drug is also formulated with paracetamol as a MIGRAINE treatment under the brand name Paramax.

metolazone a diuretic drug similar to the thiazide group used to treat high blood pressure (HYPERTENSION). A brand name is Metenix.

Metopirone a brand name for METYRAPONE.

metoprolol a cardioselective beta-blocker drug used to treat ANGINA PECTORIS, heart irregularities, high blood pressure (HYPERTENSION) and MIGRAINE. Brand names are Betaloc and Lopressor. The drug is also formulated with the diuretic HYDROCHLORO-THIAZIDE under the brand name Co-Betaloc.

Metosyn a brand name for FLUOCINONIDE.

metr- *combining form denoting* the womb.

metralgia pain in the womb.

metrifonate an organophosphorus CHOLINESTERASE inhibitor drug used to kill the worms in SCHISTOSOMIASIS, especially Schistosoma haematobium.

metritis inflammation of the womb (uterus), strictly involving both the muscle (MYOMETRIUM) and the lining (ENDOMETRIUM).

metrocolpocele undue downward protrusion of the womb (uterus) causing downward displacement of the vagina.

Metrogel a brand name for METRONIDAZOLE formulated for external use only.

Metrogyl a brand name for METRONIDAZOLE.

Metrolyl a brand name for the antibiotic drug METRONIDAZOLE.

metronidazole an ANTIBIOTIC drug effective against *Trichomonas vaginalis* and *Entamoeba histolytica* as well as many other organisms. It is especially useful in the treatment of amoebic dysentery and amoebic liver abscesses as well as ANAEROBIC infections. The drug is on the WHO official list. Brand names are Acea Gel, Elyzol, Flagyl, Metrosa and Zidoval. The drug is also formulated with the antifungal drug nystatin under the brand name Flagyl Compak and, for external use only, under the brand names Anabact, Metrogel, Metrotop and Rozex.

metrorrhagia bleeding from the womb (uterus) other than during the normal menstrual period.

metrorrhoea any abnormal discharge from the womb (uterus).

metrosalpingitis inflammation of the womb (uterus) and the Fallopian tubes.

Metrotop a brand name for METRONIDAZOLE formulated for external use only.

metyrapone an ALDOSTERONE inhibitor drug used to treat aldosterone-induced OEDEMA and CUSHING'S syndrome. A brand name is Metopirone.

mexiletine an antiarrhythmic drug drug used in the treatment or prevention of severe heart irregularity arising in the VENTRICLES. A brand name is Mexitil.

Mexitil a brand name for MEXILETINE.

MFCM *abbrev. for* Member of the Faculty of Community Medicine.

MFCMI *abbrev. for* Member of the Faculty of Community Medicine of Ireland.

MFHom *abbrev. for* Member of the Faculty of Homoeopathy.

MFOM *abbrev. for* Member of the Faculty of Occupational Medicine.

MFPaedRCPI *abbrev. for* Member of the Faculty of Paediatrics, Royal College of Physicians of Ireland.

MFPHM *abbrev. for* Member of the Faculty Public Health Medicine.

MFPM RCP (UK) *abbrev. for* Member of the Faculty Pharmaceutical Medicine Royal College Physicians UK.

MGDF *abbrev. for* megakaryocyte growth and development factor. See THROMBOPOIETIN.

MGDS *abbrev. for* Member in General Dental Surgery.

MHC *abbrev. for* MAJOR HISTOCOMPATIBILITY COMPLEX.

MHyg *abbrev. for* Master of Hygiene.

MIBiol *abbrev. for* Member of the Institute of Biology.

micelles tiny aggregates of fatty acids and monoglycerides formed by the detergent action of the bile acids on digested fats so that these materials can be made soluble and absorbed into the LACTEALS of the intestinal VILLI.

MICGP *abbrev. for* Member of the Irish College of General Practitioners.

miconazole an imidazole antifungal drug. It can be taken by mouth or given by intravenous injection in severe SYSTEMIC fungus infections and is used as an oral preparation for mouth infections. The drug is on the WHO official list. A brand name is Daktarin. The drug is also formulated for external use with benzoyl peroxide for the treatment of ACNE under the brand name Acnidazil; with hydrocortisone as

Daktacort; and as a lacquer for dentures under the brand name Dumicoat. A vaginal preparation for the treatment of thrush is available under the brand name Gyno-Daktarin.

micro- *combining form denoting* very small, abnormally small or pertaining to microscopy.

microalbuminuria the presence of almost undetectable traces of the protein albumin in the urine.

microaneurysms 1 minute, but dangerous, widenings (dilatations) of arteries often in the brain, in the region of the THALAMUS, believed to be an important cause of CEREBRAL HAEMORRHAGE. These are distinct from the berry aneurysms on the external arteries that also cause cerebral haemorrhage.
2 tiny dilatations on retinal capillaries seen with the ophthalmoscope in cases of DIABETIC RETINOPATHY.

microarray a collection on a chip of thousands of biological probes such as DNA single-strand sequences, protein-detecting molecules, or any other biologically-identifying material, that can be used to survey a specimen for the presence of a target gene or substance. Binding to the target substance can be made to cause fluorescence to occur at the unique spot or spots on the array and the chip can then be read by a scanner and the result displayed on a computer monitor. See also DNA MICROARRAYS.

microbe any microscopic organism but especially a bacterium or virus capable of causing disease. The word is almost synonymous with, but slightly upmarket from, the term 'germ'.

microbicide any agent capable of killing MICROBES. The term has, however, recently been applied specifically to any intravaginal, topical gel preparation for use by women to reduce their likelihood of acquiring HIV infection during sexual intercourse with husbands or others. The first candidate microbicide, nonoxynol-9, was shown to damage vaginal epithelial cells and actually encourage infection. Research for a safe and effective microbicide continues and includes the development of agents blocking CD4 binding sites, inhibitors of GP41-medicated fusion, prevention of HIV take up by dendritic cells and conventional pharmacological attack on HIV replication.

microbiology the study of microorganisms. The list that follows highlights the key entries related to microbiology in the dictionary: abacterial, antibacterial, aspergillus, bacteraemia, bacteria, bacterial culture, bactericidal, bacteriology, medical bacteriology, adenovirus, alphaviruses, arbovirus, arenavirus, bunyavirus, Chandipura virus, coronavirus, Coxsackie viruses, cytomegalovirus infection, Ebola virus disease, ECHO virus, enteroviruses, epidermophyton, Epstein-Barr virus, filterable virus, flavivirus, hantavirus disease, helper virus, herpes viruses, human metapneumovirus, human herpesvirus, inactivated viruses, leptospira, lyssavirus, MRSA, nanobacteria, Norwalk virus, orthomyxoviruses, papillomavirus, papovavirus, parvoviruses, picornavirus, poxviruses, protozoa, retrovirus, rhinoviruses, small round viruses, spirochaete, streptococcus, staphylococcus, togavirus, sterilization, trichophyton, viruses, virus interference.

microbubbles tiny bubbles of gas, used as a contrast medium in ULTRASOUND SCANNING, which are introduced into the vascular system or the Fallopian tubes to enhance the images obtained.

microcephaly abnormal smallness of the skull. Microcephaly often reflects poor brain development and is usually associated with MENTAL RETARDATION.

microcheilia abnormally small lips.

microcyte a red blood cell of very small diameter.

microcytic anaemia ANAEMIA in which the red blood cells are significantly smaller than normal. This is a feature of iron deficiency anaemia.

microfilaria the microscopic embryonic forms of various nematode worms that parasitize humans and animals. Microfilaria circulate in their millions in the blood and in the lymph vessels of people suffering from FILARIASIS. When taken up by a blood-sucking insect, microfilaria mature into the larval form of the worm within the body of the insect.

microgamete 1 the male sex cell or spermatozoon. The OVUM is the macrogamete. 2 the motile male sex cell of the malarial parasite.

microglia neurological connective tissue MACROPHAGES. Compare MACROGLIA.

microglossia having an abnormally small tongue.

micrognathia having an abnormally small upper or lower jaw.

micrographic surgery microscopic surveillance of the entire surgical margin of an excised tumour, such as a basal cell carcinoma, to endure that it has been completely removed.

Microgynon 30, Microgynon 30 ED brand names for low-dose oral contraceptive pills containing ETHINYOESTRADIOL (ethinylestradiol) and LEVONORGESTREL.

microinfarct a very small INFARCT. Microinfarcts become important when multiple.

micromastia having abnormally small breasts.

micrometastases small collections of cancer cells, discernible only on microscopic examination, occurring in the lymph nodes of people with cancer. They may occur in treated cancer patients and identify a high-risk group among those previously deemed to be free of the disease.

micromelia having abnormally small arms or legs. Compare PHOCOMELIA.

Micronor a low-dose oral contraceptive containing NORETHISTERONE.

Microvar a low-dose oral contraceptive containing the PROGESTOGEN drug levonorgestrel.

micronutrients dietary substances necessary for health but required only in very small quantities. Vitamins and minerals.

microphthalmos the state of having an abnormally small eyeball. In severe degrees there is usually a gross defect of vision.

micropsia perception of objects as much smaller than they in fact are. This may be caused by an abnormal separation of the cones of the centre of the retina (so that widely-spaced points on the image are interpreted by the brain as being closer together) or may be a hallucination from drugs or disorders of brain function.

microRNA very short segments of RNA involved in RNA INTERFERENCE and recently shown to be important elements in the development of plant structure. Many genes that code for microRNA have been found in many species including *H. sapiens*. There is much current speculation into their role in human development.

microscopic colitis a collective term for collagenous colitis and lymphocytic colitis.

Once considered rare gastrointestinal disorders, these conditions are now known to be relatively common and should be considered in the differential diagnosis of persistent watery diarrhoea without blood. Most cases resolve spontaneously but treatment with budesonide and bismuth subsalicylate may be necessary.

Microsporum a genus of fungus that causes TINEA.

microsporidiosis a protozoal infection caused by various organisms of the *Microsporidia* genus. Most human cases have occurred in people with AIDS. Human cells are infected when microsporidian spores impale them with a hollow tube through which DNA is passed into the host cell. Different species affect different organs. The clinical features include diarrhoea, urinary tract infection, rhinitis, sinusitis, corneal stromal infection and infection of the bile passages. Treatment is with oral albendazole and fumagillin eye drops for corneal ulceration.

microsurgery surgery in which the operation field is magnified 2 to about 40 times by means of an operating microscope. Appropriately miniaturized operating instruments are used. This method allows a high degree of precision in the cutting, approximation and stitching (suturing) of small parts and is widely used by ophthalmologists, ENT surgeons and vascular surgeons. To a lesser extent, microsurgery is employed in gynaecology and urology.

microtome an instrument for cutting very thin slices from a block of tissue set in wax, or frozen, for microscopic examination after mounting on a slide and staining.

Microval a brand name for LEVONORGESTREL as an oral contraceptive.

microvilli the millions of tiny, hair-fine, finger-like protrusions on the surface cells of EPITHELIUM which greatly increase the effective surface area so as to facilitate absorption. Microvilli occur especially on the secretory and absorptive surfaces, and are formed by extensions of the cell membrane. They have a central core of ACTIN filaments bound together with the protein VILLIN.

microwave diathermy a method of effecting deep heating of tissues, such as muscles, to promote healing.

micturating cystogram an X ray taken while the subject is actually urinating. The urine contains a dye opaque to X-rays. The method

can provide information about abnormalities of the bladder and of the urine tubes entering it (URETERS) and leaving it (URETHRA). It is especially useful in investigating reflux flow of urine back up the ureters from the bladder in children.

midazolam a BENZODIAZEPINE drug given by intravenous injection as a sedative for minor surgery or to induce general anaesthesia. A brand name is Hypnovel.

middle ear the narrow cleft within the temporal bone lying between the inside of the ear drum and the outer wall of the inner ear. The middle ear is lined with mucous membrane, contains the chain of three auditory OSSICLES and is drained into the back of the nose by the EUSTACHIAN TUBE. It is a common site of infection, which gains access by way of the tube. Middle ear infection is called OTITIS MEDIA. Also known as the tympanic cavity.

mid-life crisis a psychological upset, sometimes affecting people in middle age, who feel that their lives have become meaningless and devoid of satisfaction. This may lead to injudicious sacrifice of established achievement and a damaging change of lifestyle.

Midrid a brand name for ISOMETHEPTENE.

midwifery the nursing speciality concerned with the conduct of antenatal care, labour and childbirth. Midwifery differs from OBSTETRICS to the extent that it is concerned primarily with the normal. Complications and undue difficulties are managed or supervised by doctors specializing in obstetrics.

mifepristone a progesterone antagonist drug also known as RU-486. When given in early pregnancy mifepristone causes the detachment of the blastocyst, the production of prostaglandins that prompt contraction of the womb and softening of the cervix. The result is abortion of the conceptus. A brand name is Mifegyne.

Migard a brand name for FROVATRIPTAN.

migraine a particular form of headache caused by widening (dilatation) of some of the arteries of the scalp and brain, usually on one side. The widening is preceded by partial closure of these arteries (spasm) and this often causes temporary disturbance of brain function. Most commonly, this takes the form of an expanding, one-sided blank area in the field of vision, with a sparkling (scintillating) jagged border. Such an episode usually lasts for about 20 min. Other neurological disturbances may occur, such as weakness or loss of sensation on the face or down one side of the body or speech or comprehension defects. The headache that follows these effects may be severe and there is nausea and sometimes vomiting and great intolerance to light. Migraine is treated with various drugs including ergotamine tartrate, beta-blockers such as PROPRANOLOL, antidepressants such as amitryptyline, and the serotonin antagonist METHYSERGIDE. The term migraine comes from the words 'hemi-cranial', meaning half-head.

Migraleve a brand name for the antihistamine BUCLIZINE formulated with PARACETAMOL and CODEINE.

Migril a brand name for a mixture of the anti-MIGRAINE drugs ERGOTAMINE, CAFFEINE and CYCLIZINE.

MIH *abbrev. for* Master of Industrial Health.

MIHL *abbrev. for* music-induced hearing loss; a condition that can afflict both rock and classical musicians in which loss of the ability to hear notes of high pitch is associated with TINNITUS.

Mikulicz's disease see SJÖGREN'S DISEASE. (Johann von Mikulicz-Radecki, Polish-born 1850–1905, German surgeon).

miliaria a prickling skin eruption caused by blockage of sweat gland ducts and due to excessive sweating, especially in unacclimatized people in the tropics. Also known as prickly heat.

miliary tuberculosis an acute form of TUBERCULOSIS that occurs if a focus of tuberculosis erodes a vein so that tubercular material is scattered throughout the whole body to set up new foci of infection. There is high fever, fast pulse, drenching sweats, rapid loss of weight and anaemia and, unless effective treatment is quickly given, death within days or a few weeks.

milk the secretion of the breast (MAMMARY GLAND) of any mammal. Cow's milk differs from human milk, mainly in the composition of the fats. Human milk fats contain a higher proportion of unsaturated fatty acids that provide more resistance to bowel organisms than those in cow's milk. Human milk also contains maternal antibodies that provide the baby with protection against many organisms, until it is able to produce its own.

milk-alkali syndrome an uncommon condition caused by excessive intake of alkaline medication and calcium. Levels of blood calcium rise and the metal is deposited in various tissues including the kidneys. The blood becomes more alkaline. Kidney failure can occur.

milk, witches' see WITCHES' MILK.

Miller-Abbott tube a tube with a double bore and a balloon at the end, that is passed into and through the stomach and allowed to be carried by PERISTALSIS into the bowel to locate an obstruction and allow clearance by aspiration. (Thomas Grier Miller, American physician, b. 1886, and William Osler Abbott, 1902–43, American physician).

Miller-Fisher syndrome a rare variant of the GUILLAIN–BARRÉ SYNDROME featuring paralysis of eye movements (ophthalmoplegia), ATAXIA and AREFLEXIA.

milrinone a PHOSPHODIESTERASE INHIBITOR drug. A brand name is Primacor.

mind and body an association long regarded as a Cartesian duality of disparate entities, after the work of René Descartes (1596–1650) but now recognized by most medical scientists as aspects of a unity. The prevailing view, today, is that the manifestations of the mind are wholly the result of neurological (mainly brain) activity and that, given sufficiently detailed knowledge of the structure and function of the nervous system, the association between function of the nervous system and corresponding mental capacity will be seen to be complete. Mental processes involve widespread brain function and are not localized to single brain areas. The existence of the mind-body problem has been dismissed by some philosophers, especially Gilbert Ryle (1900–76), as an example of a category error.

mineralocorticoids hormones from the outer layer (cortex) of the adrenal gland that promote retention of sodium and excretion of potassium in the urine. ALDOSTERONE is the most powerful mineralocorticoid. Compare GLUCOCORTICOIDS.

minerals chemical elements required in the diet, usually in small amounts, to maintain health. Apart from iron and calcium, deficiency is comparatively rare. The essential minerals are calcium, iron, magnesium, copper, selenium, phosphorus, fluorine, potassium, sodium and zinc.

minimal access surgery see LAPAROSCOPIC SURGERY.

minimally invasive coronary bypass surgery the performing of a coronary artery bypass operation by LAPAROSCOPIC SURGERY without stopping the heart or using a cardiopulmonary bypass machine. The left internal mammary artery is connected (anastomosed) to the left anterior descending coronary artery. The operation is appropriate only for a blockage of this artery near the upper part of the heart.

minimally invasive surgery see LAPAROSCOPIC SURGERY.

Minims a brand name for a range of eye drop preparations dispensed in sterile, single-dose, snap-off plastic vials. The current range of 19 preparations have replaced the former undesirable practice of using the same multi-dose bottle of eye drops for more than one patient. Minims are used for a range of ophthalmic purposes including dilatation (cyclopentolate) and constriction (pilocarpine) of pupils; treatment of bacterial infections (gentamicin) and GLAUCOMA (pilocarpine); temporary paralysis of the focusing muscle ring (cyclopentolate); anaesthetizing of the cornea (amethocaine, proxymetacine); corneal epithelial staining for erosions (Rose Bengal) and for ulcers and foreign bodies (fluoresceine) and to conduct aplanation tonometry (proxymetacine and fluoresceine); and the control of inflammation (dexamethasone).

Minims benoxinate a brand name for OXYBUPROCAINE.

Minims Chloramphenicol a brand name for CHLORAMPHENICOL.

Minims fluorescein a brand name for FLUORESCEIN.

Minims lignocaine fluorescein a brand name for FLUORESCEIN eyedrops compounded with a local anaesthetic.

Minims metipranol a brand name for METOPRANOL.

Minims phenylephrine a brand name for PHENYLEPHRINE.

Minims pilocarpine a brand name for PILOCARPINE.

Minims prednisolone a brand name for PREDNISOLONE.

Minims proxymetacaine a brand name for PROXYMETACAINE.

Minims proxymetacaine fluorescein a brand name for FLUORESCEIN compounded with a local anaesthetic.

Minims Rose Bengal a brand name for ROSE BENGAL.

Minims tropicamide a brand name for TROPICAMIDE.

Minitran a brand name for GLYCERYL TRINITRATE.

Minimata disease an epidemic of neurological disorders that occurred in Minimata, Japan, in 1953-56, and was eventually shown to be caused by MERCURY POISONING from contact with the effluent from a PVC factory.

Minnesota tube a tube used to suck out secretions from the OESOPHAGUS when bleeding from varicose veins at the lower end (OESOPHAGEAL VARICES) is being controlled by balloon TAMPONADE.

Minocin a brand name for MINOCYCLINE.

minocycline a TETRACYCLINE antibiotic used to treat ACNE and general infections. Brand names are Aknemin and Minocin.

Minodiab a brand name for GLIPIZIDE.

minor surgery any surgical operation of short duration and minimal risk. Most minor surgery is performed under local anaesthesia.

minoxidil a VASODILATOR drug used in the treatment of high blood pressure (HYPERTENSION). Used externally on the scalp, the drug has a somewhat exaggerated reputation as a hair-restorer and must be used continuously if any advantage gained is to be retained. A brand name is Loniten and, for external use to restore hair, Regaine or Rogaine.

Minulet a brand name for ETHINYLOESTRADIOL (ethinylestradiol) formulated with the PROGESTOGEN drug GESTODENE as an oral contraceptive.

mio- *prefix denoting* narrowing, reduction or diminution.

miosis constriction of the pupil.

miotic a drug that constricts the pupil.

miracidium the first-stage larva of a fluke such as *Schistosoma* species *Fasciolopsis* or *Chlonorchis* species. Miracidia are released into water in human excreta and invade particular water snails in which the second-stage larvae (sporocysts) form. These release thousands of cercariae, the form that can pass through the skin to infect humans.

Mirena a brand name for a T-shaped

intrauterine contraceptive system with a hormone reservoir that slowly releases LEVONORGESTREL, providing five-year, contraception.

mirtazapine an antidepressant drug that acts by increasing the release of serotonin and noradrenaline. A brand name is Zispin.

miscarriage a spontaneous ABORTION. Spontaneous ending of a pregnancy before the fetus is mature enough to survive even with the best supportive care.

misfolded proteins see CHAPERONES.

misophonia dislike of sound. See also HYPERACUSIS.

misoprostol a PROSTAGLANDIN drug used to treat peptic ulcers especially those caused by NON-STEROIDAL ANTI-INFLAMMATORY DRUGS. Brand names are Cytotec and Mifegyne. The drug is also formulated with DICLOFENAC under the brand name Arthrotec, and with NAPROXEN under the brand name Napratec, for the treatment of RHEUMATOID ARTHRITIS.

missed abortion death of the fetus which remains in the womb (uterus) for weeks or months. The uterus ceases to enlarge and the cervix remains tightly closed. Pregnancy tests may give equivocal results for several weeks after the death of the fetus but ultrasound scans can reveal the condition. The uterus is cleared surgically.

missense mutation a mutation caused by a change in a nucleotide sequence that changes a codon specifying a particular AMINO ACID into one that specifies a different amino acid.

mistura a pharmacological mixture to be taken by mouth as medication. If used in a prescription, the term is usually abbreviated to 'Mist.' Now that the public is no longer content to be kept in ignorance by the deliberate use of medical Latin, such terms are rapidly becoming obsolete.

mithramycin a drug that reduces bone metabolism and can be useful in the treatment of PAGET'S DISEASE and HYPERCALCAEMIA.

mitochondria one of the class of important tiny elements (ORGANELLES) in the cytoplasm of nucleated (eukaryotic) cells. They may be rod-shaped, spherical, branched or ring-shaped. Mitochondria have double-layered walls, the inner layer being deeply infolded to form compartments. They contains genes and RIBOSOMES and are the site of cell respiration.

Their many functions include the Krebs cycle, metabolism of fatty acids, amino acids and steroids, pyruvate oxidation, and the production of energy in the form of adenosine triphosphate (ATP). MITOCHONDRIAL DNA is transmitted only from the mother and, apart from mutations, remains unchanged through the generations. Mitochondria are believed to have developed from bacteria that colonized primitive eukaryotic cells more than a billion years ago, thereby providing them with aerobic metabolism.

mitochondrial DNA a small circular DNA molecule of which all MITOCHONDRIA in cells have several copies. It contains 16,569 base pairs and 37 genes. Being present in the cytoplasm of the cell, is transmitted exclusively by the mother. A mature ovum contains about 100,000 copies of mitochondrial DNA; sperm contains none. The genome has been completely sequenced. Its main function is to code for enzymes needed by the mitochondrion. The sites of common mutations, especially deletions, are known as a number of diseases caused by these defects in the mitochondrial DNA. See MITOCHONDRIAL DNA DISEASES.

mitochondrial DNA diseases diseases caused by mutations in MITOCHONDRIAL DNA (mtDNA) or by nuclear DNA mutations affecting components in mitochondrial processes. Because both mitochondrial and nuclear genes may be involved, inheritance may be maternal or Mendelian. They are all rare. Pure mitochondrial diseases caused by point mutations include LEBER'S HEREDITARY OPTIC NEUROPATHY; RAGGED RED FIBRES; mitochondrial encephalomyopathy with lactic acidosis and stroke-like episodes (MELAS); and neurogenic weakness with ataxia and retinitis pigmentosa (NARP). Major rearrangements of mitochondrial DNA cause the KEARNS-SAYRE PHENOTYPE; chronic progressive external ophthalmoplegia; PEARSON'S SYNDROME; and excessive ageing.

mitogen 1 any agent that promotes cell nuclear division (MITOSIS). Mitogens are important in genetic research and technology. Pokeweed mitogen, derived from the plant *Phytolacca americana*, is a powerful mitogen of B LYMPHOCYTES.
2 any substance that non-specifically causes lymphocytes to proliferate.

mitosis the division of a cell nucleus to produce two daughter cells having identical genetic composition to the parent cell. First the long strands of CHROMATIN replicate and coil up to form dense chromosomes with the two copies (chromatids) joined at the CENTROMERE so that they appear X-shaped. At the same time, the envelope of the cell nucleus disrupts (prophase). Then two sets of strand-like microtubules (the spindle) appear, radiating from each end of the cell to the centre, the metaphase plate, and the chromosomes align themselves on the plate with the centromeres at the equator (metaphase). The copies of each chromosome (chromatids) now separate and move to opposite poles of the spindle (anaphase). Finally, the cell separates into two, the chromatin uncoils and the nuclear envelope of each reforms (telophase).

mitotic index the percentage of cells in a population that are actually undergoing MITOSIS. The mitotic index is a measure of the reproductive or growth activity of a tissue.

Mitoxana a brand name for IFOSFAMIDE.

mitozantrone mitoxantrone, a CYTOTOXIC anti-cancer drug. A brand name is Novantrone.

mitral incompetence failure of complete closure of the MITRAL VALVE of the heart, often as a result of damage by RHEUMATIC FEVER or coronary artery disease. The result is regurgitation of blood into the left ATRIUM when the VENTRICLE contracts so that the heart has to work harder to maintain the circulation. This leads to compensatory thickening of the muscle (heart enlargement) and sometimes HEART FAILURE. Valve replacement may be necessary.

mitral stenosis narrowing of the MITRAL VALVE of the heart. This is usually the result of damage from RHEUMATIC FEVER. The narrowing imposes a back pressure on the blood coming from the lungs and an early sign is breathlessness. The left ATRIUM enlarges and may beat irregularly (ATRIAL FIBRILLATION) and clots may form in the atrium. Disablement from reduced exercise tolerance may be severe and surgery may be required to widen or replace the damaged valve.

mitral valve the valve on the left side of the heart lying between the upper and lower chambers (ATRIUM and VENTRICLE). It has two cusps and is said to resemble a Bishop's mitre.

mitral valve disorders see MITRAL STENOSIS, MITRAL INCOMPETENCE and MITRAL VALVE PROLAPSE.

mitral valve prolapse a condition of the mitral valve known as the floppy valve syndrome and present in about one person in twenty. It causes a characteristic heart murmur but is usually of no consequence. Occasionally mitral valve prolapse may lead to valve leakage, chest pain, pulse irregularity, BACTERIAL ENDOCARDITIS and, rarely, HEART FAILURE.

mittelschmerz pain or discomfort in the lower abdomen felt by women at the time of OVULATION, between menstrual periods. The cause is uncertain but is thought to be either stretching of the Graafian follicle or irritation of the PERITONEUM from blood or follicle fluid. The term is German for 'middle pain'.

Mivacron a brand name for MIVACURIUM.

mivacurium a non-depolarizing muscle-relaxant drug used by anaesthetists. The drug acts withing 3–4 minutes and its effect lasts for about 15 minutes. Mivacurium is rapidly broken down by CHOLINESTERASE in the blood. A brand name is Mivacron.

mixed connective tissue disease a condition that combines some of the features of SYSTEMIC LUPUS ERYTHEMATOSUS, POLYMYOSITIS and progressive SYSTEMIC SCLEROSIS. The blood contains high levels of ANTINUCLEAR ANTIBODY. There are skin changes similar to DERMATOMYOSITIS, swelling of the fingers with RAYNAUD'S phenomenon, muscle weakness and arthritis involving several joints. The condition responds well to treatment with corticosteroid drugs and the outlook is favourable.

mixed venous oxygen saturation (SvO2) the balance between oxygen delivery and extraction, and a measure of the adequacy of oxygen delivery to the tissues. Tissue HYPOXIA may occur even when heart rate, blood pressure and central venous pressure are normal. Knowledge of the SvO_2 has been shown to be valuable in any condition or state in which tissue hypoxia is possible. The normal range is 65% to 75%. Unfortunately, its measurement requires a pulmonary artery catheter, the safety of which has been questioned.

Mixtard a brand name for a preparation of INSULIN with a prolonged action.

MLCO *abbrev. for* Member of the London College of Osteopathy.

MLCOM *abbrev. for* Member of the London College of Osteopathic Medicine.

MLD *abbrev. for* minimum lethal dose. This is the smallest quantity known to have caused death.

Mmed *abbrev. for* Master of Medicine.

MmedSc *abbrev. for* Master of Medical Science.

MMF *abbrev. for* Member of the Medical Faculty.

MMR vaccination a protective active immunization against measles, mumps and rubella that should be routine for all children unless a strong medical reason contraindicates it. Concern was raised in 1998 that MMR vaccination could lead to an intestinal disorder that allows the absorption of otherwise non-permeable peptides capable of causing autism and other developmental problems. The evidence was reviewed by the Joint Committee on Vaccination and Immunization and no case was found for abandoning a vaccine of proved effectiveness and safety.

MMSA *abbrev. for* Master of Midwifery Society of Apothecaries.

MMSC *abbrev. for* Master of Medical Science.

MND *abbrev. for* MOTOR NEURON DISEASE.

MO *abbrev. for* Master of Obstetrics.

Mobiflex a brand name for TENOXICAM.

mobile phones see CELLULAR TELEPHONES.

mobilization the process of relieving stiffness or restoring the full range of movement in a joint or a person, usually after illness or injury or after prolonged forced immobility. Local mobilization after fractures, joint or joint capsule disorders or other injuries may require PHYSIOTHERAPY or even manipulation under anaesthesia.

MobstG *abbrev. for* Master Obstetrics & Gynaecology.

moclobemide a reversible MONO-AMINE OXIDASE INHIBITOR drug used to treat severe depression and social phobia. A brand name is Manerix.

modafinil a non-amphetamine (amfetamine) nervous system stimulant used to treat NARCOLEPSY. A brand name is Provigil.

Modalim a brand name for CIPROFIBRATE.

modality 1 a type or mode, especially of sensation, of the senses or of medical treatment. 2 a quality that denotes mode, mood or manner.

Modecate a brand name for the tricyclic antipsychotic drug FLUPHENAZINE.

Moditen a brand name for FLUPHENAZINE.

Modrasone a brand name for ALCLOMETASONE.

Modrenal a brand name for TRILOSTANE.

Moducren a brand name for HYDROCHLOROTHIAZIDE formulated with AMILORIDE and TIMOLOL.

Moduret 25 a brand name for HYDROCHLOROTHIAZIDE formulated with AMILORIDE.

Moduretic a brand name for a mixture of the potassium-sparing DIURETIC drug AMILORIDE and the thiazide diuretic HYDROCHLOROTHIAZIDE.

Mogadon a brand name for the BENZODIAZEPINE hypnotic drug NITRAZEPAM. There is anecdotal evidence that the safety of this drug was tested on moggies – hence the name.

MOH *abbrev. for* Medical Officer of Health.

molality a measure of concentration equal to the number of moles (see MOLE 2.) of solute in 1000 g of solvent.

molar one of the 12 back grinding teeth. From the Latin *mola*, a grindstone.

molarity the concentration of a solution expressed in terms of the weight of dissolved substance in grams per litre divided by its molecular weight.

molar solution a solution of such concentration that the number of grams of it dissolved in 1 litre is equal to its molecular weight.

molar pregnancy see HYDATIDIFORM MOLE.

Molcer a brand name for an ear wax softening preparation containing DOCUSATE SODIUM.

mole 1 a coloured (pigmented) birth-mark (naevus). Hairy moles may be disfiguring but are never dangerous. Moles seldom undergo malignant change, but any alteration is size, shape or colour should be reported at once. Moles are easily removed under local anaesthesia. See also MALIGNANT MELANOMA. 2 the basic unit of amount of substance; the amount that contains the same number of entities as there are atoms in 0.012 kg of carbon-12. The entity nay be an atom, a molecule, an ion, and so on. From the German *molekül*, a molecule.

molecular biology the study of cellular phenomena, and especially genetics, at a molecular or chemical level. As knowledge has progressed the term has become more and more synonymous with 'biology', for, today, biology aims at nothing less than a full understanding of the functioning of living things in terms of the nature and interactions of their molecules. The list that follows highlights the key entries related to molecular biology in the dictionary: ABC transporter proteins, acid-sensitive ion channels, actin, actin binding proteins, active transport, amino acids, aminotransferases, cap binding protein, chromatin, cytochemistry, cytokines, cytology, cytoplasm, cytoskeleton, cytosol, DNA helicases, DNA polymerases, DNA replicase, endocytosis, enzyme, eukaryote, excision enzyme, exocytosis, exoenzyme, intermediate-filament proteins, membrane-protein ion channels, misfolded proteins, mitochondria, mitochondrial DNA, passive transport, plasma membrane, polymerase chain reaction, prokaryote, proteins, protein synthesis, proteoglycans, proteomics, receptor, repressor protein, restriction enzyme, signal transduction, single strand binding proteins, telomeres, topoisomerases.

molecular chaperones see CHAPERONES.
molecular genetics a now out-dated term with its implication that a serious study of genetics is possible at other than a molecular level. Even those whose interest in genetics is limited to heredity can no longer pursue their discipline without becoming involved in MOLECULAR BIOLOGY.
molgramostin a granulocyte and MACROPHAGE colony stimulating factor used to treat white cell deficiency. It is prepared by recombinant DNA techniques (GENETIC ENGINEERING). A brand name is Leucomax.
Molipaxin a brand name for TRAZODONE.
molluscum contagiosum a virus infection of the skin featuring groups of painless, small, white, hemispherical, pearl-like lumps, 2 to 3 mm in diameter, each with a central dimple. Molluscum contagiosum is caused by a pox virus and is acquired by direct or indirect contact. Treatment is by squeezing out the cheesy contents of the lumps and touching the centres with phenol.
molsidomine see LINSIDOMINE.
mometasone a CORTICOSTEROID drug used as a nasal spray to treat hay fever and in a berath-

acuated inhaler to treat ASTHMA. Brand names are Nasonex and Asmanex. The drug is also formulated for external use under the brand name Elocon for the treatment of PSORIASIS and ATOPIC ECZEMA.
Monckeberg's sclerosis an age-related degenerative disorder of the muscle coat of medium-sized arteries with severe hardening from CALCIFICATION. The condition causes some rise in systolic blood pressure but is otherwise unimportant. (Johann George Monckeberg, 1877–1925, German physician).
Mondor's disease thrombophlebitis of the antero-lateral thoraco-abdominal wall. The condition is three times as common in women as in men and may affect the breast. It presents as a linear, cord-like lesion and is usually benign and self-limiting.
Mongolian spot a bluish-black pigmented birthmark (NAEVUS) occurring on the buttocks or lower part of the back, especially in coloured children. Mongolian spots are caused by a local accumulation of the normal skin pigment (melanin). They have usually disappeared by the age of about 4.
mongolism see DOWN'S SYNDROME.
moniliasis see CANDIDIASIS.
Monistat a brand name for a cream containing MICONAZOLE.
Monit a brand name for ISOSOBIDE MONONITRATE.
monitoring close surveillance or supervision, especially of people liable to suffer a sudden and dangerous deterioration in health. Monitoring involves checks of various parameters such as pulse rate, temperature, respiration rate, the condition of the pupils, the level of consciousness, the degree of appreciation of pain and various blood gas concentrations such as oxygen and carbon dioxide. Long-term instrumental display of the ELECTROCARDIOGRAM is also common in monitoring and this may also be recorded for diagnostic purposes, using computer analysis.
monkeypox a disease of primates in Central Africa caused by a virus similar to the virus that caused the now eradicated SMALLPOX. Some cases have been transmitted from monkeys to humans
mono- *combining form denoting* single or alone.
monoamine oxidase MAO, one of a group of enzymes found in brain cells, in peripheral

adrenergic and dopaminergic nerve endings and in the intestinal wall and liver. These enzymes play an important part in the breakdown of the neuro-transmitters NORADRENALINE, DOPAMINE and serotonin (5-hydroxytryptamine). Non-selective inhibition of these enzymes will elevate mood. Selective MAO-A enzymes act on serotonin; selective MAO-B inhibitor drugs act on phenylethylamine in the glial cells of the brain and elsewhere. The selective MAO-A inhibitor drugs are used to treat DEPRESSION and ANXIETY; selective MAO-B inhibitors are used to treat Parkinsonism.

monoamine oxidase inhibitors drugs that interfere with the action of the enzyme monoamine oxidase. Examples of non-selective MAO inhibitor drugs are isocarboxazid (Marplan) and phenelzine (Nardil).

monoamine oxidase-A inhibitors drugs used to treat major DEPRESSION and social phobias. An example is moclobemide (Manerix).

monoamine-oxidase-B inhibitors drugs used to treat PARKINSONISM. An example is selegiline (Eldepryl, Zelapar).

monoarthritis inflammation of a single joint.

monoblast the precursor of the MONOCYTE normally found only in the bone marrow.

Mono-Cedocard a brand name for ISOSOBIDE MONONITRATE.

monochromasia complete absence of any perception of colour. Monochromasia is very rare. There is an absence or severe deficiency of cones in the RETINA and VISUAL ACUITY is poor. A person with this defect is called a monochromat.

Monoclate-P a brand name for FACTOR XIII.

monoclonal of a group of cells derived from a single cell, all having the same GENOTYPE. Of a single CLONE of cells.

monoclonal antibodies ANTIBODIES (immunoglobulins) produced by hybrid B lymphocyte tumours (myelomas). The type of antibodies produced depend on the selection of the B cell. These can be fused to cultured mouse, or even human, myeloma cells to form immortal tumours (hybridomas) – clones of cells that continue indefinitely to generate large quantities of the particular antibody produced by the B cell. The availability of quantities of almost any desired antibody has major diagnostic, therapeutic and research implications and monoclonal antibody production is one of the most important biotechnological advances of the century. Monoclonal antibodies can be made that will seek out and recognize cancers anywhere in the body, and this offers a number of intriguing possibilities for treatment.

monocular vision vision with one eye only, even if both are capable of seeing. In such a case, vision is suppressed in one eye, often to avoid seeing double.

monocyte a large white blood cell with a round or kidney-shaped nucleus. There are no granules in the CYTOPLASM. The monocyte migrates to the tissues where it becomes a MACROPHAGE.

monocytopenia a reduction in the number of MONOCYTES in the circulating blood.

monocytosis an abnormal increase in the numbers of MONOCYTES in the blood. This occurs in severe TUBERCULOSIS and MALARIA.

monolayer a sheet of cells only one cell thick.

Monomax a brand name for ISOSOBIDE MONONITRATE.

monomer one of the chemical groups many of which are repetitively linked together to form a POLYMER.

mononeuropathy a disorder affecting a single nerve. This may be due to nerve compression, as in the CARPAL TUNNEL SYNDROME, the THORACIC OUTLET SYNDROME or SATURDAY NIGHT PALSY, or other trauma or to DIABETES.

Mononine a brand name for FACTOR IX.

mononuclear cell a cell with a single spherical or near-spherical nucleus, as distinct from one with a lobed nucleus as in the case of the polymorphs. The mononuclear cells include LYMPHOCYTES, MONOCYTES and immature GRANULOCYTES. An unhelpful and obsolescent designation dating from a period prior to the detailed differentiation of cells of the immune system.

mononuclear phagocyte system blood MONOCYTES and tissue MACROPHAGES.

mononucleosis any condition featuring an abnormal number of monocytes in the blood. See also GLANDULAR FEVER (infectious mononucleosis).

monoplegia paralysis of a single muscle or group of muscles or of a single limb.

monorchism having only one testicle in the scrotum. This is usually due to failure of descent of one testicle from the abdomen and occurs in about 1 boy in 50. An undescended testicle remains sterile and is much more prone to cancer than normal.

monosaccharide the simplest form of sugar. Monosaccharides are classified by the number of carbon atoms in the molecule. They may thus be trioses, tetroses, pentoses, hexoses, etc. The commonest monosaccharide in the body is GLUCOSE, which is a hexose, with six carbons.

monosodium glutamate the sodium salt of glutamic acid produced by acids or enzyme action on vegetable protein such as wheat gluten or soya bean. Monosodium glutamate is used as a culinary seasoning and flavouring agent and is believed to be responsible for the CHINESE RESTAURANT SYNDROME. Also known as Ajinomoto, Vetsin, Chinese seasoning, Accent or Zest.

monosomy the absence of one complete AUTOSOMAL chromosome of a pair. This is a lethal condition. Compare TRISOMY as in DOWN'S SYNDROME.

monospot test a rapid screening antibody test for glandular fever (infectious mononucleosis).

Monotard a brand name for a form of INSULIN with prolonged action.

Monotrim a brand name for TRIMETHOPRIM.

mons a mound or rounded eminence, especially the mons pubis (or veneris), the hairy mound of fatty tissue covering the junction of the pubic bones in adult females.

montelukast a drug that binds to the receptors for certain leukotrienes thus blocking both phases of the ASTHMA response. It is used in the treatment of asthma that shows an inadequate response to inhaled steroids. A brand name is Singulair.

mood disorders see DEPRESSION, MANIA and MANIC-DEPRESSIVE ILLNESS.

moon faced pertaining to the full-cheeked, hamster-like appearance caused by excessive doses of corticosteroid drugs or by excessive production of the natural adrenal cortical hormone in CUSHING'S SYNDROME. Also known, inelegantly, as 'cushingoid'.

Moore-Federman syndrome a rare familial disorder featuring short stature, abnormal stiffness and limitation of movement of joints, liver enlargement, thickened skin, and hoarseness of the voice. Intelligence is normal. Also known as acromicric dysplasia. (Reported by W.H. Moore and D.D. Federman in *Archives of Internal Medicine* in 1965).

moracizine a drug intended for use only by expert cardiologists to control dangerous irregularities in the ventricular heart beat (ventricular arrhythmias). A brand name is Ethmozine.

morbid anatomy the branch of pathology dealing with the visible structural changes caused in the body by disease and injury and discernible at postmortem examination.

morbidity the state of being diseased or suffering.

morbidity rate the number of cases of a disease occurring in a given number (usually 100,000) of the population. The annual morbidity figure for a disease, in a particular population, is the number of new cases reported (incidence) in the year.

morbilli MEASLES.

Morcap SR a brand name for MORPHINE.

moribund dying.

morning-after pill see EMERGENCY CONTRACEPTION.

morning sickness vomiting or retching of pregnancy. A common symptom occurring from the 6th to the 12th week. It usually occurs soon after waking but seldom has any effect on health or on the pregnancy and almost always stops before the 14th week. See also HYPEREMESIS GRAVIDARUM.

moron a person of a mild to moderate degree of learning difficulty (mental retardation). A person with an IQ of between 50 and 70. The term is not used in medicine. From the Greek *moros*, stupid.

morpheme the smallest element of speech that conveys either factual or grammatical information. Compare with PHONEME which is a speech sound that serves to distinguish one word from another.

morphine a powerful pain-killing and NARCOTIC drug used to control persistent pain that cannot be relieved by lesser drugs. It can be taken by mouth or given by injection. Morphine has a valuable effect on the emotional response to pain and in relieving the anxiety associated with the contemplation of the implications of severe pain. It is a respiratory depressant and is never given in cases of head injury or in other conditions in which respiration may be prejudiced. When appropriately prescribed addiction is unlikely. The drug is on the WHO official list. Brand names are Morcap SR, MST Continus, MXL, Oramorph, Sevredol and Zomorph. The drug is also formulated with the anti-emetic cyclizine under the brand name Cyclimorph.

morphoea patchy skin hardening and atrophy (SCLERODERMA). The normal skin constituents, such as sweat glands and hair follicles, are replaced by fibrous tissue. The affected areas are usually round or oval, but may take the form of bands or stripes, and the surrounding skin may be pinkish or violet. There is no effective treatment for morphoea but ointments can be helpful.

morphogenesis the origin and development of the form and structure of the body.

Morquio's syndrome an AUTOSOMAL RECESSIVE form of MUCOPOLYSACCHARIDOSIS (Type IV) featuring clouding of the CORNEA, a short spine causing dwarfism, failure of normal development of the teeth and disease of the aortic valve of the heart. (Luis Morquio, 1867–1935, Uruguayan paediatrician).

mortality rate death rate. The ratio of the total number of deaths from one or any cause, in a year, to the number of people in the population. Crude mortality is the number of deaths in a year per thousand total population. The age-specified mortality rate is the number of deaths occurring in a year in people of a particular age or in a particular age-range. See also INFANT MORTALITY.

morula an early stage in the development of the embryo at which it consists of a solid spherical ball of apparently identical cells.

mosaic gene see DISCONTINUOUS GENE.

mosaicism the state in which two or more genetically different types of cell occur in the same individual. Although the cells are all derived from the same fertilized egg, they do not all possess the same number of chromosomes. In about 1% of cases of DOWN'S SYNDROME there are two different cell lines, one normal and the other with an additional chromosome 21 (trisomy 21). The effect of mosaicism varies with the proportion of cells containing abnormal chromosomes. Compare CHIMERA.

mosquitos any flies (diptera) of the family *Culicidae*. Mosquitos of medical importance are found in the genera *Anopheles* (transmit MALARIA and FILARIASIS), *Aedes* (transmit YELLOW FEVER, DENGUE and filariasis), *Culex* (transmit ENCEPHALITIS and filariasis) and *Mansonia* (transmit filariasis).

mossy foot a severe infection of the foot with pigmented fungi such as *Fonsecaea pedrosoi* or *Phialophora verrucosa* acquired by the penetration of the skin by splinters from decaying timber. The skin shows warty, mossy nodules that may ulcerate and become secondarily infected. Also known as chromoblastomycosis or chromomycosis.

Motens a brand name for LACIDIPINE.

Motifene a brand name for DICLOFENAC.

Motilium a brand name for the ANTI-EMETIC drug DOMPERIDONE.

motion sickness nausea or vomiting induced by any sustained, repetitive, passive movement of the body in any vehicle of transportation. There is abdominal discomfort, pallor, sweating, salivation, depression, nausea, vomiting, apathy, loss of appetite and sometimes a loss of the will to live. The cause is unknown, but it is related to repetitive stimulation of the inner ear balancing mechanisms. Motion sickness is treated with small doses of atropine or hyoscine, or antihistamine drugs such as cyclizine (Valoid) or promethazine (Avomine). The word nausea derives from the Greek word *naus*, a ship.

Motival a brand name for FLUPHENAZINE formulated with NORTRIPTYLINE.

motor 1 causing movement.
2 carrying nerve impulses that stimulate muscles into contraction or cause other responses such as gland secretion. From the Latin *movere*, to move.

motor cortex the part of the surface layer of each hemisphere of the main brain (cerebrum) in which voluntary movement is initiated. These areas can be mapped out to show which parts of them are responsible for movement of any particular parts of the body. The map resembles a distorted and inverted human figure.

motor neuron, motor neurone a nerve carrying MOTOR impulses. The upper motor neurons have their cell bodies in the surface layer (CORTEX) of the brain and their axons running down the spinal cord. The lower motor neurons have their cell bodies in a column at the front of the spinal cord and their axons running out of the cord in the spinal nerves.

motor neuron disease a rare disorder of

unknown cause in which MOTOR nerve cells suffer gradual and progressive destruction. The condition is rare before the age of 40 and affects men twice as often as women. The initial symptoms depend on which neurons are first involved and include difficulty in swallowing and speaking, or wasting and weakness of the small muscles of the hands spreading to involve the forearms and later the legs. Progressive worsening leads to widespread paralysis of the whole body. Intellectual function is never affected. There is no known treatment. Also known as motor neurone disease.

Motrin a brand name for the non-steroidal anti-inflammatory drug (NSAID) IBUPROFEN.

mould any fungus that forms multicellular, filamentous colonies. Most moulds are harmless. Some, such as the common mould *Penicillium notatum*, secrete useful antibiotics, but some can cause allergic disease, such as FARMER'S LUNG, cork worker's lung, cheesewasher's lung and malt worker's lung.

mountain sickness a syndrome caused by reduced oxygen tension in the atmosphere at heights above about 3000 m, especially in people who proceed too quickly to high altitudes. There is deep breathing, a rapid pulse, loss of appetite, greatly reduced capacity for physical or mental work, headache, nausea, weakness, dizziness and insomnia. The vision may be affected by retinal bleeding. The chief danger is from fluid in the lungs (PULMONARY OEDEMA) and brain swelling (cerebral oedema). Either may be fatal unless rapidly corrected by administration of oxygen or an immediate descent to a lower altitude. DIURETIC drugs and DEXAMETHASONE can help to reduce oedema.

mouth-to-mouth resuscitation maintenance of an oxygen supply in a person unable to breath spontaneously by periodic inflation of the lungs by blowing into the mouth or nose. This is done 16 to 20 times a minute and is verified by watching the chest rise and fall. Also known as the 'kiss of life'.

mouth ulcers painful white, grey or yellow open sores occurring anywhere on the inside of the lip or cheek or on the floor of the mouth. Most are of unknown cause, are harmless and soon resolve. Ulcers that do not disappear in a few days may be dangerous and should be reported. Also known as aphthous ulcers or canker sores.

mouthwashes mainly harmless fluids used to rinse out the mouth, leaving it feeling pleasantly refreshed for a few minutes. They serve little or no medical purpose and are no substitute for good mouth hygiene and regular dental attention.

Movelat a brand name for MUCOPOLYSACCHARIDE POLYSULPHATE.

Movicol a brand name for POLYETHYLENE GLYCOL.

Moxacin a brand name for AMOXACILLIN.

moxibustion a primitive form of treatment in which a cone of dried leaves is burned close to the skin. Apart from a minor local irritant effect in promoting an increased blood supply to the area, moxibustion is of no medical value and has no place in scientific medical practice.

moxifloxacin a fluoroquinolone wide-spectrum ANTIBIOTIC with activity against both Gram positive and Gram negative organisms. A brand name is Avelox.

moxisylyte a selective ALPHA-ADRENORECEPTOR BLOCKING DRUG given by injection into the penis to treat impotence. A brand name is Opilon.

moxonidine a drug that causes arteries to relax by influencing the action of the sympathetic nervous system. It is used to treat high blood pressure (HYPERTENSION). A brand name is Physiotens.

M protein a constituent of the streptococcal cell wall which confers virulence on Type A streptococci by its anti-phagocytic action. M protein forms large and damaging aggregates with fibrinogen in blood and tissues and is the molecular basis of the streptococcal toxic shock syndrome. The M protein-fibrinogen aggregates form powerful ligands for integrin receptors on polymorphs, thus activating these cells into the production of toxic metabolites and destructive enzymes.

MPH *abbrev. for* Master of Public Health.

MPS *abbrev. for* Member of the Pharmaceutical Society.

MPSI *abbrev. for* Member of the Pharmaceutical Society of Ireland.

MPSY *abbrev. for* Master of Psychiatry.

MpsychMed *abbrev. for* Master of Psychological Medicine.

MRACGP *abbrev. for* Member of theRoyal Australasian College of General Practitioners.

MRACO *abbrev. for* Member of the Royal Australasian College of Ophthalmologists.

MRACP *abbrev. for* Member of the Royal Australasian College of Physicians.

MRACR *abbrev. for* Member of the Royal Australasian College of Radiologists.

MRad (D) *abbrev. for* Master of Radiodiagnosis.

MRad (I) *abbrev. for* Master of Radiotherapy.

MRANZCP *abbrev. for* Member of the Royal Australian & New Zealand College of Psychiatrists.

MRC *abbrev. for* Medical Research Council.

MRCGP *abbrev. for* Member of the Royal College of General Practitioners.

MRCOG *abbrev. for* Member of the Royal College of Obstetricians and Gynaecologists.

MRCP *abbrev. for* Member of the Royal College of Physicians.

MRCPA *abbrev. for* Member of the Royal College of Pathologists of Australasia.

MRCPath *abbrev. for* Member of the Royal College of Pathologists.

MRCPI *abbrev. for* Member of of the Royal College of Physicians of Ireland.

MRCPsych *abbrev. for* Member of the Royal College of Psychiatrists.

MRCS *abbrev. for* Member of the Royal College of Surgeons.

MRCVS *abbrev. for* Member of the Royal College of Veterinary Surgeons.

MRI *abbrev. for* MAGNETIC RESONANCE IMAGING.

MRO *abbrev. for* Member of the Register of Osteopaths.

MRSA *abbrev. for* methicillin-resistant *Staphylococcus aureus*. Over 90% of hospital strains of *S. aureus* are penicillin-resistant – a matter for great concern as MRSA are responsible for many deaths. Initially occurring mainly in hospitals, MRSA infections with organisms carrying powerful staphylococcal toxin genes have now spread into the community and are becoming common there. These staphylococci have an acquired DNA sequence that confers resistance to all beta-lactam antibiotics. The sequence produces an enzyme PBP2A which enables them to continue to synthesize their cell walls even if their normal penicillin-binding proteins are inactivated by methicillin. The crystal structure of PBP2A has now been established. This may be an important step in the solution of the problem.

MRSH *abbrev. for* Member of the Royal Society of Health.

MS *abbrev. for* MULTIPLE SCLEROSIS or Master of Surgery.

MSA *abbrev. for* Member of the Society of Apothecaries.

Msc *abbrev. for* Master of Science.

MSCD *abbrev. for* Master of Dental Science.

MSRG *abbrev. for* Member of the Society of Remedial Gymnasts.

MSSC *abbrev. for* Master of Surgical Science.

MSMF *abbrev. for* Member of the State Medical Faculty.

MST Continus a brand name for MORPHINE.

Mucaine a brand name for a preparation containing ALUMINIUM HYDROXIDE and MAGNESIUM HYDROXIDE.

mucin a glycoprotein that is the main constituent of MUCUS. The term is also used as a generic name for the substance used as a drug formulated with xylitol as artificial saliva under the brand name is Saliva Orthana.

muco- *combining form denoting* MUCUS or MUCOUS MEMBRANE.

mucocoele a usually harmless cyst-like body filled with MUCUS. Mucocoeles occur in various parts of the body when mucus secreted by a MUCOUS MEMBRANE is unable to escape though normal channels. They may cause local damage by compressing or displacing other structures.

Mucogel a brand name for a preparation containing ALUMINIUM HYDROXIDE and MAGNESIUM HYDROXIDE.

mucopolysaccharide POLYSACCHARIDEs containing amino sugars or that are polymers of MONOSACCHARIDES in which one of the –OH groups is replaced by an NH_2 group. Mucopolysaccharides are important structural materials in the body forming the ground substance of many connective tissues in which fibrous proteins are embedded. Now more commonly called glycosaminoglycans.

mucopolysaccharide polysulphate a drug formulated with SALICYLIC ACID as a cream or gel for external application in minor muscle and joint disorders. A brand name is Movelat.

mucopolysaccharidoses a range of inherited errors of MUCOPOLYSACCHARIDE metabolism each due to a deficiency of a specific enzyme leading to the abnormal deposition of mucopolysaccharides in the tissues. These disorders feature dwarfism, facial coarseness, mental retardation, bone and joint abnormalities, retinal degeneration, GLAUCOMA, clouding of the cornea, and other effects.

There are at least seven varieties.

mucopurulent containing MUCUS and PUS.

mucormycosis a serious fungus infection involving especially the nose and sinuses caused by one of several fungi including *Absidia*, *Rhizopus* and *Mucor* species.

mucosal alloimmunization see ALLOREACTIVE LYMPHOCYTES.

mucous membrane the lining of most of the body cavities and hollow internal organs such as the mouth, the nose, the eyelids, the intestine and the vagina. Mucous membranes contain large numbers of goblet-shaped cells that secrete mucus which keeps the surface moist and lubricated.

mucous patches shallow, white-based ulcers with narrow red margins occurring in the mouth, throat and genitalia of 30% of people in the secondary stage of acquired SYPHILIS.

mucus a slimy, jelly-like material, chemically known as a MUCOPOLYSACCHARIDE or GLYCOPROTEIN, produced by the goblet cells of MUCOUS MEMBRANES. Mucus has important lubricating and protective properties. It prevents acid and enzymes from digesting the walls of the stomach and intestines. It traps fine particulate matter, including smoke, in the lungs. It lubricates swallowing and the transport of the bowel contents. It facilitates sexual intercourse.

Multiceps a dog tapeworm occurring in South and East Africa, the larval stage of which can infect humans causing cysts in the brain in a manner similar to HYDATID DISEASE.

multigene family a collection of genes, usually but not necessarily situated together, that have either a common or associated function or have similar nucleotide sequences.

multigravida a woman who has had at least two pregnancies.

multipara a woman who has carried at least two babies to a viable stage or who has delivered more than one live baby.

multiple myelomatosis see MYELOMATOSIS.

multiple personality a rare psychiatric dissociative disorder in which a person appears to have two or more distinct and often contrasting personalities at different times, with corresponding differences in behaviour, attitude and outlook. This condition is quite distinct from SCHIZOPHRENIA.

multiple births the production of more than one individual in a single parturition. Twins occur in about one in every 84 births in Britain, and about one in 300 pregnancies results in identical twins. Multiple births may occur as a result of the near-simultaneous release and fertilization of more than one ovum, or from the fertilization of a single ovum which then separates into two or more parts from each of which a new individual develops, all having identical genetic constitution. Non-identical (dizygotic or fraternal) twins may be of the same or of different sex and are no more alike than any other two siblings. Each has his or her own PLACENTA and set of membranes. Identical (monozygotic) twins share a placenta and often compete for nourishment so that they are of unequal weight when born. Multiple pregnancies are shorter than single pregnancies. Triplets and higher number births are biologically rare. Triplets have a natural frequency of about one in 7000 births. They are more common as a result of the use of anti-infertility drugs that induce multiple ovulation.

multiple pregnancy a pregnancy with more than one fetus.

multiple polyposis a dominant hereditary condition in which large numbers of POLYPS of MUCOUS MEMBRANE occur in the colon and rectum. These appear in adolescence and some of them invariably become malignant within about 15 years. The usual treatment is to remove the colon and rectum.

multiple sclerosis a disease of the central nervous system of uncertain cause that damages nerve fibre insulation (myelin) in a random and patchy manner causing a wide range of neurological defects. About 1 person in 2000 is affected and the course and severity are very variable. Plaques of DEMYELINATION, visible on MRI scanning, may cause loss of vision, numbness, partial paralysis, VERTIGO or incoordination. Episodes of such defects tend to last for days or weeks and to be followed by apparent recovery. There are often long periods of normality, but repeated episodes may cause permanent disability in about half the cases. It has been shown that increased sunlight exposure during childhood and early adolescence is protective against the disease, and there is evidence of a significant but small relationship between stress and exacerbations of the disease. The effect appears to relate to helper

T cell changes. Early immune therapy and the use of interferons can be helpful. The drug COPOLYMER-1 offers hope of reducing the relapse rate. See also ANTIMYELIN ANTIBODIES.

mummification drying and shrivelling of the whole or part of the body.

mumps an acute paramyxovirus infection, spread by droplet transmission and most commonly affecting children. It causes fever, MALAISE and swelling of the salivary glands in the cheeks (the PAROTID GLANDS) producing a hamster-like appearance. Mumps in adult men is commonly associated with painful inflammation of one or both testicles (ORCHITIS). Sterility from this cause is rare. There is no effective treatment but an attack of mumps confers permanent immunity.

Munchausen's syndrome the systematic practice of deliberate and calculated simulation of disease so as to obtain attention, status and free accommodation and board. People engaging in this activity study medical textbooks and report a plausible list of symptoms of a usually serious condition so as to elicit medical interest and admission to hospital. They have a preference for surgical conditions and often display an unusual number of operation scars – a circumstance that may give the game away. Detection is inevitable and is followed by the disappearance of the 'patient'. Baron Munchausen was the hero of the outrageously implausible pseudo-autobiographical tales of the novelist and criminal psychopath Rudolf Eric Raspe. The syndrome was so named, and first described, by Richard Asher in his book *Talking Sense*, published in 1972.

Munchausen's syndrome by proxy illness or injury in a child caused by a parent or other person in charge who purports the disorders to be spontaneous. The child is commonly brought, often repeatedly, for medical attention and, if suspicion is raised, any responsibility for the child's medical condition is strenuously denied. Separation from the parent or person *in loco parentis* leads to recovery of the child's disorder. The commonest caused conditions are seizures, rashes, apparent respiratory failure, rashes, bleeding, diarrhoea and vomiting and near-coma. All of these are brought about by such means as partial suffocation, pressure on the neck, the administration of drugs,

poisoning, the application of blood or the use of anticoagulants such as warfarin rat poison. Covert closed-circuit TV monitoring has been used to detect the crime.

mupirocin a broad-spectrum antibiotic used externally on the skin and as a nasal ointment to treat carriers of staphylococci. Brand names are Bactroban and Bactroban nasal.

mural on the wall of a hollow organ or structure.

mural thrombus a blood clot formed within the blood and attached to the wall of a blood vessel or to the lining of a chamber of the heart. Mural thrombi are liable to break loose and form dangerous EMBOLI.

murine pertaining to mice and rats.

murine typhus an acute but comparatively mild disease featuring fever, headache, muscle aches and a slightly raised MACULAR skin rash. It is caused by *Rickettsia mooseri*, harboured by rats, and transmitted to humans by the flea *Xenopsylla cheopis*.

murmur a purring or rumbling sound of variable pitch heard through a STETHOSCOPE especially over the heart or over a narrowed or compressed artery. Murmurs are caused by turbulence in blood flow and often imply disease such as heart valve narrowing or incompetence. See also HEART SOUNDS.

Murphy's sign tenderness and rigidity under the ribs on the right side (right hypochondrium) that increases on breathing in. (John Benjamin Murphy, 1857–1916, American physician).

Murray valley fever a togavirus infection, transmitted by mosquitos and causing ENCEPHALITIS or a haemorrhagic fever. An example of an arthropod-borne (arbo) virus infection.

MUS, *acronym for* MEDICALLY-UNEXPLAINED SYMPTOMS.

muscarine a poison produced by the mushroom *Amanita muscaria*. Muscarine is chemically related to acetylcholine

muscarinic producing the effects of post-ganglionic cholinergic stimulation of the parasympathetic nervous system. Having an effect similar to that of the mushroom poison MUSCARINE. Compare NICOTINIC.

muscle a tissue consisting of large numbers of parallel elongated cells with the power of shortening and thickening so as to approximate their ends and effect movement. Up to 50% of the body weight consists of muscle, most being attached to bone in such a way that muscle contraction causes joints to bend (flex) or straighten (extend). Muscle fibres convert chemical energy into mechanical energy. There are three kinds of muscle – striped (striated) or voluntary muscle; smooth or involuntary muscle occurring in the walls of arteries, the intestines and the urinary tract; and heart muscle (MYOCARDIUM), a network (syncytium) of muscle fibres that contract regularly and automatically without external stimulus.

muscle biopsy a method of diagnosis of muscle disorders in which a small sample of muscle is removed for microscopic and sometimes electron microscopic examination. Muscle biopsy can provide valuable information on conditions such as MUSCULAR DYSTROPHY, RHEUMATOID ARTHRITIS, MALNUTRITION, ALCOHOLISM and various endocrine disorders. Electron microscopy can reveal important abnormalities in the ultrastructure of muscle cells, especially in the MITOCHONDRIA.

muscle disorders see CARDIOMYOPATHY, CLAUDICATION, COMPARTMENT SYNDROME, CRAMPS, DERMATOMYOSITIS, FIBROIDS, MUSCLE SPASM, MUSCULAR DYSTROPHY, MYASTHENIA GRAVIS, MYOCARDITIS, MYOMA, TETANY and TRICHINOSIS.

muscle relaxants drugs that reduce muscle tension or cause temporary paralysis. Muscle relaxants (neuromuscular blocking agents) such as TUBOCURARINE, SUXAMETHONIUM, PANCURONIUM and GALLAMINE are widely used in modern anaesthesia and allow smaller and safer doses of general anaesthetic drugs to be used. Mild sedative drugs, such as the BENZODIAZEPINES, also act to relax muscle tension induced by anxiety.

muscle spasm abnormally sustained and usually powerful contraction of a muscle. This may result from disorder in the muscle itself, from irritation to the nerve supplying it or from removal of the normal inhibiting influence on muscle contraction provided by nerve connections from the brain. Damage to these connections is common in CEREBRAL PALSY (spastic paralysis) or after STROKE or head injury and a spastic condition of the muscles results.

muscular dystrophy one of a group of hereditary muscle disorders that feature gradual, progressive muscle degeneration leading to increasing weakness and disability. Duchenne dystrophy is a RECESSIVE sex-linked condition and is thus almost confined to males. It affects first the leg and buttock muscles and progresses usually to a fatal outcome in the mid-teens. The muscles appear bulkier than normal (pseudohypertrophy). The limb girdle type of dystrophy has a recessive inheritance and affects initially the shoulder and hip muscles. It usually causes severe disability within about 20 years. The facio-scapulo-humeral type has a dominant inheritance and weakens the muscles of the face, upper back and upper arm. It progresses very slowly and does not necessarily shorten life. There is no known treatment for muscular dystrophy. See also DYSTROPHIN.

musculature the muscle system of the body or the intrinsic muscles of a part of the body.

Muse a brand name for ALPROSTADIL.

musicians' overuse syndrome severe, disabling pain and loss of speed, accuracy and agility from functional disturbance in the muscles used in playing musical instruments. This occurs from overwork or excessive practising, especially if there is faulty technique. The affected muscles become swollen and there may also be some loss of feeling in the part. Treatment involves strict limitation of playing time and the use of well-designed supports for instruments. It may sometimes be necessary to give up playing for weeks or months.

mustine chlormethine, a drug used to treat some cases of HODGKIN'S DISEASE. It is very toxic and is liable to cause severe vomiting.

mutagen any agent capable of changing the structure of DNA without immediately killing the cell concerned. Any surviving MUTATION may be perpetuated to all descendants of the cell. Mutagens include ionizing radiation such as ultraviolet light, X-rays, gamma rays and cosmic rays and a wide range of chemical substances including the tars in cigarette smoke.

mutant any organism or cell with a gene or genes that have suffered a MUTATION.

mutation any persisting change in the genetic material (DNA) of a cell. Mutations most commonly involve a single gene but may affect a major part, or even the whole of, a chromosome or may change the number of chromosomes (genomic mutation). A nonsense mutation is one that alters the sequence of bases in a CODON so that no amino acid is coded. Many mutations have an unfavourable effect on the cell concerned and are not passed on, but non-lethal mutations are replicated in daughter cells. Mutation in a cell in the GONADS that gives rise to a SPERMATOZOON or an egg (OVUM), will be passed on to a clone of sperms or eggs and one of these may take part in fertilization so that the mutation is passed on to every cell in the body of the future individual, including the GERM CELLS. New mutations occurring in the sex cells (germ line mutations) may thus lead to hereditary abnormalities. Mutations in body cells (somatic mutations) cannot do this but can cause cloned abnormalities including cancers. See also FRAME SHIFT MUTATION, INSERTION MUTATION, INVERSION MUTATION, LEAKY MUTATION, LETHAL MUTATION, MISSENSE MUTATION, POINT MUTATION, NONSENSE MUTATION.

mutation rate the number of instances of a particular gene mutation occurring in a population in one generation.

mutator protein an antiviral factor found in human cells that converts one codon in DNA so that it codes for the amino acid uracil instead of cytosine. Uracil replaces cytosine in RNA. When HIV infects cells it makes a DNA copy of its own RNA to insert into the host DNA. The mutator protein offers the possibility of developing drugs that could interfere with the replication of infecting viruses.

mutism inability or refusal to speak. There are many possible causes including deafness from birth, mental retardation, severe DEPRESSION, SCHIZOPHRENIA, HYSTERIA, brain tumour and HYDROCEPHALUS.

MXL a brand name for MORPHINE.

my-, myo- *combining form denoting* muscle.

myalgia muscle pain, especially if persistent and associated with a long-term (chronic) muscle disorder. Myalgia is a feature of POLYMYOSITIS, DERMATOMYOSITIS and POLYMYALGIA RHEUMATICA. See also epidemic myalgia (BORNHOLM DISEASE).

myalgic encephalomyelitis (ME) see CHRONIC FATIGUE SYNDROME.

myambutol see ETHAMBUTOL. Myambutol was formerly a brand name for ethambutol but is now a generic name.

myasthenia muscle weakness. Myasthenia is a

feature of widespread cancer.

myasthenia gravis an autoimmune disease caused by an abnormal antibody that affects the sites (myoneural junctions) at which motor nerves stimulate muscles to contract by releasing the NEUROTRANSMITTER acetylcholine. The effect is a rapidly worsening weakness of muscles with use. There is drooping of the eyelids, double vision, difficulty in swallowing, coughing and speaking and general weakness of the limbs. Treatment is by the use of drugs that antagonize the enzyme (acetylcholinesterase) that breaks down acetylcholine. These include NEOSTIGMINE and PYRIDOSTIGMINE. Removal of the thymus gland can be helpful as can removal of the antibodies from the blood (PLASMAPHERESIS).

mycetoma a hard tumour-like mass of fungus, or of bacteria that form fungus-like colonies, in the foot or leg. There are multiple channels (sinuses) that discharge pus. The condition is confined to people living in poor conditions in the tropics. Surgical drainage and antibiotics may succeed, but amputation is often the only resource.

Mycifradin a brand name for NEOMYCIN.

Myciguent a brand name for an ointment containing the antibiotic NEOMYCIN.

myco- *combining form denoting* fungus. From the Greek *muces*, fungus.

Mycobacterium a genus of ACID FAST bacteria that contains a number of species causing TUBERCULOSIS in humans and other animals and HANSEN'S DISEASE in humans. Species of medical importance include *Mycobacterium tuberculosis*, *Mycobacterium leprae* and *Mycobacterium ulcerans*.

Mycobacterium ulcerans an organism, of the same genus as those causing TUBERCULOSIS and HANSEN'S DISEASE (leprosy), that causes gross and extensive necrotic lesions called Buruli ulcer in affected people in endemic areas, mainly in West Africa.

Mycobutin a brand name for RIFABUTIN.

mycology the science or study of fungi. Medical mycology is limited to the study of fungi that infect or affect humans and to those from which useful drugs can be derived.

mycophenolate mofetil an IMMUNO-SUPPRESSANT DRUG used to help to prevent rejection of the donated organ after kidney grafting. A brand name is Cellcept.

Mycoplasma a genus of very small micro-organisms, about the size of some viruses but capable of independent existence. Unlike bacteria they have no cell walls. *Mycoplasma pneumoniae* causes outbreaks of PNEUMONIA in institutions. *Mycoplasma hominis*, is often present harmlessly in the mouth or vagina but is believed to be a cause of URETHRITIS and SALPINGITIS. Mycoplasma infections respond to TETRACYCLINE and ERYTHROMYCIN.

mycosis any disease caused by a fungus.

mycosis fungoides a malignant tumour of T lymphocyte origin (lymphoma) affecting the skin and causing multiple flat growths that remain confined to the skin for many years. Spread to the lymph nodes and internal organs may occur at a late stage. Anticancer treatment is sometimes needed. The condition has nothing to do with fungus and was named before its true nature was known.

Mycostatin a brand name for NYSTATIN.

Mydriacyl tropicamide, a brand name for eye drops containing TROPICAMIDE.

mydriasis widening (dilatation) of the pupil of the eye, usually as a result of instillation of a mydriatic drug, such as ATROPINE or CYCLOPENTOLATE.

myel-, myelo- *combining form denoting*
1 the spinal cord.
2 the bone marrow.
3 MYELIN.

myelin the fatty, white material forming a sheath around most nerve fibres and acting as an insulator. See DEMYELINATION.

myelinated possessing a MYELIN sheath.

myelin sheath see MYELIN.

myelinolysis disruption and loss of the myelin sheath of nerves. Demyelination.

myelitis 1 inflammation of the spinal cord. This may be due to a virus infection such as POLIOMYELITIS, may follow a virus infection elsewhere in the body, may be caused by DEMYELINATION or by SYPHILIS or may be due to occlusion of small spinal arteries. The effect depends on the part, and extent, of the cord involved. Transverse myelitis affects the whole cross-section of the cord and causes paralysis of the body below the affected level. Recovery is variable, but may be complete.
2 inflammation of the bone marrow. See also OSTEOMYELITIS.

myeloblast the bone marrow cell from which the whole series of granular white blood cells (GRANULOCYTES) derives. Up to 3% of bone marrow cells are myeloblasts.

myeloblastosis the presence of an abnormally large number of MYELOBLASTS in the blood (myeloblastaemia) and other tissues, suggesting acute myelogenous LEUKAEMIA.

myelocele see MENINGOMYELOCELE.

myelocoele the narrow central canal of the spinal cord.

myelocyte an immature white blood cell normally found in the bone marrow.

myelodysplasia see MYELODYSPLASTIC SYNDROME.

myelodysplasic syndrome a group of uncommon bone marrow disorders featuring reduced blood cell production with abnormal granular white cells, especially the neutrophil polymorphonuclear leukocytes, and resulting in ANAEMIA which is very difficult to treat. The neutrophils have reduced activity against organisms, so there is increased risk of infection. The syndrome affects the elderly and tends to progress to acute myeloid LEUKAEMIA. Bone marrow transplantation can produce long-term remission in younger patients.

myelofibrosis progressive replacement of the blood-forming tissue of the bone marrow with fibrous tissue. New sites of blood cell formation occur in other parts of the body, especially the liver and the spleen and the latter is usually greatly enlarged. There is lassitude, weight loss and a tendency to dangerous rupture of the spleen from minor trauma. Also known as myelosclerosis.

myelography an X-ray examination of the interior of the bony spinal canal after a fluid opaque to X-rays (contrast medium) has been injected into the SUBARACHNOID SPACE by LUMBAR PUNCTURE. The method readily shows abnormal protrusions into the canal, as from intervertebral discs, tumours of the spinal cord and nerve root disorders. Safer and less invasive imaging methods such as CT SCANNING and MRI are replacing myelography.

myeloid pertaining to the bone marrow.

myeloid leukaemia a form of LEUKAEMIA in which the cells present in abnormal numbers are derived from primitive precursors, in the bone marrow, of the white blood cells.

myeloma a tumour derived from a lymphocyte. See LYMPHOMA.

myelomalacia softening of the spinal cord.

myelomatosis multiple myeloma, a malignant disorder of antibody-producing PLASMA CELLS. Plasma cells derive from a single selected B lymphocyte and produce a single monoclonal antibody (immunoglobulin). In myelomatosis, large quantities of monoclonal immunoglobulin are produced as a kind of cancer in the bone marrow that progressively replaces the blood-forming tissue and absorbs bone causing areas of OSTEOPOROSIS. There is widespread bone pain and crippling spontaneous fractures and the effects of anaemia and thickening of the blood from excessive globulins. This may affect brain function. The urine may contain considerable quantities of immunoglobulin (Bence Jones protein). Treatment is with anticancer drugs such as MELPHALAN, with total body irradiation followed by restoration of the bone marrow with autologous haematopoietic stem cells. THALIDOMIDE with DEXAMETHASONE has proved effective and the drug bortezomib is considered promising.

myelomeningocele see MENINGOMYELOCELE.

myelosclerosis see MYELOFIBROSIS.

myiasis infestation of the skin, wounds or body apertures by fly larvae. Fly-blown and maggotty wounds are common in the tropics and the infestation does little harm. The African tumbu fly deposits eggs through the intact skin and the larva grows into an adult fly that then emerges. Bot fly egg larvae, deposited by mosquitos, penetrate the skin. Some fly larvae gain access to the sinuses around the nose and can cause severe damage.

Mylanta a brand name for a mixture of ALUMINIUM HYDROXIDE, MAGNESIUM HYDROXIDE and SIMETHICONE.

Myleran a brand name for BUSULPHAN (busulfan).

Mynah a brand name for the anti-TUBERCULOSIS drug ETHAMBUTOL and for other anti-tuberculosis drugs.

myo- *combining form denoting* muscle.

myocardial infarction (MI) the death and coagulation of part of the heart muscle deprived of an adequate blood supply by coronary artery blockage in a HEART ATTACK. See also INFARCTION. Established major risk factors for MI are raised plasma low density lipoprotein cholesterol; decreased high density lipoprotein cholesterol; smoking; and high blood pressure.

Risk factors of secondary importance include physical inactivity; obesity; and increased plasma glucose. Currently suspected risk factors include inflammatory markers such as C-reactive protein, interleukins and serum amyloid A; and procoagulant markers such as homocyteine, tissue plasminogen activator, plasminogen activator inhibitor and lipoprotein A. Possible trigger factors include a surge of sympathetic activity and exposure to particulate air pollution. Genetic factors remain uncertain.

Myocardial stunning a reversible state of left ventricular dysfunction featuring chest pain, dyspnoea, ECG changes, and sometimes hypotension or heart failure requiring supportive measures. The condition may be precipitated by sudden severe emotional stress and in these cases the levels of catecholamines may be up to 30 times normal.

myocarditis inflammation of the heart muscle. This may result from bacterial or viral infection, from RHEUMATIC FEVER, from DIPHTHERIA toxin, from TRYPANOSOMIASIS (CHAGAS' DISEASE) or from nutritional deficiency. See also CARDIOMYOPATHY.

myoclonus a sudden, brief, involuntary muscle contraction usually causing a jerk of a limb. This occurs most commonly as a normal phenomenon in people half asleep but myoclonic contractions are a feature of EPILEPSY and of many other brain diseases.

Myocrisin a brand name for SODIUM AUROTHIOMALATE.

myoglobin the muscle cell equivalent of the haemoglobin of the blood. Myoglobin acts as a temporary oxygen store from which oxygen is drawn as the muscle requires it.

myoglobinuria the presence of MYOGLOBIN in the urine. This may occur when there is an excessive rate of breakdown of muscle (rhabdomyolysis) with release of myoglobin into the blood.

myokymia one of a range of conditions featuring involuntary, fine, twitching or rippling of muscle fibres. The common eyelid twitch, or fasciculation, is an example of myokymia.

myology the science and study of muscle.

myoma a BENIGN tumour of muscle.

myometritis inflammation of the MYOMETRIUM.

myometrium the muscle wall of the womb (uterus).

myopathy any disease or disorder of muscle. The myopathies include congenital or acquired conditions such as the muscular dystrophies, inflammatory muscle disorders and metabolic and drug-induced disorders.

myopia short-sightedness. A condition in which the optical power of the eye is too great in relation to the distance from the lens to the RETINA. Only diverging rays from near objects focus sharply. Myopia is corrected by weakening (concave) lenses. The derivation is uncertain but probably relates to 'muscular eye' – a reference to the tendency of myopes to screw up their eyelids so as to stop down the optics and improve distance vision.

myosarcoma a malignant tumour of muscle. See also SARCOMA.

myositis inflammation of muscle. This may occur as a result of a Coxsackie virus infection as in BORNHOLM'S DISEASE, or it may be a feature of DERMATOMYOSITIS, or a response to the parasitic worm Trichinella spiralis that settles in muscle, or an AUTOIMMUNE reaction affecting the external eye muscles in thyroid disease.

myositis ossificans a rare, usually familial, inflammatory disease of muscle in which CALCIFICATION occurs followed by the formation of bony tissue within the affected muscles.

myotonia congenita a dominant genetic disease in which the affected person has great difficulty in relaxing muscles after they have been contracted. A grasp can be released only slowly and with great difficulty and the tightly shut eyes may take many seconds to open again. The condition gradually improves with age.

myotonic dystrophy see DYSTROPHIA MYOTONICA.

myringo- *combining form denoting* the eardrum.

myringitis inflammation of the eardrum (tympanic membrane).

myringoplasty 1 surgical repair of a hole (perforation) in an eardrum. 2 a repair operation involving the drum and the chain of small bones (the auditory ossicles) in the middle ear.

myringotomy surgical cutting (incision) of the eardrum. This may be done to allow discharge of pus from the middle ear or, more commonly, to insert a grommet in cases of 'glue ear' (secretory OTITIS MEDIA) to drain the middle ear and relieve deafness.

Mysoline a brand name for the ANTICONVULSANT drug primidone, used in the control of EPILEPSY.

Mysteclin a brand name for a mixture of the ANTIFUNGAL drug NYSTATIN and the antibiotic TETRACYCLINE.

mythopoiesis the internal fabrication of mythic events or false memories that may subsequently be revealed or acted out in multiple personalities, trances, 'demonic possession', seemingly psychic phenomena or conviction of their reality.

myxo- *combining form denoting* mucus.

myxadenitis inflammation of mucous glands.

myxoedema the general effects of severe underactivity of the thyroid gland (HYPOTHYROIDISM). These include dry, yellow, cold, scaly, thickened and coarse skin, scanty hair, loss of the eyebrows, lethargy, marked slowing of body and mind, absence of menstrual periods, accumulation of mucoid deposits in the body, ANGINA PECTORIS, ANAEMIA and HEART FAILURE. A frank PSYCHOSIS with delusions and hallucinations may occur. Death may result from failure to maintain body temperature. Most of these effects can be prevented or reversed by giving thyroid hormone.

myxoid of a mucin-rich constitution.

myxoma a rare, benign, jelly-like tumour consisting of soft mucoid material, mainly hyaluronic acid. Myxomas may affect muscles, especially in the shoulder and thigh and sometimes occur within one of the chambers of the heart. A myxoma in this situation may cause blood clot EMBOLI or may interfere with the normal flow of blood. If necessary, a cardiac myxoma may be removed surgically.

n

nabumetone a NON-STEROIDAL ANTI-INFLAMMATORY DRUG used to treat arthritis and other painful conditions. A brand name is Relifex.

NAD *abbrev. for* nothing abnormal detected.

NADH *abbrev. for* nicotinamide adenine dinucleotide

nadolol a non-selective beta-blocker drug that acts on all beta-adrenergic receptor sites. A brand name is Corgard.

Naegleria fowleri infection a rare but severe protozoal infection causing destructive changes in the brain and meninges (necrotizing amoebic meningoencephalitis). Most infected people have a history of swimming in warm fresh water, or at a spa 2 to 14 days before the onset. The organism gains access to the brain by way of the cribriform plate at the upper part of the nose. The infection mimics bacterial meningitis and the true diagnosis is usually missed. There is high fever, neck stiffness, coma, convulsions and death within a few days of onset. Autopsy shows brain softening. The only effective drug is Amphotericin B given intravenously and into the cerebrospinal fluid.

naevus any coloured growth or mark on the skin present at birth. A birthmark. From Latin *naevus*, a spot or blemish.

nafarelin a GONADORTOPHIN RELEASING HORMONE analogue drug used to treat ENDOMETRIOSIS and infertility. A brand name is Synarel.

naftidrofuryl an artery-widening drug used to improve the blood supply to the brain and to the limbs. A brand name is Praxilene.

nail 1 a protective and functional plate of a hard, tough protein, KERATIN, lying on the back surface of the last PHALANX of each finger and toe.

2 a steel rod used surgically to secure bone fragments in apposition.

nail disorders see SUBUNGUAL HAEMATOMA, ONYCHOLYSIS, PARONYCHIA and TINEA.

nailing internal fixation of an ununited fracture of bone by means of a metal rod, often in the marrow cavity (intramedullary nailing).

nalbufine an opiate drug used to control moderate to severe pain. A brand name is Nubain.

Nalcrom a brand name for CHROMOGLYCATE.

nalidixic acid a quinolone antibiotic drug, effective against GRAM NEGATIVE bacilli, including Proteus species, and much used for urinary infections. The drug is on the WHO official list. Brand names are Negram and Uriben.

Nalorex a brand name for NALTREXONE.

nalorphine a narcotic antagonist drug so similar in structure to MORPHINE that it occupies morphine receptor sites on cell membranes and prevents morphine from acting. A small dose of the drug, given to a morphine addict, can induce withdrawal symptoms within a matter of minutes.

naloxone a narcotic antagonist drug similar to NALORPHINE, chemically related to MORPHINE, and used as an antidote to narcotic poisoning. The drug is on the WHO official list. A brand name is Narcan.

naltrexone a narcotic antagonist used as a maintenance therapy in former narcotic addicts. A brand name is Nalorex.

nandrolone decanoate a male sex hormone with ANABOLIC properties. The drug is sometimes used also to stimulate blood cell production in APLASTIC ANAEMIA. A brand name is Deca-Durabolin.

nanism DWARFISM due to arrested development.

nano- *prefix denoting* one thousand millionth (one billionth).

nanobacteria micro-organisms less than 0.1 (micrometre) long and surrounded by a mineralized shell, that were first described in mid-1998. It is claimed that cells infected with these bacteria develop mineral deposits and suggested that they may be the cause of kidney stones and a range of other diseases that feature calcification. Critics have suggested that these are simply normal bacteria that have shrunk and become calcified. Further study is required.

nanogram one billionth of a gram.

nanomedicine the application to medicine of very small structures, of size between 1 and 100 nanometres. A nanometer is a billionth (one thousand millionth) of a meter and has the symbol nm. Potentially, the possibilities of nanotechnology applied to medicine are very great and include the delivery of drugs and genes into cells; the production of nanoinstruments of hitherto impossible precision; and the use of nanorobots to carry out procedures in any part of the body. Nanomedicine is already an established fact and is being taken seriously by governments and scientific bodies. At the end of 2002 the US National Institutes of Health initiated a four-year program of nanoscience and technology in medicine, and the British Royal Society and Royal Academy of Engineering are currently studying the benefits and risks.

nanometre one billionth of a metre.

nanoparticles particles of very small size that are being exploited increasingly in medicine as in other sciences. Nanoparticles have recently been developed as delivery vehicles for drugs and for gene therapy. One unexpected finding emerging from this research is that nanoparticles of cerium oxide only 5 nanometres in diameter inserted into nerve cells in culture appear to increase the three week life of these cells to about six months. It is speculated that they are having a useful effect in mopping up damaging FREE RADICALS.

nanosecond one billionth of a second.

nanotechnology the application of the science of manipulation at an atomic level. The practical applications of the ability to move single atoms so as to construct molecules, materials, structures and even functioning machines at an atomic level. Nanotechnology is currently at a germinal stage but is expected to have extensive applications in medicine. See also MAGNETIC NANOPARTICLES.

nape the back of the neck.

nappy rash skin irritation in the nappy area from ammonia formed from the breakdown of urea, from irritating faeces or from thrush (CANDIDIASIS).

naphazoline an ADRENERGIC drug that causes small blood vessels to constrict and thus reduces congestion in mucous membranes. It may be taken as a nasal spray. A brand name is Antistin Privine.

Naprogesic a brand name for NAPROXEN.

Naprosyn a brand name for NAPROXEN.

naproxen a NON-STEROIDAL ANTI-INFLAMMATORY DRUG (NSAID). Brand names are Naprosyn, Nycopren, Synflex and, formulated with the prostaglandin drug MISOPROSTOL, Napratec.

naratriptan a SEROTONIN agonist drug used to treat MIGRAINE. It is believed to act by narrowing the brain arteries that are widened during a migraine attack. A brand name is Naramig.

Narcan a brand name for NALOXONE.

narcissism possession of an exaggerated and exhibitionistic need for admiration and praise and an overweening conviction of one's own merits and attractiveness. *Narcissus*, a character in Greek mythology, was a youth who fell in love with his own reflection in a pond.

narco- *combining form denoting* numbness, narcosis or stupor. From Greek *narke*, numbness.

narcoanalysis psychoanalysis carried out while the patient is in a drowsy state induced by drugs such as sodium amytal or THIOPENTONE (thiopental). The vogue for narcoanalysis seems to have passed, but there is a suggestion of renewed interest in the USA.

narcolepsy a disorder featuring an overwhelming tendency to fall asleep when relaxing or free from stimulating demands. People with narcolepsy may drop off many times a day and sleep for minutes to hours. The cause is unknown. Driving a car may be dangerous.

narcosis a state of unconsciousness that may range from sleep to deep, irreversible coma. In most cases narcosis is caused by a drug.

narcotic a drug which, in appropriate dosage, produces sleep and relieves pain. Overdosage of narcotics may cause coma and death. Most narcotics are derived from opium or are synthetic substances chemically related to morphine.

Nardil a brand name for the antidepressant drug PHENELZINE.

narrow-angle glaucoma a condition of raised fluid pressure within the eye resulting from obstructed access of aqueous humour to the drainage channel (the trabecular meshwork) at the root of the IRIS. This occurs because the angle between the iris and the back of the CORNEA is narrower than normal and can easily close, especially when the pupil is wide and the iris consequently bunched up.

nares the plural of NARIS.

Naropin a brand name for ROPIVACAINE.

naris a nostril. Either of the two external openings of the nasal cavity.

Nasacort a brand name for TRIAMCINOLONE.

nasal pertaining to the nose.

nasal bones the two variably-sized, flat and roughly rectangular plates of bone forming the bridge of the nose. Each nasal bone is attached to the FRONTAL BONE above, the MAXILLA to the side and to the ETHMOID internally.

nasal cannulae soft plastic tubes that can be fitted comfortably into the nostrils for the administration of OXYGEN to patients. Nasal cannulae have advantages over masks in that they do not interfere with eating and spectacle wearing and avoid rebreathing of carbon dioxide.

nasal conchae see TURBINATES.

nasal congestion swelling (OEDEMA) of the mucous membrane lining the nose, usually as a result of inflammation from a common cold virus infection or from HISTAMINE released as an allergic response to tree or grass pollen grains. Nasal congestion can be relieved temporarily by decongestant drugs.

nasal discharge any watery, PURULENT or blood-stained fluid tending to run from the nose. Nasal discharge usually comes from the mucous membrane of the nose or sinuses but after a head injury may come from inside the skull and consist of cerebrospinal fluid.

nasal obstruction interference with the free passage of air through either side of the nose from any cause. Causes of obstruction include

swelling of the mucous membrane (NASAL CONGESTION), nasal POLYPS, NASOPHARYNGEAL CARCINOMA or foreign bodies.

nasal septum the thin, central partition that divides the interior of the nose into two passages. The septum consists of a thin plate of bone, behind, and a thin plate of cartilage in front. Both are covered with MUCOUS MEMBRANE. Deflection of the septum to one side (deviated septum) is common and usually harmless.

nasion the centre of the junction (suture) between the nasal and the frontal bones. The centre of the bridge of the nose.

naso- *combining form denoting* nose or nasal.

nasogastric tube a narrow, soft rubber or plastic tube that can easily be passed through the nose and down the gullet (oesophagus) into the stomach. Nasogastric tubes are used to withdraw samples of the stomach contents or to supply liquid nutrition to people too ill to swallow. Also known as a Ryle's tube.

nasolacrimal canal the bony groove or conduit from the lacrimal bone through the MAXILLA that carries the NASOLACRIMAL DUCT.

nasolacrimal duct the membranous passage that carries the overflow of tears from the LACRIMAL SAC to the interior of the nose, opening just under the lower TURBINATE. Blockage of the nasolacrimal duct causes a persistently watering eye.

nasopharynx the space at the back of the nose, above and behind the soft palate. Normally this space is continuous with the space at the back of the mouth, but in swallowing it is shut off from the oropharynx by the soft palate pressing against the back wall. On the back wall of the nasopharynx are the openings of the EUSTACHIAN TUBES and, in childhood, the ADENOIDS.

natal 1 pertaining to birth.
2 pertaining to the buttocks.

nates the buttocks.

National Service Framework an agenda for change and development of healthcare provision for children, young people and maternity services. It prescribes eleven standards for care and includes better consultation with children and families, a more holistic approach and child- and family-centred services based on their specific needs.

Natrilix a brand name for the thiazide DIURETIC drug INDAPAMIDE.

natriuresis excretion of sodium by the kidneys.

natriuretic peptide a PEPTIDE present in the blood and raised in quantity in people with long-term (chronic) HEART FAILURE. It arises in the upper chambers of the heart, probably as a result of stretching, and causes blood vessels to widen and the output of urine to increase. By increasing output of urinary sodium and, with it, water, it helps to relieve the OEDEMA that is a feature of HEART FAILURE. Also known as atrial natriuretic factor. B-type natriuretic peptide is released by ventricular muscle cells and is used as a therapeutic agent in heart failure. It is also used as a biomarker for differential diagnosis of breathlessness and for preclinical assessment of heart failure.

Natulan a brand name for the anticancer drug PROCARBAZINE.

natural antibodies antibodies in the serum to red blood cell antigens that are not present in the body of the same individual. Natural antibodies are not derived from previous exposure to antigens. They determine the blood groups.

natural childbirth a term used to encourage the concept that having a baby should be a normal and natural process rather than a medical or surgical event, operation or emergency. A clear understanding of what is involved and informed instruction on the nature and cause of pain in labour, together with exercises in relaxation and cooperation, has made labour less difficult and painful, and more rewarding, for millions of women. It has not, however, made childbirth either easy or painless.

natural immunity the ability to resist infection that does not depend on prior experience of the invading organism and the resultant production of antibodies or amendment or selection of LYMPHOCYTES. Natural immunity is a general and non-specific resistance to infection possessed by all healthy individuals. Also known as natural resistance.

natural killer cells a class of large, granular lymphocytes that bind directly to cells bearing foreign ANTIGENS and kill them. Natural killer cells do not require prior exposure of the immune system to the antigen and kill their victims by programmed cell death (apoptosis).

natural philosophy an obsolescent term for physics.

natural remedies substances of claimed medical value derived directly from plants or other natural sources. The view that natural remedies are in some way superior to those developed scientifically is mistaken. Many useful drugs in the pharmacopoeia are derived from natural sources but these have been purified and assayed so that accurate and safe dosage becomes possible. Most readily available and useful natural remedies have been exploited in this way and the search for other useful natural drugs continues. Some natural remedies have been found to be dangerous. Many of those on sale are of little value.

natural selection the Darwin-originated principle that individuals of a species happening, by normal genetic rearrangement or by mutation, to possess inherited characteristics with survival value relative to a particular environment are more likely to survive long enough to reproduce and increase the numbers having these characteristics. Natural selection occurs quickly in rapidly reproducing micro-organisms. (Charles Darwin, 1809–82, English naturalist).

nature versus nurture the perennial argument as to whether heredity or environment is more influential in determining the outcome of any individual's development. It is now apparent that the two are so intimately inter-related in their effects as to be almost inseparable.

naturopathy a system of folk medicine that claims that all disease can be cured by restriction to a largely vegetarian diet free from all contaminants and drugs. Such a regimen, if possible, might well promote health but there are many causes of disease other than dietary and many environmental hazards are unavoidable.

nausea the unpleasant feeling of sickness that often precedes vomiting. From the Greek *naus*, a ship.

navel the depressed scar in the centre of the abdomen left when the UMBILICAL CORD drops off and the opening into the abdomen heals. The medical term is umbilicus.

Navelbine a brand name for VINORELBINE.

navicular the outermost of the wrist (CARPAL) bones on the thumb side in the nearest row. The bone is roughly boat-shaped, hence the name, which is derived from the Latin *navis*, a boat. Also known as SCAPHOID.

Navidrex a brand name for thiazide DIURETIC drug cyclopenthiazide.

Navoban a brand name for TROPISETRON.

near point the shortest distance from the eye at which fine detail can be sharply perceived. Except in short-sighted (myopic) people, the near point moves progressively further away with age. Reading glasses will generally be needed when the near point exceeds about 40 cm.

near-sightedness see MYOPIA.

nebula a cloudy spot on the CORNEA of the eye. A central nebula can severely interfere with clear vision.

nebulizer a form of inhaler used mainly in the control and treatment of ASTHMA. Nebulizers deliver an aerosol of the active drug in water or other vehicle. Some are electrically operated.

Necator a genus of hookworms that parasitize the small intestine. The commonest species to affect humans is *Necator americanus*. Infection with this worm is common in Africa, Central and South America and the Pacific.

neck any narrowing or constriction in a body or part. A cervix.

neck, broken SEE BROKEN NECK.

neck rigidity abnormal difficulty and discomfort in bending the head forward because of sustained contraction (spasm) of the neck and spinal muscles. Neck rigidity is an important sign of MENINGITIS.

necr-, necro- *combining form denoting* death.

necrobiosis natural death of cells and tissues occurring in the midst of healthy tissue. Natural cell death as opposed to death from disease or injury.

necromania an abnormal desire for the company of a dead body or dead bodies, often the body of a loved one.

necrophilia the desire for, or practice of, sexual intercourse with a dead person. This somewhat limiting propensity is described as a psychosexual disorder (paraphilia) in which arousal is possible only if the object of sexual interest is dead.

necrophobia an abnormal fear of death or of corpses.

necropsy an autopsy, or postmortem examination, of a body.

necrosis the structural changes, such as those of GANGRENE, that follow death of a body tissue. The most obvious changes are in the cell nuclei which become shrunken and condensed (pyknosis) and no longer take a basic stain. Cell CYTOPLASM becomes more homogeneous and spaces (vacuoles) develop.

necrospermia a high proportion of dead sperm in the seminal fluid. This is a cause of sterility.

necrotic pertaining to the death of tissue (NECROSIS).

necrotizing enterocolitis a dangerous disorder featuring patches or diffuse area of tissue death (necrosis) in the small or large intestine especially in premature infants but also sometimes in full-term babies. It is most likely to affect babies that are unwell, especially those with congenital heart disease or the respiratory distress syndrome. A severe infection with the organism CLOSTRIDIUM DIFFICILE is often present and there is gas production with 30% of hydrogen that balloons out the abdomen. Some cases have been ascribed to interference with the oxygen free radicals used by phagocytes to perform their immunological function by overdosage with the antioxidant vitamin E.

necrotizing fasciitis an uncommon but severe form of tissue damage caused by a streptococcus of Group A. There is widespread inflammation of the layer of fatty tissue under the skin and the effect is so intense that the tissue appears, in places, almost to be 'eaten away'. The condition features severe pain, marked general upset and intense redness of the overlying skin. Surgical exploration shows grey, swollen fat that can be stripped out easily with the finger. Surgical shock and failure of various organs, such as the kidneys, may occur and the outcome, in inadequately managed or late treated cases is often fatal. Treatment is by massive doses of antibiotics, early radical surgery to remove infected tissue and exposure to high oxygen concentrations in a special chamber (see HYPERBARIC OXYGEN TREATMENT). Inadequate treatment results in a mortality of 30%–60%.

nedocromil an anti-inflammatory drug used to treat hay fever, seasonal allergic CONJUNCTIVITIS and bronchial asthma. Brand names are Rapitil, Tilade and Tilarin.

needle exchange programmes an effective public health measure to reduce the prevalence of conditions such as AIDS and hepatitis B that are often spread among intravenous drug abusers by sharing needles. About half of new HIV infections are now caused by needle sharing. New sterile syringes and needles are supplied free of charge to discourage the practice. Many studies have shown that this is a valuable measure that does not encourage illegal drug usage but, up to early 1998, the USA, almost alone among developed countries, continued to ban it.

needle-free insulin delivery system a device that projects a fine jet of INSULIN solution at such high pressure that it penetrates the skin, delivering insulin subcutaneously. A nozzle is placed against the skin and the device fired.

needlestick injury the actual or potential harm caused by accidentally pricking oneself with a needle after giving an injection or taking blood. Needlestick injury has acquired greater significance since AIDS and HEPATITIS B have become so prevalent. Medical personnel routinely discard 'sharps' into special safe containers without first re-sheathing hypodermic needles. Sheathing readily leads to pricking.

nefopam a painkilling drug. A brand name is Acupan.

negative feedback a control entity in which part of the response to the stimulus, acting in opposition to it, is applied to the stimulus. In other words, in a system with an input and an output, a proportion of the output signal, which must be in opposite phase to the input signal, is carried back to join and modify the input signal, reducing the effect of distortional changes caused by the system. The feedback signal is usually much smaller than the input stimulus, but exerts a powerful stabilizing and linearizing effect on the whole system. Negative feedback, long used to improve the stability and quality of electronic circuits, is now known to be an important principle in a wide range of biological and physiological systems.

Negram a brand name for NALIDIXIC ACID.

Neisseria a genus of small, aerobic, GRAM NEGATIVE micro-organisms occurring in pairs (diplococci) that includes *Neisseria gonorrhoea*, the cause of GONORRHOEA and *Neisseria meningitidis* the cause of epidemic cerebrospinal MENINGITIS. (Albert Ludwig Siegmund Neisser, 1855–1916, German dermatologist).

nelfinavir a protease inhibitor drug used in combination with other antiretroviral drugs to treat HIV infections. The drug is on the WHO official list. A brand name is Viracept.

Nelson's syndrome a late complication of removal of both adrenal glands for CUSHING'S SYNDROME. A rapidly growing, invasive tumour of the PITUITARY GLAND occurs, releasing hormones that produce intense brown pigmentation of the skin. (Don H. Nelson, American physician, b. 1925).

nemat-, nemato- *combining form denoting* thread-like, as in NEMATODE worms. The term derives from the Greek *nema*, a thread.

nematocyst a coiled, tube-like stinging organ of various coelenterates, such as jellyfish. The nematocyst injects a chemical paralyzant.

nematodes unsegmented, threadlike worms of the phylum *Nematoda*. Many nematodes are parasitic on humans. They include the whipworm *Trichuris trichuria*, the muscle worm *Trichinella spiralis*, the intestinal parasite *Strongyloides stercoralis*, the hook worms *Ancylostoma duodenale* and *Necator americanus*, the threadworm *Enterobius* or *Oxyuris vermicularis*, the roundworm *Ascaris lumbricoides*, the filarial worms and the puppy dog worm *Toxocara canis*.

neo- *combining form denoting* new.

Neoclarityn a brand name for DESLORATADINE.

Neo-Cortef a brand name for a preparation, for external use, containing the anti-inflammatory drug HYDROCORTISONE and the antibiotic NEOMYCIN.

Neo-Cytamen a brand name for HYDROXOCOBALAMIN.

neologism 1 a newly coined word or phrase. 2 a meaningless word used by a psychotic person.

Neo-Medrol a brand name for a skin preparation containing the steroid drug METHYLPREDNISOLONE and the antibiotic NEOMYCIN.

Neo-Mercazole a brand name for CARBIMAZOLE.

neomycin an aminoglycoside ANTIBIOTIC drug derived from a strain of *Streptomyces fradiae*. Neomycin can be given by mouth to destroy organisms in the bowel or can be used in solution to irrigate the bladder. It is poorly absorbed into the bloodstream. It is much too toxic to be given by injection and can have seriously damaging effects on hearing and on the kidneys. The drug is widely used as a surface application in ointments with other ingredients such as steroids. A brand name is Nivemycin. Preparations of neomycin with a corticosteroid, for external use, include Audicort, Betnovate-N, Dermovate-NN, Maxitrol, Neo-Cortef, Synalar-N, Tri-Adcortyl and Vistamethasone N. The drug is also formulated with the antibiotics polymyxin and gramicidin and with the antifungal drug nystatin.

neonatal pertaining to a new-born baby.

neonate a new-born baby.

neonaticide the killing of a baby in the first 24 hours of its life.

neonatologist a doctor specializing in the management, assessment, diseases and intensive care of newborn babies, especially those that are of low birth weight and those with congenital abnormalities. After the first 4 weeks of life, care may pass to a general paediatrician.

neoplasia the process of tumour formation.

neoplasm a collection of cells, derived from a common origin, often a single cell, that is increasing in number and expanding or spreading, either locally or to remote sites. A tumour. Neoplasms may be BENIGN or MALIGNANT. The term literally means a new growth. See also CANCER.

neoplastic pertaining to a NEOPLASM.

Neoplatin a brand name for CISPLATIN.

neostigmine an ANTICHOLINESTERASE drug used in the treatment of MYASTHENIA GRAVIS. Neostigmine interferes with the enzyme that breaks down the neurotransmitter ACETYLCHOLINE and so prolongs its action. The drug is on the WHO official list. A brand name is Robinul neostigmine.

nephr-, nephro- *combining form denoting* the kidney.

nephrectomy surgical removal of a kidney. This may be necessary because of injury and severe bleeding, cancer, severe infection, malfunctioning from loss of blood supply or multiple stones. If the other kidney is healthy there is no apparent functional disadvantage from nephrectomy. One kidney provides ample kidney function to maintain health and allow full physical activity.

nephritic 1 pertaining to the kidneys.
2 pertaining to NEPHRITIS.

nephritis inflammation of the kidney. See also GLOMERULONEPHRITIS.

nephrology the study of the structure, function and disorders of the kidney.

nephroblastoma a malignant tumour of the kidney arising, usually in childhood, from primitive kidney-forming (nephroblastic) tissue. Also known as WILM'S TUMOUR.

nephrocalcinosis the presence of calcification or actual stones within the substance of the kidney.

nephrolithiasis stones in the kidney.

nephrolithotomy surgical removal of a stone (calculus) from the kidney.

nephropathica epidemica a form of haemorrhagic fever with a special tendency to affect the kidneys, that occurs in Scandinavia. It is caused by a Hantaan virus carried by small rodents and may lead to kidney failure. With effective treatment, recovery may be expected.

nephropathic cystinosis a rare autosomal recessive LYSOSOMAL STORAGE DISEASE in which cystine crystals are deposited widely throughout the body. Kidney damage may be severe with passage of large quantities of urine containing amino acids and glucose. There is acidosis of the blood with low phosphate and potassium levels and vitamin D-resistant rickets.

nephropathy any disease of the kidney involving observable change.

nephropexy surgical fixation of a floating kidney by stitching the capsule to the back wall of the abdomen.

nephrosis see NEPHROTIC SYNDROME.

nephrostomy an opening into the kidney for the purpose of draining urine by way of a tube.

nephrotic syndrome a kidney disorder in which protein, never normally found in the urine, is excreted in such quantities that blood levels may be depleted and the OSMOTIC PRESSURE of the blood reduced. This leads to accumulation of fluid in the body tissues (oedema). The nephrotic syndrome may follow kidney damage from GLOMERULONEPHRITIS or DIABETES or it may be caused by severe high blood pressure (HYPERTENSION), poisoning or adverse reactions from drugs. The condition is treated with DIURETIC drugs to get rid of the accumulated fluid in the tissues.

nephrotomy a surgical incision into a kidney.

nephrotoxicity the liability of a substance, such as a drug, to cause damage to the kidneys. A nephrotoxic effect is more likely if existing kidney damage reduces the rate of excretion of the toxic agent so that it acts for longer periods on the kidneys.

Nerisone a brand name for DIFLUCORTOLONE VALERATE.

nerve a pinkish-white, cord-like structure consisting of bundles of long fibres (AXONS) of nerve cells and fine blood vessels held together by a connective tissue sheath. Individual fibres are usually insulated with a layer of white fatty material called myelin. The larger nerves contain both MOTOR and SENSORY fibres. Twelve pairs of nerves arise directly from the brain. These are called cranial nerves and carry impulses subserving smell, eye movement, vision, facial movement and sensation, all other sensation in the head, hearing, taste, movements of the soft palate, tongue and neck muscles, and control of the heartbeat and the secretion of stomach acid. 31 pairs of nerves emerge from the spinal cord. These control all the other muscles of the body and carry impulses for sensation from all parts of the body to the spinal cord and thence to the brain.

nerve block an important method of producing an area of ANAESTHESIA by preventing nerve impulses from the area from passing to the brain. This may be done at any point along the nerve carrying sensory information from the area by injecting an anaesthetic drug around it. Nerve block anaesthesia is widely used in all forms of surgery.

nerve deafness hearing loss resulting from damage to the transducers in the inner ear (Organ of Corti) or to the acoustic nerve connections to the brain, rather than from mechanical interference with the transmission of sound vibrations to the inner ear (conductive deafness).

nerve gases powerful pharmacological agents, usually produced as volatile liquids that operate after inhalation or after absorption through the skin. Nerve gases were developed from the organophosphorus insecticides and are inhibitors of the enzyme cholinesterase. Cholinesterase inhibition prevents the breakdown of acetylcholine which thus continues to act strongly causing strong parasympathetic effects. There is extreme salivation, nausea, vomiting and diarrhoea, sweating, giddiness and tightness in the chest. The pupils of the eyes constrict and the vision

blurs. Breathing fails and there are convulsions, coma and death. Very small doses can be fatal. See also ANTICHOLINESTERASE.

nerve growth factor a peptide substance that stimulates growth and differentiation of NEURONES in the sympathetic and sensory nervous system. Nerve growth factor has been found effective in promoting the healing of corneal ulcers due to loss of the sensory innervation of the cornea. Corneal transparency has been restored by this means.

nerve impulse the wave-like progression of electrical depolarization that passes along a stimulated nerve fibre. The nerve impulse results from a movement of positive and negative ions across the membrane of the fibre.

nervous breakdown a popular and imprecise term used to describe any emotional, neurotic or psychotic disturbance ranging from a brief episode of hysterical behaviour to a major psychotic illness such as SCHIZOPHRENIA.

nervous habit see TICS.

nervous system the controlling, integrating, recording and effecting structure of the body. The nervous system is also the seat of consciousness, of the intellect, of the emotions and of all bodily satisfaction. The central nervous system consists of the brain and spinal cord. The peripheral nervous system consists of the massive ramification of nerves running to every part of the body outside the brain and cord.

Netillin a brand name for NETILMICIN.

netilmicin an AMINOGLYCOSIDE antibiotic drug derived from gentamicin. It is slightly less likely to damage the kidneys than gentamicin and is often effective against organisms resistant to that drug. A brand name is Netillin.

nettle rash see URTICARIA.

Neulactil a brand name for PERICYAZINE.

Neulasta a brand name for PEGFILGRASTIM.

Neupogen a brand name for FILGRASTIM.

neur-, neuro- *prefix denoting* nerve.

neuralgia pain experienced in an area supplied by a sensory nerve as a result of nerve disorder that results in the production of pain impulses in the nerve. Neuralgia may be caused by injury to the nerve, nerve inflammation (neuritis) from any cause, such as virus infection, or by nerve abnormality of unknown origin. Neuralgia is often episodic and may be triggered by a minor stimulus such as a light touch to the area supplied by the nerve. See also TRIGEMINAL NEURALGIA and POSTHERPETIC PAIN.

neural networks artificial electronic or software systems that can simulate some of the neurological functions including a crude form of vision. In conjunction with expert software systems neural networks are expected to prove important in medicine in the future.

neural tube defects see SPINA BIFIDA and ANENCEPHALY. See also FOLIC ACID.

neuraminidase inhibitors drugs used to treat INFLUENZA. Examples are oseltamivir (Tamiflu) and zanamivir (Relenza).

neurapraxia a peripheral nerve injury featuring temporary failure of conduction of impulses, usually due to compression without severance.

neurasthenia a state of constant fatigue, loss of motivation and energy and often insomnia and muscle aches associated with general and persistent unhappiness. In the present state of knowledge, and in the absence of any evidence of a cause, the state described as neurasthenia is considered not to be of organic origin and, in particular, to have nothing to do with nerve function.

neurectomy surgical removal of part of a nerve.

neurilemma an outer covering of flattened cells that surrounds the MYELIN sheath of the nerve fibres (axons) of the larger peripheral nerves. Neurilemma also covers the axons of non-myelinated nerve fibres. Also known as the sheath of Schwann.

neurilemmoma a benign tumour of NEURILEMMA (Schwann cells) that may occur in any peripheral or CRANIAL NERVE or in a nerve of the sympathetic nervous system. Although non-malignant, neurilemmomas of such nerves as the acoustic nerve can be dangerous.

neuritis inflammation of a nerve. This may be due to virus infection, loss of blood supply, mechanical injury, autoimmune disorder, vitamin deficiency, poisoning, or other poorly understood causes, such as the DEMYELINATION occurring in MULTIPLE SCLEROSIS. Some of these conditions involve pathological processes other than inflammation and should more properly be described as neuropathy rather than neuritis.

neuroanatomy the study of the structure of the nervous system and its relation to function. A knowledge of neuroanatomy is a prerequisite

for the diagnosis of neurological diseases and for the accurate location of the LESION causing the disorder.

neuroblast a cell in the embryo that gives rise to nerve cells.

neuroblastoma a highly malignant tumour derived from the cells that normally develop into nerve tissue. The tumour is composed of small, darkly staining cells often arranged around a central core of tangled fibrillary material to form rosettes. The neuroblastoma occurs mainly in the ADRENAL MEDULLA of children under the age of 4.

neurocirculatory asthenia a vague syndrome featuring breathlessness, palpitations, pain in the chest, ready fatiguability and a tendency to faintness. The term is imprecise as the condition is primarily caused by anxiety. Also known as EFFORT SYNDROME or DA COSTA'S SYNDROME.

neurocysticercosis involvement of the nervous system with the larvae of the tapeworm *Taenia solium*. The disease is widespread in the developing world where it is by far the commonest cause of late-onset EPILEPSY and of HYDROCEPHALUS in adults. See also CYSTICERCOSIS. Effective and cheap treatment with the drugs albendazole and praziquantel is available, but reliable diagnosis demands CT scanning or MRI, and these facilities are at a premium in the Third World.

neurocyte a nerve cell (NEURONE).

neurodermatitis skin damage and thickening caused by scratching, usually without an organic basis. Also known as LICHEN SIMPLEX.

neuroepithelioma a tumour of primitive nerve tissue similar to a NEUROBLASTOMA. Neuroepitheliomas may occur in the central nervous system, in the RETINA as RETINOBLASTOMAS, or may affect the OLFACTORY NERVE or occasionally peripheral nerves.

neurofibromatosis a genetic disease of dominant inheritance or caused by new mutations, featuring multiple soft tumours of the fibrous sheaths of nerves in the skin and elsewhere. There may be hundreds of these. The central nervous system may be involved with tumours in the brain or spinal cord. Mental retardation, usually mild, occurs in some cases. Also known as von Recklinghausen's disease. (Friedrich Daniel von Recklinghausen, 1833–1910, German pathologist).

neurofibrosarcoma see NEUROSARCOMA.

neurogenic of a lesion caused by interruption of the nerve supply.

neurogenic bladder a disorder of urinary bladder control due to damage to the spinal cord or to the nerves supplying the bladder. Voluntary control is lost but the bladder may empty itself automatically after filling.

neurogenic shock a severe drop in blood pressure and a reduction in the return of blood to the heart, resulting from widespread dilation of blood vessels caused by injury or disorder of the nervous system.

neuroglia the network of branched cells and fibres that forms the supporting connective tissue of the central nervous system. Certain brain tumours arise from neuroglial cells.

neuroglobin an oxygen-transport material in the brain, analogous to HAEMOGLOBIN in the blood and MYOGLOBIN in the muscles. Neuroglobin is a small protein of 151 amino acids. It is thought to have a neuroprotective effect in cerebral ischaemia, but its full function remains unelucidated.

neuroleptanaesthesia a form of light general anaesthesia in which drugs that block the normal responses to pain are also used. In some cases muscle relaxant drugs may be needed. The method is inherently stress-free.

neuroleptic 1 capable of bringing about emotional quietening without impairing consciousness. Capable of modifying abnormal psychotic behaviour.
2 any drug having these effects.

neuroleptic malignant syndrome a rare and sometimes fatal disorder related to the use of any NEUROLEPTIC drug in any dosage. It features high fever, sweating, severe rigidity of muscles, wide swings of blood pressure, incontinence, confusion and coma.

neuroleptoanalgesia a state of indifference to, or reduced appreciation of, pain brought about by the use of NEUROLEPTIC and ANALGESIC drugs. Consciousness is retained. Neuroleptanalgesia allows surgery to be performed without inducing general or local anaesthesia.

neurologist a doctor trained in NEUROLOGY, who specializes in the ANATOMY and PHYSIOLOGY of the nervous system and in the diagnosis and treatment of its disorders. Neurologists are learned diagnosticians and do not engage in operative treatment.

neurology the medical speciality concerned with the nervous system and its disorders. The list that follows highlights the key entries related to neurology in the dictionary: acute brain syndromes, alpha motor neurones, brain, brain abscess, brain damage, brain death, brain fever, brain haemorrhage, brain imaging, brain sand, brainstem, brain tumour, Doppler brain examination, entrapment neuropathy, epilepsy, ganglioneuroma, hindbrain hernia headache, hydrocephalus, interneuron, ischaemic neuropathy, Jacksonian epilepsy, Korsakov's psychosis, lead polyneuropathy, lower motor neuron disease, motor neuron disease, multiple sclerosis, neuralgia, neural tube defects, neuritis, neuroblastoma, neurofibromatosis, neurologist, neurology, neuroma, neuromyelitis optica, neuron, neurosurgery, neurosyphilis, optic neuritis, organic brain syndrome, polyneuritis, retrobulbar neuritis, subdural haematoma, trigeminal neuralgia.

neuroma a non-malignant (benign) tumour of nerve tissue consisting of a mass of nerve fibres. Although neuromas do not spread remotely their location, especially within the skull, may cause danger by compressing local structures. An acoustic neuroma is a tumour of the 8th CRANIAL NERVE.

neuromodulator a substance that, while not affecting the rate of firing or conduction of nerve impulses, can change the effect on a nerve of other neurotransmitters. Neuromodulators can control neurotransmitter synthesis or the amounts of neurotransmitter released in response to other stimuli. Adenosine is an example of a neuromodulator.

neuromyelitis optica an acute nervous system disorder featuring DEMYELINATION of the tracts in the nerve tracts in the spinal cord and both optic nerves. The condition occurs about a week after an attack of measles or chickenpox or may follow vaccination. There is headache, vomiting, stiff neck, paralysis and blindness and the death rate is high. In those who survive, recovery is often surprisingly complete. Also known as Devic's disease. (Eugene Devic, 1858–1930, French physician).

neuron, neurone the functional unit of the nervous system. A neurone is a single cell having a very long, fibre-like extension, called

433

an axon, and one or many short extensions called dendrites. The axon may be 100,000 times as long as the diameter of the cell body – some are as long as 1 m. Nerve impulses are moving zones of electrical depolarization and these travel outwards along the axon from the cell body. Incoming impulses travel to the cell body along the dendrites. Neurones interconnect with each other at specialized junctions called SYNAPSES, situated mainly between the end of an axon of one neurone and the cell body or the dendrites of another. Many neurones receive as many as 15,000 synapses, some more. Most synapses are interneurones connecting with other nerve cells, rather than with muscles or glands.

neuronal ceroid lipofuscinoses a group of rare autosomal recessive neurodegenerative disorders characterized by the abnormal accumulation of the pigmented material LIPOFUSCIN in tissues. The group forms the commonest neurodegenerative disorder of childhood. There is progressive destruction of retinal cell function with visual loss and deterioration of general brain function. The disease may start in early infancy, childhood or in adult life. In the latter case vision is retained but there is slow progressive dementia.

neuronitis inflammation of a NEURON.

Neurontin a brand name for GABAPENTIN.

neuropathology the study of disease changes occurring in the tissues of the nervous system.

neuropathy any NEURON disorder. Neuropathy occurs in CANCER, in DIABETES, in LEPROSY, in vitamin deficiency states, and may occur from genetic causes, from poisoning, from glue sniffing, from disorders of the AUTONOMIC NERVOUS SYSTEM and from nerve pressure.

neuropharmacology the study of drugs that act on the nervous system.

neurophysins a group of proteins found in the rear lobe of the PITUITARY GLAND and thought to be carriers for the hormones OXYTOCIN and VASOPRESSIN and to be concerned in their storage.

neurophysiology the study of the function of the nervous system.

neuropsychiatry the branch of medicine concerned with the effects on mind and behaviour of organic disorders of the nervous system. Neuropsychiatrists must be well versed in two formerly quite distinct disciplines – neurology and psychiatry.

neuroradiology the speciality concerned with the diagnosis of neurological disease by X-ray and associated methods of examination.

neurorrhaphy joining a cut nerve by stitching the ends together.

neurosarcoma a malignant tumor arising from the cells of Schwann in the sheaths of nerve fibres. Also known as a malignant schwannoma.

neurosclerosis hardening of nerve tissue.

neurosis any long-term mental or behavioural disorder, in which contact with reality is retained and the condition is recognized by the sufferer as abnormal. Attempts have been made to prohibit the term as pejorative and insulting but these have failed mainly because of a more complete and humane understanding of the subject and of the plight of neurotic sufferers. A neurosis essentially features anxiety or behaviour exaggeratedly designed to avoid anxiety. Defence mechanisms against anxiety take various forms and may appear as PHOBIAS, OBSESSIONS, COMPULSIONS or as sexual dysfunctions. In recent attempts at classification, the disorders formerly included under the neuroses have, possibly for reasons of political correctness, been given new names. The general term, neurosis, is now called anxiety disorder; hysteria has become a somatoform or conversion disorder; amnesia, fugue, multiple personality and depersonalization have become dissociative disorders; and neurotic depression has become a dysthymic disorder. These changes are helpful and explanatory but ignore the futility of euphemism. Psychoanalysis has proved of little value in curing these conditions and Freud's speculations as to their origins are not now widely accepted outside Freudian schools of thought. Neurotic disorders are probably best regarded as being the result of inappropriate early programming. Cognitive behaviour therapy seems effective in some cases.

neurosurgery the discipline concerned with the diagnosis and treatment of disorders of the nervous system that can be relieved or cured by surgical intervention. Neurosurgery is concerned mainly with head injury involving internal bleeding; tumours of the brain or spinal cord; disorders of the spinal skeleton affecting the spinal cord; abnormalities of the arteries of the nervous system, such as aneurysms around the base of the brain;

congenital disorders such as hydrocephalus or spina bifida; and abscesses of the nervous system following infection.

neurosyphilis any syphilitic infection of the nervous system. This is usually a late (tertiary) manifestation of untreated SYPHILIS, but may occur in adolescence. Its effects are widespread and include TABES DORSALIS, general paralysis of the insane (general paresis or GPI), dementia and involvement of the blood vessels of the brain and the brain coverings (meningovascular syphilis).

neuroticism the state of a person persistently and excessively prone to anxiety and to a preoccupation with self rather than with the external world. Neuroticism often involves HYPOCHONDRIASIS. See also NEUROSIS.

neurotomy the surgical cutting of a nerve, usually in the hope of relieving pain. This is seldom justified nowadays, is not always effective and will usually have serious side effects.

neurotransmitters a range of small-molecule chemical substances released by EXOCYTOSIS from a nerve ending on the arrival of a nerve impulse. Neurotransmitters are specific to particular neurons. They interacts with receptors on adjacent structures to trigger off a response, either excitatory or inhibitory. The adjacent structure may be another nerve, a muscle fibre or a gland. The main neurotransmitters are acetylcholine, glycine, glutamate, dopamine, noradrenaline, adrenaline, serotonin, histamine and GABA (gamma-amino-butyric acid). With the exception of the adrenalines all the neurotransmitters are AMINO ACIDS or derivatives of amino acids.

neurotrophic ulcer a pressure sore occasioned by loss of sensation and growth (trophic) disturbances resulting from nerve disorder.

neurotropic being attracted to, or having an affinity for, nerve tissue. Various toxic substances and some viruses are neurotropic.

neutraceuticals foods that are said to benefit health. See HEALTH FOOD.

neutral 1 neither acid nor alkaline. Having a pH of 7.
2 in the context of pharmacological INSULIN the term refers to soluble insulins that have not been formulated so as to prolong their action. Neutral insulins include those described as Rapid, Actrapid and Velosulin.

Neutrexin a brand name for TRIMETREXATE.

neutron therapy a form of radiation therapy (radiotherapy) involving bombardment of a part of the body with a stream of high velocity or slow neutrons.

neutropenia a reduction in the numbers of NEUTROPHIL POLYMORPHS (polymorphonuclear leucocytes) in the blood. This may prejudice the body's ability to resist infection.

neutropoenia see NEUTROPENIA.

neutrophil a white blood cell of the granulocyte group, with a multilobed (polymorph) nucleus and numerous granules in the CYTOPLASM that stain neither red with eosin nor blue with basic dyes. Neutrophils are the major circulating PHAGOCYTES of the granulocyte group. Compare EOSINOPHIL and BASOPHIL.

neutrophil exudation the movement of neutrophil polymorphs out of the blood capillaries into the tissue spaces. The polymorphs squeeze through narrow spaces in the capillary walls by amoeboid action.

neutrophilia an increased number of NEUTROPHIL white cells (leucocytes) in the blood. This is often an indication of an infection somewhere in the body.

nevirapine a non-nucleoside reverse transcription inhibitor drug used in combination with other antiretroviral drugs to treat HIV infections. The drug is on the WHO official list. A brand name is Viramune.

newton the unit of force required to accelerate a mass of 1 kg by 1 m per second per second. 1 N is equal to 100,000 dynes. (Sir Isaac Newton, 1642–1727, English mathematician, alchemist and physicist).

new variant CJD see CREUTZFELDT-JAKOB DISEASE.

NHI *abbrev. for* National Health Insurance.

NHS *abbrev. for* National Health Service.

NHS Direct a branch of the NHS that provides reliable medical information and advice to the general public. The web site (www.nhsdirect.nhs.uk) includes a useful medical encyclopedia. NHS Direct offers telephone consultation with experienced nurses.

niacin nicotinamide, one of the B group of vitamins. Nicotinic acid. Niacin is present in liver, meat, grains and legumes. It is a constituent of coenzymes involved in oxidation-reduction reactions. Deficiency causes PELLAGRA. Niacin is being used in the treatment of high blood cholesterol levels. The drug is on the WHO official list.

nicardipine a CALCIUM CHANNEL BLOCKER drug used to treat ANGINA PECTORIS and high blood pressure (HYPERTENSION). A brand name is Cardene.

NICE *acronym for* the National Institute for Clinical Excellence. This is a Government body tasked with the duty of determining the best forms of medical treatment. NICE was set up in April 1999 and is a part of the National Health Service. Its function is to provide patients, health professionals and the general public with reliable guidance on current best medical practice.

nickel dermatitis a severe allergic eczema caused by direct contact of the skin with the metal nickel. With the decline in nickel plating of articles such as watch straps, underwear fastenings and spectacle frames, the condition has become rare.

nickel poisoning poisoning with the highly toxic volatile liquid nickel carbonyl, which is a hazard to workers in the nickel industry. The condition features severe weakness, headache, dizziness, nausea and vomiting. The vapour causes lung OEDEMA with cough, chest pain, rapid breathing and blueness of the skin (cyanosis). Nickel can cause cancer of the nasal passages and sinuses (NASOPHARYNGEAL CARCINOMA).

niclosamide a drug used to remove tapeworms. Unlike earlier treatments, it is free from major side effects. The drug is on the WHO official list. A brand name is Yomesan.

nicorandil a POTASSIUM CHANNEL ACTIVATOR drug used to treat ANGINA PECTORIS. A brand name is Ikorel.

Nicorette a brand name for under-the-tongue tablets, chewing gum or artificial cigarettes containing NICOTINE. This is intended to make the abandonment of cigarette smoking a less painful procedure. Such measures are no real substitute for simple resolution and the acceptance of a brief period of suffering.

nicotinamide see NIACIN.

nicotine a highly poisonous alkaloid drug derived from the leaves of the tobacco plants *Nicotiana tabacum* and *Nicotiana rustica*. Large doses are fatal. Very small doses are obtained by inhaling the smoke from burning tobacco and this is done for the sake of the desired slight stimulant and mood-elevating effect and to alleviate nicotine withdrawal symptoms. Nicotine increases the heart rate and raises the blood pressure by narrowing small arteries. This effect can be dangerous. Nicotine, in the doses acquired by smokers, is comparatively harmless but the other constituents of tobacco smoke are responsible for an enormous burden of human disease. Nicotine is dispensed in the form of dummy cigarettes, skin patches and chewing gum so that people who wish to stop smoking may still, for a time, continue to enjoy the perceived advantages. The drug is also used as an insecticide.

nicotinic having the effects of acetylcholine and other nicotine-like substances on autonomic ganglia and the neuromuscular junctions of voluntary muscle. Compare MUSCARINIC.

nicotinic acid see NIACIN.

nicotinic receptors ACETYL CHOLINE receptors that also respond to NICOTINE. These receptors are at nerve-muscle junctions and in the autonomic nervous system.

nicoumalone acenocoumarol, an ANTICOAGULANT drug of the coumarin group. A brand name is Sinthrome.

Nidazol a brand name for METRONIDAZOLE.

NIDDM *abbrev. for* non-insulin dependent diabetes mellitus; a form of diabetes in which insulin production is inadequate or the body has become resistant to insulin.

nidus a localized collection, or focus, of infective organisms. From the Latin *nidus*, a nest.

Niemann-Pick disease an autosomal recessive hereditary disease in which the absence of an enzyme causes defective metabolism of SPHINGOMYELIN. A sphingolipidosis. There is abnormal accumulation of sphingomyelin causing enlargement of the liver and spleen, anaemia and severe neurological damage leading to physical and mental retardation and often death in early childhood. At least six varieties, having differing prognoses, have been described. Some have onset in adult life and do not affect the nervous system. The gene was identified in 1997. (Albert Neimann, 1880–1921, German paediatrician; and Ludwig Pick, 1868–1935, German physician).

nifedipine a CALCIUM CHANNEL BLOCKER drug used to control the symptoms of ANGINA PECTORIS and to treat high blood pressure

(HYPERTENSION). It has a powerful effect in widening (dilating) arteries, including the coronary arteries, and this improves the blood supply to the heart muscle. The drug, however, causes flushing, headache, skin itching and dizziness. It is often used in combination with a BETA-BLOCKER. Nifedipine has been used effectively to prevent high altitude lung oedema, a feature of mountain sickness. The drug is on the WHO official list. Brand names are Adalat, Adipine MR, Angiopine MR, Cardilate MR, Coracten, Fortipine LA, Tensipine MR and Unipine XL.

Niferex a brand name for IRON POLYSACCHARIDE COMPLEX.

nifurtimox a drug used in the treatment of South American trypanosomiasis (CHAGAS' DISEASE). The drug is effective against the causal agent *Trypanosoma cruzi* but its use is associated with side effects such as nausea, vomiting, loss of appetite, abdominal pain, muscle and joint aches, headache and vertigo. The drug is on the WHO official list.

night blindness moderately reduced to severely defective vision in dim light. Night blindness (nyctalopia) occurs in many people with no objectively discernible eye disorder, but is common in short-sighted people, in those with vitamin A deficiency and in the early stages of degenerative diseases of the RETINA including RETINITIS PIGMENTOSA.

nightmare a frightening dream occurring during rapid eye movement (REM) sleep often connected with a traumatic prior event such as an assault or a car accident. Nightmares may be caused by withdrawal of sleeping tablets. The Anglo-Saxon word *maere* means an evil male spirit or incubus intent on sexual intercourse with a sleeping woman, but nightmares seldom have a sexual content.

night sweat drenching perspiration occurring at night or during sleep. Night sweats may be a feature of any feverish illness but do not indicate any particular diagnosis.

night terrors sudden attacks of severe panic occurring during deep non-REM sleep and associated with very high heart rates, rapid respiration and often screaming. There is a sense of suffocation, imprisonment in a small space or a conviction of impending death. Night terrors occur most often around the age of 5.

night waking see SLEEPWALKING.

NIH *abbrev. for* the National Institutes for Health. This is an American government-sponsored body, the principal interest of which to the general public is the excellent web site (www.nih.gov) providing reliable medical information.

nihilism 1 a psychotic delusion of one's non-existence or of the non-existence of the world. 2 extreme pessimism about the effectiveness of any form of medical treatment, especially of the use of drugs (therapeutic nihilism).

nikethamide an ANALEPTIC drug used in the treatment of light coma, drowsiness and inadequate depth of respiration. It can raise the level of consciousness in comatose patients so that they can be encouraged to cough and bring up bronchial secretions.

Nilstat a brand name for the antifungal drug NYSTATIN.

nimodipine a CALCIUM CHANNEL BLOCKER drug used to minimise brain damage after subarachnoid haemorrhage. A brand name is Nimotop.

Nipent a brand name for PENTOSTATIN.

nipple the conical or cylindrical projection from the breast that is surrounded by a darker areola. The female nipple is larger than that of the male and is perforated by the ducts of the milk-secreting segments of the breast.

nipple disorders see PAGET'S DISEASE OF THE NIPPLE, INVERTED NIPPLE.

niridazole a drug used in the treatment of SCHISTOSOMIASIS. It is highly effective against the *Haematobium* variety but because of its side effects it has been largely replaced by other drugs such as PRAZIQUANTEL.

nisoldipine a CALCIUM CHANNEL BLOCKER drug used to treat angina pectoris and high blood pressure (HYPERTENION). A brand name is Syscor MR.

nit a louse egg. Each egg is glued to the shaft of a hair very close to the skin surface. Most nits will not be removed by combing unless this fact is borne in mind. Nit-picking is not recommended.

Nitradisc a brand name for a preparation of the angina-relieving drug GLYCERYL TRINITRATE.

Nitrados a brand name for NITRAZEPAM.

nitrazepam a long-acting BENZODIAZEPINE hypnotic drug, widely used to promote sleep in insomnia. A brand name is Mogadon.

nitric oxide nitrogen monoxide (NO), one of the eight oxides of nitrogen consisting of a single nitrogen atom and a single oxygen atom. In 1987 nitric oxide was found to be an important physiological mediator, a relaxant of smooth muscle in the walls of blood vessels that was derived from the inner lining (endothelium) of blood vessels. Later it was shown that nitric oxide was far more than simply an endothelium-derived relaxing factor (EDRF). Three different enzymes synthesize nitric oxide, from endothelium, nerves and macrophages and the NO produced has actions all over the body. Nitric oxide is involved in controlling blood pressure; in the phagocytic action of MACROPHAGES; in inhibiting PLATELET aggregation and hence blood clotting; in limiting the development of ATHEROSCLEROSIS; in controlling the heart action; in relaxing the smooth muscle in the air tubes of the lungs and the walls of the intestine; in a range of brain functions; and in promoting penile erection (see SILDENAFIL).

nitric oxide synthase one of three enzymes that catalyze the synthesis of NITRIC OXIDE in blood vessel ENDOTHELIUM, nerve fibres and MACROPHAGES. These enzymes are coded for, respectively, on chromosomes 7, 12 and 17. They act by splitting off a nitrogen atom from the amino acid L-arginine which is then combined with an oxygen atom from molecular oxygen to form NO.

Nitro-bid a brand name for a preparation of the angina-relieving drug GLYCERYL TRINITRATE.

Nitrocine a brand name for NITROGLYCERINE.

Nitro-Dur a brand name for GLYCERYL TRINITRATE.

nitrofurantoin a drug that damages bacterial DNA and is used to treat urinary tract infections. The drug is on the WHO official list. Brand names are Furadantin, Macrobid and Macrodantin.

nitrofurazone a drug used in the treatment of sleeping sickness (African trypanosomiasis).

nitrogen an inert, colourless and odourless gas constituting about 80% of the atmosphere. The element is present in all proteins and occurs in the urine in the form of urea. Under pressure, considerable nitrogen will dissolve in the blood. The release of gaseous nitrogen in the blood in bubbles that can block small arteries is the chief danger in too sudden decompression in divers.

nitrogen balance the difference between the amounts of nitrogen taken into and lost by the body. Nitrogen is taken in mainly in the form of protein and is mainly lost in urea in the urine.

nitrogen dioxide a toxic oxide of nitrogen that in concentrations of over about 100 parts per million will cause irritation of the nose and throat, watering of the eyes, cough, headache, and nausea and vomiting. UK occupational exposure safe limits are 5 ppm for 15 minutes and 3 ppm for an 8 hour day.

nitrogen mustard a drug used in the treatment of cancer. Nitrogen mustard is an ALKYLATING AGENT.

nitrogen narcosis the toxic effects on the brain of the high concentrations of nitrogen occurring in the blood in divers breathing air at depths of 30 m or more. This effect is different from decompression sickness. There is a sense of detachment from reality, loss of concentration and slowing of mental processes. The condition is relieved by ascending to about 10 m.

nitroglycerine see GLYCERYL TRINITRATE.

Nitrolate a brand name for a preparation of the angina-relieving drug GLYCERYL TRINITRATE.

Nitrolingual a brand name for GLYCERYL TRINITRATE.

Nitromin a brand name for GLYCERYL TRINITRATE.

Nitronal a brand name for GLYCERYL TRINITRATE.

nitroprusside a drug used in the emergency treatment of high blood pressure (HYPERTENSION). Given by controlled infusion into a vein it is the most effective known means of reducing dangerously high pressure. It must, however, be used with great care and its effects closely monitored.

nitrosamines nitrosylated secondary amines some of which can cause cancer by decomposing to form ALKYLATING AGENTS.

nitroso-redox balance the balanced interaction between the production of nitric oxide and that of superoxide. Upset of this balance plays a fundamental role in cell and organ failure.

nitrosureas a range of drugs used in the treatment of cancers. The nitrosureas are ALKYLATING AGENTS. Some nitrosureas are also capable of causing cancer.

nitrous oxide a weak anaesthetic and painkilling (analgesic) gas widely used as a vehicle for more potent anaesthetic agents in the maintenance of general anaesthesia. Also known as 'laughing gas'. The drug is on the WHO official list.

Nivaquine a brand name for CHLOROQUINE.

Nivemycin a brand name for NEOMYCIN.

nizatidine an H$_2$ RECEPTOR ANTAGONIST drug used to prevent and treat peptic ulcers. Brand names are Axid and Zinga.

Nizoral a brand name for KETOCONAZOLE.

NMDA receptor antagonists drugs used in the hope of improving the mental condition of people with Alzheimer's disease and delaying progress. An example is memantine (Ebixa).

NMDA receptors receptors for the NEUROTRANSMITTER n-methyl D-aspartate. This is a glutamate transmitter. Abnormally high levels of NDMA are thought to lead to neural dysfunction.

NMR *abbrev. for* nuclear magnetic resonance, the original term for what is now styled MAGNETIC RESONANCE IMAGING (MRI). NMR is said to have been dropped because of popular, but erroneous, association with nuclear radiation.

nocardiosis infection by the soil bacterium *Nocardia asteroides* and other species of the same genus. Nocardiosis often affects the foot and features persistent discharging abscesses (MADURA FOOT). In people with reduced resistance to infection (immunodeficiency) abscesses occur in the lungs and in other parts of the body, including the bowels and the brain. Treatment is with antibiotics.

noci- *combining form denoting* pain or injury.

nociceptors nerve endings selectively responding to painful stimuli. Stimulation of nociceptors causes the sensation of pain.

noct-, nocti- *combining form denoting* night.

noctalbuminuria the excretion of protein into the urine, occurring only during the night. Compare ORTHOSTATIC ALBUMINURIA.

nocturia passing urine during the night. One definition, that of the International Continence Society, stipulates two or more voids during the night. Normally, the stimulus of a filling bladder is insufficient to awake a person and prompt him or her to get up to urinate, but rapid or excessive filling, or undue bladder awareness, will do so. This may result from immoderate fluid intake, PROSTATE enlargement, CYSTITIS, DIABETES, DIURETIC drugs or insomnia.

nocturnal emission spontaneous ejaculation, with orgasm, occurring during sleep, often at the climax of an erotic dream. The phenomenon is experienced from time to time by most males with restricted sexual opportunities who do not regularly masturbate. Also known as a 'wet dream'.

nocturnal enuresis involuntary urination during night-time sleep. Bedwetting.

nodal tachycardia a type of heart rate abnormality occurring for periods of a few seconds to a day or so in which the heart beats at a rate of 140–220 per minute. The condition may affect otherwise normal hearts and causes faintness and breathlessness. Treatment is needed for prolonged attacks. Also known as supraventricular tachycardia.

nodes of Ranvier narrow gaps between the ends of the segments of myelin that insulate single nerve axons. (Louis Antoine Ranvier, 1835–1922, French pathologist).

nodular goitre a swelling of the thyroid gland that features multiple, small, hard lumps. Simple multinodular goitre may be due to long periods of iodine deficiency. A single nodule in the thyroid should be considered potentially malignant and should be removed for examination.

nodule a small, solid knot-like lump of tissue occurring anywhere in the body. Nodules in the skin are easily felt. The term implies nothing about the nature of the lump.

noesis a psychological term for the process by which information is derived. The cognitive process. Cognition. From the Greek *noesis*, understanding.

no-fault compensation system indemnification of the victims of medical accidents and mishaps in which no legal claim can exist against doctors or medical institutions. Such a system has been introduced in France.

Nolvadex-D a brand name for TAMOXIFEN.

nomenclature a system of names used in a science or other discipline.

noma see CANCRUM ORIS.

non- *prefix-denoting* not.

non-accidental injury see CHILD ABUSE.

non-gonococcal urethritis see NONSPECIFIC URETHRITIS.

non-nucleoside reverse transcriptase inhibitors NNRTIs, drugs used to treat HIV infections in combination with other drugs.

Examples are efavirens (Sustiva) and nevirapine (Viramune).

nonoxynol-9 a SURFACTANT spermicidal drug intended for use in conjunction with barrier contraceptives. It is available as a foam, pessary, gel, or cream. Brand names are Delfen, Double Check, Ortho-Forms, Duragel, Gynol II and Ortho-Creme.

nonsense codon one of the three nucleotide triplets (codons), UAG, UAA or UGA that mark an end point to a particular protein synthesis. U is the base uracil; A is the base adenine; and G is the base guanine.

nonsense mutation a POINT MUTATION which changes a CODON that specifies an amino acid into a termination codon – one that marks the position where translation of a messenger RNA sequence should stop. The result is a gene with a segment lopped off. Such a gene will code for a protein that may have missing amino acids and may thus be functionally defective.

non-specific 1 not attributable to any definite causal organism.
2 of a drug, having a general, as distinct from a particular, effect.

non-specific immune response an immediate protective responses of the immune system that does not require previous exposure to the invader.

non-specific urethritis a term formerly used to refer to a sexually transmitted infection of the urethra not caused by GONORRHOEA. Most cases are now known to be caused by the organism *Chlamydia trachomatis*.

non-steroidal anti-inflammatory drugs (NSAIDs) a range of drugs with painkilling and inflammation-reducing properties that act by inhibiting the enzyme cyclo-oxygenase that converts the fatty acid arachidonic acid to PROSTAGLANDINS. The latter are a common cause of pain and the inhibition of their production relieves pain, but prostaglandins also have desirable effects, hence some of the unwanted side-effects of NSAIDs. The range of NSAIDs includes ASPIRIN, BENORYLATE (benorilate), DIFLUNISAL, FENBUFEN, FENOPROFEN, IBUPROFEN, NAPROXEN, DICLOFENAC, INDOMETHACIN (indometacin), PHENLYBUTAZONE and PIROXICAM.

non-steroidal aromatase inhibitors drugs used to treat advanced breast cancer. Examples are aminoglutethimide (Orimeten), anastrozole

(Arimidex) and letrozole (Femara).

non-union failure of a fracture to form new bone and to regain bony continuity. Non-union may lead to the development of a fibrous or cartilaginous false joint (PSEUDARTHROSIS).

non-verbal communication transmission of information from person to person without the use of words, as by gesture, bodily attitude, expression, exclamation, and so on.

Nootropil a brand name for PIRACETAM.

noradrenaline norepinephrine, an important adrenergic NEUROTRANSMITTER released by POSTGANGLIONIC adrenergic nerve endings and secreted by the MEDULLA of the adrenal gland. Noradrenaline acts chiefly on alpha-adrenergic receptors and causes constriction of arteries and a rise in the blood pressure. This is a SYMPATHOMIMETIC action. One of the catecholamines. A brand name is Levophed.

noradrenaline reuptake inhibitor one of a class of drugs that function by increasing the available amount of the neurotransmitter NORADRENALINE at synapses. This is achieved by interfering with the normal physiological reuptake mechanism that brings about the removal of noradrenaline from the synaptic gap. Selective noradrenaline reuptake inhibitors can have a useful antidepressive effect. They include AMITRIPTYLINE, CLOMIPRAMINE, DOXEPIN, IMIPRAMINE, AMOXAPINE, MAPROTILINE and NORTRIPTYLINE.

noradrenergic/serotonergic enhancers drugs used to treat depression. An example is mirtazipine (Zispin).

Norcuron a brand name for VECTURONIUM.

Norditropin a brand name for SOMATOTROPIN.

norelgestromin a progestogen drug used in conjunction with ETHINYLOESTRADIOL (ethinylestradiol) as an oral or patch contraceptive.A brand name is Evra.

norethandrolone a synthetic ANABOLIC STEROID similar in chemical structure to TESTOSTERONE.

norethisterone a PROGESTOGEN drug used to treat excessive menstrual bleeding, painful menstruation, ENDOMETRIOSIS and metastatic breast cancer. The drug is on the WHO official list. Brand names are Primolut N and Utovlan. The drug is also widely used in combination with an oestrogen as an oral contraceptive. It is formulated with ETHINYLOESTRADIOL (ethinylestradiol) under such brand names as

Binovum, Brevinor, Loestrin 20, Norinyl-1, Otho-Novin 1/50, Ovysmen, Synphase and Trinovum; and with oestradiol (estradiol) valerate under the brand names Climagest and Climesse.

norfloxacin a quinolone antibacterial drug used to treat urinary tract infections. A brand name is Utinor.

Norgalax a brand name for DOCUSATE SODIUM.

norgestrel a PROGESTOGEN drug used as an oral contraceptive. A brand name is Neogest.

Norimin a brand name for ETHINYLOESTRADIOL (ethinylestradiol) formulated with a PROGESTOGEN drug as an oral contraceptive.

Norimode a brand name for LOPERAMIDE.

Norinyl-1 a brand name for MESTRANOL in combination with NORETHISTERONE as an oral contraceptive.

Normacol Plus a brand name for FRANGULA formulated with the bulking agent sterculia.

normal distribution Gaussian distribution, a distribution which when expressed graphically is bell-shaped. The distribution to which many frequency distributions of biological variables, such as height, weight, intelligence, etc correspond.

Normison a brand name for TEMAZEPAM.

normoblast a nucleated red blood cell precursor showing the features of normal red cell development, as distinct from those of the MEGALOBLAST.

normothermia a body temperature within normal limits. The term is used mainly in contexts in which hypothermia is a possibility or a risk.

Norplant a brand name for a now-withdrawn implantable long-term, reversible contraceptive containing LEVONORGESTREL. Some women may have Norplant in situ until the year 2005. Special precautions are necessary for their removal.

Norprolac a brand name for QUINAGOLIDE.

nortriptyline a tricyclic antidepressant drug. A brand name is Allegron. The drug is also formulated with the phenothiazine drug fluphenazine under the brand name Motival.

Norval a brand name for the antidepressant drug manserin.

Norvir a brand name for RITONAVIR.

Norwalk virus a small round structured virus (SRSV), 23–35 nm in diameter, responsible for a considerable number of cases of gastroenteritis, some associated with infected shellfish. The virus was first described as the causal agent for an epidemic of diarrhoea and vomiting in Norwalk, Ohio, USA.

nose a term used both for the externally visible part and for the internal nasal air passages. The nose is the normal entry route for inspired air, which is warmed, moistened and cleaned. Chemical particles in the air stimulate the nerve endings of the olfactory nerves in the roof of the nasal cavity, giving rise to the sensation of smell.

nose fracture a break in the short nasal bone forming the upper third of the nose. Such a fracture commonly results from external violence and may feature visible deformity or obstruction to breathing on one side from deviation of the NASAL SEPTUM. Broken noses are moulded back into shape by manipulation under anaesthesia. A plaster cast may be needed for 2 or 3 weeks.

nose reshaping alteration of the appearance of the nose for cosmetic purposes. This is a common cosmetic operation and is performed internally so that no visible scars result. The nasal cartilages are pared and reshaped and sometimes bone is chiselled away. Also known as rhinoplasty.

noso- *combining form denoting* disease. From the Greek *nosos*, disease.

nosocomial of disease pertaining to, or acquired in, a hospital. The term is used especially to refer to infections more likely to occur in hospital than out of hospital. From Greek *nosokomion*, a hospital.

nosology the science of the classification of diseases. There have been suggestions that nosology may sometimes be influenced by factors other than the purely terminological and the need for accurate description. If, for instance, most mood disorders are actually a combination of anxiety and depression (see COTHYMIA), it is unsatisfactory to assert that these are two different diseases requiring different drug treatments. From the Greek *nosos*, disease.

nostril one of the paired openings into the NOSE that contains hairs which can trap gross particulate matter in the inhaled air.

nostrum a medicine, especially a patent, secret and often QUACK remedy.

notexin a phospholipase enzyme from snake

venom that attacks muscle cells and motor nerve terminals. It has been proposed for the treatment of upper lid droop (blepharoptosis) in mitochondrial myopathy, to encourage the proliferation of satellite muscle cells, which contain mostly normal mitochondria.

notifiable disease any disease, especially a communicable condition, required by law to be reported to a central medical authority by the doctor who diagnoses it.

notochord a rod-like structure, present in early development, derived from the MESODERM and giving rise to the spine. In the adult, the notochord is represented by the pulpy centres (nucleus pulposus) of the intervertebral discs.

Novantrone a brand name for MITOXANTRONE.

novobiocin an antibiotic drug formerly of importance in the treatment of infections with staphylococci resistant to other antibiotics but now largely replaced by beta-lactamase resistant penicillins.

Novoseven a brand name for EPTACOG ALFA (FACTOR VIIA).

noxious harmful to health.

Noxyflex S a brand name for NOXYTHIOLIN.

noxythiolin an antifungal and antibacterial drug used to treat PERITONITIS. A brand name is Noxyflex S.

Nozinan a brand name for the antipsychotic drug METHOTRIMEPRAZINE (levomepromazine).

NSAIDs *abbrev. for* NON-STEROIDAL ANTI-INFLAMMATORY DRUGS.

Nubain a brand name for the narcotic analgesic NALBUPHINE.

nuchal rigidity SEE NECK RIGIDITY.

nuchal translucency test a method of ultrasound detection of fetuses with a chromosomal abnormality, especially Down's syndrome. The examination consists of the assessment of small collections of fluid at the back of the neck and spine of the fetus that increase translucency. About three-quarters of cases of Down's syndrome can be detected in this way.

nuclear energy energy released mainly as heat, light and ionizing radiation as a result of changes in the nuclei of atoms. Nuclear energy is released during the spontaneous decay (fission) of naturally occurring radioactive substances and during atomic fusion reactions, as in the sun. It is also released in such devices as nuclear reactors and nuclear weapons.

nuclear envelope the double membrane, with perforations (pores), surrounding a cell NUCLEUS. The outer membrane extends into the ENDOPLASMIC RETICULUM. The pores allow transport of macromolecules in both directions.

nuclear magnetic resonance (NMR) see MAGNETIC RESONANCE IMAGING (MRI).

nuclear medicine the medical specialty based on the use of radioactive substances for diagnosis and treatment of disease. Radioactive isotopes can be incorporated into a wide range of compounds that can be given by mouth or by injection. Specific radioactive elements or compounds containing them are selectively concentrated in different organs, or in particular disease tissues, and their distribution and local concentration in the body can then be detected and measured by an instrument called a GAMMA CAMERA. Certain cancers, for instance, can be detected anywhere in the body and appropriate treatment directed to every site of the disease.

nuclear pores openings in the NUCLEAR ENVELOPE allowing chemical messenger communication between the nucleus and the cytoplasm of the cell.

nuclear radiation radiation and particles coming from the nuclei of radioactive atoms during radioactive decay and nuclear reactions. Alpha particles are the nuclei of helium atoms, beta particles are high-speed electrons, X-rays and gamma rays are electromagnetic radiations of wavelength progressively shorter than visible light. Nuclear radiations differ in penetration, beta particles being least penetrative and the gamma rays most. Ionizing radiations can dislodge linking electrons from molecules, such as those of DNA, and cause damaging changes. In general, radiations are most destructive to cells most rapidly dividing.

nuclear sclerosis hardening of the central part of the internal crystalline lens of the eye. This is commonly a stage in the development of CATARACT and may lead to unexpected short-sightedness (index MYOPIA) so that reading may, for a time, be possible without glasses.

nuclease any one of several enzymes that break down NUCLEIC ACIDS.

nucleate possessing a NUCLEUS.

nucleic acid DNA or RNA. A very long polymer molecule made up of MONOMERS of either deoxyribonucleotides or ribonucleotides, joined by PHOSPHODIESTER BONDS. Nucleic acids constitute the chromosomes of almost all living cells and, by virtue of the order of the contained purine and pyrimidine BASE PAIRS, manifest the genetic code.

nucleolus a small, dense rounded body found in the nucleus of most cells. The nucleolus generates RIBOSOMES and is the site of the transcription of ribosomal RNA. The size and number of nucleoli in a cell nucleus vary with the amount of protein synthesized by the cell.

nucleoside a molecule compounded of a purine or pyrimidine base attached to a sugar (ribose or deoxyribose). The genetic code in DNA and RNA depends on the order of the nucleosides. A nucleoside is a NUCLEOTIDE without the phosphate group.

nucleoside reverse transcriptase inhibitors drugs used to treat HIV infections in combination with other drugs. Examples are abacavir (Ziagen), didanosine (Videx, Videx EC), lamivudine (Combivir, Epivir), stavudine (Zerit), zalcitabine (Hivid) and zidovudine (Retrovir). The brand Trizivir contains abacavir, lamivudine and zidovudine.

nucleoside analogue a drug that resembles a NUCLEOSIDE and that can be taken up in place of the natural nucleosides in viruses so as to form DNA that is fragile and susceptible to breakage. Drugs of this class, which include IDOXURIDINE, FAMCICLOVIR, DIDANOSINE and PENCICLOVIR, require the action of an enzyme carried by the target virus, before they become functional.

nucleosome the structural subunit of CHROMATIN consisting of about 200 BASE PAIRS and a barrel-shaped core of eight histone protein molecules (an octamer).

nucleotide a molecule formed from the bonding of a purine or a pyrimidine base with a sugar and a mono-, di- or tri-phosphate group. Compare NUCLEOSIDE. Four different nucleotides may polymerize to form DNA. They are 2´-deoxyadenosine 5´-triphosphate; 2´-deoxyguanosine 5´-triphosphate; 2´-deoxycytidine 5´-triphosphate; and 2´-deoxythymidine 5´-triphosphate. These lengthy names are commonly abbreviated to dATP, dGTP, dCTP and dTTP. Even this is too clumsy when printing out the sequence of nucleotides in a length of DNA. In that case they are abbreviated to A, G, C and T (for adenine, guanine, cytosine and thymine). In RNA the sugar is not 2´-deoxyribose, but ribose itself. Also one of the RNA bases differs from that in DNA. Thymine is replaced by uracil. So the nucleotides of RNA are adenosine 5´-triphosphate; guanosine 5´-triphosphate; cytidine 5´-triphosphate; and uridine 5´-triphosphate. These are abbreviated to ATP, GTP, CTP and UTP or simply A, G, C and U.

nucleotide reverse transcriptase inhibitors drugs used to treat HIV infections in combination with other antiviral medication. An example is tenofovir disoproxil (Viread).

nucleus 1 of a body cell, the central structure consisting of the tightly bundled genetic material DNA surrounded by a nuclear membrane.
2 of an atom, the central core of protons and, except in the case of hydrogen, neutrons which is surrounded by a rapidly moving cloud of electrons, widely separated from it. The forces which bind together the protons and neutrons are immensely powerful and it is these forces which are released in an atomic explosion. From the Latin *nucleus*, a nut or kernel.

nucleus pulposus the pulpy core of the INTERVERTEBRAL DISC, that is surrounded by the ANNULUS FIBROSUS. Degeneration of the annulus and/or undue vertical stress may lead to some of the nucleus pulposus being squeezed (prolapsed) through the annulus. This usually occurs at the back of the disk and the prolapsed material may press on the nerve roots entering and leaving the spinal cord, causing severe pain and sometimes muscle weakness. The imprecise lay term for this process is 'slipped disk'.

nuclide an artificially produced radioactive isotope of an element. Many of these are used in medicine as tracers or for RADIOTHERAPY.

Nuelin SA a brand name for THEOPHYLLINE.

null cells a group of large granular LYMPHOCYTES that falls into neither the T cell nor the B cell category. The group includes the NATURAL KILLER CELLS and the KILLER CELLS.

null hypothesis in statistics, the assumption that one variable has no effect on another variable, or that only one hypothesis can possibly account for a phenomenon. The assumption that there are no differences in two population in matters relevant to the current investigation. In a clinical trial of a new treatment the null hypothesis might be that the proportion of patients improved by it was the same as the proportion improved by the existing standard treatment. See HYPOTHESIS TEST.

nullipara a woman who has never given birth to a viable child.

null mutation a mutation that eliminates the function of the affected gene. In many cases the null mutation is a complete deletion of the gene.

nummular coin-shaped.

Nurofen a brand name for a range of products containing IBUPROFEN.

nurse a health care professional who is the most immediate ancillary to the medically qualified members of the profession. The responsibility of the nurse extends far beyond that of providing assistance to doctors. She, or he, has a responsibility for many things, including continuing personal medical education; ensuring the well-being and safety of patients; assisting in their recovery from illness and the promotion of positive health; care of the unconscious patient; care of the elderly and the dying; respect for patients' rights, privacy and confidentiality; and the formation and maintenance of an ethical basis of behaviour. In UK, student nurses are required to undergo a specified period of training in a hospital approved by General Nursing Council and to pass an examination before qualifying for registration as a Registered General Nurse (RGN) with the United Kingdom Central Council for Nursing, Midwifery, and Health Visiting. The scope of nursing is rapidly expanding as many qualified nurses are now university graduates.

nurse-anaesthetist a nurse trained to administer general anaesthetics. Once common in the USA but not adopted in the UK, the nurse-anaesthetist has been largely replaced by specialist anaesthetists who are medically qualified. Nurse anaesthetists worked under the supervision of specialists. Increasing demands for medical services are prompting a re-appraisal of the concept of the nurse anaesthetist.

nurse hierarchy the administrative and clinical levels in the nursing profession. Domestic ward work is done by Health Care Assistants who do not have a nursing qualification. A nurse working for her or his RGN (see NURSE) is called a student nurse. After qualifying the nurse may become a staff nurse and may then advance to become a Team Leader or Ward Manager (informally, Sister). Above the Team Leaders is the Hospital Manager (formerly Matron) or the Director of Nursing Services.

nursing the application of medical and humanitarian principles, by a person ancillary to the medical profession, so as to maintain health and fitness, assist in recovery from mental or physical illness or injury, relieve pain or distress or ease the process of dying.

nurse practitioner a fully qualified and experienced nurse who carries out most or all of the functions of a medically qualified general practitioner, referring patients who need emergency or specialist care to appropriate doctors or facilities. Experience in the USA suggests that the idea is feasible. The nursing profession in both UK and USA has responded warmly to the idea but there has been some medical opposition.

nurse-prescribing a change in medical practice in 1994, authorized by *The Medicinal Products: Prescribing by (Nurses Act (1992)* that allows registered nurses, health visitors and midwives to prescribe drugs from within an agreed formulary. Nurses who have completed the extended nurse prescribing course are entitled to prescribe hundreds of drugs, many of which are prescription-only medication. From April 2003, nurses were empowered to prescribe more products and treat a wider range of conditions than ever before.

nursing process a formal description of the actions involved in nursing, that forms the basis of most nursing in the UK and the USA. The stages in the process consist of obtaining information about the patient; using this information to identify problems and determine objectives; writing a nursing care plan; providing the planned care; and assessing the effectiveness of the care provided.

nurse specialist a qualified nurse who has undergone additional training in a particular medical speciality allowing her or him to manage cases of a particular disease or condition, applying knowledge and skills in that context that may, in many cases exceed those of a General Practitioner. The nurse specialist cadre has become well established in the UK in recent years and now includes nurse specialists in asthma, colorectal surgery, diabetes, hypertension and cardiovascular disorders, incontinence, smoking control, stoma care, well woman management, vaccination and travel prophylaxis, and wound care. Colorectal nurse specialists may sub-specialize in endoscopy, cancer chemotherapy, pelvic floor dysfunction, and behavioural therapy.

nutation nodding of the head, usually involuntary.

nutmeg liver a term used by pathologists to describe the appearance of the cut surface of the liver in conditions of persistent blood congestion, as in failure of the right side of the heart.

nutmeg psychosis an acute psychiatric disorder featuring agitation, hallucinations, excitement, thought disorder, a sense of impending death, brought on by the ingestion of one to three whole nutmegs or and equal number of teaspoonsful of grated nutmeg. Nutmeg from the tree *Myristica fragrans* is a toxic substance, which, in a dosage of as little as 5 g, may cause flushing, fast pulse, fever, dry mouth, amphetamine (amfetamine)-like effects and the ingestion of large quantities of fluid to the point of water overload and even epileptiform seizure.

nutrient anything that nourishes. Any physiologically valuable ingredient in food.

nutrition 1 the process by which substances external to the body are assimilated and restructured to form part of the body or are consumed as a source or energy.
2 the study of the dietary requirements of the body and of the amounts of water, carbohydrates, fats, proteins, vitamins, minerals and fibre needed for the maintenance of health.

nutritional anaemia anaemia resulting from nutritional deficiency, especially of protein and iron.

nutritional oedema abnormal fluid retention in the tissues (oedema) resulting especially from lack of protein in states of starvation or malnutrition. Oedema can, however, occur in starvation even if the blood levels of albumin

are not lowered.

nutritionist a person who specializes in the study of NUTRITION and especially in the applications of the principles of nutrition in the maintenance of health and the treatment of disease.

Nutrizym GR a brand name for PANCREATIN.

nyctalopia inability to see well in conditions of poor illumination. NIGHT BLINDNESS. From the Greek *nyktos*, night, *alaos*, blind and *ops*, the eye.

nymphomania excessive desire by a woman for copulation. The concept of nymphomania is largely a fiction, engendered in less liberal days by male wish-fulfilment fantasy or by puritanical and censorious contemplation of healthy female sexuality.

nystagmus persistent, rapid, rhythmical, jerky or wobbling movement of the eyes, usually together. The movement is usually transverse and most commonly of a 'sawtooth' pattern with a slow movement in one direction followed by a sudden recovery jerk in the other. This kind of nystagmus is often CONGENITAL and, in this case, although associated with some reduction in visual acuity, is usually of little significance. Nystagmus may also be pendular or, when vision is very poor, of a searching type. Acquired nystagmus is always of significance as it implies an acquired disorder of the nervous system.

Nystan a brand name for NYSTATIN.

nystatin a drug used in the treatment of fungus infections, such as thrush (CANDIDIASIS). Nystatin is useful for external infections only as it is not absorbed when given by mouth and is too toxic to be given by injection. The drug is on the WHO official list. A brand name is Nystan. Nystatin is produced in various formulations with other drugs such as NEOMYCIN (Gregoderm), METRONIDAZOLE (Flagyl Compak), TRIAMCINOLONE (Tri-Adcortyl), OXYTETRACYCLINE (Terra-Cortril Nystatin) and the steroid CLOBETASONE (Trimovate).

O

oat-cell carcinoma a highly malignant form of lung cancer in which the cells are small, undifferentiated and rapidly spreading. About a quarter of lung cancers are oat-cell carcinomas. At the time of diagnosis the tumour is usually found to have spread remotely and the outlook is very poor. Cigarette smoking is the principle cause.

obesity excessive energy storage in the form of fat. This occurs when food intake exceeds the requirements for energy expenditure. Obesity is a hazard to health and longevity and increases the risk of high blood pressure (HYPERTENSION), DIABETES, various cancers, osteoarthritis, foot trouble and depression.

obesity mediators see GLP-1, LEPTIN, OB GENE and OREXIN.

ob gene a gene on chromosome 7 that codes for the cytokine LEPTIN which is produced in adipose tissue and which exercises control over food intake and energy expenditure. Ob is an abbreviation of 'obesity'.

objective the lens in a microscope nearest to the object being examined.

obligate able to survive only in a particular environment. Used especially of certain parasites.

ob receptor one of a family of LEPTIN receptors on the choroid plexus of the brain through which the cytokine appears to enter the brain to perform its function of switching off appetite.

obsession a compulsive preoccupation with an idea or an emotion, often unwanted or unreasonable, and usually associated with anxiety.

obsessive-compulsive disorder a psychiatric disorder featuring frequent bouts of anxiety associated with intrusive thoughts or feelings with little relevance to events (obsessions), or recurrent strong promptings to perform an act, such as washing one's hands (compulsions), logically recognized as unnecessary or irrelevant. These thoughts or promptings are so frequent and intrusive as to cause distress or disability. There is often depression and sometimes suicide. Treatment is with tricyclic antidepressant drugs or behaviour therapy. It is claimed that the disorder can be cured by cognitive behaviour therapy.

obstetrician a doctor specializing in the conduct of childbirth and possessing the skills, knowledge and experience required to ensure that this is achieved with the minimum risk to mother and baby. From the Latin *obstetrix*, a midwife.

obstetrics the branch of medicine concerned with childbirth and with the care of the woman from the onset of pregnancy until about 6 weeks after the birth, when the reproductive organs have returned to normal. The list that follows highlights the key entries related to obstetrics in the dictionary: abortion, abruptio placentae, amniotic fluid, antenatal care, dystocia, epidural anaesthesia, episiotomy, fetal distress, fetal alcohol syndrome, hyperemesis, induction of labour, labour, maternal mortality, meconium, miscarriage, placenta, placenta praevia, pregnancy, prematurity, puerperium, puerperal sepsis, stillbirth, multiple births, ultrasound.

obstetrical analgesia the use of drugs to relieve the pain of childbirth. Drugs commonly used include PETHIDINE often combined with sedatives such as promethazine, nitrous oxide and TRICHLOROETHYLENE inhalation, and anaesthetic drugs given as an EPIDURAL block.

obstetrical forceps wide, open-bladed traction forceps, the blades of which can be separated and applied individually to the sides of the head of the fetus and then interlocked. Forceps are sometimes used in cases of difficult or unduly prolonged labour. A commonly used alternative is the VENTOUSE.

obstetric ultrasound a widely used and safe method of imaging used during pregnancy for many purposes. These include the confirmation of pregnancy, the detection of abortion, the diagnosis of ECTOPIC PREGNANCY, the diagnosis of multiple pregnancy, the detection of fetal abnormalities, of malplacement of the PLACENTA and of excessive uterine fluid and the diagnosis of HYDATIDIFORM MOLE.

obstructive airway disease a general term for any condition in which the movement of normal quantities of oxygen from the atmosphere to the blood is prejudiced. The term 'chronic obstructive airway disease' (COAD) is usually limited to chronic BRONCHITIS and EMPHYSEMA.

obstructive jaundice JAUNDICE caused by any process in the liver or bile ducts that prevents the normal outflow of bile. Obstructive jaundice is commonly caused by GALLSTONES (large duct obstruction) or a cancer of the head of the PANCREAS, or by disease processes that occlude the small bile ducts within the liver, such as HEPATITIS and CIRRHOSIS (small duct obstruction). Unrelieved obstruction causes ever-deepening jaundice.

obstructive sleep apnoea the periodic cessation of breathing or a substantial reduction in breathing caused by temporary blockage of the airway by the tongue or respiratory collapse of the lower throat during sleep. After 10–90 seconds lack of oxygen alerts the brain and the person wakes. This may happen up to 400 times in one night and may damage health or even cause a stroke. A major factor is obesity.

obtundity a state of reduced consciousness.

obturation closure of an opening.

obturator any device, object or anatomical structure that closes or obstructs an opening or cavity.

obturator foramen a large opening on each side of the pelvis below and in front of the socket for the hip bone (the ACETABULUM).

obturator muscles the obturator externus and obturator internus muscles that cover the outer surface of each side of the front of the pelvis. The tendons of these muscles pass behind the hip joint and are inserted into the top of the femur. They rotate the thigh outwards.

Occam's razor a principle in science and philosophy, much applied in medicine, that one should try to account for an observed phenomenon in the simplest possible way and should not look for multiply explanations of its different aspects. For instance, a range of symptoms and signs occurring together should always, if possible, be attributed to a single disease rather than to several different diseases occurring simultaneously. (William of Occam, ca. 1290–1349, English philosopher).

occipital bone the curved, shield-shaped bone forming the lower rear part of the skull.

occipital lobe the rear lobe of the main brain (cerebral hemisphere). The occipital lobe is concerned with vision.

occiput the back of the head.

Occlusal a brand name for SALICYLIC ACID.

occlusion 1 closing off or covering of an opening, or obstruction to a hollow part. 2 the relationship of the biting surfaces of the teeth of the upper and lower jaws. 3 the deliberately covering of one eye for periods of weeks or months in the treatment of AMBLYOPIA in children.

occult concealed or hidden, especially of traces of blood in the faeces or sputum which can be detected only by special tests.

occupational diseases diseases resulting from the effects of work. Occupational diseases are those caused by exposure to toxic, irritating or cancer-inducing substances, or to unusual physical conditions of heat, cold, noise, vibration, atmospheric or gas pressure or radiation of any kind. Certain occupational diseases are NOTIFIABLE by law.

occupational hearing loss damage to hearing as a result of sustained high levels of noise or vibration, or exposure to agents such as organic solvents that have a direct toxic effect on the hair cell mechanism of the inner ears. Noise and such toxic agents can potentiate each other in producing permanent hearing loss.

occupational medicine the branch of medicine concerned with people at work and the effects of work on health and of health on the ability to work. It is essentially a branch of preventive or environmental medicine based on a knowledge of working conditions and a concern to detect and remedy work hazards. One of the weapons of occupational medicine is legislation and one of its main preoccupations is to ensure that existing legislation is complied with. The list that follows highlights the key entries related to occupational medicine in the dictionary: anthracosis, byssinosis, bagassosis, baker's itch, bird-fancier's lung, contact dermatitis, farmer's lung, occupational diseases, occupational hearing loss, occupational medicine, occupational therapy, quartz dust silicosis, silicosis, skin allergy.

occupational therapist a person engaged in OCCUPATIONAL THERAPY.

occupational therapy the teaching and supervision of specially selected occupations to the sick and injured in order to exercise mind and body, arouse and sustain interest, promote confidence and overcome disability. The aim of occupational therapy is the inculcation of new work interests leading to complete rehabilitation.

ochre codon one of the three CODONS that causes termination of protein synthesis. A stop codon. It is the triplet UAA (uracil, adenine, adenine).

ochre mutation any mutation that changes a codon to the stop OCHRE CODON.

ochronosis persistent joint disease associated with blue or brownish discoloration of the joint cartilages occurring in patients with ALKAPTONURIA.

Ockham's razor see OCCAM'S RAZOR.

octreotide an hormone inhibitor analogue of the natural substance SOMATOSTATIN. Octreotide has a much longer effective time of action than somatostatin and is selective in its action on secretion of growth hormone, GASTRIN, SECRETIN and MOTILIN. It is also effective against various tumours of the ENDOCRINE system. A brand name is Sandostatin.

Ocufen a brand name for FLURBIPROFEN.

ocular 1 pertaining to the eye.
2 the eyepiece of an optical device such as a microscope.

ocular melanocytosis a congenital eye disorder featuring diffuse hyperplasia of melanocytes causing darkening of the iris of the affected eye especially at the pupil margin, brownish discolouration of the episclera, darkening of the fundus, and an increased risk of developing melanomas and GLAUCOMA.

oculist 1 an OPHTHALMOLOGIST.
2 an ophthalmic OPTICIAN (optometrist).

oculogyric crisis a sustained, fixed, maximal turning of the eyes in one direction, usually upwards, that persists for periods of minutes or hours. The phenomenon is characteristic of the type of PARKINSONISM that follows ENCEPHALITIS or is induced by drugs.

oculomotor nerve the third of the paired cranial nerves arising directly from the brainstem. This nerve supplies four of the six small muscles that move the eye, the muscle that elevates the upper lid and the circular muscles of the iris. Paralysis of an oculomotor nerve causes the pupil to be enlarged, the lid to droop and the eye to be unable to turn inwards.

Ocusert a brand name for a device that leaches PILOCARPINE into the conjunctival sac, for the treatment of GLAUCOMA.

ODA abbrev. for Operating Department Assistant.

odont, odonto- combining form denoting teeth.

odontoblast a specialized connective tissue cell, lying in the outer surface of the dental pulp, that produces DENTINE.

odontoid process a strong tooth-like process projecting upwards from the front arch of the second vertebra of the neck (the axis bone) around which the first vertebra rotates to allow the head to turn to either side.

odontology the study of the structure, growth, function and diseases of the teeth.

Odrik a brand name for TRANDOLAPRIL.

-odynia suffix denoting pain.

oedema excessive accumulation of fluid, mainly water, in the tissue spaces of the body. Oedema may be local, as at the site of an injury, or general. It often affects specific organs, such as the brain or the lungs. It may be caused by injury, allergy, starvation, HEART FAILURE, kidney failure or disease – especially the NEPHROTIC SYNDROME, liver disease – CIRRHOSIS, hormonal changes in the menstrual cycle, varicose veins or poisoning. General oedema is often treated with DIURETIC drugs.

oedipus complex the Freudian belief that much psychiatric disorder, especially the 'psychoneuroses', are caused by the persisting effects, including unresolved guilt feelings, of the child's unconscious wish to kill the parent of the same sex and to have sexual intercourse with the parent of the opposite sex. The notion was one of the central tenets of Freudian dogma but is no longer widely held. Freud derived the term from the name of the swollen-footed, mythical hero of Sophocles' tragedies who was nailed up by his feet as a baby (hence the swelling) but who survived to kill his father and marry his mother. See also FREUDIAN THEORY.

oesophageal varices varicose veins, often large, occurring at the lower end of the gullet (oesophagus) in conditions such as CIRRHOSIS of the liver in which there is severe restriction to the flow of blood from the intestine to the liver in the PORTAL VEIN. Such varices may bleed dangerously and this is treated by means of compression with a balloon and by injections which cause the blood in the veins to clot.

oesophagitis inflammation of the gullet (OESOPHAGUS). The commonest cause is reflux of acid into the oesophagus from the stomach (reflux oesophagitis).

oesophagoscopy direct visual examination of the interior of the OESOPHAGUS usually by means of a flexible, fibreoptic ENDOSCOPE but sometimes using a rigid tube. Oesophagoscopy is an important method of examination in cases of suspected cancer, in narrowing (stricture) and in PHARYNGEAL POUCH.

oesophagostomiasis infection with species of the NEMATODE worm parasite Oesophagostomum. This resembles a hookworm but may cause a granulomatous mass on the lining of the intestine resembling a tumour. The condition has been reported mainly in Uganda.

oesophagus the gullet. The oesophagus is a muscular tube, about 24 cm long, extending from the throat (pharynx) to the STOMACH. Just above the stomach it passes through the DIAPHRAGM. In swallowing, food is carried down by repetitive controlled contractions of the muscular walls, known as PERISTALSIS. Immediately above the stomach the wall of the oesophagus shows an increased tendency to contract, thus forming a muscle ring known as the cardiac SPHINCTER. This normally closes after swallowing, to prevent regurgitation of the stomach contents.

oesophagus disorders see HEARTBURN, PHARYNGEAL POUCH, HIATUS HERNIA, REFLUX OESOPHAGITIS, OESOPHAGEAL VARICES.

oestradiol estradial, a natural oestrogen drug that can be taken by mouth as a HORMONE REPLACEMENT THERAPY and to control menopausal symptoms. Brand names are Climaval, Ellest Solo, Menorest, Progynova, Sandrena, Vagifem and Zumenon. Preparations of oestradiol (estradiol) for external use as a transdermal patch include Estelle Solo MX 40, Estraderm MX, Evorel, Fematrix 40 and Femseven. The drug is also used externally in a vaginal ring to treat post-menopausal vaginitis, under the brand name Estring.

oestriol estriol, an OESTROGEN used to treat infertility due to inadequate penetration of the cervical mucus by spermatozoa. A brand name is Ovestin.

oestrogen one of a group of steroid sex hormones secreted mainly by the ovaries, but also by the testicles. Oestrogens bring about the development of the female secondary sexual characteristics and act on the lining of the uterus, in conjunction with progesterone, to prepare it for implantation of the fertilized OVUM. They have some ANABOLIC properties and promote bone growth. Oestrogens are used to treat ovarian insufficiency and menopausal symptoms, to limit postmenopausal OSTEOPOROSIS, to stop milk production (lactation) and to treat widespread cancers of the PROSTATE gland. They are extensively used as oral contraceptives. Brand names are Premarin and, with Norgestrel, Prempac-C.

oestrogen receptors chemical groups to which oestrogens bind and which are commonly found in substantial quantities on breast cancers. The oestrogen receptor status of a woman with breast cancer is important because the prognosis is much worse in women with high levels of oestrogen receptor alpha than in those with oestrogen alpha negative cancers. The status can easily and cheaply be determined by gene expression micro array analysis. 70% to 80% of breast cancers are oestrogen receptor alpha positive. TAMOXIFEN, which has substantially reduced breast cancer mortality, is now regarded as an oestrogen receptor modulator.

Oestrus a genus of flies whose larvae can parasitize humans and animals. The larvae can attach themselves with hooks to the CONJUNCTIVA and may cause serious damage to the eye.

ofloxacin an antibacterial drug. Brand names are Exocin for an eye drop preparation and Tarivid to be taken by mouth for general infections. The drug is on the WHO official list.

Ogilvie's syndrome acute colonic pseudo-obstruction resulting in massive dilatation of the bowel in the absence of any luminal blockage. The condition, which may be life-threatening, is a form of local adynamic ileus and most commonly follows surgical procedures. It is thought to be caused by excessive sympathetic stimulation, parasympathetic malfunction, or both.

-oid *suffix denoting* like.

ointment a semisolid, viscous material consisting of one or more substances with medicinal properties thoroughly mixed with a suitable base. Ointment bases may be of hard paraffin, emulsions of oil in water (aqueous creams), vegetable oils, wool fat (lanolin) or other substances. Ointments are used on the skin and in the eyes.

olanzapine a thienobenzodiazepine drug used to treat SCHIZOPHRENIA. it is similar to CLOZAPINE. A brand name is Zyprexa.

Olbetam a brand name for ACIPIMOX.

olecranon the hook-shaped upper end of one of the forearm bones (the ulna) that projects behind the elbow joint, fitting into a hollow on the back of the lower end of the upper arm bone (humerus) and forming the point of the elbow. The olecranon prevents over-extension of the elbow.

olestra a non-digestible fat substitute that was given approval by the US Food and Drug Administation (FDA) in 1996 but which does not appear to be the final solution to the obesity problem. About 20% of those eating it are said to have abdominal symptoms such as cramping or diarrhoea. There is also concern that Olestra might inhibit the absorption of fat-soluble antioxidant carotenoids.

olfaction the sense of smell or the act of smelling.

olfactory pertaining to the sense of smell.

olfactory nerves the nerves of smell and the first of the 12 paired CRANIAL NERVES arising directly from the brain. The olfactory nerves lie on the floor of the front section of the cranial cavity and run forward, close together, over the roof of the nose. From their terminal bulbs many tiny, hair-like filaments pass down through perforated bony plates (cribriform plates) into the upper part of the nose. Tiny particles of odorous material dissolved in the nasal secretions can be detected by the olfactory nerve endings with great sensitivity and discrimination.

oligo- *combining form denoting* little, few or an abnormally small quantity of.

oligocythaemia a deficiency of the cellular elements of the blood.

oligodendrocyte a connective cell of the central nervous system (glial cell) that participates in the formation of the myelin sheaths of nerve cell axons.

oligodendroglioma a slowly growing tumour of the nervous system derived from neural connective tissue cells, the oligodendroglial cells. The cells of the tumour are small, well-defined 'halo cells' with round nuclei and clear CYTOPLASM.

oligohydramnios a rare deficiency of AMNIOTIC FLUID. This is associated with poor function of the PLACENTA, fetal growth retardation and congenital abnormalities.

oligomenorrhoea abnormally infrequent menstrual periods. Often the interval between periods exceed 40 days.

oligometric protein a protein consisting of only a small number of identical POLYPEPTIDE subunits. Also known as oligomer.

oligophrenia mental deficiency.

oligospermia an abnormally low concentration of sperms in the seminal fluid. Fertile semen contains about 100 000 000 sperms per ml. Semen with less than about 20 000 000 sperms per ml is likely to be infertile.

oliguria an abnormally small output of urine. In health, the urinary output varies from 700 ml to 2 l. Oliguria is usually caused by inadequate fluid intake or increased fluid loss in sweating or diarrhoea. A more serious cause of oliguria is KIDNEY FAILURE, either acute or, less often, following long-term kidney disease.

olive 1 a smooth, oval swelling on each side of the upper part of the MEDULLA caused by the underlying olivary nucleus. These nuclei connect with each other and with the CEREBELLUM.
2 the smooth, elliptical tip of a vein stripper,

used in the treatment of VARICOSE VEINS.

olmesartan medoxomil a selective
ANGIOTENSIN II RECEPTOR antagonist drug used
to treat high blood pressure. The drug is
effective on a once-a-day dosage. It is a prodrug
that is converted to olmesartan by esterases
present in the intestine and portal vein blood.

Olmetec a brand name for OLMESARTAN
MEDOXOMIL.

Olmsted's syndrome a severely disfiguring
but localized autosomal dominant disorder of
the palms of the hands and the soles of the feet.
There is gross overproduction of the outer
horny layer of the epidermis (hyperkeratosis)
with tight constriction bands around the bases
of the fingers and toes that may lead to
spontaneous amputation. The syndrome also
features short stature and laxity of the joints.
First described by H.C. Olmstead in 1927.

olopatadine an ANTIHISTAMINE drug
formulated as eye drops and used to relieve and
control the symptoms of seasonal allergic
CONJUNCTIVITIS. A brand name is Opatanol.

olsalazine a salicylate drug used to treat
ulcerative colitis. A brand name is Dipentum.

-oma suffix denoting a tumour.

omega-3 marine triglycerides fish oils
containing the omega-3 polyunsaturated fatty
acids eicospentaenoic and docosahexaenoic
acids. A third type of omega-3 fatty acid, alpha
linoleic acid, is derived mainly from vegetable
oils. There is good evidence that fish oils are
protective against coronary heart disease and
have value after heart attacks. They are also used
to treat patients with abnormally high blood fat
(triglyceride) levels who are at risk of heart
attacks. A brand name for the oils, used as a
drug in capsule form, is Maxepa.

omentum one of two double folds of
PERITONEUM, the greater and lesser omenta,
that hang down like aprons from the liver
and stomach over the coils of small intestine.
The omenta usually contain fat and are often
effective in sealing down and localizing areas of
inflammation of the peritoneum (PERITONITIS).
Also known as the epiploon.

omeprazole the first of the class of proton
pump inhibitor drugs used to control the
production of stomach acid and treat stomach
and duodenal ulcers and especially the
ZOLLINGER-ELLISON SYNDROME. OMEPRAZOLE
can be effective in cases that have failed to

respond to H-2 receptor blocker drugs such as
RANITIDINE. The drug is long-acting and need
only be taken once a day. A brand name is
Losec.

omni- prefix denoting all.

omnivorous eating food of both animal and
vegetable origin, as in the case of most people.

Omnopon a brand name for PAPAVERETUM.

omphal- combining form denoting the
umbilicus. From the Greek omphalos, the navel.

omphalitis inflammation of the umbilicus.

omphalocele herniation of some of the
abdominal contents into the umbilical cord.

omphaloproptosis abnormal protrusion of
the umbilicus.

onanism an obsolescent term for
MASTURBATION or COITUS INTERRUPTUS.

oncho- combining form denoting a swelling,
mass or tumour. From the Greek onkos, a lump.

onchocerciasis a tropical parasitic disease,
mainly of West Africa, caused by the
microfilarial worm Onchocerca volvulus. The
filarial forms of the worm are spread by the
biting blackfly Simulium damnosum, which
breeds only in turbulent rivers – hence the
alternative term river blindness. Onchocerciasis
causes lumps or nodules under the skin, each
containing at least one male and one female
adult worm. After impregnation, the female
worm releases millions of microscopic
microfilaria which migrate under the skin and
enter the eyes where, on dying they set up a
severe and destructive inflammation that leads
to irremediable blindness. The microfilaria also
often block lymph channels and cause
ELEPHANTIASIS. Treatment is with drugs such as
diethylcarbamazine and suramin to kill the
worms. This may cause severe reactions.

onco- combining form denoting a tumour.

oncogenes genes that contribute to cancerous
changes in cells. Oncogenes are mutations of
normal cell genes and must work together to
cause cancer. Similar or identical genes are
found in viruses known to be able to cause
cancer. If one of the three virus genes – gag, pol
or env – is replaced by an oncogene, such as ras,
the virus becomes capable of causing cancer.
The normal ALLELES of the oncogenes are called
proto-oncogenes.

oncogenesis the process of the origination of
a tumour.

oncology the study of the causes, features and

treatment of cancer. An oncologist is a cancer specialist.

oncolysis destruction or breakdown of a tumour, either spontaneously or as a result of treatment.

Oncovin a brand name for the anticancer drug VINCRISTINE.

OND *abbrev. for* Ophthalmic Nursing Diploma.

ondansetron a serotonin antagonist drug used to relieve nausea and vomiting caused by anticancer chemotherapy and radiotherapy and to prevent sickness after surgery. A brand name is Zofran.

One-alpha a brand name for ALFACALCIDOL.

onomatomania an obsessive, repetitious intrusion of word or phrase into the thoughts.

ontogeny the development of an individual organism of a species from fertilization to maturity.

onyali a form of THROMBOCYTOPENIC PURPURA of unknown origin occurring from time to time in Africa. A striking feature is the appearance of large blood-filled blisters on the tongue and inner surfaces of the cheeks.

onychia inflammation of the growing area (matrix) of the nail. This inevitably results in loss of the nail.

onycho- *combining form denoting* a finger- or toenail or claw.

onychogryphosis abnormal changes in finger- or toenails so that they resemble talons. This may occur spontaneously or as a result of repeated injury or CANDIDIASIS. The term derives from the name of the mythological griffon.

onycholysis loosening or separating of the nail from its bed.

onychomycosis fungus infection of the nails, usually by Candida or epidermophyton species.

onychorrhexis longitudinal striation of the nail.

onychosis any disorder of the nails.

O'nyong-nyong fever an ARBOVIRUS infection caused by togaviruses spread by mosquitos mainly in Africa. The condition causes an illness similar to DENGUE with fever, headache, irritating rash and severe pain in the joints. Also known as joint-breaker fever.

oo- *combining form denoting* an egg (ovum).

oocyesis an ECTOPIC PREGNANCY occurring in the ovary.

oocyst a structure that develops on the outer wall of the mosquito's stomach from the fertilized malarial parasite. The parasite divides

repeatedly within the oocyst which rapidly fills up with the infective form of the parasite (SPOROZOITES) until it bursts, releasing the sporozoites into the body cavity of the mosquito to be passed on to humans.

oocyte a cell in the OVARY that undergoes MEIOSIS to produce an OVUM. In meiosis the 46 chromosomes are reduced to half the normal number (HAPLOID), so that the full complement can be restored by a haploid contribution from the sperm. Primary oocytes develop in the ovaries of the fetus but only a fraction of these will ever give rise to OVULATION. Secondary oocytes divide to form the mature OVUM but the second maturation division occurs only after the ovum has been fertilized by a sperm.

oogenesis the production of egg cells (ova) in the ovaries and their preparation for release and fertilization. Oogenesis starts in the fetal ovary with the formation of OOGONIA. These divide by MEIOSIS to form OOCYTES.

oogonia the precursors of OOCYTES in the OVARY derived from primordial female germ cells that have migrated to the site of the ovaries.

ookinete the highly motile fertilized form of the malarial parasite that bores through the lining of the mosquito's stomach to form the OOCYST.

oophor- *combining form denoting* the OVARY.

oophoralgia pain in the ovary. See also MITTELSCHMERZ.

oophorectomy surgical removal of one or both ovaries. Removal of one OVARY has little effect, but loss of both causes sterility and has secondary effects from a reduction in sex hormone production, especially OESTROGEN.

oophoritis inflammation of an OVARY.

oophoroma any tumour of the OVARY.

oophoron obsolete term for the OVARY. From the Greek roots *oon*, an egg and *phoros*, bearing.

Okazaki fragments short segments of DNA, 1000 to 2000 bases long, that later join up to form continuous lengths of DNA. Okazaki fragments occur in replicating DNA in both prokaryotes and eukaryotes. They form up on the 'lagging' strand during replications and join by ligation. (Reiji Okazaki, Japanese geneticist.).

Opatanol a brand name for OLOPATADINE.

open-angle glaucoma a condition in which the pressure of the fluid within the eye is increased to a damaging degree, but in which there is no apparent mechanical obstruction to the outflow of fluid through the normal drainage channel. This is the common type of GLAUCOMA, symptomless until a late stage and responsible for much avoidable blindness. Also known as chronic simple glaucoma.

open reading frame in RNA, a sequence of base pair triplets (codons) with no introns, which is translatable into a protein.

operable capable of being effectively treated by a surgical procedure.

operant conditioning a method of behaviour therapy in which a response is reinforced or suppressed, whenever it occurs, by immediate reward or punishment.

operating microscope a binocular, low-powered microscope with coaxial lighting and foot controls for focus, zoom magnification and X and Y shift used by surgeons to permit a degree of surgical precision not otherwise obtainable. Operating microscopes are most used by OPHTHALMOLOGISTS, ENT SURGEONS, VASCULAR SURGEONS and GYNAECOLOGISTS.

operating theatre a room, or suite of rooms, designed for the safe performance of surgical operations. Much consideration is given in the design to minimizing the risk of infection. Walls and floors are commonly covered with washable material and are washed daily. Materials liable to build up charges of static electricity are avoided. Ventilation is arranged so as to avoid air contamination and exhaled anaesthetic gases are vented. Intense but shadowless illumination is provided by special lamps. X-ray and scan viewing boxes are often built into the walls. Ancillary rooms include changing rooms, scrub rooms, sterilizing rooms, anaesthetic rooms and recovery rooms.

operation any act or performance. A surgical operation is a procedure, usually performed with instruments, but sometimes with the hands only, intended to effect some beneficial change. Most surgical operations are carried out under anaesthesia, which may be local or general.

operator gene the first gene in an OPERON. The operator gene controls the transcription of the genes in the operon.

operculum a covering membrane, flap or lid of tissue, especially in the brain, or over an erupting tooth.

operon a row of consecutive genes on a chromosome that operates as a functional unit. The structural genes in the operon are preceded by two regulatory sites occupied by regulatory genes, the promoter and the operator. These are essential for the expression of the operon. The genes in an operon have related functions that occur sequentially. All the genes in the operon are turned on and off together. All are transcribed into one large segment of MESSENGER RNA.

Ophthaine a brand name for PROXYMETACAINE.

Ophthalin a brand name for SODIUM HYALURONATE.

ophthalm-, ophthalmo- *combining form denoting* the eye.

ophthalmia an obsolescent term for any inflammatory eye disorder.

ophthalmia neonatorum eye inflammation occurring in the newborn baby as a result of infection acquired during birth. The condition may be due to GONORRHOEA and this, unless treated, may lead to blindness. Routine prophylactic antibiotic eye drops are often used to prevent such an outcome.

ophthalmic digital imaging systems a system in which a retinal or corneal camera or slit lamp ophthalmic microscope is coupled to a personal computer so that an immediate, high-resolution, colour digital bit-mapped image of all visibly-accessible parts of the eye may be displayed on the computer monitor for convenient study and may be saved for clinical record-keeping and training purposes. The system, which runs under familiar Windows 98 software, has been described as the most important advance in ophthalmic imaging since the advent of the retinal camera.

ophthalmitis eye inflammation. The term is usually qualified to indicate the nature or site of the inflammation, as in SYMPATHETIC OPHTHALMITIS.

ophthalmodynamometry a method of assessing the pressure in the arteries within the eye by exerting measurable external pressure on the globe and noting, through an OPHTHALMOSCOPE, the point at which the internal vessels collapse.

ophthalmologist a doctor who specializes in OPHTHALMOLOGY.

ophthalmology the combined medical and surgical speciality concerned with the eye and its disorders. The practice of ophthalmology involves a mastery of ophthalmic optics, of the structure, function and diseases of the eyes, of the associated neurological systems concerned with vision, of the range of general conditions that affect the eyes and of the microsurgical skills and techniques used in the treatment of many ophthalmic conditions. The list that follows highlights the key entries related to ophthalmology in the dictionary: age-related macular degeneration, astigmatism, blepharitis, blepharoptosis, cataract, colour blindness, conjunctivitis, dendritic ulcer, ectropion, epiphora, floaters, glaucoma, hypermetropia, iris, lacrimation, lagophthalmos, meibomian cyst, myopia, pinguecula, pterygium, pupil, retinal detachment, retinitis pigmentosa, retinopathy, squint, stye, visual field defect, uveitis.

ophthalmoplegia paralysis of the muscles within the eye or of the external muscles that move the eye. The latter is sometimes referred to as external ophthalmoplegia.

ophthalmoscope an instrument capable simultaneously of illuminating and allowing observation of the inside of the eye. The direct ophthalmoscope is held as close as possible to the eye; the indirect ophthalmoscope is used at a short distance and requires the use of a separate hand-held image-forming lens.

ophthalmotonometer see TONOMETER.

-opia, -opsia *combining form denoting* a specified form of vision.

opiates any narcotic drugs containing opium or an opium derivative or having opium-like properties, used to relieve severe pain associated with anxiety. Examples are morphine (Oramorph, Sevredol, Morcap SR, Morphgesic SR, MST Continus, MXL), diamorphine, methadone (Physeptone), fentanyl (Sublimaze), buprenorphine (Temgesic, Transtec), dihydrocodeine (DF 118 Forte, DHC Continus), codeine (Galcodine), pholcodine (Galenphol), meptazinol (Meptid), loperamide (Norimode), nalbuphine (Nubain), oxycodone (Oxynorm), hydromorphone (Palladone), papaveretum and pethidine.

opiate analogues drugs that simulate the effect of OPIATES and are used to relieve moderate to severe pain associated with anxiety. An example is tramadol (Dromadol SR, Dromadol XL, Tramake, Zydol SR and Zydol XL).

Opilon a brand name for THYMOXAMINE (moxisylyte).

opis-, opistho- *combining form denoting* back or backwards.

opisthognathous having receding jaws.

opisthorchiasis infection with the liver fluke *Opisthorchis felineus* whose intermediate hosts are snails and freshwater fish. The condition is commonest in the Far East, especially Thailand and the effects are similar to those of CLONORCHIASIS.

opisthotonus spasmodic, powerful contractions of the back and rear neck muscles causing the body to arch backwards so that the heels approximate to the head. This is a feature of TETANUS, severe MENINGITIS, strychnine poisoning and some brainstem disorders.

opportunistic infection infection by organisms not normally causing infection because they are usually excluded by the body's defence mechanisms. Opportunistic infections may occur when these mechanisms are temporarily or permanently malfunctioning, as in states of IMMUNODEFICIENCY such as AIDS, HYPOGAMMAGLOBULINAEMIA or those caused by immunosuppressive drugs. They may occur in people on long courses of antibiotics and in those who have prolonged intravenous therapy. Other causes include cancer, prolonged debilitating diseases, alcoholism, DIABETES, CIRRHOSIS of the liver and severe burns. Opportunistic organisms include *Pneumocystis carinii*, CYTOMEGALOVIRUS, *Candida albicans* and herpes simplex.

-opsis *combining form denoting* something resembling that specified.

opsoclonus a rare ophthalmic disorder featuring involuntary jerky (saccadic) eye movements in random directions. Opsoclonus should not be confused with NYSTAGMUS in which the movements are periodic and uniform. The disorder most commonly affects infants with neuroblastoma. In adults it may be related to other malignancies or to neurological infections. It is often associated with myoclonus and ataxia.

opsonin one of a number of substances, especially an antibody, naturally present in the blood that bind to the surface of bacteria to make them more readily susceptible to attack and destruction by PHAGOCYTES.

opsonization the process by which bacteria or other antigen-bearing entities are rendered attractive to PHAGOCYTES by the binding of

OPSONIN to their surface.

-opsy *combining form denoting* examination.

opt- *combining form denoting* the eye or vision.

optical activity the property of some substances in solution of causing of a ribbon-like beam of polarized light projected through the solution to twist through a small angle. Some substances cause rotation of the beam to the left (levorotatory), some to the right (dextrorotatory). Some optically active drugs are more potent in one form than in the other; a few are almost inert in one rotatory form.

optic atrophy permanent degeneration, with loss of the component nerve fibres, of the optic nerve. This causes variable degrees of permanent visual loss. Optic atrophy may be hereditary or due to many causes including injury, pressure from a growing pituitary tumour, methanol poisoning, MULTIPLE SCLEROSIS, GLAUCOMA or RETINITIS PIGMENTOSA.

optic chiasma the junction of the two OPTIC NERVES lying under the brain. In the chiasma optic nerve fibres from the inner half of each RETINA cross over. Those from the outer half do not. Thus fibres from the inner half of each retina run out of the chiasma in close association with fibres from the outer half of the retina on the other side. The two optic tracts so formed run into the brain. This arrangement ensures that input to both eyes from the right field of vision causes signals that pass to the left half of the brain, and vice versa.

optic disc the small circular area at the back of the eye at which all the nerve fibres from the retina come together to form the optic nerve.

optic disc oedema swelling of the head of the optic nerve, as seen with an OPHTHALMOSCOPE at the inside of the back of the eye. Optic disc oedema may be a sign of optic nerve inflammation but commonly indicates a rise in the pressure within the skull from any cause, such as a brain tumour. It is thus a sign of high clinical significance. Also known as PAPILLOEDEMA.

optician 1 a person qualified to test vision, examine the eyes and prescribe glasses and contact lenses (ophthalmic optician).
2 a person qualified to fit spectacle frames, to make the measurements necessary to ensure that spectacle lenses are properly centred in the frames, and to fit contact lenses (dispensing optician).

optic nerves the 2nd of the 12 pairs of CRANIAL NERVES which emerge directly from the brain. The optic nerves are bundles of about one million nerve fibres originating in the RETINAS and connecting these to the brain. Each nerve passes through a channel in the bone at the back of the eye sockets (orbits) to reach the inside of the skull and to join with, and partially cross over, its fellow in the OPTIC CHIASMA.

optic neuritis inflammation of the optic nerve. This is sometimes due to infection but is most commonly due to DEMYELINATION as in MULTIPLE SCLEROSIS. There is tenderness on pressure on the eye and on extremes of movement but the most striking effect is loss of vision over the central part of the field of vision of the eye on the affected side. Recovery, in about 6 weeks, is usual but there may be some permanent loss of visual acuity or colour sensitivity. There is no effective treatment.

Opticrom a brand name for CROMOGLYCATE (cromoglicate).

optic tract the part of the nerve pathway for visual impulses lying between the OPTIC CHIASMA and the first set of connections (SYNAPSES) in the brain – the lateral geniculate body. If an optic tract is destroyed half of the field of vision of each eye is lost. The field loss in each eye is on the side opposite to the damaged tract.

optimal most favourable or desirable.

optometer an automatic machine for determining the REFRACTION of the eye. Also known as a refractometer.

optometrist the American equivalent of ophthalmic OPTICIAN.

Orabet a brand name for antidiabetic drug METFORMIN.

Oradexon a brand name for DEXAMETHAZONE.

oral pertaining to the mouth.

oral contraceptive a drug or combination of drugs taken by mouth for the purpose of preventing pregnancy. Most oral contraceptives must be taken by women. They contain oestrogens and/or PROGESTOGENS and act by preventing the ovaries from producing eggs (ova). They also have some effect in making the lining of the womb less suitable for implantation of the ovum and may make the mucus in the canal of the cervix less easily passable by sperms. Oral contraceptives are second after sterilization in effectiveness in avoiding pregnancy. Risk attributable to oral contraceptives is very small among non-smokers but there are certain categories, notably women with thrombophilia from genetic mutations, in which the risk is slightly increased. The increased risk of breast cancer has been greatly exaggerated. It amounts to no more than roughly 1 additional case per 20,000 women. Also known as 'the pill'. See also CONTRACEPTION.

Oraldene a brand name for HEXETIDINE.

oral rehydration salt formulations solutions of sodium chloride, and other salts such as sodium bicarbonate, sodium citrate dihydrate, sodium lactate and potassium chloride, often with glucose, given by mouth to treat dehydration. Such solutions have saved many lives especially in children. These preparations are on the WHO official list.

oral sex any sexual activity in which the mouth is substituted for the vagina. One consequence of this practice is the confusion between the strains of the virus herpes responsible for oral and genital herpes. Formerly, these were, respectively herpes simplex 1 and herpes simplex 2. The matter is no longer so simple.

oral stage the first and most primitive of Freud's proposed stages of psychosexual development, in which the mouth is said to be the focus of the libido and the primary source of satisfaction. Such ideas no longer command widespread respect.

Oramorph a brand name for MORPHINE.

Orap a brand name for the antipsychotic and movement disorder drug PIMOZIDE.

orbicular 1 circular or spherical.
2 circular and flat.

orbicularis oculi the flat, circular, SUBCUTANEOUS muscle that surrounds each eye and that, on contraction, causes the eye to 'screw up'.

orbicularis oris the SPHINCTER muscle surrounding the mouth used to close the mouth and purse the lips.

orbit the bony cavern in the skull that contains the eyeball and OPTIC NERVE, the muscles that move the eye, the LACRIMAL GLAND, a quantity of fat and various arteries, veins and nerves.

orbital cellulitis inflammation of the soft tissues in the bony cavern which encloses and protects the eyeball. There is great pain, swelling of the eyelids, bulging of the CONJUNCTIVA and often protrusion of the eyeball. Urgent antibiotic treatment, and sometimes surgical drainage of pus, are needed.

orbitotomy a surgical opening into the ORBIT.

orbiviruses double-stranded RNA viruses that cause Colorado tick fever.

orchi- *combining form denoting* the testicle.

orchidalgia pain in the testicle. This may be a REFERRED PAIN from a stone in the ureter.

orchidectomy surgical removal of a testicle. This may be necessary for cancer of the testicle. Removal of both testicles is often done to reduce secretion of the male sex hormone testosterone in the treatment of a sex-hormone dependent cancer of the PROSTATE GLAND that has spread to other parts of the body. Also known as orchiectomy.

orchidopexy an operation to bring an undescended testicle down into the scrotum and to fix it in place. A testicle left in the abdomen will become sterile and may be more liable to develop cancer. The operation should ideally be done before the age of three.

orchidotomy a surgical incision into the testicle, usually for the purpose of BIOPSY.

orchitis inflammation of the testicle. This occurs in at least 20% of men who contract mumps after puberty. Apart from this, the condition is rare. The affected testicle is swollen, exquisitely tender and acutely painful and there is usually high fever. The condition settles in 3 to 7 days. Orchitis may be followed by atrophy of the testicle, but sterility is uncommon unless both are affected. There is no specific treatment for orchitis.

orciprenaline a non-selective beta-adrenoceptor agonist that can be used as a heart stimulant. A brand name is Alupent.

orexin one of a pair of centrally-acting neuropeptides produced by the lateral hypothalamus where the sensation of hunger is mediated. Rats given orexin will eat about ten times the normal amount of food and rats starved for 48 hours have more than twice the normal concentrations of orexin. There are also specific receptors for the two orexins. These facts are being exploited in the design of drugs that can both stimulate and reduce appetite.

Orelox a brand name for CEFPODIXIME.

orf a pox virus infection of sheep and goats that occasionally spreads to humans causing a fluid-filled blister on the hand or arm that may persist for weeks.

organ any part of the body consisting of more than one tissue and performing a particular function.

organelle any one of the bodies forming the internal functional components, or 'little organs', of the cell. The organelles include MITOCHONDRIA, the GOLGI APPARATUS, the ENDOPLASMIC RETICULUM, RIBOSOMES, LYSOSOMES and the CENTRIOLES.

organic 1 pertaining to animals or plants, rather than to non-living matter.
2 pertaining to an organ of the body.
3 caused by a pathological change in bodily structure rather than by a purely mental process.
4 of a chemical compound (other than carbon dioxide or its salts or carbon monoxide), containing carbon.
5 of food, grown without the use of artificial fertilizers.

organic brain syndrome any psychiatric disorder secondary to brain damage arising from disease or injury. The condition most commonly features irritability, confusion, impaired judgment, deterioration in personal habits, defective intellectual function and DEMENTIA.

organic chemistry the chemistry of carbon compounds.

organism any living animal or plant.

organ of Corti a spiral structure on the inner surface of the basilar membrane of the COCHLEA that contains a large series of sensory receptors that respond to sound vibrations of different frequencies and stimulate appropriate nerve impulses subserving hearing. (Marquis Alfonso Corti, 1822–88, Italian anatomist).

organon, organum a system of rules, principles or methods used in scientific investigation.

organophosphorous poisoning poisoning with compounds used as insecticides and as war nerve gases because of their powerful action in preventing CHOLINESTERASE from breaking down the neurotransmitter ACETYLCHOLINE. The effect of these agents are to produce excessive cholinergic activity – salivation, nausea, vomiting, diarrhoea, perspiration, small pupils, twitching, convulsions and death. ATROPINE, that blocks cholinergic nerve endings is the mainstay of treatment. Cholinesterase

reactivators such as obidoxime and other oximes are also useful.

orgasm the sequence of bodily, and especially genital, processes, occurring at the climax of sexual intercourse, and involving the pleasurable release of heightened muscle tension followed by the decline of TUMESCENCE in erectile tissue. Most sexual activity becomes focused on the achievement of orgasm – an inherent property making for species survival.

orgasmolepsy sudden widespread bodily relaxation and transitory loss of consciousness occurring during an ORGASM.

oriental sore LEISHMANIASIS of the skin. This is a tropical condition caused by the single-celled microscopic parasite Leishmania tropica and transmitted by the bite of the sandfly. It occurs in Mediterranean areas, China, and parts of India, but is spreading to the west Mediterranean holiday resorts. At the site of the bite, usually on the face, arms or legs, a red papule develops which enlarges to 2–10 cm in diameter and which may ulcerate. Small satellite papules commonly develop. The condition persists for 3 months to 3 years, then heals leaving a depressed, often disfiguring, scar.

origin the point or area of attachment of a muscle that remains mainly fixed when the muscle contracts. Compare INSERTION.

orlistat an anti-obesity pill that acts in the intestine by inhibiting the action of intestinal fat-splitting enzymes (lipases) so that up to one third of dietary fat is excreted in the faeces. Orlistat was approved by the Food and Drug Administration (FDA) in 1997.

Ornithodorus a genus of soft ticks that transmit RELAPSING FEVER.

ornithosis see PSITTACOSIS.

oropharynx the part of the PHARYNX at the back of the mouth and extending down to the top of the OESOPHAGUS.

Oroxine a brand name for the thyroid hormone THYROXINE.

Oroya fever a severe and often fatal form of BARTONELLOSIS.

orphan drugs a drug used to treat a rare disease and for which the market is so small that manufacturers have little incentive to go to the expense of producing them. In 1983 US legislation provided financial incentives, in the form of tax credits and 7 year exclusive rights, to firms willing to produce such drugs. This has been effective and, by mid-2003, 229 orphan drugs were available.

orphan genes isolated solitary genes situated remotely from their usual cluster site.

orphenadrine a drug used to relieve muscle spasm, especially in Parkinson's disease. Brand names are Biorphen and Disipal.

ortho- *combining form denoting* straight, upright, corrective or normal.

orthochromatic of a tissue for microscopic examination, taking stain normally.

orthodontics the dental speciality concerned with the correction of irregularities of tooth placement and in the relationship of the upper teeth to the lower (occlusion). Teeth can readily be permanently moved by sustained pressure using braces, springs, wires and harnesses.

orthognathous having the lower jaw correctly aligned with the upper so that it neither protrudes nor recedes.

orthomyxoviruses single-stranded RNA viruses that cause INFLUENZA.

orthopaedic collar a firm supportive collar used in the treatment of various neck conditions such as arthritis or inflammation of the neck bones (cervical SPONDYLOSIS). Orthopaedic collars are seldom worn for more than about 2 months at a time.

orthopaedics the branch of surgery concerned with correction of deformity and restoration of function following injury to, or disease or congenital abnormality of, the skeletal system and its associated ligaments, muscles and tendons. The term derives from the Greek for a 'straight child', not 'straight foot', as is commonly thought. The list that follows highlights the key entries related to orthopaedics in the dictionary: arthritis, bone cancer, cartilage, fibromyalgia, fracture, joint replacement, joints, ligament, osteoarthritis, osteochondritis, osteomyelitis, rheumatoid arthritis, sprain, subluxation, tendon.

orthopaedic surgeon a doctor specializing in the treatment of fractures, dislocations, joint disorders of all kinds, back problems generally, foot bony disorders, congenital defects of the skeleton and many other conditions. Increasingly the orthopaedic surgeon is concerned with the replacement of damaged and degenerate joints with prosthetic devices, especially artificial hip and knee joints.

orthophoria a state of perfect alignment of the two eyes even when they are deprived of the assistance of the binocular reflexes that maintain alignment. In orthophoria, the eyes remain in alignment even when one is covered. See also ESOPHORIA and EXOPHORIA.

orthopnoea difficulty in breathing when lying down.

orthoptics a discipline, ancillary to OPHTHALMOLOGY, concerned mainly with the management of squint (STRABISMUS) in childhood and the avoidance of AMBLYOPIA. See also ORTHOPTIST.

orthoptist a person trained in the diagnosis of inapparent squint; in the measurement of the angle of squint; in assessing the visual acuity in young children; determining the degree to which the child is able to perceive simultaneously with the two eyes (binocular vision); and diagnosing ABNORMAL RETINAL CORRESPONDENCE. Othoptists work to avoid or overcome AMBLYOPIA largely by the judicious covering for variable periods of the better-seeing eye (occlusion). They use a range of optical instruments in their work.

orthosis an appliance worn on the body to reduce or prevent deformity or to provide support, relieve pain and facilitate movement.

orthostatic pertaining to the erect posture.

orthostatic albuminuria the presence of small amounts of albumin in the urine in the absence of demonstrable kidney disease. The condition occurs rarely in young people. Urine formed during the night while the affected person is recumbent is free from albumin. Orthostatic (or postural) albuminuria is not believed to be of significance.

orthotics the branch of medicine dealing with the use of supportive mechanical devices. See also ORTHOSIS.

Orudis a brand name for KETOPROFEN.

Oruvail a brand name for KETOPROFEN.

Oruvail gel a brand name for KETOPROFEN formulated for external use.

os a bone or a mouth.

-ose *suffix denoting* characterized by or full of.

oseltamivir phosphate a prodrug of oseltamivir carboxylate, an inhibitor of neuraminidase enzymes on the surface of influenza viruses. These enzymes are essential for the release of the viruses from infected cells and thus the proliferation throughout the body. The drug is used to treat and prevent influenza A and B. A brand name is Tamiflu. Resistance to this drug from mutations of the neuraminidase gene was reported in 2003.

Osgood-Schlatter disease a knee disorder most common in early adolescent boys. It is caused by repetitive tension on the upper part of the front of the main lower leg bone (tibia) by the strong tendon of the front thigh muscles (quadriceps). This occurs as the knee is straightened against resistance as in climbing and cycling, and softening occurs in the protrusion on the bone into which the tendon is inserted, causing pain, muscle spasm and disability. The condition is treated by rest or, in severe cases, by immobilizing the knee in a plaster. (Robert Bayley Osgood, 1873–1956, American surgeon; and Carl Schlatter, 1864–1934, Swiss surgeon).

-osis *suffix denoting* a process or activity, an increase in, a disease or pathological process, or a non-inflammatory process.

Osler's nodes painful swellings in the skin of the fingertips probably caused by disease of small blood vessels (VASCULITIS) that occur as an occasional feature of INFECTIVE ENDOCARDITIS. (Sir William Osler, 1849–1919, Canadian-born British physician).

osmole the standard unit of osmotic pressure. The osmole is equal to the molecular weight of the dissolved substance expressed in grams divided by the number of particles or IONS into which each molecule of the substance dissociates in solution.

osmolality the property of a solution that depends on its concentration in osmolal units. See OSMOLE.

osmolar having a concentration of 1 OSMOLE per litre.

osmolarity the concentration of a solution in OSMOLAR units.

osmoreceptors cells in the HYPOTHALAMUS that monitor the concentration of solutes in the blood. An abnormal increase, as occurs in dehydration, stimulates the release of VASOPRESSIN from the PITUITARY gland. This acts on the kidney to reduce water loss.

osmosis the automatic movement of the fluid part of a solution through a membrane, separating two quantities of the solution, in such a direction as to dilute the solution of higher concentration. The membrane is permeable to the liquid but not to the dissolved substance. Such a membrane is said to be semipermeable and membranes of this kind occur widely in the body. Osmosis is an important principle on which much of physiology is based.

osseo- *combining form denoting* bone.

osseointegrated dental implant a method of permanently fixing individual artificial teeth. A titanium or titanium alloy screw is inserted directly into the bone of the upper or lower jaw as an implant to which the artificial tooth is secured.

osseous composed of, containing or resembling bone.

ossicle a small bone, especially one of the tiny bones, the auditory ossicles, in the middle ear that link the ear-drum to the inner ear. From the outside-in, the auditory ossicles are the malleus, the incus and the stapes.

ossification the process of conversion of other tissues into bone. Most bone forms from CARTILAGE but some is laid down by other connective tissue (membranous bone). Ossification may also occur in tissues that have been the site of disease such as long-term inflammation.

Ossopan 800 a brand name for HYDROXYAPATITE.

ost-, osteo- *combining form denoting* bone.

osteitis inflammation of bone. See also OSTEOMYELITIS.

osteitis deformans SEE PAGET'S DISEASE.

osteitis fibrosa cystica a disorder characterized by many large bone cysts filled with fibrous tissue. These are readily visible on X-ray. The condition is due to generalized bone demineralization due to an increased output of PARATHYROID hormone (HYPERPARATHYROIDISM).

osteoarthritis a common form of persistent degenerative joint disease involving damage to the cartilaginous bearing surfaces and sometimes widening or remodelling of the ends of the bones involved in the joint. RHEUMATOID FACTOR is not present in the blood. Osteoarthritis is an age-related condition and affects especially those joints that have previously been damaged.

osteoarthropathy any disease involving bones and joints.

osteoarthrosis see OSTEOARTHRITIS.

osteoblast a bone-building cell. Osteoblasts are continuously active remodelling bone that has been broken down by OSTEOCLASTS.

osteochondritis inflammation of both bone and cartilage, usually of unknown cause and often affecting children or adolescents. See also OSTEOCHONDRITIS DISSECANS.

osteochondritis dissecans an inflammatory disorder of joints in which small fragments of cartilage or bone are released into the interior of the joint, causing swelling, pain and limitation of movement. In some cases loose bodies may have to be removed.

osteochondroma a bony protrusion capped with cartilage, occurring most commonly at the ends of long bones. These are thought to be disorders of bone growth rather than tumours, but occasionally malignant change supervenes.

osteochondrosis see OSTEOCHONDRITIS.

osteoclasia the process of dissolution and resorption of bone prior to its regeneration.

osteoclasis deliberate surgical fracture of bone to correct deformity.

osteoclast 1 a giant cell containing many nuclei and capable of bone destruction and absorption. Osteoclasts work in conjunction with OSTEOBLASTS in the process of normal bone growth and in bone repair after fractures. 2 a surgical instrument used to fracture bone.

osteoclastoma a benign but aggressive tumour of bone causing a large, thin-walled cyst usually near the end of a long bone and often leading to unexpected fracture. The tumour contains many giant cells similar to normal OSTEOCLASTS. Also known as giant cell tumour of bone. The bone cysts can be scraped out (curetted) but recurrence is common.

osteocyte a bone cell.

osteodystrophy defective bone formation.

osteogenesis bone formation.

osteogenesis imperfecta any one of a range of hereditary connective tissue diseases featuring excessive fragility of bone and frequent spontaneous fractures. The condition is often associated with blueness of the whites of the eyes (scleras), opalescent teeth and deafness. Also known as osteitis fragilitans or brittle bone disease.

osteogenic sarcoma see OSTEOSARCOMA.

osteogenin an extract from bone that has been used experimentally to induce muscle, cartilage

and other soft tissue to transform into bone. Osteogenin is a glycoprotein that can transform muscle flaps placed in moulds into cancellous bone matching the exact shape of the mould.

osteoid resembling bone.

osteology the science and study of bones.

osteolysis reabsorption or demineralization of bone.

osteoma a BENIGN tumour of bone, largely confined to the skull and jawbone. Osteomas often arise in a sinus or in the ORBIT, are slow-growing and can be removed if causing cosmetic or other problems.

osteomalacia bone softening as a result of defective mineralization, usually occurring because of defective calcium absorption from vitamin D deficiency. Osteomalacia is commoner in women than in men. The softened bones may distort or bend under the body weight. The condition is treated with vitamin D.

osteomyelitis an infection of all elements of bone, including the PERIOSTEUM and the bone marrow, usually with staphylococci (see STAPHYLOCOCCUS). The disease is commonest in children, and causes fever and severe pain at the affected site. Intensive antibiotic treatment is necessary to avoid a long-term problem with abscess formation and death of an isolated piece of bone (sequestrum formation).

osteo-odonto-keratoprosthesis an artificial cornea used as a last resource to restore vision to people whose corneas have been rendered opaque by dry-eye disease or chemical injury that precludes successful corneal grafting. A tooth is removed and a section cut from it. This is drilled and a plastic lens cemented into the hole. The tooth section is then buried under the skin until it has acquired a soft tissue surround. It is then sutured into a hole cut in the opaque cornea.

osteopathy a system of medical practice that includes many orthodox principles but central to which is the notion that health depends on the proper relationship of the structures of the body to each other. Much emphasis is placed on the importance of the function of the spinal column as a whole and of the relationship of its component bones to each other and to the pelvis and the limb bones. Osteopathic treatment is manipulative and is aimed at freeing and loosening joints and re-establishing proper relationships. Osteopaths in UK are now formally registered as practitioners.

osteopetrosis a group of hereditary bone disorders featuring increased density ('marble bones') but increased fragility ('osteosclerosis fragilis'). In some cases excessive bone growth can cause pressure effects on nerves passing through bony canals. The condition is due to a defect of bone resorption by OSTEOCLASTS SO that osteoblastic bone synthesis proceeds unchecked. It can sometimes be treated by bone marrow transfusion to provide normal osteoclasts. Also known as Albers-Schonberg disease after Heinrich Ernst Albers-Schönberg (1865–1921) who was professor of radiology at Hamburg.

osteophyte a bony outgrowth occurring usually adjacent to an area of articular cartilage damage in a joint affected by OSTEOARTHRITIS. Osteophytes are also common around the intervertebral discs of the spine.

osteoporosis a form of bone atrophy involving both the COLLAGEN scaffolding and the mineralization. It is thought to be due to predominance of reabsorption of bone over natural bone formation. It is commonest in women after the menopause and tends to be progressive, giving rise to the risk of fractures from minimal trauma. Osteoporosis has many causes, the most important being long-term disuse and loss of sex hormones. Other causes include overactivity of the thyroid and parathyroid glands, CUSHING'S SYNDROME, malnutrition and prolonged treatment with corticosteroid drugs. The progress of osteoporosis can be reduced in women by HORMONE REPLACEMENT THERAPY and by calcium supplements. In some cases fluoride or ANABOLIC STEROIDS are recommended. Other drugs that can help to minimize osteoporotic damage include tamoxifen, raloxifene and alendronate.

osteoprotegerin (OPG) a secreted protein which inhibits OSTEOCLAST differentiation. The cytokine TRANCE binds to osteoprotegerin.

osteosarcoma a highly malignant form of bone cancer that affects mostly young people between the ages of 10 and 20. The tumour is commonest at the lower end of the thigh bone (femur) or the upper end of the shin bone (tibia) causing swelling and sometimes pain, local warmth and tenderness. A characteristic 'sun-ray' effect of bone spicules is often visible on X-ray. Early spread to other parts of the body (METASTASIS) is common and unexplained pain or swelling at either of these sites should always be investigated without delay. In confirmed cases, urgent treatment is necessary if life is to be saved.

osteosclerosis any abnormal bone thickening resulting in an increase in bone density. See also OSTEOPETROSIS.

osteotome a strong surgical chisel or other instrument used to cut bone.

osteotomy surgical cutting or sectioning of bone.

ostium an opening or mouth.

OT *abbrev. for* Occupational Therapist.

ot-, oto- *combining form denoting* the ear.

otalgia pain in the ear.

OTC *abbrev. for* over the counter. This refers to drugs or other remedies that may be purchased from a pharmacist without a doctor's prescription.

otic pertaining to the ear.

otitis externa inflammation of the skin of the ear canal or of the external ear (pinna). This is commonly the result of infection with one of a variety of organisms such as staphylococci, herpes viruses, and fungi of various kinds, including the thrush fungus Candida albicans.

otitis media inflammation in the middle ear cavity. This usually results from spread of infection from the nose or throat by way of the EUSTACHIAN TUBE. In acute suppurative otitis media there is rapid production of pus with a pressure rise that causes the eardrum to bulge outwards. In chronic suppurative otitis media, there is a hole (perforation) in the drum and usually a persistent discharge (otorrhoea). Secretory otitis media, or 'glue ear', is persistent and insidious and mainly affects children causing unsuspected deafness and educational disadvantage. All forms of otitis media respond well to expert treatment. Glue ear is usually treated by the insertion of grommets in the drum to promote middle ear drainage.

otocyst the precursor, in the MESODERM of the head of the embryo, of the membranous LABYRINTH of the inner ear.

otolith one of the many tiny calcareous particles found in the utricle and sacculus of the inner ear. These move under gravitational and accelerative forces causing stimulation of hair cells and the production of nerve impulses that provide the brain with information about the position and movement of the head.

otology the surgical speciality concerned with the study of the structure, function and disorders of the ears and the treatment of ear disease.

-otomy *suffix denoting* a surgical incision into.

otomycosis fungus infection of the external ear. A form of OTITIS EXTERNA.

otoplasty any plastic surgical operation to correct cosmetically unacceptable ears. Otoplasty for prominent, bat-like ears, or for 'lop ears' is usually performed in childhood.

otorhinolaryngology the surgical speciality concerned with the diseases of the ear, nose and throat. Also known as otolaryngology.

otorrhoea discharge from the ear. See also OTITIS EXTERNA, OTITIS MEDIA.

otosclerosis a hereditary bone disease affecting the freedom of vibration of the footplate of the inner auditory OSSICLE (the stapes) in the oval window in the wall of the inner ear. Progressive immobilization of the bone interferes with the transmission of vibrations from the ear drum and leads to progressive deafness. The condition can usually be effectively treated by a microsurgical operation.

otoscope an instrument for illuminating and examining the external ear canal and the ear drum (tympanic membrane). Also known as an auriscope.

ototoxicity damage to ear function by the poisoning effects of drugs or other agents. These can affect both hearing and balancing mechanisms. Ototoxic effects can be caused by large doses of AMINOGLYCOSIDE antibiotics such as STREPTOMYCIN, GENTAMICIN, or NEOMYCIN, by some diuretic drugs such as FRUSEMIDE (furosemide), by QUININE, aspirin and other salicylates. Kidney damage that delays excretion of ototoxic agents increases the danger.

Otrivine-Antistin a brand name for ANTAZOLINE and XYLOMETAZOLINE.

Ottawa ankle rules an accurate clinical procedure for excluding the diagnosis of ankle and mid-foot fractures and reducing the number of unnecessary X-rays. Essentially, the rules are based on the presence or absence of bony tenderness and the ability or inability to bear weight. Analogous rules have been formulated for knee and head injuries.

outpatient a patient receiving medical attention in a medical facility who does not occupy a bed overnight.

ovalocytosis 1 a change in a small proportion of red blood cells to an elliptical form occurring in various forms of anaemia.
2 a hereditary condition in which most of the red blood cells are of oval shape. It is usually BENIGN but sometimes causes HAEMOLYTIC ANAEMIA.

oval window the oval opening in the outer wall of the inner ear in which the footplate of the inner of the three AUDITORY OSSICLES, the stapes, is free to vibrate.

ovari- *combining form denoting* the OVARY.

ovarian agenesis failure of the ovaries to develop.

ovarian cysts usually benign, fluid-filled closed sacs growing from an OVARY. They may contain watery fluid or a mucoid material. Some are caused by ENDOMETRIOSIS and may contain altered blood. Ovarian cysts are common and may be symptom-free, but some grow to a considerable size and may simulate obesity or pregnancy. These may lead to varicose veins or piles (haemorrhoids) or may cause breathlessness and abdominal discomfort. Large cysts cause trouble mainly by their bulk, but may cause severe complications if they become twisted and their blood supply is cut off or if they rupture or become infected. In such cases, and when cysts are caused by endometriosis, surgical treatment is usually necessary.

ovarian dysmenorrhea DYSMENORRHEA originating in disorder in an OVARY.

ovarian hyperstimulation syndrome ovarian enlargement, the production of multiple ovarian cysts, increased capillary permeability with generalized oedema and intravascular fluid depletion, SHOCK, and sometimes even death. The syndrome, which is uncommon, is caused by gonadotropin medical treatment to stimulate ovulation. Rarely, it may occur spontaneously during pregnancy as a result of a mutation in the gene for the follicle-stimulating hormone receptor.

ovarian remnant syndrome persistent pelvic pain, either constant or cyclical, occurring within five years after surgery for removal of the womb and both ovaries. The amount of residual ovarian tissue may be very small but an estimation of pituitary follicle-stimulating hormone may show the presence of functioning ovarian tissue. Treatment is by surgery, which may be technically difficult because of residual adhesions. There is a risk of damage to ureters or bladder.

ovariectomy see OOPHORECTOMY.

ovary one of the paired female gonads, situated in the pelvis, one on each side of the womb (uterus), just under and inward of the open ends of the FALLOPIAN TUBES. Ovaries are almond-shaped and about 3 cm long. They are the site of egg (OVUM) formation and release one or more ova each month about 14 days before the onset of the next menstrual period. This is called ovulation. See also OOCYTE, OOGONIA.

overdose a quantity of a drug well in excess of the recommended dose.

overt obvious.

over-the-counter drugs drugs that can be purchased from a pharmacy without prescription. The list of drugs formerly obtainable only on prescription but now freed from that restriction is growing apace. Contrary to the previous situation, many effective remedies are now available in UK over-the-counter. They include corticosteroid ointments, antihistamines, imidazole creams, H-2 antagonist drugs, nicotine patches and the anti-herpes drug aciclovir.

Ovestin a brand name for the oestrogen drug OESTRIOL (estriol).

oviduct the FALLOPIAN TUBE.

Ovranette a brand name for LEVONORGESTREL, a PROGESTOGEN drug formulated with ETHINYLOESTRADIOL (ethinylestradiol) as an oral contraceptive.

ovulation the release of an OVUM from a mature Graafian follicle in the OVARY. Ovulation occurs about half way between the beginning of consecutive menstrual periods, usually about 14 days before the expected date of onset of the next period.

ovum the female gamete or ovum which, when fertilized by a spermatozoon, can give rise to a new individual. The egg is a very large cell, compared with other body cells, and contains only 23 chromosomes, half the normal number (haploid). Like most other cells ova contain many mitochondria each containing many copies of mitochondrial DNA. This DNA is not present in sperms.

ovum donation the provision of human eggs (ova) by harvesting from living donors, cadavers or aborted fetuses. Donated ova could be used to relieve infertility or for research purposes. The topic is highly controversial and has aroused strong reactions in both directions.

Ovysmen a brand name for ETHINYLOESTRADIOL (ethinylestradiol) formulated with a PROGESTOGEN drug as an oral contraceptive.

oxalosis a rare hereditary metabolic disorder in which calcium oxalate is deposited in the tissues. The condition is caused by the deficiency of the enzyme D-glycerate dehydrogenase.

oxaluria abnormal excretion of oxalic acid or oxalates in the urine.

oxamniquine a drug used in the treatment of SCHISTOSOMIASIS. It is on the WHO official list.

oxazepam a BENZODIAZEPINE tranquillizing drug.

oxazolidinones ANTIBIOTIC drugs used to treat infections for which commoner antibiotics are unsuitable or ineffective. An example is linezolid (Zyvox).

oxerutins a bioflavonoid drug used to treat oedema from poor venous drainage. A brand name is Paroven.

oxicams a class of NON-STEROIDAL ANTI-INFLAMMATORY DRUGS used to treat arthritis. Examples are piroxicam (Feldene), meloxicam (Mobic), tenoxicam (Mobiflex) and lornoxicam (Xefo).

oxidative phosphorylation the process of cellular respiration occurring within the MITOCHONDRIA and responsible for the production of adenosine triphosphate (ATP). In this process energy derived from the oxidation of hydrogen, to form water, is transferred to ATP.

oxidative stress the widespread effects of oxygen FREE RADICALS on any part of the body.

oxidoreductases a group of enzymes that promote oxidation-reduction reactions. The group includes some enzymes also known as dehydrogenases and oxidases.

oximeter a device for measuring or monitoring the oxygenated fraction of the haemoglobin in the circulating blood. Oximeters use photoelectric methods to detect colour differences in blood of different oxygen saturation. They are valuable aids to safety and are widely used in operating theatres and in intensive care units. See also PULSE OXIMETER.

Oxis Turbohaler a brand name for an inhaler charged with EFORMOTEROL (formoterol) as a breath-actuated powder for the relief of ASTHMA.

oxitropium an ANTICHOLINERGIC drug used from an inhaler to treat ASTHMA and chronic obstructive lung disease. A brand name is Oxivent.

Oxivent a brand name for OXITROPIUM.

oxpentifylline pentoxifylline, a xanthine drug that relaxes smooth muscle and is used to improve blood flow in peripheral blood vessel disorders. A brand name is Trental.

oxprenolol a beta blocker drug used to treat ANGINA PECTORIS, high blood pressure (HYPERTENSION) and disorders of heart rhythm. Brand names are Slow-Trasicor and Trasicor.

oxy- *combining form denoting* sharp.

oxybuprocaine benoxinate, a local anaesthetic drug used as eyedrops to effect rapid anaesthetization of the cornea for pressure measurement in glaucoma (tonometry), foreign body removal and other purposes. A brand name is Minims benoxinate.

oxybutynin an anticholinergic antispasmodic drug used to treat urinary urgency, frequency and incontinence and bed-wetting in children. Brand names are Cystrin, Ditropan and Lyrinel XL.

oxycephaly a skull abnormality causing the head to assume a conical or peaked appearance. Oxycephaly is due to premature closure of the irregular junctions on the side of the skull between the bones of the vault (the coronal or lambdoidal sutures). Also known as tower head.

oxygen a colourless, odourless gas, essential for life, that constitutes about one fifth of the earth's atmosphere. Oxygen is required for the functioning and survival of all body tissues, and deprivation for more than a few minutes is fatal. The respiratory system captures oxygen from the atmosphere and passes it to the blood by means of which it is conveyed to all parts of the body. Oxygen is needed for the fundamental chemical process of oxidation of fuel to release energy. This series of reactions is known as oxidative phosphorylation and involves the synthesis of the universal energy carrier ATP (ADENOSINE TRIPHOSPHATE) in the inner membranes of the MITOCHONDRIA of the cells.

Oxygen is on the WHO official list.

oxygen concentrators portable devices containing molecular sieves of silica and alumina through which air is forced. The sieves selectively adsorb nitrogen and carbon dioxide from the air to give an output of 95% of medically acceptable oxygen and 5% of the inert gas argon. These concentrators deliver oxygen to patients in their own homes at a small fraction of the cost of oxygen in cylinders.

oxygen therapy treatment in which the inhaled air contains a much higher concentration of oxygen than normal atmospheric air. Oxygen therapy is appropriate for conditions in which the oxygen concentration in the blood is reduced for any reason. It is also used to improve the oxygen supply to the tissues even when the haemoglobin of the blood is fully saturated. It achieves this by increasing the amount of oxygen dissolved in the blood plasma. Oxygen is given by light plastic masks or by soft tubes fitting comfortably into the nostrils (NASAL CANNULAE).

oxyhaemoglobin the bright red, oxygenated form of HAEMOGLOBIN in the red blood cells, in which a molecule of oxygen has attached itself reversibly to the iron atom in the haemoglobin molecule. Oxyhaemoglobin transports oxygen from the lungs to the tissues.

oxyntic cells cells in the glands of the lining of the stomach that secrete hydrochloric acid and INTRINSIC FACTOR. Also known as parietal cells.

oxyphenbutazone a non-steroidal anti-inflammatory drug limited to external use in ointment form. A brand name is Tanderil.

oxytetracycline a broad-spectrum tetracycline antibiotic derived from the mould-like bacterium *Streptomyces rimosus*. The drug is effective against a range of GRAM POSITIVE and GRAM NEGATIVE organisms including Rickettsiae and is widely used to treat ACNE (but not in its role as an antibiotic). Oxytetracycline is formulated for external use with steroids and other ingredients under the brand names Terra-Cortril, Terra-Cortril-Nystatin and Trimovate.

oxytocic 1 hastening delivery of a baby by inducing contraction of the womb muscles. 2 a drug that hastens childbirth.

oxytocin an OXYTOCIC hormone produced by the pituitary gland. The hormone promotes contraction of the womb and is used as a drug in obstetrics to bring on labour at term and to augment slow labour. It is given by intravenous infusion. The drug is on the WHO official list. A brand name is Syntocinon.

oxyuriasis THREADWORM infection.

ozaena inflammation and atrophy of the mucous membrane lining of the nose, with discharge, crusting and a foul smell, of which the sufferer is usually unaware. The condition is now rare.

ozone a gas consisting of molecules in which three atoms of oxygen are linked together. Concentrated ozone is a blue explosive liquid. Even in low concentrations the gas is poisonous and highly irritating. The ozone layer in the stratosphere, between 10 and 50 km above the earth's surface, is produced continuously by the action of ultraviolet radiation from the sun and forms a protective barrier, cutting down the intensity of the ultraviolet component in sunlight. Without the ozone layer we would suffer serious biological effects from solar radiation, including a large increase in the incidence of skin cancer. Atmospheric ozone is broken down by the catalytic action of chloro-fluoro-carbons (CFCs) and other substances.

Recent studies have shown that ozone is involved in the oxidative stress production of ATHEROSCLEROSIS in arteries. Cholesterol is converted by ozone to 5,6-secosterol which is cytotoxic and induces the formation of foam cells in the presence of low-density lipoproteins.

p

p21 an anticancer protein of the class of cyclin-dependent kinase inhibitors. Cyclin-dependent kinases are enzymes that have been described by Elizabeth Finkel as 'the engines that drive the cell-cycle past its various control checkpoints.' Inhibition of these enzymes provides a way of controlling rapidly-reproducing cells such as cancer cells. High levels of p21 are found in ageing cells.

p53 a gene that induces production of p21. A tumour suppressor gene, the absence or mutation of which can greatly increase the probability that cancer will develop. When DNA damage, as from anticancer drugs, occurs in normal cells the expression of p53 is increased. The gene may then act to protect the cell by halting the cell cycle so that the DNA damage can be repaired, or, if the DNA damage is too severe, p53 can kill the cell by APOPTOSIS so that the defective DNA is not passed on. Mutations in p53 have been found in a range of cancers including those of the breast, colon, ovary, bladder and oesophagus. They have also been found to be associated with failure to respond to anticancer drugs.

PABA *abbrev. for* para-aminobenzoic acid, a substance with the property of absorbing ultraviolet light. Sometimes used in lotions as a sunscreen.

pabulum any substance that provides NOURISHMENT.

pacemakers electronic devices that deliver regular short pulses of electricity to promote contraction of the heart muscle in people with a defect in the heart's conduction system (heart block). Pacemakers may be external or internal (implanted), the latter being buried under the skin of the chest and having an electrode that runs into the heart through a large vein. The rate of the electrical impulses varies with the demands on the heart or can be programmed from the outside by radio signals. External pacemakers are used in the emergency treatment of heart block until more permanent arrangements can be made.

pachy- *combining form denoting* thick.

pachydermatous abnormally thick-skinned.

pachymeningitis inflammation of the DURA MATER.

pachyonychia abnormal thickness of the nails.

pacing controlling the rate of an activity, especially the heart rate, usually by electronic devices, such as PACEMAKERS.

Pacinian corpuscle a specialized encapsulated ending of a sensory nerve occurring in the deep layers of the skin. Pacinian corpuscles respond to touch and heavy pressure. (Filippo Pacini, 1812–83, Italian anatomist).

paclitaxel a TAXANE anticancer drug used mainly to treat ovarian cancer and widespread breast cancer. A brand name is Taxol.

paed-, paedo- *combining form denoting* child.

paediatrics the medical speciality concerned with all aspects of childhood diseases and disorders and with the health and development of the child in the context of the family and the environment. The list that follows highlights the key entries related to paediatrics in the dictionary: bottle feeding, breast feeding, chickenpox, child abuse, coeliac disease, congenital heart disease, cleft lip and palate, cystic fibrosis, dentition, diarrhoea, encephalitis, febrile convusion, leukaemia, malnutrition, measles, MMR vaccination, mumps, meningitis, neural tube defects, phenylketonuria, respiratory distress syndrome, rhesus factyor disease, rheumatic fever, roseola infantum, rubella, shaken baby syndrome, sudden infant death syndrome.

paedomorphism retention by the adult of juvenile characteristics.

paedophilia recurrent sexual urges towards a prepubertal child by a person over the age of 16 and at least five years older than the child. If manifested, these urges, which constitute criminal sexual molestation, usually involve fondling of the genitals and oral intercourse. Vaginal or anal intercourse is relatively infrequent except in cases of incest. Active paedophilia is not a medical or psychiatric condition; it is a crime universally condemned. The Internet has become a vehicle both for the promulgation of paedophilic graphics and for the promotion of paedophilic contacts.

Paget's disease a bone disease affecting up to 3% of the elderly population and involving mainly the skull, the collar bones (clavicles) the spine, the pelvis and the leg bones. The affected areas become warm with softening and increased bone growth with distortion. Skull thickening and enlargement may cause headache and compression of the CRANIAL NERVES. Legs may become bowed, spinal changes may cause compression of the cord and paralysis and fractures may occur spontaneously. Paget's disease is thought to be due to a virus infection of OSTEOCLASTS. It is treated with pain-relieving drugs and with the thyroid hormone calcitonin, which decreases the rate of bone turn-over and allows more calcium and phosphorus to be lost in the urine. (Sir James Paget, 1814–99, English surgeon).

Paget's disease of the nipple a slowly growing cancer of a milk duct of the breast that presents as a form of ECZEMA affecting the nipple. Diagnosis is by BIOPSY and treatment is by local surgical removal. (Sir James Paget, 1814–99, English surgeon).

pain an unpleasant or distressing localized sensation caused by stimulation of certain sensory nerve endings called nociceptors, or by strong stimulation of other sensory nerves. Nociceptors are stimulated by the chemical action of substances, such as prostaglandins, released from local cells damaged by injury or inflammation. Whatever the site of nerve stimulation, pain is usually experienced in the region of the nerve endings. Referred pain is pain experienced at a site other than that at which the causal factor is operating. Pain impulses pass to the brain via a series of control 'gates' analogous to those in computers and these can be modulated by other nerve impulses. Pain commonly serves as a warning of bodily danger and leads to action to end it. Pain is best treated by discovering and removing the cause. It is a complex phenomenon with many components – somatic, emotional, cognitive and social.

The management of acute, self-limiting pain is not the same as long-term pain. The latter requires treatment by a multidisciplinary team in a pain clinic. ANALGESIC drugs can be used to target specific receptors and should not be withheld until pain is severe but given repeatedly in expectation of pain. Pain may be relieved by drugs self-administered on an as-required basis; by electrical stimulation of the skin; ACUPUNCTURE; massage; cold sprays; LOCAL ANAESTHETIC injections; or even, in extreme cases and rarely, by permanent nerve destruction by alcohol injection or by surgical severance. From the Latin *poena*, punishment. See also ENDORPHINS.

painful arc syndrome an inflammatory disorder of a tendon or BURSA around the shoulder joint in which pain occurs when the arm is lifted between 45° and 160° from the side of the body. The condition can be relieved by local injections of corticosteroid drugs.

pain dysfunction syndromes see CHRONIC PAIN SYNDROMES.

painkillers see ANALGESICS.

Painstop a brand name for a mixture of the painkiller drugs PARACETAMOL and CODEINE.

palatal 1 pertaining to the palate.
2 of phonation, produced with the front of the tongue near or against the hard palate.

palate the partly hard, partly soft partition that forms the roof of the mouth and separates it from the nose. The hard palate consists of a plate of bone, part of the MAXILLA, covered with mucous membrane. The soft palate, attached to the back of the hard palate, is a small flap of muscle and fibrous tissue enclosed in a fold of mucous membrane. It can press firmly against the back wall of the PHARYNX, sealing off the opening to the nose during swallowing and when one is blowing out through the mouth.

palatine pertaining to the palate.

palilalia the repetition of words or phrases with increasing rapidity. Palilalia is a feature of an organic brain disorder.

palinopsia the persistent perception of a visual image for some time after the direction of gaze has been moved so that the original image is superimposed on another. Multiple identical images (polyopia) may be perceived. The cause of this rare symptom remains uncertain but some cases are epileptic phenomena affecting the non-dominant occipito-temporal cortex.

Palladone a brand name for HYDROMORPHONE.

palliative treatment treatment that relieves symptoms but does not cure their cause.

pallor undue paleness of the skin, observable also in certain mucous membranes, such as the CONJUNCTIVA and the lining of the mouth. Transient pallor may result from constriction of the blood vessels near the surface. Longer-term pallor may be due to ANAEMIA or lack of exposure to sunlight. Permanent pallor may be caused by ALBINISM.

palmar pertaining to the palm of the hand. Compare PLANTAR.

palpable able to be felt.

palpation examination by feeling with the fingers and hands.

palpebral pertaining to the eyelids.

palpitation abnormal awareness of the action of the heart, because of rapidity or irregularity. Irregularity is most commonly due to EXTRASYSTOLES each of which causes a brief sense of stoppage. Other causes include ATRIAL TACHYCARDIA and ATRIAL FIBRILLATION.

palsy an obsolete term for PARALYSIS, retained for historical reasons in a few cases such as those of BELL'S PALSY and CEREBRAL PALSY.

Paludrine a brand name for the antimalarial drug proguanil.

palliative care the application of specialist knowledge to the relief of severe suffering, physical or mental, in people in whom such relief cannot be achieved by cure of disease or disorder. Palliative care is now a recognized specialty mainly exercised in hospices and in large hospitals with cancer units. It is not, however, necessarily limited to those with no prospect of recovery.

pallidotomy a neurosurgical operation that involves incision into or partial destruction of the globus pallidus, one of the nuclei at the base of the brain. This radical procedure has been found effective in PARKINSON'S DISEASE and severe tardive dyskinesia.

Pamergan P100 a brand name for PETHIDINE formulated with PROMETHAZINE.

pamidronate a BISPHOSPHONATE drug that prevents bone reabsorption by interfering with the action of osteoclasts. The drug has been used to treat cancer bone metastases and multiple myeloma. A brand name is Aredia.

pan- *combining form denoting* all, or the whole of.

panacea a mythical universal remedy or cure-all. See also QUACKERY.

Panadeine a brand name for a mixture of PARACETAMOL and CODEINE.

Panadol a brand name for a range of products containing PARACETAMOL.

panagglutinin an AGGLUTININ capable of agglutinating red blood cells of any blood group.

Panamax a brand name for the painkilling drug PARACETAMOL.

panarthritis inflammation of several joints.

pancarditis inflammation of all parts of the heart – the lining (endocardium), the muscle (myocardium) and the surrounding sac (pericardium).

pancoagulation destruction of the whole of the periphery of the retina by multiple laser burns in the treatment of DIABETIC RETINOPATHY.

Pancoast's tumour any tumour situated in the lower part of the neck which, because of its location, involves certain structures to cause a characteristic group of physical signs. These may include pain in and around the region caused by spread of the tumour to the lung covering (pleura) the ribs and the spine; weakness in the arm from damage to nerves in the armpit; hoarseness of the voice due to involvement of the nerves to the LARYNX; and HORNER'S SYNDROME from damage to the sympathetic chain of nerves in the neck. Pancoast's tumour is commonly an advanced lung cancer (bronchial carcinoma). (Henry Khunrath Pancoast, 1875–1939, American radiologist).

pancreas a dual function gland situated immediately behind the STOMACH with its head lying within the loop of the DUODENUM, into which the duct of the pancreas runs. The pancreas secretes digestive enzymes capable of breaking down carbohydrates, proteins and fats into simpler, absorbable, compounds. It is also a gland of internal secretion (an endocrine gland). The endocrine element consists of the Islets of Langerhans, specialized cells that monitor blood and produce four hormones – INSULIN, GLUCAGON, SOMATOSTATIN and a pancreatic polypeptide of unknown function. See also DIABETES.

Pancrease a brand name for PANCREATIN.

pancreas transplant a method of treating DIABETES by grafting healthy pancreatic tissue from a donor. Unfortunately, the immunosuppressive treatment needed to prevent graft rejection is currently more dangerous than diabetes. Several thousand successful transplants have, however, been achieved in diabetics who required immunosuppression for other purposes, usually kidney transplants.

pancreatectomy removal of all or part of the pancreas. This may be done to treat pancreatic cancer, various endocrine tumours of the pancreas or PANCREATITIS.

pancreatic diarrhoea diarrhoea resulting from deficiency of pancreatic digestive enzymes so that the stools contain large quantities of undigested fats and proteins.

pancreatic juice the clear, alkaline fluid that passes along the pancreatic duct into the DUODENUM and contains enzymes that are able to break down proteins, carbohydrates and fats into simpler and absorbable substances.

pancreatin a preparation of pancreatic digestive enzymes that can be taken by mouth. This may be required by people who have had a PANCREATECTOMY or whose pancreatic enzyme production is inadequate. Brand names are Creon, Nutrizym GR, Pancrease and Pancrex V.

pancreatitis inflammation of the pancreas. This may be a sharp, severe illness (acute pancreatitis) or a recurrent disorder (chronic pancreatitis). Acute pancreatitis is often due to blockage of the outflow from the gland by a gallstone stuck in the common outlet of the pancreatic and bile ducts, with digestion of the pancreatic tissue by its own enzymes. There is sudden severe pain in the abdomen, nausea, vomiting and shock. Chronic pancreatitis is usually related to heavy alcohol consumption. X-ray or CT scan shows that the pancreas is full

of cysts, many of them filled with chalky stones. Attacks are short, severe and tend to recur. Extensive damage to the pancreas may result and this can cause DIABETES. Continued drinking by people with chronic pancreatitis carries a high mortality.

pancreatography any method of imaging of the pancreas and its ducts, as by the use of X-ray contrast medium, CT SCANNING or ULTRASOUND SCANNING.

pancreolauryl test a non-invasive test of pancreatic function that depends on the ability of pancreatic enzymes to split a substance given by mouth, the products of which can be detected in the urine.

Pancrex a brand name for PANCREATIN.

pancytopenia an abnormal decrease in the numbers of the cellular elements in the blood and of the PLATELETS.

pandemic a world-wide EPIDEMIC.

panencephalitis an ENCEPHALITIS involving the grey and white matter simultaneously. A very severe form affecting children is caused by a MYXOVIRUS (subacute sclerosing panencephalitis).

panic attack the episode characteristic of the PANIC DISORDER.

panic disorder a condition featuring recurrent brief episodes of acute distress, mental confusion and fear of impending death. The heart beats rapidly, breathing is deep and fast and sweating occurs. Overbreathing (hyperventilation) often makes the attack worse. These attacks usually occur about twice a week but may be more frequent and they are especially common in people with AGORAPHOBIA. The condition tends to run in families and appears to be an ORGANIC disorder with a strong psychological component. Treatment is with antidepressant drugs, especially the tricyclic group, and MONOAMINE OXIDASE INHIBITORS. Cognitive behaviour therapy can also be helpful.

panniculitis inflammation and NECROSIS of the layer of fat under the skin especially in the abdomen. Nodular formation is common. Panniculitis is associated with trauma especially the trauma of repeated injections. It is also associated with a range of pancreatic disorders, including pancreatic cancer, and with multiple joint disorders (polyarthropathy). On microscopic examination, nodules of panniculitis show empty ('ghost') fat cells.

pannus a membrane of fine blood vessels and fibrous tissue that spreads down over the cornea in TRACHOMA and other inflammatory corneal disorders causing loss of vision. A similar membrane can affect the inner linings of joints.

panophobia fear of everything.

panophthalmitis inflammation involving all the tissues of the eyeball. Panophthalmitis usually ends in blindness.

Panoxyl a brand name for BENZOYL PEROXIDE in a preparation used to treat ACNE.

Pantheline a brand name for PROPANTHELINE.

pantoprazol a PROTON PUMP INHIBITOR drug used to treat peptic ulceration and other disorders due to excess stomach acid. A brand name is Protium.

pantothenic acid one of the B group of vitamins and a constituent of coenzyme A which has a central role in energy metabolism. Deficiency is rare.

panuveitis inflammation of the entire UVEAL TRACT – the iris, the ciliary body and the CHOROID.

papain a mixture of enzymes found in pawpaws. Papain includes the protein-splitting enzyme chymopapain and this makes it useful for breaking down organic debris and so cleaning up wounds and ulcers. Chymopapain is used to break down material extruded from the pulpy nuclei of intervertebral discs (chemonucleolysis).

papaveretum a mixture of purified opium alkaloids. Papaveretum has the same painkilling and narcotic properties as MORPHINE and is mainly used for surgical premedication. Also known as Omnopon. A brand name of the drug combined with ASPIRIN and PAPAVERETUM is Aspav. The drug should not be confused with PAPAVERINE.

papaverine an opium derivative used as a smooth muscle relaxant and to treat heart irregularities following a heart attack. Papaverine has been used to treat organic impotence by direct injection into the corpora cavernosa of the penis.

papilla a small, nipple-like projection.

papillary muscles the finger-like muscular processes arising from the floors of the VENTRICLES of the heart to which are attached the strings (chordae tendineae) that tether the cusps of the atrioventricular valves.

papilloedema swelling and protrusion of the OPTIC DISC at the back of the inside of the eye. This is visible by means of an OPHTHALMOSCOPE and is an important indication of a rise in the pressure within the skull. Raised pressure is transmitted along the sheaths of the optic nerves. Papilloedema is always serious and may indicate a brain tumour or other major disorder. Early observation of papilloedema may be life-saving.

papilloma a benign tumour of skin or mucous membrane in which epithelial cells grow outward from a surface around a connective tissue core containing blood vessels. Papillomas may be flat or spherical with a narrow neck (pedunculated) and occur on the skin, in the nose, bladder, larynx or breast. Most skin papillomas are WARTS.

papillomatosis widespread formation of numerous papillomas.

papillomatous of the character of, or pertaining to, a PAPILLOMA.

papillomavirus any virus of the *Papillomavirus* genus of the *Papovaviridae* family. These viruses cause various kinds of warts, including venereal warts. Papillomavirus infections are thought to be the probable reason for the higher incidence of cancer of the cervix in women with many sexual partners.

PAPNET an automated neural net cervical smear test used to supplement smear examination by human pathologists. PAPNET checks every cell, comparing it with a normal standard. It then selects the 128 that are most abnormal and displays them on a monitor where they are checked by an expert. The system has been able to identify abnormal cells previously reported as normal up to 12 years before a positive diagnosis was reached.

papovavirus a member of the family of viruses that includes the human wart (papilloma) viruses.

Pap smear a popular term for the cervical smear test. A method of screening women for the earliest signs of cancer of the neck (cervix) of the womb. A wooden or plastic spatula is used gently to scrape some surface cells off the inner lining of the cervix and these are then spread on a microscope slide, stained and examined by a pathologist skilled in CYTOLOGY. (George Nicholas Papanicolaou, 1884–1962, Greek-born American anatomist).

papule any small, well-defined, solid skin elevation. Papules are usually less than 1 cm in diameter and may be smooth or warty. From the Latin *papula*, a pimple.

para- *prefix denoting* alongside, beyond, apart from, resembling or disordered.

para-aminosalicylic acid (PAS) a drug formerly widely used to treat pulmonary TUBERCULOSIS but now superceded by more effective antibiotics. The drug is on the WHO official list.

paracentesis surgical puncturing of a body cavity with a needle for the purpose of removing fluid. This may be done either to obtain a sample for diagnostic purposes or to relieve symptoms caused by excessive fluid accumulation.

paracetamol a drug widely used to relieve pain and reduce fever. The drug does not irritate the stomach, as ASPIRIN does, but overdose causes liver and kidney damage and may cause death from liver failure. 15 g or more is potentially serious. The victim remains well for a day or two and liver failure develops between the third and fifth day. The drug is on the WHO official list. Brand names are Alvedon, Calpol Disprol Paediatric, Infadrops, Medinol and Salzone. Preparations that include paracetamol include Cosalgesic, Distalgesic, Domperamol, Fortagesic, Kapake, Midrid, Migraleve, Paradote, Paramax, Remedeine and Solpadol.

paracrine pertaining to the chemical transmission of information through an intercellular space. Compare ENDOCRINE and EXOCRINE.

Paradex a brand name for a mixture of DEXTROPROPOXYPHENE and PARACETAMOL.

paradigm 1 a human being's mental model of the world, which may or may not conform to that of others but is often stereotypical.
2 in the philosophy of science, a general conception of the nature of scientific operation within which a particular scientific activity is undertaken. Paradigms are, of their nature, persistent and hard to change. Major advances in science – such, for instance, as the realization of the concept of the quantum or the significance of evolution in medicine – involve painful paradigmic shifts which some people, notably the older scientists, find hard to make.

Paradote a brand name for METHIONINE in combination with paracetamol as an antidote.

paradoxical chest movement an apparent inward movement of part of the chest wall on inspiration that may occur as a result of extensive rib fractures and a collapsed underlying lung.

paradoxical embolus an EMBOLUS arising in a vein which is able to reach the general (systemic) arterial circulation by passing through a defect in the inner wall of the heart, such as a PERSISTENT FORAMEN OVALE, to reach the left side.

paraesthesia numbness or tingling of the skin. 'Pins-and-needles' sensation.

paraffinoma a tumour-like swelling caused by an inflammatory reaction to prolonged exposure to paraffin, including liquid paraffin.

paragonimiasis infection, usually of the lungs, with the fluke parasite *Paragonimus westermani* usually acquired by eating raw crabs or crayfish. The condition is commonest in south-east Asia.

parainfluenza an infection with a parainfluenza virus. This is usually no more than a common cold, but sometimes parainfluenza viruses cause serious illnesses featuring CROUP and PNEUMONIA.

paraldehyde a rapidly acting drug used by injection to control severe excitement, delirium, mania or convulsions.

paralexia a disorder causing great difficulty in reading aloud and featuring transposition of words or substitution of meaningless sounds for some words or syllables.

Paralgin a brand name for the painkiller PARACETAMOL.

paralysis temporary or permanent loss of the power of movement of a part of the body (motor function). Paralysis may be due to damage to the nerves tracts or peripheral nerves carrying motor impulses to the muscles to cause them to contract or may be due to disorders of the muscles themselves. In the former case, the damage is most commonly within the brain or the spinal cord. Paralysis of one half of the body is called HEMIPLEGIA. Paralysis of the legs and lower part of the body is called PARAPLEGIA. Paralysis of all four limbs is called QUADRIPLEGIA.

paralysis agitans an alternative term for PARKINSON'S DISEASE.

Paramax a brand name for METOCLOPRAMIDE formulated with paracetamol.

paramedic any health-care worker other than

a doctor, nurse, or dentist. The ranks of the paramedics include trained ambulance personnel, first aiders, laboratory technicians, PHYSIOTHERAPISTS, OCCUPATIONAL THERAPISTS, ORTHOPTISTS and RADIOGRAPHERS. See also PROFESSIONS ALLIED TO MEDICINE.

parametric of data that are normally distributed, the distribution curve being symmetrically bell-shaped. Data that are not normally distributed are said to be skewed and the bell shape of the curve is distorted.

parametric test a test or trial that depends on the assumption that the date involved are normally distributed.

parametrium the connective tissue lying between the two layers of the BROAD LIGAMENT of the womb and separating the CERVIX from the bladder.

parametritis inflammation of the PARAMETRIUM.

paramnesia a memory disturbance in which fantasy is recollected as experience. Paramnesia often has elements of DEJA VU.

paramyxoviruses a family of viruses resembling the myxoviruses and responsible for causing PARAINFLUENZA, MUMPS, MEASLES and respiratory syncytial disease in infants.

paranaesthesia anaesthesia of the body below the level of the waist. Compare PARAPLEGIA.

paraneoplastic syndromes syndromes caused by the secretion into the blood of the products of cancers, usually polypeptide hormones, which affect parts remote from the tumours. Thus, lung cancers can secrete ANTIDIURETIC HORMONE or ACTH and cause confusing effects.

paranoia a delusional state or system of DELUSIONS, usually involving the conviction of persecution, in which intelligence and reasoning capacity, within the context of the delusional system, are unimpaired. HALLUCINATIONS or other mental disturbances do not occur. Less commonly there may be delusions of grandeur, of the love of some notable person, of grounds for sexual jealousy or of bodily deformity, odour or parasitization. Many hypotheses have been advanced to explain paranoia, but the cause is unknown. Because the delusional state usually provides the subject with essential psychological sustenance, treatment is very difficult.

paranomia a form of APHASIA in which objects or people are incorrectly named.

paraparesis partial paralysis of both legs and sometimes of the lower part of the trunk.

paraphasia a DYSPHASIA in which speech is fluent but often meaningless or irrelevant and contains incorrectly substituted words. This is a feature of Wernicke's dysphasia.

paraphilia any deviation from what is currently deemed to be normal sexual behaviour or preference. Thus, paraphilia may include BESTIALITY, EXHIBITIONISM, FETISHISM, HOMOSEXUALITY, MASOCHISM, PAEDOPHILIA, SADISM, TRANSVESTISM AND VOYEURISM.

paraphimosis constriction of the neck of the bulb (GLANS) of the penis, following retraction of a very tight foreskin (PREPUCE), of such degree as to interfere with the return of blood by the veins. The gland and prepuce become greatly swollen and the condition worsens. Treatment involves compressing the glans so that the prepuce can be pulled forward. This may be assisted by injection of an enzyme, hyaluronidase, to aid the dispersion of OEDEMA fluid. Later CIRCUMCISION is indicated.

paraphrenia a well-organized system of paranoid delusions affecting elderly people. The personality is relatively unaffected and there is little in the way of mood disorder. Hallucinations may or may not be present. Many psychiatrists, notably in the USA, make no distinction between paraphrenia and late-onset paranoid SCHIZOPHRENIA.

paraplegia paralysis of both lower limbs. Paraplegia caused by damage to the spinal cord is also associated with paralysis of the lower part of the trunk and loss of normal voluntary bladder and bowel control. In spastic paraplegia there is constant tension in the affected muscles often leading to fixed deformities. In flaccid paraplegia the muscles remain limp. Paraplegia may be hereditary or caused by birth injury, injury or disease of the brain or spinal cord or sometimes the peripheral nerves, as in alcoholic or dietary polyneuropathy, or by HYSTERIA or old age. See also PARAPARESIS.

paraplegic walking the use of various methods of leg splinting with passive movement powered by the arms, sometimes assisted by electrical stimulation of paralysed muscles, so as to achieve a form of walking movement for paraplegic people. The method is still experimental.

paraprotein an abnormal plasma protein such as the MONOCLONAL ANTIBODY in MULTIPLE MYELOMA.

parapsychology the attempted study, by scientific methods, of a range of real or imagined phenomena not explicable by science. The subjects of parapsychology include EXTRASENSORY PERCEPTION, telepathy, clairvoyance, spoon-bending and the movement of objects without physical force (telekinesis). The history of science has been a long and painful struggle to escape from the realms of magical thinking and superstition and many scientists are concerned at the possible dangers of conferring a kind of respectability and plausibility on matters which they consider to be without scientific basis.

paraquat a highly poisonous defoliant weedkiller that can cause progressive lung damage, respiratory failure and kidney failure. The poison can be absorbed through the skin. Charcoal or Fuller's earth are useful antidotes.

parasitaemia the presence of parasites in the blood.

parasite an organism that lives on or in the body of another living organism, and depends on it for nutrition and protection. Ectoparasites live on the surface, endoparasites live inside. Parasites do not contribute to the host's welfare and are often harmful. Human parasites, which cause thousands of diseases, include VIRUSES, BACTERIA, FUNGI, PROTOZOA, WORMS, FLUKES, TICKS, LICE, BUGS, some burrowing FLIES and LEECHES.

parasiticide any agent that kills PARASITES.

parasitology the study of organisms which use other organisms as their living environment. Medical parasitology is concerned mainly with the larger, usually visible, parasites of humans such as the various worms and the external parasites (ectoparasites). Bacteria, viruses and protozoa, although parasites, are so important as to require separate disciplines and are not normally included in medical parasitology.

Paraspen a brand name for the painkiller PARACETAMOL.

parasuicide an apparent attempt at suicide, usually by self-poisoning, in which the intent is to draw attention to a major personal problem rather than to cause death.

parasympathetic nervous system one of the two divisions of the AUTONOMIC NERVOUS SYSTEM. The parasympathetic system leaves the central nervous system in the 3rd, 7th, 9th and 10th CRANIAL NERVES and from the 2nd to the 4th SACRAL segments of the spinal cord. Parasympathetic action constricts the pupils of the eyes, promotes salivation and tearing, slows the heart, constricts the BRONCHI, increases the activity of the intestines, contracts the bladder wall and relaxes the SPHINCTERS and promotes erection of the penis. See also SYMPATHETIC NERVOUS SYSTEM.

parasympathomimetic any effect similar to that produced by stimulation of the parasympathetic nervous system, especially the effect of CHOLINERGIC drugs. See also SYMPATHOMIMETIC.

parathion a highly poisonous organo-phosphorous, cholinesterase inhibitor, agricultural insecticide. See also ORGANO-PHOSPHOROUS POISONING.

parathyroidectomy removal of one or more PARATHYROID GLANDS. This may be necessary in the condition of hyperparathyroidism.

parathyroid glands four, yellow, bean-shaped bodies, each about 0.5 cm long, lying behind the THYROID GLAND, usually embedded in its capsule. The parathyroids secrete a hormone, parathyroid hormone (parathormone or PTH), into the blood if the level of calcium in the blood drops. This hormone promotes the release of calcium from the bones, controls loss in the urine and increases absorption from the intestine, thus correcting the deficiency in the blood. Maintenance of accurate levels of blood calcium is more important, physiologically, than the strength of the bones. Secretion of abnormal quantities of PTH from a parathyroid tumour can lead to bone softening. Underaction of the parathyroids causes a dangerous drop in the blood calcium.

paratyphoid fever an infectious disease, closely similar to but milder than, TYPHOID. It is caused by the organism *Salmonella paratyphi* and is spread in the same ways as *Salmonella typhi*.

parecoxib a pro-drug of the cyclo-oxygenase-2 (COX-2) inhibitor VALDECOXIB and is used to relieve post-operative pain. A brand name is Dynastat.

parenchyme parenchyma, the functional tissue of an organ, as distinct from its purely structural elements.

parenchymal pertaining to, or resembling, the functional elements of an organ or tissue, rather than to its structural parts (matrix).

parenchymal jaundice JAUNDICE due to liver cell damage rather than to mechanical obstruction to the passage of the bile.

parenteral of drugs or nutrients, taken or given by any route other than by the alimentary canal. Parenteral routes include the intramuscular and the intravenous.

parenteral nutrition intravenous feeding. This is required when the normal (enteral) route cannot be used. Early attempts at intravenous feeding via peripheral veins invariably led to severe THROMBOPHLEBITIS within a matter of hours because of the strong sugar solutions used. A central venous cannula had therefore to be used. Developments in design of cannulas and new feeding solutions, with calorie-rich lipids in place of strong sugar concentrations, amino acids and weaker carbohydrates may, it is hoped, allow safe peripheral vein feeding.

parenting the process of caring for, nurturing and upbringing of a child.

paresis WEAKNESS or reduction in muscle power, as compared with complete PARALYSIS.

parietal pertaining to the wall or outer surface of a part of the body. From Latin *parietem*, a wall or partition.

parietal bone one of two large bones of the vault of the skull lying between the FRONTAL and OCCIPITAL bones on either side and forming the sides and top.

parietal cells large cells in the lining of the stomach that secrete hydrochloric acid. Also known as oxyntic cells.

parietal lobe the major lobe in each half of the brain (cerebral hemisphere) that lies under each parietal bone.

Parkinsonism an obsolescent term for PARKINSON'S DISEASE of known causation.

Parkinson's disease a SYNDROME featuring involuntary tremor of the hands with 'pill-rolling' finger movements, muscle rigidity and slowness of movements. The face becomes mask-like, the speech slow and the voice quiet and monotonous. Hand-writing becomes minute. There is difficulty in starting to walk and a tendency for the body to incline forwards. Steps are short and tottering, as if the affected person were falling forwards. Cognitive loss and psychiatric changes may occur. Parkinson's disease affects about 1 person in 100 over age 60 and becomes progressively more common with advancing age. It is due to brain changes in the area of the connections between the SUBSTANTIA NIGRA and the CORPUS STRIATUM, with loss of pigment and dopamine-producing cells. There are intraneuronal Lewy bodies. It may be a side effect of certain drugs, such as various phenothiazine or designer drugs or the effects of various poisons such as carbon monoxide. It may be caused by brain tumours, ENCEPHALITIS and repeated head injuries, as from boxing. In 2% of cases there is a mutation in the gene LRRK2 that codes for the protein dardarin, and this mutation is present in 5% of familial cases and 7% of autosomal dominant disease. Most cases remain idiopathic. Treatment is by dopamine replacement using the drug levodopa and other drugs which stimulate dopamine receptors in the brain. Unilateral pallidotomy may be useful in some cases. The status of fetal cell implantation treatment remains uncertain. Also known as paralysis agitans. (James Parkinson, 1755–1824, London physician).

Parlodel a brand name for BROMOCRIPTINE.

paronychia infection of the skin fold at the base or side of the nail. Acute paronychia is usually caused by common bacteria such as *Staphylococci* and often progresses to abscess formation. Persistent (chronic) paronychia is usually caused by the thrush yeast fungus *Candida albicans*.

parotid glands the largest of the three pairs of SALIVARY GLANDS. Each parotid is situated over the angle of the jaw, below and in front of the lower half of the ear and has a duct running forward through the cheek to open on the inside of the mouth at about the level of the upper molar teeth.

parotid gland disorders see MIXED SALIVARY TUMOUR, MUMPS, PAROTITIS and SJOGREN'S SYNDROME.

parotitis inflammation of the parotid glands, usually as a feature of MUMPS.

paroxetine a SEROTONIN RE-UPTAKE INHIBITOR drug. A brand name is Seroxat.

paroxysm 1 a sudden attack, such as a seizure, convulsion or spasm.
2 a sudden worsening of a disorder.

paroxysmal nocturnal haemoglobinuria a rare disease featuring episodic HAEMOLYSIS that occurs during the night when a decline in the pH of the blood triggers activation of complement components. The release of haemoglobin into the blood causes the morning urine to be black. The condition also features thrombosis and this may involve the hepatic vein causing the BUDD-CHIARI SYNDROME.

paroxysmal tachycardia a heart disorder featuring apparently spontaneous episodes of rapid heartbeat, in excess of 100 per minute. The condition may be caused by drugs, anaemia, HEART FAILURE, thyroid gland over-activity and conduction defects within the heart.

Parstelin a brand name for a mixture of TRANYLCYPROMINE and TRIFLUOPERAZINE.

parthenogenesis the development of an unfertilized egg into an adult organism. Virgin birth. This occurs naturally in bees and ants and in some animal species development of an ovum can be induced chemically or by pricking with a fine glass fibre. The result is a clone of the mother cell identical in all respects. Only females can be produced by parthenogenesis, as no Y chromosome is present. If achieved, human parthenogenesis would make men biologically redundant. Very early human embryos derived only from ova have been produced experimentally by a parthenogenetic technique using chemicals that changed the concentration of ions in the ova.

partial-birth abortion an abortion in which a live fetus is partially delivered but is then killed before the delivery is completed. The concept has aroused fierce controversy as the procedure is considered by many to be indistinguishable from infanticide. It is, however, performed only when it is medically necessary to protect the life or health of the mother and, in such cases, is usually protected by law.

partial beta-agonists cardio-selective beta-blocking drugs used to treat mild to moderate hypertension. An examples is celiprolol (Celectol).

partial opioid agonists drugs used for the short-term relief of moderate pain. An example is meptazinol (Meptid).partially selective beta-agonists,

partial reinforcement the process of inter-mittently re-strengthening of a CONDITIONED REFLEX by repetition of the association between the unconditioned and the conditioned stimuli.

Partobulin a brand name for ANTI-D IMMUNOGLOBULIN.

parturition the process of giving birth.

parrot fever PSITTACOSIS.

parulis a gumboil. An abscess in the tooth socket.

parvoviruses a family of viruses that cause RUBELLA-like illnesses, transient joint pain and, in sickle cell disease, a failure of production of blood cells. Parvovirus B19 enjoys worldwide infectivity by droplet and has been spread in blood products. It causes Fifth disease, arthralgia and inflammatory arthritis, transient aplasia of red blood cells, miscarriage and hydrops fetalis. IMMUNOGLOBULINS are an effective treatment.

passive euthanasia a form of euthanasia in which medical treatment that could keep a dying patient alive for a time is withdrawn.

passive immunity immunity, especially to specific infections, resulting from the acquisition of ANTIBODIES, either by injection or by transfer through the PLACENTA or ingestion in the breast milk.

passive smoking inhaling cigarette smoke exhaled by others. It has been shown that the rate of lung cancer in non-smokers rises significantly if they are regularly exposed to other people's cigarette smoke. At least 10 separate studies have shown an increase of up to 30% in the risk of lung cancer among non-smokers living with smokers, compared with non-smokers living with non-smokers.

passive transport the movement of dissolved material through a biological membrane in the direction of fluid flow and without the expenditure of energy. Compare ACTIVE TRANSPORT.

pasteurization a method of destroying infective micro-organisms in milk and other liquid foods. The liquid is rapidly heated to about 78 °C and maintained at that temperature for fifteen seconds. It is then rapidly cooled to below 10 °C. (Louis Pasteur, 1822–1895, French pioneer of bacteriology).

past-pointing a physical sign in disease of the CEREBELLUM in which, if the eyes are closed, a pointing finger overshoots its intended mark towards the side of the cerebellar damage.

patella the knee cap. The patella is a large triangular SESAMOID bone lying on front of the knee joint within the tendon of the QUADRICEPS FEMORIS group of muscles.

patella disorders see CHONDROMALACIA PATELLAE and OSGOOD-SCHLATTER'S DISEASE.

patent 1 open or unobstructed.

2 a term still sometimes applied to proprietary medication, as in patent medicine. From Latin *patent*, open.

patent ductus arteriosus a congenital heart defect in which the ductus arteriosus, which, during fetal life allows blood to bypass the lungs, fails to close at or soon after birth. The ductus arteriosus lies between the AORTA and the PULMONARY ARTERY. Persistent patency is often of minor degree. The result of a widely patent ductus may be inadequate oxygenation of the blood with breathlessness and strain on the heart which has to work harder than normal to provide an adequately oxygenated circulation. Treatment, if necessary, is initiated by use of the drug indomethacin (indometacin). If this fails, the abnormally retained connection may be tied off.

patent foramen ovale persistence of the normal fetal opening in the internal wall of the heart (the FORAMEN OVALE) after birth.

paternity tests tests designed to confirm or deny the claim that a man is the father of a particular child. When the man is not the father, this can be confirmed by normal blood-grouping tests in 97% of cases. Blood-group and tissue typing (HLA) tests cannot prove that a particular man is the father, but they can offer strong supportive evidence. Genetic finger-printing can prove paternity beyond any doubt.

pathergy the appearance of a papular or pustular lesion around a point on the skin at which a sterile substance was injected 24 to 48 hours before.

pathogen any agent that causes disease, especially a micro-organism.

pathogenesis the mechanisms involved in the development of disease. Compare AETIOLOGY.

pathogenic able to cause disease.

pathognomonic of a symptom or physical sign that is so uniquely characteristic of a particular disease as to establish the diagnosis.

pathological pertaining to disease or to the study of disease (PATHOLOGY).

pathological gambling an addiction to the state of excitement experienced while gambling. There is progressive preoccupation with betting and a need to increase the size of wagers to achieve the desired mental effect. The syndrome includes lying to conceal losses, stealing and rationalising the theft as temporary borrowing. If gambling is prevented there is irritability, restlessness and even physical symptoms.

pathology the branch of medical science dealing with bodily disease processes, their causes, and their effects on body structure and function. Subspecialties in pathology include morbid anatomy, histopathology, haematology and clinical chemistry. Practitioners of forensic pathology apply all these disciplines to criminal investigation. The list that follows highlights the key entries related to pathology in the dictionary: abscess, adenoma, adhesion, agenesis, arteritis, amyloid, anaplasia, aneurysm, aplasia, antibody, apoptosis, atelectasis, atheroma, atherosclerosis, atopy, atrophy, autoimmunity, autopsy, benign, calcification, callus, carcinogenesis, carcinoma, cancer, cellulitis, chronic, coarctation, cyst, degeneration, demyelination, ectasia, erythema, exudate, fibrosis, fistula, free radicals, granuloma, haematology, histopathology, hyaline, hypertrophy, inflammation, keratosis, lesions, malignant, metastasis, morbib anatomy, papilloma, phagocyte, polyp, pus, rejection, septic, teratoma, ulcer, virulence.

pathophysiology the discipline concerned with the effects of disease on body function.

-pathy *suffix denoting* perception, feeling or suffering.

patient-controlled analgesia a method of pain control in which the patient cooperates. An intravenous drip is set up and the patient has a small control unit with a button which, when pressed, inserts a small dose of a drug such as morphine, into the infusion fluid. Overdosage cannot occur. A disadvantage is the need to urinate at frequent intervals.

patient's charter a document produced by the Department of Health in 1992, and revised in 1995, that affirms the Government's acknowledgement of certain rights for patients (see PATIENTS' RIGHTS) and its expectations of the achieving of certain standards in patient care. The charter deals with such matters as waiting list times for surgery; waiting times for outpatient appointments after referral; waiting times in routine clinics and in Accident and Emergency Departments; waiting times for provision of a bed after a decision to admit to hospital.

patients' rights the entitlement of patients, especially those in hospital, to considerate and respectful care, to information about what is being done to them or what is proposed and to knowledge of the diagnosis and probable outlook (prognosis). Patients are especially entitled to all information necessary to enable them to give informed consent to any surgical operation or other form of treatment, especially if associated with risk. Patients have a right to refuse treatment and to be informed of the probable consequences. They are entitled to privacy and confidentiality over their medical details and may not be included in any form of medical trial or experiment without their full knowledge and consent. Patients may discharge themselves from hospital at any time, but may be required to sign a document to the effect that they understand the possible consequences.

Paul-Bunnell test a test for antibody to sheep's red blood cells that is specific for glandular fever (INFECTIOUS MONONUCLEOSIS) (John Rodman Paul, American physician, b. 1893; and Walls Willard Bunnell, 1902–66, American physician).

patulous spreading apart or expanded.

Pavacol-D a brand name for PHOLCODINE.

PC *abbrev. for* Pharmaceutical Chemist.

PCO₂ the concentration of carbon dioxide in the blood. This is a sensitive indication of the efficiency or level of ventilation of the lungs. Hyperventilation causes a drop in PCO_2; underventilation causes a rise.

PCR *abbrev. for* POLYMERASE CHAIN REACTION.

PDA *abbrev. for* PERSONAL DIGITAL ASSISTANT.

peak expiratory flow measurement a test widely used to determine the presence, and assess the degree, of any kind of obstruction to the air passages. The method is especially valuable in the assessment of ASTHMA and chronic BRONCHITIS and of the response to treatment. The instrument used is called a peak flow meter and this measures the maximum flow rate of air on the strongest possible forced expiration through a wide nozzle. See also FORCED EXPIRATORY VOLUME.

peanut allergy an often severe form of ALLERGY in which up to one-third of sufferers experience ANAPHYLAXIS. Peanut allergy is not more common than other food allergies, all of which are rare, affecting about 1 person in 100,000 per year. It is becoming commoner, however, and is liable to be more severe than most, and is especially dangerous in asthmatic children. Peanut proteins may be found in such diverse foodstuffs as chocolate spread and scotch eggs. The allergy has been shown to be significantly associated with intake of soya milk or soya formula and with the use of skin preparations containing peanut oil. The increasing incidence is thought to be due to unduly early exposure of babies to peanut butter after weaning.

Pearson's syndrome a severe MITOCHONDRIAL DNA disease caused by high levels of rearrangement of mtDNA in all tissues. The syndrome features sideroblastic anaemia, lactic acidosis or liver dysfunction, or both, and the possibility to progress to the KEARNS-SAYRE PHENOTYPE.

peau d'orange an orange-skin-like dimpling of an area of the skin, affecting especially the breast and caused by LYMPHOEDEMA occurring in certain kinds of cancer.

pectinate having teeth like a comb.

pectoral muscles the group of muscles, consisting of the pectoralis major and minor on either side, covering the upper ribs on either side of the front of the chest. The pectoral muscles help to control the shoulder-blade (scapula) and, through it, to move the arm forward and down, and, acting directly on the arm, to pull it towards the body.

pederasty anal intercourse, especially with a boy.

pediculosis any kind of louse infestation.

pedigree a family tree, showing the members who have suffered from hereditary disorder, prepared for purposes of genetic diagnosis and research.

peduncle a stalk-like bundle of fibres, especially nerve fibres that connects different parts of the central nervous system.

pedunculated on a stalk. Compare with SESSILE.

PEEP *abbrev. for* positive end-expiratory pressure. This is a method of mechanical ventilation, for people with respiratory failure or adult RESPIRATORY DISTRESS SYNDROME, used to try to maintain adequate oxygenation of the blood.

peeping Tom a person who derives sexual

pleasure and arousal from secretly watching others in a state of undress or engaged in sexual activity. A voyeur. The term derives from the legend of Tom the tailor of Coventry who was the only person to look at the naked Lady Godiva, and lived to regret it, being instantly struck blind. See also VOYEURISM.

pegfilgastrim a drug used to treat low white cell counts (NEUTROPENIA) resulting from cancer treatment with cytotoxic drugs. Pegfilgastrim is human granulocyte colony stimulating factor (G-CSF) produced by recombinant DNA technology. A brand name is Neulasta.

pegvisomant an analogue of human growth hormone that has been genetically-modified to act as a growth hormone antagonist. The hormone is produced by an *E. coli* recombinant DNA method. The drug is highly selective for the growth hormone receptor and is used to treat ACROMEGALY in patients who have responded inadequately to surgery or radiation.

Pel-Ebstein fever a fever occurring in episodes lasting for a few days and separated by intervals of days or weeks. This type of fever is said to be a feature of Hodgkin's disease. (Pieter Klasses Pel, 1852–1919, Dutch physician; and Wilhelm Ebstein, 1836–1912, German physician).

pellagra a disease caused by deficiency of the B vitamin NIACIN. It may occur in alcoholics who derive their entire caloric needs from alcohol. The disease features DIARRHOEA, a sunburn-like blistering and cracking skin disorder (dermatitis) and, in severe cases, brain involvement leading to delirium and eventual DEMENTIA. Pellagra responds dramatically to niacin by mouth or injection often within a day or two.

pelvic examination direct examination of a woman's external genitalia and manual examination of the internal pelvic organs, via the vagina or sometimes the rectum.

pelvic girdle the ring of bones at the lower end of the spine with which the legs articulate. Compare shoulder girdle. See also PELVIS.

pelvic infection infection of the organs in the pelvis, especially the reproductive organs of the female. Pelvic infection in the female commonly results in blockage of the Fallopian tubes and sterility.

pelvic inflammatory disease persistent infection of the internal reproductive organs

of the female. This may be due to a sexually transmitted disease or may follow childbirth or an ABORTION.

pelvimetry the measurement or assessment of the outlet of the female pelvis. This is done so as to anticipate possible difficulty in delivery of the baby.

pelvis 1 the basin-like bony girdle at the lower end of the spine with which the legs articulate. The pelvis consists of the SACRUM and COCCYX, behind, and the INNOMINATE bones on either side. Each innominate bone is made up of three bones – the pubis, the ilium and the ischium. **2** any funnel-shaped structure such as the pelvis of the kidney.

pemphigoid a rare, persistent, autoimmune skin disease featuring large blisters that are sometimes intensely itchy. Compare PEMPHIGUS. Treatment is with corticosteroid or immunosuppressant drugs.

pemphigus a serious skin disease featuring blisters on the skin and mucous membranes of the mouth and sometimes the nose. These blisters may be induced by minor pressure and rupture easily, leaving raw areas that readily becoming infected. Widespread pemphigus can lead to serious functional skin loss and life-threatening infection. Treatment is with corticosteroid or other immunosuppressant drugs. These often have to be given for long periods.

Penbritin a brand name for AMPICILLIN.

penciclovir a NUCLEOSIDE ANALOGUE drug used to treat cold sores (herpes simplex infection) of the lips. A brand name is Vectavir.

pendulous hanging loosely or suspended so as to be able to swing or sway.

penetrance the frequency with which a GENE manifests its effect. Failure to do so may result from the modifying effect of other genes or from environmental influences. A single hereditable dominant or recessive characteristic is either penetrant or not. Penetrance is measured as the proportion of individuals in a population with a particular genotype who show the corresponding PHENOTYPE.

penicillamine a drug used to treat severe RHEUMATOID ARTHRITIS not responding to nonsteroidal anti-inflammatory drugs (NSAIDs). Penicillamine is a CHELATING AGENT and is also used to treat poisoning with metallic salts or disorders such as WILSON'S DISEASE. The drug is on the WHO official list. Brand names are Distamine and Pendramine.

penicillinase an enzyme present in some bacteria, especially STAPHYLOCOCCI, that inactivates penicillins, by HYDROLYSIS of the beta-lactam bond, so that the organisms possess resistance to the drug. Also known as beta-lactamase.

penicillins an important group of antibiotic drugs. The original natural penicillin was derived from the mould *Penicillium notatum* but the extensive range of penicillins in use nowadays is produced synthetically. The original penicillins was penicillin G (Crystapen), which had to be given by injection. This was followed by the phenoxymethyl derivative, penicillin V, which could be taken by mouth. The semisynthetic penicillins followed from the discovery that 6-aminopenicillanic acid could be obtained from cultures of *Penicillium chrysogenum*. The penicillin molecule contains a beta-lactam ring and many organisms produce an enzyme, beta-lactamase, that can inactivate the drug by breaking this ring. Side chains are added to the basic molecule to try to frustrate the action of this enzyme. Penicillins act by interfering with the synthesis of the walls of bacteria.

Penicillium one of a range of common blue-green moulds of the genus *Penicillium*, that grow on decaying fruits and ripening cheese. *Penicillium* species such as *P. notatum* and *P. rubrum* were originally studied by Fleming in investigating the properties of the antibiotic penicillin. (Alexander Fleming, 1881–1955, Scottish bacteriologist).

penile implant one of a range of prostheses inserted into the penis so that men suffering from organic impotence can achieve a form of erection and enjoy sexual intercourse.

penile warts fleshy, cauliflower-like warts occurring on the penis as a result of a sexually transmitted PAPILLOMAVIRUS infection.

penis the male organ of copulation containing the URETHRA through which urine and seminal fluid pass. The normally flaccid penis becomes enlarged and erect by virtue of three longitudinal cylindrical bodies of spongy tissue into which blood can flow under pressure under the influence of sexual excitement or other stimuli. One of these bodies, the corpus spongiosum, surrounds the urethra. The other

two, the corpora cavernosa, lie side by side above the corpus spongiosum. Erection physiology is mediated partly by nitric oxide.

penis disorders see BALANITIS, HYPOSPADIAS, IMPOTENCE, PARAPHIMOSIS, PENILE WARTS, PEYRONIE'S DISEASE, PHIMOSIS and PSEUDOHERMAPHRODITISM.

penis envy the Freudian concept that all women have a repressed wish to have a penis and resent the fact that they are incomplete men. The idea is no longer taken seriously.

pentaerythitol tetranitrate a drug used to relieve the symptoms of ANGINA PECTORIS. A brand name is Mycardol.

Pentacarinat a brand name for PENTAMIDINE.

pentagastrin test a test of the acid production by the stomach. An injection of a synthetic pentapeptide substance, pentagastrin is given, and an hour later the fasting stomach contents are withdrawn through a nasogastric tube.

pentamidine a drug used in the treatment of PNEUMOCYSTIS CARINII PNEUMONIA and TRYPANOSOMIASIS. It was the exceptional demand for pentamidine in 1981 that heralded the onset of the AIDS pandemic. The drug is on the WHO official list. A brand name is Pentacarinat.

Pentasa a brand name for MESALAZINE.

pentazocine a synthetic painkilling drug with actions similar to those of MORPHINE. A brand name is Fortral.

pentose a sugar with five carbon atoms in each molecule. The 'backbone' of DNA on each side of the helix consists of a chain of pentose sugars alternating with phosphate groups. The sugar in DNA is 2-deoxyribose, and in RNA is ribose. The NUCLEOTIDE chain is formed by linking the 5´ position of one pentose ring to the 3´ position on the next via a phosphate group. 5´ and 3´ are used to indicate the ends of a DNA fragment and the directions in which the 'backbones' run.

pentostatin an ADENOSINE DEAMINASE INHIBITOR anticancer drug. A brand name is Nipent.

pentosuria a benign autosomal recessive disease in which more than a gram of a pentose sugar, L-xylulose, is excreted in the urine daily. The disease, which is due to a defect in the enzyme NADP-xylitol dehydrogenase, is largely limited to Ashkenazi Jews. The condition is harmless except that the urine sugar may lead to an incorrect diagnosis of DIABETES.

Pentothal the former brand name for the rapid-acting barbiturate drug THIOPENTONE SODIUM (thiopental) commonly used to induce general anaesthesia. The drug is now known as Intraval.

pepsin a digestive ENZYME whose precursor PEPSINOGEN is secreted by cells in the stomach lining. Pepsin breaks down protein to PEPTIDES. See also PEPTIDASE.

pepsinogen a biochemically inert substance produced by the cells of the stomach lining (gastric mucosa) that is converted to PEPSIN by the action of hydrochloric acid.

peptic ulcer an area on the inner mucosal surface of the STOMACH, DUODENUM or OESOPHAGUS in which stomach acid and digestive ENZYMES have acted as to erode the surface and expose the underlying layers of muscle. Infection with *Helicobacter pylori* organisms is important, especially in the case of duodenal ulcer. In extreme cases perforation occurs. Peptic ulcers are treated by eradication of *H. pylori* with METRONIZADOLE or clarithromycin and the use of proton pump inhibitor drugs such as OMEPRAZOLE or HISTAMINE receptor blocker drugs such as CIMETIDINE or RANITIDINE (Zantac) which reduce acid production. Sometimes a protective drug such as sucralfate may be used. See also ZOLLINGER-ELLISON SYNDROME.

peptidase an enzyme that hydrolyses (see HYDROLYSIS) protein fragments (PEPTIDES), breaking them down to AMINO ACIDS.

peptide a chain of two or more AMINO ACIDS linked by peptide bonds between the amino and carboxyl groups of adjacent acids. Large peptides, containing many amino acids, are called polypeptides. Chains of linked polypeptides, are called PROTEINS. Peptides occur widely in the body. Many HORMONES are peptides.

peptide antibiotics a class of antibiotics that rapidly kill bacteria by the disruption of their membranes. Gramicidin and polymyxin have been available for many years for external use but thousand of new compounds in this class of cationic peptides are being tested.

peptide bond a covalent bond formed between amino acids during protein synthesis. The OH- on a carbon atom links with the H- on a nitrogen atom to form a water molecule which is given off as each peptide bond is formed.

Amino acids linked by peptide bonds form dipeptides, tripeptides or polypeptides.

peptide YY$_{3-36}$, PYY an intestinal hormone fragment that is produced during digestion and passes to the hypothalamus to signal satiety. When given by intravenous injection it reduces appetite and food intake for about 12 hours. Research has shown that obese people have much lower levels of PYY$_{3-36}$ than non-obese people.

peptidyl transferase the enzyme that catalyzes the formation of PEPTIDE BONDS during the synthesis of a polypeptide (translation).

peptones various protein derivatives obtained by acid or enzyme HYDROLYSIS of protein and used as nutrients or culture media.

percentile one of 100 equal parts in an ordered sequence of statistical data. Thus, for instance, the 93rd percentile is the value that equals 93% of those in the series. If a value in a range of values falls in the 20th percentile, there are 19 lower and 80 higher. The method is widely used to record and check such parameters as the extent of body growth at a particular age.

perception the reception, selection, organization and interpretation of sensory data. Perception is greatly influenced by previous experience and the stored data accumulated from such experience.

percussion a technique used in examining the chest or the abdomen. A finger of one hand is pressed firmly on the part and tapped briskly with a finger of the other hand. The quality or resonance of the sound produced indicates whether the underlying area is air-filled, fluid-filled or solid.

percutaneous through the skin, especially in relation to the use of needles, CANNULAS or CATHETERS inserted for any purpose.

percutaneous coronary angioplasty the correction of narrowing or blockage of a branch of a coronary artery by means of a balloon catheter passed through the skin and into an artery, along which it is threaded to the site of the procedure.

percutaneous transluminal renal angioplasty a treatment for narrowing of the artery supplying the kidney with blood (the renal artery) of such a degree that the function of the kidney is prejudiced. The widening of the artery is achieved by means of a balloon catheter similar in design to those used in the coronary artery. Recoil narrowing can be prevented by means of a STENT.

percutaneous transtracheal ventilation an emergency, life-saving means of providing an oxygen supply using a 16 gauge plastic catheter sheathed needle and positive pressure ventilation. The catheter needle is passed directly through the skin in the middle of the front of the neck until the catheter is in the windpipe. The needle is then withdrawn and the positive pressure machine connected to the catheter.

Percutol a brand name for GLYCERYL TRINITRATE in a formulation for absorption through the skin.

Perfan a brand name for ENOXIMONE.

perforation a hole through the full thickness of the wall of an organ or tissue made by disease, injury or deliberate surgical act.

perforin a molecule produced by cytotoxic T cells and natural killer cells which forms a pore in the membrane of the attacked cell resulting in LYSIS and cell death. A similar process can be brought about by COMPLEMENT.

perfusion 1 the passage of blood or other fluids through the body.
2 the effectiveness with which a part, such as the brain, is supplied with blood.

pergolide a drug that simulates the action of dopamine and is used to treat PARKINSON'S DISEASE. A brand name is Celance.

Pergonal a brand name for MENOTROPHIN.

peri- *prefix denoting* round about, surrounding.

Periactin a brand name for CYPROHEPTADINE.

periadenitis inflammation of the tissues around a gland or a lymph node.

periarteritis inflammation of the outer coat of an artery and of the surrounding tissues.

periarteritis nodosa see POLYARTERITIS NODOSA.

pericarditis inflammation of the membranous bag surrounding the heart (the PERICARDIUM). Pericarditis may be associated with an accumulation of fluid (pericardial effusion) in the pericardial sac or with adhesions between the layers of the sac. Either may embarrass the heart action. Treatment may involve withdrawing fluid through a needle or surgery to relieve constriction.

pericardium the double-layered membranous sac that completely envelops the heart. The inner layer is attached to the heart and the outer layer to the DIAPHRAGM and the back of the breastbone (sternum). The two layers are separated by a thin film of lubricating fluid.

pericholangitis inflammation of the biliary system in the liver.

perichondritis inflammation of the PERICHONDRIUM.

perichondrium the fibrous connective tissue that covers cartilage surfaces, apart from the bearing surfaces (articular cartilages) of joints.

pericranium the PERIOSTEUM covering the outer surface of the skull.

pericyazine a PHENOTHIAZINE DERIVATIVE drug used to treat psychotic disorders. A brand name is Neulactil.

perikaryon 1 the PROTOPLASM surrounding the nucleus of a cell.
2 the cell body of a neuron containing the nucleus.

perilymph the fluid, similar to CEREBRO-SPINAL FLUID, that lies in the space between the membranous and bony labyrinths of the internal ear.

perimetry a test, performed on each eye separately, to measure how far vision extends around the point at which the subject is looking. This is called the field of vision and it may be reduced in conditions such as GLAUCOMA or brain tumour. The eye under examination must gaze directly ahead while each observation of peripheral vision is made. Electronic devices can be used to ensure this.

perimysium a sheath of connective tissue surrounding and separating bundles of muscle fibres.

perinatal pertaining to the period immediately before and after birth. For statistical purposes, the perinatal period is defined as the period from the 28th week of pregnancy to the end of the 1st week after birth. Perinatal mortality is the number of babies born dead together with the number dying during the first week after birth.

perinatology the study of the care of the pregnant woman, the developing fetus and the new-born baby, and especially of those cases in which risk is anticipated from conditions known to endanger the life or health of the fetus or mother.

perindopril an ANGIOTENSIN CONVERTING ENZYME INHIBITOR drug used to treat HEART

FAILURE and high blood pressure (HYPERTENSION). A brand name is Coversyl.

perinephrium the connective and fatty tissue surrounding the kidney.

perineum that part of the floor of the PELVIS that lies between the tops of the thighs. In the male, the perineum lies between the anus and the scrotum. In the female, it includes the external genitalia.

perineurium a sheath of connective tissue surrounding and separating nerve fibre bundles.

period see MENSTRUAL PERIOD.

periodic fever 1 a rise of temperature occurring repeatedly at intervals.
2 an AUTOSOMAL RECESSIVE inherited condition causing recurrent attacks of fever. Also known as familial Mediterranean fever.

periodicity 1 recurring at intervals or in cycles.
2 of DNA, the number of base pairs in one complete turn of the double helix. The periodicity of DNA is about 10.

periodontal disease any disorder of the periodontium (the tissues surrounding and supporting the teeth). The most common type of periodontal disease is chronic gingivitis (inflammation of the gums), which, if untreated, leads to periodontitis (inflammation of the periodontal membranes around the base of the teeth and erosion of the bone holding the teeth).

periodontics the dental speciality concerned with the management of diseases of the PERIODONTIUM, especially GINGIVITIS and PERIODONTITIS.

periodontitis inflammation of the PERIODONTIUM. This may be centred mainly around the root of the tooth (apical periodontitis) or may be a persistent (chronic) condition affecting the whole periodontium as a complication of severe gum inflammation (gingivitis). Treatment of apical periodontitis is by drilling to drain any pus present and filling. Chronic periodontitis requires scrupulous attention to tooth hygiene, scaling, cleaning and sometimes removal of excessive gum tissue.

periodontium the layer of fibrous, supportive connective tissue between the root of the tooth and the tooth socket. For practical convenience, dentists extend this definition to include the CEMENTUM, the gum surrounding the neck of the tooth and the bone of the socket (alveolar bone).

perionychia inflammation in the tissue surrounding the nail.

periosteum the tissue that surrounds bone. Periosteum has an inner bone-forming (osteoblastic) layer, a middle fibrous layer and an outer layer containing many blood vessels and nerves.

periostitis inflammation of the PERIOSTEUM most commonly as a result of injury. There is swelling, pain and tenderness.

periotic situated around the ear.

peripheral nerve entrapment syndromes a range of disorders caused by pressure on nerves situated in confined spaces as under anatomical tunnels over bone. They include CARPAL TUNNEL SYNDROME, SATURDAY NIGHT PALSY, TARSAL TUNNEL SYNDROME and THORACIC OUTLET SYNDROME.

peripheral nervous system the entire complex of nerves that leave the confines of the brain and the spinal cord (the central nervous system) to supply the muscles, skeleton, organs and glands. The CRANIAL NERVES, the spinal nerves and the AUTONOMIC NERVOUS SYSTEM.

peripheral vascular disease disease of the major blood vessels supplying the limbs, especially diseases such as ATHEROSCLEROSIS, diabetic large vessel disease, Raynaud's disease and THROMBOANGIITIS OBLITERANS, that result in narrowing of vessels and restriction of blood supply. Advanced peripheral vascular disease tends to lead to GANGRENE and is difficult to treat. Avoidance of smoking is one of the most important measures. Arterial reconstructive surgery to bypass affected vessels or ENDARTERECTOMY may help.

periphlebitis inflammation of the outer coat of a vein (adventitia) and/or of the surrounding tissues.

peristalsis a coordinated succession of contractions and relaxations of the muscular wall of a tubular structure, such as the OESOPHAGUS, small intestine or the URETER, producing a wave-like pattern whose effect is to move the contents along.

peritoneal cavity the potential space between the layers of the PERITONEUM.

peritoneal dialysis a method of reducing the levels of waste products in the blood in cases of kidney failure, as an alternative to the use of an artificial kidney dialysis machine. Fluid is repeatedly run into the PERITONEAL CAVITY of the ABDOMEN through a CANNULA, allowed to reach equilibrium with the blood, and then removed and discarded.

peritoneoscope a LAPAROSCOPE. An ENDOSCOPE that can be passed into the peritoneal cavity through a small incision in the abdominal wall so as to allow inspection of the PERITONEUM. Gas is used to separate the loops of bowel.

peritoneum the double-layered, serum-secreting membrane that lines the inner wall of the ABDOMEN and covers, and to some extent supports, the abdominal organs. The fluid secreted by the peritoneum acts as a lubricant to allow free movement of organs such as the intestines. The peritoneum contains blood vessels, lymph vessels and nerves. From the Greek *peri*, round about, and *teinein*, to stretch.

peritonitis inflammation of the PERITONEUM. This is most commonly due to perforation of the bowel, with the release of infected material into the peritoneal cavity, and is always serious. Causes of perforation include ruptured APPENDIX, PEPTIC ULCER, DIVERTICULITIS, SALPINGITIS, CHOLECYSTITIS or SEPTICAEMIA. Treatment usually involves emergency surgery to deal with the cause and clean out any infected material, supplemented by antibiotics and fluid infusions.

peritonsillar abscess see QUINSY.

permanent teeth the 32 teeth forming the second set that begins to appear (erupt) after the shedding of the primary or 'milk' teeth at about the age of 6. The permanent tooth complement of each jaw consists of four biting teeth (incisors) at the front, flanked by two eye teeth (canines), four premolars and six grinding teeth (molars). The 'wisdom teeth' are the pair of third molars that often do not erupt until well into adult life.

perleche inflammation, with fissuring, at the angles of the mouth.

permethrin a drug used externally in a hair rinse to get rid of head lice. The drug is on the WHO official list. A brand name is Lyclear.

pernicious anaemia a condition featuring abnormal red blood cells which are larger than usual and with less than the normal amounts of HAEMOGLOBIN. Pernicious anaemia is due to a failure of absorption of vitamin B_{12} (cobalamin) which is necessary for normal DNA synthesis in the bone marrow and

elsewhere. Absorption of B_{12} requires a factor normally produced by the stomach (the intrinsic factor) and this is absent in pernicious anaemia as a result of an autoimmune inflammation of the lining of the stomach. Pernicious anaemia features tiredness, lassitude, breathlessness, PALPITATIONS, dizziness, PALLOR, a smooth, sore tongue, diarrhoea, a yellow tint in the skin, an enlarged SPLEEN, numbness in the fingers and toes and sometimes DEMENTIA. Treatment is by injections of hydroxycobalamin.

pernio see CHILBLAINS.

peroneal pertaining to the outer side of the leg or to the FIBULA.

peroneal muscular atrophy a rare genetic muscle disorder featuring wasting of the muscles of the extremities of the limbs. The foot and calf muscles waste leaving the upper muscles intact so that the legs come to resemble inverted bottles. The arms may be similarly affected. Progression is slow and although walking is affected, severe disability is rare. There is no effective treatment. Also known as Charcot-Marie-Tooth disease. (Jean-Martin Charcot, 1925–93, French neurologist; Pierre Marie, 1853–1940, anatomist, neurologist, painter, sculptor and pupil of Charcot; and Howard Henry Tooth, 1856–1926 English neurologist, who described the condition independently of the Frenchmen).

peroneus any one of the muscles that take origin from the FIBULA and are inserted into the bones of the foot. The peroneal muscles assist in walking and in everting the raised foot.

peroxisomal diseases a range of rare genetic disorders due to the absence of PEROXISOMES or their enzymes. They include Zellweger syndrome, infantile REFSUM'S DISEASE and neonatal adrenoleukodystrophy. They all feature a form of retinal degeneration (retinal dystrophy).

peroxisomes membrane-bound cell organelles containing oxidative enzymes concerned in the detoxification of various molecules and in the breakdown of fatty acids to acetyl-CoA.

perphenazine a phenothiazine derivative drug used in the treatment of SCHIZOPHRENIA and other psychotic conditions. It is also used to relieve severe vomiting and control persistent hiccups. A brand name is Fentazin.

Persantin a brand name for the antiplatelet

drug DIPYRAMIDOLE, used to prevent THROMBOSIS.

perseveration 1 the involuntary continuation or repetition of an activity, action or verbal or other response.

2 the continuing, unchanged perception of a scene for a short time after the direction of gaze has changed. This form of perseveration usually indicates organic brain damage.

persistent foramen ovale failure of the hole in the wall between the two upper chambers of the heart to close fully at birth. This opening is necessary during fetal life so that blood can bypass the lungs, but changes in pressure normally cause it to close after birth. In some cases a small opening remains, but this is usually harmless.

persistent vegetative state a condition that has proved difficult to define because of uncertainties as to the real meaning of 'consciousness', 'awareness' and 'wakefulness'. Patients in a persistent vegetative state can breathe without mechanical assistance. Heart, kidney and intestinal functions are normal and the bladder and bowels empty automatically. At times they appear to be awake. They will respond to painful stimuli by opening their eyes, moving their limbs, breathing more quickly, and occasionally grimacing. The type and degree of brain damage indicates, however, that they cannot perform any of the higher neurological or mental functions known to be essential for any mental processes or appreciation of their situation.

personal digital assistant (PDA) a light-weight, hand-held and pocketable computer that has become important in medicine as in many other strongly information-based disciplines. PDAs use the familiar Windows environment and can communicate with other PDAs using wireless or infra-red networks. They are invaluable for rapidly accessing information of all kinds including patients' records; consulting medical textbooks and medical databases; for internet access, diary, timetable and calendar purposes; and for running application software such as word processors and spreadsheets.

personality the totality of a person's mental and behavioural characteristics as modified by experience and education. Personality defines a unique, recognizable individual and is developed as a result of the interaction of the inherited elements and the life-time environment.

personality disorders a group of behaviour patterns manifesting a general failure to adapt appropriately to social conventions. Personality disorders usually result in impaired social interaction and often lead to unhappiness and occupational failure. In some cases there is insight into the problem, but many people appear unaware of anything unusual in their personalities. Personality disorders fall into different groups. Their characteristics include a consistent failure to conform to accepted standards of behaviour, eccentric or histrionic conduct, inappropriate suspiciousness, coldness of manner, narcissistic preoccupation with self, exaggerated self-importance, undue dependency on others, rigidity of habit and extreme lack of self-confidence. Attempts at treatment by counselling or behaviour therapy are seldom very successful.

personality tests tests, usually in the form of elaborate and lengthy questionnaires, that purport to classify people according to personality traits or types. They are used for psychological research and to assess suitability for various forms of employment. The value of these tests has not been established.

perspiration sweating.

Perthes' disease inflammation at the growing upper end (EPIPHYSIS) of the thigh bone (femur) probably due to interference with the blood supply in the area. Perthes' disease is commonest in children and causes pain in the thigh and groin, limping and restriction of movement at the hip joint. Treatment is by rest and splinting and occasionally surgery. (Georg Clemen Perthes, 1869–1927 German surgeon).

pertussis see WHOOPING COUGH.

pes cavus see CLAW FOOT.

pes planus FLAT FOOT.

pessary 1 a device, often ring-shaped, that is placed in the vagina to support the womb or other pelvic organs.

2 a vehicle for medication that is placed in the vagina. Medicated pessaries are often made of cocoa butter which melts under body heat. They contain drugs to treat vaginal disorders, such as thrush (CANDIDIASIS) or TRICHOMONIASIS, or spermicides for contraceptive purposes.

pestle a club-shaped tool, used in a mortar, for

grinding or mashing material.

petechiae tiny, flat red or purple spots in the skin or mucous membranes caused by bleeding from small blood vessels. Petechiae are a feature of the bleeding disorder PURPURA.

pethidine a synthetic NARCOTIC painkilling drug somewhat less powerful than morphine. Pethidine is widely used during childbirth and as a PREMEDICATION. Overuse may lead to addiction. The drug is on the WHO official list. A brand name of pethidine in a formulation with promethazine is Pamergan P100.

petit mal a minor form of EPILEPSY. Petit mal attacks are almost entirely confined to children and adolescents. There is a momentary unappreciated loss of awareness and social contact but the child does not fall and may even continue automatically with some activity, such as cycling. Attacks may be very frequent and may severely interfere with education. Petit mal can be controlled with anticonvulsant drugs.

Petri dish a shallow circular dish of glass or plastic with an identically shaped, loose-fitting cover, used to grow micro-organisms on a layer of culture medium. The design of the dish was suggested by an assistant of Louis Pasteur. (Richard Julius Petri, 1852–1921, German bacteriologist).

petrosal pertaining to, or near, the inner part of the temporal bone (the petrous portion) that surrounds the inner ear. From the Latin *petrosus*, rocky.

PET scanning POSITRON EMISSION TOMOGRAPHY. This is a diagnostic imaging technique based on the detection of gamma rays produced by the annihilation of positively charged electrons (positrons) emitted by specially prepared radioactive substances that have been injected intravenously. Substances labelled with oxygen-15, fluorine-18, carbon-11 or nitrogen-13 are most commonly used. PET scanning provides uniquely valuable images of tissues showing local metabolic activity, especially in the brain, the rate of glucose and oxygen consumption at various sites, blood flow, neurotransmitter activity and the fate of drugs. Positron-emitting substances have a very short half-life and must be prepared on site in a cyclotron. This limits the application of the technique.

Peutz-Jeghers syndrome a rare AUTOSOMAL DOMINANT genetic disorder in which large numbers of small polyps grow on the lining of the intestine, and small, flat, brown spots appear on the lips and in the mouth. Unlike MULTIPLE POLYPOSIS this condition rarely progresses to cancer. Complications are uncommon. (John Law Augustine Peutz, 1886–1957, Dutch physician, and Harald Jos Jeghers, American physician, b. 1904).

Pevaril, Pevaril TC brand names for the antifungal drug ECONAZOLE.

-pexy *combining form denoting* a fixing, securing or making fast.

peyote a Mexican cactus of the species *Lophophora williamsii* from the flowering heads of which the hallucinogenic drug mescaline is prepared.

Peyronie's disease a disorder of the penis in which the organ is bent at an angle when erect. This is the effect of local thickening and indistensibility of the fibrous tissue sheath. The thickening may extend into the erectile tissue and the condition is liable to interfere with sexual intercourse. The cause is unknown and the treatment difficult. Corticosteroid injections may help and surgical removal of the thickened areas may be tried. (Francois de la Peyronie, 1678–1747, French surgeon).

PGD *abbrev. for* PREIMPLANTATION GENETIC DIAGNOSIS.

pH an expression, widely used in medicine, of the acidity or alkalinity of a solution. pH is the logarithm to the base 10 of the concentration of free hydrogen ions in moles per litre, expressed as a positive number. The pH scale ranges from 0 to 14. Neutrality is 7. Figures below 7 indicate acidity, increasing towards zero; figures rising above 7 indicate increasing alkalinity. The pH of body fluids, in health, is accurately maintained between about 7.3 to 7.5. Below this range the condition of acidosis exists; above it, alkalosis. Both are dangerous.

phaeochromocytoma a rare ADRENALINE-secreting tumour of the inner part of an ADRENAL gland or occurring in similar tissue elsewhere in the body. The resulting excessive levels of adrenaline in the blood cause a severe and sometimes dangerous rise in the blood pressure as well as other distressing effects such as emotional upset, a rapid pulse, palpitations, nausea, vomiting and headache. Treatment is by surgical removal of the tumours.

-phage *suffix denoting* one that eats, as in MACROPHAGE.

phage a BACTERIOPHAGE.

phagocyte an AMOEBOID cell of the immune system that responds to contact with a foreign object, such as a bacterium, by surrounding, engulfing and digesting it. Phagocytes occur widely throughout the body wherever they are likely to be required. Some wander freely throughout the tissues. They include macrophages and neutrophil polymorphonuclear leukocytes ('polymorphs'). From the Greek *phago*, eating and *kutos*, a hollow or receptacle.

phagocytosis the envelopment and destruction of bacteria or other foreign bodies by PHAGOCYTES.

phagosome the vacuole, formed within a PHAGOCYTE, that surrounds material that has been taken up by cell membrane invagination. A phagosome may fuse with a lysosome to provide digestive enzyme.

phakoemulsification a method of CATARACT surgery in which the opaque lens is broken up within its capsule into tiny particles by ultrasonic vibration of a fine probe inserted into the eye. At the same time irrigation fluid is passed into and out of the capsule carrying with it the emulsified lens matter. Following complete removal of the lens in this way a replacement plastic lens is slipped into the capsule. If a foldable soft lens is used, the entire procedure may be conducted through a very short incision which does not require to be stitched. Considerable technological advances in recent years have made the procedure safer and more reliable.

phakomatoses a group of disorders that involve developmental abnormalities of tissue of ectodermal origin – tissue that gives rise to the skin and the nervous system. The three principal phakomatoses are TUBEROUS SCLEROSIS, VON HIPPEL-LINDAU DISEASE and the STURGE-WEBER SYNDROME.

phalanges the small bones of the fingers and toes. Fingers have three phalanges; the thumbs and big toes have two.

phalanx a finger or toe bone. Plural PHALANGES.

phallic pertaining to the PHALLUS.

phallus 1 the penis.

2 any object symbolizing the penis.

phantom limb a powerful sense that a limb which has been amputated is still present. The effect is due to nerve impulses arising in the cut nerves in the stump. These can only be interpreted as coming from the original limb.

pharmaceutical 1 any DRUG intended for medicinal use.

2 pertaining to medicinal drugs or to the preparation and use of drugs (pharmaceutics).

pharmaco-economics the application of health economics to the selection and supply of medical drugs, with special reference to cost-effectiveness in prescribing. The topic, which includes such matters as measures to promote the prescription of generic drugs rather than the higher-priced branded equivalent trade, has become increasingly important as medical cost escalate.

pharmacogenomics the recognition of the fact and significance of human genetic variability in relation to drug action and its application to medical treatment. Genetic variability affects drug absorption, distribution, metabolism and excretion. As a result, many drugs which work very well in some people work poorly in others. At present, the best doctors can do is to prescribe a drug and then wait and see how well the patient responds. Fuller knowledge of pharmacogenomics will, in the future, allow more reliable treatment and avoid expensive waste.

pharmacokinetics the study of how DRUGS are absorbed into, distributed and broken down in, and excreted from, the body.

pharmacology the science of drugs. Pharmacology is concerned with the origins, isolation, purification, chemical structure and synthesis, assay, effects, uses, side effects, relative effectiveness of drugs and the influence of genetic factors on drug action. It thus includes, among other disciplines, genetics, organic chemistry, pharmacokinetics, therapeutics and toxicology. The list that follows highlights the key entries related to pharmacology in the dictionary: adrenergic-blocking drugs, adrenolytic drug therapy, analeptic drugs, analgesic drugs, anorectic drugs, anti-androgen drugs, antibiotic drugs, antibiotic resistance, anticoagulant, antidepressant, antiemetics,antiepileptic drugs, antifungal, antihelminthic, antihistamine, antihypertensive, anti-inflammatory, antileukotreines, antimalarials, antimicrobial, antimycotic, antineoplastic, antioxidants, antiparkinsonism drugs, antiperspirant, antiprotozoals,antipruritic, antipsoriatics, antipsychotic, antipyretic, antirabies serum, antirachitic, antirheumatic, antispasmodic, antitetanus immunoglobulin,anti-tetanus serum, antitoxin, antitussive, antivenene, antivenom, antiviral, beta-lactam antibiotics, beta-lactam inhibitors, cytotoxic antibiotics, cytotoxic drugs, cytotoxic immunosuppressants, drug idiosyncrasy, drug tolerance, erythropoietic drugs, fertility drugs, generic drug, hypoglycaemic drugs, immunosuppressant drugs, laxative drugs, non-steroidal anti-inflammatory drugs.

pharmacopoeia a book, known as a formulary, that lists and describes the characteristics of drugs used in medicine. The major pharmacopoeias, such as the *British Pharmacopoeia* (BP), the *Pharmaceutical Codex* and the *Extra Pharmacopoeia*, are large volumes dealing with all important drugs and offering a semiofficial guide to pharmacists, doctors and others as to their uses and disadvantages. A revised version of *The British National Formulary*, an 800-page paperback book, is published every six months by the British Medical Association and the Royal Pharmaceutical Society of Great Britain. It is also available on the Internet.

pharmacy 1 the process of preparing, compounding and dispensing drugs, usually to the prescription of a doctor.

2 a place where these activities are performed.

Pharmorubicin a brand name for EPIRUBICIN.

pharyngeal diverticulum see PHARYNGEAL POUCH.

pharyngeal pouch a blind-ending sac of mucous membrane, bulging backwards and downwards from a point near the junction of the PHARYNX and the OESOPHAGUS, through a weakness in the muscle wall. The pouch fills with food causing persistent discomfort, a sense of incomplete swallowing and some danger that food may enter the LARYNX. Treatment is by surgical removal and repair of the wall deficit.

pharyngitis inflammation of the PHARYNX causing a sore throat and discomfort in swallowing, and often enlarged LYMPH NODES in the neck. Pharyngitis is most commonly caused by virus infection as part of a common cold, but is sometimes caused by bacteria, such as streptococci, *Corynebacterium diphtheriae* or

other organisms. Persistent pharyngitis may be caused by smoking or excessive drinking of strong alcohol. Very severe pharyngitis may endanger life by causing OEDEMA of the LARYNX. Treatment is necessary in severe or persistent cases and antibiotics may be given after a throat swab has been taken for bacterial culture.

pharynx the common passage to the gullet (OESOPHAGUS) and the windpipe (TRACHEA) from the back of the mouth and the back of the nose. The pharynx is a muscular tube lined with MUCOUS MEMBRANE, and consists of the NASOPHARYNX, the OROPHARYNX and the LARYNGOPHARYNX.

pharynx disorders see PHARYNGITIS and PHARYNGEAL POUCH.

-phasia *suffix denoting* a speech disorder, as in aphasia.

Phazyme a brand name for the silicone preparation DIMETHICONE (dimeticone), used to treat indigestion from intestinal gas.

PhD *abbrev. for* Doctor of Philosophy.

phenazines drugs used to treat leprosy. An example is clofazimine (Lamprene).

phencyclidine a drug of abuse, commonly known as ANGEL DUST. Also known as PCP.

phenelzine an ANTIDEPRESSANT drug of the MONOAMINE OXIDASE INHIBITOR group. A brand name is Nardil.

Phenergan a brand name for PROMETHAZINE.

phenindione an ANTICOAGULANT drug that can be taken by mouth. Now little used because of allergic side effects. A brand name, no longer used in the UK, is Dindevan.

phenobarbitone phenobarbital, a BARBITURATE drug now used mainly as an ANTICONVULSANT. Phenobarbitone is no longer used as a sedative or HYPNOTIC. The drug is on the WHO official list. A brand name is Luminal.

phenocopy a PHENOTYPE or disorder caused by non-genetic factors that mimics, and may be mistaken for, a genetic disorder.

phenothiazines an important group of drugs derived from a molecule with a three-ring structure in which two benzene rings are linked by a sulphur and a nitrogen atom. They are widely used to treat serious mental (PSYCHOTIC) illness and to relieve severe nausea and vomiting. Phenothiazines are divided into three groups. Group I contains drugs such as chlorpromazine (Largactil), methotrimeprazine (Nozinan) and promazine. Group II includes thioridazine (Melleril), pericyazine (Neulactil) and pipothiazine (Piportil Depot). And group III contains prochlorperazine (Stemetil, Buccastem), perphenazine (Fentazin), fluphenazine (Modicate, Moditem, Motival), trifluoperazine (Stelazine) and amitriptyline (Triptafen).

phenothrin a drug used to eliminate head and pubic lice. A brand name is Full Marks.

phenotype 1 the observable appearance of an organism which is the result of the interaction of its genetic constitution and its subsequent environmental experience.

2 any identifiable structural or functional feature of an organism. Compare GENOTYPE.

phenoxybenzamine an alpha-adrenergic blocker drug with a powerful and persistent action, used to treat bladder neck obstruction and the effects of the adrenaline-producing tumour, the PHAEOCHROMOCYTOMA. A brand name is Dibenyline.

phenoxymethylpenicillin a synthetic PENICILLIN. A brand name is Crystapen V. The drug is on the WHO official list.

phentermine a drug with an AMPHETAMINE (amfetamine)-like action used for appetite control in obesity. A brand name is Duromine. There is evidence that phentermine may be associated with heart valve disease and pulmonary hypertension.

phentolamine an alpha-ADRENERGIC BLOCKING DRUG used in the treatment of PHAEOCHROMOCYTOMA. A brand name is Rogitine.

phenylalanine one of the 20 AMINO ACIDS from which proteins are constructed. Phenylalanine is an essential amino acid and cannot be synthesized in the body; it must be provided in the diet.

phenylbutazone a non-steroidal anti-inflammatory drug (NSAID) once widely used but now available for use in hospitals only because of its tendency to cause HEART FAILURE from fluid retention and severe blood disorders. It is used, under specialist supervision, in cases of ANKYLOSING SPONDYLITIS.

phenylephrine a SYMPATHOMIMETIC drug used as eye drops to dilate the pupils for ophthalmic examination of the interior of the eyes. A brand name is Minims phenylephrine.

phenylketonuria an AUTOSOMAL RECESSIVE inherited deficiency of the liver enzyme phenylalanine hydroxylase that converts the amino acid phenylalanine into tyrosine. Phenylalanine and its toxic derivatives accumulate in the body and can cause brain damage with mental retardation, unexpectedly fair hair, blue eyes and a musty body odour. The disease is caused by some of more than 500 mutations of the gene that codes for phenylalanine hydroxylase. A co-factor, tetrahydrobiopterin is also involved in the conversion and it has been discovered that in mild cases of phenylketonuria this substance can significantly lower the blood levels of phenylalanine. Babies are screened at birth by the Guthrie test and about 1 in 10,000 is found to have the condition. A diet free from phenylalanine can prevent harm from developing, so breast feeding must be avoided and special diets provided.

phenytoin an ANTICONVULSANT drug widely used as a long-term suppressant of major EPILEPSY. The drug is on the WHO official list. A brand name is Epanutin.

pheromone an odorous body secretion that affects the behaviour of other individuals of the same species, acting as a sex attractant or in other ways. Pheromones are important in many animal species but, until recently, were thought to be unimportant in humans. It has now been shown, however, that the timing of ovulation in women can be controlled by pheromones from the armpit. This is believed to be the explanation of the fact that women living together will frequently develop synchronized menstrual cycles.

Philadelphia chromosome an acquired chromosomal defect in which the long arm of chromosome 22 is deleted and attached (translocated) to another chromosome, usually number 9. Clones of cells with this defect cause chronic myeloid LEUKAEMIA.

-philia *suffix denoting* a tendency or attraction towards.

-philiac *suffix denoting* one that has a tendency toward.

phimosis tightness of the FORESKIN (prepuce) of such degree as to prevent retraction. This may be congenital or the result of inflammation. Severe phimosis that interferes with urination is an indication for CIRCUMCISION. From the Greek *phmoun*, to gag or muzzle.

phleb-, phlebo- *combining form denoting* vein.

phlebitis inflammation of a vein. This is usually associated with clot formation so the condition is often described as THROMBOPHLEBITIS.

phlebography X-ray imaging of veins after injection of a liquid opaque to radiation. Also known as venography.

phlebolith a stone (calculus) in a vein.

phlebothrombosis blood clotting in a vein in the absence of veininflammation (phlebitis).

Phlebotomus a genus of sandfly that transmits LEISHMANIASIS (KALA AZAR) and SANDFLY FEVER.

phlebotomus fever an acute viral infection, transmitted by the fly *Phlebotomus papatosii* and characterized by fever, pains in the head and eyes, inflammation of the CONJUNCTIVA, LEUKOPENIA and general malaise. Also known as sandfly fever.

phlebotomy cutting into, or puncture of, a vein, usually for the purpose of removing blood.

phlegm see SPUTUM.

PHLS *abbrev. for* Public Health Laboratory Service.

phlycten a small, greyish, blister-like growth on the CORNEA or CONJUNCTIVA occurring as an immunological reaction to TUBERCULOSIS organisms.

-phobia *combining form denoting* abnormal fear of.

phobia an inappropriate, irrational or excessive fear of a particular object or situation, that interferes with normal life. Phobias may relate to many objects including reptiles or insects, open spaces or public places (agoraphobia), crowds, public speaking, performing or even eating in public and using public toilets. Exposure causes intense anxiety and sometimes a PANIC ATTACK. Treatment is by cognitive behaviour therapy.

phobophobia fear of developing a phobia. The term is in the dictionaries but, like may other alleged phobias, was probably invented by a lexicographer.

phocomelia a major, congenital limb defect featuring absence of all long bones so that the hands or feet are attached directly to the trunk and resemble flippers. Spontaneous cases of phocomelia are rare but the condition occurred in many children whose mothers were given thalidomide early in their pregnancy.

pholcodine an opioid drug used mainly for cough suppression. Brand names are Galenphol and Pavacol-D.

phoneme one of the many sounds in speech that distinguish the meaning of one word from another, as in the case of 'b' and 'w' which distinguish, for instance, 'bed' and 'wed' in English.

phonetics the branch of linguistics concerned with the study of the speech sounds (phonemes) of a language and their classification and representation.

phono- *combining form denoting* sound or voice.

phonocardiograph an instrument that converts heart sounds, especially heart murmurs, into a permanent graphic record for analysis.

phonophobia fear of sound. See also HYPERACUSIS.

phosphatase an enzyme that removes phosphate groups from a molecule.

phosphates salts or esters of phosphoric acids or salts or esters containing a phosphorus atom. Most of the body phosphate is combined with calcium in the bones and teeth but an important fraction occurs in the blood and in all cells. Phosphates help to stabilize the pH of the blood and other tissue fluids and occur in the ADENOSINE TRIPHOSPHATE (ATP) which stores and releases energy in cells. They are also important groups in the structure of DNA and RNA NUCLEOTIDES.

phosphodiesterase inhibitors drugs used to prevent inactivation of the cell messenger CYCLIC AMP and thereby increase its stimulating effect on the heart. It is useful to strengthen the heart's action in certain cases of HEART FAILURE. Examples are enoximone (Perfan) and milrinone (Primacor).

phosphodiesterase type 4 inhibitors a class of drugs that act to increase intracellular concentrations of CYCLIC AMP and have a broad range of anti-inflammatory activity. These drugs are showing promise in the treatment of asthma and chronic obstructive pulmonary disease (COPD). They include roflumilast and cilomilast.

phosphodiesterase type 5 inhibitors drugs used to treat impotence. Examples are SILDENAFIL (Viagra), tadalafil (Cialis) and VARDENAFIL (Levitra).

phosphodiester bond the chemical linkages

that join up the sugar, base and phosphate NUCLEOTIDES of DNA and RNA into polynucleotide strands. The subunits of the strand are triphosphate nucleosides, but when a number of these join up (polymerize) under the action of the enzyme DNA polymerase, two of the phosphates are cleaved off leaving only one phosphorous atom between each pair of adjacent sugar molecules. The two ester (diester) bonds in each linkage are Carbon–Oxygen–Phosphorus from the 5′-carbon on one sugar *and* Carbon–Oxygen–Phosphorus from the 3′-carbon on the next. The hydroxyl (–OH) on the 3′-carbon is also lost.

phot-, photo- *combining form denoting* light.

photic pertaining to light.

photocoagulation destruction of tissue by the heating effect of intense focused white light or by the use of a laser. It is widely used by ophthalmic surgeons to treat disorders of the RETINA, especially DIABETIC RETINOPATHY and areas of retinal degeneration that threaten to lead to retinal detachment.

photodynamic therapy a treatment in which a photosensitizing drug is given intravenously, followed by a local targeted irradiation by light. The method is being used effectively with laser light in selected cases of age-related macular degeneration.

photomicrograph a photograph made through a microscope.

photo-onycholysis separation of a fingernail from its base following exposure to light. Light exposure alone is unlikely to cause ONYCHOLYSIS, but the condition has been reported following the use of the antibiotic doxycycline for prophylaxis of LYME DISEASE after tick bites.

photophobia undue intolerance to light. This is a feature of certain eye disorders, especially corneal abrasions or ulcers, IRIDOCYCLITIS and congenital glaucoma. It also occurs in MIGRAINE and MENINGITIS.

photopsia visual sensations of light originating in the eyes or the nervous system and due to stimulation of the retinas or visual nerve pathways other than by light. Mechanical stimuli from traction on the retina by the VITREOUS BODY can cause photopsia. They are examples of entoptic phenomena. Also known as phosphenes.

photoreceptors specialized cells, such as the rods and cones of the RETINA, that originate nerve impulses when stimulated by light.

photosensitivity a state in which an abnormal reaction occurs on exposure to sunlight. The commonest reaction is a skin rash occurring as a combined effect of light and some substance that has been eaten or applied to the skin. Such substances are called photosensitizers and include various drugs, plant derivatives, dyes or other chemicals. Avoidance of either or both elements is important.

phototherapy treatment with light, especially in conjunction with a sensitizing drug such as the psoralen methoxalen. This is known as PUVA (psoralen ultraviolet-A) therapy and is useful in the management of PSORIASIS. Ultraviolet therapy is sometimes used in the treatment of ACNE, and blue light is used to treat babies with JAUNDICE due to liver inadequacy. This alters BILIRUBIN in the skin to a form that can be excreted in the urine.

-phrenia *combining form denoting* the mind or the DIAPHRAGM.

phrenic pertaining to the mind or to the DIAPHRAGM.

phrenic nerves the two main nerves supplying the DIAPHRAGM and thus controlling breathing. Each phrenic nerve arises from the 3rd, 4th, and 5th cervical spinal nerves and passes down through the chest to supply one side of the diaphragm.

phrenology a theory, taken seriously for a time in the 18th century, that human characteristics were reflected in the relative growth of parts of the brain and that these could be detected by palpation of the skull bumps which, it was claimed, conformed to the shape of the brain.

phthisis wasting or consumption. An outmoded term for pulmonary TUBERCULOSIS.

Phyllocontin a brand name for AMINOPHYLLINE.

phylogeny the evolutionary history ending in a species.

phylum the taxonomic group below kingdom and above class.

Physeptone a brand name for METHADONE.

physical medicine a branch of medicine concerned with the treatment and rehabilitation of people disabled by injury or illness. Apart from specialist doctors, the discipline involves PHYSIOTHERAPISTS,

OCCUPATIONAL THERAPISTS and SPEECH THERAPISTS.

physician 1 a person qualified and licensed to practice medicine.
2 a doctor specializing in a medical, as distinct from a surgical, speciality.

physician-assisted suicide see DOCTOR-ASSISTED SUICIDE.

physiology the study of the functioning of living organisms, especially the human organism. Physiology includes biochemistry but this is such a large discipline that it is followed as a separate speciality. Together with anatomy and pathology, physiology is the basis of medical science. The list that follows highlights the key entries related to physiology in the dictionary:

absolute refractory period, ab sorption, acclimatization, accommodation, acetylcholine, acetyl coenzyme A, actin, actin binding proteins, action potential, active transport, adenosine triphosphate (ATP), adenylate cyclase, agonist, anaerobic, angiotensin, ATPase, autonomic nervous system, baroreceptor, beta cells, blood-brain barrier, buffers, carbonic anhydrases, carotid body, carotid sinus, catabolism, coagulation, collagen, collagenases, contraction, corticotrophin, cortisol, cyclic AMP, diastole, dopamine, emission, endocytosis, endothelins, endothelium, erection, excitatory amino acids, free radicals, G proteins, glycogen, homeostasis, interleukins, ligand, micelles, meiosis, mitosis, myoglobin, osmosis, peroxisomes, pituitary gland, preganglionic, secretin, thyroid-stimulating hormone, urea, urease, vasomotor, vasopressin.

Physiotens a brand name for MOXONIDINE.

physiotherapist a person engaged in the practice of PHYSIOTHERAPY.

physiotherapy the treatment discipline ancillary to medicine that uses physical methods such as active or passive exercises, gymnastics, weight-lifting, heat treatment, massage, ultrasound, short-wave diathermy and HYDROTHERAPY. Physiotherapists aim to restore the maximum possible degree of function to any disabled part of the body and are also much concerned with patient motivation. See also PHYSICAL MEDICINE.

physostigmine a CHOLINESTERASE inhibitor drug used to constrict the pupil of the eye and lower the pressure within the eye in GLAUCOMA. It is also used to treat poisoning with ANTICHOLINERGIC drugs. It is derived form the Calabar bean *Physostigma venenosum*. Also known as eserine.

phyto- *combining form* meaning plant or vegetation.

phytomenadione a VITAMIN K derivative used to treat haemorrhagic disease in new-born babies. The drug is on the WHO official list. A brand name is Konakion.

phyto-oestrogens a range of naturally-occurring oestrogen-like substances derived from plants and present in the diet. Phyto-oestrogens have anticancer properties. Research has shown, for instance, that the risk of breast cancer is substantially lower in women with high levels of phyto-oestrogens, as measured by urinary secretion of these substances, than in those with a low intake. The main phyto-oestrogens are isoflavonoids (which are high in soya products) and lignans (which are high in whole grains, fruit, vegetables and berries). It has been found that the phyto-oestrogen genistein, found in soya, binds preferentially to the oestrogen receptors occurring mainly in the cardiovascular system rather than in those in the breast and uterus. This has encouraged the hope that phyto-oestrogens might be valuable in controlling atherosclerosis and osteoporosis without increasing the risk of cancer.

phytopharmaceuticals drugs derived from plants.

phytophilia a healthy dietary preference leading to an emphasis on vegetables and fruit rather than animal and dairy products.

phytotherapy medical treatment based on plant extracts and products. Many important drugs are derived from plants but, in scientific medicine, these are purified and assayed and their effect is known and can be predicted. Treatment using crude plant extracts can be dangerous because of the wide and uncontrolled range of potency involved in seemingly identical samples of the same plant. A diet based on a high intake of vegetables and fruit is to be recommended on strong scientific evidence as a means of reducing the risk of cancer, heart attacks and strokes.

pia mater the delicate, innermost layer of the MENINGES. The pia follows the convolutions of the brain, dipping into the SULCI.

pica a craving for, and the eating of, unsuitable material such as sand, earth, chalk or coal. Pica is commoner during pregnancy than at other times and may occur in cases of iron-deficiency anaemia. Also known as paroxia.

Pick's disease chronic constrictive PERICARDITIS. (Friedel Pick, 1867–1926, Polish ENT specialist).

Pickwickian syndrome the association of obesity, excessive sleepiness, abnormally shallow breathing and SLEEP APNOEA. The syndrome is related to defective control of respiration and long-term lack of oxygen in the blood. It is named after the fat boy Joe in *The Pickwick Papers* of Charles Dickens.

picornavirus a family of small, single-strand RNA viruses that includes the polioviruses, the RHINOVIRUSES, the coxsackie viruses and the enteroviruses. From the Italian *piccolo*, small, and RNA.

PID *abbrev. for* prolapsed intervertebral disc or pelvic inflammatory disease.

piebaldism 1 VITILIGO.

2 partial ALBINISM.

3 a rare hereditary disease in which there are patchy areas of skin with no pigment.

pigeon chest a deformity in which the chest is peaked forward, seen in people who have suffered from severe asthma from infancy. Also known as pectus carinatum.

pigeon fancier's lung a form of allergic alveolitis caused by repeated inhalation of pigeon dust in pigeon lofts. Acute attacks feature cough, breathlessness, fever, shivering and a feeling of illness. The condition may become chronic and may progress to severe deterioration in lung function. Adequate mask protection and the use of protective clothing can reduce the risk.

pigeon toes a mainly cosmetic defect in which the leg or foot is rotated inwards.

pigmentation coloration of any part of the body, especially the skin. Normal pigmentation of skin, hair and eyes is occasioned by the presence of melanin – a brown or black pigment produced by cells called melanocytes. Abnormal pigmentation may occur from local or general loss of melanin. ALBINISM is caused by a general deficiency of melanin. Other causes of abnormal pigmentation include skin disease, pregnancy (see CHLOASMA), ADDISON'S DISEASE,

CUSHING'S SYNDROME, JAUNDICE and HAEMOCHROMATOSIS.

piles the common name for HAEMORRHOIDS.

pill see ORAL CONTRACEPTIVE.

pilo- *combining form denoting* hair.

pilocarpine a drug used in the form of eye-drops to treat GLAUCOMA. Pilocarpine causes extreme constriction of the pupils so that traction is exerted on the root of the iris so as to open up the drainage channels for aqueous humour. The drug is on the WHO official list. Brand names are Minims pilocarpine, Pilogel, Salagen, Sno Pilo, and, in the form of a sustained-release insert placed behind an eyelid and left for a week at a time, Ocusert Pilo.

Pilogel a brand name for PILOCARPINE.

pilonidal sinus a depression or pit in the skin in the upper part of the cleft between the buttocks that often contains hairs. The origin is unclear but the condition is thought to be due to hairs burrowing into the skin as a result of the movement of the buttocks. Pilonidal sinuses can become infected and surgical opening and exposure may be necessary.

piloerection hair 'standing on end' under the influence of the tiny pilomotor muscles attached to the hair follicles in the skin.

Pilopt a brand name for eye drops containing PILOCARPINE.

pilose hairy.

pilosebaceous pertaining to the hair follicles and their associated sebaceous glands.

pimecrolimus a skin-selective inflammatory CYTOKINE inhibitor used to treat atopic ECZEMA. A brand name is Ekidel.

pimozide a long-acting phenothiazide antipsychotic drug of the diphenylbutylpiperidine group that is also used in the treatment of the GILLES DE LA TOURETTE'S SYNDROME. A brand name is Orap.

pimple a PUSTULE or PAPULE commonly occurring in adolescents and young adults suffering from ACNE.

pinch graft a small, circular, full-thickness skin graft obtained by pinching up a cone of skin with a needle or pulling up on a hair, and cutting it free. Pinch grafts give a poor cosmetic result and are now seldom used.

pindolol a BETA-BLOCKER drug used in the treatment of ANGINA PECTORIS, high blood pressure (HYPERTENSION) and heart irregularity. A brand name is Visken.

pineal gland a tiny, cone-shaped structure within the brain, whose sole function appears to be the secretion of the hormone melatonin. The amount of hormone secreted varies over a 24-hour cycle, being greatest at night. Control over this secretion is possibly exerted through nerve pathways from the retina in the eye; a high light level seems to inhibit secretion. The exact function of melatonin is not understood, but it may help to synchronize circadian (24-hour) or other biorhythms. The pineal gland is situated deep within the brain, just below the back part of the corpus callosum (the band of nerve fibres that connects the two halves of the cerebrum). In rare cases, it is the site of a tumour.

pinguecula a small, flat, yellowish spot, sometimes raised and fatty-looking, on the CONJUNCTIVA over the exposed areas of the white of the eye. Pingueculas are almost universal in people living in tropical areas and, if large and protuberant, may lead to the development of PTERYGIUM.

pink-eye see CONJUNCTIVITIS.

pink puffer a facetious term sometimes used by doctors to describe patients breathless from CHRONIC lung disease but still able to maintain sufficient oxygenation of the blood to avoid CYANOSIS. Compare BLUE BLOATER.

pinna the visible external ear. The pinna consists of a skin flap on a skeleton of cartilage. It has comparatively little effect on the acuity of hearing. Also known as the auricle.

pinocytosis the process in which cells engulf fluid to form tiny clear spherical containers (vacuoles) which then move through the cell cytoplasm, sometimes acting as scavenging vehicles to be discarded through another part of the cell membrane.

pins-and-needles sensation PARAESTHESIA. This is usually due to a temporary interference with the normal conduction of nerve impulses along a sensory nerve, often from sustained pressure on the nerve. It may also be caused by any NEUROPATHY.

pinta a skin disorder caused by *Treponema carateum* an organism closely related to the spirochaete causing SYPHILIS. The disease is not sexually transmitted and is confined to under-developed areas of central and south America. It features a scaly, raised spot that slowly enlarges and becomes surrounded by satellite spots. Up to a year later there is a secondary stage with a widespread rash that leads to loss of skin pigment. Pinta is treated with penicillin.

pinworms see THREADWORMS.

piperacillin a broad-spectrum PENICILLIN.

Pipelle a proprietary name for a device used to obtain a sample of endometrium without DILATATION AND CURETTAGE. It consists of a flexible polypropylene sheath with a soft, rounded end, containing an inner piston. The blunt end, which has a perforation near the tip, is passed through the cervix into the womb and the piston drawn sharply back. In this way a small core sample of tissue is obtained. The end of the sheath is then cut off and sent to a laboratory for histological examination. The procedure can often be performed without anaesthesia.

piperazine an ANTHELMINTIC drug used to get rid of ROUNDWORMS and THREADWORMS. The drug paralyses the worms which are then passed with the faeces. A brand name for the drug formulated with the laxative senna is Pripsen.

pipothiazine pipotiazine, a phenothiazine antipsychotic drug that can be given by depot injection for the maintenance treatment of SCHIZOPHRENIA.

piracetam a drug that simulates the action of the NEUROTRANSMITTER GABA and is used to treat MYOCLONUS. A brand name is Nootropil.

pirenzepine a drug formerly used to cut secretion of acid by the stomach in the treatment of PEPTIC ULCER but now discontinued.

Piriton a brand name for the ANTIHISTAMINE drug CHLORPHENIRAMINE (chlorphenamine).

piroxicam a non-steroidal anti-inflammatory drug (NSAID) used mainly to control symptoms in the various forms of ARTHRITIS. A brand name is Feldene.

pisiform 1 resembling a pea.
2 the pea-shaped bone of the wrist near the lower end of the ULNA.

Pitressin a brand name for argipressin, a synthetic form of VASOPRESSIN.

pitting oedema OEDEMA that allows visible but temporary indenting of the skin by finger pressure.

pituitary dwarfism stunted growth due to deficiency of pituitary growth hormone during the early years of life. This is now seldom allowed to occur as treatment with growth hormone is readily available.

pituitary gland the central controlling gland in the ENDOCRINE system. The pituitary is a pea-sized gland that hangs by a stalk from the underside of the brain and rests in a central bony hollow on the floor of the skull. The pituitary stalk emerges immediately under the HYPOTHALAMUS and there are numerous connections, both nervous and hormonal, between the hypothalamus and the gland. The pituitary releases many hormones that regulate and control the activities of other endocrine glands as well as many body processes. Hormonal feedback information from the various endocrine glands to the hypothalamus and the pituitary ensures that the pituitary is able to perform its control function effectively. See also ADRENOCORTICOTROPIC HORMONE, ANTIDIURETIC HORMONE, FOLLICLE-STIMULATING HORMONE, LUTEINIZING HORMONE, MELANOCYTE-STIMULATING HORMONE, OXYTOCIN, PROLACTIN, and THYROID-STIMULATING HORMONE.

pityriasis any skin condition featuring bran-like scaling of the skin.

pityriasis alba a common form of ECZEMA causing pinkish plaques that resolve to leave fine, scaly, pale patches. The condition affects children and adolescents and clears up spontaneously.

pityriasis rosea a common, mild skin disease, probably caused by a virus, and featuring flat, oval, reddish, scaly spots in the line of skin creases. A single prominent 'herald' patch usually occurs on the trunk or an arm about a week before the outbreak. The rash lasts for 6 to 8 weeks and then clears up without treatment. Itching may call for calamine lotion or antihistamine drugs.

pityriasis versicolor a common fungus infection of the outer layer of the skin (the EPIDERMIS) that causes white, brown, or salmon-coloured flaking patches. The condition may be inapparent until the unaffected skin becomes tanned by the sun. Treatment is by antifungal creams or lotions.

pizotifen an antihistamine drug used in the treatment of severe MIGRAINE. A brand name is Sanomigran.

PKU test PHENYLKETONURIA test.

placebo 1 a pharmacologically inactive substance made up in a form apparently identical to an active drug that is under trial. Both the placebo and the active drug are given, but the subjects are unaware which is which. This is done for the purpose of eliminating effects due to purely psychological causes. 2 a harmless preparation prescribed to satisfy a patient who does not require active medication. From the Latin *placere*, to please. See also PLACEBO EFFECT.

placebo effect the often significant, but usually temporary, alteration in a patient's condition, following the exhibition of a drug or other form of treatment, which is due to the patient's expectations or to other unexplained psychological effects, rather than to any direct physiological or pharmacological action of the drug or treatment. The placebo effect has done much to foster the reputation of many valueless forms of treatment.

placenta the part of the early developing EMBRYO, that differentiates to form an organ attached to the lining of the womb and provides a functional linkage between the blood supplies of the mother and the fetus. This allows for the passage of oxygen and nutrients from the mother to the fetus. The placenta is connected to the fetus by the UMBILICAL CORD and is discharged from the womb after the birth of the baby. Also known as afterbirth.

placenta accreta a placenta with abnormally deep penetration of the CHORIONIC VILLI into the wall of the womb. After delivery of the baby, the placenta does not separate and come away as normal but is retained. HYSTERECTOMY is sometimes necessary.

placental-blood transplantation the use of umbilical cord blood as a source of haematopoietic stem cells and progenitor cells to restore bone marrow function in patients whose bone marrow has ceased to form blood cells as a result of disease, especially leukaemia. The procedure has been found useful even if the donor is unrelated to the recipient.

placenta praevia a PLACENTA situated in the lower part of the womb near the cervix, or wholly or partially covering the outlet. Such placement may make normal delivery impossible and inevitably result in separation and vaginal bleeding when labour starts. Placenta praevia can be detected by ultrasound scanning and in such cases the baby is usually delivered by Caesarean section around the 38th week.

placoid plate-like.

plague a serious infectious disease endemic in rats and spread to humans by rat fleas. Plague is caused by the organism *Yersinia pestis* and takes two main forms, bubonic and pneumonic. The latter is a complication of bubonic plague and can be spread by coughed droplets.
Bubonic plague features high fever, shivering, severe headache, painful swelling of the LYMPH NODES (buboes), especially in the groins, armpits and neck, seizures and, in untreated cases, death. SEPTICAEMIA and pneumonic plague are especially dangerous complications. Treatment is with antibiotics such as STREPTOMYCIN, TETRACYCLINE or CHLORAMPHENICOL. These reduce the mortality to less than 5%. Also known as the 'black death'.

plagiocephaly a skull deformity in which the major dimension is on a diagonal because of premature closure of the SUTURES on one side.

Planequil a brand name for the antimalarial drug hydroxychloroquine.

planes of the body imaginary, two-dimensional surfaces used for anatomical description. The sagittal plane is a vertical plane that cuts the body into right and left halves. The coronal plane is a vertical plane that separates the front half of the body from the back. The transverse plane cuts the body horizontally at any level.

plantar pertaining to the sole of the foot. Compare PALMAR.

plantar fasciitis an inflammatory disorder of the strong sheet of white fibres under the shin of the sole of the foot that helps to maintain the longitudinal arch. Plantar fasciitis may be caused by unaccustomed athletic activity, sudden weigh gain or unsuitable footwear. It is the commonest cause of pain under the heel but will usually resolve without treatment.

plantar wart an ordinary wart (verruca) occurring on the sole of the foot and forced into the skin by pressure from the weight of the body.

plaque 1 an area of ATHEROMA found in the inner lining of arteries in the disease of ATHEROSCLEROSIS.
2 a sticky mixture of food debris, saliva and bacteria that persists around the necks of uncleaned teeth and is the main cause of tooth decay.

Plaquenil a brand name for HYDROXY-CHLOROQUINE.

plasma 1 the fluid in which the blood cells are suspended.
2 blood from which all cells have been removed. Plasma contains proteins, electrolytes and various nutrients and is capable of clotting.

plasma cell one of a number of large oval cells, cloned from a selected B LYMPHOCYTE, that synthesize large quantities of the required IMMUNOGLOBULIN (antibody).

plasma expander any substance used to increase the volume of the fluid component of circulating blood. The commonest plasma volume expander is donated human plasma obtained from anticoagulated whole blood. Other plasma expanders include dextran solution, fresh whole blood, and a range of electrolyte solutions.

plasmapheresis a method of reducing the concentration of unwanted substances, especially destructive ANTIBODIES and IMMUNE COMPLEXES in the blood. Blood is withdrawn and the cells are removed and suspended in a PLASMA substitute. It is then retransfused. The method is used mainly in such conditions as MYASTHENIA GRAVIS, GOODPASTURE'S SYNDROME and severe complicated cases of SYSTEMIC LUPUS ERYTHEMATOSUS.

plasma membrane the membrane that defines the boundary of a cell.

plasma proteins the proteins present in blood plasma. They include albumin, the range of IMMUNOGLOBULINS and prothrombin and fibrinogen necessary for blood clotting. Plasma proteins help to maintain the OSMOTIC PRESSURE of the blood and hence the blood volume.

plasmid a ring-shaped, double-stranded, piece of DNA in bacterial cells that contains genes extra to those in the chromosome. Plasmid genes code for characteristics such as toxin production and the factors that cause antibiotic resistance. Plasmids are convenient vehicles for the introduction of new genes into organisms in recombinant DNA technology (genetic engineering).

plasmin a protein-splitting enzyme in the blood that dissolves FIBRIN clots.

plasminogen the precursor to PLASMIN.

plasminogen activation system the cascade that regulates the conversion of plasminogen to the proteinase plasmin. It involves a urokinase-type plasminogen activator, a tissue-type activator and at least two inhibitors.

Plasmodium a genus of sporozoa parasites that invade red blood cells. The genus includes the four parasites that cause MALARIA.

plasmolysis shrinkage or dissolution of the protoplasm in a cell.

plaster cast see CAST.

plaster of Paris a white powder of dried calcium sulphate dihydrate which, mixed with water, gives off heat and hardens. Reinforced with loose bandage it forms a strong and useful support (CAST) or dental mould.

-plastic *combining form denoting* forming, developing or growing.

plastic surgery any surgical procedure designed to repair or reconstruct injured, diseased or malformed tissue so as to restore normal appearance and function. Compare COSMETIC SURGERY.

Platamine a brand name for CISPLATIN.

platelet a fragment of the CYTOPLASM of a MEGAKARYOCYTE 2–4 mm in diameter. Each megakaryocyte produces 1000 to 3000 platelets, which are present in large numbers in the blood – 50,000 to 300,000 per cu. mm. Platelets survive for about 10 days and play an essential part in blood clotting. Platelet plasma membranes contain a range of glycoproteins by means of which they bind to different materials including collagen, fibrinogen and von Willebrand factor. Platelets are by no means the passive tissue fragments they were formerly thought to be. They carry many granules and a canalicular system by which the granules are released. They also have a dense tubular membrane system in which prostaglandins and thromboxanes are synthesized. Platelet granules contain heparin-neutralizing factor, von Willebrand factor, smooth muscle growth factor and fibrinogen. Deficiency of platelets is known as thrombocytopenia.

platelet activating factor a factor which, like PROSTAGLANDINS and LEUKOTRIENES, is released from cell membranes. It is a potent cause of INFLAMMATION and an activator of several cell types of the immune system. It is rapidly destroyed and its effect is local.

platelet-associated autoantibodies see ANTIPLATELET ANTIBODIES.

platelet disorders a range of disorders that includes intrinsic platelet abnormalities, both congenital and acquired, and the disorders caused by a deficiency of platelets (thrombocytopenia) or an excess (thrombocytosis). Several syndromes include thrombocytopenia, platelet membrane disorders or giant platelets. Platelet disorders may be of genetic origin or may be acquired and may involve reduced platelet production or increased platelet consumption.

platelet glycoprotein receptor one of a range of receptors on blood platelets that bind glycoproteins. Platelet glycoprotein receptor IIb/IIIa binds fibrinogen, thereby promoting platelet aggregation and the formation of a blood clot within a blood vessel. This receptor can be blocked by various substances such as HIRUDIN or a number of synthetic drugs such as tirofiban.

Platosin a brand name for the anticancer drug cisplatin.

platy- *combining form denoting* flat or broad.

platysma the broad, flat muscle lying immediately under the skin of the neck, from the shoulders to the point of the chin. The action of the platysma is to tighten the skin of the neck, pull down the corners of the mouth and lower the jaw.

platyspondylia a rare congenital abnormal flatness of the bodies of the vertebrae of the spine.

platyhelminth a member of the phylum of flatworms that includes flukes, TAPEWORMS, and schistosomes. See LIVER FLUKE and SCHISTOSOMIASIS.

pleasure any enjoyable or agreeable emotion or sensation, to the pursuit of which most people, who are free to do so, devote their lives.

pleasure principle the tendency to seek immediate gratification of instinctual desires and to avoid pain. In the Freudian model, this primitive id reaction is gradually modified by the reality principle, a more mature ego function. See also FREUDIAN THEORY.

Plendil a brand name for FELOPIDINE.

pleo- *combining form denoting* excessive or multiple.

pleocytosis an abnormal increase in the number of cells in the CEREBROSPINAL FLUID.

pleomorphism taking different physical forms. Also known as polymorphism.

pleoptics a method of treatment for AMBLYOPIA, especially for those cases in which the wrong part of the retina is being used (eccentric fixation). The method forces the subject to use the central, highly sensitive part (the fovea).

Plesmet a brand name for FERROUS GLYCINE SULPHATE.

Pletal a brand name for CILOSTAZOL.

plethoric having a ruddy complexion from widening of blood vessels under the skin or, rarely, from POLYCYTHAEMIA.

plethysmography a method of assessing the volume of blood flowing through a limb or other body part by measuring the change in volume, using strain gauges, air cuffs, impedance electrodes or other methods.

pleura the thin, double-layered membrane that separated the lungs from the inside of the chest wall. The inner layer is attached to the lung and the outer to the inside of the chest cavity. A film of fluid between the two layers provides lubrication to allow smooth movement during breathing.

pleural disorders see PLEURAL EFFUSION, PLEURISY and PNEUMOTHORAX.

pleural effusion an excessive accumulation of fluid between the layers of the PLEURA that may compress the underlying lung. This may be caused by lung infections such as PNEUMONIA or TUBERCULOSIS, by lung or pleural cancers or by HEART FAILURE. Treatment is that of the underlying cause and the excess fluid may have to be removed through a needle.

pleurisy inflammation of the PLEURA. This is usually caused by a virus infection or as a secondary effect of an underlying lung infection, such as PNEUMONIA. There is dull pain that becomes severe and stabbing on inspiration. There is no specific treatment for viral pleurisy or viral pneumonia. Bacterial pneumonia will usually respond to antibiotics.

pleurodynia see BORNHOLM DISEASE.

plexus any interlacing network, as of nerves, blood or lymph vessels. The solar plexus is a network of AUTONOMIC nerve fibres lying on the abdominal AORTA.

plication folding or tucking, usually as a surgical procedure on a hollow organ to reduce its size.

-ploid *combining form denoting* some multiple of a chromosome set, as in haploid, diploid, triploid.

ploidy the number of copies of the set of chromosomes in a cell. A normal diploid cell with two copies has a ploidy of two; a haploid cell with one copy, such as an ovum or a spermatozoon, has a ploidy of one.

plumbism lead poisoning.

Plummer-Vinson syndrome difficulty in swallowing from webs of tissue that form across the upper oesophagus, sore tongue, spoon-shaped fingernails (koilonychia) and severe iron-deficiency ANAEMIA. The syndrome mainly affects middle-aged women. Treatment of the anaemia usually resolves the syndrome. (Henry Stanley Plummer, 1874–1937, American physician; and Porter Paisley Vinson, 1890–1959, American surgeon).

pluripotentiality the ability of stem cells to differentiate into almost all cells that arise from the three germ layers but not to form placenta or supporting structures. See also UNIPOTENTIALITY.

plutonium a highly poisonous, radioactive metallic element produced from uranium in atomic breeder reactors and used as a fissile element in nuclear weapons. Plutonium concentrates in the bones where it remains for many years.

PMO *abbrev. for* Principal Medical Officer.

PMS *abbrev. for* PREMENSTRUAL SYNDROME.

PMT *abbrev. for* premenstrual tension. See PREMENSTRUAL SYNDROME.

pneumaturia air or gas in the urine. This usually indicates that an abnormal connection (a fistula) has occurred between the COLON and the bladder.

Pneumo- *prefix denoting* the lung.

pneumoconiosis any of a group of conditions in which a mineral dust, such as asbestos, bauxite, coal dust, diatomite, granite dust, quartz, silicon or talc, has accumulated in the lungs. The significance depends on the material and the particle size. Pneumoconiosis may cause severe lung damage with scarring (FIBROSIS) that may interfere with lung function. It may also lead to secondary HEART FAILURE and an increased risk of TUBERCULOSIS and lung cancer. See ANTHRACOSIS, ASBESTOSIS, SILICOSIS, SIDEROSIS.

pneumocystis pneumonia a lung infection with the microorganism *Pneumocystis carinii*. This is an OPPORTUNISTIC INFECTION largely limited to people with AIDS. There is fever, cough and breathlessness from severe impairment of lung function from fluid in the air sacs. Pneumocystis pneumonia is a common terminal event in AIDS. Intensive antibiotic treatments may control the infection but recurrence is common.

pneumoencephalography a method of X-ray examination of the VENTRICLES of the brain in which the CEREBROSPINAL FLUID is replaced by air. This very unpleasant procedure has been rendered obsolete by CT SCANNING and MRI.

pneumohaemothorax the presence of air and blood in the PLEURAL cavity. Also known as haemopneumothorax.

pneumonectomy surgical removal of a lung. This is sometimes done to treat cancer limited to one lung.

pneumomycosis any lung disease caused by a fungus.

pneumonia inflammation of the lower air passages (bronchioles) and air sacs (alveoli) of the lungs due to contact with irritant or toxic material or to infection with any of a wide spectrum of micro-organisms, including viruses, RICKETTSIA, bacteria, fungi and microscopic parasites. Pneumonia is commonest at the extremes of life and is a common terminal event in the elderly. Pneumonia features fever, chills, shortness of breath, and a cough with greenish or blood-stained sputum. PLEURISY is a common complication. The treatment depends on the nature of the cause. Antibiotics are often effective. See also LOBAR PNEUMONIA and BRONCHOPNEUMONIA.

pneumonic plague a severe and often fatal complication of bubonic PLAGUE in which the infection spreads to the lungs. Unlike bubonic plague, pneumonic plague can spread directly from case to case.

pneumonitis inflammation of the lungs from any cause, including ALLERGY. See PNEUMONIA.

pneumopericardium the presence of air in the pericardial sac.

pneumoperitoneum air in the PERITONEAL CAVITY.

pneumothorax the presence of air in the normally potential space between the two layers of the PLEURA (the pleural cavity). This may occur spontaneously from the rupture of a CONGENITAL bleb on the inner layer, or may result from air access from the outside through a wound. Pneumothorax causes the collapse of the lung on the same side. In minor cases there is recovery without treatment, but the air may have to be withdrawn through a tube.

PO₂ the concentration of OXYGEN in the blood. This commonly measured parameter is an important indicator of the efficiency with which oxygen is transferred from atmosphere to blood. When PO₂ drops, respiration is automatically stimulated.

pod-, podo- *combining form denoting* the foot.

podagra GOUT, especially of the great toe.

podiatry chiropody. Currently the usage is mainly American.

podophyllotoxins a range of powerful substances derived from the mandrake root (*Podophyllum peltatum*). Podophyllotoxins act as TOPOISOMERASE inhibitors causing breaks in DNA strands. Ironically in view of John Donne's famous reference to mandrake, podophillotoxins are also used locally to treat genital WARTS in both sexes. Brand names of preparations for the latter purpose are Condyline and Warticon.

podophyllotoxin derivatives drugs used to treat CANCER. An example is etoposide (Etopophos, Vepesid).

podophyllum resin a drug used externally to destoy WARTS. The drug is on the WHO official list. A brand name is Posalfilin.

POEM *acronym for* Patient-Oriented Evidence that Matters. This is a summary published weekly in the British Medical Journal of valid research deemed to be important to patients.

POEMS syndrome a SYNDROME named as an acronym for Polyneuropathy (a disorder of peripheral nerves), Organomegaly (enlarged organs – liver and spleen), Endocrinopathy (endocrine gland hormonal disorders), M-proteins (Monoclonal IMMUNOGLOBULIN increase) and Skin changes (pigmentation, thickening, sweating, hairiness and FINGER CLUBBING). The condition is rare in Britain but many cases have been reported in Japan.

poikilo- *combining form denoting* varied or variegated.

poikilocytosis a condition in which the red blood cells (erythrocytes) are distorted.

point mutation the replacement of one NUCLEOTIDE with another. This need not necessarily cause any change in the protein produced by the affected gene because 18 of the 20 amino acids have more than one coding triplet of base pairs (codon). Glycine, for instance, is coded for by GGA, GGU, GGG and GGC.

This redundancy feature of the genetic code arises because the four bases, taken three at a time, allow 64 triplets to code the 20 amino acids and the three stop codons. It is called degeneracy.

poison any substance capable, in small amounts, of damaging the structure or function of living organisms or of causing their death. The virulence of a poison is assessed by the smallness of the dose required to produce its effect and by the severity of the effect. Many of the most poisonous substances act by interfering with fundamental cell enzyme systems. Bacterial toxins are amongst the most poisonous substances known.

pokeweed mitogen an agent, useful for promoting MITOSIS especially in B lymphocytes, derived from the North American plant, *Phytolacca americana*.

pol a viral gene which, in retroviruses, acts in conjunction with the gag gene to direct the formation of gag-pol MESSENGER RNAS.

polar of a molecule or chemical group whose electric charges are separated so that one end is positive and one negative (forming a dipole). Cell plasma membranes are made of a double layer of phosopholipid molecules each containing a polar head group with a strong affinity for water (hydrophilic) and a non-polar hydrocarbon tail that avoids water (hydrophobic). The polar head groups in both layers are oriented outwards in the membrane so as to form both free surfaces. So the term 'polar' is used to refer to a hydrophilic chemical group, and 'non-polar' refers to a hydrophobic group.

polio *abbrev. for* POLIOMYELITIS.

poliomyelitis an infectious disease, affecting mainly children and young adults, caused by one of three strains of polioviruses and spread by faecal contamination. The illness caused is usually mild and unimportant but the virus may attack the brain and spinal cord leading to extensive and fatal paralysis. In most cases polio causes no more than a few days of slight fever, sore throat, headache and vomiting. In some cases, however, stiffness of the neck and back, muscle aching and twitching occur and the condition progresses to paralysis. The use of polio vaccines (the spread of which has also been assisted by faecal contamination) has virtually eliminated the disease in developed countries. Also known as infantile paralysis.

pollenosis a general term for the allergic responses to atmospheric pollen grains from trees, grasses, flowers or weeds. See ALLERGIC RHINITIS.

poly- *combining form denoting* many, much or excessive.

polyacrylic acid a substance used to formulate artificial tears and supplied as eye drops for the relief of dry eye syndromes. A brand name is Viscotears.

polyandry marriage to more than one man, simultaneously.

polyarteritis nodosa an inflammatory disease of medium-sized arteries, causing nodular swellings (aneurysms) along the length of the affected vessels. The condition is due to a disturbance of the immune system sometimes triggered by the hepatitis B virus. There is loss of appetite and weight, obstruction to the blood flow causing raised blood pressure, muscle weakness and sometimes gangrene. Involvement of the CORONARY ARTERIES may cause a heart attack. Treatment is with large doses of corticosteroid drugs. Also known as periarteritis nodosa.

polyarthritis ARTHRITIS affecting many joints.

Polybactrin a brand name for a mixture of the antibiotics bacitracin, NEOMYCIN and polymyxin. For external use.

polycoria more than one pupillary opening in a single iris.

polychlorinated biphenyl PCB. Any one of a family of industrial pollutants known to be capable of inducing cancer.

polyclinic a clinic that covers a range of medical and surgical specialties.

Polycrol a brand name for a mixture of the ANTACID drugs aluminium hydroxide and magnesium oxide and the antifoaming agent DIMETHICONE (dimeticone).

polycyclic aromatic hydrocarbons compounds found in the particulate content of diesel exhaust, tobacco smoke, smoked food, whisky, coal tar anti-dandruff shampoos and other elements in the human environment that have been suspected, but not proved, of being capable of causing cancer.

polycystic kidney a genetically determined condition in which both kidneys are greatly enlarged and contain large numbers of cysts. Kidney function is prejudiced and most affected people suffer kidney failure or other serious

complications by middle age. See also
AUTOSOMAL POLYCYSTIC KIDNEY DISEASE.

polycystic ovary a condition of unknown
origin featuring enlargement of the ovaries
with multiple cysts. It ranges from simple,
symptomless ovarian cysts detected as an
unexpected finding or ultrasound examination,
to a major endocrine upset known as the
POLYCYSTIC OVARY SYNDROME.

polycystic ovary syndrome polycystic
ovarian syndrome, a complex of signs and
symptoms commonly associated with
POLYCYSTIC OVARY. There is obesity, menstrual
upset, infertility from anovulation, ACNE and a
male distribution of body hair from hormonal
disturbances. Insulin resistance appears to be
an important causal factor. Possible late
manifestations include DIABETES, high blood
pressure (HYPERTENSION), heart disease and
cancer of the womb lining (endometrial
carcinoma). Treatment is by increased exercise
and improved diet to promote weight loss, and
use of the drugs METFORMIN and clomifene.

polycythaemia an abnormal increase in the
number of red blood cells as a result of
increased red cell production by the bone
marrow. This occurs naturally in people living
at high altitudes (secondary polycythaemia) but
may occur for no apparent reason (polycythaemia
vera) causing flushed skin, headaches, high
blood pressure (HYPERTENSION) and blurred
vision. STROKE is a common complication.
Treatment is by regular bloodletting
(venesection) sometimes supplemented by
the use of anticancer drugs or radioactive
phosphorus. An American study reports that
low-dose aspirin can safely prevent thrombotic
complications in people with this disease. A gene
for polycythaemia vera was reported in 1998.

polydactyly the possession of more than the
normal number of fingers or toes.

polydipsia excessive thirst leading to excessive
fluid intake. This is a feature of untreated severe
DIABETES MELLITUS and of DIABETES INSIPIDUS.

polyethylene glycol a substance used with
other ingredients to be used as a laxative.
Brand names are Klean-prep and Movicol.

Polyfax a brand name for a mixture of the
antibiotics bacitracin and polymyxin B,
used externally.

polygamy marriage to more than one spouse,
simultaneously.

polygeline a plasma substitute blood volume
expander used to treat SHOCK from blood loss,
burns, peritonitis, pancreatitis and crush
injuries. A brand name is Haemaccel.

polygraph an instrument that simultaneously
records changes in various physiological
parameter such as pulse rate, respiration rate,
blood pressure and skin resistance changes from
sweating. These sensitively reflect alterations in
the emotions and the device is used to detect
deception in answers to questions. A 'lie
detector'.

polygyny marriage to more than one woman,
simultaneously.

polyhydramnios excess amniotic fluid in the
womb (uterus) during pregnancy. The main
effects are discomfort and breathlessness. The
uterus is larger than normal for the stage of the
pregnancy. Withdrawal of excess fluid through a
needle passed through the abdominal wall can
provide temporary relief. Compare
OLIGOHYDRAMNIOS.

polymastia having more than two breasts.

polymer a chain molecule made up of
repetitions of smaller chemical units or
molecules called monomers. Polysaccharides,
for instance, are long chains made up of
repeated units of simpler sugars such as
monosaccharides. Proteins are polymers of
AMINO ACIDS. Polymerization is the process of
causing many similar or identical small chemical
groups to link up to form a long chain. From
Greek, *poly*, many and *meros*, a part.

polymerase any enzyme that promotes the
linkage of a number of similar or identical
chemical subunits into repetitive long-chain
molecules (polymers), especially of NUCLEOTIDES
to form DNA or RNA. Derivation as in POLYMER
with the -ase suffix denoting an enzyme.

polymerase chain reaction an important
technique for rapidly producing large numbers
of copies of any required sequence of DNA. DNA
is separated by heat into its two strands, small
molecules called primers are attached to the
sequences at either end of the target sequence,
and an enzyme, DNA polymerase, is used to
build a new strand of the section between the
primers. This becomes a template for the
production of further strands and in twenty
cycles a million copies are made. The polymerase
chain reaction is one of the most powerful
techniques currently in use in biological

science. The American biochemist inventor of the process, Karry B. Mullis, was awarded the Nobel Prize for Chemistry in 1993.

polymerization the formation of POLYMERS from monomers.

polymorph the common abbreviated term for polymorphonuclear neutrophil leukocyte, the small phagocytic white cell of the immune system present in enormous numbers in the blood and the tissues. Polymorphs are amoeboid and highly motile scavengers of foreign material especially antigen-bearing bacteria and other antigenic material to which antibodies have been bound. See also POLYMORPHIC.

polymorphism 1 occurring in many different shapes.
2 in genetics, the existence of different ALLELES of the same gene in different genomes. See also RESTRICTION FRAGMENT LENGTH POLYMORPHISM.

polymorphic occurring in a variety of shapes, as in the case of the nucleus of the neutrophil polymorphonuclear leukocyte (POLYMORPH).

polymorphonuclear having a lobed nucleus of varying lobe number or shape. The term is used of three classes of LEUKOCYTES, neutrophil, basophil and eosinophil.

polymyalgia rheumatica an uncommon disease of the elderly causing muscle pain and stiffness in the hips, thighs, shoulders, and neck. The cause is uncertain. A striking feature is the difficulty in getting out of bed in the mornings. Corticosteroid drugs are effective. Some affected people also suffer from TEMPORAL ARTERITIS and may require urgent treatment with corticosteroid drugs to prevent blindness.

polymyositis a rare, inflammatory, AUTOIMMUNE disease of muscles causing pain, tenderness and muscle weakness. Polymyositis is often associated with skin changes (DERMATOMYOSITIS) and responds to treatment with corticosteroid drugs.

polymyxins a group of five POLYPEPTIDE antibiotic drugs active against various GRAM NEGATIVE bacteria. They are used almost exclusively as external applications in ointments and eye and ear drops because of their toxicity if taken internally.

polyneuritis any inflammatory disorder affecting peripheral nerves.

polyopia the perception of multiple images of a single object.

polyp any growth or mass of tissue projecting,

usually on a stalk, from a surface, especially a mucous membrane. Polyps commonly occur on the lining of the nose, the LARYNX, the intestine and the cervix of the womb. Most polyps are BENIGN but some become MALIGNANT. Surgical removal is generally easy.

polypectomy surgical removal of a POLYP.

polypeptide a molecule consisting of a chain of AMINO ACIDS linked together by peptide bonds. A POLYMER of amino acids that may form part of a protein molecule. Polypeptides link together to form proteins.

polyphagia the state of having an excessive or pathological desire to eat.

polypharmacy a mildly facetious term for the generally disapproved practice of prescribing several different drugs to one person at the same time. Polypharmacy increases the risk of unwanted side effects and of dangerous interactions between different drugs.

polypill a proposed medication, to be taken daily, consisting of a STATIN drug to lower blood cholesterol, small doses of three drugs to control blood pressure, 0.8 mg of folic acid to reduce blood homocysteine, and 70 mg of aspirin to reduce the clotting tendency of the blood. The principal targets of this combination are heart attacks and strokes, and the proposers estimate that people who take the polypill will have reduced their risk of these disasters by 80% and will enjoy substantially prolonged lives. The idea has aroused much controversy.

polyploid having more than twice the normal HAPLOID number of chromosomes. See also DIPLOID.

polyposis coli a rare, inherited disorder of the colon in which between 100 and 1000 polyps occur on the lining of the colon and rectum. Cancerous change in some of these is almost inevitable by the age of 40 and it is usual to remove the colon, and sometimes the rectum, to prevent this.

polyprotein a large gene product that is split into two or more independent proteins.

polyribosome a cluster or string of ribosomes held together by a molecule of messenger RNA.

polyserositis widespread inflammation of serous membranes, with discharge of serum, occurring especially in the upper abdomen. Polyserositis is a feature of COLLAGEN DISEASES.

polysomnography the simultaneous monitoring, during sleep, of a number of parameters in a patient. These include electroencephalogram, electrocardiogram, electromyogram, rapid eye movements, chest excursion, mouth and nose air entry rates, blood oxygen saturation and the frequency and loudness of snoring.

Polytar a brand name for COAL TAR.

polythiazide a thiazide diuretic used to relieve oedema and treat high blood pressure (HYPERTENSION). A brand name is Nephril.

polyubiquitination the process of tagging proteins destined for degradation by attaching a chain of UBIQUITIN molecules to them. Such tagged proteins are then taken up by PROTEASOMES and enzymatically degraded to peptides.

polyunsaturated pertaining to long chain carbon compounds, especially fatty acids, that contain many carbon to carbon double bonds (unsaturated bonds).

polyuria the formation of abnormally large quantities of urine. See also POLYDIPSIA.

polyvidone an ocular lubricant used to treat dry eye syndromes. A brand name is Oculotect.

POMC *abbrev. for* PROOPIOMELANOCORTIN.

pompholyx a form of acute ECZEMA in which itchy blisters occur on the palms of the hands (cheiropompholyx) and/or on the soles of the feet (podopompholyx). The cause is usually inapparent but there may be an allergy. Astringent lotions or corticosteroid creams may help.

pons 1 any anatomical structure joining two parts or bridging between them.
2 the middle part of the BRAINSTEM, lying below the cerebral peduncles of the midbrain and above the MEDULLA OBLONGATA. From the Latin *pons*, a bridge.

Ponstan a brand name for MEFENAMIC ACID.

Pontiac fever a disease associated with organisms of the *Legionella* genus and characterized by sudden fever, headache, painful muscles and debility. It does not, however, like LEGIONNAIRES' DISEASE, progress to pneumonia nor is it contagious.

popliteal pertaining to the hollow surface behind the knee joint.

popliteus muscle a short diagonally placed muscle running from the outer side of the lower end of the thigh bone (femur) to the back of the upper part of the main lower leg bone (TIBIA). It action is to rotate the femur on the tibia, or vice versa.

Porcine Biphasic a brand name for INSULIN.

pore a tiny opening, especially opening in the skin through which sweat or sebaceous secretion (SEBUM) pass to the surface. Most of the sebaceous pores are also hair follicles.

porencephaly the presence of one or more abnormal cavities within the substance of the brain, usually communicating with a lateral VENTRICLE. The cavity of a lateral ventricle may extend to the surface of the cerebral hemisphere. The condition may result from brain tissue destruction or maldevelopment.

Pork Mixtard a brand name for pig INSULIN.

Pork Insulatard a brand name for pig INSULIN.

porphyria any of several inherited disorders in which substances called porphyrins accumulate in the body because of a deficiency of certain ENZYMES. Porphyrins are components formed in the course of the synthesis of HAEMOGLOBIN. The effects are numerous. There may be extreme sensitivity to sunlight, sweating, rapid heart rate, abdominal pain, vomiting, constipation, paralysis and other nervous system disturbances including psychotic disorders. In some cases the effects are mainly on the skin and include blistering, scarring and baldness, especially on exposure to light. Treatment is difficult and varies with the different types. Avoidance of sunlight is often important.

portal pertaining to an entrance or gateway, especially to the porta hepatis, the fissure under the liver at which the PORTAL VEIN, the hepatic artery and the hepatic bile ducts pass through.

portal hypertension increased blood pressure in the PORTAL VEIN, that carries blood from the intestines and spleen to the liver. The commonest cause is CIRRHOSIS of the liver. The rise in pressure in the veins at the lower end of the oesophagus causes them to become stretched and irregular (varicose) and there is a real danger of severe bleeding from these oesophageal varices. This can be controlled by the use of balloons inserted into the oesophagus and then inflated. Injections of hardening solution into the varices to close them off (sclerotherapy) may be helpful. A blood shunting operation is sometimes performed.

portal vein the large vein that carries blood from the intestines, the STOMACH, the lower end of the OESOPHAGUS and the SPLEEN into the liver. After a meal the portal vein contains large quantities of digested nutrients.

port-wine stain a flat, permanent, purple-red birthmark caused by a benign tumour of small skin blood vessels. A capillary HAEMANGIOMA. Port-wine stains can be treated by skin grafting or with laser burns.

Posalfilin a brand name for PODOPHYLLUM RESIN with SALICYLIC ACID.

position effect the effect on the expression of a gene resulting from its translocation to a different part of the genome. A gene may, for instance, be inactivated if moved to a region that is permanently in a highly condensed condition (heterochromation).

positivism a school of philosophy that rejects value judgements, metaphysics and theology and holds that the only path to reliable knowledge is that of scientific observation and experiment.

positron emission tomography see PET SCANNING.

post- *prefix denoting* after.

postcode lottery a situation in which the standard of medical care available to the public varies from area to area, depending on the funding policies of various health boards, and other factors. Government legislation has been drafted to try to avoid this inequality.

postcode prescribing variations in the availability of medication depending on where patients live, and which treatments their health board is willing and able to provide.

postcoital contraception the use of any measure to prevent pregnancy after sexual intercourse has occurred. Such measures are not strictly contraceptive as they are likely to act after conception has occurred. They include taking two high-dose contraceptive pills as soon as possible and then 12 hours later; the taking of a single dose of mifepristone; and the insertion of a copper-releasing IUCD. Mifepristone is currently not licensed anywhere outside China for postcoital contraception. Also known as emergency contraception or the 'morning after pill'.

postconcussional syndrome a spectrum of symptoms occurring after what appears to be a relatively minor head injury with brief loss of consciousness and little or no immediate memory loss (retrograde or post-traumatic amnesia). The syndrome includes headache, depression, loss of concentration and the power of attention, memory loss, anxiety, dizziness

and low tolerance to noise. These symptoms may persist for a year or longer.

postencephalitic Parkinsonism PARKINSONISM occurring as a sequel to ENCEPHALITIS LETHARGICA.

posterior pertaining to the back of the body or a part. Dorsal. Compare ANTERIOR.

posterior leucoencephalopathy syndrome a serious brain disorder featuring oedema of the white matter of the rear parts of the cerebral hemispheres demonstrable on CT scanning and magnetic resonance imaging. The syndrome features headache, visual disturbances, vomiting, confusion and seizures, and the possible causes include eclampsia, severe hypertension and treatment with immunosuppressive drugs such as CYCLOSPORIN (ciclosporin), INTERFERON ALFA, and TACROLIMUS. Also known as the posterior reversible encephalopathy syndrome (PRES).

postganglionic pertaining to the nerve cells and fibres arising from the ganglia of the AUTONOMIC NERVOUS SYSTEM. Compare PREGANGLIONIC.

postherpetic pain persistent pain experienced in an area previously affected by SHINGLES. Postherpetic pain may last for years and is a severe burden to the elderly victim. Early use of ACYCLOVIR during an attack of shingles can minimize the damage to sensory nerves that causes the pain.

posthitis inflammation of the FORESKIN (prepuce).

posthypnotic suggestion a command to a hypnotized person to perform a specified action after restoration from the hypnotic state.

postmaturity the state in which a pregnancy lasts longer than two weeks beyond the normal 40 weeks from the first day of the last menstrual period.

postmortem examination see AUTOPSY.

postmyocardial infarction syndrome see DRESSLER'S SYNDROME.

postnasal drip an intermittent trickle of watery nasal discharge or mucus from the back of the nose into the throat. The excess secretion usually results from inflammation of the mucous membrane of the nose, as in RHINITIS from any cause.

postnatal occurring subsequent to birth.

postnatal care care of the mother for the period of about 6 weeks after delivery of a baby.

postnatal depression depression affecting the mother after childbirth. This is common and may vary from a mild sadness to a severe psychotic depressive illness with strong suicidal and sometimes infanticidal tendencies. Antidepressant drugs may be necessary.

postoperative after surgery.

postpartum following childbirth.

postpartum depression see POSTNATAL DEPRESSION.

postpartum haemorrhage excessive blood loss after childbirth usually from the site to which the PLACENTA was attached. This may happen if the womb fails to contract normally after delivery of the placenta. Blood transfusion may be necessary and drugs, such as ergometrine, are given to stimulate uterine contractions.

post-polio syndrome a complex of fatigue, weakness, muscle and joint pain and intolerance to cold occurring in people decades after recovering muscle strength by energetic therapy following an attack of POLIOMYELITIS.

postprandial after a meal.

post-traumatic stress disorder an anxiety disorder caused by the major personal stress of a serious or frightening event such as injury, assault, rape or exposure to warfare or a natural or transportational disaster. The reaction may be immediate or delayed for months. There are nightmares, insomnia, 'flash-backs' in which the causal event is vividly relived, a sense of isolation, guilt, irritability and loss of concentration. Emotions may be deadened or depression may develop. Most cases settle in time, but support and skilled counselling may be needed. Some persist for a lifetime.

postural drainage a method of disposing of sputum or other secretions by positioning the body so that gravity helps to carry them into a position from which they can be coughed out or otherwise drained away. Chest postural drainage may be assisted by gentle thumps with a cupped hand.

postural hypotension a drop in the blood pressure caused by standing or by rising suddenly. The brain is temporarily deprived of a full blood supply. This is a common cause of fainting.

postural stridor noisy breathing related to a particular posture, when a posture (such as raising the arms) causes indirect pressure on the larynx or trachea. This can occur from a cervical mass such as a goitre or tumour.

posture the relationship of different parts of the body to each other and to the vertical. In youth, posture is fully under voluntary control. Faulty posture tends to become permanent and may affect health as well as appearance.

post-viral fatigue syndrome an ill-defined and controversial disorder more commonly, if erroneously, called MYALGIC ENCEPHALITIS. The condition may follow a virus infection and features severe fatigue, limitation of activity, muscle aching and emotional disturbance. The condition is not caused by brain inflammation as the name implies and there is controversy as to whether it is of organic origin but there is no questioning the distress and disablement of the sufferers. Now often called chronic fatigue syndrome.

Potaba a brand name for AMINOBENZOIC ACID.

potassium an important body mineral present in carefully-controlled concentration. Potassium is necessary for normal heart rhythm, for the regulation of the body's water balance and for the conduction of nerve impulses and the contraction of muscles. Many diuretic drugs result in a loss of potassium from the body and this can be dangerous. Supplementary potassium is often included in the formulation of these preparations. Potassium may also be given as a separate supplement in such preparations as Kay-Cee-L or Slow-K.

potassium channel activator one of a new class of drugs that greatly enhances the movement of potassium ions through channels in cell membranes. The action on the membranes of smooth muscle cells in arterial walls is to cause hyperpolarization so that the cells' sensitivity to the normal stimuli to contraction is reduced. The muscle fibres are thus relaxed and the arteries widened. Drugs in this class are useful in improving the blood supply to the heart muscle in ANGINA PECTORIS. A typical drug in this group is nicorandil (Icorel).

potassium chloride a drug used to treat potassium deficiency. The drug is on the WHO official list. A brand name is Kay-Cee-L.

potassium iodide a drug used in the pre-operative management of HYPERTHYROIDISM, in the treatment of the fungal infection cutaneous SPOROTRICHOSIS, and to treat iodine deficiency. The drug is on the WHO official list.

potassium permanganate a soluble compound that gives a skin-staining, deep purple solution with antiseptic and astringent properties. Now little used.

potato nose a popular term for the condition of RHINOPHYMA in which overgrowth of sebaceous tissue and blood vessels causes a bulbous deformity. A feature of some cases of ACNE ROSACEA.

potency 1 the ability of a man to obtain an erection and so perform sexual intercourse.
2 the strength of a drug based on its effectiveness to cause change.
3 the claimed increase in the power of homeopathic remedies (see HOMEOPATHY) with increasing dilution and shaking.

pothead a slang term for a habitual MARIJUANA smoker.

Pott's disease tuberculosis of the spine, with collapse of one or more vertebrae, so as to produce a sharp angulation and a hump-back. Also known as spinal caries. (Sir Percivall Pott, 1714–88, English surgeon).

Pott's fracture an ankle break (fracture) in which the delicate outer bone of the leg (the fibula) breaks and the main bone (the tibia) either dislocates, with rupture of the ligament on the inner side, or fractures. Treatment involves manipulation of the bones into position under anaesthesia and immobilization of the foot, ankle and lower leg in a cast for 8 to 10 weeks.

pouch of Douglas the space, lined with PERITONEUM, between the womb and the rectum. (James Douglas, 1675–1742, Scottish anatomist).

poultice a warm pack, usually of kaolin wrapped in soft fabric, applied in the hope of reducing local inflammation and pain. Poultices are of relatively little value and are now seldom used.

povidone-iodine an antiseptic drug suitable for application to the skin or, in the form of pessaries, to the vagina. It is also used as a mouthwash or gargle to treat mouth infections. Brand names are Betadine and Inadine.

Powergel a brand name for KETOPROFEN formulated for external use.

pox 1 any of the various infectious diseases, such as CHICKENPOX or cowpox, that cause blistering skin rashes. Some are caused by POXVIRUSES. Chickenpox is caused by a HERPES virus.
2 a slang term for SYPHILIS, which is not a pox.

poxviruses the largest viruses, just visible by light microscopy, these were responsible for SMALLPOX and now cause cowpox (VACCINIA), orf and MOLLUSCUM CONTAGIOSUM, but not CHICKENPOX.

Prader-Willi syndrome a genetic disorder caused by a small deletion from the long arm of chromosome 15. At birth the baby is very floppy and initial physical development is very slow. Later in childhood there is a rapid increase in weight and obesity. Older children may show severe obsessive-compulsive behaviour problems, temper tantrums and stubborn indiscipline. The face is narrow with a thin upper lip and down-turned mouth. The genitalia are underdeveloped, especially in males, and puberty is delayed. (A. Prader and H. Willi are Swiss paediatricians who described the syndrome in 1956. They were anticipated by almost 100 years by Langdon Down (1828–96) who described a case in detail in 1864 and whose syndrome is even better known).

Pragmatar a brand name for a mixture of coal tar, the skin-softening agent SALICYLIC ACID and sulphur.

pragmatism 1 action determined by the need to respond to immediate necessity or to achieve a particular practical result, rather than by established policy or dogma.
2 the philosophic principle that the truth and meaning of an idea is entirely relative to its practical outcome.

Pramin a brand name for METOCLOPRAMIDE.

Praminil a brand name for IMIPRAMINE.

pramoxine pramocaine, a local anaesthetic drug used as a surface application in conjunction with HYDROCORTISONE to treat irritating haemorrhoids. A brand name for the combination is Proctofoam HC.

prandial referring to a meal, or to the effects of a meal. Prandial insulin is insulin given in the attempt to mimic the response of endogenous insulin to food intake.

pravastatin one of the class of statin cholesterol-lowering drugs. A brand name is Lipostat. See STATINS.

Praxilene a brand name for the VASODILATOR drug NAFTIDROFURYL.

praxis 1 action.
2 the ability to perform skilled actions.

praziquantel an ANTHELMINTIC drug used to dispose of tapeworms. The drug is on the WHO official list. A brand name is Cysticide.

prazosin a drug that widens arteries (VASODILATOR) and is used in the treatment of high blood pressure (HYPERTENSION), HEART FAILURE and RAYNAUD'S PHENOMENON. The drug is on the WHO official list. A brand name is Hypovase.

PRCA *abbrev. for* PURE RED CELL APLASIA.

pre- *prefix denoting* before, preceding or prior to.

precancerous any condition tending to proceed to cancer, to be associated with the development of cancer, or to carry a significant risk of CANCER.

preclinical 1 pertaining to the incubation period of a disease or to the period before signs and symptoms occur.
2 the period of training of a medical student in the basic medical sciences before access to patients is allowed.

precocious puberty the onset of physical sexual maturity at an abnormally early age, arbitrarily set at prior to 6 years for girls and 7 years for boys. If there are signs of unusually rapid development of the secondary sexual characteristics or growth before 8 in girls or 9 in boys, precocious puberty should be suspected.

Precortisyl Forte a brand name for PREDNISOLONE.

Pred Forte a brand name for PREDNISOLONE.

Predenema a brand name for PREDNISOLONE.

Predfoam a brand name for PREDNISOLONE.

prediabetes a syndrome in severely obese children featuring impaired glucose tolerance, insulin resistance, fat accumulation within muscle cells and in the abdomen, and a high risk of diabetic complications from Type II diabetes.

predisposition a special susceptibility to a disease or disorder, as by the action of direct or indirect genetic or environmental factors.

Prednesol a brand name for PREDNISOLONE.

prednisolone a semisynthetic corticosteroid drug derived from the natural steroid hormone cortisol and used in the treatment of a wide range of inflammatory disorders. Prednisolone may be given by mouth or injection, but many preparations are formulated for application to the skin or the eyes or ears and the drug may also be given as an enema. The drug is on the WHO official list. Brand names are Deltacortril, Deltastab, Minims Prednisolone, Precortisyl Forte, Pred Forte, Predenema, Predfoam, Prednesol, and Predsol.

prednisone a synthetic corticosteroid drug used to reduce inflammation and relieve symptoms in rheumatoid arthritis, ulcerative colitis and many other conditions. A brand name is Decortisyl.

Predsol a brand name for PREDNISOLONE.

Predsol-N a brand name for NEOMYCIN with PREDNISOLONE, for external use.

pre-eclampsia a syndrome of high blood pressure (HYPERTENSION), fluid accumulation in the tissues (OEDEMA) and protein in the urine (albuminuria) that becomes apparent in the second half of pregnancy. Pre-eclampsia is primarily a placental disorder with damage to the inner lining (endothelium) of placental blood vessels. Oxygen FREE RADICALS cause endothelial cell damage, and may lead to reduced NITRIC OXIDE production, so that blood vessel widening (vasodilatation) is interfered with. Pre-eclampsia is a warning of the dangerous complication of ECLAMPSIA – a condition of seizures carrying a high maternal and fetal mortality. A major reason for antenatal care is to monitor for pre-eclampsia and to treat the condition, induce labour or perform a Caesarean section. It has been shown that abnormally high levels of circulating angiogenic factors such as vascular endothelial growth factor and soluble fms-like tyrosine kinase 1 predict the development of pre-eclampsia.

prefrontal pertaining to the front part of the frontal lobe of the brain.

prefrontal leucotomy, prefrontal lobotomy a surgical operation to cut the white fibres that connect the PREFRONTAL lobes of the brain to the THALAMUS. This operation is now rarely performed.

Pregaday a brand name for FERROUS FUMARATE in conjunction with FOLIC ACID.

preganglionic pertaining to the nerves of the spinal cord that connect to the chains of ganglia of the AUTONOMIC NERVOUS SYSTEM lying alongside the spine.

pregnancy the state of a woman during the period from fertilization of an ovum (conception) to the birth of a baby or termination by ABORTION.

pregnancy disorders see ABORTION, ANTEPARTUM HAEMORRHAGE, MISCARRIAGE, OLIGOHYDRAMNIOS, POLYHYDRAMNIOS, PRE-ECLAMPSIA, PREMATURITY and RHESUS INCOMPATIBILITY.

pregnancy-induced hypertension any rise in blood pressure brought about by pregnancy and unaccompanied by protein in the urine or endothelial activation as indicated by a rise in circulating cellular fibronectin. Hypertension in pregnancy will, however, always raise the possibility of PRE-ECLAMPSIA.

pregnancy tests tests on urine or blood for the presence of human chorionic gonadotrophin, a hormone produced by the PLACENTA and thus occurring only during pregnancy. Urine pregnancy tests are about 97% accurate if positive and about 80% accurate if negative.

Pregnyl a brand name for CHORIONIC GONADOTROPHIN.

preimplantation genetic diagnosis the use of genetic analysis in the course of IN VITRO FERTILIZATION to ensure that a baby does not possess a known genetic defect of either parent. After analysis of the embryos formed, only those free of defect are implanted in the mother's womb.

prejudice the maintenance of an adverse opinion about a person or class of persons in spite of evidence to the contrary. This is a common characteristic of the human being and is linked with the habit of arguing illogically from the particular to the general and the tendency to irrational chauvinism.

premalignant precancerous.

Premarin a brand name for a preparation of conjugated oestrogens. The name is said to derive from the source – pregnant mare's urine.

premature ejaculation the occurrence of a male orgasm at such an early stage in sexual intercourse as to deprive both partners of satisfaction. Premature ejaculation is usually due to sexual inexperience or over-excitement.

prematurity birth of a baby before the 37th week of pregnancy gestation or of a baby weighing less than 2500 g, regardless of the gestation period.

premedication drugs given an hour or so before a surgical operation to relieve pain and anxiety and to reduce the dose of anaesthetic needed. Atropine or an atropine-like (anticholinergic) drug is often also given to dry up respiratory secretions and protect the heart against undue slowing.

premenstrual tension see PREMENSTRUAL SYNDROME.

premenstrual syndrome a group of physical and emotional symptoms that may affect women during the week or two before the start of each menstrual period. The cause of the syndrome remains unclear. It features irritability, depression, fatigue, tension, headache, breast tenderness, a sense of abdominal fullness and pain, fluid retention and backache. Various treatments may have to be tried before relief is obtained. Suggested remedies include diuretic drugs, modification of diet, vitamin B$_6$, EVENING PRIMROSE OIL, progesterone or oral contraceptives.

premenstrual dysphoria disorder a syndrome affecting some women during the period from about a week before the start of menstruation to about three days after and featuring marked swings of mood, depression and self-critical thoughts, anger, irritability, crying, fatigue, increased appetite and sometimes a craving for high-carbohydrate foods. The disorder is often severe enough to disrupt normal social activity. The condition has been most effectively treated with selective serotonin re-uptake inhibitor drugs such as fluoxetine (Prozac), but some sufferers require hormone treatment with an oral contraceptive.

Premique, Premique Cycle brand names for MEDROXYPROGESTERONE formulated in conjunction with conjugated oestrogens for post-menopausal hormone replacement therapy.

premolars the four pairs of permanent grinding teeth situated on either side of each jaw between the CANINES and the MOLARS.

prenatal existing or occurring before birth.

Prepidil a brand name for DINOPROSTONE (Prostin E2).

prepuce see FORESKIN.

presbyacusis progressive loss of hearing for the higher frequencies that occurs with age. Presbyacusis is a sensorineural type of deafness probably caused by several factors. From the Greek *presbys*, an old man, and *akousis*, hearing.

presbyopia progressive loss of focusing power of the eyes associated with loss of elasticity of the internal (crystalline) lenses. The condition is closely age-related and the effect is to make close work, such as reading, increasingly difficult. The term derives from the Greek *presbys*, an old man, and *ops*, an eye.

Prescal a brand name for ISRADIPINE.

prescription an instruction to a pharmacist, written by a doctor, to dispense a stated quantity of a particular drug in a specified dose. A prescription also contains instructions to the patient indicating how the drug is to be taken, how often, and for how long. These are usually computer-printed on the label by the pharmacist.

Preservex a brand name for ACECLOFENAC.

pressure points places where major arteries lie near the surface and over bones. Direct pressure applied to these points can limit the blood flow and control severe bleeding as a first aid measure in cases of injury.

pressure sores see BEDSORES.

Prestim a brand name for a mixture of the thiazide DIURETIC drug bendrofluazide (bendroflumethiazide) and the beta-blocking drug TIMOLOL.

prevalence the number of people suffering from a particular disease at any one time in a defined population. Prevalence is usually expressed as a rate per 100,000 of the population. Compare INCIDENCE.

preventive medicine the branch of medicine concerned with the prevention of disease by any means. These include public education in health matters, immunization, safe food legislation and inspection, the provision of safe water supplies and measures to limit dangerous practices such as smoking.

Priadel a brand name for LITHIUM.

priapism persistent, usually painful erection of the corpora cavernosa of the penis without sexual interest. Priapism results from the failure of blood to drain from the penis and may lead to permanent damage from blood clotting. Urgent treatment is needed to withdraw the blood through a wide-bore needle or to obtain detumescence by other means. From the Greek *Priapos*, the god of procreation.

prickly heat an irritating skin disorder caused by excessive sweating so that the skin becomes waterlogged, the ducts of the sweat glands blocked and sweat is forced into the skin. The condition settles if the affected person can be kept cool by air conditioning or frequent cool showers. Also known as miliaria rubra.

prilocaine a local anaesthetic drug normally given by injection. A brand name is Citanest. The drug can also be applied in a cream for surface anaesthesia under the brand name EMLA.

Primacor a brand name for the PHOSPHODIESTERASE INHIBITOR drug MILRINONE.

primaquine a drug used in the treatment of

Plasmodium vivax and Plasmodium ovale MALARIA. The drug is on the WHO official list.

primary 1 occurring as an initial, rather than as a secondary, event or complication.
2 originating within the affected organ or tissue, rather than having spread from another source.
3 the first of several diseases to affect a part.
4 of unknown cause.

primary angioplasty immediate intervention, with minimal delay, to restore the patency of the coronary arteries after a heart attack. Primary angioplasty is an alternative to attempts to remove the occluding blood clot by enzymatic fibrinolysis – which is not without danger. It calls for a preliminary angiogram and may be performed by balloon catheter angioplasty with or without the insertion of a stent, or by other means. Enthusiasts for the method claim that the results are markedly superior to other forms of heart attack treatment.

primary immune response the weak initial reaction caused by the first encounter of a 'naïve' lymphocyte with a particular antigen. Antibodies are nor detectable for several days then rise to a (low) peak concentration and then fall again. If now there is a second challenge with the same antigen, there is a more rapid and much higher rise in the level of antibodies. This is the secondary immune response.

primary immunodeficiency disorders see GENETIC IMMUNODEFICIENCY DISORDERS.

primary progressive aphasia an atypical form of DEMENTIA featuring progressive loss of the language function without severe memory loss, loss of visual and spacial skills or deterioration in behaviour. The defect is essentially one of word comprehension so that there is inexorable loss of the ability to find an appropriate word or name objects (anomia) or to employ normal syntax. The condition is associated with focal degeneration in the speech areas on the left temporal lobe of the brain, but it is not considered to be a subset of Alzheimer's disease.

primary systemic vasculitis a range of disorders of blood vessel walls featuring inflammation and cell death (necrosis) with thickening and nodular protrusions. The group includes polyarteritis nodosa, Wegener's granulomatosis, the CHURG-STRAUSS SYNDROME and KAWASAKI DISEASE.

primary teeth the first set of teeth to appear, usually beginning to erupt around the age of 6 months. There are 20 primary teeth consisting of 8 incisors, 4 canines and 8 molars. Also known as deciduous or milk teeth. Compare PERMANENT TEETH.

Primaxin a brand name for CILASTATIN.

primer 1 a short RNA sequence paired with one DNA strand that provides a free 3'–OH end on which synthesis of a deoxyribonucleotide chain can start.
2 the short nucleotide sequence used to start the POLYMERASE CHAIN REACTION (PCR) process.

primidone an ANTICONVULSANT drug used in the treatment of EPILEPSY. A brand name is Mysoline.

primigravida a woman pregnant for the first time.

Primolut N a brand name for NORETHISTERONE.

Primoteston a brand name for TESTOSTERONE.

Primperan a brand name for the ANTIEMETIC drug metoclopramide.

primum non nocere a dictum, universally-respected among doctors, to the effect that one's first concern should be to do no harm to the patient.

Prioderm a brand name for a preparation containing MALATHION for external use.

prion a protease-resistant sialoglycoprotein that is a normal constituent of the brain. Abnormal forms of the protein are now generally accepted as the causal agents in CREUTZFELDT-JAKOB DISEASE (CJD) and bovine spongiform encephalopathy (BSE). The protein was isolated by Stanley Prusiner in 1982, the term prion (an abbreviation of 'proteinaceous infectious particle') being proposed by Prusiner to make the point that it was not a virus. Prion protein (PrP) is found in high concentration in brains affected with spongiform encephalopathy, and forms AMYLOID deposits in these brains. This structurally simple, seemingly-infectious agent of simpler constitution than any virus, is capable of causing a severe and invariably fatal disease of the nervous system. Prions resist sterilization by normal methods and have been spread on surgical instruments and in donated human growth hormone. Prusiner was awarded the Nobel Prize in 1998 for his work on prions. See also PRION PROTEIN DISEASE.

prion disease see PRION PROTEIN, PRION PROTEIN DISEASE and CREUTZFELDT-JAKOB DISEASE.

prion protein disease one of a number of transmissible diseases, including CREUTZFELDT-JAKOB DISEASE, Gerstmann-Strussler syndrome and KURU, all of which feature a SPONGIFORM ENCEPHALOPATHY. They are all associated with an abnormal form of a normal cell protein called PRION PROTEIN. They feature plaques of AMYLOID in the brain tissue and the prion protein is the main constituent of these plaques.

Pripsen a brand name for a mixture of the ANTHELMINTIC drug PIPERAZINE and the laxative senna.

pro- *prefix denoting* forward, first, to, towards the front or preceding. It may or may not be a coincidence that hundreds of drug names, especially brand names, have this prefix. More than 50 of the names of those currently being commonly prescribed, start with 'pro-' and the practice appears to be spreading to the naming of products outside pharmacology.

probability see P-VALUE.

proband the presenting patient of a group with an identical or similar disorder, especially the member of a family first found to have an inheritable disorder. Also known as propositus.

probang an instrument once used to remove foreign bodies blindly from the larynx or esophagus. Now rendered obsolete by the development of endoscopic techniques.

Pro-Banthine a brand name for the antispasmodic drug propantheline.

probe any slender, usually blunt-ended instrument used to explore a passageway, cavity or wound.

probenecid a drug used to prevent kidney damage during treatment with the antiviral drug cidofovir.

probiotic a single or mixed culture of live micro-organisms used therapeutically to improve the properties of the indigenous microflora. *Lactobacilli* and *Bifidobacterium* species are commonly employed as probiotics. They are claimed to be useful as a protective against colonic cancer, to reduce blood cholesterol levels, improve lactose digestion and relieve vaginal infections and secondary cystitis.

problem-orientated medical records medical records organized on the basis of presenting problems, that distinguish between objective and subjective information, and that maintain a historical summary of both active and inactive problems.

pro-brain natriuretic peptide an inactive prohormone peptide released from stretched cardiac muscle cells. The prohormone is split into the active BNP and the inactive n-terminal fragment. Levels of the latter have been found to be an effective prognostic marker of the long-term mortality risk in people with coronary artery disease.

procainamide a local anaesthetic-like drug used intravenously to control heart irregularities by its action to diminish the excitability of the conducting bundles in the heart muscle. The drug is on the WHO official list. A brand name is Pronestyl.

procaine a local anaesthetic drug now largely replaced by others that are more quickly effective or of more persistent action.

procaine penicillin procaine benzylpenicillin, a depot form of penicillin, given by deep intramuscular injection, that can provide effective concentrations of the drug for up to 24 hours. Benzylpenicillin can, however, no longer be relied on to be effective against organisms formerly highly sensitive to it. The drug is on the WHO official list.

procarbazine an anticancer drug used especially in the treatment of LYMPHOMAS. The drug is on the WHO official list. A brand name is Natulan.

prochlorperazine a PHENOTHIAZINE derivative antipsychotic drug used to treat SCHIZOPHRENIA and MANIA and to relieve nausea and vomiting. Brand names are Buccastem and Stemetil.

procidentia displacement (PROLAPSE) especially of the womb (uterus), from its normal position. In procidentia the uterus descends through the VAGINA to a varying degree and must be retained in place either by a PESSARY or by a surgical repair.

proctalgia fugax sudden short attacks of severe cramping pain in the RECTUM, probably caused, in most cases, by anxiety-related muscle spasm.

proctitis inflammation of the RECTUM. This causes pain, bleeding and often a discharge of mucus and pus. Proctitis is commonly associated with ULCERATIVE COLITIS, CROHN'S DISEASE, DYSENTERY or sexually transmitted diseases in people engaging in anal intercourse. The treatment is directed to the cause.

proctology the branch of medicine concerned with the disorders of the lower (sigmoid) colon, the rectum and the anus.

proctoscopy direct visual examination of the ANUS and RECTUM either by means of a short rigid metal tube (a proctoscope) or by using a flexible, fibreoptic ENDOSCOPE. Both are inserted through the anus.

procyclidine an ANTICHOLINERGIC drug used to treat PARKINSON'S DISEASE. Brand names are Arpicolin and Kemadrin.

prodrome a symptom or sign that precedes the start of a disease and gives early warning. KOPLIK'S SPOTS are a prodrome of MEASLES and the AURA is a prodrome of an epileptic seizure or an attack of MIGRAINE.

prodrug a substance which, after metabolic action in the body, is coverted to an active drug.

proenzyme a protein that can give rise to an enzyme.

professions allied to medicine a general title for a range of disciplines that offer medicine a wide spectrum of specialized knowledge and skills. The allied professions work in close association with clinicians to promote the recovery and welfare of patients. They include BIOMEDICAL ENGINEERING, CHIROPODY, DIETETICS, medical physics, OCCUPATIONAL THERAPY, ORTHOPTICS, ORTHOTICS, PHYSIOTHERAPY, prosthetics, RADIOGRAPHY and SPEECH THERAPY. The term 'paramedic' may be applied to some or all of these.

Proflex a brand name for IBUPROFEN in a preparation for external use.

progeria premature ageing. There are two types: Hutchinson-Gilford syndrome and Werner's syndrome. In the former, a child of 10 may show all the characteristics of old age – baldness, grey hair, wrinkled skin, loss of body fat and degenerative diseases of the arteries. In the latter, the disease starts in adult life and runs a rapid course over about 10 years. Both types are now believed to result from single spontaneous gene mutations. In HG syndrome the mutation is in the gene coding for lamin A, an important structural protein. In Werner's syndrome the mutation is in a helicase – a gene that unwinds double-strand DNA into two single strands. From the Greek *pro*, before and *geras*, old age.

Progesic a brand name for the non-steroidal anti-inflammatory drug (NSAID) fenoprofen.

progesterone the hormone secreted by the CORPUS LUTEUM of the ovary and by the PLACENTA. Progesterone acts during the menstrual cycle to predispose the lining of the womb (endometrium) to receive and retain the fertilized ovum. During pregnancy, progesterone from the placenta ensures the continued health and growth of the womb and promotes the growth of the milk-secreting cells of the breasts. Progesterone-like substances (progestogens) are widely used in medicine and are common constituents of oral contraceptives. The hormone is used to treat menstrual symptoms and infertility and as an adjunct to oestrogen in post-menopausal hormone replacement therapy (HRT). Brand names are Crinone, Cyclogest and Gestone.

progestogen one of a group of drugs chemically and pharmacologically similar to the natural hormone PROGESTERONE. They are used in oral contraceptives to interfere with ovulation, to alter the womb lining so that it is less receptive to a fertilized egg and to make the mucus in the cervix less readily penetrable by sperms. They are also used to treat menstrual disorders and cancers that are being promoted by oestrogens.

proglottid one of the segments of a tapeworm, containing both male and female reproductive organs. The proglottides increase in size progressively as they become remote from the head of the worm.

prognathism abnormal protrusion of either jaw, especially the lower.

prognosis an informed medical guess as to the probable course and outcome of a disease. Prognosis is based on a knowledge of the natural history of the disease and of any special factors in the case under consideration.

Progout a brand name for ALLOPURINOL.

progressive multifocal leucoencephalopathy a rare brain disorder featuring widespread patches of DEMYELINATION and changes in the supportive (glial) cells suggestive of a papova virus infection. There is severe brain damage and the condition usually progresses to death within a few weeks.

progressive muscular atrophy see MOTOR NEURON DISEASE, MYOPATHY and MUSCULAR DYSTROPHY.

progressive supranuclear palsy an uncommon neurodegenerative disorder that starts in middle and late life and is often misdiagnosed as Parkinson's disease. The disease features Parkinsonism, partial paralysis of eye movement, reduced blinking rate and postural insecurity with poor balance and a tendency to fall over. About 15% have a degree of progressive cognitive loss with apathy and emotional lability.

progressive systemic sclerosis see SYSTEMIC SCLEROSIS.

proguanil an antimalarial drug mainly used for prevention (as a PROPHYLACTIC). A brand name is Paludrine. The drug is on the WHO official list. Formulated in conjunction with ATOVAQUONE, it is produced under the brand name Malarone.

Progynova a brand name for OESTRADIOL (estradiol).

prohormones molecules that are split by enzymes to form hormones. Most are proteins of at least moderate size. Peptide hormones cannot be directly synthesized because cells cannot produce proteins below a particular size.

prohormone convertases enzymes that cleave prohormones to yield active hormones.

prokaryote, procaryote a class of primitive single-cell living organisms, containing the bacteria and the blue-green algae, and so called because the members do not possess a discrete nucleus with a nuclear membrane. The genome is merely dispersed throughout the cell. All nucleated cells and organisms are said to be eukaryotic or eucaryotic.

prolactin one of the PITUITARY GLAND hormones. Prolactin stimulates the development and growth of the breasts (mammary glands) and helps to start and maintain milk production at the end of pregnancy.

prolactinoma a benign tumour of the PITUITARY GLAND that secretes large quantities of the hormone PROLACTIN. The tumour can cause blindness by pressing on the OPTIC CHIASMA and may be suspected because of unexpected milk production (lactation). Treatment is by surgery or by drugs.

prolapse the downward displacement, or movement to an abnormal position, of a body part or tissue. Common examples are prolapse of the uterus (PROCIDENTIA), prolapse of the RECTUM and prolapse of the pulpy centre of an intervertebral disc.

prolapsed intervertebral disc the backward expression of the pulpy centre (NUCLEUS PULPOSUS) of an intervertebral disc as a result of degenerative changes in the outer fibrous portion of the disc (the annulus fibrosus). Disc pulp is likely to press on adjacent spinal nerve roots causing severe pain and sometimes weakness in leg muscles. Also known as 'slipped disc'.

Proleukin a brand name for ALDESLEUKIN.

proliferation multiplication. The process of increasing in number by reproduction.

Proluton a brand name for HYDROXYPROGESTERONE HEXANOATE.

promazine a phenothiazine derivative antipsychotic drug used as a sedative. A brand name is Sparine.

promethazine an ANTIHISTAMINE drug used to relieve itching, to control motion sickness and as a sedative. The drug is on the WHO official list. A brand name is Phenergan.

promiscuity a loose term for sexual promiscuity – a common pattern of behaviour in which sex is valued for its variety and immediate gratifications rather than as one of the important bases for a long-term relationship. Some psychologists equate promiscuity with social immaturity; others hold it to be unrelated. Promiscuity has always carried penalties of some kind, often in the form of sexually transmitted diseases such as gonorrhoea, herpes and Chlamydial infections. In an AIDS context, these have become much more significant.

promoter in genetics, a nucleotide sequence to which RNA polymerase must bind before the process of transcription can start. The promoter is located UPSTREAM of the gene it regulates.

pronation the act of turning to a face down (prone) position, or of rotating the horizontal forearm so that the palm of the hand faces the ground. The opposite movements are called supination.

prone lying with the front of the body downward. Face downward. Compare SUPINE.

Pronestyl a brand name for the ANTIARRHYTHMIC drug PROCAINAMIDE.

proofreading in genetics, the correction, performed by DNA polymerase, of mistakes in the incorporation of nucleotides in a sequence, the corrections being made after individual units have been added to the chain.

proopiomelanocortin (POMC) the prohormone from which ACTH, beta-lipotropin, and beta-ENDORPHIN are produced by cleavage. POMC is found most abundantly in the pituitary

and hypothalamus, but also occurs in the sex glands and elsewhere.

propafenone a drug used to treat heart irregularities (arrhythmias). A brand name is Arythmol.

propamidine an antibacterial drug used externally in the form of eye drops to treat eye infections. A brand name is Golden Eye.

propantheline an antispasmodic drug used to relieve bowel spasm and to treat the IRRITABLE BOWEL SYNDROME and urinary incontinence caused by an irritable bladder. A brand name is Pro-Banthine.

Propecia a brand name for FINASTERIDE.

prophase the first stage in cell division by MITOSIS and MEIOSIS, during which CHROMATIN coils up to form chromosomes.

prophylactic and any act, procedure, drug or equipment used to guard against or prevent an unwanted outcome, such as a disease.

Propine a brand name for DIPIVEFRIN.

propofol a general anaesthetic drug given by injection. A brand name is Diprivan.

propranolol a beta-blocker drug used to treat anxiety, MIGRAINE, high blood pressure (HYPERTENSION), ANGINA PECTORIS and heart irregularities (cardiac arrhythmias). The drug is on the WHO official list. Brand names are Beta-Prograne, Inderal and Syprol.

proprietary 1 privately or exclusively owned, as of the right to manufacture and sell a particular drug or to use a particular drug name.

2 patented for production by one company only.

proprioception awareness of the position in space, and of the relation to the rest of the body, of any body part. Proprioceptive information is essential to the normal functioning of the body's mechanical control system and is normally acquired unconsciously from sense receptors in the muscles, joints, tendons and the balance organ of the inner ear.

proptosis abnormal protrusion of the eyeball. Also known as EXOPHTHALMOS. Proptosis is cause by any process that increases the bulk of the soft tissues in the ORBIT behind the eyeball.

propyliodone a contrast medium used for the X-ray examination of the respiratory tract. The drug is on the WHO official list.

propylthiouracil a drug used to treat over-activity of the thyroid gland (HYPERTHYROIDISM). The drug is on the WHO official list.

Proscar a brand name for FINASTERIDE.

prosencephalon the forebrain.

prostacyclin a short-acting hormone produced by the lining of blood vessels (ENDOTHELIUM) and by the lungs, that limits the aggregation of PLATELETS and is probably of major importance in preventing THROMBOSIS. Prostacyclin has a half-life of only 2–3 minutes.

prostaglandins a group of unsaturated fatty acid mediators occurring throughout the tissues and body fluids. They are generated from cell membrane ARACHIDONIC ACID by the action of phospholipase A$_2$ and function as hormones. They have many different actions. They cause constriction or widening of arteries, they stimulate pain nerve endings, they promote or inhibit aggregation of blood PLATELETS and hence influence blood clotting, they induce abortion, reduce stomach acid secretion and relieve asthma. They can both stimulate and inhibit immune responses. Some painkilling drugs, such as aspirin, act by preventing the release of prostaglandins from injured tissue.

prostaglandin drugs synthetic PROSTAGLANDINS used to induce labour or procure ABORTION, to treat PERSISTENT DUCTUS ARTERIOSUS and to relieve PEPTIC ULCER.

prostate see PROSTATE GLAND.

prostate cancer the most common cancer in men, with an incidence that increases with age. At autopsy, 30% of men over 50 and 75% of men over 80 have a prostate cancer, usually unsuspected. Most cases are adenocarcinomas arising from the ACINAR processes of the gland. Small local lymph node metastases of prostate cancer can be detected by MRI scanning especially if magnetic iron nanoparticles have been given by intravenous injection beforehand. There is growing evidence that the regular consumption of whole tomatoes is protective against the disease. Studies suggest that this effect is not only caused by the content of the carotenoid lycoprene. Most prostate cancers are androgen-dependent but metastases may later become androgen-refractory. Drug treatments for the latter with docetaxel and prednisolone have recently been developed.

prostatectomy an operation to remove an enlarged PROSTATE GLAND or to remove enough of it to relieve urinary obstruction. Prostatectomy is usually performed via the urine tube (urethra) using an instrument called a resectoscope which incorporates a heated wire used to cut away unwanted tissue. This is called transurethral prostatectomy (TURP). Total prostatectomy is performed to treat cancer of the prostate.

prostate gland a solid, chestnut-like organ situated under the bladder surrounding the first part of the urine tube (urethra) in the male. The prostate gland secretes part of the seminal fluid.

prostate gland disorders see PROSTATIC HYPERPLASIA, PROSTATISM, PROSTATE CANCER, and PROSTATITIS.

prostate screening routine examination and PROSTATE-SPECIFIC ANTIGEN testing in a population of men in whom there is no particular reason to suppose that any individual has prostate cancer. The proposal has aroused prolonged controversy.

prostate-specific antigen (PSA) an enzyme produced by the epithelial cells of the prostate gland, whether healthy or malignant, to liquefy the seminal fluid. Small quantities of PSA enter the bloodstream and the levels can be measured. Raised levels imply an increase in the bulk of prostate tissue and can thus be used as a marker for PROSTATIC HYPERPLASIA or prostate cancer. PSA levels below 4 nanograms per decilitre are, in general, considered normal, but do not preclude cancer. Levels above 10 ng/dl suggest a 70% risk of prostate cancer. The test is made more sensitive for men with levels below 10 ng/d by noting the ratio of free PSA to PSA complexed with antichymotrypsin. If free PSA is 25% or more of total PSA and the gland feels normal, biopsy is considered unnecessary. A free PSA of 15% or less suggests cancer. The opinion is growing among experts that the PSA is a less reliable test for prostate cancer than was formerly thought. See also PSA VELOCITY.

prostatic hyperplasia increase in the size of the inner zone of the PROSTATE GLAND. This commonly occurs, for no obvious reason, in men over 50 and leads to interference with the outflow of urine. The condition is treated by PROSTATECTOMY.

prostatism a group of symptoms resulting from enlargement of the PROSTATE GLAND. They include urgency to urinate, undue frequency of urination, a weak urinary stream and burning pain on urination.

prostatitis inflammation of the prostate gland.

This is commonly caused by bacterial infection which may be sexually acquired. There is pain on passing urine, increased frequency of urination and sometimes discharge. In severe cases there may be fever. Prolonged treatment with antibiotics may be needed.

prosthesis any artificial replacement for a part of the body. Prostheses may be functional or purely cosmetic and may be permanently installed internally or worn externally. The range of prosthetic devices is wide – from artificial eyes and legs to heart valves and testicles.

Prostigmin a brand name for NEOSTIGMINE.

Prostin E2 a brand name for DINOPROSTONE.

prostitution sale of sex, most commonly by women. This may be a part-time or full-time private enterprise or one organized on a small or large scale by pimp, brothel-keepers or call-girl ring organizers. In general, the lot of the prostitute is not a happy one and most of the girls involved are driven by economic necessity into an unpleasant and often dangerous trade. Many of them are unable to sustain more conventional employment. The legal status of prostitution varies considerably from country to country and even within a country. Prostitution is legal, for instance, in Nevada, but illegal in other American states. Most male prostitutes offer services to other men, but a few (gigolos) cater for women.

Prosulf a brand name for PROTAMINE SULPHATE.

protamine sulphate an antidote to the anticiagulant HEPARIN. The drug is on the WHO official list. A brand name is Prosulf.

protamine zinc insulin a slow-release form of insulin with an action lasting for 12–24 hours. A brand name is Humulin Zn.

protanopia partial colour blindness with defective perception of red.

Protaphane a brand name for a form of INSULIN.

protease one of a range of protein-splitting enzymes. One focus of current interest in proteases is in their role in breaking down tissue barriers in the spread of cancer. High concentrations of the activator of one of these proteases has been found to be associated with a poor outlook in cancers of the colon and rectum.

protease inhibitor one of a range of drugs that interfere with the action of the enzyme protease used by HIV to activate the synthesis of its polymer protein coat. These drugs slow the progression of the infection and lengthen life. An undesirable direct or indirect effect is the abnormal laying-down of body fat and high levels of lipids in the blood, which may lead to coronary artery disease and strokes. Brand names are indinavir, ritonavir and saquinavir.

proteasome a large, cylindrical protein complex of several sub-units, present in the cytoplasm and nucleus of all cells and an essential component in cell metabolism. The function of the proteasome is to act as a kind of shredder, degrading unwanted proteins that have been tagged for destruction with UBIQUITIN chains. It strips proteins of their ubiquitin, unfolds them and catalyzed them to peptides. Proteasomes have aroused much interest as therapeutic targets in cancer. The proteasome 26S is involved both in the induction and repression of APOPTOSIS. See also POLYUBIQUITINATION.

proteins large molecules consisting of up to thousands of AMINO ACIDS linked together by peptide bonds to form polypeptides which, in turn, are linked to form proteins. These long chains of amino acids are often folded in specific ways. Fibrous proteins, such as COLLAGEN, are formed from spiral strand polypeptides. They are insoluble and constitute much of the structure of the body. Globular proteins are soluble and include the ENZYMES, many of the hormones and the blood proteins such as haemoglobin and the IMMUNOGLOBULINS (antibodies). Conjugated proteins contain other constituents such as sugars (glycoproteins) and lipids (lipoproteins).

protein S a natural anticoagulant the deficiency of which causes an increased risk of blood clotting within the vessels (thrombosis) and embolism. Protein S deficiency may be of genetic origin or may have other causes. It has been suggested that women with low free protein S may be at increased risk of thrombo-embolism if they are using oral contraceptives.

protein folding the process by which proteins acquire their normal, energetically-favourable, three-dimensional form. The folding has long been believed to be specified by the amino acid sequence, but recent research suggests that proteins may fold into abnormal shapes by mechanisms not yet determined. Abnormal folding results in loss of normal protein function but also in proteolytic degradation and the accumulation of fragments that form insoluble plaques in the various organs including the brain and the liver. This is believed to be the way in which the characteristic plaques and fibrillary tangles of ALZHEIMER'S DISEASE occur.

protein synthesis the construction of protein molecules from AMINO ACIDS. This occurs in the cell CYTOPLASM on the basis of the GENETIC CODE in the DNA. Sections of DNA that code for the particular protein are first transcribed to MESSENGER RNA and this passes out of the cell nucleus to the cytoplasm. There, one or more ribosomes attach themselves to one end of the mRNA molecule and move along it to effect transcription, using, in the process, the sequence of RNA bases to indicate which amino acids should be selected from the cell pool and in what order. In this way the correct amino acids are linked together to form polypeptides and these are then joined to form the particular protein.

proteinuria the passage of more than minimal amounts of protein in the urine. This usually indicates kidney disease, such as GLOMERULO-NEPHRITIS or the NEPHROTIC SYNDROME, but may also occur in MULTIPLE MYELOMATOSIS or other conditions in which the amount of protein in the blood is excessive.

proteoglycans bimolecule complexes of proteins and GLYCOSAMINOGLYCANS with a high proportion of carbohydrate (up to 96%) to protein. They are structural components of connective tissues and lubricants, help in the adhesion of cells to the extracellular matrix, and bind factors that promote cell proliferation.

proteolytic able to split protein molecules into polypeptides and amino acids, as of enzymes such as PEPSIN and CHYMOTRYPSIN. Proteolysis occurs by HYDROLYSIS of peptide bonds.

proteome the totality of all the proteins in an organism such as the human body.

proteomics the study of the proteome – the proteins expressed by the approximately 22,000 genes in the GENOME or by a cell. The form and quantity of the proteins produced by a cell cannot be fully predicted from DNA or RNA analysis alone. This is because of the controls and the many modifications that can occur in the stages between transcription and protein formation. Thus the totality of the

genes can result in at least several hundred thousand different proteins. Proteomics includes the study of the factors that cause this multiplication. The discipline is being applied effectively to cancer studies.

Proteus a genus of GRAM NEGATIVE, rod-shaped bacteria that frequently cause urinary infections or ENTERITIS. A common species is *Proteus vulgaris*.

Prothiaden a brand name for the tricyclic antidepressant drug dothiepin (dosulepin).

prothionamide protionamide, a drug used in the treatment of TUBERCULOSIS resistant to commoner drugs.

Protium a brand name for PANTOPRAZOL.

prothrombin a soluble protein in the blood that is converted to the insoluble form thrombin, under the action of the enzyme prothrombinase, at the end of the cascade of events involved in blood clotting. Thrombin is the main ingredient of the blood clot.

prothrombin time a test for blood clotting defect due to deficiency of clotting factors I (fibrinogen), II (prothrombin) V (proaccelerin), VII (serum prothrombin conversion acclelerator), or X (Stuart-Prower factor). The test determines the ratio between the time taken for the treated patient's blood sample to clot and the time taken for a standard control sample. Prothrombin time estimation is important in bleeding disorders and when oral ANTICOAGULANT drugs (which are antagonists of vitamin K) are being used. Vitamin K is necessary for the formation of several of the clotting factors. A deficiency of platelets does not affect the prothrombin time.

proto- *combining form denoting* first, earliest or primitive.

protocol a plan for the conduct of a clinical trial or a course of treatment.

proton pumps systems of enzymes that transport hydrogen ions across membranes, using energy in the process. Proton pumps that produce hydrochloric acid in the stomach derive their energy from hydrolysis of ATP.

proton pump inhibitor one of a class of drugs that interfere with the action of the proton pump responsible for the synthesis of hydrochloric acid in the parietal cells of the stomach lining. The proton pump is the enzyme H^+, K^+ -ATPase and this can be blocked by drugs such as OMEPRAZOLE (Losec).

proto-oncogene any gene capable of becoming a cancer-producing gene (an oncogene). Proto-oncogenes have important functions in the normal cell, but, by mutation or by the acquisition of genetic control elements from oncoviruses they can lose their normal regulatory functions and lead to uncontrolled multiplication.

Protopic a brand name for TACROLIMUS.

protoplasm the whole of the internal substance of the living cell, consisting of the material surrounding the nucleus (the CYTOPLASM) and the nuclear material (nucleoplasm).

protoporphyrin a porphyrin occurring in the course of the synthesis of HAEMOGLOBIN. Excess of this porphyrin, protoporphyria, causes intense itching, swelling and redness of the skin on exposure to sunlight and leads to a strikingly weatherbeaten appearance.

Protostat a brand name for METRONIDAZOLE.

protozoa primitive, single-celled, microscopic animals able to move by amoeboid action or by means of CILIA or whip-like appendages (flagellae). Many protozoa are parasitic on humans and are of medical importance. These include the organisms that cause AMOEBIASIS, BALANTIDIASIS, CRYPTOSPORIDIOSIS, GIARDIASIS, ISOSPORIDIOSIS, LEISHMANIASIS, MALARIA, SLEEPING SICKNESS, TOXOPLASMOSIS and TRICHOMONIASIS.

Provera a brand name for the PROGESTOGEN drug METHYLPROGESTERONE.

Provigil a brand name for MODAFINIL.

Pro-Viron a brand name for the male sex hormone drug MESTEROLONE.

provitamin a substance that is converted in the body to a VITAMIN.

provocative test a method of obtaining diagnostic information by deliberately provoking a characteristic disease reaction.

proximal pertaining to any point on the body nearer to, or nearest to, the centre. The upper arm is proximal to the hand and is the proximal part of the arm. Compare DISTAL.

proxymetacaine a local anaesthetic drug used as eyedrops for ophthalmic procedures. Brand names are Minims proxymetacaine and Ophthaine.

Prozac a brand name for FLUOXETINE. This widely used mood-controlling drug can interact dangerously with drugs of the MAO inhibitor group and some other antidepressants.

prurigo a widespread, itchy skin rash sometimes secondary to constant scratching but often of no obvious local cause.

pruritus itching. The term is often linked with a word that indicates the site, as in pruritus ani or PRURITUS VULVAE.

pruritus vulvae persisting itching of the external genitalia in women.

Prussian blue a solution of potassium ferric hexacyanoferrate, used to treat thallium poisoning and to remove radiocaesium from the body.

PSA see PROSTATE-SPECIFIC ANTIGEN.

PSA velocity the rate of rise in the level of prostate-specific antigen. An increase in the level by more than 2.0 nanograms per millilitre in the year prior to the diagnosis of prostate cancer suggests a relatively high risk of death from the disease in spite of radical prostatectomy.

pseud-, pseudo- *prefix denoting* false.

pseudarthrosis a false fibrous joint that may form at the site of an ununited fracture. Occasionally a pseudarthrosis is deliberately induced to allow movement after the failure of a hip replacement operation.

pseudocyesis the occurrence of the signs and symptoms of pregnancy when no pregnancy exists. This may sometimes be a manifestation of an overwhelming desire for conception in an infertile woman.

pseudodementia severe depression in an elderly person that mimics DEMENTIA. About 10% of those assumed to be demented are, in fact, suffering from a treatable depression that may respond well to antidepressant drugs.

pseudoephedrine a decongestant drug used to relieve nasal stuffiness (congestion) and contained in many cold remedies. A brand name is Galpseud. It is also formulated with antihistamine drugs under the brand names Dimotane and Sudafed.

pseudoepidemic an outbreak, usually in a closed community or an institution, of a disorder with no demonstrable physical cause. Pseudoepidemics are probably a form of HYSTERIA induced by group suggestibility and the conviction that the condition is contagious. As a rule the symptoms are vague and minor. This term is an example of what happens when words are coined without regard to the etymology of their constituents. 'Epidemic' means 'among the people' so there is nothing 'pseudo' about such outbreaks.

pseudogenes the stable and inactive, long-term consequences of earlier mutations that occurred during the process of evolution. Pseudogenes might be considered as analogues of fossils in geology.

pseudogout acute arthritis resulting from the deposition of calcium pyrophosphate dihydrate crystals in a joint. The symptoms are closely similar to those of GOUT and the cause is unknown. Occasionally it occurs as a complication of HYPERPARATHYROIDISM or HAEMOCHROMATOSIS. Treatment is with non-steroidal anti-inflammatory drugs (NSAIDs).

pseudohermaphroditism a congenital abnormality of the GENITALIA in which they resemble those of the opposite sex. The testes and ovaries (gonads) are, however, those of the genetically correct sex.

Pseudomonas a genus of GRAM NEGATIVE bacteria widely found in nature and responsible for much decomposition of organic matter. *Pseudomonas* species, especially *P. aeruginosa*, cause many serious, especially OPPORTUNISTIC, infections and produce a bluish-green pus.

pseudomucinous cystadenoma a benign tumour of the ovary filled with mucinous material.

psilocybin a powerfully hallucinogenic phosphorylated tryptamine present in the fungi contaminating some types of mushrooms, especially in *Psilocybe mexicana*. It is a powerful hallucinogenic drug with properties similar to those of LSD.

psittacosis an acute, infectious influenza-like disease caused by the organism, *Chlamydia psittaci*, acquired by humans from birds by inhaling dust from their droppings. It affects mainly pigeon fanciers, poultry farmers and pet shop workers. There is fever, headache, sore throat, cough, muscle pain, lethargy and depression. Treatment is with tetracycline antibiotics.

psoas muscle a two-part muscle running from the front of the lower spine to the margin of the pelvis (psoas minor) and to the front of the top of the thigh bone (femur) (psoas major). Its action is to raise the thigh forwards.

psoralen drugs a plant derivative (coumarin) which, when applied to the skin or taken internally, increases the tendency of the skin to pigment under the action of ultraviolet light.

This effect is exploited in the treatment of PSORIASIS and other skin conditions. See also PUVA.

psoriasis a common skin disease featuring obvious, dull red or salmon-pink, oval, thickened patches covered with silvery scales. These may occur anywhere on the body and vary greatly in number. The condition may be complicated by ARTHRITIS. The cause is unknown. Psoriasis is treated by exposure to sunlight or ultraviolet light. PUVA is effective. COAL TAR, dithranol or corticosteroid ointments are used as is the CYTOTOXIC drug METHOTREXATE.

psych- *prefix denoting* mind, mental, psyche.

psyche the mind, as opposed to, or in contradistinction to, the body.

psychedelic drugs see HALLUCINOGENIC DRUGS.

psychiatry the branch of medicine concerned with the management of mental illness and emotional and behavioural problems. Compare psychology. The list that follows highlights the key entries related to psychiatry in the dictionary: alcoholism, anorexia nervosa, antidepressant drugs, anxiety, bipolar disorder, bulimia, depersonalization, depression, drug addiction, electroconvulsive therapy, group psychotherapy, hypochondriasis, hypomania, hysteria, mania, mental retardation, neurosis, organic brain syndrome, paranoia, personality disorders, phobia, psychosis, psychotherapy, SADS, schizophrenia, sex therapy, stress, suicide.

psychoanalysis 1 a purported treatment for psychiatric disorders in which the patient is encouraged to reminisce freely about his or her past life while the analyst silently interprets these free associations in the light of FREUDIAN THEORY. Success is said to be unlikely unless the subject falls in love with the analyst (transference). Classical psychoanalysis involves sessions of about an hour, up to six times a week, for several years.
2 a dogmatic theory of human behaviour.

psychodrama a technique in PSYCHOTHERAPY in which the subject acts out relevant incidents or adopts particular roles, so allowing the expression of troublesome emotions or the contemplation of deep conflicts.

psychogenic of mental rather than of physical origin. The term is usually applied to symptoms or disorders thought to be due to problems of social or personal adjustment rather than to organic disease.

psychogeriatrics the psychiatry of old age. This became an official speciality in the British National Health Service in 1989.

psychology the scientific study of behaviour and its related mental processes. Psychology is concerned with such matters as memory, rational and irrational thought, intelligence, learning, personality, perceptions and emotions and their relationship to behaviour.

psychometry the measurement of psychological functions, including correlative ability, memory, aptitudes, concentration and response to logical puzzles. Intelligence has never been adequately defined and so there are no tests for pure intelligence.

psychoneuroimmunology the discipline concerned with the effect of the emotions on the immune system and hence on the development of disease. Psychoneuro-immunology is not predicated on the proposition that the mind and the body are discrete entities that interact via the hypothalamic-pituitary-adrenal axis; it is based on the growing recognition that mental and physical events are so inextricably inter-related that nothing of importance can happen to one without affecting the other.

psychoneurosis see NEUROSIS.

psychopathology the study of the nature of abnormal mental processes and their effects on behaviour.

psychopath a person whose behaviour suggests indifference to the rights and feelings of others. A person in whom prior experience has induced an antisocial personality disorder.

psychopharmacology the study of drugs that affect the state of the mind and the behaviour.

psychosexual disorders a range of conditions affecting the mental and emotional attitudes to sexuality and which may interfere with normal sexual responses. They include IMPOTENCE, PREMATURE EJACULATION, non-organic DYSPAREUNIA, TRANSSEXUALISM, and various SEXUAL DEVIATIONS. Many of these conditions respond well to expert treatment.

psychosis one of a group of mental disorders that includes SCHIZOPHRENIA, major AFFECTIVE DISORDERS, major PARANOID states and organic mental disorders. Psychotic disorders manifest

some of the following: DELUSIONS, HALLUCINATIONS, severe thought disturbances, abnormal alteration of mood, poverty of thought and grossly abnormal behaviour. Many cases of psychotic illness respond well to antipsychotic drugs in the sense that these drugs, while they are being taken, often induce a state of docility, acquiescence, apparent mental normality and conformity with social norms readily acceptable to medical staff and relatives.

psychosomatic 1 pertaining to the relationship between the mind and the body.
2 pertaining to the apparent effect of mental and emotional factors in contributing to physical disorders. These definitions imply the possibly untenable assumptions enshrined in the long-held view (Cartesian dualism) that the mind and the body are distinct, separable entities.

psychosurgery any brain operation performed to relieve severe mental illness. Developments in drug therapy have reduced the need for psychosurgery, and the cruder forms, such as a prefrontal lobotomy, are now obsolete. More precise methods, employing stereotaxic surgery, are still sometimes used to relieve dangerous depression or anxiety or to treat disabling obsessive-compulsive disorder. Parts of the temporal lobe of the brain are sometimes removed to treat temporal lobe EPILEPSY.

psychotherapy any purely psychological method of treatment for mental or emotional disorders. There are many schools of psychotherapy but results appear to depend on the personal qualities, experience and worldly wisdom of the therapist rather than on the theoretical basis of the method. Currently the most fashionable, and seeming successful, school is that of cognitive behaviour therapy.

psychotropic analgesic nitrous oxide the use of inhaled nitrous oxide, without producing general anaesthesia, as a measure to assist in the management of drug and alcohol withdrawal. Nitrous oxide acts on opioid systems in the nucleus accumbens to regulate dopamine accumulation there. This is said to be directly related to the withdrawal state. Also known as PAN.

psychotropic drugs drugs that effect the state of the mind, including sedatives, TRANQUILLIZERS, ANTIPSYCHOTIC drugs and HALLUCINOGENIC drugs.

PTC124 a drug similar to gentamicin that has been developed to treat genetic diseases in which a mutation causes a premature stop in a gene so that the full normal protein product is not produced. PTC124 binds to a component in the transcription process allowing it to continue past the stop point. The phenomenon was first noted with gentamicin and the new drug has been developed to be safer than this antibiotic and more easily absorbed. Trials on mice with CYSTIC FIBROSIS and muscular dystrophy have produced encouraging results. About a third of genetic diseases are caused by a premature STOP MUTATION.

pterygium a wing-shaped thickening of the CONJUNCTIVA that extends over the visible area of the white of the eye and across on to the CORNEA. Pterygium is common in tropical areas and is due to ultraviolet light damage from exposure to sunlight or to local corneal drying. Pterygium usually recurs following surgical removal. Also known as web-eye or *duffir* (Arabic).

pterygoid 1 wing-shaped.
2 pertaining to two processes attached like wings to the body of the SPHENOID bone in the skull.

ptomaine poisoning a mistaken and now obsolete term for food poisoning. Ptomaines occur in decaying proteins but the poisoning is caused by bacteria.

ptosis drooping of the upper eyelid. Ptosis may be a congenital weakness of the lid elevating muscle or may result from later injury or disease, such as MYASTHENIA GRAVIS, STROKE or a brain tumour. Ptosis can be corrected by surgery once the cause has been dealt with.

ptyalin the salivary enzyme MALTASE.

ptyalism excessive salivation from any cause, such as mercury or organophosphorous poisoning, mouth irritation, OESOPHAGITIS or PEPTIC ULCER.

puberty the period during which the sexual organs change from the infantile to the adult form, the SECONDARY SEXUAL CHARACTERISTICS develop and the bodily structure assumes adult proportions. Body weight may double during puberty. Puberty usually occurs between the ages of about 10 and 15 and is often associated with emotional upsets as the individual comes to terms with his or her new-found sexuality. Puberty is initiated by PITUITARY GLAND

hormones called GONADOTROPHINS. These stimulate the testes and ovaries to produce sex hormones.

pubes the pubic hair or the PUBIC region of the body.

pubic pertaining to the pubic bone (os pubis) at the front of the pelvis or to the region at the central point at the front of the lowest part of the abdomen at which the inner aspects of the two pubic bones normally lie in close apposition.

pubic lice see LICE.

pubic symphysis the mid-line cartilaginous joint between the inner surfaces of the pubic bones.

pubic symphysis diastasis separation of the two pubic bones at the PUBIC SYMPHYSIS. This may occur in the course of major injury or in the course of giving birth to a large baby when the pelvic ligaments have become lax under the influence of hormones. Pubic diastasis in childbirth causes pain in the region which may last for weeks, and which is made made worse by weight bearing.

publication bias the tendency to publish reports of research that appears to support a hypothesis and to refrain from publishing findings that do not, thereby creating opinions about the truth of the hypothesis that may be unduly optimistic.

public health the branch of medicine concerned with prevention of disease and the promotion of health in populations by organizing efficient systems of sanitation, by controlling communicable diseases, by ensuring safety in the workplace, by public health education and by the provision and organization of medical, nursing and ancillary health services. An extensive organization of agencies exists to administer public health. The list that follows highlights the key entries related to public health and preventive medicine in the dictionary: contact tracing, electronic smart health cards, food additives, food irradiation, food poisoning, health, health care practitioner, health education, hygiene, infectious diseases, Medical Officer of Health, MMR vaccination, preventive medicine, public health, Public Health Laboratory Service, vaccination, water-borne infection, World Health Organization.

Public Health Laboratory Service a department of the National Health Service consisting of over 50 laboratories in Britain that provide all necessary facilities for diagnosis and testing in cases of suspected infectious disease.

pudenda the external genitalia. From the Latin *pudere*, to be ashamed.

pudendal block a form of local anaesthesia used during childbirth, especially to allow painless forceps delivery. Injections of a local anaesthetic drug are given either through the side walls of the vagina or through the skin on either side of the LABIA MAJORA into the area on either side of the vagina.

puerperal sepsis infection in the female genital tract within 10 days of childbirth, MISCARRIAGE, or ABORTION. There is fever, pain in the lower abdomen and an ill-smelling vaginal discharge. The main site of infection is the raw area on the inside of the womb previously occupied by the PLACENTA but infection may spread to the Fallopian tubes causing SALPINGITIS and sterility or may progress to cause PERITONITIS and SEPTICAEMIA. Treatment is with antibiotics and the surgical removal of any remaining products of conception.

puerperium the period after childbirth when the womb (uterus) and VAGINA are returning to their normal state.

Pulmicort a brand name for the corticosteroid drug bursonide.

pulmonary pertaining to the lungs.

pulmonary alveolar proteinosis a rare disease featuring the accumulation of proteinaceous material in the alveoli of the lung. Sufferers are unusually susceptible to pulmonary infections, sometimes with opportunistic organisms. The disease may be congenital or acquired, and there are indications that the latter may be an autoimmune disorder.

pulmonary anthrax a serious form of ANTHRAX caused by inhalation of dust containing the spores of *Bacillus anthracis*. After an initial mild phase lasting for a few days, there is a severe illness with breathlessness, oedema of the chest and neck, shock and usually death within 24 hours.

pulmonary aspergillosis infection of the lung with Aspergillus fungi. This produces an illness resembling TUBERCULOSIS.

pulmonary embolism occlusion of a main lung artery or one of its branches by an EMBOLUS, usually a large blood clot that has been carried in the bloodstream from a deep leg or pelvic vein where it has formed as a result of PHLEBITIS. A large pulmonary embolism is usually fatal and is a much-feared complication of recent surgery or pregnancy with prolonged immobilization and inadequate movement of the limbs. Moderate-sized emboli cause chest pain, breathlessness, dizziness from low blood pressure and coughing up of blood. Repeated small emboli may cause PULMONARY FIBROSIS or PULMONARY HYPERTENSION. Treatment is with an anticoagulant drug to reduce the clotting ability of the blood and with thrombolytic drugs to help to dissolve the clots. In a massive pulmonary embolism life may sometimes be saved by an emergency operation to remove the clot.

pulmonary fibrosis scarring of lung tissue from any cause, such as PNEUMOCONIOSIS, previous PNEUMONIA or TUBERCULOSIS or repeated attacks of PULMONARY EMBOLISM. Fibrosis interferes with the efficient transfer of oxygen from the atmosphere to the blood and causes breathlessness. There is no specific treatment, short of a lung transplant, but progress can often be slowed.

pulmonary function tests a range of tests of the efficiency of the lungs and of diagnostic procedures to detect lung disease. They include tests of chest expansion, air lung volume, the maximum volume of air that can be expired (vital capacity), the peak air flow rate achievable (see PEAK FLOW METER) and tests of blood concentrations of oxygen and carbon dioxide.

pulmonary hypertension abnormally high blood pressure in the arteries supplying the lungs. This occurs if the resistance to blood flow though the lungs is increased, as by PULMONARY FIBROSIS, so that the heart has to pump more strongly. Pulmonary hypertension causes the right side of the heart to enlarge and perhaps, eventually to fail. Endothelin-1 is known to have an important role in the disease.

pulmonary incompetence failure of efficient closure of the heart valve at the beginning of the PULMONARY ARTERY. This is an uncommon heart valve defect and, as a rule, is not, in itself, particularly serious.

pulmonary oedema accumulation of fluid in

the lungs, usually as a result of failure of the left side of the heart to pump away, sufficiently quickly, the blood returning from the lungs (left HEART FAILURE). Pulmonary oedema may also be caused by inhalation of irritant gases or to any disorder causing generalized oedema. There is severe breathlessness usually worse when lying flat (ORTHOPNOEA), a productive cough and sometimes blood-tinged sputum. Treatment is with DIURETIC drugs and attention to the cause.

pulmonary stenosis narrowing of the heart valve at the outlet of the right VENTRICLE (the pulmonary valve). The condition is nearly always present at birth (congenital) and causes heart enlargement and a diminished blood flow through the lungs with breathlessness and sometimes enlargement of the liver. The seriousness depends on the degree of narrowing. Enlargement of the opening of the valve with a balloon catheter or by open heart surgery may be needed.

Pulmozyme a brand name for DORNASE ALFA.

pulp 1 the soft tissue in the middle of each tooth that contains blood vessels and nerves.
2 the soft tissue, the NUCLEUS PULPOSUS, in the centre of each INTERVERTEBRAL DISC.

pulpectomy the removal of the entire dental PULP of a tooth. Pulpectomy is a necessary preliminary to root-canal treatment.

pulpotomy removal of part or all of the part of the pulp of a tooth within the crown. This is necessary usually because of infection resulting from tooth decay and is done before the tooth is filled to seal off the enamel.

pulse the rhythmic expansion of an artery from the force of the heart beat. In health, the pulse is regular, moderately full and at a rate of between about 50 and 80 beats per minute.

pulseless disease see TAKAYASU DISEASE.

pulse oximeter a device for the continuous monitoring of the blood oxygen levels, both by visible and audible means, during general anaesthesia. This is a major aid to patient safety as a very small drop in blood oxygenation is immediately apparent, alerting the anaesthetist to investigate the cause. A small transducer device is clipped to, or pushed over, a finger of the patient and connected to the main equipment by a light cable.

pulsus alternans alternating strong and weak pulse beats. Pulsus alternans is a sign of failure of the left side of the heart (left ventricular failure).

pulsus bisferiens a pulse with a double peak. This is suggestive of a narrowing and leakage of the heart valve at the beginning of the AORTA.

punch-drunk pertaining to the state of brain damage resulting from repeated blows to the head as are sustained in boxing. A punch-drunk person has slow mental processes, slurred speech and impaired concentration. Recovery is unlikely.

punctuation codon a CODON that marks the start or the end of a gene.

pupil the circular opening in the centre of the iris of the eye. The pupil becomes smaller (constricts) in bright light and widens in dim light under the action, respectively of its circular and radial muscle fibres.

pupil disorders see ADIE'S PUPIL, ARGYLL ROBERTSON PUPIL, COLOBOMA and IRITIS.

pure red cell aplasia a severe failure of production of red blood cells by the bone marrow with normal production of other blood cells. The result is a temporary or persistent severe anaemia. The condition may be caused by some virus infections, some drugs, cancers, rheumatoid arthritis and systemic lupus erythematosus.

purgative a strong laxative drug.

purines a group of nitrogen-containing compounds that includes adenine and guanine, the bases whose sequence forms the genetic code. An excess of purines can cause GOUT.

Puri-Nethol a brand name for the anticancer drug MERCAPTOPURINE.

Purkinje cells nerve cells with very large, pear-shaped bodies and a profuse collection of dendrites that are found in the middle layer of the surface zone (cortex) of the CEREBELLUM. (Johannes Evangelista von Purkinje, 1787–1869, Czech polymath and physiologist).

Purkinje fibres the large specialized heart muscle fibres that form the impulse conducting system that coordinates the heart beat (atrial and ventricular contraction).

purpura any of a group of bleeding disorders that cause visible haemorrhage into the skin in the form of tiny spots (petechiae), local bruises (ecchymoses) or widespread areas of discolouration. There are many different types and causes of purpura. These include the effects of old age, allergy (see HENOCH-SCHONLEIN PURPURA), a deficiency of blood platelets

(THROMBOCYTOPENIA) from various causes, SCURVY, AUTOIMMUNE disorders or SEPTICAEMIA. Treatments vary with the cause.

purulent pertaining to PUS.

purse-string suture a surgical stitch used to close an opening in an internal structure or to narrow a passage. A single strand is inserted, in an in-and-out manner around the opening and the two ends brought out close together. The ends are then pulled tight so that the opening is closed or narrowed, and are then tied. The purse-string suture is widely used in surgery. It is, for instance, used after invagination of the appendix stump in an appendix operation; it is used to prevent miscarriage in cervical incompetence; and it has been used to control rectal prolapse in children.

pus a yellowish or green viscous fluid consisting of dead white blood cells, bacteria, partly destroyed tissue and protein. Pus is formed at the site of bacterial infection but may occur in sterile situations as a result of inflammation from other causes.

pustule a small skin elevation or pimple containing PUS and often forming in a hair follicle. Many, but not all, are caused by skin infection. ACNE pustules are caused by the irritation of SEBUM within the skin.

putamen the outer shell of the lentiform nucleus of the BASAL GANGLIA of the brain.

PUVA *abbrev. for* PSORALENS and ultraviolet A.

p-value the probability, expressed as a number, that a particular effect or association is real or that a given statement or hypothesis is true. If a trial has *n* possible outcomes and *m* of these are the desired outcome, then the probability (p) of obtaining the desired outcome is m/n. If all the outcomes are as desired then $m = n$ and $p = 1$. If none are as desired $p = 0$. So p is a measure that will alwys range from 0 to 1.

PWA *abbrev. for* person with AIDS.

py-, pyo- *combining form denoting* PUS.

pyarthrosis severe joint inflammation with pus in the joint fluid.

pyaemia 'blood poisoning' caused by the presence of pus-forming organisms in the blood. Pyaemia is usually associated with multiple abscesses throughout the body.

pyel-, pyelo- *combining form denoting* the pelvis of the kidney.

pyelitis see PYELONEPHRITIS.

pyelography SEE UROGRAPHY.

pyelolithotomy an operation involving cutting into a kidney to remove a stone (calculus). LITHOTRIPSY, using ultrasonic waves to break up stones, has made this operation less often required.

pyelonephritis inflammation of the pelvis and of the substance of the kidney. This is usually caused by bacterial infection spreading up from the bladder. Acute pyelonephritis causes high fever, shivering and pain in the loin. Repeated or long-term (chronic) attacks may cause permanent damage to the kidney, with high blood pressure (HYPERTENSION) and eventual kidney failure. The condition is treated with antibiotics.

pyle- *combining form denoting* the PORTAL VEIN.

pylephlebitis inflammation of the PORTAL VEIN.

pyloric stenosis narrowing of the muscular outlet from the stomach (the pylorus) so that the passage of food into the DUODENUM is obstructed. The condition may be CONGENITAL, calling for an urgent operation to relieve the obstruction, or may be acquired as a result of repeated attacks of ulceration in the area. In this case, PYLOROPLASTY may be needed. Pyloric stenosis is occasionally caused by cancer of the stomach.

Pylorid a brand name for RANITIDINE BISMUTH CITRATE.

pyloroplasty an operation to widen the PYLORUS so as to allow free passage of food from the STOMACH into the intestine.

pylorospasm spasm of the PYLORUS.

pylorus the narrowed outlet of the stomach where it opens into the DUODENUM. At the pylorus, the muscular coats of the stomach wall are thickened to form a strong muscle ring (a SPHINCTER) capable of closing and opening to control the movement of food.

pyoderma gangrenosum a rare disease featuring areas of gangrene of the skin, mainly affecting the legs. In spite of the name, the condition is not of infective origin. It occurs in a small percentage of people with ULCERATIVE COLITIS.

pyorrhoea 1 a flow of PUS.
2 PERIODONTITIS with discharge of pus from the tooth sockets.

pyr-, pyro- *combining form denoting* fire, heat or fever.

Pyralvex a brand name for ANTHRAQUINONE GLYCOSIDES.

pyramidal tract the great inverted pyramid of motor nerve fibres descending from the motor cortex of the cerebrum through the internal capsule and down into the brainstem where the fibre bundles on each side cross to the other side. This is why a STROKE on the right side causes paralysis on the left side of the body.

pyramidal tract signs signs of damage to a PYRAMIDAL TRACT as may occur in STROKE. They include weakness or paralysis on one side of the body, increased tension in the affected muscles (SPASTICITY), increased tendon reflex jerks and a BABINSKI reflex.

pyrantel an anthelmintic drug used to treat intestinal worm infestations, especially ROUNDWORMS and THREADWORMS. The drug is on the WHO official list.

pyrazinamide an ANTITUBERCULOSIS drug that diffuses well into the CEREBROSPINAL FLUID and is used to treat tuberculous MENINGITIS. The drug is on the WHO official list. A brand name, with other antituberculosis drugs, is Rifater.

pyrazolones a group of non-steroidal anti-inflammatory drugs that includes PHENYLBUTAZONE and azapropazone.

pyrexia fever.

pyrexia of uncertain origin persistent or recurrent fever for which no cause can be found.

pyridostigmine a CHOLINERGIC drug used in the treatment of MYASTHENIA GRAVIS. The drug is on the WHO official list. A brand name is Mestinon.

pyridoxine one of the B_6 group of vitamins. The drug is on the WHO official list.

pyrimethamine a drug used in the treatment of MALARIA and TOXOPLASMOSIS. The drug is on the WHO official list. Brand names are Daraprim and, with other antimalarial drugs, Fansidar and Maloprim.

pyrimidine a nitrogenous base compound. Two pyrimidines, cytosine and thymine, are the DNA bases which, with two PURINES, form the genetic code. A third pyrimidine, uracil, takes the place of thymine in RNA.

pyrithioxine a vitamin B_6 derivative said to be useful in the management of senile DEMENTIA and behavioural disorders in children.

Pyrogastrone a brand name for a mixture of the antacid drugs aluminium hydroxide, the antifoaming agent alginic acid and the ulcer-protective drug carbenoxolone.

pyrogen any substance that causes fever. Endogenous pyrogens are proteins, such as interleukin-1, released by white blood cells in response to bacterial or viral infections. These act on the temperature-regulating centre in the brain, effectively resetting the thermostat at a higher level and causing the muscles to contract repeatedly and rapidly (shivering) so as to raise body temperature.

pyromania a compulsion to start fires.

pyrosis see HEARTBURN.

pyuria the presence of abnormal numbers of white blood cells (pus cells) in the urine. Pyuria usually indicates inflammation in the kidney or bladder, usually from infection.

pyrvinium an ANTHELMINTIC drug used mainly in the treatment of THREADWORMS.

PZI Hypurin a brand name for protamine zinc INSULIN.

q

Q fever an INFLUENZA-like illness caused by the rickettsial organism *Coxiella burnetti* found in the excreta and especially in the PLACENTAS of farm animals. There is high fever, headache, muscle aches and a form of PNEUMONIA causing cough and pain in the chest. Most affected people recover well but prolonged illness is associated with liver and heart complications.

qid *abbrev. for quater in die*, meaning four times a day. This abbreviation is often used in prescriptions under the signature – the part giving the directions to the patient.

qinghao an old Chinese remedy that has finally been accepted by Western medicine. Extracts of the sweet wormwood *Artemisia annua* are effective against the most dangerous malarial parasite *Plasmodium falciparum* in pateines who have become resistant to chloroquine. Artemisinins act on the malarial parasite by blocking one of the enzymes necessary for pumping the correct quantity of calcium into its cell membrane.

QRS complex the part of the electro-cardiograph tracing corresponding to the contractions of the main chambers of the heart (the ventricles). The Q wave is a short downwards deflection, the R wave a conspicuous upwards stroke and the S wave a return to below the level of the base-line.

qs *abbrev. for quantum sufficit*, or *quantum satis*, meaning a sufficient quantity. This abbreviation was often used in prescription writing.

quack a person fraudulently claiming medical knowledge or skills or attempting to sell fraudulent remedies.

quadrantectomy a limited operation for breast cancer in which only the quadrant of the breast containing the cancer is removed.

Quadrantectomy is now less often performed than LUMPECTOMY.

quadrantopia loss of a quarter segment of the field of vision, usually the corresponding upper segment in the fields of both eyes. Quadrantopia is due to a destructive LESION in the OPTIC RADIATIONS on one side of the brain.

quadri- *combining form denoting* four.

quadriceps muscles the bulky muscle group on the front of the thigh, consisting of four muscles arising from the thigh bone (femur), and from the front of the pelvis. These muscles end in a stout tendon which incorporates the kneecap (patella) and is attached to a bony ridge on the upper end of the front of the main bone of the lower leg (tibia). The quadriceps group powerfully straighten the knee.

quadrigemina pertaining to the four bodies, the corpora quadrigemina, or colliculi, on the roof of the fourth ventricle of the midbrain. The upper pair of quadrigeminal bodies are concerned with visual tracking and the lower pair are associated with hearing.

quadriparesis weakness in the muscles of all four limbs and of the trunk.

quadriplegia paralysis of the muscles of both arms, both legs and of the trunk. Quadriplegia results from severe spinal cord damage in the neck, usually as a result of a fracture-dislocation, but sometimes as a result of neurological disease.

qualm a sudden feeling of nausea or faintness.

quantum dots highly fluorescent nanoparticles that show promise in the field of cellular imaging. Dots with monoclonal antibodies attached have been produced which can target and image cancerous cells in living animals.

quarantine isolation of a person who has been

exposed to an infectious disease so as to prevent spread. From the Italian *quarantina*, 40 – a period of days longer than the incubation period of most diseases, other than RABIES.

quartan recurring on the fourth day, as in the case of the fever in quartan MALARIA.

quartz glass a glass of pure silica, transparent to ultraviolet light.

quartz lamp a mercury vapour lamp with a quartz bulb that emits strong ultraviolet radiation.

quartz dust silicosis a particularly severe and rapidly developing form of SILICOSIS occurring in stonemasons and other workers exposed to quartz dust for periods of as short as a few months.

quaternary ammonium compounds compounds in which the four hydrogen atoms of the ammonium radical are replaced by organic radicals. They are used as antiseptics.

Queckenstedt's test a test used to detect a block in the circulation of CEREBROSPINAL FLUID in the spinal canal. While performing a LUMBAR PUNCTURE and measuring the pressure in the CSF, one of the jugular veins is briefly compressed. The pressure in the CSF should rise if there is no obstruction. (Hans Heinrich Georg Queckenstedt, 1876–1918, German physician).

quetiapine a dibenzothiazepine antipsychotic drug used to treat SCHIZOPHRENIA. A brand name is Seroquel.

Queensland tick typhus a mild to moderate infectious disease occurring in rural north eastern Australia, caused by *Rickettsia australis* and transmitted by the tick *Ixodes holocyclus*. The condition is very similar to ROCKY MOUNTAIN SPOTTED FEVER and features an obvious spot at the site of the bite which heals slowly, fever, enlarged lymph nodes and a generalized rash involving the palms and the soles. Most cases recover completely.

queer a slang term referring to male homosexuality.

quickening perception by the mother-to-be of movements of the fetus in the womb. In first pregnancies this is usually noticed around the 20th week, but, with experience, quickening may be recognized as early as the 16th week.

quiescent of a disease, inactive or dormant.

quinacrine a yellow acridine dye useful in studying chromosomal structure because of its property of fluorescing when bound to certain regions of chromosomes. Also known as mepacrine. Quinacrine was once widely used to prevent malaria and to remove tapeworms.

quinagolide a drug with properties similar to those of DOPAMINE used to treat infertility in women with excess levels of the hormone prolactin. A brand name is Norprolac.

quinalbarbitone secobarbital, a barbiturate drug used for brief periods of treatment of insomnia in people addicted to barbiturates. A brand name is Seconal Sodium.

quinapril an ANGIOTENSIN CONVERTING ENZYME INHIBITOR (ACE inhibitor) drug used to treat HEART FAILURE and high blood pressure (HYPERTENSION). A brand name is Accupro.

Quinate a brand name for QUININE.

Quinbisul a brand name for QUININE.

quinghaosu a Chinese herbal drug used for 2000 years to treat MALARIA. The active ingredient is a sesquiterpene lactone that greatly reduces the number of malarial parasites in the blood. The mode of action is unknown but is being investigated and trials of the drug have recently started in the West.

quinidine a drug derived from QUININE and used to control irregularity or excessive rapidity of the heart beat by depressing the excitability of the muscle. The drug is on the WHO official list. A brand name is Kinidin Durules.

quinine the first drug found to be effective in the prevention and treatment of MALARIA. Quinine was originally derived from the bark of the cinchona tree. It is still used to treat CHLOROQUINE-resistant malaria but is no longer used as a PROPHYLACTIC. The drug is on the WHO official list.

Quinoctal a brand name for QUININE.

quinolones a group of synthetic antibiotic drugs that includes nalidixic acid, oxfloxacin and enoxacin. These drugs act by inactivating an enzyme, DNA gyrase, necessary for replication of the organisms.

Quinsul a brand name for QUININE.

quinsy an abscess between the TONSIL and the underlying wall of the throat (pharynx). Quinsy is almost always secondary to acute TONSILLITIS and features great pain, high fever, difficulty in swallowing and speaking and excessive salivation. The soft palate is pushed across towards the other side. Quinsy is treated by surgical incision to release the pus.

quotidian fever a fever occurring every day. This may occur in a patient suffering from a mixed malarial infection with overlapping effects.

quintuplets five babies born in a single gestation. Quins were once rare but since the introduction of fertility drugs that promote multiple ovulation they have become more common.

r

rabbit fever see TULARAEMIA.

rabid pertaining to, or suffering from, RABIES.

rabies a nervous system disease that affects many different animals. Rabies is a brain inflammation (encephalitis) caused by a lyssavirus, a member of the rhabdovirus family, that enters the nervous system at the site of a bite by a rabid animal. The time taken for the virus to reach the brain and cause the disease varies with the distance of the bite from the brain, and may be from 10 days to 3 or 4 months. Rabies starts with fever, headache, neck stiffness, anxiety and disorientation. Soon there is acute fear of swallowing because of violent spasms of the throat and diaphragm causing gagging, choking and extreme panic. Seizures, delusions and hallucinations then occur, followed by coma and death, usually within a week of the start of the severe symptoms. Careful cleaning of bites and the use of human antirabies globulin and rabies vaccine can prevent the disease. There is no specific treatment for the established encephalitis. Also known as hydrophobia on account of a principal symptom.

rabies immunoglobulin an antibody preparation given both intramuscularly and at the site of the bite to people who have been attacked by an animal in a country in which rabies is endemic. Rabies vaccine is also given. The drug is on the WHO official list.

rabies vaccines human diploid cell vaccine or purified chick embryo cell vaccine used either as a prophylaxis for people at special risk, or for people who have been attacked by an animal in a region in which rabies is endemic. The drug is on the WHO official list.

racemose having a structure of clustered parts, especially of a gland. From the Latin *racemosus*, clustered, as in *racemus*, a bunch of grapes.

rachi- *combining form denoting* spine or spinal cord. From Greek *rachis*, the spine.

rachitic affected by rickets.

rad a unit of dosage of absorbed ionizing radiation. The rad is equal to 0.01 joule of absorbed energy per kilogram of the exposed tissue or other material.

RADC *abbrev. for* Royal Army Dental Corps.

radial 1 branching out, like rays, from a point. 2 pertaining to the RADIUS bone or its associated artery or nerve.

radial keratotomy an eye operation in which eight or more radiating cuts are made in the outer zone of the CORNEA so as to produce scars that flatten the curvature and reduce short sight (MYOPIA). The results are uncertain and the operation has been criticised. It has been largely replaced by excimer laser corneal reshaping.

radial nerve one of the main nerves of the arm and hand. The radial nerve is a mixed motor and sensory nerve. It supplies the forearm muscles that straighten the flexed wrist and conveys sensation from the back of the forearm and hand.

radiation the emission and almost instantaneous propagation of electromagnetic waves ranging in wavelength from thousands of metres (radio waves) to millionths of millionths of millimetres (gamma rays). Radiation of long wavelength may cause body atoms and molecules to vibrate but does not, so far as is known, significantly damage them (non-ionizing radiation). Very short wavelength radiation, such as X-rays and gamma rays (ionizing radiation), however, can knock out linking electrons from molecules, causing them to separate into smaller charged bodies or chemical groups called ions, or FREE RADICALS. Ionizing radiation can damage any body molecules, including DNA, and this may kill cells or alter their genetic structure. Such mutations in surviving cells may lead to cancer. At the same time, rapidly dividing cancer cells are more susceptible to the effects of ionizing radiation than normal cells. This is the basis of RADIOTHERAPY.

radiation burn a burn caused by local over-exposure to RADIATION.

radiation sickness the effects of major doses of ionizing RADIATION on the whole body. The symptoms and rapidity of onset depend on the dose taken. They include nausea and vomiting, bloody diarrhoea, bleeding into the skin, the effects of severe ANAEMIA, hair loss and sterility. Very large doses, of 30 to 100 GRAY, cause rapid onset of abdominal symptoms with anxiety, disorientation, coma and death within a few days from damage to the nervous system. Radiation sickness is caused by the production of large numbers of damaging FREE RADICALS.

radiation therapy see RADIOTHERAPY.

radic-, radicul-, radiculo- *combining form* denoting root.

radical surgery extensive and often mutilating surgery designed to remove all the diseased tissue, usually cancerous. From the Latin *radix*, a root.

radicle any small structure resembling a root. From the Latin *radicula*, diminutive of radix, a root.

radicular cyst a cyst of the PERIODONAL tissue at the root of a tooth.

radiculitis inflammation of a nerve root.

radiculoneuropathy disease of peripheral spinal nerves and their roots, as in SHINGLES.

radio- *combining form denoting* radiation.

radioactive marker a compound containing a radio-isotope atom whose movement through a chemical reaction can be monitored by virtue of the radiation emitted.

radioactivity 1 spontaneous emission of RADIATION.
2 the radiation emitted by unstable atomic nuclei or in the course of a nuclear reaction. Radioactivity includes alpha particles (helium nuclei), beta particles (high speed electrons), neutrons and gamma rays.

radiobiology the study of the effects of radiation, especially ionizing radiation, on living organisms.

radiodermatitis skin degeneration following exposure to excessive dosage of ionizing RADIATION.

radiography the use of X-radiation to produce images that can help in diagnosis. Radiography includes the use of CT SCANNING, which is an X-ray technique, RADIONUCLIDE SCANNING and, by courtesy, magnetic resonance imaging (MRI). Compare RADIOLOGY.

radioimmunoassay any method of measuring the extent of linkage between ANTIGEN and ANTIBODY in which one or other of these is labelled with a radioactive substance (radionuclide). Measurement of radiation can be remarkably precise.

radioisotope scanning see RADIONUCLIDE SCANNING.

radiolabelling a method of tagging and following the movement of a molecule by incorporating into it a radioactive atom. In genetics, radiolabelling is commonly used for the purposes of HYBRIDIZATION PROBING.

radiologist a doctor who specializes in medical imaging and who is skilled in the interpretation of X-ray, CT scan, MRI, PET scan and RADIONUCLIDE SCANNING films. He or she is a specialist in nuclear medicine, familiar with the use of radioactive isotopes and with electronic imaging and intensifying methods, and an expert in the insertion of arterial and cardiac CATHETERS. Radiologists also practice RADIOTHERAPY.

radiology the medical specialty concerned with the use of radiation for diagnosis and treatment. The list that follows highlights the key entries related to radiology in the dictionary: bone scanning, CT scanning, Doppler ultrasound scanning, gallium scan, isotope scanning, PET scanning, radiography, radioisotope scanning, radioisotope scanning, radiolabelling, radiologist, radiology, radionuclide scanning, radiopaque, radiotherapy, radium, thyroid scanning,ultrasonography, ultrasound scanning, X-ray, X-ray therapy.

radionuclide scanning a method of body imaging using elements that emit radiation (radionuclides) and which are incorporated into compounds that concentrate in certain parts of the body or in diseased areas. The location of the radionuclide is shown on an image produced by a device called a GAMMA CAMERA. The method can, for instance, reveal cancer, both primary growths and unexpected METASTASES, especially in the brain.

radiopaque offering major resistance to the passage of X-rays. Radiopaque substances, such as barium sulphate and iodine-containing liquids, are commonly used to outline hollow structures, especially in the intestinal canal and the urinary system. See also BARIUM MEAL and intravenous or retrograde UROGRAPHY.

radiotherapy the medical specialty concerned with the treatment, almost exclusively of cancer, by ionizing radiation. Radiation affects cancerous cells more than normal cells and can be directed accurately by shielding, collimation and other means. The size and timing of the dosage is calculated to cause maximal damage to the tumour and the minimal damage to the patient. Radiotherapy sources include high voltage X-ray machines, linear accelerators and powerful radioactive isotopes such as cobalt 60. Isotopes may be inserted directly into tumours in tubes or needles or may be placed in close proximity.

radium a naturally radioactive element with a half-life of 1620 years which decays into the radioactive gas radon. Radium was once widely used in RADIOTHERAPY but has now been largely replaced by caesium 137 and other radionuclides.

radius one of the two forearm bones, the other being the ULNA. The radius is on the thumb side and lies parallel to the ulna when the palm is facing forward. When the hand is rotated so that the thumb turns inward, the upper end of the radius rotates on a boss on the lower end of the upper arm bone (HUMERUS) but the lower end crosses over the ulna.

radius fracture see COLLES' FRACTURE.

RADS *eponym for* reactive airways dysfunction syndrome. This is a non-specific form of ASTHMA that typically occurs as a result of massive exposure to a severe respiratory irritant.

Rafen a brand name for IBUPROFEN.

ragged red fibres a feature of several MITOCHONDRIAL DNA disorders in which a high proportion of the muscle fibres contain structurally and functionally abnormal mitochondria. When stained and examined under the microscope these fibres appear red and ragged. The finding is commonly associated with slowly progressive weakness of the muscles of the limbs, defects of ocular movements, abnormally rapid tiredness on exertion, and a marked rise in the levels of lactic acid in the blood on exertion or even at rest.

rales abnormal rattling sounds accompanying the breath sounds and heard through a STETHOSCOPE during examination of the chest. They are caused by air passing through fluid or mucus in the small air tubes (bronchioles). Compare RHONCHI.

raltitrexed a folate analogue drug used in the palliative treatment of advanced cancer of the colon or rectum. A brand name is Tomudex.

RAMC *abbrev. for* Royal Army Medical Corps.

ramipril an ANGIOTENSIN CONVERTING ENZYME inhibitor drug that has been shown to be capable of greatly extending life after heart attack. The drug is especially useful in the condition of dilated cardiomyopathy and in reducing the risk of heart attack and stroke in predisposed persons. A brand name is Tritace.

ramose many-branched.

ramus a branch or subdivision arising from the division (bifurcation) of a blood or lymphatic vessel or a nerve.

ranitidine an H-2 (histamine-2) receptor antagonist drug used to reduce acid secretion in cases of peptic ulceration. A band name is Zantac. See also RANTITIDINE BISMUTH CITRATE.

rantitidine bismuth citrate a drug that combines the properties of RANITIDINE with the protectant action of BISMUTH. A brand name is Pylorid.

ranula a translucent, saliva-filled cyst under the tongue caused by obstruction of the duct of one of the salivary glands, usually by a salivary stone (calculus). Treatment is by opening the cyst and stitching the edges of the incision to keep it open (MARSUPIALIZATION).

rape sexual intercourse with a woman who does not, at the time, consent to it, or who is asleep, and would not have given consent, or unconscious. It is rape if consent was obtained by fraud or threats or if physical force was used to effect intercourse against the woman's will. The man must know that the woman does not consent. It is also rape if the woman is incapable of understanding what she is consenting to. Some degree of vaginal penetration, however slight, is necessary. Marriage is no defence to rape. Rape of a man, by a man, is a defined offence in many American States.

raphe a seam. The line or ridge of union between two mirror-image or symmetrical body parts.

Rapifen a brand name for ALFENTANIL.

Rapilysin a brand name for RETEPLASE.

Rapitil a brand name for NEDOCROMIL.

rasburicase an enzyme used to treat hyperuricaemia and prevent kidney failure in people with widespread cancer. A brand name is Fasturtec.

rash any inflammatory skin eruption of reasonable extent and of whatever cause.

ras proto-oncogenes genes in humans and many other animals that influence cell differentiation. Mutations of ras genes may contribute to one third of all cases of cancer.

rat-bite fever either of two diseases transmitted by the bite of a rat or by ingestion of contaminated milk. They are sodoku, occurring mainly in Japan, and caused by *Spirillum minor*, and Haverhill fever, caused by *Streptobacillus moniliformis*, occurring mainly in North America. Both feature painful inflammation at the site of the bite, fever, spleen and lymph node enlargement and lymph vessel inflammation (LYMPHANGITIS) and a dusky red, slightly raised, sparse rash. Haverhill fever also sometimes causes multiple joint ARTHRITIS. Both diseases respond well to penicillin and other antibiotics.

rationalism a general term for the group of philosophic schools that reject received or authoritarian wisdom and dogmatic religion and hold that knowledge is to be obtained only from observation and the application of logic to data so derived. Rationalism does not necessarily exclude religious beliefs, but tends to do so.

rationing see MEDICAL RATIONING.

rauwolfia dried extracts from the plant Rauwolfia serpentina that contains the alkaloid RESERPINE, a sedative and tranquilizing drug that also lowers blood pressure.

Raynaud's disease a disorder of the small arteries of the fingers and toes affecting mainly young women. The cause is unknown. Exposure to cold causes these arteries to narrow so that blood flow is greatly reduced and the digits become cold and white. There is burning pain and numbness. The pallor is followed by blueness (CYANOSIS) and, on warming, by redness as the arteries open and the blood floods in again. The long-term effect may be permanent arterial blockage with GANGRENE at the tips of the affected fingers or toes. People with Raynaud's disease must avoid cold and cigarette smoking and can be helped by the use of drugs to relax the smooth muscle in the walls of the arteries. (A.G. Maurice Raynaud, 1834–81, French physician).

Raynaud's phenomenon the term given to the symptoms of RAYNAUD'S DISEASE when the cause is known. Raynaud's phenomenon may be caused by any form of narrowing arterial disease, such as ATHEROSCLEROSIS, Buerger's disease (THROMBOANGIITIS OBLITERANS), EMBOLISM, THROMBOSIS, diabetic large vessel disease, RHEUMATOID ARTHRITIS or SYSTEMIC LUPUS ERYTHEMATOSUS. It may also be caused by repetitive strain or strong vibration or artery-constricting drugs or poisons. The treatment is the management of the cause.

Raynaud's sign the characteristic white, blue and red colour changes of arterial spasm in the fingers and toes. See RAYNAUD'S DISEASE.

RCAMC *abbrev. for* Royal Canadian Army Medical Corps.

RCM *abbrev. for* Royal College of Midwives.

RCN *abbrev. for* Royal College of Nursing.

RCNT *abbrev. for* Registered Clinical Nurse Teacher.

RCOG *abbrev. for* Royal College of Obstetricians & Gynaecologists.

RCP *abbrev. for* Royal College of Physicians.

RCS *abbrev. for* Royal College of Surgeons.

RCT *abbrev. for* randomised clinical trial.

reading frame an imaginary window through which base pairs can be inspected three at a time, and which provides a way in which a nucleotide sequence can be viewed as three different sets of CODONs only one of which is correct.

reason the faculty by which new information is derived from old, judgement exercised and argument pursued.

RDA *abbrev. for* recommended daily allowance. The daily intake of a particular nutrient considered adequate to maintain health. RDAs are decided upon by various official nutritional committees and tend to be diverse in detail.

reaction time the interval between the application of a stimulus and the first sign of a response.

reactive hyperaemia a brief increase in blood flow following restoration of the blood supply to a part after occlusion.

reaginic antibody an antibody, usually of the IgE class, that binds to MAST CELLS in people prone to acute ANAPHYLACTIC (Type I hypersensitivity) reactions. In association with the ANTIGEN, such as pollen grains, reaginic antibody causes release from the mast cells of HISTAMINE, LEUKOTRIENES, PLATELET ACTIVATING FACTOR and other agents responsible for the allergic reaction. Also known as reagin.

rebound phenomenon the inability to prevent large over-shoot movements of a limb when resistance to strong muscle contraction is suddenly removed. This is a sign of cerebellar dysfunction.

rebound tenderness a clinical sign of inflammation somewhere in the intestine, as in APPENDICITIS. Gentle but increasing pressure is applied to the front of the abdomen, remote from the suspected site, and then suddenly released. A definite pain, felt in another part of the abdomen suggests disease there.

re- *prefix denoting* again or back or backward.

reboxetine a selective NORADRENALINE REUPTAKE INHIBITOR antidepressant drug. A brand name is Edronax.

receding chin congenital underdevelopment of the lower jaw bone (mandible) of cosmetic importance only. Various plastic operations are possible. Also known as retrognathism.

receptor 1 any structure on or penetrating a plasma cell membrane or other membrane, capable of binding a specific external substance, such as a HORMONE, CYTOKINE, STEROID or NEUROTRANSMITTER, and, as a result, effecting a response within the cell. Plasma membrane receptors commonly respond by releasing a 'second messenger' within the cell. 2 a sensory nerve ending capable of receiving stimuli of various kinds and responding by the production of nerve impulses. The receptor has gradually come to be recognized as one of the fundamentally important entities in physiology, pathology, pharmacology and medical science generally.

recession surgical retroplacement of a part,

especially the insertion of a muscle so as to weaken its action.

recessive pertaining to an alternative form of a gene (ALLELE) that produces an effect only when carried by both members of the pair of homologous chromosomes (only when HOMOZYGOUS). People with heterozygous alleles for a condition are called carriers. A recessive gene has no effect in the presence of a DOMINANT allele either because of its inactivity or because of the absence of a product.

recessive lethal a gene that has a lethal effect when present in both loci (homozygous).

recombinant pertaining to an organism, chromosome or segment of DNA produced by genetic material from more than one source.

recombinant DNA DNA produced by the artificial linkage, in the laboratory or factory, of DNA from different sources. See also GENETIC ENGINEERING.

recombinant protein a protein synthesized in a cell from DNA into which the gene sequence that codes for the protein has been artificially introduced. Recombinant proteins can be produced in large quantities by GENETIC ENGINEERING.

recombination the formation in offspring of a combination of two or more genes that differs from the arrangement of these genes in either parent. This is the result of the exchange of segments of DNA during the germ cell divisions that resulted in the formation of paternal sperms and maternal ova.

recombination repair the process of making good a gap in one strand of DNA by plugging it with a homologous strand taken from another length of double helix.

recon the smallest genetic unit capable of recombination.

recovery room a room adjoining an operating theatre, in which patients who have undergone surgical operations are kept under close surveillance until safely recovered from general anaesthesia.

recreational drugs a dubious term that trivialises the dangers and serious social implications of the use of drugs such as COCAINE, AMPHETAMINE (amfetamine), various HALLUCINOGENIC DRUGS and MARIJUANA.

recruitment 1 activation of an increasing number of responsive cells as the size of the stimulus increases.

2 an unpleasant blasting sensation experienced by people with sensorineural deafness when exposed to loud noises.

rectal pertaining to the RECTUM.

rectal bleeding release of blood from a disease process in the RECTUM, such as cancer, rectal polyps, AMOEBIC DYSENTERY, ULCERATIVE COLITIS or DIVERTICULITIS. Blood on the stools usually arises from a less serious cause, such as HAEMORRHOIDS but should never be ignored.

rectal cancer a malignant tumorous growth starting in the lining of the RECTUM and growing around the inside of the bowel, protruding into the interior or invading the wall. This is one of the commonest of all cancers. Its symptoms and signs include a change in the bowel habit with early morning urgency and a repeated strong desire to empty the bowel, difficulty in defaecation, a sense of incomplete evacuation and the passage of mucus and blood. Treatment is by surgical removal of the affected segment of bowel. A temporary or permanent COLOSTOMY may be necessary.

rectal examination an important method of examination performed with a gloved, lubricated finger. Rectal examination can reveal thrombosed internal piles, ano-rectal abscesses, benign or cancerous enlargement of the PROSTATE GLAND, rectal polyps, RECTAL CANCER, abnormalities of the CERVIX of the womb, enlargement of the ovaries or inflammation in the APPENDIX.

rectal prolapse a turning inside-out of the RECTUM so that the mucous membrane lining is seen to protrude, to a variable degree, from the ANUS. In complete prolapse the whole thickness of the bowel protrudes as a thick cylindrical mass with the lining on the outside. Prolapse in women tends to follow childbirth with resulting weakness of the floor of the pelvis. Treatment is by an operation to tighten the muscle ring around the anus (the anal sphincter) or to fix the rectum in place internally.

Recklinghausen's disease see NEUROFIBROMATOSIS.

rectocele bulging forward (prolapse) of the RECTUM into the vagina.

rectopexy an operative procedure to secure in place a rectum liable to PROLAPSE.

rectum the 12.5 cm long, very distensible terminal segment of the large intestine, situated immediately above the anal canal. In spite of its name (*rectus* is Latin for straight), the rectum is curved and follows the hollow of the SACRUM. Its lining is smooth and the whole of the inside is accessible to the examining finger (SEE RECTAL EXAMINATION). Movement of bowel contents into the rectum causes the desire to defaecate.

rectus any of several straight muscles, such as the central vertical muscle on either side of the midline of the abdomen (the rectus abdominis), the rectus femoris on the front of the thigh or the four rectus muscles that move the eyeball. From the Latin *rectus*, straight.

recumbent lying down or reclining.

recurrent laryngeal nerves branches of the vagus, the 10th pair of cranial nerves. The recurrent laryngeal nerves leave the main trunk low in the neck, especially on the left side, and run up again to supply the muscles of larynx concerned with phonation. One of these nerves is commonly involved in neck cancer, the first sign of which may be severe loss of voice from paralysis of one vocal cord.

red blood cell SEE ERYTHROCYTE.

red eye see CONJUNCTIVITIS.

redout temporary reddening of the field of vision caused by exposure to reversed gravitation forces so that blood is forced into the head.

Redoxon a brand name for vitamin C (ascorbic acid).

reduction the restoration of a displaced or broken part of the body to its proper position or alignment by manipulation or other surgical procedure. Reduction of bone fractures involves energetic pulling (traction) under anaesthesia to correct overlap, and local moulding pressure to realign the bone.

reduction division see MEIOSIS.

Reduviidae a family of hemipterous insects that includes the bugs, known as assassin, kissing or cone-nosed bugs, that transmit *Trypanosoma cruzi*, the cause of CHAGAS' DISEASE.

Reed-Sternberg cell a giant cell with paired, mirror-image nuclei that is a diagnostic feature of HODGKIN'S LYMPHOMA and distinguishes it from non-Hodgkin's lymphoma. (Dorothy M. Reed, 1874–1964, American pathologist; and Karl von Sternberg, 1872–1935, Austrian pathologist).

re-epithelialization the usually final healing stage of a wound in which the surface layer

(EPITHELIUM) regenerates from the edges to cover the wound site.

refeeding syndrome the tendency to develop dangerous illness usually within four days of resuming normal eating after a prolonged period of starvation. Low insulin production during starvation with breakdown of body fat and protein result in loss of intracellular electrolytes, especially phosphate. The shift to a carbohydrate metabolism causes increased insulin production which stimulates cellular uptake of phosphate from the blood. Low serum phosphate depletes ATP and causes rhabdomyolysis, respiratory and heart failure, hypotension, seizures and death. Monitoring of serum phosphate and intravenous phosphate supplementation are required.

referred pain pain felt in a place other than the site of the causal disorder. Stimulation of a sensory nerve at any point, including its root ganglion (as in SHINGLES), always causes a sensation in the area of the peripheral distribution of the nerve. Referred pain also arises because nerves running to a particular segment of the spinal cord may come from widely separated points, and impulses coming from one of these areas may be interpreted as coming from the other. Stimulation from an inflamed gall bladder, for instance, causes pain in the right shoulder, the pain of ANGINA PECTORIS is felt in the arms and neck, and pain from a URETER is often felt in the testicle.

reflex 1 an automatic, involuntary and predictable response to a stimulus applied to the body or arising within it.
2 the point of light reflected from a curved smooth surface, such as the CORNEA.

reflex bladder a urinary bladder no longer under voluntary control that empties automatically from time to time under the control of a local spinal reflex. This is a common sequel to severe spinal cord injury or disease.

reflexology a form of alternative or complementary therapy based on the hypothesis that the body contains channels of 'life force' similar to the meridians of ACUPUNCTURE. These terminate in the feet and practitioners of the method claim to be able to detect blockage in the channels by feeling the feet and toes. Massage and manipulation of the feet is then performed to unblock the channels

and, allegedly, cure disorders caused by the blocked channels.

reflex sympathetic dystrophy a condition commonly following injury to a limb, that features pain, tenderness, swelling, abnormal blood flow, disorders of sweating, involuntary movements and atrophic structural changes in tissue known a trophic changes. Also known as Sudeck's atrophy, complex regional pain syndrome and algodystrophy. (Paul Hermann Martin Sudeck, 1866–1919, German professor of surgery).

reflux movement of fluid or semifluid material in a direction opposite to the normal. Regurgitation. Examples are reflux of acid material from the STOMACH into the OESOPHAGUS, of urine from the bladder up the URETERS to the kidneys or of the abnormal movement of blood back through a leaking (incompetent) valve in the heart.

reflux oesophagitis inflammation of the lining at the lower end of the gullet from abnormal upwards movement of acidic stomach contents. This is the cause of the symptom of heartburn.

Refolinon a brand name for FOLINIC ACID.

refraction 1 the bending of light rays that occurs when they pass obliquely from a transparent medium of one density to one of another density.
2 the assessment of the optical errors of the eyes so that appropriate correcting spectacles can be prescribed.

refractory period the period immediately following the passage of a nerve impulse or the contraction of a muscle fibre during which a stimulus, normally capable of promoting a response, has no effect.

Refsum's disease a rare autosomal recessive degenerative disorder due to a gene mutation on chromosome 10 that causes a deficiency of the enzyme phytanoyl-CoA hydroxylase. The disease features widespread demyelination of nerves, RETINITIS PIGMENTOSA with hight blindness, ICHTHYOSIS of the skin, loss of the sense of smell, deafness, and poor balance from cerebellar dysfunction. Infantile Refsum disease is caused by a mutation of the gene on chromosome 7 for phytanic acid alpha-hydroxylase. It features impaired peroxisomal function with accumulation of phytanic acid and other substances.

Regaine Rogaine, a brand name for MINOXIDIL in a preparation for external use as a hair restorer.

regenerative cell therapy a form of treatment purporting to rejuvenate the skin or even the whole person by the injection of tissues taken from other animals. There is no evidence that these treatments are of any advantage. Also known as 'monkey gland' therapy.

regimen any system or course of treatment, especially one involving special diet or exercise.

regional block anaesthesia a form of local anaesthesia in which loss of sensation is achieved in a part or region of the body by injecting an anaesthetic drug at a remote point around the nerves carrying sensory impulses from the area.

regional ileitis see CROHN'S DISEASE.

registrar in UK, a specialist in training for a medical consultancy who is above the level of Trainee or Senior House Officer, and below the level of Senior Registrar.

regression 1 a psychoanalytic term implying a return to childish or a more primitive form of behaviour or thought, as from a genital to an oral stage.
2 a psychological term denoting a temporary falling back to a less mature form of thinking in the process of learning how to manage new complexity. Cognitive psychologists view such regression as a normal part of mental development.
3 a statistical term defining the relationship two variables such that a change in one (the independent variable) is always associated with a change in the average value of the other (the dependent variable).

Regulan a brand name for ISPAGHULA.

regulator gene a gene that codes for RNA or for a protein whose function is to controls the expression of one or more other genes.

regurgitation see REFLUX.

rehabilitation 1 restoration of the physically, mentally or socially disabled to a normally functional life.
2 the specialty of physical medicine which is concerned with such restoration.

reiki a complementary medical therapy in which the practitioner allegedly channels energy into the patient in order to encourage healing or restore wellbeing. As in some other forms of complementary medicine the term 'energy' here has a fluid definition.

reimplantation the reattachment of an amputated body part or the restoration of a dislodged tooth to its socket.

reinfection another infection after full or partial recovery from an earlier infection with the same organism.

reinforcement a term used in learning theory and in behaviour therapy that refers to the strengthening of a tendency to respond to particular stimuli in particular ways. In classical conditioning, the occurrence or deliberate introduction of an unconditioned stimulus along with a conditioned stimulus; in operant conditioning, a reinforcer is a stimulus, such as a reward, that strengthens a desired response.

Reiter's syndrome a disorder affecting mainly young men and featuring a non-gonococcal discharge from the penis, ARTHRITIS, CONJUNCTIVITIS and sometimes UVEITIS or a skin rash. The condition is thought to be an abnormal response to infection and is almost confined to people of the tissue type HLA B-27. There is no specific remedy and recurrences after the first attack are common. (Hans Conrad Julius Reiter, 1881–1969, German physician).

relapse the reappearance or worsening of a disease after apparent recovery or improvement.

relapsing fever an infection with organisms from the *Borrelia* genus of SPIROCHAETES transmitted by the bite of a louse or an *Ornithodorus* tick. Epidemics are common in times of war, famine or civil disorder. The infection causes a sharp rise of fever with shivering, headache, muscle aches, vomiting and PHOTOPHOBIA. The fever and symptoms continue for 3–6 days and may end fatally, but usually settle down completely only to recur 7–10 days later. Each recurrence tends to be shorter and milder than the previous. Treatment is with antibiotics but these must be given cautiously as death of the spirochaetes causes a severe and sometimes fatal reaction.

relative erythrocytosis an increase in the concentration of red blood cells resulting from a reduction in the volume of the fluid part of the blood.

relaxant anything, but especially a drug, that induces muscle relaxation or relieves tension. Relaxant drugs are widely used in general anaesthesia so as to avoid the necessity for deep levels of unconsciousness. They include TUBOCURARINE, SUXAMETHONIUM and DANTROLINE.

relaxin a polypeptide found in the corpus luteum of various mammals that softens the neck of the womb (cervix) and relaxes the pubic joint of the pelvis to ease childbirth. Relaxin has not been proved to occur in humans.

releasing hormones hormones secreted by neurones in the hypothalamus which control the production of hormones by the PITUITARY GLAND.

Relestat a brand name for EPINASTINE HYDROCHLORIDE.

Relifex a brand name for NABUMETONE.

religion an entity of wide human significance encompassing doctrinal, historical, literary, devotional, experiential, behavioural and transcendental elements. It is concerned with man's relationship to God, however perceived. Religion may be formalized in dogma or entirely free and individual. It may be a matter of indifference or of the most central importance. Its influence on health may be beneficial, negligible or malign. Religion has been one of the major causes of human suffering and a source of immense consolation to millions. It has brought out the direst cruelty and the most benevolent and altruistic conduct. By their nature, religious beliefs cannot be validated in the manner of scientific facts and must always be matters of faith and unsupported belief. Doctors have a duty to respect the religious beliefs of their patients.

Relpax a brand name for ELETRIPAN.

remediable capable of being remedied.

remedial curative. Pertaining to, or providing, a remedy.

remission a marked reduction in the severity of the symptoms or signs of a disease, or its temporary disappearance.

remifentanil a narcotic painkiller used during the induction or maintenance of general anaesthesia. The use of painkillers during general anaesthesia is not, as it may seem, pointless. Painful stimuli act on the autonomic nervous system causing effects that can interfere with the smooth conduct of the anaesthetic and the post-operative period. A brand name is Ultiva.

REM sleep rapid eye movement sleep. This occurs during about 20% of the sleeping time

and features constant movement of the eyeballs, twitching of the muscles and erection of the penis in men. REM sleep is deep and is associated with dreaming. It is necessary for health.

renal pertaining to the kidneys.

renal calculus SEE KIDNEY STONES.

renal colic severe, periodic pain in the loin usually caused by the spasmodic muscular efforts of the tube from the kidney to the bladder (the ureter) to force an obstructing body, such as a kidney stone (calculus), downwards. Renal colic may also be caused by blood clots in the ureter.

renal disorders SEE KIDNEY DISORDERS.

renal dwarfism failure of body growth as a result of persistent kidney disease in childhood.

renal failure SEE KIDNEY FAILURE.

renal pelvis the conical cavity lying on the inner side of the kidney into which all urine secreted by the kidney runs. The renal pelvis is connected directly to the ureter.

renal rickets loss of mineralization of bone occurring in severe kidney disease in which the kidney is unable to convert vitamin D to its active form. The resulting failure of absorption of calcium from the intestine leads to low blood calcium and its withdrawal from bone. See also RICKETS.

renal transplant SEE KIDNEY TRANSPLANT.

reniform kidney-shaped.

renin an enzyme produced by the kidney in conditions of abnormally low blood pressure. Renin catalyses the release of angiotensinogen I from a blood globulin, and this, in turn, is converted to angiotensin II by a converting enzyme found in the lung. Angiotensin II causes the adrenal glands to secrete the hormone aldosterone which acts on the kidneys to reduce the loss of sodium in the urine. The increased blood sodium raises the blood pressure. See also ACE INHIBITORs.

renoprotection measures taken to prevent damage to the kidneys from any cause, IATROGENIC or otherwise.

Reopro a brand name for the drug ABCIXIMAB.

reovirus any of a group of double-stranded RNA viruses which occur in the respiratory and digestive tracts of healthy individuals but which may cause infantile diarrhoea (rotaviruses) and Colorado tick fever (orbiviruses). A part-acronym from 'Respiratory', 'Enteric', 'Orphan'.

reperfusion injury the damage, and loss of function, that commonly occurs in the heart muscle when, after a heart attack, the flow of blood to the muscle is restored. Reperfusion injury is generally agreed to be due mainly to the action of oxygen FREE RADICALS. It is also known as myocardial stunning.

repetitive strain injury a disorder of motor function caused by any often-repeated activity that is persisted in beyond a particular threshold, especially if the activity involves an inherently awkward or uncomfortable position of the body. RSI particularly affects musicians, keyboard operators, cleaners, packers and machine operators. There is acute pain and cramp-like stiffness, and sometimes total inability to continue in the associated occupation. Initially, the condition explicitly, and by definition, excluded all disorders of known cause, but this led to many legal and other difficulties, and accounts now list numerous causes. RSI is, however, often stress-related and in many cases no muscular, tendon or neurological abnormality can be found, except that affected people often have raised thresholds for the appreciation of vibration. In some cases it appears analogous to WRITER'S CRAMP. Changes in the proportions of the different types of muscle fibres and an increase in the number of muscle cell MITOCHONDRIA have been described. The condition is usually managed by rest and rationed periods of work.

Replenine a brand name for blood clotting FACTOR IX.

repolarization restoration of the resting polarized state in a muscle or nerve fibre. Polarization implies a balanced electrical charge on either side of the fibre membrane, being, in the resting state, negative on the inside and positive on the outside. In depolarization the charges are locally reversed.

repressed of a gene that is inhibited from transcription by the bonding to it of a REPRESSOR PROTEIN.

repression 1 inhibition of transcription at a particular site on DNA or MESSENGER RNA by the binding of REPRESSOR PROTEIN to the site. 2 the prevention of the synthesis of certain enzymes by bacterial products.

repressor gene a gene that codes for a repressor protein.

repressor protein a protein that binds to an operator gene on DNA to inhibit its transcription into MESSENGER RNA, or that binds to RNA to prevent its translation.

reproduction any process by which an organism gives rise to a new individual. Most biological reproduction is cellular and asexual and occurs by chromosomal duplication followed by elongation and splitting of the cell into two individual cells identical to the parent. Sexual reproduction is more complex and involves the production of specialized body cells called gametes which have experienced two stages of shuffling and redistribution of chromosomal segments and a reduction to half the full number of CHROMOSOMES (haploid). In the fusion of the male and female gametes, sperm and egg respectively (fertilization), the full complement of chromosomes is made up. The potential new individual now has a GENOME different from that of either parent and will differ in many respects. A fertilized ovum divides rapidly and repeatedly, but the reproduced cells do not usually separate, but continue to duplicate and specialize until a new individual is formed. Sometimes, after the first or second division, the reproduced cells separate to form genetically identical siblings.

reproterol a BETA-ADRENOCEPTOR stimulating drug used to treat ASTHMA. A brand name is Bronchodil.

Requip a brand name for ROPINIROLE.

resection surgical removal of any part of the body or of diseased tissue.

resectoscope a surgical instrument that is passed along the male URETHRA to allows a view of the inside of the bladder and of an enlarged PROSTATE GLAND. The resectoscope incorporates an electrically heated wire loop used to cut away redundant prostate tissue so as to allow the free outflow of urine.

reserpine a RAUWOLFIA alkaloid that decreases the concentration of the neurotransmitter 5-hydroxytryptamine in the nervous system and has a sedative, ANTIHYPERTENSIVE and tranquillizing effect. The drug is on the WHO official list.

resorcinol a drug used externally that softens and helps to remove the horny outer layer of the skin. A keratolytic drug. A brand name for a preparation containing resorcinol is Eskamel.

Resperdal a brand name for RISPERIDONE.

respiration 1 breathing.

2 the whole process by which oxygen is transferred from the atmosphere to the body cells and carbon dioxide is moved from the cells to the atmosphere. Respiration is vital to life and cessation for more than a few minutes is fatal. See also CHEYNE-STOKES RESPIRATION.

respirator 1 any mechanical device used to maintain the breathing and the supply of air or oxygen to the lungs. Most modern respirators are of the intermittent positive pressure type. **2** a filtering device that covers the face and removes toxic elements form the inspired air.

respiratory arrest cessation of breathing.

respiratory distress syndrome a condition of impeded passage of oxygen through the lungs into the blood caused by increased fluid in the lungs or by the failure of the lungs to inflate fully after birth. Adult respiratory distress syndrome may be caused by infection, inhalation of irritant fluids or gases, partial drowning, breathing high oxygen concentrations, narcotic overdose and by various drugs. In premature newborn babies the syndrome is the result of the deficiency of a surfactant wetting agent which lowers the surface tension of the fluid in the lung air sacs and allows easy expansion of the lungs. Treatment is by administration of oxygen, sometimes under pressure, and the inhalation of NITRIC OXIDE.

respiratory rate the number of breaths per minute.

respiratory tract infections see BRONCHIOLITIS, BRONCHITIS, COMMON COLD, CROUP, LARYNGITIS, PHARYNGITIS, PNEUMONIA, SINUSITIS and TONSILLITIS.

Respolin a brand name for SALBUTAMOL.

Resprim a brand name for CO-TRIMOXAZOLE.

Restandol a brand name for TESTOSTERONE.

restenosis relapse to the narrowed state, as may happen in a coronary artery following successful widening by balloon angioplasty. Stenting is commonly used to prevent restenosis.

resting membrane potential the voltage difference between the inside and the outside of a cell when no stimulus is applied.

restless legs syndrome nocturnal aching of the legs which are constantly moved about in an attempt to achieve comfort and which cause insomnia. The aching, may be associated with muscular cramps, which interfere with sleep

and may affect pregnant women or people with kidney disease. Examination is negative and special nerve conduction tests and muscle biopsies are normal. Recent research suggests that an abnormality of central dopamine production may be responsible. Good results have been obtained with levodopa, pramipexole, or pergolide. Also known as Ekbom's syndrome.

restriction enzyme one of the many enzymes that break DNA at specific sites. These enzymes are extensively used in research and in GENETIC ENGINEERING. Also known as restriction endonucleases.

restriction fragment length polymorphism (RFLP) variations within a species in the lengths of fragments of DNA caused by RESTRICTION ENZYMES. The variations are caused by mutations that either abolish the normal sites of breakage or create new ones, characteristic of the mutations. RFLP analysis may allow genetic abnormalities to be detected, often before birth, even if the location of the mutated gene or genes is unknown.

restriction map a diagram of the sites on DNA that are cut by different RESTRICTION ENZYMES.

resuscitation 1 restoration of a stable physiological condition to a person whose heart action, blood pressure or body oxygenation have dropped to critical levels. **2** active measures to treat shock.

RET *abbrev. for* rearranged during TRANSFECTION.

retardation a state of backwardness or delayed development, especially of the intellectual functions. Learning difficulty or mental deficiency.

rete a mesh or network, as of blood vessels. From the Latin *rete*, a net.

rete testis a network of cords in the testicle that canalize to become the SEMINIFEROUS TUBULES in which the spermatozoa develop.

retention cyst a CYST resulting from obstruction of the outlet channel of a gland so that the normal secretion accumulates and expands and compresses adjacent tissue to form a capsule.

reteplase a drug that dissolves blood clots. A fibrinolytic drug used in the early stages of a heart attack to try to restore patency to a coronary artery branch that has been blocked by a blood clot. A brand name is Rapilysin.

reticular net-like.

reticular formation a network of islets of grey matter, consisting of large and small nerve cells and their connections, scattered throughout the brainstem and extending into the THALAMUS and HYPOTHALAMUS. The formation receives information from many other parts of the brain and is concerned with alertness and direction of attention to external events, as well as sleep. It has a major effect on the sensory and motor systems.

reticulo- *combining form denoting* a net or a net-like structure.

reticulocyte an immature red blood cell (ERYTHROCYTE) that contains a network that can be stained blue with basic dyes. Reticulocytes appear in the circulation at times of increased red cell formation.

reticulocytosis a greater than normal proportion of RETICULOCYTES in the blood. This indicates an increased rate of red cell formation, as during the treatment of ANAEMIA or following HAEMORRHAGE.

reticuloendothelial system an obsolescent term for the widespread system of protective MACROPHAGE (phagocyte) cells and endothelial cells found in the bone marrow, liver, spleen and elsewhere. The cells of the reticulo-endothelial system include HISTIOCYTES, MONOCYTES, the KUPFFER CELLS of the liver and lung macrophages.

reticulosarcoma an obsolete term for non-Hodgkin's LYMPHOMA.

reticulum any netlike structure of the body.

Retin-A a brand name for TRETINOIN.

retina the complex membranous network of nerve cells, fibres and photoreceptors that lines the inside of the back of the eye and converts optical images formed by the lens system of the eye into nerve impulses. The retina contains colour-blind but very sensitive rods and colour-sensitive cones and a computing system that refines the signals produced by these. The impulses leave each retina by way of about one million nerve fibres that form the optic nerve.

retinaculum a fibrous band, strap or ligament that holds another part in place. The flexor retinaculum prevents the flexor tendons from springing away from the front of the wrist when it is bent.

retinal the aldehyde found in visual pigments,

such as visual purple. Also known as retinaldehyde.

retinal disorders see CENTRAL SEROUS RETINOPATHY, MACULAR DEGENERATION, RETINAL DETACHMENT, RETINAL HAEMORRHAGE, RETINITIS PIGMENTOSA, RETINOBLASTOMA, RETINOPATHY, TOXOCARIASIS and TOXOPLASMOSIS.

retinal detachment separation of part or all of the retina from the underlying CHOROID by an accumulation of fluid. Retinal detachment usually follows the development of a hole or a tear (rhegmatogenous detachment) and is commonest in people with severe MYOPIA or who have had a crystalline lens removed for CATARACT. The condition is painless and presents with the perception of flashing lights and dark spots and the appearance of a black curtain covering part of the field of vision. Treatment involves the application of low temperature (cryopexy) to cause sterile inflammation, and the indenting of the white of the eye over the detachment by stitching on a silicone rubber sponge.

retinal haemorrhage bleeding into the RETINA from any cause, such as diabetic RETINOPATHY, severe high blood pressure (HYPERTENSION) or occlusion of a retinal vein. Retinal haemorrhage obscures vision to a degree that depends on its severity. The cause must be investigated and, if possible, treated.

retinal vein occlusion blockage of the central vein of the RETINA or one of its branches, usually by a THROMBOSIS. The vision is severely affected in central vein occlusion but less so with a branch occlusion. There is no specific treatment but firm massage of the eye may help at an early stage.

retinitis inflammation of the RETINA.

retinitis pigmentosa a slow degenerative disorder of the rods and cones of the RETINAS of both eyes with migration of pigment from the retinal pigment layer. Initially, this causes night blindness only but later there is progressive loss of an ever-enlarging area of the peripheral field of vision. Retinitis pigmentosa varies greatly in age of onset and severity. It usually has a hereditary basis but spontaneous cases occur. There is no known treatment. This condition is not inflammatory and the term is inappropriate. A small proportion of cases are due to a gene mutation that prevents retinaldehyde from being converted to the form used by retinal photoreceptors. Some recessive forms are caused by mutations in ABCA4 GENES. Also known as tapetoretinal degeneration or pigmentary retinopathy.

retinitis proliferans the extension of new blood vessels and fibrous tissue following bleeding into the VITREOUS body from the RETINA in diabetic RETINOPATHY. This tends to lead to RETINAL DETACHMENT and blinding of the eye. Microsurgical removal of the whole VITREOUS body together with the proliferative tissue is sometimes successful.

retino- *combining form denoting* RETINA.

retinoblastoma a highly malignant tumour of the RETINA affecting babies and young children and usually presenting as a squint (strabismus) or as a visible whiteness in the pupil. In one-third of cases both eyes are affected. Retinoblastoma can spread to all parts of the body and early removal of the affected eye is often advised. If there is tumour in both eyes, radiotherapy is given to the less severely affected eye. Retinoblastoma is a genetic disorder inherited as an autosomal dominant. There is evidence that the genetic basis for retinoblastoma is loss of a tumour-suppressor gene on chromosome 13. Loss of the homologous normal retinoblastoma gene is also necessary for the tumour to develop. Because of the genetic basis it is important for other young children in the family to be examined by an ophthalmologist.

retinoids a class of compounds containing 20 carbon atoms and related to RETINAL and vitamin A. They include retinol, TRETINOIN, isotretinoin, etretinate, acitretin and arotinoid. Retinoids bind to cell nuclear retinoid receptors and the latter bind to DNA. The effect of the retinoids is to promote transcription of DNA in much the same way as do steroids and thyroid hormone. They have a wide range of biological actions and have been found useful in ACNE, certain skin cancers, PSORIASIS, skin ageing and other skin disorders. Retinoids taken in the first three weeks of pregnancy are liable to cause abortion or serious fetal defects. For this reason the use of systemic retinoids in women is strictly controlled.

retinol the common form of vitamin A found in animal and fish livers and other foods of animal origin. It is easily converted in the body into

RETINAL. The drug is on the WHO official list.

retinopathy any non-inflammatory disease of the RETINA. Retinopathies include CENTRAL SEROUS RETINOPATHY, DIABETIC RETINOPATHY, HYPERTENSIVE RETINOPATHY, retinopathy of prematurity (see RETROLENTAL FIBROPLASIA), RETINITIS PIGMENTOSA and retinopathy caused by drugs such as CHLOROQUINE and ETHAMBUTOL.

retinoschisis local splitting of the retina into two layers with an intervening space.

retinoscope an optical instrument used to determine the state of refraction of the eye by RETINOSCOPY. It is not an instrument for examining the retina but a means of producing a light that is reflected from the retina. The direction of the movement of this light varies with the refraction and with lenses held in front of the eye.

retinoscopy an objective method of quantitative determination of optical errors in the eye so that correcting glasses may be prescribed.

Retinova a brand name for TRETINOIN.

retirement the period, demonstrably dangerous to health and longevity, after the permanent cessation of work.

RET oncogene a proto-oncogene on chromosome 10 that codes for one of the tyrosine kinase receptors. Several mutations are known and all of them are associated with thyroid tumours. A number of children living in the Chernobyl region at the time of the power station disaster have been found to have rearrangements of the RET oncogene. Thyroid cancers, normally very rare in children are now occurring much more frequently than usual.

retractor an instrument used, often in pairs, to hold surgical incisions open or to keep tissue out of the way of the operating surgeon.

retro- *combining form denoting* back, backward or behind.

retrobulbar neuritis inflammation of the OPTIC NERVE, caused most commonly by demyelinization, as in MULTIPLE SCLEROSIS, but also by local sinus infections. Retrobulbar neuritis causes a central blank in the field of vision of the affected eye, but recovery is usual after about 6 weeks.

retrograde amnesia loss of memory for a period before the time of a head injury. In general, the more severe the injury and the longer the period of loss of memory after the injury, the longer will be the retrograde amnesia.

retrograde ejaculation the passage of seminal fluid into the bladder during the male ORGASM. This is due to failure of closure of the internal urethral sphincter as a result of injury during prostatectomy, damage to the sympathetic nerves in the region during local surgery, spinal injury or diabetic neuropathy. Infertility may result but various measures may be used to overcome this.

retrolental fibroplasia an eye disorder affecting premature babies who have been exposed to unduly high concentrations of oxygen in incubators. It is a form of retinopathy in which fronds of new blood vessels and strands of fibrous tissue extend into the vitreous gel behind the lens, seriously interfering with vision and leading, later, to RETINAL DETACHMENT. Early treatment with a freezing probe (cryopexy) can prevent retinal detachment.

retroperitoneal behind the peritoneal membrane of the abdomen.

retroperitoneal fibrosis inflammatory scarring of tissues at the back of the abdominal cavity. The condition may be caused by drugs such as practolol and methysergide but usually occurs for no known reason. It may cause obstruction of the ureters and kidney failure.

retroperitoneal lymph node dissection surgery to remove the lymph nodes behind the peritoneum. This has been found an effective measure in certain cases of testicular cancer that have spread to the lymph nodes. In non-seminomatous cancer the cure rate by this means has approached 98%.

retrosternal behind the breastbone.

retroversion a turning or tilting backward or the state of being turned or tilted back.

retroverted uterus a UTERUS that lies in line with the long axis of the vagina or at an angle that slopes back from this axis. Normally, the uterus is inclined forward at about a right angle to the vagina. Retroversion is the condition of about 20% of women and is not, in itself, considered to be in any way harmful.

Retrovir an antiviral drug with some useful effect against the RETROVIRUS HIV that causes AIDS. Also known as AZT (azidothymidine) and ZIDOVUDINE.

retrovirus a virus with a GENOME consisting of a single strand of RNA from which DUPLEX DNA is synthesized under the catalytic influence of an enzyme called reverse transcriptase. This is the reverse of the much more common DNA to RNA process. The AIDS virus HIV is a retrovirus.

Rett syndrome a brain disorder affecting only girls and, from the age of 9–36 months, causing progressive loss of recently acquired skills, such as speech and walking, repetitive writhing (athetoid) movements, epileptic seizures, AUTISM and gradual disablement. Brain examination shows a significant reduction in the profusion of the dendritic trees in layers 3 and 5 of the frontal and inferior temporal cortices. The visual cortex remains unaffected. The cause remains obscure but is thought to be the result of a fresh mutation rather than an inherited genetic defect. (First described in 1966 by the Austrian physician Andreas Rett).

revalidation a process by which all doctors working in the United Kingdom can, at intervals of five years, be reassessed for the purposes of maintaining their license to practice. Revalidation may be achieved in two ways – by appraisal by superiors in general practice (GPs) or hospital, or by the independent submission of evidence that the doctor is working in accordance with acceptable principles of practice. In both cases the necessary standards are those laid down in the GENERAL MEDICAL COUNCIL's booklet GOOD MEDICAL PRACTICE.

Revanil a brand name for LYSURIDE (lisuride).

reverse transcriptase an enzyme that allows certain viruses, notable HIV, to synthesize double strand DNA from a single strand of RNA so that it can be incorporated into the genome of the host cell. Such viruses are called retroviruses.

reverse transcriptase inhibitors a range of drugs that interfere with the process by which retroviruses, such as HIV, convert their RNA genomes into duplex DNA which can then be incorporated into the DNA of the attacked cell. By delaying this process the progress of a retroviral infection can be slowed. Brand names are lamivudine, stavudine, zalcitabine and zidovudine.

reward deficiency syndrome a name for a relative failure of the dopaminergic system which plays a major part in brain-reward mechanisms. The syndrome, which has been linked to dysfunction of the D_2 dopamine receptors, includes various conditions, such as drug and alcohol abuse, smoking, obesity, pathological gambling and attention deficit hyperactivity disorder, in which the subject seems to be unusually concerned to achieve reward. The D_2 dopamine receptor gene is on chromosome 11 and has multiple allelic forms. Variants have been correlated with these and other reward-seeking behaviours.

Reyataz a brand name for ATAZANAVIR.

Reye's syndrome a severe childhood disorder that may follow a virus infection such as chickenpox, rubella, influenza or a herpes simplex, or echovirus infection. Reye's syndrome features HEPATITIS and dangerous swelling of the brain that may lead to coma and death. The condition is strongly associated with the use of aspirin and this should no longer be routinely given to children. Treatment involves removal of fluid from the brain. (Ralph Douglas Kenneth Reye, 1912–77, Australian physician).

RFN *abbrev. for* Registered Fever Nurse.

RG *abbrev. for* Remedial Gymnast.

RGN *abbrev. for* Registered General Nurse.

RHA *abbrev. for* Regional Health Authority.

rhabdo- *combining form denoting* rod-shaped or striped.

rhabdomyo- *combining form denoting* striped muscle.

rhabdomyolysis breakdown of muscle with release of MYOGLOBIN. This is usually the result of a severe crushing injury but may occur in severe and persistent exertion; dopaminergic blockade or withdrawal of dopaminic agents; low potassium, sodium or phosphate levels; the use of statin drugs; or following a virus infection of muscle. The condition causes weakness or temporary paralysis but full recovery is usual except in cases of severe injury. The condition may occur in MCARDLE'S DISEASE.

rhabdomyosarcoma a rare and often highly malignant tumour of muscle affecting people at both extremes of life. Treatment is by surgical removal, RADIOTHERAPY and anticancer drugs.

rhabdovirus one of a family of bullet-shaped, single-strand RNA viruses that includes the RABIES virus and the vesicular STOMATITIS virus.

rheology the study of the deformation and flow of matter in tubes and elsewhere. Rheology has become important in studies of blood flow in vessels.

rhesus factor Rh factor. A group of antigens occurring on red blood cells in a proportion of people, the most important of which was first found in a rhesus monkey. The gene locus for the Rh factor is on one end of the long arm of chromosome 1. See RHESUS FACTOR DISEASE.

rhesus factor disease a severe blood disorder caused by incompatibility between the blood group of the fetus and that of the mother. The rhesus factor is acquired by dominant inheritance and is present is 85% of the population. The danger arises if the mother is rhesus negative and the father rhesus positive and passes this on to the fetus. When the fetus is rhesus positive, its red blood cells act as ANTIGENS causing the mother to produce ANTIBODIES against them. The danger is minimal in the first pregnancy but increases thereafter as antibody levels rise. In the most severe cases, the fetus may die in the womb. If born alive, the baby is deeply jaundiced with an enlarged liver and spleen and a low haemoglobin level. Treatment is by an exchange transfusion, via the UMBILICAL CORD, immediately after birth or even while still in the womb. Rhesus negative women can be prevented from developing antibodies by being given an anti-D GAMMAGLOBULIN.

rheumatic carditis inflammation of any part of the heart resulting from rheumatic fever. The commonest type is rheumatic endocarditis in which the heart lining, and especially one or more heart valves, are involved.

rheumatic fever a disease caused by an ANTIGEN present on certain strains of STREPTOCOCCI which is closely similar to an antigen on the muscle fibres of the heart and elsewhere. Antibodies are produced by the body and these attack the heart and other parts. Joint involvement is fleeting and unimportant but damage to the heart valves and sometimes the nervous system is permanent. Possible sequels are heart valve leakage (incompetence) or narrowing (stenosis) and 'St Vitus' dance' (SYDENHAM'S CHOREA). Rheumatic fever and subsequent damage can be avoided by treating streptococcal infections with penicillin. Sydenham's chorea is helped by tranquillizer drugs and sedatives.

rheumatism a common term for pain and stiffness in joints and muscles as well as for major disorders such as RHEUMATOID

ARTHRITIS, OSTEOARTHRITIS and POLYMYALGIA
RHEUMATICA.

rheumatoid arthritis a general disease
affecting women more often than men and,
in severe cases, causing progressive joint
deformity, joint destruction and disability. The
small joints of the fingers and hands are most
seriously affected but the condition can spread
to involve the wrists, elbows, shoulders and
other joints. The disease is believed to be
triggered by an infection that prompts the
immune system to form damaging aggregates of
ANTIGEN and ANTIBODY (IMMUNE COMPLEXES).
The antibodies IgM, IgG and IgA (rheumatoid
factors), and antibodies to COLLAGEN and cell
nuclei, are present in the blood. Pro-
inflammatory CYTOKINES, especially TUMOUR
NECROSIS FACTOR are involved. Rheumatoid
arthritis causes loss of appetite and weight,
lethargy, muscle and tendon pain, nodules
under the skin and often severe eye
inflammation. There are many complications
including ANAEMIA, PERICARDITIS, VASCULITIS
and RAYNAUD'S PHENOMENON. Treatment is
limited to control of inflammation and
complications and the relief of pain by means
of rest, splintage, physiotherapy and anti-
inflammatory and painkilling drugs.
Immunosuppressive drugs can be helpful and
Penicillamine and gold are also widely used.
See also STILL'S DISEASE (juvenile rheumatoid
arthritis).

rheumatoid factors the antibodies
(immunoglobulins) present in the blood in
cases of RHEUMATOID ARTHRITIS. These are
IgM, IgG and IgA autoantibodies to the
patient's own IgG.

rheumatoid spondylitis see ANKYLOSING
SPONDYLITIS.

rheumatology the medical specialty concerned
with the causes, PATHOLOGY, diagnosis, and
treatment of diseases affecting the joints,
muscles, and connective tissue.

Rheumox a brand name for AZAPROPAZONE.

rhin-, rhino- *combining form denoting* nose.

rhinencephalon the part of the brain
concerned with smell.

rhinitis inflammation of the mucous
membrane lining of the nose. Rhinitis is one of
the commonest of human complaints and is a
major feature of the common cold and of hay
fever (ALLERGIC RHINITIS). The membrane

becomes swollen, so that the air flow is partly
or wholly obstructed, and its glands become
overactive causing excessive mucus production
and a watery discharge. Vasomotor rhinitis is
the result of a disturbance of the nervous
control of blood vessels in the mucous
membrane. Hypertrophic rhinitis, with
thickening and persistent congestion of the
membrane, is the result of long-term
inflammation or repeated infection. Atrophic
rhinitis features shrinkage and loss of the
mucous membrane, with dryness, crusting
and loss of the sense of smell.

rhinogenous originating in the nose.

Rhinolast a brand name for AZELASTINE.

rhinology the medical and surgical specialty
concerned with the structure, functions and
diseases of the nose.

rhinophyma a form of ROSACEA, affecting
elderly men and causing a bulbous deformity
(potato nose) with readily visible enlarged skin
pores, extreme oiliness of the skin from
sebaceous over-secretion and permanent
redness from wide dilation of small blood
vessels. Treatment involves paring down the
excess tissue with a scalpel so as to restore the
nose to more normal dimensions. Skin grafting
is unnecessary and healing is rapid.

rhinoplasty any cosmetic operation to alter the
shape of the nose.

rhinorrhea watery discharge from the nose.
This is usually due to RHINITIS, but following a
head injury with a fracture of the base of the
skull, a persistent drip from the nose may be
due to leakage of CEREBROSPINAL FLUID from
the brain cavity.

rhinosinusitis inflammation of the lining of
the nose and of the sinuses surrounding the
nose. This may be allergic as in ALLERGIC
RHINITIS, infective, hormonal, occupational or
emotional in origin.

rhinosporidiosis a fungus disease caused
by *Rhinosporidium seeberi* that causes fungal
polyps in the nose and swellings in the
surrounding tissues. These can be removed
surgically. The condition occurs in India, East
Africa and South America.

rhinoviruses a group of PICORNAVIRUSES that
are the major cause of the common cold. There
are well over a hundred distinguishable types.

rhizotomy surgical division of a root, especially
that of a nerve.

Rh negative lacking the rhesus factor on the red blood cells.

rhodopsin the retinal rod photoreceptor pigment. Also known as visual purple.

rhonchi continuous wheezing sounds of low or high pitch heard with a STETHOSCOPE when listening to the breath sounds. Rhonchi are caused by partial obstruction of the smaller breathing tubes in the lungs (bronchioles) by swelling of the lining or by the presence of thick mucus.

RHV *abbrev. for* Registered Health Visitor.

rhythm method an unreliable method of contraception based on an attempt to predict, and avoid, the part of the menstrual cycle on which OVULATION is most likely to occur.

rhytidectomy a ridiculous term used by cosmetic surgeons for a face lift operation. Skin is freed from the underlying tissue, pulled tight and the excess cut off. A disingenuous and inappropriate derivation from the Greek *rhytis*, a wrinkle and *ektome*, a cutting off.

ribs the flat, curved bones that form a protective cage for the chest organs and provide the means of varying the volume of the chest so as to effect respiration. There are 12 pairs of ribs, and each pair articulates with a vertebra in the spine, at the back. The upper 10 pairs are joined to cartilages connected to the breastbone at the front, but the 11th and 12th pairs are free at the front (floating ribs).

ribavirin an antiviral drug effective against a range of both DNA and RNA viruses including the herpes group and those causing hepatitis, and several strains of influenza.

riboflavin vitamin B_2. The drug is on the WHO official list.

ribonuclease an enzymes that promotes the HYDROLYSIS of ribonucleic acid (RNA).

ribonucleic acid see RNA.

ribose a pentose sugar that is a component of nucleic acids.

ribosomal RNA (rRNA) ribonucleic acid that is a permanent structural feature of RIBOSOMES.

ribosome a spherical cell ORGANELLE made of RNA and protein which is the site of protein synthesis in the cell by linking amino acids into chains. Ribosomes may be free or may be attached to the endoplasmic reticulum. During translation, ribosomes attach to MESSENGER RNA molecules and travel along them, synthesizing polypeptides as they go.

ribosome binding site the base sequence on a MESSENGER RNA molecule to which a RIBOSOME attaches.

riboswitches 1 the mechanism that regulates gene expression (the turning on and off of genes) by means of a set of molecular switches. 2 a therapeutic procedure to control gene expression using self-cleaving catalytic RNA to achieve mRNA self-destruction or preservation. The structure of RNA can readily be altered by the binding on of small molecules or oligonucleotides.

ribozyme one of a unique class of RNA molecules that can act as cleaving enzymes in addition to storing genetic information. This is a notable exception to the general rule that all enzymes are proteins. Ribozymes form complementary base pairs in the normal manner but can cleave segments of nascent RNA during the splicing process of the formation of mature RNA transcripts of DNA. Ribozymes can be used in various ways as treatment modalities.

ricin a highly poisonous substance found in the castor oil bean *Ricinis communis*.

rickets a disorder of bone mineralization in children caused by vitamin D deficiency, both nutritional and skin-synthesised, and the resulting failure of absorption of calcium from the intestine. As a result of diminished deposition of calcium and phosphorus in the bones there is weakening and softening. There may be bowing of the legs, curvature of the spine, squaring-off and flattening of the skull, delay in the eruption of teeth with softening of the enamel and an increased tendency to bone fracture. Rickets is essentially a problem of the developing world where its is promoted by cultural patterns involving covering of the female skin, over-long breast-feeding by vitamin-D deficient mothers, geberal nutritional deficiency and possibly genetic factors. The disease is treated with vitamin D and a calcium-rich diet. The equivalent disease in adults is OSTEOMALACIA.

Rickettsia a micro-organism intermediate in size between the largest viruses and the smallest bacteria. *Rickettsiae* are spread by ticks and small insects, and cause TYPHUS, Q FEVER, and ROCKY MOUNTAIN SPOTTED fever. The eponymous discoverer of the genus died of typhus while investigating the cause. (Howard

Taylor Ricketts, 1871–1910, American pathologist).

rickettsial pox a disease caused by *Rickettsia akari* and spread by mites from domestic mice. It occurs almost exclusively in New York and Philadelphia. There is a small blister (papule) at the site of the bite which then breaks down to form a scab (eschar) and is followed by fever, muscle aches and then a papular rash that crusts but heals without causing scars.

rictus a facial contortion or grimace of pain.

Ridaura a brand name for AURANOFIN.

Riedel's thyroiditis a rare thyroid gland disorder featuring irregular localized stony hard areas and widespread FIBROSIS without signs of inflammation. Also known as Riedel's struma or woody thyroiditis. (Bernhard Moritz Karl Ludwig Riedel, 1846–1916, German surgeon).

rifabutin a drug used to treat tuberculosis of the lungs and to prevent the development of lung TB in AIDS patients. A brand name is Mycobutin.

Rifadin a brand name for RIFAMPICIN.

rifampicin an antibiotic drug used mainly to treat TUBERCULOSIS and LEPROSY, but also LEGIONNAIRES' DISEASE, PROSTATITIS, ENDOCARDITIS and OSTEOMYELITIS. Rifampicin acts by inhibiting transcription of bacterial nucleic acid. It interferes with the action of oral contraceptives. The drug is on the WHO official list. Brand names are Rifadin and Rimactane.

rifater a brand name for a formulation of RIFAMPICIN and ISONIAZID. The drug is on the WHO official list.

rifinah a brand name for a formulation of RIFAMPICIN and ISONIAZID. The drug is on the WHO official list.

Rift Valley fever a disease occurring mainly in South Africa and caused by an arbovirus normally infecting sheep and goats. It is transmitted by mosquito bite and causes a DENGUE-like illness sometimes complicated by JAUNDICE, haemorrhages, RETINOPATHY and MENINGOENCEPHALITIS. There is no specific treatment.

rigidity sustained muscle tension causing the affected part of the body to become stiff and inflexible. Rigidity may be due to muscle injury, neurological disease such as PARKINSON'S DISEASE, underlying inflammation as in PERITONITIS, or arthritis in an adjacent joint. See also SPASTICITY.

rigor a violent attack of shivering causing a rapid rise in body temperature.

rigor mortis the stiffening of muscles which occurs after death as a result of the coagulation of muscle by accumulating lactic acid. Rigor usually starts about 3 or 4 hours after death and is usually complete in about 12 hours. It may start much earlier, sometimes almost immediately, if the subject was engaged in strenuous activity or was fevered or suffering convulsions before death. It passes off as enzymes break down and soften the muscles over the course of the next 2 or 3 days.

riluzole an antiglutamate drug used to slow the rate of progress and prolong life in AMYOTROPHIC LATERAL SCLEROSIS. A brand name is Rilutek.

Rimactane a brand name for RIFAMPICIN.

Rimactazid a brand name for a formulation of RIFAMPICIN and ISONIAZID.

Rimso-50 a brand name for a solution of DIMETHYLSULFOXIDE (DMSO).

Rinatec a brand name for IPRATROPIUM BROMIDE.

Ringer's solution a solution in water of sodium chloride, potassium chloride and calcium chloride of such concentration as to be ISOTONIC to blood and tissue. Ringer's solution is used for local (topical) applications. (Sydney Ringer, 1835–1910, British physiologist).

ringing in the ears see TINNITUS.

ringworm see TINEA.

Rinstead a brand name for a range of preparations containing CHLOROXYLENOL.

river blindness see ONCHOCERCIASIS.

risk assessment a study of a patient, taking into account all known relevant factors, done for the purpose of trying to determine the probability that a person will develop a particular disease or, if the disease is already present, the probability that the person will suffer exacerbation of it or death from it.

risperidone a benzisoxazole antipsychotic drug used to treat SCHIZOPHRENIA and other psychotic disorders. The drug acts by interfering with serotonin and dopamine receptors. A brand name is Resperidal.

risus sardonicus a characteristic facial expression, as of a sardonic grin, caused by spasm of the muscles of the forehead and the corners of the mouth in acute TETANUS.

Ritalin a brand name for METHYLPHENIDATE.

ritodrine a drug that relaxes the muscles of the womb and is used to prevent the onset of premature labour. A brand name is Yutopar.

ritonavir a PROTEASE INHIBITOR drug used in combination with other drugs to treat AIDS. The drug is on the WHO official list. A brand name for ritonavor with lopinavir is Kaletra.

rituximab a MONOCLONAL ANTIBODY anticancer drug used to treat non-Hodgkin's lymphomas. A brand name is Mabthera.

rivastigmine an ANTICHOLINESTERASE INHIBITOR drug used in the early stages of dementia with Lewy bodies (DLB) in the hope of improving mental performance. An unknown proportion of people with Alzheimer's disease have DLB and can benefit from anticholinesterase inhibitor drugs.

Rivotril a brand name for CLONAZEPAM.

RM *abbrev. for* Registered Midwife.

RMN *abbrev. for* Registered Mental Nurse.

RMO *abbrev. for* Regimental Medical Officer or Resident Medical Officer.

RN *abbrev. for* Registered Nurse.

RNA *abbrev. for* ribonucleic acid. This molecule, in common with DNA and MITOCHONDRIAL DNA, carries coded instructions for the synthesis of specific proteins from AMINO ACIDS. RNA may be a double chain like DNA but in the cell usually exists as a single polynucleotide chain, like one strand of the double helix of DNA. Whereas in most cells DNA carries the permanent, inheritable code for cell reproduction, RNA most commonly acts as a transcriber or as MESSENGER RNA (mRNA) carrying the code elsewhere, as to the RIBOSOMES in cells where proteins are actually formed. In some viruses, however, the inherited code for replication occurs in the form of RNA. TRANSFER RNA (tRNA) picks up and carries amino acids to the ribosomes to be inserted in the correct sequence of the protein. Ribosomes contain ribosomal RNA (rRNA) and proteins.

RNA interference (RNAi) a pathway that blocks gene expression by degrading RNA. RNA interference occurs naturally against viruses and to control gene activity and has attracted much attention for its potential as a therapeutic process. It involves an attack on MESSENGER RNA using small RNA molecule fragments (siRNA) that matches part of the sequence of the target gene. In the search for effective artificial RNA interference methods, arbitrary short sequences

have often been found to fail because they are 'decoyed' by other genes in the genome. MicroRNAs have been shown to be important in the development of flower structure and may also be important in animal development. RNAi has been used in genetic research in determining the function of genes.

RNA polymerase an enzyme that catalyses the joining of appropriate NUCLEOTIDES to form a molecule of RNA, using DNA as a template.

RNA replicase an enzyme that catalyses the synthesis of RNA, using RNA as a template. The enzyme is used by RNA viruses for their replication within a cell.

Rnase RIBONUCLEASE.

RNA transcript an RNA complementary copy of a gene. The RNA transcript is always longer than the gene because the RNA polymerase also transcribes a leader segment prior to the gene code and a trailer segment after it.

RNT *abbrev. for* Registered Nurse Tutor.

Roaccutane a brand name for ISOTRETINOIN.

Robaxin a brand name for METHOCARBAMOL.

Robinul a brand name for GLYCOPYRRONIUM BROMIDE.

Robinul neostigmine a brand name for GLYCOPYRRONIUM BROMIDE compounded with NEOSTIGMINE.

robotics the branch of technology concerned with the development of machines capable of performing complex tasks of a kind normally limited to humans. Robotic machines of limited function controlled by computer have now become commonplace in the manufacturing industries, but the expected development of anthropomorphic or humanoid robots, in the manner predicted by the writer Karel Capek in his 1921 novel Rossum's Universal Robots, has not been fulfilled in any but a trivial sense. Robotics is now impinging on surgery and is likely to be important in the future.

robotic surgery a technology to use robotic devices, based on the engineering principles of those used in automobile manufacture, which promises to improve the precision and ease of surgery. Robotic arms have for some time been used to replace surgical assistants holding retractors, and more advanced devices are now in use. Telemanipulations systems exist by which the surgeon's hand movements are accurately reproduced within the patient's body. Internal mammary artery, coronary artery bypass surgery has been performed successfully on the beating heart using such a device with an internal 3-D camera and ventilation of the right lung only.

Rocatrol a brand name for CALCITRIOL.

Rocephin a brand name for CEFTRIAXONE.

Rocky Mountain spotted fever an acute infectious disease caused by the organism *Rickettsia rickettsii* and transmitted by the bite of an Ixodid hard tick from small rodents and dogs. The disease occurs mainly in south-eastern USA and South America. About a week after the bite there is fever, headache, nausea, muscle aches, loss of appetite and irritability and a rash of small round pink spots which spreads all over the body becoming darker. Most cases are mild, with fever for about 2 weeks, but some progress to an illness of great severity involving widespread haemorrhages and gangrene of the fingers, ears or genitalia and death within a week of onset. In these cases, prompt treatment with CHLORAMPHENICOL or a TETRACYCLINE antibiotic may be life-saving. Also known as tick typhus.

rocuronium bromide a non-DEPOLARIZING muscle relaxant drug used in general anaesthesia. A brand name is Esmeron.

rodent ulcer see BASAL CELL CARCINOMA.

roentgenography see X-RAYS and RADIOLOGY.

rofecoxib a COX-2 selective cyclo-oxygenase inhibitor NSAID used for the symptomatic treatment of OSTEOARTHRITIS and RHEUMATOID ARTHRITIS. A brand name is Vioxx. This drug was withdrawn from the market in 2004 when it was found that users suffered an increased risk of heart attack and stroke.

Roferon-A a brand name for INTERFERON ALFA-2a.

Rogitine a brand name for PHENTOLAMINE.

Rohypnol a brand name for FLUNITRAZEPAM. This drug has, in recent years, acquired an unpleasant reputation as a means of facilitating rape. It is subject to prescription requirements under the Misuse of Drugs Act and is not prescribable under the NHS.

role-playing 1 the acting out of a pattern of behaviour considered appropriate to one's social, educational or professional position or to one's current health status.
2 the adoption of a role foreign to one's normal situation.

rolfing a form of COMPLEMENTARY MEDICINE whose practitioners claim to be able to realign, or correct, the structural integration of the soft tissues of the body by deep massage so as to release tension that has accumulated in muscles, ligaments and tendons. The process is claimed also to release emotional memories retained in the muscles and other tissues so as to cure psychological problems. Medical scientists are sceptical.

Romana's sign closure of one eye as a result of a firm, reddish swelling in the upper eyelid in CHAGAS' DISEASE. (Cecilio Romana, Argentinian physician, b. 1899).

Romberg's sign a tendency to sway or fall while standing upright with the feet together, the arms stretched out and the eyes closed. A positive Romberg's sign suggests disease of the balancing mechanism in the inner ear or of its nerve connections or a loss of sensory information about the position of the legs (proprioception), usually from disease of the sensory tracts in the spinal cord. (Moritz Heinrich von Romberg, 1795–1873, German physician).

root canal the pulp cavity in the root of a tooth.

root-canal treatment a procedure designed to save a tooth with dead or irremediably diseased pulp. An opening is drilled into the tooth through the crown, the entire pulp and all diseased tissue is removed and a temporary antibiotic filling is inserted. A few days later the temporary filling is removed, the cavity is sealed with paste and the hole in the crown definitively filled with AMALGAM.

ropinirole a drug with dopamine-like action used to treat PARKINSON'S DISEASE. A brand name is Requip.

ropivacaine an aminoamide local anaesthetic drug similar to BUPIVACAINE but with a less toxic effect on the heart and a reduced tendency to block the function of motor nerves. A brand name is Naropin.

Rorschach test see INK BLOT TEST. (Hermann Rorschach, 1884–1922, German-born Swiss psychiatrist).

rosacea a persistent skin disorder of unknown cause, affecting especially the area of the face around and above the nose and the below eyes (the 'butterfly' area). The main features are redness from small dilated blood vessels, acne-like PUSTULES and thickening and oiliness of the skin. The corneas may be affected and, in men,

RHINOPHYMA may develop. Rosacea may be kept under control by a small daily dose of the antibiotic tetracycline. Tetracycline antibiotics or METRONIDAZOLE gel or cream may be applied to the skin. Rosacea is not an infection.

rose bengal a biological stain that can be applied to the cornea as eye drops to reveal subtle damage to the outer layer (epithelium). A brand name is Minims Rose Bengal.

roseola infantum a common disorder of small children of unknown cause. Roseola has been transmitted by filtered blood but no virus has, so far, been demonstrated. There is high fever for three days, enlarged lymph nodes, and, as the fever settles, a very transient pink rash similar to that of RUBELLA. The rash may last for less than a day and is easily missed. Complete recovery without treatment is the rule. Also known as 'sixth disease' or exanthem subitum.

roseola typhosa the rose-coloured rash of TYPHUS or TYPHOID.

Rose-Waaler test a test for RHEUMATOID FACTORS in RHEUMATOID ARTHRITIS. Sheep or human red blood cells coated with rabbit antired cell antibody are clumped together (agglutinated) in the presence of rheumatoid factors. (George Gibson Rose, b. 1922, American researcher; and Erik Waaler, 20th century Norwegian biologist).

rosuvastatin a long-acting statin drug (see STATINS). A brand name is Crestor.

rotator cuff the tendinous structure around the shoulder joint consisting of the tendons of four adjacent muscles blended with the capsule of the joint. Tearing or degeneration of any of these fibres may cause the common, painful and disabling rotator cuff syndrome in which there may be inability to raise the arm in a particular direction. Surgical repair may be necessary.

rotaviruses see REOVIRUSES.

Rotor syndrome mild JAUNDICE with an apparently normal liver which appears to be temporarily affected in its ability to take up and store BILIRUBIN. The outlook is excellent. (Arturo B. Rotor, Phillipine physician.).

roughage dietary fibre, consisting of polysaccharides such as celluloses, pectins and gums for which no digestive enzymes are present in the intestinal canal. Roughage is effective in treating CONSTIPATION, DIVERTICULITIS and the IRRITABLE BOWEL SYNDROME, and may reduce the probability of developing cancer of the colon.

rouleau a stacked collection of red blood cells, like a roll of coins. Rouleau formation suggests an increase in immunoglobulins in the blood.

round window the membranous, elastic opening in the outer wall of the inner ear that allows free movement of the fluid within the COCHLEA of the inner ear when sound vibrations are conveyed to it by the AUDITORY OSSICLES.

roundworms common nematode intestinal parasites, especially *Ascaris lubricoides* which inhabit the small intestine and live for about a year. Roundworm eggs are acquired by fecal contamination of food or fingers. If the worms are present in sufficient numbers there may be abdominal discomfort, pain, nausea, vomiting, loss of appetite and disturbed sleep. Roundworms are easily dislodged by means of anthelmintic drugs such as piperazine, levamisole or mebendazole.

Rowatinex a brand name for a mixture of the essential oils anethol, camphene, pinenes, borneol, fenchone and cineole used to treat urinary stones.

royal jelly a foodstuff secreted by worker bees for the nutrition of larvae and queen bees and sold at high prices. There is no reason to suppose that royal jelly has any medicinal value.

Royal Society of Medicine a unique British medical society of which full Fellowship is available to all registered medical, dental and veterinary practitioners. The RSM is independent of government or of any university. It does not train medical students or award degrees but it is deeply concerned with post-graduate medical education. It contains 40 speciality sections covering all disciplines, each with a distinguished consultant as President, and holds 400 meetings each year. Fellows have the right to attend any meeting in any discipline. The premises are at 1 Wimpole Street, London where, among other facilities, the largest medical library in Britain is to be found.

Rozex a brand name for METRONIDAZOLE formulated for external use only.

RRC *abbrev. for* Royal Red Cross.

RSCN *abbrev. for* Registered Sick Children's Nurse.

RSI *abbrev. for* repetitive strain injury, a form of OVERUSE INJURY.

rubber dam a perforated sheet of rubber that is

pushed over one or more teeth during certain dental procedures to acts as a barrier to prevent inhalation of debris or contamination of the operation site by saliva.

rubefacient any substance that reddens the skin by dilating the skin blood vessels. Rubefacients are sometimes included in liniments but are of little medical value.

rubella a common infectious disease caused by a respiratory virus. Rubella has an incubation period of up to 3 weeks, during which the virus spreads to lymph nodes, especially those in the back of the neck. The illness is mild and often consists of no more than a slight fever, swollen nodes and a scattered rash of slightly raised red patches. Rubella is notorious for its effects on the fetus, especially during the early months of pregnancy, when it can cause congenital heart disease and other physical malformations, CATARACT, deafness and mental retardation. An attack confers life-long immunity but all seronegative young girls and women should be vaccinated unless already pregnant and should be protected from pregnancy for 3 months after vaccination. Also known as German measles.

rubeola an alternative term for MEASLES.

rugae folds, wrinkles or creases, as in the skin of the scrotum.

rumination voluntary regurgitation of food from the stomach which is then again chewed and swallowed. Rumination sometimes occurs in mentally disturbed people.

rump the buttocks.

rupture a popular term for an abdominal HERNIA.

Rx a symbol used as the heading of a prescription for medicine or a medical appliance. An abbreviation of the Latin *recipe*, take thou.

Rynacrom a brand name for CROMOGLYCATE (cromoglicate).

Rynacrom Spray a brand name for a CROMOGLYCATE (cromoglicate) nasal spray.

Rythmodan a brand name for DISOPYRAMIDE.

S

Sabia virus an arenavirus first isolated in Sao Paulo, Brazil. Infections are usually acquired by exposure to infected rodent excreta and give rise to muscle pain, stiff neck, headache and a dangerous haemorrhagic fever with liver necrosis. The antiviral drug ribavirin is effective.

Sabin vaccine an effective oral vaccine used to immunize against POLIOMYELITIS. This vaccine contains live attenuated viruses that spread by the fecal-oral route in the manner of the original disease, thus effectively disseminating the protection. It was produced in 1955 and has been highly successful. (Albert Bruce Sabin, 1906–93, Russian-born American bacteriologist).

Sabril a brand name for VIGABATRIN.

sac any bag-like organ or body structure.

saccades rapid intermittent eye movements made as the attention switches from one point to another.

saccharine a sweetening agent with no caloric or nutritional value, that is excreted unchanged in the urine. It is said to be 550 times sweeter than sugar.

saccular aneurysm a sac-like ballooning in the wall of an artery that communicates with the vessel by a relatively small opening.

sacral pertaining to the SACRUM.

sacralgia pain in the sacrum usually from pressure on a spinal nerve.

sacralization 1 congenital fusion of the lowest lumbar vertebra to the top of the SACRUM; a harmless condition.
2 a surgical procedure to fuse the lowest lumbar vertebra to the sacrum in the treatment of SPONDYLOLISTHESIS.

sacro- *combining form denoting* SACRUM.

sacroiliac joints the firm ligamentous junctions between the sides of the SACRUM and the two outer bones of the pelvis (iliac bones). Normally the sacro-iliac joints are semi-rigid, but in late pregnancy they relax a little to allow easier childbirth. See also RELAXIN.

sacroiliitis inflammation of the sacroiliac joint.

sacrum the large, triangular, wedge-like bone that forms the centre of the back of the PELVIS and the lower part of the vertebral column. The sacrum consists of five fused, broad vertebrae and terminates in the tail-like COCCYX.

sadism a form of deviant sexuality in which pleasure and sexual arousal are derived from the infliction, or contemplation, of another's pain. From the name of the Marquis de Sade (1740–1814), a French writer of pornographic pseudophilosophy. Compare MASOCHISM.

sadomasochism a sexual deviation in which arousal is achieved by inflicting pain (SADISM) or by experiencing pain or abuse of various kinds (MASOCHISM).

SADS *abbrev. for* 1 seasonal affective disorder syndrome in which the mood changes according to the season of the year and which is treated by exposure to bright light.
2 sudden adult death syndrome: the sudden death of an apparently healthy adult, for which no cause can be found at postmortem.

safe period the part of the menstrual cycle in which coitus cannot result in fertilization because of the absence of an ovum. As a basis for contraception the term is far from appropriate.

safe sex measures taken to try to minimize the risk of sexually transmitted disease, especially AIDS. These include the avoidance of promiscuity, fidelity to the partner, the use of condoms and non-penetrative sexual activity.

sage the plant *Salvia officinalis* long claimed to promote health and long life, the extract of which (LEMON BALM) has recently shown some promise of improving the state of patients with ALZHEIMER'S DISEASE. Cur moriartur homo, ciu salvia crescit in horto? (Why die when you have sage in the garden?)

sagittal 1 pertaining to the SUTURE that joins the two parietal bones of the skull.
2 pertaining to the SAGITTAL PLANE. From the Latin *sagitta*, an arrow.

sagittal plane the front-to-back longitudinal vertical plane that divides the upright body into right and left halves.

Saizen a brand name for SOMATOTROPIN.

Salagen a brand name for PILOCARPINE.

Salamol Steri-Neb a brand name for SALBUTAMOL.

Salazopyrin a brand name for the drug SULPHASALAZINE used to treat RHEUMATOID ARTHRITIS, ULCERATIVE COLITIS and CROHN'S DISEASE.

Salbulin a brand name for SALBUTAMOL.

salbutamol a BRONCHODILATOR drug used to treat ASTHMA, CHRONIC BRONCHITIS and EMPHYSEMA. It is also sometimes used to relax the muscle of the womb and prevent premature labour. The drug is on the WHO official list. Brand names are Aerolin Autohaler, Airomir, Asmasal, Salamol Steri-Neb, Ventmax SR, Ventodisks, Ventolin and Volumax.

salicylates a group of anti-inflammatory, mildly ANALGESIC and fever-reducing (antipyretic) drugs that includes aspirin, sodium salicylate and BENORYLATE (benorilate).

salicylic acid a drug that softens and loosens the horny outer layer of the skin (the epidermis) and is used in the treatment of various skin disorders such as ACNE, PSORIASIS, ICHTHYOSIS, WARTS and CALLOSITIES. The drug is on the WHO official list. Brand names are Acnisal, Occlusal, Pyravlex, and Verugon. Numerous skin preparations contain salicyclic acid in conjunction with other ingredients.

salicylism toxicity from overdosage doses with salicylates.

saline a solution of salt (sodium chloride) in water. Normal saline is a solution with the same concentration of salt as body fluids and is suitable for infusion into a vein. Also known as physiological saline.

saliva a slightly alkaline, watery fluid secreted into the mouth by the SALIVARY GLANDS. Saliva contains the digestive enzyme amylase capable of breaking down starch to simpler sugars. Saliva keeps the mouth moist, dissolves taste particles in food so that they can stimulate the taste buds on the tongue and lubricates food during mastication to assist in swallowing.

Saliva Orthana a brand name for a MUCIN preparation.

salivary glands three pairs of glands that open into the mouth to provide a cleaning, lubricating and digestive fluid. The largest pair, the parotid glands, lie in the cheek in front of the ear. The other two pairs, the sublingual and the submandibular glands are in the floor of the mouth.

salivary gland disorders see MIXED PAROTID TUMOUR, MUMPS and SJÖGREN'S SYNDROME.

salivation the production of saliva. Excessive salivation is a feature of mouth ulcers and other causes of mouth irritation, PARKINSON'S DISEASE, nerve gas poisoning, organophosphorus insecticide poisoning, mercury poisoning, RABIES and overactivity of the parasympathetic nervous system.

Salk vaccine a killed virus anti-POLIOMYELITIS vaccine. (Jonas Salk, American microbiologist, b. 1914).

salmeterol an adrenaline-like drug used to treat ASTHMA. A brand name is Serevent.

Salmonella a genus of bacteria containing over 2000 strains, no longer considered to be separate species. Some have species-specific infectivity. About half of the strains are known to cause FOOD POISONING in humans. Salmonella organisms also cause TYPHOID and PARATYPHOID fevers. Common contaminants of food include *Salmonella typhimurium*, *S. hadar*, *S. enteritidis* and *S. virchow*. (Daniel E. Salmon, American pathologist, 1850–1914).

salmonellosis infection with SALMONELLA organisms.

Salofalk a brand name for MESALAZINE.

salping-, salpingo- *combining form denoting* the FALLOPIAN TUBE or the EUSTACHIAN TUBE.

salpingectomy surgical removal of one or both of the FALLOPIAN TUBES.

salpinges the Fallopian tubes. The singular is salpinx.

salpingitis inflammation of a FALLOPIAN TUBE, usually as a result of infection that has spread from the vagina or womb (uterus). Salpingitis may be caused by chlamydial infection, GONORRHOEA or an infection acquired after childbirth.

salpingo-oophoritis inflammation of the FALLOPIAN TUBES and OVARIES.

salpingo-oophorectomy surgical removal of one or both of the Fallopian tubes and one or both ovaries.

salt 1 any substance that dissociates in solution into ions of opposite charge.
2 common salt, sodium chloride (NaCl).

salve an ointment.

sandflies delicate, small, long-legged biting flies of the families *Psychodidae* and *Simuliidae*. Sandflies can cause annoying bites, especially after dark and transmit LEISHMANIASIS, SANDFLY FEVER and BARTONELLOSIS.

sandfly fever an influenza-like illness of short duration caused by a bunyavirus transmitted by the bite of the sandfly *Phlebotomus papatasii*. The disease occurs in the Mediterranean region and Middle East and features fever for 3 days, headache, CONJUNCTIVITIS and a drop in the white cell count in the blood (leukopenia).

Sandimmun a brand name for CYCLOSPORIN (ciclosporin).

Sandostatin a brand name for OCTREOTIDE.

Sandrena a brand name for OESTRADIOL (estradiol).

sane of sound mind. This is a legal rather than a medical term, as in the case of 'insanity'. The lawyers are forced by their trade to assume that a person must either be sane or insane; the doctors are not so sure.

sanguine of a ruddy complexion.

sanguineous pertaining to blood.

sanitary pertaining to health and hygiene.

sanitary protection pads or tampons used to avoid blood staining of clothing during the menstrual period.

sanitation measures concerned with the protection or promotion of public health, especially those relating to the disposal of sewage.

Sanomigran a brand name for PIZOTIFEN.

sapon-, *combining form denoting* soap.

saponaceous having soap-like properties.

saponification hydrolysis of a fat by an alkali to form a soap and an alcohol, usually glycerol.

Sapphic pertaining to female homosexuality. From the Greek female poet *Sappho* who lived on the island of Lesbos.

sapr-, sapro- *prefix denoting* decay or putrefaction.

sapraemia septicaemia.

saprogenic causing, or resulting from, putrefaction.

saprophyte an organism that lives on and derives its nourishment from dead or decaying organic matter.

saquinavir a PROTEASE INHIBITOR drug used in conjunction with other anti-HIV drugs to treat AIDS. Saquinavir acts by blocking the enzyme aspartic protease, so preventing the cleavage of GAG and gag-pol polyproteins into functional proteins. The result is the production of immature and non-infectious viral particles. The drug is on the WHO official list. A brand name is Invirase.

sarc-, sarco- *prefix denoting* flesh or striped muscle.

sarcoid 1 pertaining to or resembling flesh.
2 SARCOIDOSIS.

sarcoidosis a disease of unknown cause featuring GRANULOMAS in many parts of the body, especially in the lymph nodes, liver, lungs, skin and eyes. Sarcoidosis mainly affects young adults. Symptoms include fever, muscle and joint pain, ARTHRITIS, breathlessness and eye inflammation. There are enlarged lymph nodes in the neck and elsewhere, purplish swellings on the legs (erythema nodosum), a purplish rash on the face and areas of numbness. Treatment, when necessary, is with corticosteroid drugs. Most cases recover fully within 2 years without treatment.

sarcolemma a delicate membrane surrounding a striped muscle fibre.

sarcoma one of the two general types of cancer, the other being CARCINOMA. Sarcomas are malignant tumours of connective tissue such as bone, muscle, cartilage, fibrous tissue and blood vessels. Sarcomas are named after the parent tissue and include osteosarcoma, myosarcoma, chondrosarcoma, fibrosarcoma and angiosarcoma. KAPOSI'S SARCOMA is a tumour of blood vessels.

sarcomatosis multiple SARCOMA-like growths occurring in various parts of the body.

sarcomere the structural unit of a striped muscle fibre (myofibril).

sarcoplasm the cytoplasm of muscle cells.

Sarcoptes scabei the mite that causes SCABIES.

sarcoptic mange animal SCABIES.

sarin a military and terrorist nerve gas agent that causes breathing difficulty, cyanosis, running nose, salivation, profuse sweating and vomiting, constricted pupils, major tonic-clonic convulsions, coma and death.

Saroten a brand name for AMITRIPTYLINE.

SARS *acronym for* Severe Acute Respiratory Syndrome, the epidemic lung infection that started in Guangdong province and Hong Kong in early 2003 and spread rapidly to many parts of the world. The virus is a new coronavirus and has the largest genome of any RNA virus yet found. The genome was sequenced in May 2003. SARS features fever, influenza-like symptoms, and X-ray appearances of infiltrates of variable density compatible with pneumonia. The mortality increases with age and may be as high as 50% in patients over 65. Treatment is with antiviral drugs such as ribavirin in combination with antibiotics such as levofloxacin or clarithromycin. The angiotensin-converting enzyme 2 has been identified as the receptor for the coronavirus.

sartorius a long, narrow, flat, strap-like muscle that crosses the front of the thigh obliquely from the hip to the inner side of the top of the main lower leg bone (tibia). From the Latin *sartor*, a tailor – a reference to the historic cross-legged sitting posture of the tailor, which the muscle assists in adopting.

satyriasis an almost uncontrollable male craving for sexual intercourse. The male equivalent of NYMPHOMANIA.

saturated fats fats containing FATTY ACIDS in which the carbon atoms are linked to four other atoms by single bonds.

Saventrine a brand name for ISOPRENALINE.

saw-scaled viper venom a snake venom with a powerful effect in inactivating the action of blood platelets in forming clots within the circulation. A synthetic drug tirofiban (Aggrastat) has been developed from this venom which has been shown to have a substantial advantage over the anticoagulant HEPARIN in preventing heart attacks and deaths in cases of UNSTABLE ANGINA.

scab a skin crust formed when serum leaking from a damaged area mixes with pus and dead skin and then clots.

scabies skin infestation with the mite parasite *Sarcoptes scabei* which burrows into the superficial layers, usually of the hands or wrists, to feed on dead epidermal scales and lay eggs. Scabies is acquired by direct close contact, sometimes from domestic animals with mange. There is intense itching and damage is often caused by scratching and secondary infection. Treatment with insecticide lotions such as benzyl benzoate, is effective, but all members of the family should be treated if the parasite is to be eliminated.

scald a burn caused by hot liquid or steam.

scaling removal of dental calculus from the teeth to prevent or treat PERIODONTAL DISEASE. The hard calculus is levered or scraped off with a sharp-pointed steel scaler and the teeth are polished with an abrasive.

scalp the soft tissue layers covering the bone of the vault of the skull and consisting of a thin sheet of muscle, the epicranius, a layer of connective tissue richly supplied with blood vessels and the skin.

scalpel a surgical knife. Most scalpels consist of handles of various size that can be fitted with disposable steel blades. For delicate purposes, such as ophthalmic surgery, scalpels are made very small and fine and the cutting edge may be made of ruby or diamond.

scanning optical microscopy a method of light microscopy in which the object, often a block of wet or dry tissue, is illuminated with a scanned laser beam in such a way as to bring a narrow plane into focus while leaving the remainder out of focus. Serial observations, with photographs, of different planes can be made so that cutting sections is unnecessary. A three-dimensional image can be built up. The sites of binding of fluorescence-labelled antibodies can be determined with great accuracy.

scanning techniques see CT SCANNING, DIGITAL RADIOGRAPHY, MRI, RADIONUCLIDE SCANNING, SCANNING OPTICAL MICROSCOPY and ULTRASOUND SCANNING.

scaphoid bone one of the eight bones of the wrist. The scaphoid is roughly boat-shaped and is also known as the navicular bone. Because of its shape it is more readily fractured than the other carpal bones. From Greek *skaphoidis*, a boat, and Latin *navis*, a boat.

scapula the shoulder blade. A flat, triangular bone with a prominent, near-horizontal raised spine, lying over the upper ribs of the back. At its upper and outer angle the scapula bears a shallow hollow with which the rounded head of the upper arm bone (the humerus) articulates. The spine ends in a bony process, the coracoid process, the end of which connects with the outer end of the collar bone (clavicle).

scarabiasis intestinal infection with dung beetles. This occurs mainly in children and features loss of appetite, emaciation and diarrhoea.

scarification an obsolete operation in which numerous small cuts were made in the skin so as to increase the blood flow in the underlying tissues.

scarlatina a mild attack of SCARLET FEVER.

scarlet fever an infectious disease caused by STREPTOCOCCI (see STREPTOCOCCUS) acquired by inhaled droplets. Scarlet fever usually affects children but is now comparatively uncommon. It features sore throat, headache, fever and a characteristic rash caused by bacterial toxin. This starts as myriad tiny red spots spreading from the neck and upper chest to cover the whole body. The face is flushed but a pale zone is left around the mouth (circumoral pallor). The tongue has a white coating with red spots. As the rash fades there is skin peeling. Prompt treatment with penicillin is indicated to avoid the complications of streptococcal infection – RHEUMATIC FEVER or GLOMERULONEPHRITIS.

scar tissue fibrous COLLAGEN formed by the body to repair any wound, whether on the skin or internally. If the edges of the wound are brought close together the amount of scar tissue formed is minimal.

Schering PC4 a brand name for ETHINYLOESTRADIOL (ethinylestradiol) formulated with LEVONORGESTREL as an oral contraceptive.

Schick test a skin test of susceptibility to DIPHTHERIA. (Bela Schick, 1877–1967, Hungarian-born American paediatrician).

Schilling test a test to demonstrate the failure of absorption of vitamin B_{12} due to a lack of stomach INTRINSIC FACTOR. The test is used in the investigation of PERNICIOUS ANAEMIA. Cobalt 57 radio-labelled B_{12} is given by mouth and the amount excreted in the urine over the following 24 hours is an indication of the degree of absorption. (Victor Theodore Schilling, 1883–1960, German haematologist).

Schirmer test a test of tear production and the adequacy of corneal wetting in conditions such

as SJÖGREN'S SYNDROME. A narrow strip of filter paper is bent and hooked over the lower lid with one end between the lid and the eyeball. After a few minutes, wetting should extend for at least 8 mm. (Rudolph Schirmer, 1831–96, German ophthalmologist).

-schisis *combining form denoting* a splitting or cleaving.

schistosomiasis a parasitic worm disease common in most tropical countries and acquired during immersion in water contaminated with the larval forms of schistosome worms, such as *Schistosoma mansoni*. These penetrate the skin and travel to the veins of the bowel, bladder, liver and other organs where they grow to adult size – 1 to 2.5 cm. Worm eggs are excreted in urine and faeces. Late complications of schistosomiasis include CYSTITIS, loss of normal bladder function, bladder stones, cancer of the bladder, kidney failure and CIRRHOSIS of the liver. Some species of schistosomes can cause bowel and liver upset and may involve the nervous system to cause epilepsy, paralysis, coma and death. Schistosomiasis can be avoiding by staying out of water which might be contaminated with human excreta. The drug praziquantel will kill the adult worms. The name derives from the fact that the body of the adult male worm is effectively split longitudinally to form a 'gynaecophoric canal' in which the female worm usually lies.

schiz-, schizo- *prefix denoting* split or cleft, cleavage or fission.

schizogenesis reproduction by simple division into two or more individuals (fission).

schizogony multiple fission of a unicellular organism so that many daughter organisms are formed. This occurs in the life cycle of malarial parasites.

schizoid personality a term describing people who are withdrawn, solitary, socially isolated, often appearing cold and aloof and sometimes eccentric. About 10% of people of this personality type develop overt SCHIZOPHRENIA.

schizont a stage in the life-cycle of a sporozoan parasite, especially a malarial parasite. A schizont reproduces by SCHIZOGONY producing multiple trophozoites or merozoites.

schizophrenia the commonest major psychiatric disorder affecting about 1% of Western populations and usually appearing in adolescence or early adult life. Schizophrenia is not a disease in the normal medical sense and the diagnosis is based entirely on behaviour and on the statements of the affected person. Schizophrenics are said to have DELUSIONS, HALLUCINATIONS, disordered thinking and loss of contact with reality. They indulge in non-logical free associations, appear to confuse literal and metaphorical meaning and use invented words. The cause has not been established but life case histories suggest that some schizophrenics have adopted an alternative reality as an escape from an intolerable life situation. There also appears to be some genetic basis, but this does not exclude an important environmental causation. A mutation in the serotonin receptor gene has been proposed as a cause. Schizophrenics can usually be made to conform to conventional social mores by treatment with antipsychotic drugs. Psychoanalysis has no value in the treatment of schizophrenia.

Schwann cell a NEURILEMMA cell of a nerve fibre that produces the myelin sheath. (Theodor Schwann, 1810–1882, German anatomist).

sciatica pain arising from abnormal stimulation of the SCIATIC NERVE, usually from pressure on the sciatic nerve roots from pulp material from an INTERVERTEBRAL DISC. The symptom varies from minor backache to severe pain extending down to the foot and associated with muscle weakness. The treatment is that of the cause.

sciatic nerve the main nerve of the leg and the largest nerve in the body. The sciatic nerve is a mixed MOTOR and sensory nerve. It arises from the lower end of the spinal cord and runs down through the buttock to the back of the thigh. It supplies the muscles of the hip, many of the thigh muscles, all the muscles of the lower leg and foot, and most of the skin of the leg.

SCID *abbrev. for* SEVERE COMBINED IMMUNODEFICIENCY DISORDER.

scintigraphy RADIONUCLIDE SCANNING.

scirrhous hard and fibrous, especially of malignant tumours containing dense fibrous tissue.

scler-, sclero- *combining form denoting* hard or the SCLERA.

sclera the white of the eye. The tough outer coating of dense, interwoven collagen fibrils visible through the transparent overlying CONJUNCTIVA.

scleritis inflammation of the SCLERA, usually as a feature of a general disease such as rheumatoid arthritis or as a complication of ophthalmic shingles (herpes zoster) or Wegener's granulomatosis. Treatment is with corticosteroid drugs often in the form of eyedrops.

scleroderma a rare AUTOIMMUNE disorder that may affect skin, lungs, heart, arteries, kidneys, joints and the intestines. It often causes thickening and shininess of the skin giving the face a mask-like appearance and causing stiffness of joints. RAYNAUD'S PHENOMENON is common. There may be difficulty in swallowing, breathlessness, palpitations, high blood pressure (HYPERTENSION) and muscle weakness. There is no specific treatment.

scleromalacia softening of the sclera usually as a complication of SCLERITIS complicating RHEUMATOID ARTHRITIS.

sclerosed hardened. Affected with SCLEROSIS.

sclerosing adenomatosis a breast tissue abnormality in which the milk ducts become encased in fibrous tissue, producing an effect closely similar to an invasive cancer.

sclerosis hardening of tissues usually from deposition of fibrous tissue, following persistent INFLAMMATION.

sclerosteosis a bone abnormality involving increased density.

sclerotherapy a treatment for varicose veins in which the affected veins are injected with a solution that causes inflammation of the vein lining, clotting of the contained blood and closure of the vein.

sclerotic 1 the white outer coat (sclera) of the eye.
2 pertaining to the SCLERA.

sclerotomy an incision into, or through, the sclera.

SCM *abbrev. for* State Certified Midwife.

scolex the rounded head end of a tapeworm, bearing suckers or hooks by which it attaches itself to the intestine of the host.

scolio- *combining form denoting* twisted.

scoliosis a spinal deformity in which the column is bent to one side usually in the chest or lower back regions. This may cause crowding of the ribs on one side.

scombroid poisoning a condition believed to be caused by heat-stable toxin that develops in the muscles of red meat fish, such as tuna, that have been stored without adequate refrigeration. There is a bitter taste in the mouth, a wide-spread rash, a feeling of hotness, a fast pulse rate and sometimes diarrhoea and wheezing. These effects usually settle within 12 hours. Antihistamine drugs speed up recovery but the condition is not an allergy to fish.

Scop a brand name for HYOSCINE.

scopolamine an ATROPINE-like drug used in premedication as a sedative and to dry up respiratory and salivary secretions.

scoto- *combining form denoting* darkness.

scotoma a blind spot or area in the field of vision. This may be caused by GLAUCOMA, MULTIPLE SCLEROSIS, MIGRAINE, retinal disorders or a brain tumour.

scotopia ability to see in poor light. Vision adapted to night-time conditions.

scrapie a fatal nervous system disease of sheep featuring a SPONGIFORM ENCEPHALOPATHY. Scrapie is caused by a PRION and has an incubation period of 2 to 7 years.

screening the routine examination of numbers of apparently healthy people to identify those with a particular disease at an early stage.

screw-worm fly a fly, *Cochliomyia hominivorax*, that breeds in the living tissue of mammals, usually in open wounds, producing parasitic larvae that can cause serious tissue damage or even death.

scrofula bovine TUBERCULOSIS of the lymph nodes of the neck, with or without breakdown of the skin. Milk pasteurization and herd control have reduced this once common condition to a negligible incidence in developed countries.

scrotum the skin and muscle sac containing the testicles and the start of the SPERMATIC CORD. The wrinkled appearance of the scrotal skin is due to the thin layer of DARTOS MUSCLE under the skin.

scrub typhus an acute infectious disease caused by *Rickettsia tsutsugamushi* and transmitted to men by the bite of the larval *trombiculid* mite. The disease is common in rural areas in Asia. There is a black scar at the site of the bite (tache noir), sudden fever, painful swelling of the lymph nodes, headache, eye pain, cough and a skin rash. Antibiotics are effective.

scurf an exaggerated loss (desquamation) of the surface layers of the EPIDERMIS of the skin, especially from the scalp. Dandruff.

scurvy a deficiency disease caused by an inadequate intake of vitamin C (ascorbic acid). This vitamin C is needed for the formation of stable COLLAGEN; deficiency leads to weakness of small blood vessels and poor healing of wounds, and spontaneous bleeding occurs into gums, skin, joints and muscles. Treatment with large doses of ascorbic acid is rapidly effective.

sea sickness one of the several forms of MOTION SICKNESS.

seasonal affective disorder syndrome see SADS.

seb-, sebo- *combining form denoting* fat, SEBUM.

sebaceous cyst a wen. A harmless soft swelling within the skin, consisting of an accumulation of fatty sebaceous material (SEBUM), the normal secretion of the sebaceous glands of the skin. Cysts develop when a gland opening becomes blocked. Sebaceous cysts, however large, are easily treated by a simple surgical operation.

sebaceous glands tiny skin glands that secrete an oily lubricating substance, called SEBUM, either into hair follicles or directly on to the surface of the skin.

seborrhoea excessive secretion of SEBUM. This causes an oily appearance of the skin, especially of the face, and a greasy scalp. Seborrhoea also predisposes to ACNE. The cause is uncertain, male sex hormones (androgens) are involved. Seborrhoea usually settles without treatment.

seborrhoeic dermatitis severe dandruff. Local inflammation of the skin, with redness, scales, crusting yellowish patches and itching. It affects mainly the scalp, eyebrows, beard area and groins.

sebum the secretion of the SEBACEOUS GLANDS. Sebum is chemically complex and consists mainly of triacyl glycerols, wax esters and squalene. Blackheads (comedones) are plugs of sebum, the darkened tips being due to oxidation.

Seconal sodium a brand name for the barbiturate drug QUINALBARBITONE (secobarbital).

secondary a disease or disorder that results from and follows another disease or a prior episode of the same disease. Secondary cancer is the occurrence of a METASTASIS at a site remote from that of the primary tumour. Since the tumour originated in a different tissue it may differ in character from a primary growth at the new site.

secondary immune response see PRIMARY IMMUNE RESPONSE.

second-degree burn a burn more severe than a FIRST-DEGREE BURN, with blistering, OEDEMA and destruction of the surface layers. Burns are now usually classified as partial-thickness, in which the skin can regenerate, and full-thickness, in which it cannot and grafting is usually necessary.

secretin a hormone secreted in the DUODENUM that prompts the production of PANCREATIC JUICE.

secretion the synthesis and release of chemical substances by cells or glands. Substances secreted include enzymes, hormones, lubricants, surfactants and neurotransmitters. Internal secretion is secretion into the bloodstream. External secretion may be into the intestinal canal or other organs or on to the skin. Compare EXCRETION.

secretor status the ability of an individual to secrete the water-soluble form of the ABO blood group ANTIGENS into body fluids. There is a genetically determined inability to secrete these antigens and those so affected are unduly susceptible to various bacterial and superficial fungal infections.

sectioning 1 an informal term, or euphemism, used to describe the implementation of a section of the UK Mental Health Act so that a person suffering from a psychiatric disorder can be detained (See CERTIFICATION OF INSANITY). **2** cutting a thin slice of tissue for microscopic examination.

Sectral a brand name for ACEBUTOLOL.

security object any object, such as a teddy bear, a baby blanket or a former night garment, that brings comfort and a sense of security to a young child.

Securon a brand name for the drug VERAPAMIL.

sedation the use of a mild drug to calm, alleviate anxiety and promote sleep.

sedative drugs a group of drugs that includes antianxiety drugs, sleeping drugs, antipsychotic drugs and some antidepressant drugs. See also HYPNOTIC.

SeHCAT test a test of the absorbing power of the small intestine. A synthetic bile acid (HC) is labelled with radioactive selenium (Se) and given by mouth. The degree of absorption can be calculated from the measured radioactivity in the abdomen.

seizure an episode in which uncoordinated electrical activity in the brain causes sudden muscle contraction, either local (partial seizure) or widespread (generalized seizure). Recurrent seizures are called EPILEPSY. Also known as a fit.

SELECT a double-blind, placebo-controlled trial involving 32,400 men with apparently normal prostate glands and normal PSA levels, designed to determine the value of selenium and vitamin E in preventing prostate cancer. The trial was started in 2001 and the final results will not be available until 2013.

selective digestive decontamination (SDD) the use of non-absorbable antibiotics to target potentially pathogenic organisms in the gut while leaving the normal anaerobic commensals unaffected. The purpose of SDD is to reduce the risk of transmitting dangerous infections to other patients in hospital. Antibiotics used include polymyxin B, tobramycin and amphotericin.

selective serotonin re-uptake inhibitors (SSRIs) a range of drugs that act at the clefts of synapses in the brain preventing released SEROTONIN from being removed and thus increasing its action as a NEUROTRANSMITTER. These drugs are used to treat depression, anxiety, panic disorders, agoraphobia, bulimia, obsessive-compulsive disorders and post-traumatic stress disorder syndrome. Generic names are CITALOPRAM, FLUOXETINE, FLUVOXAMINE, PAROXETINE, and SERTRALINE. Other drugs (e.g. VENLAFAXINE) are specific promoters of the action of both serotonin and noradrenaline and are termed selective noradrenaline and serotonin inhibitors (SNRIs). Doubts have been expressed as to the specificity of some of the drugs in this group for treating certain of these conditions. Brand names can be found in the generic entries.

selegiline a selective MONOAMINEOXIDASE INHIBITOR drug used in the treatment of PARKINSONISM. Selegiline is thought to retard the breakdown of DOPAMINE. Brand names are Eldepryl and Vivapril.

selenium a trace element recently found to be an essential component of the enzyme deiodinase which catalyses the production of triiodothyronine (T_3) from thyroxine (T_4) in the thyroid gland. Selenium deficiency prevents the formation of T_3.

selenium sulphide selenium sulfide, an anti-

DANDRUFF agent formulated as a shampoo. The drug is on the WHO official list. Brand names are Lenium and Selsun.

selenosis selenium poisoning.

self-image a person's conception of his or her own appearance, personality and capabilities.

self-mutilation acts of destruction of parts of one's own body, such as amputation of fingers, limbs or genitals, gouging out of eyes, and so on.

Selsun a brand name for a SELENIUM-containing shampoo used to treat DANDRUFF.

semantics the study of meaning, of the effectiveness with which thought is translated into language, and of the relationship between words and symbols and meaning.

semeiography a description of the signs and symptoms of a disease. Also semiography.

semen SEE SEMINAL FLUID.

semi- *prefix denoting* half or partial.

semicircular canals the three tubular structures of the labyrinth of the inner ear, which lie in three different planes and which contain fluid. Movement of the head leads to differential stimulation of nerve endings within the canals and provides the brain with information about orientation.

semicoma a partially comatose state in which the patient appears to be unconscious but can be roused by painful stimuli and usually makes purposeful movements.

semiconscious half-conscious.

Semi-daonil a brand name for GLIBENCLAMIDE.

semilunar *or* **semilunate** shaped like a half moon or crescent.

semilunar bone the LUNATE bone in the wrist.

semilunar valves the crescent-shaped valves, each having three cusps, situated one at the beginning of the AORTA and the other at the origin of the PULMONARY ARTERY. These valves allow blood to flow only in a direction away from the heart.

semilunate semilunar.

seminal fluid a creamy, greyish-yellow, sticky fluid that is forced out of the penis during the ejaculation that accompanies the sexual orgasm. Seminal fluid is secreted by the PROSTATE GLAND, the SEMINAL VESICLES, the lining of the sperm tubes and some small associated glands. It contains the male gametes, the SPERMATOZOA.

seminal vesicles two small, elongated, sac-like containers situated on the PROSTATE GLAND at

the point at which the VAS DEFERENS passes through to join the URETHRA. The seminal vesicles store SEMINAL FLUID until it is discharged by ejaculation.

seminiferous tubules the many, long, coiled-up, fine tubes, hundreds of which are present in each testicle and are said to total in length over 400 m. The spermatozoa develop from cells in the walls of these tubules.

seminoma a malignant tumour of the testicle, composed of cells resembling primitive germ cells. The seminoma is highly sensitive to radiotherapy.

semiotics the study of signs, including words, symbols, gestures and body language, and of their cardinal role in conveying information. Semiotic studies suggest that meaning, although it may often seem self-evident, is always the result of social conventions. Cultures can be analyzed in terms of a series of sign systems. One difficulty, perhaps responsible for a certain vagueness in discussion of the subject, is that the experts have never been able to reach full agreement on the exact definition of the central terms 'sign', 'symbol' and 'signal'.

semipermeable able to allow the passage of molecules below a certain size and to retain those above this size. Much of PHYSIOLOGY depends on the semipermeability of body membranes.

semipermeable membrane any membrane permeable to water and other liquids but which does not allow the passage of dissolved molecules larger than a certain size. The association of semipermeable membranes with solutions allows selective movement of substances into and out of various body compartments and cells and subserves the principle of OSMOTIC PRESSURE.

SEN *abbrev. for* State Enrolled Nurse.

senescent ageing. The term ought not to imply physical or mental deterioration, but often does.

Sengstaken tube a tube with two inflatable balloons near one end that is passed into the stomach and inflated to exert pressure on the lower end of the OESOPHAGUS and the upper part of the stomach. This is done to control bleeding from OESOPHAGEAL VARICES. (Robert William Sengstaken, American surgeon, b. 1923).

senile pertaining to old age. From the Latin *senilis*, old.

senile dementia see DEMENTIA.

senile eczema a form of DERMATITIS occuring in elderly people who are unable to maintain normal standards of personal hygiene and who may also suffer from dietary deficiency.

senile emphysema age-related degenerative changes in the lungs, with breakdown of the walls of the ALVEOLI.

senile gangrene tissue death affecting the extremities and caused by loss of the blood supply from age-related obstructive arterial disease.

senile vaginitis inflammation of the vagina affecting elderly women and due to thinning and atrophy of the mucous membrane from oestrogen deficiency.

senility old age, usually with the connotation of mental or physical deterioration. From the Latin *senilis*, old (which had no negative significance).

senna a stimulant laxative drug used to treat constipation. The drug is on the WHO official list. A brand name is Senokot.

Senokot a brand name for SENNA.

senopia an acquired form of MYOPIA, occurring in the elderly, that may allow reading without glasses. Senopia is due to an increase in the refractive index of the crystalline lenses in incipient CATARACT. Also known as index myopia.

sensate perceived by the senses.

sensate focus technique a method of managing male impotence and female lack of sexual interest, essentially by prohibiting coitus and encouraging sensual massage, performed in stages, until, willy-nilly, nature has its way. The formal prohibition relieves anxiety which is at the root of most cases of impotence.

sensation the conscious experience produced by the stimulation of any sense organ such as the eye, ear, nose, tongue, skin, or any internal sensory receptor.

sensitization the preliminary exposure of a person to an ALLERGEN that leads to ANTIBODY production by the immune system and, on subsequent exposure, to an ALLERGIC or hypersensitivity reaction. Immunoglobulin Type E (IgE) is the main type of antibody involved.

sensory cortex an area on the outer layer (cortex) of the CEREBRUM through the stimulation of which consciousness of sensation is mediated. The sensory cortex for pressure, pain, taste and temperature lies immediately behind the motor cortex on the side of each cerebral hemisphere, about half way back. The cortex for visual sensation is at the back, and that for sound is in the temporal lobes on either side.

sensory deprivation the effecting of a major reduction in incoming sensory information. Sensory deprivation is damaging because the body depends for its normal functioning on constant stimulation. Sensory deprivation early in life is the most damaging of all and can lead to severe retardation and permanent malfunctioning of the deprived modality.

sensorineural deafness deafness caused by any defect in the inner ear mechanism that converts sound vibrations into nerve impulses, especially the hair cells of the cochlea, or in the acoustic nerve (8th cranial nerve) or the brain. Compare CONDUCTIVE DEAFNESS.

sensory aphasia inability to appreciate the meaning of spoken or written words, gestures or signs. In speech, words are used incorrectly and do not convey the desired ideas. Sensory APHASIA is the result of brain damage, usually from STROKE.

sentinel node a lymph node presumed to be the first to which a cancer will extend by lymphatic spread. In the case of breast cancer, armpit (axillary) sentinel nodes can be identified prior to surgery by injecting serum albumin tagged with the radioactive marker technetium-99m near to a breast tumour site. Lymph drainage ensures that the radioactivity will be concentrated in the sentinel node and this is demonstrated by scintigraphy. Surgical identification of the sentinel node can also be aided using a blue dye injected into the skin. See also SENTINEL NODE BIOPSY.

sentinel node biopsy the identification and removal for examination of the SENTINEL NODE using a hand-held gamma-ray detector probe. It is claimed that examination of this single lymph node can accurately predict in 97.5% of cases whether or not a breast cancer has spread to the lymph nodes. The false negative rate is 4.6%. The method has also been used in the management of malignant melanoma. The sentinel node biopsy concept was originated by Professor Umberto Veronesi of the European Institute of Oncology, Milan, Italy.

separation anxiety excessive and

inappropriate levels of anxiety experienced by children during separation, or the threat of separation, from a parent or from a person in loco parentis.

sepsis the condition associated with the presence in the body tissues or the blood of micro-organisms that cause infection or of the toxins produced by such organisms. Sepsis varies in severity from a purely local problem to an overwhelming and fatal bacterial intoxication. Sepsis has been defined as the systemic inflammatory response to infection based on the clinical criteria of a temperature over 38 °C, a heart rate of over 90 beats per minute, a resiratory rate of over 20 per minute and a white blood cell count increase of more than 12,000 or with more than 10% immature neutrophil polymorphs. Severe sepsis is defined as sepsis associated with organ dysfunction. Severe sepsis has a mortality of up to 50%.

septal defect an abnormal opening in the central wall of the heart providing a communication from the right side to the left or vice versa. This is a developmental congenital defect and its significance varies from trivial to grave depending on its position and size. Popularly known as 'hole in the heart'.

septate having a partition (SEPTUM) or several partitions (septa).

septic pertaining to SEPSIS.

septic abortion an ABORTION complicated by infection of the lining of the womb (endometrium).

septicaemia the presence in the circulating blood of large numbers of disease-producing organisms. Septicaemia causes high fever, shivering, headache and rapid breathing and may progress to delirium, coma and death. Treatment is with antibiotics and sometimes transfusion. Also known as blood poisoning. See also SEPTIC SHOCK.

septic embolus an EMBOLUS containing bacteria.

septic shock a dangerous condition caused by damage to immune cells, the endothelium of blood vessels and the malfunction of most of the organs of the body by the uncontrolled production of potent CYTOKINES mainly by bacterial pathogens. These include tumour necrosis factor and interleukin-1 which are produced as a response to the toxins of bacteria

in the course of SEPTICAEMIA. Small blood vessels become leaky and so much fluid is lost into the tissue spaces that the normal circulation cannot be maintained and the blood pressure drops. This is called shock and it is similar in effect to shock from other causes such as severe blood loss or severe burns. Urgent treatment with antibiotics, transfusion and organ support is necessary to save life.

septoplasty an operation to correct a deviation to one side of the central partition of the nose (the nasal SEPTUM).

Septrin a brand name for a combination of TRIMETHOPRIM and SULPHAMETHOXAZOLE. Also known as Co-trimoxazole.

septum any thin dividing wall or partition within or between parts of the body.

sequela a sequel. Any condition or state that follows a disease, disorder, or injury, especially one that is a consequence of it. A COMPLICATION. The term is most often used in the plural form – sequelae.

sequestration separation and physiological isolation of a portion of dead tissue from surrounding healthy tissue. The commonest example of sequestration is the formation of a bony SEQUESTRUM as a complication of OSTEOMYELITIS.

sequestrum a piece of dead, often detached, bone lying within a cavity or abscess. Sequestra usually form as a result of long-term OSTEOMYELITIS.

Serc a brand name for the drug betahistidine used in the treatment of MÉNIÈRE'S DISEASE.

Serdolect a brand name for SERTINDOLE.

Serenace a brand name for the tranquillizing drug HALOPERIDOL.

Serepax a brand name for OXAZEPAM.

Seretide 500 a brand name for an inhaler containing SALMETEROL and FLUTICASONE. Seretide was approved for the treatment of COPD in mid-2003.

serine a non-essential amino acid found as a component of most proteins. It is a precursor of choline, glucine, cysteine and pyruvate. Serine is present in most diets but most of the body serine is synthesized.

sermorelin a growth hormone releasing factor used as a drug to treat growth failure. A brand name is Geref.

sero- *prefix denoting* SERUM or serotherapy.

serodiagnosis diagnosis based on the findings

of an examination of the blood serum of a patient, especially for ANTIBODIES.

serology the branch of laboratory medicine concerned with the investigation of blood SERUM with special reference to its antibody (immunoglobulin) content. Detection of antibodies and ANTIGENS is of considerable medical importance especially in diagnosis.

Serophene a brand name for the drug CLOMIPHENE (clomifene), used in the treatment of infertility.

seropurulent composed of SERUM and PUS.

Seroquel a brand name for QUETIAPINE.

serotherapy treatment of disease by the injection of human or animal serum containing antibodies.

serotonin 5-hydroxytryptamine (5-HT). A NEUROTRANSMITTER and HORMONE found in many tissues, especially the brain, the intestinal lining and the blood platelets. Serotonin is concerned with controlling mood and levels of consciousness. Its action is disturbed by some hallucinogenic drugs and imitated by others. It constricts small blood vessels, cuts down acid secretion by the stomach and contracts the muscles in the wall of the intestine.

serotonin syndrome a potentially dangerous reaction to drug administration or drug interactions that involve excessive serotonergic agonism. The effects range from mild to life-threatening and include AKATHISIA, tremor, altered mental states, agitation, clonus, muscular hypertonicity, hyperthermia and death. Many drugs have been found to be implicated and these are not limited to the selective serotonin re-uptake inhibitors.

serotype 1 a subgroup of a genus of micro-organisms identifiable by the ANTIGENS carried by the members.

2 a category into which material is placed, based on its serological activity, especially in terms of the antigens it carries or the antibodies it produces in the body.

sertindole a phenylindole antipsychotic drug used to treat SCHIZOPHRENIA. A brand name is Serdolect. This is one of the few drugs with the distinction of having been withdrawn and then reintroduced (with stated precautions).

sertraline a SELECTIVE SEROTONIN RE-UPTAKE INHIBITOR drug used to treat depression and severe premenstrual syndrome. A brand name is Lustral.

serum the clear, straw-coloured fluid that separates from blood when it is allowed to clot and then to stand. Serum is blood less the red cells and the proteins which form the clot. It contains many substances in solution including sodium, potassium, calcium, magnesium, chloride, bicarbonate, phosphate, albumin, globulins, amino acids, carbohydrates, vitamins, hormones, urea, creatinine, uric acid and bilirubin.

serum albumin one of the soluble protein fractions of blood serum. Albumin is important in maintaining the OSMOTIC PRESSURE of the blood.

serum dependence the necessity for the presence of factors contained in serum before cells can be grown in culture.

serum globulin one of the soluble protein fractions of blood serum. Most of the serum globulins are ANTIBODIES (immunoglobulins).

serum hepatitis HEPATITIS B.

serum shock an acute allergic (ANAPHYLACTIC) reaction occurring after the injection of foreign serum into a person who has become sensitized to it by previous exposure.

serum sickness a brief allergic reaction that may develop after an injection of an antiserum of animal origin. In serum sickness, the immune system produces antibodies to substances in the serum and these may form IMMUNE COMPLEXES which cause inflammation in various tissues.

sesamoid bone a bone lying within a tendon to assist in its mechanical action and to bear pressure. The most conspicuous sesamoid bone is the knee cap (patella).

sessile having no stalk, flat and wide-based. Compare PEDUNCULATED.

setting sun sign persistent downward deviation of the eyes without a corresponding lowering of the upper lids, so that the corneas appear to descend behind the edge of the lower lids. This is a sign of raised pressure within the skull as occurs in infants with HYDROCEPHALUS.

severe combined immunodeficiency disorder (SCID) a congenital immuno-deficiency of both T and B LYMPHOCYTES. The condition is due to a genetic defect that causes a defect in the recombinase enzymes essential for the production of T and B cell receptors. As a result neither of these classes of lymphocytes can become immunologically functional and the affected child is gravely susceptible to infections of all kinds.

sevoflurane a recently-introduced volatile, non-irritant, pleasant-smelling inhalational general anaesthetic that causes rapid induction and from which recovery is also rapid.

Sevredol a brand name for MORPHINE.

sex 1 gender, as genetically determined.
2 the condition of being male or female.
3 the urge or instinct manifesting itself in behaviour directed towards copulation.
4 the genitalia.
5 a popular term for COITUS.

sex cell a GAMETE.

sex chromosomes the pair of chromosomes that determines gender. The other 22 pairs of chromosomes are known as autosomes. Women have two sex chromosomes of similar appearance called X chromosomes (XX). Men have one X chromosome and another, much smaller chromosome, called a Y (XY). Sperms have half the normal complement of chromosomes (haploid) and contain either an X or a Y. If an X chromosome effects fertilization the result will be a female, if a Y, a male.

sex gland a testis or ovary. A gonad.

sex hormones HORMONES that bring about the development of bodily sexual characteristics and regulate sperm and egg production and the menstrual cycle. There are steroids of three main types – androgens (male), oestrogens (female) and PROGESTOGENS that prepare women for, and maintain, pregnancy.

sex-linkage inheritance in which the gene for the condition is carried on one of the X or Y sex chromosomes. Recessive sex-linked conditions almost always affect males, are carried on the male X chromosome and thus cannot be transmitted directly from father to son. The best-known sex-linked recessive condition is haemophilia. Y-linked conditions are rare; the Y chromosome is very small and carries few genes.

sex-linked see SEX-LINKAGE.

sexology the study of sexual behaviour, especially in humans.

sex pilus see BACTERIAL CONJUGATION.

sex reassignment surgery surgical treatment to alter the external appearance in the direction of the opposite sex. It is rarely performed but is sometimes justified in the case of people with ambiguous genitalia or in the case of some TRANSSEXUALS who are convinced that they are of the wrong anatomical sex.

sex selection the determination of the sex of a future individual before conception by the separation of sperms bearing Y chromosomes (male) from those bearing X chromosomes (female). Such techniques are still experimental and uncertain and raise major ethical issues.

sextan occurring every 6 days, especially of MALARIA.

sex therapy specialized methods of treatment for problems such as erectile dysfunction (impotence), premature ejaculation, anorgasmia (failure to achieve orgasm), VAGINISMUS, sexual phobias and DYSPAREUNIA. See also SENSATE FOCUS TECHNIQUE, SEXUAL DISORDERS.

sextuplets six SIBLINGS delivered at one birth.

sexual pertaining to sex, sexuality, the sexes, reproduction, erotic desires or activity, the sex organs or the union of male and female GAMETES.

sexual abuse subjection of any person, but especially a minor, to sexual activity likely to cause physical or psychological harm. See also CHILD ABUSE, RAPE.

sexual deviation an arbitrary term whose meaning varies with the attitudes and views of the user. Few, however, would exclude from its definition SADISM, SADOMASOCHISM, PAEDOPHILIA, BESTIALITY, sexual exhibitionism, sexual FETISHISM, VOYEURISM, telephone scatologia, FROTTEURISM and COPROPHILIA.

sexual disorders see ANORGASMIA, IMPOTENCE, KRAUROSIS VULVAE, PEYRONIE'S DISEASE, PREMATURE EJACULATION, SEXUAL DEVIATION, SEXUALLY TRANSMITTED DISEASES and VAGINISMUS.

sexual intercourse 1 the totality of the physical and mental interplay between humans in which the explicit or implicit goal is bodily union and, ideally, the expression of love and affection.
2 COITUS.

sexuality 1 the structural differences between male and female.
2 a person's sexual attitudes, drive, interest or activity.
3 all the emotions, sensations, behaviour patterns and drives connected with reproduction and with the use of the sex organs.
4 (Freudian) all drives connected with bodily

satisfaction. See also HETEROSEXUALITY, HOMOSEXUALITY and BISEXUALITY.

sexually transmitted infections (STI, STD) a growing problem in Britain and elsewhere in the world. Between 1999 and 2004 in the UK, figures for gonorrhoea rose 78%, for chlamydial infections 73% and for syphilis 374%. The list that follows highlights the key entries related to sexually transmiited infections in the dictionary: Acquired immune deficiency syndrome, amoebiasis, candidiasis, chancroid, chlamydial infections, crab lice, *gardnerella vaginalis* infection, genital herpes, genital warts, genital thrush, giardiasis, gonorrhoea, hepatitis, granuloma inguinale, lymphogranuloma venereum, non-specific urethritis, scabies, syphilis, trichomoniasis, yaws.

Sezary syndrome a rare condition featuring a malignant spread of excessive numbers of abnormal T LYMPHOCYTES in the blood, with enlarged lymph nodes and deposits in the skin, liver and spleen. There are red, scaly patches on the skin extending to form a widespread, itchy and flaking rash, hair loss and distortion of the nails. The condition is thought to be caused by a retrovirus, HTLV-I. Treatment is with anticancer drugs and RADIOTHERAPY. (Albert Sezary, 1880–1956, French physician).

shaken baby syndrome the association in a small baby of unexplained fractures of long bones and blood clot under the main membrane surrounding the brain (subdural haematoma). These injuries, which are caused by whiplash and rotational movement of the head caused by violent shaking in the course of child abuse, may lead to irritability, convulsions, coma and death. Legal developments have led to the questioning of the evidential basis for the syndrome and it is now accepted that no single sign, such as subdural or retinal haemorrhage, or even a combination of such signs are, in themselves, sufficient to establish criminal activity.

shaking palsy PARKINSON'S DISEASE.

shame a distressing emotion involving a strong sense of having transgressed against a social or moral code. Shame is always relative to current mores or to the upbringing of the person concerned.

sharp any medical instrument with a sharp point or edge, especially an injection needle or a disposable scalpel, that, handled carelessly may inflict injury or dangerous infection on the user.

sheath 1 an enveloping structure or part, usually tubular.

2 a condom.

Sheehan's syndrome the effects of destruction of the front part of the PITUITARY GLAND by loss of its blood supply (infarction) following severe bleeding from the womb after delivery of a baby (postpartum haemorrhage). There is failure of milk production, loss of body hair, absence of menstruation, lethargy and other effects of underaction of the endocrine glands. (Professor Harold Leeming Sheehan, 1900–86, English physician).

shell shock see POST-TRAUMATIC STRESS DISORDER.

shiatsu ACUPRESSURE.

shigellosis a form of dysentery caused by *Shigella flexneri* or *Shigella sonnei* and acquired from food contaminated with the excreta of infected people or carriers. There is fever, nausea, abdominal pain, spasms of the rectum, and diarrhoea up to twenty or more times a day. The stools are streaked with mucus and blood. Small children often die of DEHYDRATION and fluid infusions may be needed. The antibiotic tetracycline is effective.

shin the front part of the leg below the knee and above the ankle. The surface of the TIBIA that lies close under the skin.

shinbone the TIBIA.

shingles herpes zoster. A disease caused by the reactivation of an earlier infection with chicken-pox (varicella-zoster) viruses which have lain dormant, often for years, in the sensory nerve ganglia near the spinal cord. On reactivation the viruses produce an acute inflammation of the ganglion and this causes pain and a typical rash of small blisters in the area supplied by the nerve. Most often this occurs in a strip on one side of the trunk, but shingles may also affect the face above and below one eye. If the eye is involved vision may be affected. Shingles is often followed by intractable pain that may last for years. The drug ACYCLOVIR (Zovirax), given early can minimize severity. From the Latin *cingulum*, a girdle.

shin splints a popular term for pain in the lower leg muscles and bones occurring in runners and football players and made worse by exertion. Causes include COMPARTMENT SYNDROME, muscle tear, MYOSITIS, PERIOSTITIS or tendon inflammation.

ship fever TYPHUS.

Shirodkar suture a circular stitch to control CERVICAL INCOMPETENCE.

shivering a rapid succession of contractions and relaxations of muscles and an important means of heat production in the body. The temperature rise in high fever is caused mainly by shivering.

SHO *abbrev. for* Senior House Officer.

SHMO *abbrev. for* Senior Hospital Medical Officer.

shock 1 a syndrome featuring low blood pressure, a prejudiced blood supply to important organs such as the brain and heart, and low kidney output. Causes of shock include severe blood loss, burns, severe infection, allergy, heart damage from CORONARY THROMBOSIS and head injury. Untreated shock may be rapidly fatal. The main element in treatment is the rapid restoration of the circulating blood volume by transfusion and the use of the drug VASOPRESSIN to help to maintain the blood pressure.
2 a temporary state of psychological overburdening from severe mental distress, often associate with stupefaction.

shock therapy see ELECTROCONVULSIVE THERAPY.

short bowel syndrome a disorder caused by the necessary surgical removal of a segment of intestine. It features weight loss, diarrhoea, fatty stools (steatorrhoea), and deficiencies of sodium, potassium and trace elements (hyponatremia, and hypokalemia). Affected people must eat several small meals a day, of readily-absorbed, finely chopped or ground foods supplemented by vitamins and minerals.

short-sightedness see MYOPIA.

shoulder-blade see SCAPULA.

shoulder-hand syndrome a condition of unknown cause featuring pain, stiffness and disability in the shoulder and the hand on one side. There is wasting of the muscles and the hand may become hot, sweaty and swollen. Spontaneous recovery is usual but this may take up to two years.

shunt any bypassing or sidetracking of flow, especially of fluid such as blood or cerebrospinal fluid. A shunt may be the result of disease or may be surgically induced, or inserted as a prosthesis, to effect treatment.

Shy-Drager syndrome a rare degenerative disorder of the autonomic nervous system affecting elderly people. Men are affected more often than women and the cause is unknown. The syndrome features dizziness on standing up (postural hypotension), Parkinsonism, incontinence of urine and impotence. There is no specific treatment. (George Milton Shy, 1919–67, American physician; and Glen A. Drager, 1917–67, American neurologist).

SI units SI is *abbrev. for* Systeme Internationale. SI units are now almost universally used in medicine. They include the metre for length, the kilogram for weight, the mole for amount of substance in a solution, the joule for energy and the pascal for pressure. These units are qualified by decimal multipliers or divisors such as mega- (a million), kilo- (a thousand), deci- (a tenth), centi- (a hundredth), milli- (a thousandth), micro- (a millionth), nano- (a thousand millionth), pico- (a million millionth), and femto- (a thousand million millionth). SI units were initially adopted by US doctors and then abandoned.

SIADH *abbrev. for* Syndrome of Inappropriate Antidiuretic Hormone. This is a condition in which excessive production of ADH (also known as vasopressin) by the PITUITARY GLAND results in water retention and low levels of sodium. The syndrome occurs in various serious diseases, especially cancer.

sial-, sialo- *combining form denoting* saliva or salivary gands.

sialadenitis inflammation of a salivary gland.

sialagogue anything that increases the flow of saliva.

sialogram an X-ray image of the duct of a salivary gland after injection of a radio-opaque liquid contrast medium. The process is known as sialography.

sialolithiasis stones (calculi) in the salivary glands or ducts.

Siamese twins identical (monozygous) twins that have failed fully to separate after the first division of the ovum and remain partially joined together at birth. The junction is usually along the trunk or between the two heads. From the male twins, Chang and Eng, born in Siam in 1811.

Siberian tick typhus a mild form of TYPHUS occurring in northern Asia, caused by *Rickettsia siberica* and transmitted by ticks of the *Dermacentor* and *Haemaphysalis* genera.

sib a SIBLING.

sibilant 1 hissing.

2 a speech sound, such as 's', 'sh' or 'z'.

3 a sibilant consonant.

sibling any member of a group of related brothers or sisters.

sibling rivalry strong competition or feelings of resentment between SIBLINGS, especially between an older child and a new baby. Sibling rivalry may persist throughout life.

sibutramine an antiobesity drug that acts on the nervous system in a manner similar to that of Prozac so that the patient is able to feel satisfied with smaller amounts of food. The drug is not recommended for people under 18 and is used for a maximum period of one year. It is prescribed mainly for those with a body mass index (BMI) of 30 or over. Brand name Reductil.

sicca syndrome dryness of the mouth and eyes from inadequate secretion of saliva and tears occurring in the absence of a connective tissue disorder. See also SJÖGREN'S SYNDROME.

sick building syndrome a varied group of symptoms sometimes experienced by people working in a modern office building and attributed to the building. Symptoms include fatigue, headache, dryness and itching of the eyes, sore throat and dryness of the nose. No convincing explanation has been offered.

sick headache a headache accompanied by nausea.

sickle cell anaemia an inherited blood disease mainly affecting black people and those of Mediterranean origin. The basic defect is in the HAEMOGLOBIN molecule of the red blood cells, which is abnormal (haemoglobin S) and deforms in conditions of low oxygen tension causing the red cells to become sickle-shaped (sickling) and to rupture readily. The HETEROZYGOUS form is comparatively mild; the HOMOZYGOUS form is severe and dangerous and an incidental illness can bring on a sickling crisis calling for prompt and energetic treatment.

sickling crisis an acute episode in homozygous sickle cell disease in which a massive breakdown of red blood cells occurs with widespread severe pain from blockage of small blood vessels by sickled red cells. Some cases involve great enlargement of the liver or spleen and gross anaemia, others may affect the lungs with severe breathlessness and pleuritic pain, or the brain causing a stroke. Skilled and energetic management in hospital is mandatory for the sickling crisis.

sickling test the observation of a blood film, mixed with a solution of sodium metabisulphite, under the microscope. If haemoglobin S is present the red cells will assume a sickle shape within 20 minutes. See also SICKLE CELL ANAEMIA.

sick sinus syndrome abnormal functioning of the natural pacemaker, the SINOATRIAL NODE of the heart. This causes episodes of slowing or speeding or even short periods of heart stoppage. An artificial pacemaker may be fitted.

Siddha medicine a system of medicine practised in Tamil areas of Southeast India and by Tamil-speaking people elsewhere. The system is based on humoral concepts of wind, bile and phlegm and on diagnosis by the analysis of the pulse and the appearance of the urine. The darker the urine, the more severe the disease. It includes yogic practices, faith in the miraculous alchemical properties of mercury and sulphur, and the prolongation of life through rejuvenating treatments especially the regulation of the breathing. It is believed that eternal youth is to be achieved by 21,600 respirations a day.

side effect any effect of a drug or other treatment additional to the required effect. Most side-effects are unwanted and some are dangerous.

sidero- *combining form denoting* iron.

sideroblast a developing red blood cell with free iron granules in its CYTOPLASM. This is normal. Iron granules in the MITOCHONDIA and forming a ring around the nucleus are characteristic of SIDEROBLASTIC ANAEMIA.

sideroblastic anaemia rare disorders which may be hereditary or acquired and which features disordered iron metabolism. Clinically, they resemble other anaemias but treatment with iron makes things worse. Transfusion with red cell concentrates may be necessary. Vitamin B$_6$ (pyridoxine) is sometimes effective.

siderofibrosis FIBROSIS caused by iron deposits in the body.

siderosis any condition in which there is an excessive accumulation of iron in the body.

siderosis bulbi the damaging eye condition that follows retention of an iron-containing intraocular foreign body. Iron in the eye leads to a spectrum of damage affecting the iris, lens, retina and optic nerve. Outlook for vision may be poor unless the foreign body is removed.

SIDS *abbrev. for* SUDDEN INFANT DEATH SYNDROME.

sievert the SI UNIT of equivalent absorbed dose of ionizing radiation. Compare RAD.

Sigmacort a brand name for HYDROCORTISONE.

sigmoid *or* **sigmoidal** 1 S-shaped.
2 pertaining to the SIGMOID COLON.

sigmoid colon the S-shaped lower end of the colon extending down from about the level of the brim of the pelvis to the RECTUM. Sigma is the Greek letter S.

sigmoiditis INFLAMMATION of the sigmoid part of the colon.

sigmoidoscopy a method of direct, visual examination of the inside of the rectum and lower colon using either a straight metal tube or a fibre optic ENDOSCOPE. In either event the instrument used is called a sigmoidoscope.

sign an objective indication of disease, perceptible by an external observer. Compare SYMPTOM.

signal transduction the common process by which the binding of a molecule to a receptor on a cell plasma membrane results in the transmission of a signal within the cell (second messenger) to trigger off a biochemical pathway in the cell.

sildenafil citrate an oral therapy for impotence in men. During sexual stimulation nitric oxide is released in the corpora cavernosa of the penis. Nitric oxide activates the enzyme guanylate cyclase, which leads indirectly to higher levels of cyclic guanosine monophosphate. This relaxes smooth muscle in the corpora cavernosa so that blood can flow in easily under arterial pressure. The monophosphate is, however, broken down by a phosphodiesterase enzyme (type 5) which limits its action. Sildenafil is a selective inhibitor of this type of enzyme resulting in prolonged action of cyclic guanosine monophosphate and a more substantial and better-sustained erection. The drug has its maximal effect about an hour after ingestion. It is said to have no effect in the absence of sexual stimulation. The drug potentiates the blood pressure-lowering effect of nitrates and should not be taken by patients using organic nitrates in any form. Other side effects include headache and transient blue-green colour perception defect. Men taking the drug should avoid grapefruit juice and should be aware of the other possible interactions. It should be avoided by those thought to be at risk of heart attacks. A brand name is Viagra.

silent mutation a change in DNA that has no effect.

silent site in a gene, one of the positions at which a mutation does not change the product.

silicone any polymeric (long-chain), organic compounds of silicon and oxygen in which each silicon atom is linked to an alkyl group. Silicones may be produced as oils, greases or rubbers. Silicone rubber (Silastic) is a valuable prosthetic surgical structural material as it is inert and permeable to oxygen and well tolerated by the tissues.

silicosis a persistent and damaging lung disease caused by long-term inhalation of silica-containing dusts. See also PNEUMOCONIOSIS.

Silkis a brand name for CALCITRIOL.

silver nitrate an astringent drug formerly used in solution to treat various conditions such as CONJUNCTIVITIS, OTITIS EXTERNA and cervical erosion. It causes black staining and is now seldom used in the Western world. The drug is on the WHO official list.

silver sulfadiazine a drug used to treat infected leg ulcers, burns, skin graft donor sites and pressure sores (bedsores). The drug is on the WHO official list. A brand name is Flamazine.

Simeco a brand name for a mixture of ALUMINIUM HYDROXIDE, MAGNESIUM HYDROXIDE and SIMETHICONE.

simethicone a silicone-based material with antifoaming properties used in the treatment of flatulence and often incorporated into antacid remedies.

Simmonds' disease underactivity of the pituitary gland with resultant inadequacy of hormone production by the other endocrine glands. There is lassitude, loss of body hair, loss of sexual interest, abnormally low blood pressure, MYXOEDEMA and intolerance to cold. Panhypopituitarism. Compare SHEEHAN'S SYNDROME. (Morris Simmonds, 1855–1925,

Danish-born German pathologist).

simvastatin a statin drug used to treat raised blood cholesterol levels. A very large seven-year trial of the drug suggested that it reduces the chances of a heart attack or a stroke by one third. A brand name is Zocor. See STATINS for an account of the drug's action.

Sindbis fever an African togavirus infection spread by mosquitoes, and similar to O'NYONG-NYONG FEVER.

Sinemet a brand name for LEVODOPA in combination with carbidopa.

Sinequan a brand name for the tranquillizing drug DOXEPIN.

sinew a popular term for a TENDON.

singer's nodes small, polyp-like swellings or nodules on the vocal chords resulting from overuse of the voice in an unnatural manner. Singer's nodes cause hoarseness and loss of phonation and must be removed surgically. Vocal training can prevent recurrence.

single strand binding proteins proteins that keep single strands of DNA apart during replication. They do so by attaching to the separated strands at the point of separation (the replication fork) so as to seal them off from each other and prevent immediate re-linking.

Singulair a brand name for MONTELUKAST.

singultus see HICCUP.

sinoatrial node a small area of specialized muscle cells in the upper right chamber of the heart (right atrium) that acts as the natural pacemaker of the heart, setting the rate, in conjunction with other controlling influences, and transmitting impulses throughout the heart muscle.

Sinthrome a brand name for NICOUMALONE (acenocoumarol).

sinus 1 one of the paired mucous membrane-lined air cavities in a bone, specifically the frontal sinuses in the forehead, the maxillary sinuses (antrums) in the cheek bones, the multicelled ethmoidal sinuses on either side of the upper part of the nose and the sphenoidal sinuses in the base of the skull. **2** any wide blood channel such as the venous sinuses in the MENINGES. **3** any tract or FISTULA leading from a deep infected area to a surface.

sinus bradycardia a slow, regular, heart rate resulting from a low rate of pacing by the SINOATRIAL NODE. The heart rate is less than 60 beats per minute. Sinus bradycardia is a normal, healthy feature of high physical fitness but may also occur in conditions such as HYPOTHYROIDISM in which the metabolic rate is reduced. It may also be caused by beta-blockers and other drugs.

sinusitis inflammation of the mucous membrane linings of one or more bone cavities (SINUSES) of the face. This almost always results from infection. There is a feeling of fullness or pain in the forehead, cheeks or between the eyes, fever and general upset. Treatment may involve surgical drainage and antibiotics.

sinus tachycardia a fast regular, heart rate caused by a high rate of pacing by the SINOATRIAL NODE. This is a normal feature of exertion and may be caused by anxiety, fever, HYPERTHYROIDISM and other disorders.

situs inversus an uncommon mirror-image reversal of the organs of the trunk. The heart points to the right, the LIVER and APPENDIX are on the left and the stomach and spleen on the right. Situs inversus is seldom of medical significance, but may confuse diagnosis until detected. See also DEXTROCARDIA.

SIV *abbrev. for* simian immunodeficiency virus. This is an organism, similar to HIV, that affects monkeys.

Sjögren's syndrome an immunological disorder causing reduced secretion of many body glands as a result of damage by antibodies to body tissues (autoantibodies). This causes severe dryness of the eyes, mouth and vagina. The syndrome is commonly associated with other immunological disorders, such as RHEUMATOID ARTHRITIS, SYSTEMIC LUPUS ERYTHEMATOSUS and MYASTHENIA GRAVIS. There is no specific treatment but relief can be obtained from artificial tears, moistening mouth sprays and vaginal lubricants. (Henrik Samuel Conrad Sjögren, b. 1899, Swedish ophthalmologist).

skatole 3-methylindole, the substance in faeces that confers the smell. It is a breakdown product of bile and can be prepared by the action of potassium hydroxide on egg albumin. It attracts dung flies but, for evolutionary reasons connected with the bacterial content of faeces, repels humans. See also INDOLE.

skeletal pertaining to the SKELETON.

skeleton the framework of usually 206 articulated bones that give the body its general shape, and provides support and attachments for the muscles. The skeleton also provides varying degrees of protection for the internal organs (see Fig. 1).

Skelid a brand name for TILUDRONIC ACID.

skewed of data that are not normally distributed. See PARAMETRIC.

skia- *combining form denoting* a shadow.

skiascope a RETINOSCOPE.

skiascopy RETINOSCOPY.

skin the body's outer covering. The skin is a major organ, of area 5–6 m². It is self-regenerating, self-lubricating and self-repairing and provides heat regulation. It is sensitive to touch, pressure, pain and temperature. It protects against solar radiation and bacterial infection and synthesizes vitamin D. The lower layer, the true skin (corium) is living, the outer layer (epidermis) has an external layer of dead, flattened horny cells.

skin ache syndrome a persistent and debilitating disorder of unknown cause in which pain is brought on by pressing on or pinching certain small areas of the skin. The most common sites appear to be the knee, over the shoulder blade and the abdominal wall skin. The pain is abolished by the injection of a local anaesthetic under the 'trigger' point and this is often permanently curative.

skin allergy see ATOPIC ECZEMA, DERMATITIS and URTICARIA.

skin biopsy a portion of diseased skin removed for laboratory analysis, usually under local anaesthesia.

skin cancer one of various malignant conditions of the skin such as MALIGNANT MELANOMA, BASAL CELL CARCINOMA, SQUAMOUS CELL CARCINOMA, PAGET'S DISEASE OF THE NIPPLE, MYCOSIS FUNGOIDES and KAPOSI'S SARCOMA.

skin disorders see ACNE, BASAL CELL CARCINOMA, BOILS, CARBUNCLES, CELLULITIS, COLD SORES, CUTANEOUS HORNS, DERMATITIS, ECZEMA, EPIDERMOPHYTOSIS, HAEMANGIOMA, IMPETIGO, KERATOACANTHOMA, KERATOSIS, MALIGNANT MELANOMA, NAEVUS, NAPPY RASH, PRICKLY HEAT, PSORIASIS, PURPURA, PUSTULES, ROSACEA, SCABIES, SCAR, SEBACEOUS CYST, SHINGLES, SQUAMOUS CELL CARCINOMA, TINEA, VITILIGO, WARTS and XANTHELASMA.

skin flap a surgically delineated area of full-thickness skin, attached at a broad base and moved to an adjacent position to cover a bare area or make good a deficit in tissue.

skinfold thickness measurement a method of assessing the amount of fat under the skin by means of special calipers, sprung to exert a standard pressure and fitted with a scale. Skinfold thickness measurements may more accurately assess obesity than weighing.

skin graft the transference of an area of skin from one part of the body to another. A plastic surgical technique used to repair areas of deficient skin. Skin grafts may be split-skin or full-thickness or may have attached blood vessels that are rejoined by microsurgery to vessels at the new location.

Skinoren a brand name for AZELAIC ACID.

skin peel a cosmetic procedure to improve the appearance of the facial skin by removing small wrinkles, scars, freckles and other blemishes. A paste containing carbolic acid is used.

skin tests investigations to determine allergic sensitivity to various substances by injecting small quantities into or under the skin or by applying the substance under patches (patch tests).

skin tumours see SKIN DISORDERS.

skull the bony skeleton of the head and the protective covering for the brain. The part of the skull that encloses the brain is called the cranium.

SLE *abbrev. for* SYSTEMIC LUPUS ERYTHEMATOSUS.

sleep the natural, regular, daily state of reduced consciousness and METABOLISM that occupies about one-third of the average person's life. Sleep requirements vary considerably in health, between about 4 and 10 hours in each 24 hour period. The purpose of sleep is unknown but prolonged deprivation is harmful, causing depression and mental disturbances, including hallucinations.

sleep apnoea repetitive periods without breathing, occurring during sleep and lasting for 10 seconds or longer. Most cases are due to over-relaxation of the muscles of the soft palate, in heavy snorers, which sag and obstruct the airway. Obesity is a common factor. Less commonly, the condition is due to disturbance of the brain mechanisms that maintain respiration.

sleeping drugs a group of drugs used to promote sleep. The group includes many BENZODIAZEPINE drugs, some ANTIHISTAMINE drugs, antidepressant drugs and chloral hydrate. The BARBITURATE drugs, once widely used for this purpose, have fallen into disrepute.

sleep paralysis a feeling, experienced for a few seconds when falling asleep, of being unable to move. This is a feature of NARCOLEPSY but may affect healthy people.

sleeping sickness 1 ENCEPHALITIS LETHARGICA. 2 TRYPANOSOMIASIS.

sleep terror a childhood phenomenon featuring sudden screaming, an appearance of severe agitation, apparent inability to recognize faces or surroundings, return to sleep and no subsequent memory of the event. Sleep terror appears to be harmless and ceases in adolescence. Also known as night terror.

sleepwalking a state of dissociated sleeping and waking common in children, especially boys, and lasting usually for only a few minutes, in which the child gets out of bed and moves about. Sleepwalking in childhood is never purposeful and is of little importance so long as danger from falls is avoided. The child should be guided gently back to bed. Sleepwalking in adults usually has a hysterical basis.

sling a support, usually of folded cloth, to immobilize and rest the arm. Slings are used either as a first-aid measure or to place the arm in an appropriate position for the healing of a fractured collar bone (CLAVICLE). A sling may also be used to rest an arm which has sustained soft tissue injury or which is severely infected.

slipped disc see PROLAPSED INTERVERTEBRAL DISC.

slipped epiphysis separation at the junction between the shaft of a long bone and the growing sector at the end (the EPIPHYSIS). This usually results from a fall or applied force. An undisplaced epiphysis heals rapidly without ill effect, but, otherwise, careful REDUCTION is necessary to avoid disturbance of growth.

slit-lamp a low-power, binocular microscope with an intense light source, used to examine the internal structures of the front part of the eye and, by means of special eye contact lenses, the VITREOUS BODY and the RETINA.

Slo-phyllin a brand name for THEOPHYLLINE.

slough 1 dead tissue cast off or separated from its original site. 2 the casting off of dead tissue.

Slow-Fe Folic a brand name for FERROUS SULPHATE in conjunction with FOLIC ACID.

Slow-K a brand name for a POTASSIUM preparation.

Slow-Trasicor a brand name for OXPRENOLOL.

slow viruses a loose term applied to the presumptive causal agents of some nervous system diseases with an INCUBATION PERIOD measured in years. These were formerly thought to include CREUTZFELDT-JAKOB DISEASE, KURU, possibly a form of ALZHEIMER'S DISEASE and, in animals, SCRAPIE and bovine SPONGIFORM ENCEPHALOPATHY, but these conditions are now known to be caused by PRIONS rather than by viruses. Because of its long incubation period, AIDS is more appropriately designated a slow virus disease.

Slozem a brand name for DILTIAZEM.

Smad a family of eight proteins that participate in tumour suppression in conjunction with transforming growth factor-beta (TGF-). Smad 1,2,3,5 and 8 are receptor-activated; Smad 4 is a co-mediator; and Smad 6 and 7 are inhibitory. The absence of Smad 3 is a feature of acute T cell lymphoblastic LEUKAEMIA. The term is derived from the proteins' homology to *Caenorhabditis elegans* Sma and drosophila MAD proteins.

small cell carcinoma see OAT CELL CARCINOMA.

small bowel see SMALL INTESTINE.

small intestine the longest, but narrowest part of the intestine. The part in which digestion and absorption of food is performed. The small intestine extends from the outlet of the stomach (the PYLORUS) to the CAECUM at the start of the large intestine (COLON), and consists of the DUODENUM, the JEJUNUM and the ILEUM.

smallpox a severe, highly infectious virus disease with the unique distinction of having been eradicated. Smallpox was spread mainly by droplet infection and caused fever, headache, muscle aches and a severe blistering rash that left deep pitted scars. The mortality was sometimes as high as 20%. The destruction of the last samples of the virus was finally approved in 1994. Of nearly half a million American service personnel vaccinated against smallpox between December 2002 and May 2003 there was one case of encephalitis and 37 cases of myopericarditis. An American plan to vaccinate half a million health care workers against smallpox in 2003 was a failure when fewer than 40,000 accepted vaccination. The plan was prompted by fears of bioterrorism.

small round viruses a heterogeneous group of poorly-characterized small viruses of about 25–35 mn in diameter. They are divided into small round structured viruses (SRSV) and small round non-structured viruses. They include the Norwalk agent and are known to be responsible for many cases of food poisoning and gastroenteritis.

smear a thin film of tissue, cells, blood or other material spread on a transparent slide for microscopic examination.

smegma accumulated, cheesy-white, sebaceous gland secretions occurring under the foreskin of an uncircumcised male with poor standards of personal hygiene. Smegma becomes infected, foul-smelling and irritating and can cause local inflammation. It has been said to be CARCINOGENIC to sexual consorts but this has not been proved. Associated papillomaviruses may be the cause.

smell one of the five senses. Smell is mediated by airborne chemical particles that dissolve in the layer of mucus on the upper part of the nose lining and stimulate the endings of the olfactory nerve twigs. The olfactory system is capable of distinguishing a large number of distinct odours.

Smith-Petersen nail a three-flanged stainless steel nail used to secure fractures of the neck of the thigh bone (FEMUR). The nail is hammered into the outer side of the bone so that it passes through the neck with the tip lying in the spherical head. Early mobilization of the patient is then possible. (Marius Smith-Petersen, 1886–1953, Norwegian-born American surgeon).

SMO *abbrev. for* Senior Medical Officer.

smooth muscle the unstriped involuntary muscle occurring in the walls of blood vessels, the intestines and the bladder, and controlled by the AUTONOMIC NERVOUS SYSTEM and by HORMONES.

snake oil a general informal term for a fraudulent PANACEA.

SNAP *abbrev.* for SCORE FOR NEONATAL ACUTE PHYSIOLOGY.

sneezing a protective reflex initiated by irritation of the nose lining and resulting in a blast of air through the nose and mouth that may remove the cause. The vocal cords are tighly approximated, air in the chest is compressed and the cords suddenly separated.

Snellen's chart test a standard vision-testing chart of letters of diminishing size, used at the standard distance of 6 m. The eyes are tested one at a time and the result recorded in terms of the lowest line that can be correctly read. (Hermann Snellen, 1834–1908, Dutch ophthalmologist).

Sno Phenicol a brand name for CHLORAMPHENICOL antibiotic eye drops.

snoring a noise caused by vibration of the soft palate and other soft tissue in the upper airway by turbulent air flow. Snoring occurs during sleep usually when the mouth is open and is thus commonest when the snorer is lying on the back or when the nose is blocked. Snoring is never heard by the person causing the sound. Snoring may be treated by oral appliances to advance the mandible, by surgical palatoplasty or by hypnotherapy.

snow blindness the popular term for actinic keratopathy – damage to the outer layer of the corneas (the EPITHELIUM) from the effects of prolonged exposure to solar ultraviolet light. There is a temporary inability to keep the eyes open because the corneal nerves are painfully stimulated by the moving lids and there is tearing and BLEPHAROSPASM. If the eyes are kept shut the corneal epithelium regenerates in a day or two.

social anxiety disorder social phobia, a phobic disorder featuring disabling and distressing embarrassment, anxiety and humiliation experienced in social contexts, especially in public. The condition is commoner than was formerly supposed and the true prevalence has been masked by under-diagnosis because of the shame and reticence of the sufferers. Currently, the most effective treatment involves cognitive behaviour therapy supplemented by the use of selective serotonin reuptake inhibitor drugs such as paroxetine (Seroxat), sertraline (Lustral) or fluvoxamine (Faverin).

sociopathy an earlier term for what is now called ANTISOCIAL PERSONALITY DISORDER.

Sodium Amytal a brand name for AMYLOBARBITONE (amobarbital).

sodium aurothiomalate a gold preparation given by injection for the treatment of RHEUMATOID ARTHRITIS. A brand name is Myocrisin.

sodium bicarbonate baking soda. An antacid drug used to relieve indigestion, heartburn and the pain of peptic ulcer. Sodium bicarbonate is not a preferred antacid as it leads to the production of carbon dioxide and 'rebound' acid production.

sodium calcium edetate a CHELATING AGENT used to treat poisoning with lead and other heavy metals. The drug is on the WHO official list. A brand name is Ledclair.

sodium chloride common salt. A compound ubiquitous in the body. Used in the preparation of SALINE. The drug is on the WHO official list.

sodium clodronate a drug that prevents bone loss by interfering with the cells (osteoclasts) that break down bone. Brand names are Bonefos and Loron.

sodium cromoglycate sodium cromoglicate, a drug used to treat hay fever (ALLERGIC RHINITIS), allergic CONJUNCTIVITIS, food allergy and allergic ASTHMA. Cromoglycate stabilizes the MAST CELL membrane and prevents the release of HISTAMINE. Brand names are Cromogen, Hay-Crom, Intal, Intal Syncroner, Nalcrom, Opticrom, Pliva Pharma Hayfever Eye Drops, and Vivicrom.

sodium fluoride a fluoride supplement drug used to strengthen children's developing teeth in regions of low water fluoride content. Fluoride supplements are contraindicated when the water fluoride content exceeds 0.7 parts per million. The drug is on the WHO official list. Brand names are Endekay, Fuoregard and Fluor-a-day.

sodium fusidate an antibacterial drug used both generally and for local application. A brand name is Fucidin.

sodium hyaluronate a viscous, gel-like material used in ophthalmic surgery to protect the important inner lining of the cornea and maintain the front chamber of the opened eye. The drug is also used OSTEOARTHRITIS as a replacement for synovial fluid and to treat some forms of cystitis. Brand names are Cystistat, Ophthalin, Orthovisc, Supartz and Suplasyn.

sodium hydrogen carbonate sodium bicarbonate, baking soda, a drug used in solution to correct metabolic and respiratory acidosis. The drug has also been used to neutralize gastric acidity and to alkalinize the urine. Used as an antacid it produces carbon dioxide. The drug is on the WHO official list.

sodium lactate, compound solution a solution given by intraveous infusion to correct electrolyte imbalance. The drug is on the WHO official list.

sodium nitrite a drug used in the treatment of cyanide poisoning in conjunction with SODIUM THIOSULPHATE. The drug is on the WHO official list.

sodium nitroprusside a drug used to treat a dangerous rise in the blood pressure (hypertensive crisis), to produce controlled hypotension during anaesthesia, and to treat heart acute or chronic heart failure. The drug is on the WHO official list.

sodium pentothal a rapid-acting BARBITURATE drug used for the induction of general anaesthesia.

sodium perborate an antiseptic drug used as a mouthwash. A brand name is Bocasan.

sodium picosulphate sodium picosulfate, a stimulant laxative drug used to treat constipation. A brand name is Laxoberal.

sodium salicylate an ANALGESIC drug used to treat RHEUMATIC FEVER. It has no advantages over aspirin (acetyl salicylic acid) and the same adverse effects.

sodium tetradecyl sulphate a sclerosing substance that can be injected into segments of emptied varicose veins so as to close them off and relieve symptoms. A brand name is Fibro-vein.

sodium thiosulphate a drug used to treat cyanide poisoning in conjunction with sodium nitrite. Sodium nitrite produces methaemo-globinaemia and the cyanide ions convert methaemoglobin to cyanmethaemoglobin. As this slowly dissociates, the thiosulphate converts it to non-toxic thiocyanate which is excreted in the urine. The drug is on the WHO official list.

sodium valproate an anticonvulsant drug used to treat EPILEPSY. A brand name is Epilim.

sodomy 1 anal copulation with a male.
2 anal or oral copulation with a woman.
3 copulation with an animal. Also known as buggery.

Sofradex a brand name for eye or ear drops or ointment containing DEXAMETHASONE, FRAMYCETIN and GRAMICIDIN.

Soframycin a brand name for the antibiotic drug FRAMYCETIN.

soft palate the mobile flap of muscle covered with mucous membrane that is attached to the rear edge of the hard palate. The soft palate seals off the cavity of the nose from the mouth during swallowing.

soft-tissue injury damage to skin, muscle, ligament or tendon.

soiling inappropriate discharge of faeces after the age of about 3 or 4. Soiling is usually accidental. Compare ENCOPRESIS.

solar pertaining to the sun or to the SOLAR PLEXUS.

solar dermatitis any skin disorder caused by exposure to the sun, other than sunburn. Some forms of solar dermatitis are precancerous.

solar plexus a large network of autonomic nerves situated behind the stomach, around the coeliac artery. It incorporates branches of the VAGUS NERVE and the splanchnic nerves and sends branches to most of the abdominal organs. Also known as the coeliac plexus. The term derives from the sun-like appearance of the radiating branches.

Solcode a brand name for a mixture of ASPIRIN and CODEINE.

Solian a brand name for AMISULPRIDE.

Solone a brand name for PREDNISOLONE.

Solprin a brand name for ASPIRIN.

Solu-Cortef a brand name for HYDROCORTISONE.

Solu-Medrone a brand name for METHYLPREDNISOLONE.

Solvazinc a brand name for ZINC SULPHATE.

solvent abuse deliberate inhalation of vapour from various organic solvents for the sake of their intoxicant effect. The effects include loss of full awareness, incoordination, hallucinations and unconsciousness. Many deaths have occurred from asphyxiation and brain, liver and kidney damage are common. Also known as glue sniffing.

somat-, somato- *combining form denoting* the body.

somatic 1 pertaining to the body (soma), as opposed to the mind (psyche).
2 pertaining to general body cells that divide by MITOSIS, as distinct from ova and spermatozoa that are formed by MEIOSIS. All the body cells except those in the ovaries and testes that produce ova and spermatozoa.

somatic gene therapy genetic treatment that affects only the SOMATIC cells and thus is limited in its effect to the individual treated. The alternative form – genetic treatment affecting

the germ cells in the ovaries or testicles – may be perpetuated through succeeding generations. For this reason it is currently prohibited.

somatic mutation a mutation affecting SOMATIC cells that can affect only those cells and their offspring, so cannot be passed on to future generations. Such a mutation dies with the death of the individual.

somatization disorder the current term for HYSTERIA, adopted as a euphemism.

somatopsychic psychosomatic. Pertaining to both body and mind.

somatorelin a drug used to check the growth hormone function of the pituitary gland and help in the diagnosis of growth hormone deficiency. A brand name is GHRH Ferring.

somatostatins tetradecapeptides widely distributed in the body, that inhibits the secretion of many HORMONES and NEUROTRANSMITTERS. Somatostatins are secreted in the hypothalamus, elsewhere in the brain, the gastrointestinal tract, pancreas, retina, spinal cord and various endocrine glands. They have been suggested as antidotes to growth hormone in conditions such as ACROMEGALY but have a very short duration of action and results in rebound over-secretion. The drug octreotide (Sandostatin) is a somatostatin analogue.

somatotropin growth hormone produced by RECOMBINANT DNA techniques (genetic engineering) and used to treat growth defects. Brand names are Genotropin, Humatrope, Norditropin, Saizen and Zomacton.

somatotype the physical build of a person. A body type, claimed by some, with little evidence, to have a reliable correlation with personality. See also ECTOMORPH, ENDOMORPH, MESOMORPH.

somatrem a preparation of human growth hormone used to treat short stature caused by growth hormone deficiency.

Somavert brand name for PEGVISOMANT.

-some *suffix denoting* body, as in chromosome.

Sominex a brand name for the antihistamine drug PROMETHAZINE used as a sedative.

somn-, somni- *prefix denoting* sleep.

somnambulism see SLEEPWALKING.

Somophyllin a brand name for THEOPHYLLINE.

Sone a brand name for PREDNISONE.

Soneryl a brand name for the barbiturate drug BUTOBARBITONE (butobarbital).

Sonne dysentery bacillary DYSENTERY caused by the organism *Shigella sonnei*. (Carl Olaf Sonne, 1882–1948, Danish bacteriologist).

soporific 1 tending to induce sleep.
2 a sleep-inducing drug.

sorbitol a sweetening agent derived from glucose.

Sorbitrate a brand name for ISOSORBIDE DINITRATE.

sore any local breakdown of a body surface (ULCER) or septic wound.

sore throat see PHARYNGITIS and TONSILLITIS.

sorption the general term for the passive movement of liquid molecules, as by adsorption, absorption or persorption.

Sotacor a brand name for SOTALOL.

sotalol a long-acting beta-blocker drug used to treat irregularity of the heart action. Brand names are Beta-Cardone and Sotacor.

Southern blotting a method of identifying a fragment of DNA containing a specific sequence of bases. A mixture of fragments, produced by cutting DNA with restriction enzymes, is separated on a gel block by ELECTROPHORESIS. The fragments are denatured to single strand DNA and transferred, by blotting, to a nitrocellulose sheet. The position of the desired fragment can then be shown by hybridizing it with a DNA probe labelled with radioactive phosphorous that will cause a black line on an X-ray film. The method was named after its developer Edward M. Southern. A similar technique for RNA analysis has been humorously called 'Northern blotting' and the play on words has been extended to include 'WESTERN BLOTTING'.

space medicine the medical specialty concerned with the physical and mental effects of space flight. Space medicine is often practised by specialists in aviation medicine.

space sickness 1 the nausea that people can experience in the low-gravity environment of space.
2 the damage to health from exposure to prolonged low-gravity situations (such as osteoporosis and muscle weakness) or from radiation.

Spanish fly dried extract of the blister beetle, *Lytta vesicatoria*. Cantharides. This is a highly irritant and poisonous substance with an unjustified reputation as an APHRODISIAC.

Sparine a brand name for the phenothiazine antipsychotic drug PROMAZINE.

spasm involuntary strong contraction of a muscle or muscle group. Spasms may be brief or sustained (cramps) and may result from minor muscle disorders, disease of the nervous system or habit (TICS).

Spasmonal a brand name for ALVERINE CITRATE.

spastic pertaining to spasms.

spasticity rigidity in muscles causing stiffness and restriction of movement. Spasticity may or may not be associated with paralysis or muscle weakness. Spasticity with paralysis is a feature of many cases of STROKE. It occurs in SPASTIC PALAYSIS (cerebral palsy) and sometimes in MULTIPLE SCLEROSIS.

spastic colon see IRRITABLE BOWEL SYNDROME.

spastic diplegia SPASTIC PARALYSIS affecting both sides of the body equally, but usually affecting the legs more than the arms.

spastic ileus temporary obstruction of the intestine as a result of closure of a segment due to spasm of the muscles in the wall.

spastic paralysis a non-progressive loss of function of the MOTOR part of the brain, present at birth or soon after and not associated with any readily visible brain abnormality. The effects vary from the most minor disability from SPASTICITY to complete inability to walk and severe mental retardation. Also known as CEREBRAL PALSY.

spastic paraplegia paralysis of both lower limbs with muscle spasm. This may be due to diseases of the brain or spinal cord, spinal nerve roots or peripheral nerves. The condition may be hereditary.

spatula a small broad, flat, blunt instrument of wood or plastic used to press down the tongue while examining the throat or to scrape the lining of the CERVIX of the womb in a PAP SMEAR test.

spatulate shaped like a SPATULA.

speaking in tongues see GLOSSOLALIA.

specialist 1 a person devoted to a particular branch of study or practice.
2 a doctor qualified to practise in a restricted area of medicine or surgery.

specialist registrar a hospital doctor senior to a HOUSE OFFICER but junior to a consultant.

SPECT *acronym for* Single Photon Emission Computed Tomography, a type of radionuclide scanning.

spectacles pairs of simple thin lenses, usually mounted in frames and used for the correction of short sight (MYOPIA), long sight (HYPERMETROPIA), ASTIGMATISM and PRESBYOPIA.

spectinomycin an aminocyclitol antibiotic used by intramuscular injection to treat GONORRHOEA. The drug is on the WHO official list. Users should avoid Botox treatments.

specular pertaining to a mirror, as in specular reflection.

speculum an instrument of varying design used to hold open or widen a body orifice such as the ear canal, a nostril, the eyelids, the anus or the vagina so as to allow examination.

speech therapy treatment designed to help people with a communication difficulty arising from a disturbance of language, a disorder of articulation, difficulty in voice production or defective fluency of speech.

speedball a slang term for a dose of cocaine and heroin taken intravenously.

speed freak a slang term for a habitual AMPHETAMINE (amfetamine) user.

Spencer Wells artery forceps a self-retaining, scissors-like forceps fitted with a ratchet, and used to clamp bleeding arteries until they can conveniently be tied off with catgut ligatures. A haemostat. (Sir Thomas Spencer Wells, 1818–97, English ophthalmic and gynaecological surgeon).

spermat-, spermato- *combining form denoting* spermatozoa or semen.

spermatic pertaining to SPERM.

spermatic cord a cord-like structure consisting of the VAS DEFERENS surrounded by a dense plexus of veins and other blood vessels, lymphatic vessels and nerves. The spermatic cord runs upwards from the back of the testicle through the INGUINAL CANAL into the abdominal cavity where the vas leaves it to run into the PROSTATE GLAND.

spermatic fluid SEMINAL FLUID.

spermatids cells formed in the testicle, having half the normal number of chromosomes (haploid), that develop into a SPERMATOZOA without further division.

spermatocide see SPERMICIDE.

spermatocoele a cyst of the EPIDIDYMIS that contains fluid and SPERMATOZOA. Spermatocoeles are harmless unless large, when they can be removed surgically.

spermatocyte a cell of the seminiferous tubules of the testis that is converted by MEIOSIS into four SPERMATIDS.

spermatorrhoea involuntary discharge of semen without orgasm.

spermatozoa microscopic cells about 0.05 mm long occurring in millions in seminal fluid. Spermatozoa are male GAMETES, carrying all the genetic contribution from the father and bearing either an X chromosome to produce a daughter, or a Y chromosome to produce a son.

spermaturia SPERMATOZOA in the urine.

sperm count a method of determining the concentration of SPERMATOZOA in a semen sample of known dilution. Counts are done on a slide engraved with squares of known size, using a microscope. Fertility is unlikely if the count is below 20,000,000 per ml.

sperm donation seminal fluid provided by a donor for the purposes of fertilization of women whose husbands or partners are sterile. Seminal fluid can be preserved indefinitely frozen in a glycerol cryoprotectant in phials, or plastic straws and kept in liquid nitrogen sperm banks.

spermicides contraceptive preparations designed to kill SPERMATOZOA. In general, spermicides used alone are unreliable as contraceptives.

sperm injection IVF a method of in vitro fertilization in which an ovum is held steady by a suction device while a single sperm is injected directly into it through a very fine needle. The method, which was adopted to ensure fertilization in cases in which the father's sperm count is too low, has been criticized on the grounds that it may increase the likelihood of birth defects. It is suggested that it interferes with the natural selection process in which only the fittest sperms are able to penetrate the egg.

sphenoid wedge-shaped, or cuneiform. From Greek *sphenoidis*, a wedge.

sphenoid bone the wedge-shaped, bat-like central bone of the base of the skull.

spherocytosis a blood disorder in which the red cells are unusually small and spherical. In hereditary spherocytosis the red cells are fragile and burst easily, causing ANAEMIA.

sphincter a muscle ring, or local thickening of the muscle coat, surrounding a tubular passage or opening in the body. When a sphincter contracts it narrows or closes off the passageway.

sphincterotomy surgical cutting or weakening of a SPHINCTER.

sphingolipidoses a group of hereditary metabolic disorders featuring local accumulations of fatty material (glycolipids and phospholipids) in various parts of the body. These cannot be broken down further because of the absence of the necessary ENZYMES. The sphingolipidoses feature progressive degeneration of the retinal gangion cells with progressive loss of vision. See also NIEMANN-PICK DISEASE.

sphygmomanometer a mercury manometer or aneroid instrument used to measure blood pressure. See KOROTKOFF SOUNDS.

spider naevus a common, tiny skin blemish consisting of a small, central, slightly raised, bright red area from which fine red lines, like spider legs, radiate. Numerous spider naevi occur in serious liver disease, such as cirrhosis and sometimes in pregnant women or those receiving hormone replacement therapy.

spider fingers see ARACHNODACTYLY.

spin-, spino- *combining form denoting* spine, spinal or spinal cord.

spina bifida a developmental defect in the neural tube of the embryo leading to loss of the rear part of one or more of the vertebrae of the spine so that the neural tissue and the covering MENINGES can protrude to a varying degree. In spina bifida occulta there is no external protrusion and the effects are minimal. In more severe cases, the meninges bulge through the opening to form a cyst-like swelling (a MENINGOCOELE) in the lower back. In the worst cases the spinal cord is exposed (MYELOCELE) and there may be total paralysis of the lower part of the body and incontinence. Various neurological complications may occur. Spina bifida and other neural tube defects can nearly always be prevented by an adequate intake of folic acid prior to, and in the early weeks of, conception. All women liable to become pregnant should be aware of this. Recommendations are 5 mg a day for women who have previously had a baby with a neural tube defect or who have a family history of neural tube defect, and 0.5 mg a day for low risk women.

spinal anaesthesia a major form of local anaesthesia, performed by injecting an anaesthetic drug between two of the vertebrae of the lower back into the CEREBROSPINAL FLUID. This blocks nerve transmission in the adjacent spinal nerves.

spinal canal the tube-like space running the length of the VERTEBRAL COLUMN formed by the arches of the successive vertebrae through which the SPINAL CORD and its membranes pass.

spinal column see VERTEBRAL COLUMN.

spinal cord the downward continuation of the BRAINSTEM that lies within a canal in the spine (VERTEBRAL COLUMN). The cord is a cylinder of nerve tissue about 45 cm long containing bundles of nerve fibre tracts running up and down, to and from the brain. These tracts form SYNAPSES with the 62 spinal nerves that emerge in pairs from either side of the cord, between adjacent vertebrae, and carry nerve impulses to and from all parts of the trunk and the limbs.

spinal decompression an operation to relieve pressure on the spinal cord or on the nerve roots emerging from it. The commonest indication is a PROLAPSED INTERVERTEBRAL DISC.

spinal fusion a surgical procedure to effect permanent healing between the bodies of two or more adjacent VERTEBRAE. This is done to avoid dangerous movement between vertebrae arising from bone disease of various kinds.

spinal nerves the 31 pairs of combined MOTOR and sensory nerves that are connected to the spinal cord.

spinal tap see LUMBAR PUNCTURE.

spine see VERTEBRAL COLUMN.

spinothalamic tracts the nerve bundles running up the spinal cord carrying sensory impulses to the great sensory nucleus of the basal ganglia – the THALAMUS.

spinous process the rearward projection of a vertebra.

spiral computed tomography a development of CT scanning that is rapid, allows scanning of a large body volume on a single breath-hold, and provides high-quality two- and three-dimensional images. The X-ray tube rotates around the patient in a spiral, taking less than a second to complete one rotatation. Up top 60 rotations are possible. A special surface-shading display reveals astonishing detail, especially of bones.

Spiriva a brand name for TIOTROPIUM BROMIDE.

spirochaetaemia SPIROCHAETES in the blood.

spirochaete a class of fine, spiral, highly motile bacteria. The three medically most important genera are the *Treponema* which includes the causal agent of syphilis *T. pallidum*; the *Leptospira*, which includes *L. icterohaemorrhagiae*, the cause of leptospirosis; and the *Borrelia*, which include the cause of relapsing fever, *B. recurrentis*, and of Lyme disease, *B. burgdorferi*.

Spiroctan a brand name for SPIRONOLACTONE.

spirometry a lung function test used to determine the efficiency with which air passes from the atmosphere to the ALVEOLI of the lungs and carbon dioxide passes out. Spirometry can also be used to assess the maximum volume of air that can be made to pass in and out of the lungs (the vital capacity).

spironolactone a DIURETIC drug that does not lead to loss of potassium from the body. It is an antagonist of the hormone aldosterone. The drug is on the WHO official list. Brand names are Aldactone and Spiroctan.

splanchnic pertaining to the internal organs (viscera).

spleen a solid, dark purplish organ, lying high on the left side of the abdomen between the stomach and the left kidney. The spleen is the largest collection of lymph tissue in the body and contains a mass of pulpy material consisting mainly of LYMPHOCYTES, PHAGOCYTES and red blood cells. The spleen is the main blood filter, removing the products of breakdown of red blood cells and other foreign and unwanted semisolid material. It is a source of lymphocytes and a major site of antibody formation.

splenectomy surgical removal of the spleen. Formerly believed to be almost harmless, the procedure is now known to carry a number of major later risks, including an increased tendency to heart attacks and strokes and a risk of overwhelming pneumococcal infection.

spleen enlargement the spleen becomes enlarged in HAEMOLYTIC ANAEMIA, HODGKIN'S DISEASE, INFECTIOUS MONONUCLEOSIS, KALA-AZAR, LEUKAEMIA, MALARIA, non-Hodgkin's LYMPHOMA, SCHISTOSOMIASIS, SEPTICAEMIA, SYPHILIS, THALASSAEMIA, TRYPANOSOMIASIS, TUBERCULOSIS, TYPHOID and TYPHUS.

splen-, spleno- *prefix denoting* spleen.

splenic pertaining to the spleen.

splenius one of two muscles at the back of the neck, running from the back and sides of the vertebrae to the OCCIPITAL bone of the skull.

The splenius muscles rotate and extend the head.

splenomegaly SPLEEN ENLARGEMENT.

splicing in genetics, the process in a DISCONTINUOUS GENE in MESSENGER RNA of removal of INTRONS and the joining together of exons.

splint a usually temporary support or reinforcement for an injured part, often used to minimize movement at the site of injury, especially in the case of a fracture of a bone.

splinter haemorrhages small linear streaks of blood under the nails that resemble splinters. They are a feature of infective ENDOCARDITIS.

split personality a rare condition in which the subject adopts, at different times, one of two or more distinct personas. The condition may be associated with EPILEPSY and there is often a history of abuse in childhood. It is not a feature of SCHIZOPHRENIA.

spondarthritis a group of diseases that includes ANKYLOSING SPONDYLITIS, ARTHRITIS associated with ULCERATIVE COLITIS and CROHN'S DISEASE, REITER'S SYNDROME, arthritis associated with PSORIASIS, BEHÇET'S SYNDROME and WHIPPLE'S DISEASE. All feature inflammation of joints, especially of the spine, a tendency to inflammation at tendon attachments and a negative response to tests for RHEUMATOID ARTHRITIS.

spondyl-, spondylo- *combining form denoting* VERTEBRA or vertebral.

spondylitis inflammation of any of the joints between the VERTEBRAE of the spine. This may occur in OSTEOARTHRITIS, RHEUMATOID ARTHRITIS, or, more specifically, in ANKYLOSING SPONDYLITIS.

spondylolisthesis the moving forwards of a vertebra relative to the one under it, most commonly of the 5th lumbar vertebra over the top of the SACRUM. This is due to a congenital weakness (SPONDYLOLYSIS) of the bony arch that bears the facets by which the vertebrae articulate together. Spondylolisthesis causes severe backache on standing and leads to nerve pressure effects. The condition may also affect vertebrae in the neck.

spondylolysis a symptomless congenital deficiency of bone in the arch of the 5th or 4th lumbar vertebra disorder of the spine. The arch is formed of soft fibrous tissue and there is a weak link with adjacent vertebrae so that the condition of SPONDYLOLISTHESIS may occur.

spongiform encephalopathy one of a number of diseases of the nervous system featuring spongy degeneration of the grey matter of the brain, loss of nerve cells and overgrowth of the brain connective tissue cells (astrocytes). The effects are severe loss of function and death. These diseases are associated with an abnormal cellular inclusion called a PRION and which can be diagnosed by locating specific defects within the prion gene. See also CREUTZFELDT-JAKOB DISEASE and KURU.

spongioblasts embryonic cells of the neural tube that give rise to the neural connective tissue (neuroglial) cells, the astrocytes and the oligodendrocytes.

spontaneous abortion premature and unexpected expulsion of the fetus from the womb for no immediately obvious reason. See also ABORTION.

spontaneous amputation loss of an extremity as a result of a disease process causing constriction and death of tissue. See also AINHUM.

spontaneous pneumothorax sudden and unexpected incursion of air into the space between the two layers of the PLEURA so that the underlying lung collapses. The usual cause is rupture of a congenital bleb on the inner pleural layer so that air passes from the lung. In most cases the leak seals itself and the lung soon re-expands.

spor-, sporo- *prefix denoting* spore.

sporadic fatal insomnia see FATAL FAMILIAL INSOMNIA.

Sporanox a brand name for ITRACONAZOLE.

spore 1 a dormant or resting stage of certain bacteria and other organisms, capable of surviving for long periods in hostile environments and of reactivating under suitable conditions.
2 a single-celled propagative form of a fungus capable of developing into an adult.

sport-prohibited drugs a list of stimulants, narcotics, anabolic agents, diuretics and hormones prohibited by the Olympic Movement Anti-Doping Code. The list includes amphetamines (amfetamines), bromantan, caffeine (above 12 mcg/ml), carphedon, cocaine, ephedrine, certain beta agonists, diamorphine (heroin), morphine, methadone, pethidine, methandianone, nandrolone, stanozole, testosterone, clenbuterol, DHEA, androstenedione, 19-norandrostenediol, acetazolamide, frusemide (furosemide), hydrochlorothiazide, triamterene, mannitol, growth hormone, corticotrophin (corticotropin), chorionic gonadotrophin, pituitary and synthetic gonadotrophins, erythropoietin, insulin, and all corresponding releasing factors and analogues.

sporotrichosis a persistent infection caused by the plant and moss fungus *Sporothrix schenckii* and contracted by way of a skin wound or by inhalation. There is a local ulcer followed by the appearance of nodules under the skin from masses of the fungus in the adjacent lymph channels. Lung cavities may occur. Treatment is with potassium iodide solution in milk by mouth and continued for a month.

sporozoon a parasitic protozoon of the class Sporozoea, that includes the malarial parasites.

sporozoite a motile reproductive form of a SPOROZOON that has been released from an oocyst and is ready to penetrate a new host cell, as in malaria transmission.

sports medicine the branch of medicine concerned with the physiology of exercise and its application to the improvement of athletic performance and fitness, and with the prevention, diagnosis and treatment of medical conditions caused by, or related to, sporting activities of all kinds.

sporulation the production or release of spores.

spot a popular term for any small lump or inflamed area on the skin such as a PUSTULE, PAPULE, COMEDONE, CYST, MACULE, SCAB or VESICLE.

spotted fever 1 one of a range of serious Rickettsial infectious diseases, such as TYPHUS and ROCKY MOUNTAIN SPOTTED FEVER, that feature conspicuous skin rashes.
2 an epidemic form of CEREBROSPINAL MENINGITIS.

sprain stretching or a minor tear of one of the ligaments that hold together the bone ends in a joint or of the fibres of a joint capsule.

sprue a disorder in which nutrients are poorly absorbed from the intestine. See also MALABSORPTION.

sputum mucus, often mixed with PUS or blood, that is secreted by the goblet cells in the MUCOUS MEMBRANE lining of the respiratory tubes (BRONCHI and BRONCHIOLES). Excess sputum prompts the cough reflex. Also known as phlegm.

squalamine a drug extracted from the dogfish that has been claimed to be capable of killing a range of sexually-transmitted bacteria including the *gonococcus* and *Chlamydia* and of killing cells invaded by viruses.

squamous 1 scaly. Covered with, or formed of, scales.

2 pertaining to, or resembling a scale or scales.

squamous cell a flat, scaly epithelial cell.

squamous cell carcinoma a form of skin cancer related to sunlight exposure. A squamous cell cancer starts as small, firm, painless lumps occurring most commonly on the lip, ear, or back of the hand and slowly enlarging. Surgical removal and examination is important as, unlike the rodent ulcer (BASAL CELL CARCINOMA), this tumour may spread to other parts of the body, with fatal consequences.

squamous epithelium an outer layer of a surface (epithelium) that is composed of flat, scaly cells.

squint see STRABISMUS.

SRN *abbrev. for* State Registered Nurse.

ST *abbrev. for* Speech Therapist.

stable 1 of an ill person, in a currently unchanging state, neither improving nor deteriorating.

2 of a personality, not liable to mental disturbances or abnormal behaviour.

Stafoxil a brand name for the antibiotic FLUCLOXACILLIN.

stage a recognizable point or phase in the development of a progressive disease, particularly a cancer. In breast cancer, for instance, three recognizable stages might be: tumour confined to the breast tissue; tumour extended to the axillary lymph nodes; tumour widely metastasized. Compare GRADE.

staging determination of the stage to which a disease, especially a cancer, has progressed. Staging is important as an indication of the likely outcome (prognosis) and in deciding on the best form of treatment, as this may differ markedly at different stages.

staining the use of selected dyes to colour biological specimens such as cells, cell products, thin slices of tissues or microorganisms to assist in examination and identification under the microscope. See also GRAM NEGATIVE, GRAM POSITIVE.

standard deviation a measure of dispersion widely used in statistics. Standard deviation is the square root of the arithmetic average of the squares of the deviations of the members of a sample from the mean.

Stanford-Binet test a type of intelligence test on which many current tests are based. (Alfred Binet, 1857–1911, French psychologist. Test adapted at Stanford University).

stannosis an occupational lung disease caused by deposition of tin dioxide in the lung tissues. It is a hazard of tin mining.

St Anthony's fire an archaic term for ERYSIPELAS and a few other similar conditions. There was little precision in diagnosis in medieval times.

stapedectomy an operation to relieve the deafness caused by OTOSCLEROSIS.

stapes the innermost of the three tiny linking bones of the middle ear (auditory ossicles). The footplate of the stapes lies in the oval window in the wall of the inner ear and transmits vibration to the fluid in the COCHLEA.

staph *abbrev. for* STAPHYLOCOCCUS, staphylococci or staphylococcal.

Staphylex a brand name for FLUCLOXACILLIN.

staphylococcal infections see ABSCESS, BACTERAEMIA, BOIL, CARBUNCLE, ENDOCARDITIS, FOOD POISONING, OSTEOMYELITIS, SEPTIC SHOCK and STYE.

staphylococcus one of a wide range of GRAM POSITIVE, spherical bacteria of the genus *Staphylococcus*, that congregate in grape-like clusters and cause boils, septicaemia and other infections. See also STAPHYLOCOCCAL INFECTIONS.

starch a complex polysaccharide carbohydrate consisting of chains of linked glucose molecules. Amylose is a chain of 200 to 500 glucose units. Amylopectin consists of 20 cross-linked glucose molecules. Most natural starches are a mixture of these two. Starch, in the form of potatoes, rice and cereals forms an important part of the average diet and about 70% of the world's food.

Staril a brand name for FOSINOPRIL.

starvation long-term deprivation of food and its consequences. These are severe loss of body fat and muscle, changes in body chemistry with KETOSIS and constant hunger.

stasis a reduction or cessation of flow, as of blood or intestinal contents.

stasis dermatitis inflammation of the skin of the legs, resulting from stagnation of blood in the veins. This is a common feature of VARICOSE VEINS.

statins drugs of the hydroxymethyl glutaryl coenzyme A reductase inhibitor class (HMG-CoA reductase inhibitors). These drugs block the liver's production of cholesterol by competitive inhibition of the reductase coenzyme that catalyzes the rate-limiting step of cholesterol synthesis. They can lower the levels of low-density lipoproteins (LDLs) by 25–45% and a number of major trials have shown their benefits in preventing heart attacks and other effects of ATHEROSCLEROSIS. It has been established that intensive statin treatment after heart attacks provides greater protection against death than does a standard regimen. Recent research on mice has suggested that statins may have some value in MULTIPLE SCLEROSIS because of an effect of diminishing the cellular immune reponse. This growing drug class includes atorvastatin (Lipitor), cerivastatin (Liponay), fluvastatin (Lescol), pravastatin (Lipostat), rosuvastatin (Crestor) and simvastatin (Zocor). Note that the root 'statin' has proved popular with pharmacological neologists so, unfortunately, there are many other drugs, not in the HMG-CoA reductase inhibitor class, with 'statin' in their names.

statistics see VITAL STATISTICS.

status asthmaticus a dangerous and often fatal form of ASTHMA requiring emergency hospital treatment by experts. In status asthmaticus the level of oxygen in the blood rapidly drops to a critical degree. Oxygen is given under pressure together with steroid drugs and bronchodilators. Mechanical ventilation may be needed.

status epilepticus a repeated sequence of major epileptic seizures (grand mal) without recovery of consciousness between attacks. The condition is dangerous and may prove fatal unless controlled. Diazepam or more powerful drugs are given by intravenous injection.

statutory rape sexual intercourse with a girl below the age of consent.

stavudine a REVERSE TRANSCRIPTASE INHIBITOR drug used to treat HIV infections. The drug is on the WHO official list. A brand name is Zerit.

STD *abbrev for* sexually-transmitted disease. See SEXUALLY TRANSMITTED INFECTIONS.

STI *abbrev for* SEXUALLY-TRANSMITTED INFECTION.

steato- *combining form denoting* fat.

steatorrhoea excess fat in the stools, which are usually pale, bulky, oily and hard to flush away. Steatorrhoea occurs in any condition, such as PANCREATITIS or COELIAC DISEASE, in which the breakdown and absorption of fats is diminished.

Steele-Richardson-Olszewski syndrome see PROGRESSIVE SUPRANUCLEAR PALSY.

Stein-Leventhal syndrome a condition in which menstrual disturbances or absence of menstruation, sterility, obesity and a male distribution of body hair is associated with multiple cysts in the ovaries. Removal of large wedges from both ovaries is effective. (Irving F. Stein, b. 1887, American gynaecologist; and Michael Leo Leventhal, 1901–71, American obstetrician).

Steinmann pin a fine surgical nail passed through the lower end of the FEMUR or the upper end of the TIBIA and held under tension in a steel stirrup so that TRACTION can be applied in the treatment of fractures. (Fritz Steinmann, 1872–1932, Swiss surgeon).

Stelazine a brand name for the phenothiazine antipsychotic and ANTIEMETIC drug TRIFLUOPERAZINE.

stem cell a pluripotential progenitor cell from which a whole class of cells differentiate. A stem cell in the bone marrow, for instance, gives rise to the entire range of immune system blood cells (neutrophils, eosinophils, basophils, monocytes/macrophages, platelets, T cells and B cells) and the red blood cells (erythrocytes). Stem cells from umbilical cord blood have a considerable potential for medical treatment. A major research effort to produce stem cells artificially for medical purposes is under way. The genetic material from an ovum can be removed and a cumulus cell from the outside of an egg, or a fibroblast, can be inserted.

Stemetil a brand name for the phenothiazine antipsychotic drug and ANTIEMETIC prochlorperazine.

stenosis narrowing of a duct, orifice or tubular organ such as the intestinal canal or a blood vessel.

stent see STENTING.

stenting the use of a physical device, such as a tubular stainless steel or plastic mesh or coil of wire, to keep a body tube fully open. Stents are used in the CORONARY ARTERIES, the AORTA, the renal arteries, the FEMORAL ARTERIES, the intestine and elsewhere. In addition to the widespread use in arteries, self-expanding metallic stents have been successfully used to maintain patency in narrowing of urethras and bile ducts and for swallowing difficulties (dysphagia) caused by cancer of the OESOPHAGUS. Silicone rubber stents have been used in the TRACHEA and BRONCHI. Stents in arteries are liable to blockage by blood clotting. Anticoagulant treatment is required. Drug-eluting coronary stents designed to prevent restenosis are currently displacing bare-metal stents. Sirolimus appears to be the drug of choice at the time of writing.

stercorous pertaining to excrement.

sterculia a bulking agent used to treat constipation. A brand name is Normacol.

stereo- *combining form denoting* solid or three-dimensional.

stereognosis the ability to identify the shape, size and texture of objects by touch, without the benefit of sight.

stereoisomerism mirror-image molecular asymmetry. Also known as CHIRALITY. In the case of amino acids, the two forms are represented on paper with the carboxyl group of the carbon chain at the top. In the laevo (L) form, the functional groups connected to the central carbon or carbon chain are shown as projecting to the left and in the dextro (D) form they are shown projecting to the right.

stereotaxic surgery operations, especially on the brain, in which fine instruments are guided with precision to the required point by three-dimensional scanning methods.

stereopsis the normal ability to perceive objects as being solid. Stereoscopic vision.

sterile 1 free from bacteria or other microorganisms.
2 incapable of reproduction.

sterilization 1 the process of rendering anything free from living micro-organisms.
2 any procedure, such as hysterectomy, tying of the fallopian tubes, vasectomy or castration that deprives the individual of the ability to reproduce.

sternal pertaining to the STERNUM.

sternum the breastbone.

Sterofrin a brand name for eye drops containing PREDNISOLONE.

steroid 1 sterol-like.

2 any member of the class of fat-soluble organic compounds based on a structure of 17 carbon atoms arranged in three connected rings of six, six and five carbons. The steroids include the adrenal cortex hormones, the SEX HORMONES, PROGESTOGENS, BILE SALTS, STEROLS and a wide range of synthetic compounds produced for therapeutic purposes. Anabolic steroids are male sex hormones that stimulate the production of protein.

steroid drugs a large group of drugs that are derived from, resemble, or simulate the actions of, the natural corticosteroids or the male sex hormones of the body.

sterols a group of mainly unsaturated solid alcohols of the steroid group occurring in the fatty tissues of plants and animals. The sterols include CHOLESTEROL and ERGOSTEROL.

stertorous of breathing, a heavy, coarse snoring associated with a falling back of the tongue.

Ster-Zac Bath Concentrate a brand name for TRICLOSAN.

Ster-Zac Powder a brand name for HEXACHLOROPHANE (hexachlorophene) dusting powder.

Stesolid a brand name for DIAZEPAM.

stethoscope a binaural or monaural tube that conveys sounds conveniently from the body of a patient to the ears of the examining physician or other person. From the Greek *stethos*, chest and *skopein*, to look at; from which it will be seen that the name of the instrument was carelessly chosen. The careful auscultator will often close his or her eyes, the better to hear all the subtleties of body sounds, especially heart murmurs.

Stevens-Johnson syndrome a rare but severe condition involving skin and MUCOUS MEMBRANES of the eyes, mouth, nose and genitals and featuring ulceration and loss of epithelium with abnormal adhesions. A form of ERYTHEMA MULTIFORME usually caused by an adverse reaction to drugs such as the SULPHONAMIDES. (Albert Mason Stevens, 1884–1935, American paediatrician; and Frank Chambliss Johnson, 1894–1934, American paediatrician).

STICH *acronym for* Surgical Trial in Intracerebral Haemorrhage, an international randomised trial designed to compare the results of early surgery and conservative treatment in cases of spontaneous supratentorial haematomas. A trial report in 2005 suggested that early surgery offered no benefit, but technical advances in surgery are thought likely to challenge this view.

sticky ends complementary single strands of DNA protruding from the ends of a DNA fragment as a result of the cleaving of each half of the double helix at different points near to each other. Sticky ends readily provide attachment points for other pieces of DNA or for further DNA synthesis.

Stiedex LP a brand name for DESOXYMETHASONE (desoxymetasone).

Stiedex lotion a brand name for DESOXYMETHASONE (desoxymetasone).

stiff-person syndrome a rare nervous system disorder characterized by muscle pain, rigidity, spasm and severe stiffness. The condition is related to stress and is often precipitated by being startled. The disorder usually starts in one muscle group and then spreads progressively to other parts of the musculature. Often the whole of the trunk becomes involved and the spasms may become almost continuous so that the disability is severe. Sixty% of patients have autoantibodies to glutamic acid decarboxylase.

stilboestrol DIETHYLSTILBOESTROL, DES, a synthetic oestrogen drug similar in action to the natural hormone oestradiol (estradiol). Stilboestrol is used to treat cancer of the PROSTATE, some types of breast cancer and postmenopausal atrophic VAGINITIS. A brand name of a preparation used in pessary form is Tampovagan.

stillbirth birth of a dead baby. The distinction from MISCARRIAGE is arbitrary and, in Britain, is set at 28 weeks of pregnancy. Stillbirths must be registered and the cause of death established before a certificate of stillbirth can be provided and burial may take place.

Still's disease juvenile RHEUMATOID ARTHRITIS. The condition is commonly complicated by the eye disorder UVEITIS. (Sir George Frederick Still, 1868–1941, English paediatrician).

Stilnoct a brand name for ZOLPIDEM.

stimulus anything that causes a response, either in an excitable tissue or in an organism.

stitch 1 a SUTURE.
2 a brief, sharp pain in the abdomen or flank caused by severe or unaccustomed exercise, especially running.

St Louis fever a togavirus infection spread by mosquitoes and causing ENCEPHALITIS or HAEMORRHAGIC FEVER.

Stokes-Adams attacks repeated, brief episodes of loss of consciousness from inadequacy in the blood supply to the brain due to cessation or extreme slowness of the heart action. Stokes-Adams attacks occur in cases of severe ARRHYTHMIA or complete HEART BLOCK. Most cases are treated by the fitting of an artificial PACEMAKER. (William Stokes, 1804–78, Irish physician; and Robert Adams, 1791–1875, Irish surgeon).

stom-, stomato- *combining form denoting* mouth.

stoma a mouth or orifice, especially one formed surgically, as in a COLOSTOMY or ILEOSTOMY.

stomach the bag-like organ lying under the DIAPHRAGM in the upper right part of the ABDOMEN into which swallowed food passes, by way of the OESOPHAGUS. The stomach has an average capacity of about 1.75 l and secretes hydrochloric acid and the protein-digesting enzyme PEPSIN.

stomach cancer malignant change in the stomach lining. This is an insidious disease of the elderly often with few early signs so that the diagnosis may not be apparent until a late stage. Warning signs include new upper abdominal pain or discomfort, unexplained vomiting and blackening of the stools. Treatment is by surgery but the outlook is usually poor.

stomach disorders see PEPTIC ULCER, PERNICIOUS ANAEMIA, PYLORIC STENOSIS and STOMACH CANCER.

stomach pump see GASTRIC LAVAGE.

stomach ulcer see PEPTIC ULCER.

stomach washout see GASTRIC LAVAGE.

stomatitis inflammation or ulceration of the mouth.

stones see CALCULUS.

stools faeces.

stop codons three nucleotide triplets, one of which marks the end of every gene and indicates that protein synthesis ends at that point. The three stop codons are UAG (the amber codon), UAA and UGA. U is uracil, A is adenine and G is guanine.

stop mutation any mutation that changes a CODON that codes for an amino acid into a codon that codes for a 'stop'. Stop codons are

UAG (amber codon), UAA (ochre codon) and UGA (opal codon). The effect of a stop mutation is that a protein is shortened so that an abnormal form is produced. CYSTIC FIBROSIS, MUSCULAR DYSTROPHY and other genetic disorders are caused by stop mutations. See also PTC124.

storage diseases a range of metabolic disorders in which various substances accumulate in abnormal amounts in certain body tissues or organs such as the liver. See also SPHINGOLIPIDOSES.

stork bites a popular term for the small, harmless, pinkish skin blemishes that commonly occur around the eyes and on the back of the neck in new-born babies. Stork bites are benign tumours of small blood vessels (haemangiomas) and usually disappear within the first year of life.

storm a sudden worsening of the symptoms and other features of a disease. Used more often in the adjectival form 'stormy' or as the metaphor 'stormy passage'.

strabismus squint. The condition in which only one eye is aligned on the object of interest. The other eye may be directed too far inward (convergent strabismus), too far outward (divergent squint), or upward or downward (vertical squint). Squint in childhood, or any squint of recent onset, requires urgent treatment. Untreated childhood squint often leads to AMBLYOPIA. New squints in adults usually imply a disorder of the nervous system.

strain stretching or tearing of muscle fibres, usually in the course of athletic overactivity. There is swelling, pain, bruising and a tendency to muscle spasm. Treatment is by rest, STRAPPING and painkilling drugs.

strangulated hernia an intestinal hernia in which the blood supply is cut off because of compression of the vessels at the neck of the hernia.

strangulation constriction or compression of any passage or tube in the body, such as the jugular veins of the neck in manual strangulation, or the intestine in HERNIA. Strangulation may also result from twisting of a part as in VOLVULUS or torsion of the testis.

strangury a frequent, painful but unproductive desire to empty the bladder. Strangury is a feature of bladder stones, bladder cancer, CYSTITIS and PROSTATITIS.

strapping the use of adhesive tape or firm bandages to maintain the desired relationship of parts of the body or to rest an injured or inflamed part.

Strattera brand name for the drug ATOMOXETINE used to treat ATTENTION DEFICIT HYPERACTIVITY DISORDER (ADHD).

strawberry naevus a bright red, raised skin blemish that, although not present at birth, appears within the first few weeks and grows rapidly, sometimes to a large size. The strawberry naevus is a kind of HAEMANGIOMA and invariably eventually disappears.

strep *abbrev. for* STREPTOCOCCUS, streptococci or streptococcal.

strep throat a throat infection with STREPTOCOCCI.

Streptase a brand name for the blood clot dissolving enzyme drug STREPTOKINASE.

strepto- *combining form denoting* twisted, chain-like or coiled.

streptococcal infections see ENDOCARDITIS, ERYSIPELAS, GLOMERULONEPHRITIS, IMPETIGO, PHARYNGITIS, RHEUMATIC FEVER, SCARLET FEVER and TONSILLITIS.

streptococcus any of a range of spherical or ovoid bacteria of the genus *Streptococcus* that occur in chains or in pairs. See also STEPTOCOCCAL INFECTIONS.

streptodornase a protein-splitting ENZYME used externally to clean wounds. A brand name is Varidase.

streptogramins antibiotic drugs used to treat hospital-acquired infections when no other antibiotic is effective. Examples are quinupristin (Synercid), dalfoprisyin (Synercid), pristinamycin and virginiamycin.

streptokinase a protein-splitting ENZYME used as a drug to dissolve blood clot in a coronary artery so as to minimize the degree of MYOCARDIAL INFARCTION during a heart attack. It is also used to treat PULMONARY EMBOLISM. The drug is on the WHO official list. Brand names are Kabikinase and Streptase.

streptolysin a substance derived from some strains of streptococci that breaks down red blood cells (haemolysin).

streptomycin an aminoglycoside antibiotic drug used to treat some rare infections such as BRUCELLOSIS, GLANDERS, PLAGUE, TUBERCULOSIS and TULARAEMIA. It is avoided for commoner infections because of its side effects, which include deafness and TINNITUS. The drug is on the WHO official list.

stress any physical, social or psychological factor or combination of factors that acts on the individual so as to threaten his or her well-being and produce a physiological, often defensive, response. The response to stress may be beneficial, distressing or, occasionally, dangerous. Responses such as the production of ADRENALINE and CORTICOSTEROIDS, raised heart rate and blood pressure, increased muscle tension and raised blood sugar, are natural; but persistent civilized suppression of the natural physical concomitants (fight or flight) may be damaging. Most medical scientists view with scepticism the proposition that many human diseases are caused by stress. There is, however, no questioning the fact that overwhelming stress can cause physical and psychological damage. See POST-TRAUMATIC STRESS DISORDER.

stress genes a general term for genes that are induced to transcribe following exposure to DNA-damaging agents such as radiation or the action of oxygen free radicals.

stress ulcers acute stomach ulcers developing as a consequence of SHOCK, BURNS or severe illness or injury.

stretch marks a popular name for STRIAE.

striae broad, purplish, shiny or whitish lines of atrophy on the skin, most commonly affecting pregnant women, and occurring on the abdomen, breasts or thighs. Striae are due to altered COLLAGEN. Also known as stretch marks.

striated striped, grooved, or ridged.

striated muscle voluntary, skeletal muscle and heart (cardiac) muscle, characterized by microscopic transverse stripes or striation. Compare SMOOTH MUSCLE.

stricture narrowing of a body passage.

stridor noisy breathing caused by the narrowing or the partial obstruction of the LARYNX or TRACHEA.

stroke the effect of acute deprivation of blood to a part of the brain by narrowing or obstruction of an artery, usually by thrombosis (80%), or of damage to the brain substance from bleeding into it (CEREBRAL HAEMORRHAGE) (15%). Subarachnoid haemorrhage is the cause in 5%. The results of such damage are most obvious if they involve the nerve tracts concerned with movement,

sensation, speech and vision. These are situated close together, in the internal capsule of the brain, and are often involved together. There may be paralysis and loss of sensation down one side of the body or of one side of the face, loss of corresponding halves of the fields of vision, a range of speech disturbances or various disorders of comprehension or expression. In most cases a degree of recovery, sometimes considerable, may be expected. Haemorrhage into the brainstem, where the centres for the control of the vital functions of breathing and heart-beat are situated, is the most immediately dangerous to life. Diagnosis of the type of stroke is important and this requires neuroimaging of the brain.

stroke in progression brain damage caused by an obstruction to the blood supply (ischaemia) that increases progressively over the course of hours, days or weeks. Has also been defined as 'a stroke in which the neurological deficit is still increasing in severity or distribution after the patient is admitted to observation'. The condition is associated with high concentrations of glutamate in the blood and cerebro-spinal fluid.

stroma the tissue forming the framework of an organ. Compare PARENCHYMA.

strongyloidiasis a persistent intestinal infection with the small parasitic worm *Strongyloides stercoralis*, which is common in many parts of the Far East. The infection tends to be permanent by internal breeding and may cause discomfort and distention, diarrhoea, SEPTICAEMIA, MENINGITIS or severe bleeding from the lungs. Treatment is with the drug thiabendazole (tiabendazole) but repeated courses must be given.

strontium 90 a radioactive isotope of 28 years half-life that is produced in large quantities in nuclear fission reactions. It accumulates in the bones and may cause leukaemia and bone tumours.

strontium ranelate a bone-seeking drug shown in the mid-1990s to be capable of substantially reducing the risk of fractures in post-menopausal women with OSTEOPOROSIS. The drug stimulates bone formation and reduces resorption. The usefulness of the drug was shown in a large trial, the results of which were published in January 2004. Side effects are said to be minor.

structural gene a GENE that codes, as most do, for the amino acid sequence of a protein rather than for a regulatory protein.

strychnine a bitter-tasting, highly poisonous substance occurring in the seeds of *Strychnos* species of tropical trees and shrubs. Poisoning causes restlessness, stiffness of the face and neck, exaggerated sensations, extreme arching of the back (opisthotonus) and death from paralysis of breathing unless artificial ventilation is used.

Stugeron a brand name for CINNARIZINE.

stupor a state of severely reduced consciousness, short of COMA, from which the affected person can be briefly aroused only by painful stimulation.

Sturge-Weber syndrome the association of a large purple HAEMANGIOMA on one side of the face with a similar malformation of blood vessels in the brain. There may be weakness on the opposite side of the body, epileptic seizures, GLAUCOMA and sometimes mental retardation. (William Allen Sturge, 1850–1919, English physician; and Frederick Parkes Weber, 1863–1962, English physician).

St Vitus' dance see SYDENHAM'S CHOREA.

stye a small abscess caused by a STAPHYLOCOCCAL INFECTION around the root of an eyelash. Treatment is by antibiotic ointments to prevent recurrence.

styloid pointed and slender.

styloid process any pointed bony protuberance as that on the TEMPORAL BONE, the FIBULA, the RADIUS or the ULNA.

styptic causing contraction of tissues or blood vessels and tending to check bleeding.

sub- *prefix denoting* under, less.

subacute intermediate in duration between ACUTE and CHRONIC.

subacute combined degeneration of the cord a complication of PERNICIOUS ANAEMIA (vitamin B_{12} deficiency) that can be prevented by timely diagnosis and treatment. DEMYELINATION, of the sensory and motor tracts of the spinal cord and of the peripheral nerves, occurs causing progressive loss of sensation and muscle weakness with staggering (ataxia). Position sense in the legs is lost. Unless adequately treated the condition progresses to severe disablement with DEMENTIA. Treatment with hydroxycobalamin is curative in the early stages.

subarachnoid haemorrhage bleeding over and into the substance of the brain from a ruptured artery lying under the arachnoid layer of the MENINGES. The commonest cause is rupture of a pre-existing berry-like swelling (ANEURYSM) on one of the arteries or bleeding from a tumour-like malformation on an artery. Subarachnoid haemorrhage is the main cause of spontaneous STROKE in young people. There is a sudden severe headache followed by loss of consciousness or other signs of neurological damage. The death rate is high. Treatment is directed to keeping the blood pressure reasonably low, preventing blood vessels from going into spasm and preventing blood clot in an aneurysm from dissolving. Surgery is sometimes appropriate.

subarachnoid space the space between the PIA MATER and the arachnoid mater, occasioned by the fact that the pia, the innermost layer of the meninges, closely invests the surface of the brain while the arachnoid, external to it, bridges over the grooves. The subarachnoid space contains blood vessels.

subclavian 1 situated below or under the CLAVICLE.

2 pertaining to the subclavian artery or vein.

subclavian artery a short length of the major artery that branches from the aorta on the left side and from the innominate artery on the right side and continues as the axillary artery to supply the arm. The subclavian arteries also supply the brain via their vertebral branches.

subclavian steal syndrome a phenomenon caused by a partial blockage of one of the main arteries that gives branches to the head and then to the arms. Use of the arm may divert blood from the head, leading to VERTIGO, headache, uncontrollable deviation of the eyes, double vision, nausea and vomiting. There is a serious risk of STROKE.

subclinical of a degree of mildness, or of such an early stage of development, as to produce no symptoms or signs.

subconjunctival haemorrhage painless bleeding under the transparent membrane (the CONJUNCTIVA) covering the white of the eye. This causes a conspicuous bright red patch that usually reabsorbs in about two weeks. The condition is harmless.

subconscious 1 of mental processes and reactions occurring without conscious perception.

2 the large store of information of which only a small part is in consciousness at any time, but which may be accessed at will with varying degrees of success.

3 in psychoanalytic theory, a 'level' of the mind through which information passes on its way 'up' to full consciousness from the unconscious mind. Compare CONSCIOUS, UNCONSCIOUS.

subcutaneous under the skin. Many injections are given subcutaneously. An alternative term is hypodermic.

subcutaneous emphysema see SURGICAL EMPHYSEMA.

subdural haematoma a dangerous complication of head injury in which bleeding occurs from tearing of one of the blood vessels under the DURA MATER. The blood gradually accumulates to form an expanding clot which slowly compresses the brain. After recovery of consciousness from the original injury there is typically a relapse into coma some time later. Treatment, which is life-saving, involves opening the skull and tying off the bleeding vessel.

subdural haemorrhage bleeding between the DURA MATER and the underlying ARACHNOID MATER. See SUBDURAL HAEMATOMA.

sublimation deflection of socially unacceptable drives into acceptable channels so that the necessity for repression is avoided. Sublimation is a psychoanalytic concept and is considered to be a healthy feature of a mature personality.

Sublimaze a brand name for FENTANYL.

subliminal perception the reception of stimuli, often complex or verbal and usually visual, that are presented for such a short time as to be barely noticed or unnoticed. Such stimuli can, however, influence behaviour and present potential opportunities for abuse. The conclusion, now verified by physiological research, that consciousness and information transmission may involve different systems that can operate independently has major implications for psychology and philosophy and has aroused much controversy.

sublingual under the tongue.

subluxation partial or incomplete dislocation of a joint.

submaxillary pertaining to the lower jaw. Under the MAXILLA.

submicroscopic too small to be see under a visible light microscope.

submucous resection an ENT operation to relieve nasal obstruction by removing displaced cartilage and bone from under-neath the mucous membrane of a deviated central partition (septum) of the nose.

subphrenic abscess an abscess under the diaphragm.

subscapular below or on the underside of the shoulder blade (scapula).

substance a general term meaning any physical matter, or the nature of the matter of which something is made, which has, in recent years acquired a new sense. The term, in this restricted sense, is applied to any chemical, solid, jiquid or gaseous, capable of affecting the state of the mind. A psychoactive material.

substance abuse a general term referring to the non-medical and 'recreational' use of drugs such as amphetamine (amfetamine), cannabis, cocaine, methylenedioxymethamphetamine (ecstasy), heroin, lysergic acid diethylamide (LSD), organic solvents by inhalation, and so on. The term is also applied to an intake of alcohol that is likely to prove harmful. Oddly enough is not currently applied to a commonly-used substance more dangerous than most of these – tobacco.

substance use disorder a term originating in America and referring to addiction to drugs and alcohol.

substantia nigra a layer of grey matter (nerve cell bodies) containing pigmented nerve cells, that spreads throughout the white substance of the midbrain and receives fibres from the BASAL GANGLIA. DOPAMINE is produced in the substantia nigra, and loss of the pigment cells is a constant finding in PARKINSON'S DISEASE.

substrate the substance on which an ENZYME acts. Any reactant in a reaction that is catalyzed by an enzyme.

subungual under a nail.

subungual haematoma a collection of blood under a nail.

succinimides drugs used to treat epilepsy, especially absence seizures. An example is ethosuximide (Zarontin).

succussion the act of shaking violently.

sucking wound of chest an open wound in the chest wall through which air passes in and out with the respiratory movements. The air enters the pleural cavity and the underlying lung collapses. There is an urgent need for the wound to be closed and this should be done as a first aid measure.

sucralfate a drug that forms a protective coating over the stomach or duodenal lining. Sucralfate is used in the treatment of peptic ulceration. A brand name is Antepsin.

sucrose cane or beet sugar. A crystalline disaccharide carbohydrate present in many foodstuffs and widely used as a sweetener and preservative. During digestion, sucrose hydrolyses to glucose and fructose.

suction the application of negative pressure so as to withdraw fluid. Suction may be by syringe or mechanical pump and is often applied through a container which acts both as a trap and as a receptacle.

suction lipectomy a cosmetic surgical operation is which unwanted fat is removed through small incisions using a blunt-ended metal CANNULA connected to a powerful vacuum pump.

Sudafed a brand name for PSEUDOEPHEDRINE with TRIPROLIDINE.

sudamen a tiny fluid-filled VESICLE formed at a sweat pore, as in PRICKLY HEAT.

sudden infant death syndrome cot death. The sudden, unexplained death of an apparently well baby. No apparent cause is established, even after a detailed postmortem examination. Many theories have been put forward and it seems likely that a range of causes is operating, including putting babies down to sleep in the prone position. Many sudden deaths in healthy babies can be explained.

Sudeck's atrophy severe OSTEOPOROSIS with muscle atrophy and loss of the use of a hand or foot, occurring after a fracture. Recovery is usual. (Paul Hermann Sudeck, 1866–1945, German surgeon).

sudoriferous sweat-producing or secreting.

suffocation oxygen deprivation by mechanical obstruction to the passage of air into the lungs, usually at the level of the nose, mouth, LARYNX or TRACHEA.

suicide intentional self-killing. Depression is the commonest cause of suicide and severely depressed people are always at risk. Suicide is also common among alcoholics, people with SCHIZOPHRENIA and people with severe personality disorders.

sulcus a narrow fissure or groove especially one

of the furrows that separates adjacent convolutions (gyri) on the surface of the brain.

Suleo-M a brand name for a preparation containing MALATHION for external use.

sulfadoxine a SULPHONAMIDE DRUG drug used as an adjunct to CHLOROQUINE in the treatment of Falciparum MALARIA. A brand name is Fansidar.

sulfametopyrazine a SULPHONAMIDE DRUG taken weekly to control infection in chronic bronchitis. A brand name is Kelfizine W.

sulindac a non-steroidal anti-inflammatory drug (NSAID). A brand name is Clinoril.

Sulparex a brand name for SULPIRIDE.

sulphacetamide sulfacetamide, a SULPHONAMIDE DRUG limited to external use. A brand name for a vaginal cream preparation also containing sulphathiazole and sulphabenzamide, is Sultrin.

sulphadiazine sulfadiazine, a sulphonamide drug used to prevent recurrences of RHEUMATIC FEVER. The drug is on the WHO official list.

sulphadoxine with pyrimethamine sulfadoxine with pyrimethamine, a drug combination used to treat Falciparum MALARIA and TOXOPLASMOSIS. The drug combination is on the WHO official list. A brand name is Fansidar.

sulphamates drugs used to treat epilepsy. An example is topiramate (Topamax).

sulphamethoxazole sulfamethozazole, a SULPHONAMIDE DRUG used in combination with the folic acid inhibitor drug trimethoprim in the treatment of various infections, especially urinary infections. The drug combination is on the WHO official list. Brand names are Chemotrim and Septrin.

sulphasalazine sulfasalazine, a compound of a SULPHONAMIDE DRUG and 5-aminosalicylic acid used to treat RHEUMATOID ARTHRITIS, ULCERATIVE COLITIS and CROHN'S DISEASE. The drug is on the WHO official list. A brand name is Salazopyrin.

sulphinpyrazone sulfinpyrazone, a URICOSURIC drug used to reduce the frequency of attacks of GOUT. A brand name is Anturan.

sulphonamide drugs sulfonamide drugs, a large group of antibacterial drugs now largely superseded by the antibiotics except for the treatment of urinary tract infections. The group includes SULFADOXINE, SULPHACETAMIDE (sulfacetamide), sulphadiazine (sulfadiazine), sulphadimethoxine (sulfadimethoxine), sulphadimidine (sulfadimidine), sulphamethoxazole (sulfamethoxazole) and sulphathiazole (sulfathiazole).

sulphones drugs used to treat malaria, Hansen's disease and dermatitis herpetiformis. An example is dapsone.

sulphonylureas a class of drugs used in the treatment of maturity onset (Type II), non-insulin dependency DIABETES. They are taken by mouth. Also known as oral hypoglycaemic drugs. Examples are glibenclamide (Daonil, Euglucon), gliclazide (Diamicron), glimepiride (Amaryl), glipizide (Glibenese, Minodiab), gliquidone (Glurenorm) and repaglinide (Novonorm).

sulphur an element occurring in AMINO ACIDS and hence in many proteins, including COLLAGEN. Sulphur is often incorporated into ointments used in the treatment of various skin disorders such as ACNE, DANDRUFF and PSORIASIS.

sulphur dioxide an atmospheric pollution that, in industrial areas, can reach levels of 200 micrograms per cubic metre, and has been associated with increased mortality both from respiratory causes such as asthma and bronchitis and from heart attacks.

sulpiride an antipsychotic drug used to treat SCHIZOPHRENIA. Brand names are Dolmatil, Sulparex and Sulpitil.

Sulpitil a brand name for the antipsychotic drug SULPIRIDE.

Sultrin a brand name for SULPHACETAMIDE (sulfacetamide) in combination with sulphathiazole and sulphabenzamide.

sumatriptan a SEROTONIN antagonist drug that has been found effective in the symptomatic treatment of acute MIGRAINE. A brand name is Imigran.

sunburn the damaging effect of the ultraviolet component of sunlight on the skin. This varies from minor reddening to severe, disabling blistering.

sunscreens creams or other preparations used to protect the skin from the damaging effects of sunlight. Most contain para-aminobenzoic acid (PABA) which absorbs ultraviolet radiation.

sunstroke see HEATSTROKE.

super- *prefix denoting* above or excessive.

superantibody an antibody that has been chemically modified so that it is capable of binding to an antigen within a cell rather than on a cell surface. Superantibodies are thought to have potential for new forms of treatment.

superantigen one of a class of molecules that react with a substantial proportion of the whole population of T cells in the body. They include *Staphyloccocus aureus* ENTEROTOXINS. Staphylococcal enterotoxin A (SEA) is a powerful T-cell mitogen and can give rise to the release of large quantities of CYTOKINES and LEUKOTRIENES. This is believed to be one of the bases of the TOXIC SHOCK SYNDROME.

superbug an informal term for an infective micro-organism that has become resistant to antibiotics and is capable of causing serious infection. Rapid evolutionary natural selection forces have ensured that some organisms, such as *Staphylococcus aureus* and various *Enterobacteriaceae*, are now resistant to virtually all the earlier antibiotics; and resistance to a range of antibiotics has arisen in numerous other organisms including those causing bacillary dysentery, food poisoning, gonorrhoea and tuberculosis.

superciliary pertaining to the eyebrow. Literally, situated above the eyelashes.

supercoiling the secondary coiling of a DNA helix to form coiled strands. In positive supercoiling, both strands of the double helix coil together in the same direction as the coiling of the strands.

superego a psychoanalytic term for the conscience. See also FREUDIAN THEORY.

superfecundation the fertilization of more than one ovum within a single menstrual cycle by separate acts of coitus, so that twins may be born with different fathers.

superfetation the rare occurrence of two or more fetuses of different ages in a womb that are the result of fertilizations occurring in different menstrual cycles.

superficial near the surface.

superinfection a second infection, often with a fungus or virus, complicating an existing infection. The superinfecting organism is usually one which is resistant to the drugs being used in the treatment of the original infection.

superior above, higher than, with reference to the upright body. Compare INFERIOR.

superiority complex an unrealistically exaggerated belief in one's own merits. Alfred Adler (1870–1937, Austrian psychologist) suggested that in some people a superiority complex is a response to feelings of inferiority.

superjacent lying immediately above or upon something.

supernatant floating on the surface.

supernumerary more than the normal NUMBER, as in supernumerary nipples or supernumerary teeth.

superovulation the production of more than one or two ova at one time. Superovulation is common when drugs are used to stimulate ovulation in the treatment of infertility.

superoxide dismutase a natural body enzyme that converts the superoxide free radical to hydrogen peroxide, which is then catalyzed to water. The gene for superoxide dismutase is on the long arm of chromosome 21 near the Alzheimer's locus. Brain tissue is highly susceptible to free radical damage. People with Alzheimer's disease have reduced levels of superoxide dismutase.

supinator one of the forearm muscles whose action is to rotate the hand into the palm-up position.

supine lying on the back with the face upwards.

supination the act of turning the body to a SUPINE position or of turning the horizontal forearm so that the palm of the hand faces upward. Compare PRONATION.

suppository a vehicle for a drug in the form of a block of cocoa butter or gelatin of a variety of shapes and sizes that is solid at room temperature but melts at body temperature. Suppositories are placed in the vagina or rectum and release drugs either for local action or to be absorbed. They may contain antibiotics and antifungal agents, LOCAL ANAESTHETICS, CORTICOSTEROIDS, non-steroidal anti-inflammatory drugs (NSAIDs) and ANTIEMETIC drugs.

suppressor gene a GENE capable of suppressing the expression of a mutant gene at a different locus.

suppuration the production or discharge of PUS.

supra- *prefix denoting* above.

supraorbital situated above the bony eye cavern (orbit), as supraorbital artery, vein and nerve.

suprapubic referring to the region on the centre of the front wall of the abdomen immediately above the pubic bone.

suprapubic catheterization an emergency procedure offering immediate relief to a patient with a full bladder and total obstruction to urinary outflow. Under local anaesthesia a TROCAR and surrounding CANNULA are passed directly through the abdominal wall in the mid line at a point about one third of the distance from the pubis to the navel. The cannula is pushed into the bladder and the trocar removed to that urine can flow out. In children an intravenous cannula can be used.

suprarenal glands a now obsolete term for the adrenal glands.

supraspinatus syndrome the painful arc syndrome – a condition in which pain occurs when the arm is moved in the arc between about 45 and 160. The pain is caused by inflammation of the tendon of the supraspinatus muscle.

supraventricular tachycardia episodes of abnormally fast heart-rate lasting for hours or days. The rate may be as high as 300 beats per minute but is usually between 140 and 180. It is caused by fast spontaneous impulses, arising in the upper chambers of the heart, that over-ride the natural pacemaker. There may be chest pain, breathlessness, consciousness of the heart action (PALPITATIONS) and faintness. Attacks may be stopped by the VALSALVA MANOEUVRE or by the use of antiarrhythmic drugs. Sometimes electrical cardioversion is necessary.

Suprax a brand name for CEFIXIME.

sural pertaining to the calf of the leg.

suramin sodium a drug used in the treatment of TRYPANOSOMIASIS. The drug is on the WHO official list.

surface tension a property of a liquid surface, arising from unbalanced molecular cohesive forces, in which the surface behaves as if it were covered by a thin elastic membrane under tension and tends to adopt a spherical shape.

surfactant deficiency inadequate production of SURFACTANTS so that lung alveoli fail to remain adequately open. Severe cases (fatal surfactant deficiency) in newborns has recently been shown to be caused by various mutations of the ABCA3 gene.

surfactants substances that reduce SURFACE TENSION and promote wetting of surfaces. The lungs contain a surfactant to prevent collapse of the alveoli. Pulmonary surfactant is a complex mixture of proteins and lipids, and this may be deficient in premature babies leading to the RESPIRATORY DISTRESS SYNDROME (hyaline membrane disease). Surfactants can also be used to interfere with the motility of spermatozoa and so act as supplementary contraceptives with a spermicidal action. Examples of surfactant drugs are poractant (Curosurf), non-oxynol-9 (Duragel, Gynol II, Ortho-Creme) and beractant (Survanta).

surfer's nodules bony outgrowths (exostoses) on the foot and upper part of the shin caused by repeated blows from the surfboard during paddling while kneeling.

Surgam a brand name for TIAPROFENIC ACID.

surgeon a medical practitioner whose practice is limited to the diseases treated by surgical operation and who performs such treatment. General surgeons operate on almost all parts of the body but are now uncommon. The practice of specialist surgeons includes cardiovascular surgery, neurosurgery, orthopaedic surgery, ophthalmic surgery, genitourinary surgery and ear, nose and throat surgery.

surgeon's knot any one of a range of secure knots used in surgery for tying LIGATURES or SUTURES, especially a reef knot with an extra throw and an extra twist.

surgery 1 the treatment of disease, injury and deformity by physical, manual or instrumental interventions.
2 the diagnosis of conditions treated in this way.
3 the practice of operative treatment.
4 a room or suite used for medical consultation and treatment. From the Greek *cheirourgia*, hand work, as in *cheir*, hand and *ergon*, work. The list that follows highlights the key entries related to surgery in the dictionary: body contour surgery, breast plastic and reconstructive surgery, cataract surgery, cosmetic surgery, drain, endoscope, excimer laser refractive surgery, heart surgery, heart transplantation, heart valve replacement, keyhole surgery, laparoscopic surgery, minimal access surgery, minor surgery, plastic surgery, radical surgery, robotic surgery, scalpel, sex reassignment surgery, stereotaxic surgery, surgery, surgical drainage, surgical emphysema, suture, videoscopic surgery.

surgical 1 pertaining to surgery or surgeons.
2 used in surgery.
3 pertaining to diseases treated by surgical rather than by medical means.

surgical drainage provision of an easy outflow route for infected or contaminated secretions or other unwanted fluid from an operation site or an area of infection or disease. Drains include soft rubber or plastic tubes or corrugated rubber sheeting.

surgical emphysema air or gas in the tissues, most commonly in the neck as a result of leakage from a lung, injury to the OESOPHAGUS or fracture of the wall of one of the nasal SINUSES. There is a characteristic crackling effect when the affected area is pressed with the fingers. Surgical emphysema is not, in itself, harmful and the air soon absorbs if further leakage from the source is prevented.

Surmontil a brand name for the tricyclic antidepressant drug TRIMIPRAMINE.

surrogacy an agreement by a woman to undergo pregnancy so as to produce a child which will be surrendered to others. Fertilization may be by seminal fluid provided by the future adoptive father, or an ovum fertilized IN VITRO may be implanted in the surrogate mother. Surrogacy for gain is illegal in Britain and in some other countries.

Suscard Buccal a brand name for the artery-dilating drug GLYCERYL TRINITRATE (nitroglycerine).

suspensory ligament any LIGAMENT from which an organ or bodily part hangs, or by which it is supported.

Sustac a brand name for the artery-dilating drug GLYCERYL TRINITRATE (nitroglycerine).

Sustanon a brand name for the male sex hormone drug TESTOSTERONE.

sustentacular supporting.

susceptibility a more than normal tendency to contract an infection or other disease.

suture 1 a length of thread-like material used for surgical sewing or the product of surgical sewing. Sutures are made of many materials including catgut, collagen, linen, silk, nylon, polypropylene, polyester, human FASCIA LATA and stainless steel, and are available in a wide range of thicknesses. Many are provided with a suitable needle swaged on to one or both ends. See also SUTURING.
2 a fixed joint between bones of the vault of the skull.

suturing surgical stitching to close a wound or incision or to approximate parts. Suturing may be continuous or by separated stitches (interrupted suturing) and may employ absorbable SUTURES, such as collagen or catgut, or non-absorbable sutures that may have to be removed.

suxamethonium a short-acting depolarizing muscles relaxant commonly used immediately after inducing general anaesthesia to facilitate the insertion of an endotracheal tube. The drug is on the WHO official list. A brand name is Anectine.

swab 1 a folded piece of loose-woven cotton gauze, or other absorbent material, used in surgery to apply cleaning and antiseptic solutions to the skin and to mop up free blood and other fluids in the course of the operation. 2 a small sterile twist of cotton wool on the end of an orange stick used to obtain bacterial samples for culture and examination.

swallowing difficulty see DYSPHAGIA.

swamp fever see LEPTOSPIROSIS.

Swan-Ganz catheter a soft, flexible, double-bore tube with a small balloon at one end. The catheter is passed along a vein to the right ATRIUM of the heart and the balloon inflated. The force of the blood flow then carries the balloon into the right VENTRICLE and then into the PULMONARY ARTERY, allowing pressure measurements to be made. (Harold James C. Swan, American cardiologist, b. 1922, and William Ganz, American cardiologist, b. 1919).

swayback an increase in the forward curvature of the spine in the lower back region (lumbar LORDOSIS) with a compensatory increase in the backward curvature in the chest region (dorsal KYPHOSIS).

sweat glands tiny, coiled tubular glands deep in the skin that open either directly on to the surface or into hair follicles and secrete a salty liquid. Apocrine glands occur only on hairy areas and open into hair follicles. Apocrine sweat contains organic matter that can be decomposed by skin bacteria and cause odours. Eccrine glands open on the surface, especially of the palms of the hands and the soles of the feet.

sweating see HYPERHIDROSIS.

swimmer's ear see OTITIS EXTERNA.

swimmer's itch skin inflammation (dermatitis) caused by the penetration of CERCARIAE of certain schistosome worms while the subject is immersed in waters. See also SCHISTOSOMIASIS.

swollen glands a misnomer. 'Swollen glands'

are LYMPH NODES enlarged by inflammation or by infiltration with parasites or cancer. Inflammation of lymph nodes is called lymphadenitis.

sycosis barbae barber's itch. An infection of hair follicles in the beard area, usually with *Staphylococcus aureus*, acquired from infected razors or towels. Treatment is with antibiotic drugs and temporary avoidance of shaving.

Sydenham's chorea a nervous system disorder related to an attack of RHEUMATIC FEVER. The condition features restlessness, irritability, slurred speech and involuntary jerky or fidgety movements of the head, face, limbs and hands. The condition is treated by bed rest, antibiotics and sedation and usually settles in 2 or 3 months. Also known as St Vitus' dance. (Thomas Sydenham, 1624–89, English physician).

sym-, syn- *prefix denoting* together, conjointly.

symblepharon adhesion of the layer of CONJUNCTIVA lining the eyelids to the layer lining the eyeball. This results from loss of the 'non-stick' epithelial surface layers.

symbiosis a close association, of inter-dependence or mutual benefit, between two or more organisms, often of different species.

Symmetrel a brand name for AMANTADINE.

sympathectomy an operation to remove the SYMPATHETIC NERVOUS SYSTEM supply to an area in order to limit constriction of the blood vessels and thus improve the blood supply to the part.

sympathetic nervous system one of the two divisions of the AUTONOMIC NERVOUS SYSTEM, the other being the PARASYMPATHETIC. The sympathetic system causes constriction of blood vessels in the skin and intestines and widening (dilatation) of blood vessels in the muscles. It increases the heart rate, dilates the pupils, widens the bronchial air tubes, relaxes the bladder and reduces the activity of the bowel.

sympathetic ophthalmitis a persistent and damaging UVEITIS occurring in a healthy eye following a penetrating injury, or sometimes an intraocular operation, in the other eye.

sympathomimetic of any agent that simulates or stimulates the sympathetic nervous system. ADRENERGIC. Sympathomimetic action can increase the heart output by 100% over resting values. It can constrict arteries and increase the blood pressure. And it can widen the air tubes of the lungs allowing more free access of large volumes of air.

symphysis a joint in which the component bones are immovably held together by strong, fibrous cartilage. There is a symphysis between the two pubic bones at the front of the pelvis.

symptom a subjective perception suggesting bodily defect or malfunction. Symptoms are never perceptible by others. Objective indications of disease are called signs.

symptomatic abacteruria a condition, usually affecting women, in which the symptoms of a urinary infection (frequency, burning on urination and sometimes incontinence) are present, but no bacteria can be found in the urine.

symptomatology 1 the symptomatic features of particular disease or of a particular case of a disease.
2 the study of symptoms and their relation to disease.

syn- *prefix denoting* together, conjointly or joined.

Synacthen a brand name for TETRACOSACTRIN (tetracosactide).

synaesthesia the phenomenon in which stimulations of one sense modality produces the effect of stimulation of another. Thus, a person may consistently experience a particular letter of the alphabet, or a musical tone, as a particular colour.

Synalar a brand name for the steroid drug FLUOCINOLONE, used for local applications.

Synalar C a brand name for FLUOCINOLONE with the antifungal drug CLIOQUINOL.

Synalar N a brand name for FLUOCINOLONE with NEOMYCIN.

Synandone a brand name for the steroid drug FLUOCINOLONE, used for local applications.

synapse the junctional area between two connected nerves, or between a nerve and the effector organ (a muscle fibre or a gland). Nerve impulses are transmitted across a synapse by means of a chemical NEUROTRANSMITTER such as ACETYLCHOLINE or NORADRENALINE. Synapses allow impulses to pass in one direction only and single brain cells may have more than 15 000 synapses with other cells. This complexity, allowing logical 'gate' operation, partly or wholly underlies the computational and storage abilities of the brain.

Synarel a brand name for NAFARELIN.

synarthrosis an immovable junction between bones.

synchondrosis a SYNARTHROSIS in which the bones are joined by a layer of cartilage.

syncope fainting.

synaesthesia a disorder of perception in which stimulation of a sense organ produces, in addition to the normal response, a response in another part of the body, or the effect of stimulation of another sense organ.

syndactyly fusion of two or more adjacent fingers or toes. Syndactyly is usually CONGENITAL. The fusion may involve skin only allowing easy surgical separation, but in more severe cases the bones may also be fused.

syndesmosis a joint in which the bones are connected by ligaments or fibrous sheets.

syndrome a unique combination of sometimes apparently unrelated symptoms or signs, forming a distinct clinical entity. Often the elements of a syndrome are merely distinct effects of a common cause, but sometimes the relationship is one of observed association and the causal link is not yet understood. Originally, the term was applied only to entities of unknown cause but many syndromes have now been elucidated and their names retained because of familiarity. From the Greek *syn*, together, and *dromos*, a course or race.

syndrome E a condition of desensitisation to violence, loss of human sympathy, excessive arousal, obsessive ideas and compulsive repetition that enables affected individuals, nearly all men, to engage in repetitive killing of defenceless people, especially when this is done with the approval of authority. The syndrome has been observed repeatedly throughout human history. Critics have suggested that to call this entity a syndrome may be to excuse it.

synergism cooperative action, especially of groups of muscles, so as to achieve an end impossible by individual action.

Synflex a brand name for the non-steroidal anti-inflammatory drug (NSAID) NAPROXEN.

syngamy the fusion of two GAMETES. Sexual reproduction.

syngenesis sexual reproduction.

Synopessin a brand name for the drug lypressin used in the treatment of DIABETES INSIPIDUS.

Synphase a brand name for ETHINYLOESTRADIOL (ethinylestradiol) formulated with a PROGESTOGEN drug as an oral contraceptive.

synovectomy surgical removal of the SYNOVIAL

MEMBRANE. This may be done as a treatment for persistent SYNOVITIS.

synovial membrane the secretory membrane that lies within the capsule of a joint and produces the clear, sticky, lubricating synovial fluid without which smooth joint movement would be impossible. The synovial membrane covers all the internal structures of the joint except the bearing surfaces (the articular cartilages). Also known as the synovium.

synovioma a tumour, usually benign, of a SYNOVIAL MEMBRANE.

synovitis inflammation of the SYNOVIAL MEMBRANE.

synovium the SYNOVIAL MEMBRANE.

Syntaris a brand name for the corticosteroid drug FLUNISOLIDE.

Syntocinon a brand name for the womb muscle stimulating drug OXYTOCIN.

Syntometrine a brand name for ERGOMETRINE.

syphilis a sexually or congenitally transmitted disease caused by the spirochaete *Treponema pallidum*. In the adult form the first sign is the chancre – a single, small, painless, hard-edged ulcerated crater with a wet base, teeming with spirochaetes, that appears on the genitalia about 3 weeks after exposure. The local lymph nodes enlarge. The chancre heals and the spirochaetes disperse throughout the body to cause a secondary stage, featuring conspicuous skin rashes, and a tertiary stage, many years later, in which the nervous system and the larger arteries may be affected, with serious consequences. Tertiary syphilis may involve TABES DORSALIS, GENERAL PARALYSIS OF THE INSANE and ANEURYSM of the AORTA. Treatment is by a single depot dose of benzathine penicillin G which maintains bactericidal levels for weeks. Resistance to the macrolide antibiotic azithromycin has been detected. This is associated with an A to G point mutation in the 23S ribosomal RNA genes of T. pallidum. See also CONGENITAL SYPHILIS.

Syraprim a brand name for the antibacterial drug TRIMETHOPRIM.

Syrette a brand name for a squeezable tube with a hypodermic needle attached, containing a single dose of a drug, such as MORPHINE, for use in emergency or wartime situations by unskilled persons, or for self-medication.

syring-, syringo- *combining form denoting* a tube or FISTULA.

syringe an instrument, consisting of a barrel and a tight-fitting piston with a connecting rod, used to inject or withdraw fluid. The barrel is usually calibrated in fluid units and the nozzle is shaped to fit a standard range of needles. Luer-lock syringes are designed so that the needle cannot be forced off by high pressure. Most modern syringes are plastic and disposable and are pre-sterilized and supplied in sealed containers.

syringobulbia SYRINGOMYELIA affecting the MEDULLA OBLONGATA of the brainstem.

syringomyelia a rare brainstem or upper spinal cord defect in which the central canal progressively expands and damages adjacent nerve tracts. There is loss of pain and temperature sensation in the neck, shoulders and upper limbs followed by muscle wasting and loss of the sense of touch. Later, there is paralysis and SPASTICITY and progressive disablement.

Syscor MR a brand name for NISOLDIPINE.

system a group of related organs that act together to perform a common function. Body systems include the digestive system, the respiratory system, the cardiovascular system, the urinary system and the reproductive system.

systematic of each body system considered separately.

systemic 1 pertaining to something that affects the whole body rather than one part of it. 2 of the blood circulation supplying all parts of the body except the lungs. 3 of a drug taken by mouth or given by injection, as distinct from a drug applied externally.

systemic amyloidoses a group of diseases that have in common the deposition, outside the cells, of an abnormal, insoluble fibrillary protein called amyloid. In primary AMYLOIDOSIS the amyloid fibrils are monoclonal fragments of antibody (immunoglobulin) light chains. In secondary and familial amyloidoses other proteins, including apolipoprotein, fibrinogen, lysozyme and transthyretin, are involved.

systemic lupus erythematosus the form of LUPUS ERYTHEMATOSUS that affects the body generally.

systemic sclerosis a generalized CONNECTIVE TISSUE disorder featuring FIBROSIS and degeneration of the skin and the internal organs. There is severe RAYNAUD'S

PHENOMENON, swelling of the fingers, pigmentation, shiny atrophy and tightening of the skin so that the face becomes mask-like and there is difficulty in opening the mouth. There is no effective treatment.

systole the period during which the chambers of the heart (the atria and the ventricles) are contracting. Atrial systole, in which blood passes down into the ventricles, precedes the more powerful ventricular systole in which blood is driven into the arteries. Systole alternates with a relaxing period called DIASTOLE.

Sytron a brand name for the iron preparation, sodium iron edetate (sodium feredetate), used in the treatment of iron deficiency ANAEMIA.

t

tabes 1 progressive wasting or emaciation.
2 TABES DORSALIS.

tabes dorsalis degeneration of the sensory
nerve columns in the rear part of the spinal
cord caused by untreated SYPHILIS. There are
severe, stabbing 'lightning' pains in the legs or
lower trunk, unsteadiness and a characteristic
gait in which the feet are kept well apart, lifted
high and stamped forcibly. Joint damage and
foot ulcers occur and vision may be affected
by optic nerve involvement. Treatment with
penicillin can arrest the progress of the disease.
Also known as locomotor ataxia.

tabun a type of nerve gas that acts by interfering
with the enzyme acetylcholinesterase, thereby
prolonging the action of acetylcholine and
causing usually fatal overaction of the
parasympathetic nervous system.

tacalcitol a vitamin D analogue drug used to
treat PSORIASIS. A brand name is Curatoderm.

tache noire the initial sign of the tick-borne
TYPHUS fevers of Africa – a painless, raised red
area with a black centre of dead (necrotic)
tissue, that appears at the site of the tick bite.

tachy- *combining form denoting* rapid or
abnormally rapid.

tachyarrhythmia an excessively rapid and
irregular heart beat.

tachycardia a rapid heart rate from any cause.

tachypnoea abnormally fast breathing, as from
exercise, heart or lung disease or anxiety.

tacrine an acetylcholinase inhibitor drug that
has been found to be of value in 30–40% of
people with mild-to-moderate Alzheimer's
disease. The drug has been approved for use in
the USA but, because of its side effects, not in
the UK. Newer acetylcholinase inhibitors are
being developed.

tacrolimus a potent immunosuppressant
macrolide compound isolated from a
bacterium. Tacrolimus is effective in reducing
the risk of rejection of solid-organ transplants
especially liver transplants. It has been
successfully used as a monotherapy to prevent
graft rejections and has virtually eliminated
immuno-suppression-related morbidity.
It has also been found useful in ointment form
for the treatment of moderate-to-severe atopic
dermatitis in which it has been found as
effective as strong topic steroids. Brand names
are Prograf and Protopic.

tactoreceptor a sensory nerve ending that
responds to touch.

tadalafil an inhibitor of the enzyme
phosphodiesterase-5 which limits penile
erection (see SILDENAFIL CITRATE for fuller
details), used in the treatment of impotence.
The drug takes effect within half an hour,
reaches maximum blood concentration in two
hours and remains effective for up to 36 hours.
It has been available in Britain since February
2003. A brand name is Cialis.

taeniacide a drug that kills tapeworms.

taeniasis TAPEWORM infection either with
the common human tapeworm *Taenia solium*
(the pig tapeworm), *T. saginata* (the beef
tapeworm), or, in some parts of Europe, Africa
and South America, with the fish tapeworm
Diphylobothrium latum.

Tagamet a brand name for CIMETIDINE.

tailbone the COCCYX.

Takayasu disease a disease rare except in
Japan that affects young women causing an
inflammation and narrowing of the major
arteries of the upper part of the body. There
is headache, faintness, muscle wasting and

defective vision from diminished blood supply. The pulses in the upper limb can hardly be felt. Corticosteroids may help but the outlook is poor. Also known as pulseless disease or the aortic arch syndrome. (Michishige Takayasu, 1860–1938, Japanese ophthalmologist).

talcosis a lung disease caused by inhalation of talc dust and characterized by chronic induration and fibrosis.

taliped clubfooted.

talipes clubfoot. A congenital deformity affecting the shape or position of one or both feet. In talipes cavus, there is exaggeration of the curvature of the longitudinal arch. In talipes equinovarus the ankle is extended and the heel and sole turned inwards.

talus the second largest bone of the foot that rests on top of the heel bone (calcaneus) and articulates with the TIBIA and FIBULA to form the ankle joint.

Tambocor a brand name for FLECAINIDE ACETATE.

Tamiflu a brand name for OSELTAMIVIR.

Tamofen a brand name for TAMOXIFEN.

tamoxifen a drug that blocks oestrogen receptors and is useful in the treatment of certain cancers, especially breast cancer. Research involving 37,000 women has shown that tamoxifen substantially improves the survival figures after breast cancer and substantially reduces the probability of cancer in the other breast. The drug also stimulates egg production from the ovaries and can be used to treat infertility. It is on the WHO official list. Brand names are Nolvadex and Tamofen.

tampon a cylindrical mop of absorbent material placed in the VAGINA to absorb menstrual blood and allow freedom of activity during the menstrual period.

tamponade obstruction to the blood flow to or through an organ by external pressure. The term is applied most commonly to compression of the heart, usually from a collection of fluid in the pericardial sac, as in PERICARDITIS or cardiac injury. This prevents normal heart filling and leads to breathlessness and sometimes collapse from reduced heart output. Fluid can be withdrawn through a needle.

Tampovagan a brand name for STILBOESTROL (diethylstilboestrol).

tamsulosin a selective alpha-adrenergic smooth muscle relaxing drug that is used to

relieve the symptoms of enlargement of the PROSTATE GLAND. A brand name is Flomax MR.

tannic acid an antifungal drug, used externally to treat fungus infections of the skin. A brand name of a preparation containing tannic acid and other drugs is Phytex.

tantrum see TEMPER TANTRUM.

tapeworm a ribbon-like population, or colony, of joined flatworms, of the class *Cestoda*, derived from a common head (scolex) equipped with hooks or suckers by which it is attached to the lining of the intestine. Each segment, of which there may be a thousand, is called a proglottid and each contains both male and female reproductive organs. The younger, smaller proglottids release sperms which fertilize the eggs in the older, larger, proglottids. Fertilized segments break off and are passed in the faeces. If these are eaten by an animal (the intermediate host), the larvae develop, travel to the animal's muscles and form cysts, and if such animal meat is eaten, undercooked, the worm is released in the intestine, attaches itself, and the life cycle is continued. Tapeworms can be eliminated with anthelmintic drugs.

tardive dyskinesia involuntary repetitive shaking movements induced by drugs, such as the phenothiazines, that persist or become worse after the drug is withdrawn. The condition usually affects elderly people after years of treatment with the drug.

target cells red blood cells with the haemoglobin disposed as an outer ring and a small circular central mass. Target cells are seen in liver disease and in the HAEMOGLOBINOPATHIES.

tarsal 1 pertaining to the tarsal bones of the foot.
2 pertaining to the fibrous skeleton (tarsal plate) of the eyelid.

tarsal gland a MEIBOMIAN gland in the tarsal plate of the eyelid.

tarsal tunnel syndrome entrapment of the nerves to the foot by pressure from the fibrous band that restrains the tendons (the flexor retinaculum) at the ankle. The effects are weakness of the muscles of the foot and numbness. Compare CARPAL TUNNEL SYNDROME.

tarsus 1 the part of the foot between the leg and the metatarsal bones.
2 the seven bones of the tarsus

3 a fibrous plate that gives rigidity and shape to the eyelid.

tarsalgia pain in the lower part of the ankle and rear part of the foot, often as a result of flattening of the arches of the foot.

tarsorrhaphy sewing together of the eyelids after removal of strips of marginal skin so that the raw areas heal together and remain closed. Tarsorrhaphy may be performed to conceal an unsightly and blind eye, but is also used to protect the CORNEA from drying and damage in excessive protrusion of the eye (EXOPHTHALMOS). BOTULINUM TOXIN can be used as an alternative in cases in which only a few weeks' coverage is needed.

tartar see DENTAL CALCULUS.

taste one of the five special senses. Taste is mediated by specialized nerve endings on the tongue called taste buds. These can distinguish only sweet, salt, sour and bitter, but, in combination with the wide range of perceptible smells, allows an almost infinite number of flavours to be experienced.

taste bud one of the many spherical nests of cells containing specialized nerve endings distributed over the edges and base of the tongue. The taste buds respond to the crude flavours of substances dissolved in saliva. See also TASTE.

tattooing deliberate or accidental insertion of coloured material into the deeper layers of the skin. Tattooing commonly follows deep abrasions or nearby explosions. Brown or black particles buried deep in the skin cause a blue colouring. Decorative tattooing may be complicated by skin infection or allergy, HEPATITIS B, AIDS, PSORIASIS, LICHEN PLANUS and DISCOID LUPUS ERYTHEMATOSUS.

tau protein a major structural protein associated with the microtubules that form the cytoskeleton of nerve cells. An abnormal form with a shorter molecule is found in the helical filaments in senile neural plaques and in the insoluble neurofibrillary tangles of ALZHEIMER'S DISEASE. It is found in the cerebrospinal fluid of people with DEMENTIA but is present in higher concentration in Alzheimer's disease than in other forms of dementia. Abnormal tau protein binds strongly to the normal protein and the latter then become shortened by nerve cell proteolytic enzymes into the abnormal form. The latter is not split by these enzymes.

taurocholic acid one of the bile acids and an important constituent of bile. From the Greek *tauros*, a bull, from the bile of which the acid was first obtained.

tautomers structural ISOMERS that exist in equilibrium with each other. They have identical chemical formulae but their molecular structures differ slightly. A change in tautomeric form in the bases in DNA can cause a mutation as the alteration in the position of the atoms can interfere with the formation of HYDROGEN BONDS between the base pairs.

Tavegil a brand name for CLEMASTINE.

taxane one of a group of diterpene substances derived from the Pacific yew tree *Taxus brevifolia* that have been found useful in cancer treatment. Taxanes have a unique action in permanently stabilizing the microtubule assembly in cells. This prevents chromosome movement and halts cell division. One of the taxanes, PACLITAXEL has been licensed for use and has been found helpful in the treatment of cancer of the ovary resistant to other treatment. A brand name in Taxol. See also TAXOID DRUGS.

taxis movement of an organism toward or away from a stimulus.

Taxol a brand name for PACLITAXEL.

taxoid drugs anticancer drugs such as PACLITAXEL and docetaxel extracted from the needles of the yew *Taxus baccata*. These drugs enhance cellular microtubule assembly and interfere with the depolymerization of tubulin. The result is that cells cannot form the normal mitotic spindle and are unable to divide. As with most other anticancer modalities, the effect is greatest on the most rapidly-dividing cells.

Tay-Sachs disease a recessive genetic disorder, affecting mainly Ashkenazi Jews, in which the absence of an enzyme necessary for the breakdown of ganglioside in the nervous system leads to damaging accumulation of this material. The condition appears soon after birth and features blindness, deafness, progressive dementia, seizures, paralysis and death, usually before the age of 3. There is no effective treatment but the diagnosis can be made before birth by CHORIONIC VILLUS SAMPLING and termination of pregnancy considered. (Warren Tay, 1843–1927, British ophthalmologist; and Bernard Sachs, 1858–1944, American neurologist).

taxon any group of organisms constituting one of the formal categories of classification, such as a phylum, class, order, family, genus, or species. See also TAXONOMY.

taxonomy the science or principles of biological classification and the assignment of appropriate names to species.

tazarotene a RETINOID drug used externally to treat PSORIASIS. A brand name is Zorac.

tazobactam a beta-lactamase inhibitor penicillin antibiotic. A brand name is Tazocin.

Tazocin a brand name for TAZOBACTAM.

TB *abbrev. for* TUBERCULOSIS.

T-box gene family a family of genes that code for a range of transcription factors essential for normal organ development and body pattern development in both vertebrates and invertebrates. The family has a highly-conserved DNA binding feature known as a T-box.

T cell one of the two broad categories of LYMPHOCYTE, the other being the B cell group.

T-cell lymphoma see MYCOSIS FUNGOIDES.

TCP a popular over-the-counter nostrum containing phenol, halogenated phenols and sodium salicylate. TCP commands strong partisanship especially among the elderly and is widely believed to have remarkable properties, some of which must be attributed to its all-pervading aroma.

TDD *abbrev. for* Tuberculosis Diseases Diploma.

tears the secretion of the lacrimal glands. Tears consist of a solution of salt in water with a small quantity of an antibacterial substance called lysozyme. The tear film on the cornea also contains mucus and a thin film of oil.

technetium an artificial radioactive element that can be incorporated into various molecules for use in RADIONUCLIDE SCANNING.

tectum any roof-like body structure such as the back (dorsal) part of the midbrain.

teeth the instruments of biting (incisors), tearing (canines) and grinding (molars) of food. There are 20 primary teeth and 32 permanent teeth, but it is common for one or more of the third molars, at the back (the 'wisdom teeth') to remain within the gum (unerupted) until well into adult life. The permanent teeth are numbered, 1 to 8, from the centre, in each quadrant. A dentist might thus refer to an 'upper right 3' meaning the patient's top right canine tooth.

teething the eruption of the primary teeth. This usually starts around the age of 6 or 7 months and all 20 primary teeth have usually erupted within 30 months. Teething often causes fretfulness but is not a cause of fever, convulsions, diarrhoea or loss of appetite.

Tegretol a brand name for CARBAMAZEPINE.

teichopsia the scintillating scotoma of migraine. A slowly-expanding area of visual loss with a shimmering, jagged border that lasts for about 20 minutes and then fades away leaving normal vision. Teichopsia may or may not be followed by headache. Also known as 'fortification spectra', hence the Greek derivation from *teichos*, a wall, and *ops*, vision. There is anecdotal evidence that teichopsia is commoner in academics and intellectuals than in the general population.

telangiectasia a local or general increase in the size and number of small blood vessels in the skin. Often incorrectly called 'broken veins'. Telangiectasia may be present from birth but may be caused by undue exposure to sunlight or may be a feature of ROSACEA, PSORIASIS, LUPUS ERYTHEMATOSUS and DERMATOMYOSITIS.

telekinesis the alleged movement of objects other than by the application of force. Telekinesis is one of the claimed, but un-demonstrated, phenomena of parapsychology.

telemedicine medical activity in which written, audible and visual communication between doctor and patient, or between medical personnel, is conducted at long range via a communication network such as the Internet or an intranet. This communication can include tele-conferencing, teleconsultation, teleradiology, distance learning and the performing of surgical operations at a remote distance from the patient. Telemedicine broadens the scope of consultation and makes access to experts easier. It can effect considerable savings in medical costs. See also MEDICAL COMPUTING.

telemetry measurement at a distance by radio waves or other means. The method has been used in medical research and diagnosis.

teleoanalysis the process of combining different classes of data and taking evidence from different kinds of sources so as to increase knowledge of the quantitative relationship between a causal factor and the risk of a particular disease. In studies, for instance, of how maternal folic acid intake affects the incidence of neural tube defects, teleoanalysis would combine data on the effect of increased folate intake on serum folate concentration with data on the effect of the latter on the incidence of neural tube defects. Teleoanalysis should be distinguished from meta-analysis in which evidence is combined from a number of studies of the same kind. From the Greek *teleio* meaning 'perfect'.

teleology the belief that there is a purpose or design behind events or phenomena and that they are best explained in terms of their seeming purpose or end. It would, for instance, be a teleological argument to suggest that we have an immune system because, without it, we should all die from infections. Medical scientists tend to reject teleological arguments. Theological arguments are often teleological. From the Greek *tele* meaning 'far off or distant'.

telepathy communication claimed to occur without the interposition of the senses.

Telfast a brand name for FEXOFENADINE.

telomerase the enzyme that can reforms the TELOMERES at the ends of chromosomes. Telomerase is found in cancers and is able to prevent the shortening that would otherwise occur with repeated replication, thus allowing cancerous cells in culture to achieve immortality.

telomeres the sections of DNA that form the natural end of a CHROMOSOME. The points that resist union with fragments of other chromosomes. Telomeres consist of repeated groups of the base sequence TTAGGG, where T, A and G represent the bases thymine, adenine and guanine, respectively. Formation of telomeres involves the shaving-off of some junk DNA at the chromosome end. There is a limit to the number of times that this can occur and this is believed to be the reason for the upper limit in the number of times cells can reproduce. Telomere length is a function of age but there is recent evidence that it may also be an X-linked familial trait.

telophase the last phase of MITOSIS, in which the chromosomes of the two daughter cells are grouped together at each separating pole to form new nuclei.

Temaze a brand name for TEMAZEPAM.

temazepam a benzodiazepine drug used to treat insomnia. A brand name is Normison.

Temgesic a brand name for BUPRENORPHINE.

temoporfin a drug used in photodynamic therapy in the palliative treatment of advanced squamous cell carcinoma of head or neck. A brand name is Foscan.

temperature regulation the process by which body temperature is maintained within narrow limits. Blood temperature is monitored in the hypothalamus of the brain. A drop in temperature prompts closure of the skin blood vessels and shivering; a rise in temperature results in skin flushing and sweating so that heat may be lost by radiation and evaporation. In fevers, the hypothalamic thermostat is set high and shivering and skin vessel closure raise the temperature.

temper tantrum an expression of frustration by a child who is prevented from demonstrating unconstrained action. The temper tantrum is an effective weapon in the war of independence and may involve screaming, floor-rolling, head-banging and breath-holding.

temporal pertaining to the temples.

temporal arteritis a disease of the elderly in which the walls of certain arteries in the head become inflamed and thickened so that blood flow is reduced or stopped. The arteries of the temple become prominent, red and exquisitely tender. There is a serious danger that the arteries to the eyes may become affected and cause blindness. The diagnosis is assisted by a raised blood sedimentation rate. Urgent treatment with steroids is necessary to save the sight. Also known as giant cell arteritis.

temporal bone one of two bones forming part of the sides and base of the skull and containing the hearing apparatus. Each temporal bone bears the mastoid process and articulates on its under surface with the head of the jaw bone (mandible).

temporal lobe epilepsy a variety of EPILEPSY in which the effects are limited to the result of discharge in a localized part of the side of the brain. Attacks feature the perception of unpleasant noises, smells and tastes, and, in children, hyperactivity and rage. There may be grimacing, rotational movements of the head and eyes and sucking and chewing movements. Temporal lobe epilepsy is classified as a type of focal or partial seizure epilepsy.

temporomandibular joint the joint, immediately in front of the ear, between the head of the lower jaw bone (the mandible) and the under side of the temporal bone of the skull. Movement at this joint can often be seen through the skin if the mouth is opened widely.

temporomandibular joint replacement a surgical procedure to replace the hinge joint of the jawbone with a prosthesis in cases of severe limitation of mouth opening from disease or derangement of this joint.

temporomandibular joint syndrome pain in the side of the face and ear from the effects of spasm of the chewing muscles on the articulation of the jawbone (the temporo-mandibular joint) which lies just in front of the ear. The condition is usually due to emotional tension reflected in muscle contraction.

Tempra a brand name for PARACETAMOL.

ten day rule the regulation, observed in all X-ray departments, that radiological examination of the lower abdomen in women of childbearing age should be restricted to the 10 days immediately following the first day of the last menstrual period. This is to avoid irradiating a young embryo.

tenderness pain elicited by touch or pressure.

tendinitis inflammation of a TENDON, usually from injury.

tendolysis an operation to free a TENDON from adhesions to the inside of the sheath in which it moves.

tendon a strong band of COLLAGEN fibres that joins muscle to bone or cartilage and transmits the force of muscle contraction to cause movement. Tendons are often provided with sheaths in which they move smoothly, lubricated by a fluid secreted by the sheath lining. Tendons may become inflamed, or may be torn or cut.

tendon jerk a reflex contraction of the muscle to which a tendon is attached when the tendon is struck sharply so as to exert a sudden pull on the muscles. This reflex demonstrates the integrity of both the sensory and the motor nerve supply to the muscle. An exaggerated response may indicate the absence of higher nervous control on the reflex.

tendon of Achilles SEE ACHILLES' TENDON.

tendon transfer an operation to disconnect a TENDON from its normal insertion and connect it to a new site, so that its muscle can perform a different function, such as restoring movement to a paralysed part.

tenesmus a frequently recurring or continuous sense of wishing to empty the bowels. Tenesmus leads to ineffective straining and is a feature of the IRRITABLE BOWEL SYNDROME, HAEMORRHOIDS, ULCERATIVE COLITIS, DYSENTERY, POLYPS in the RECTUM, PROLAPSE of the rectum and sometimes cancer of the rectum.

tennis elbow inflammation of the bony prominence on the outer side of the elbow caused by overuse of the forearm muscle whose TENDONS are attached to this point. Treatment involves rest, temporary immobilization, the use of anti-inflammatory drugs and professional advice on playing technique. The condition has been successfully treated with botulinum toxin.

tenofovir disoproxil an antiviral drug of the nucleotide analogue reverse transcriptase inhibitor class. It is used in combination with other ani-HIV drugs mainly to treat HIV infections that have shown reduced sensitivity to other treatment regimens. A brand name is Viread.

Tenoretic a brand name for ATENOLOL.

Tenormin a brand name for ATENOLOL.

tenosynovitis inflammation of a tendon sheath, usually from overuse. There is pain, swelling, limitation of movement and a creaking sensation on movement of the tendon in its sheath. The condition is treated by rest, immobilization and injections of corticosteroid drugs around the affected tendon.

tenotomy complete or partial surgical cutting of a tendon to abolish or weaken the effect of a muscle.

tenovaginitis inflammation of the sheath surrounding a tendon.

tenoxicam a NON-STEROIDAL ANTI-INFLAMMATORY DRUG used to treat arthritis and other painful conditions. A brand name is Mobiflex.

TENS *abbrev. for* Transcutaneous Electrical Nerve Stimulation. This is a method of treating long-persistent pain by passing small electric currents into the spinal cord or sensory nerves by means of electrodes applied to the skin. The necessary equipment is miniaturized and is readily portable.

tension muscle contraction as a reflection of anxiety. Most headaches are caused in this way. Tension, and associated symptoms, can often be relieved by formal relaxation procedures.

Tensipine MR a brand name for NIFEDIPINE.

tensor a muscle that tenses a part.

terat-, terato- *combining form denoting* developmental abnormality.

teratogen any agent capable of causing a severe congenital bodily anomaly (monstrosity).

teratogenesis the production of a fetal congenital bodily abnormality.

teratology the study of the processes operating during early embryonic and fetal development that lead to major anomalies of body structure.

teratoma a tumour formed from germ cells showing various degrees of differentiation. Most teratomas occur in the ovaries or testicles. Some teratomas are benign, some malignant.

terazosin a selective alpha-adrenergic blocker drug used to treat high blood pressure and to relieve the symptoms of simple enlargement of the PROSTATE GLAND (benign prostatic hyperplasia). A brand name is Hytrin.

terbinafine an antifungal drug that acts by causing leakage of the fungal cell contents through the fungal cell wall. It is especially useful against TINEA of the skin and nails for which it is said to be more effective than clotrimazole. A brand name is Lamisil.

terbutaline a bronchodilator drug used in the treatment of ASTHMA, BRONCHITIS and EMPHYSEMA. It is also used to relax the muscle of the womb and prevent premature labour. A brand name is Bricanyl.

terfenadine a non-sedating antihistamine drug used to treat ALLERGIC RHINITIS and URTICARIA. The drug can cause heart irregularities and should not be used by people with heart or liver disease. It should not be taken with grapefruit juice which increases its bioavailability.

teriparatide a drug used to treat advanced OSTEOPOROSIS. Teriparatide consists of fragments of parathyroid hormone produced by recombinant DNA technology. These preferentially stimulate osteoblasts over osteoclasts thus increasing new bone formation. The drug is given by subcutaneous injection via a pre-filled pen injector.

terlipressin a drug that releases vasopressin over a period of hours. This is used to help to control bleeding from OESOPHAGEAL VARICES by constricting the small arteries in the intestinal tract. A brand name is Glypressin.

terminal care care of the dying.

termination codon see STOP CODON.

termination of pregnancy see ABORTION.

Terramycin a now historic brand name for the tetracycline antibiotic OXYTETRACYCLINE. The drug is now prescribed in its generic form as oxytetracycline.

Terrence Higgins Trust a charitable community-based aid organization that provides current information to HIV-infected and at-risk individuals. It was named after one of the earliest victims of AIDS in the UK.

tertian recurring on alternate days (on the third day).

tertian fever fever in MALARIA caused by the invasion of new red blood cells by Plasmodium vivax. This occurs in a 48 hour cycle.

tertiary the ordinal that follows primary and secondary, used especially when the third stage of a disease has distinct characteristics, as in SYPHILIS.

tertiary structure used mainly of a protein to refer to its three-dimensional folded shape in space. The primary structure is simply the order of the amino acids in the polypeptide chain; the secondary structure may be a coiling, the alpha helix, or a layering known as the beta-pleated sheet. The tertiary structure is determined by chemically active groups spaced along the chain that attract each other to form bonds at specific positions. The tertiary structure of proteins such as enzymes, is crucial to their function.

Tertroxin a brand name for LIOTHYRONINE SODIUM.

testicle see TESTIS.

testicular feminization syndrome a rare X-linked, genetically induced defect of the male sex hormone receptors on the surface of body cells in men. Male hormones are thus unable to act and normal male characteristics cannot develop. There is male PSEUDOHERMAPHRODITISM. The testicles are present, but undescended, the penis is rudimentary and there is a short, blind-ended vagina. The breasts may be well developed. It is usual to removed the testicles and give female sex hormones to promote full development of the nominal female sex.

testis one of the two male gonads, suspended in the scrotum by the spermatic cord. The testis, or testicle, contains the long, coiled seminiferous tubules in which the SPERMATOZOA are formed. Between the tubules are cells that secrete testosterone and other masculinizing steroid hormones and oestrogens.

testis disorders see EPIDIDYMITIS, ORCHITIS, TORSION OF TESTIS and UNDESCENDED TESTIS.

test meal a now largely superseded test for the secretion of stomach acid. A small quantity of liquid food is left in the stomach for a short period and then sucked out through a tube for analysis.

testosterone the principal male sex hormone (androgen) produced in the INTERSTITIAL cells of the TESTIS and, to a lesser extent in the OVARY. Testosterone is ANABOLIC and stimulates bone and muscle growth and the growth of the sexual characteristics. It is also used as a drug to treat delayed puberty or some cases of infertility or to help to treat breast cancer in post-menopausal women. It may be given by mouth, depot injection or skin patch. The drug is on the WHO official list. Brand names are Andropatch, Restandol, Sustanon, Testogel and Virormone.

test tube baby a popular term for a baby derived from an ovum fertilized outside the body (in vitro fertilization).

tetanus a serious infection of the nervous system caused by the organism *Clostridium tetani* which gains access to the body by way of penetrating wounds. The organism produces a powerful toxin which causes muscles to contract violently, and an early sign is spasm of the chewing muscles (trismus) so that there is great difficulty in opening the mouth ('lockjaw'). Spasm spreads to the muscles of the face and neck, producing a snarling, mirthless smile ('risus sardonicus'), and to the back muscles which become rigid. In severe cases, the back becomes strongly arched backwards. There is also fever, sore throat and headache. Death may occur from exhaustion or ASPHYXIA. Tetanus is treated with human antitetanus immunoglobulin and large doses of antibiotics or METRONIDAZOLE. A recent study of 120 patients showed that the intrathecal route for immunoglobulin was more effective than the intramuscular route. Spasms are controlled by intravenous DIAZEPAM but it may be necessary to paralyse the patient temporarily with curare and maintain respiration artificially. Tetanus is easily prevented by immunization with tetanus toxoid. Compare TETANY.

tetany muscle spasm resulting from abnormally low levels of blood calcium. This can result from a reduction in blood acidity from deliberate or hysterical over-breathing (hyperventilation) or from underaction of the PARATHYROID GLANDS. Tetany affects mainly the hands and feet, causing a claw-like effect with extension of the nearer joints and bending of the outer joints (carpopedal spasm). Compare TETANUS.

tetracaine hydrochloride a local anaesthetic drug. The preferred term for AMETHOCAINE. The drug is on the WHO official list.

tetracosactrin tetracosactide, an analogue of ACTH used as a test of adrenal function. An injection of the drug is given and the resulting rise in serum cortisol is monitored. A brand name is Synacthen.

tetracycline one of a group of antibiotic drugs originally derived from *Streptomyces* species. They are used to treat a wide range of infections including RICKETTSIAL DISEASES, CHOLERA, BRUCELLOSIS, LYME DISEASE and most of the SEXUALLY TRANSMITTED DISEASES. They have the disadvantage that they are deposited in bones and teeth and will cause permanent yellow staining of the latter if given to young children. They will similarly affect fetuses if given to women in late pregnancy. The tetracyclines have a useful effect on ACNE and ROSACEA. This does not imply that acne is an infection. Tetracyclines are effective in acne because non-pathogenic bacteria present in the sebum in acne produce enzymes that separate fatty acids from the fats and these acids cause inflammation. Tetracyclines are concentrated in sebum, while penicillins are not. Tetracyclines are on the WHO official drug list. Brand names are Achromycin, Deteclo and, for external use, Topicycline.

tetrahydroaminoacridine a drug that has been used experimentally to try to improve the situation of people with ALZHEIMER'S DISEASE.

tetrahydrobiopterin see PHENYLKETONURIA.

tetrahydrofuryl salicylate a formulation of drugs for external use that cause reddening of the skin and increase the blood flow in the underlying tissue. A rubefacient. A brand name is Transvasin.

tetrahydrolipstatin an early anti-obesity pill of the class that acts by preventing the absorption of dietary fats. Experience has shown the disadvantages of this seemingly ideal way to enjoy the best of both worlds – abdominal discomfort, loss of fat-soluble vitamins, loss of advantageous fats such as fish oils, fatty stools hard to flush, and loss of the incentive to try to control greediness.

tetralogy of Fallot see FALLOT'S TETRALOGY.

Tetralysal a brand name for LYMECYCLINE.

tetraplegia quadriplegia. Paralysis of all four limbs.

Tetrex a brand name for TETRACYCLINE.

tetrodotoxin puffer fish toxin, one of the most powerful known neurotoxins with a mortality of about 50%. There is no known antidote.

thalamus one of two masses of grey matter lying on either side of the midline in the lower part of the brain. It receives sensory nerve fibres from the spinal cord and connections from the midbrain, the eyes, the ears and the cerebral CORTEX. It sends fibres to the sensory part of the cerebral cortex. It is the collecting, coordinating and selecting centre for almost all sensory information, other than OLFACTORY, received by the body. Only part of the mass of information it receives is passed to the cortex. From the Greek thalamos, an inner chamber.

thalassaemia one of several hereditary abnormalities of synthesis of the globin chains of HAEMOGLOBIN leading to severe ANAEMIA. The disorder is common in the area surrounding the Mediterranean sea. When the abnormality is HETEROZYGOUS (thalassaemia minor), disability is minimal, but when HOMOZYGOUS (thalassaemia major), anaemia may be severe with breathlessness, jaundice, spleen enlargement and sometimes physical and mental retardation. Treatment is by blood transfusion and bone marrow transplantation. From the Greek words thelazia, the sea, and haima, blood.

thalidomide a drug (Distaval and many other brand names) that was widely advertised as a safe sedative. In 1961 it was found that, when given to pregnant women, it caused severe bodily malformation of the fetus with stunting of the limbs, which were often replaced by short flippers (phocomelia), and other congenital defects. Thalidomide is an ANGIOGENESIS inhibitor, anti-inflammatory and immunomodulator and has been found useful in the treatment of erythema nodosum leprosum, rheumatoid arthritis, Crohn's disease, HIV-associated Kaposi's sarcoma, a range of cancers, and Behçet's syndrome. It was approved by the US Food and Drug Administration (FDA) for the treatment of leprosy in 1997.

thallium a rare metallic element of which a radioactive ISOTOPE is used in RADIONUCLIDE SCANNING of the heart. Thallium scanning can reveal areas of heart muscle that are deprived of a normal blood supply as a result of coronary artery occlusion.

thanatology 1 the study of death.

2 the forensic study of the causes of death and their relation to postmortem appearances.

THC abbrev. for tetrahydrocannabinol, the active ingredient in marijuana.

theca a casing, outer covering or sheath.

thenar eminence the fleshy, muscular mass on the palm at the base of the thumb.

theophylline a bronchodilator drug used to treat asthma and to assist in the treatment of HEART FAILURE by increasing the heart rate and reducing OEDEMA by promoting excretion of urine. The drug is on the WHO official list. Brand names are Nuelin SA, Slo-Phyllin and Uniphyllin Continus. Franol is a theophylline preparation with EPHEDRINE.

therapeutic community a small local population of people of strong antisocial tendency, set up under the supervision of medical staff but in a non-clinical environment, to try to treat personality disorder. The object is to demonstrate the effects of such behaviour and to try to instil constructive patterns of conduct and improve social and interpersonal skills. Results have been promising.

therapeutics the branch of medicine concerned with treatment of disease and injury.

therapist 1 a person providing or conduct-ing any form of medical or psychological treatment. 2 a psychotherapist.

therapy treatment of disease or of conditions supposed to be diseases. The term is often qualified to limit its range, as in CHEMOTHERAPY, PHYSIOTHERAPY, PSYCHOTHERAPY, RADIOTHERAPY, HYDROTHERAPY and HYPNOTHERAPY.

therm-, thermo- combining form denoting heat.

thermocoagulation destruction of tissue by locally applied high temperatures, as in ELECTROCAUTERY or by using a high-frequency alternating current.

thermography a scanning technique in which temperature differences on the surface of the skin are represented as an image or as colour differences. Thermography readily demonstrates areas of inflammation and variations in blood supply, but has not proved particularly useful as an aid to diagnosis.

thermometer a device for registering body temperature. Thermometers may be analogue, as in the case of the common mercury expansion thermometer or colour-change devices, or may have a digital display.

thermoreceptor a sensory receptor that responds to heat.

thermoregulation the control of body temperature and its maintenance within narrow limits in spite of factors tending to change it.

thermotherapy treatment of disease by local or general application of heat. This is neither particularly useful nor widely used.

thiabendazole tiabendazole, an ANTHELMINTIC drug used to get rid of worms such as *Toxocara canis*, *Strongyloides stercoralis* and *Trichinella spiralis*.

thiazolidinediones a class of drugs used to combat INSULIN RESISTANCE in patients with Type 2 DIABETES. These drugs are insulin sensitizing agents and act by binding selectively to preoxisome-proliferator-activated gamma receptors (PPAR). These regulate gene expression in response to binding.

thioacetazone with isoniazid a drug combination that has been used in the primary treatment of pulmonary tuberculosis. The combination is on the WHO official list.

thiamine vitamin B_1. The drug is on the WHO official list. See also VITAMINS.

thienobenzodiazepines drugs used for the maintenance treatment of SCHIZOPHRENIA. An example is olanzapine (Zyprexa).

thioguanine tioguanine, a drug used in the treatment of acute myeloblastic leukaemia. A brand name is Lanvis.

thiomersal a mercurial antiseptic often used to sterilize eye drops and other solutions.

thiopentone sodium thiopental, a barbiturate drug used as a pleasant and rapid induction agent for general anaesthesia. The drug is given by slow intravenous injection. The drug is on the WHO official list. A brand name is Thiopental.

thioridazine an antipsychotic drug used to treat SCHIZOPHRENIA and MANIA. A brand name is Melleril.

thioxanthenes a class of antipsychotic drugs used mainly to treat SCHIZOPHRENIA. Examples are flupenthixol (flupentixol) (Depixol,

Fluanxol) and zuclopenthixol (Clopixol).

third generation oral contraceptives see ORAL CONTRACEPTIVE.

third ventricle the small, slit-like midline, fluid-filled space in the centre of the brain which communicates with the two large lateral ventricles, one in each hemisphere, and with the FOURTH VENTRICLE behind.

thirst the strong desire to drink, arising from water shortage (dehydration) causing an increased concentration of substances dissolved in the blood. This change is monitored by nerve receptors in the HYPOTHALAMUS in the brain, and thirst is induced by a nerve reflex.

thorac-, thoraco- *combining form denoting* chest.

thoracic pertaining to the chest.

thoracic duct the main terminal duct of the lymphatic system that runs up alongside the spine from the abdomen to the root of the neck and then discharges into the large neck veins.

thoracic outlet syndromes a group of conditions in which nerves to the arm, or the SUBCLAVIAN ARTERY, are compressed or angulated by a CERVICAL RIB, an abnormal first rib, the edges of muscles in the region or by a band of tissue running from the side of the lowest neck vertebra to the first rib. The effects include pain, tingling and numbness in the arm and hand, on the little finger border, and weakness or even atrophy of the small muscles of the hand. Surgical treatment may be needed to relieve the pressure.

thoracic surgeon a surgeon specializing in operative treatment within the chest cavity, especially on the windpipe (trachea), the lungs, the heart and the gullet (oesophagus).

thoracoplasty the removal of part of a rib or of several ribs so as to collapse the underlying lung and promote healing of disease such as TUBERCULOSIS. The method is now obsolete.

thoracotomy a surgical opening in the chest wall made to gain access to the interior. Most thoracotomies are made between the ribs but access to the heart usually involves splitting the breastbone vertically and prizing the halves apart.

thorax the part of the trunk between the neck and the ABDOMEN. The thorax contains a central compartment, the MEDIASTINUM that contains the heart and separates the two lungs. The thorax also contains the TRACHEA, the

OESOPHAGUS, a number of large arteries and veins connected to the heart. Its walls consist of the dorsal VERTEBRA, the breastbone (sternum) and the rib cage.

thought disorders a group of mental aberrations occurring in schizophrenia and various forms of dementia. They include false beliefs (DELUSIONS), memory loss, defects of attention and concentration, thought blocking and flight of ideas. Thought disorders may also be manifested by the use of word connections on the basis of phonetic resemblance rather than logic (clang associations) and by the use of meaningless or invented words (neologisms).

threadworms intestinal parasitic worms which infect at least 20% of children at any one time. *Enterobius vermicularis* is a small, white worm about 1 cm long with a blunt head and a fine, hair-like, pointed tail. Eggs are laid on the skin around the child's anus and itching causes scratching and reinfection via the mouth. Threadworms can be removed with drugs such as mebendazole or piperazine, but all the members of the family must be treated. Also known as pinworms.

threonine one of the 20 AMINO ACIDS that form proteins and an essential ingredient in the diet. The substance is used as one of the ingredients in the externally-applied antibiotic preparation Cicatrin.

thrill a coarse vibrating sensation felt with the flat of the hand on the front of the chest. Thrills are caused by severe turbulence in blood flow in the heart from valve disease or congenital heart disorder and are always audible with a STETHOSCOPE. They can be considered as exaggerated heart murmurs.

throat see PHARYNX.

throat lump see GLOBUS HYSTERICUS.

thromb-, thrombo- *combining form denoting* blood clot or THROMBUS.

thrombasthenia an obsolescent term for the condition in which blood platelets are present in normal numbers but do not function normally in their role in blood clotting. The condition may be inherited but is more commonly acquired. With the rapid growth in understanding of platelet function this term is likely to disappear.

thrombectomy surgical removal of a blood clot from an artery or vein.

thrombin an enzyme in the blood that converts fibrinogen to fibrin, thus forming a blood clot.

thromboangiitis obliterans see BUERGER'S DISEASE.

thrombocyte a blood PLATELET, one of the numerous, non-nucleated fragments derived from the large cells, the megakaryocytes, and necessary for blood clotting.

thrombocythaemia an abnormally high number of blood PLATELETS and megakaryocytes. There is an abnormal tendency to THROMBOSIS, but also to bleeding. The platelet number can be reduced by chemotherapy or radioactive phosphorus.

thrombocytopenia an abnormally low number of PLATELETS in the blood. The lower limit of normality is about 150,000 per cubic millimetre. See also THROMBOCYTOPENIC PURPURA.

thrombocytopenic purpura visible haemorrhages into the skin, mucous membranes and elsewhere resulting from a decreased number of PLATELETS (thrombocytes) per unit volume of blood. Platelets are necessary for normal clotting of the blood.

thrombocytosis an increase above normal in the number of PLATELETS (thrombocytes) in the circulating blood. The normal upper limit is about 450,000 per cubic millimetre. Thrombocytosis may be a reactive process or it may be the result of a clonal increase in the number of megakaryocytes in the bone marrow. The production of platelets from megakaryocytes requires the binding of thrombopoietin to these cells. Other (disease) processes can result in increased production of thrombopoietin. In clonal thrombocytosis, impaired binding of thrombopoietin results in an increase in free thrombopoietin and increased platelet production.

thromboembolectomy surgical removal of an EMBOLUS that arose from a blood clot (thrombus) elsewhere in the circulation.

thromboembolism an EMBOLISM caused by a dislodged THROMBUS.

thrombolytic drugs drugs that dissolve blood clots and can be useful in the treatment of THROMBOSIS or EMBOLISM affecting any part of the body. Also known as fibrinolytic drugs.

thrombophilia a tendency to blood clotting within the blood vessels (a hypercoagulable state). The condition, which may be of genetic origin results from any defect or deficiency of a natural anticoagulant such as activated protein C, antithrombin or protein S. Resistance to activated protein C is an important cause. Thrombophilia increases the probability of heart attacks, strokes and, in pregnant women, miscarriage.

thrombophlebitis inflammation of a vein (phlebitis) with resulting local clotting of the blood. In a vein near the surface, this causes redness, swelling, acute TENDERNESS and often fever and general upset. Deep vein thrombophlebitis produces similar symptoms but may also lead to the formation of a long, loose, soft, eel-like clot that can break away and cause serious or fatal plugging of the main lung arteries (PULMONARY EMBOLISM).

thromboplastin blood clotting Factor III, an obsolete term referring to what is now known to be several blood clotting factors operating together.

thrombopoietin a hormone responsible for the growth of colonies of megakaryocytes and the production of platelets. The existence of thrombopoietin has been suspected for 30 years but was realized only in 1994. In 1997 the results of a trial of polyethylene-conjugated genetically-engineered (recombinant) thrombopoietin – described as recombinant human megakatyocyte growth and development factor (PEGrHuMGDF) – was published. It was found to have a powerful stimulatory effect on PLATELET production. Thrombopoietin is the ligand for the cytokine receptor Mpl.

thrombosis clotting of blood within an artery or vein so that the blood flow is reduced or impeded. If the vessel is supplying a vital part, such as the heart muscle or the brain, and the thrombosis cuts off the flow, the result may be fatal. Thrombosis of arteries supplying limbs or organs may lead to GANGRENE. See also CORONARY THROMBOSIS and CEREBRAL THROMBOSIS.

thrombosis, cavernous sinus see CAVERNOUS SINUS THROMBOSIS.

thrombosis, coronary see CORONARY THROMBOSIS.

thrombosis, cerebral see CEREBRAL THROMBOSIS.

thrombosis, deep vein see THROMBOPHLEBITIS.

thrombotest a test of the coagulability of the blood used to monitor treatment with anticoagulant drugs. It is a modified prothrombin time test that measures Factor IX and other factors dependent on vitamin K.

thrombotic thrombocytopenic purpura a disseminated thrombotic microangiopathy similar to the childhood haemolytic-uraemic syndrome and featuring low platelet counts, haemolytic anaemia, fever, kidney damage and neurological disorders. Affected people have unusually large forms of the von Willebrand factor, and it was reported at the end of 1998 that the non-familial form is due to an inhibitor of the protease enzyme that cleaves the von Willebrand factor. The familial form is due to a deficiency of the enzyme.

thromboxane a substance similar to the prostaglandins that promotes blood clotting. Aspirin in small doses reduces the production of thromboxane by PLATELETS.

thrombus a blood clot forming especially on the wall of a blood vessel. This is commonly the result of local damage to the inner lining of the vessel (the endothelium).

thrush infection with the common fungus of the genus *Candida*, especially by the species *Candida albicans*. Thrush mainly affects the warm, moist areas of the body such as the mouth or the vagina but any part of the skin may be affected. There is persistent itching or soreness and characteristic white patches, like soft cheese, with raw-looking inflamed areas in between. Thrush also causes vaginal discharge. The condition is treated with antifungal drugs, such as CLOTRIMAZOLE, MICONAZOLE or NYSTATIN, in ointments, creams or PESSARIES.

thunderclap headache a very severe headache that occurs suddenly and without warning. Such headaches may signify several dangerous possibilities including subarachnoid haemorrhage, dissection of a vertebral or carotid artery or a cerebral venous sinus thrombosis. More commonly, the thunderclap headache implies nothing more grave than a migraine.

thymic aplasia congenital absence of the THYMUS.

thymine a pyrimidine base, one of the four whose particular sequence forms the genetic code in the deoxyribonucleic acid (DNA) molecule.

thymoma any tumour of the THYMUS gland.

Thymomas are often associated with MYASTHENIA GRAVIS and this can sometimes be cured by removal of the tumour.

thymoxamine moxisylyte, a drug that widens blood vessels (vasodilator) and may be useful in the management of RAYNAUD'S DISEASE. A brand name is Opilon.

thymus a small flat organ of the lymphatic system situated immediately behind the breastbone, that is apparent in children but inconspicuous after puberty. The thymus processes primitive LYMPHOCYTES so that they differentiate into the T cells of the immune system.

thyro- *combining form denoting* thyroid.

thyroglossal cyst a cyst formed within remnants of the THYROGLOSSAL DUCT.

thyroglossal duct a duct in the embryo that runs between the THYROID GLAND and the back of the tongue. Normally, the thyroglossal duct disappears before birth but part or all of it may persist.

thyroid cartilage the largest of the cartilages of the LARYNX, consisting of two backward-sloping, broad processes joined in front to form the protuberance in the neck known popularly as the Adam's apple.

thyroidectomy surgical removal of part, or sometimes the whole, of the THYROID GLAND. This is done to reduce the output of thyroid hormones in some cases of THYROTOXICOSIS and GOITRE, and in the treatment of thyroid cancer. After total thyroidectomy replacement thyroid hormone (thyroxine, levothyroxine) must be given.

thyroid function tests tests of the production of the thyroid hormones thyroxine (T_4), which has four iodine atoms in the molecule, and triiodothyronine (T_3), which has three. This can be done by measuring the rate at which radioactive iodine is accumulated by the gland. The amounts of the two hormones in the blood can also be measured in the laboratory using samples of serum taken from the patient. Thyroid function can be measured indirectly by assessing the rate of the body's oxygen consumption in the resting state. This is called the basal metabolic rate (BMR).

thyroid gland an ENDOCRINE GLAND, situated in the neck like a bow tie across the front of the upper part of the windpipe (trachea). The gland secretes hormones that act directly on almost all the cells in the body to control the rate of their METABOLISM.

thyroid gland disorders see CRETINISM, DYSHORMONOGENESIS, GOITRE HASHIMOTO'S THYROIDITIS, HYPERTHYROIDISM, HYPOTHYROIDISM and THYROTOXICOSIS. Other disorders include painless sporadic thyroiditis, painless postpartum thyroiditis, painful subacute thyroiditis, suppurative thyroiditis, drug-induced thyroiditis and RIEDEL'S THYROIDITIS. There are many synonyms for these various forms.

thyroiditis inflammation of the thyroid gland. See THYROID GLAND DISORDERS.

thyroid scanning a method of assessing the rate of uptake of iodine by, and the pattern of distribution in, the thyroid gland using a compound containing radioactive iodine and a GAMMA CAMERA.

thyroid-stimulating hormone the hormone, thyrotropin, produced by the PITUITARY GLAND that prompts secretion of thyroxine (levothyroxine) by the thyroid gland.

thyrotoxicosis the disorder resulting from excessive production of thyroid hormones, so that all cellular metabolic processes are accelerated. Thyrotoxicosis is much commoner in women than in men. The majority of cases are of AUTOIMMUNE origin. There is loss of weight, good appetite, a fast, irregular pulse, anxiety, inability to relax, shakiness, palpitation, sweating and dislike of hot weather and frequent bowel actions. Retraction of the upper eyelids causes a staring appearance and the eyes may protrude (EXOPHTHALMOS) from swelling of the tissues behind them. Treatment is with drugs, such as carbimazole, methimazole and thiouracil, which reduce the activity of the gland, by the use of radioactive iodine which concentrates in the gland or by surgical removal of part of the gland (partial THYROIDECTOMY).

thyrotrophin releasing hormone a hormone produced in the HYPOTHALAMUS that passes to the PITUITARY GLAND where it prompts the secretion of thyroid stimulating hormone.

thyroxine the principal thyroid hormone. Thyroxine has four iodine atoms in the molecule and is often known as T_4. The sodium salt of thyroxide (levothyroxine) is sold as a drug used to treat thyroid deficiency disorders (hypothyroidism) under the brand name Eltroxin.

tiaprofenic acid a NON-STEROIDAL ANTI-INFLAMMATORY DRUG (NSAID) of the propionic acid group, used to treat a wide range of arthritic and muscular inflammatory disorders. A brand name is Surgam.

tibia the shin bone, the stronger of the two long bones in the lower leg. The front surface of the tibia lies immediately beneath the skin. Its upper end articulates with the femur (thigh bone) to form the knee joint and the lower end forms part of the ankle joint. Its companion bone, the fibula, lies on its outer side and is attached to it by ligaments.

tibolone a synthetic sex hormone drug used to treat menopausal and post-menopausal symptoms and disorders and to reduce the tendency to osteoporosis. A brand name is Livial.

ticarcillin a penicillin antibiotic useful for its action against the organism *Pseudomonas aeruginosa*. The drug is formulated with the CLAVULANIC ACID under the brand name Timentin.

ticlopidine a thienopyridine drug that interacts with platelet glycoprotein in such a way as to inhibit platelet function. It has been found useful in preventing vein grafts from becoming occluded by thrombosis.

tics repetitive, twitching or jerking movements of any part of the face or body and occurring at irregular intervals to release emotional tension. Children are commonly affected but tics seldom persist into adult life. They do not indicate organic disorder and can be controlled by an effort of will. See also GILLES DE LA TOURETTE SYNDROME.

tic douloureux see TRIGEMINAL NEURALGIA.

ticks small, eight-legged, blood-sucking ectoparasites of the family *Ixodoidea*. Ticks can transmit LYME DISEASE, Q FEVER, RELAPSING FEVER, ROCKY MOUNTAIN SPOTTED FEVER, TULARAEMIA and VIRAL ENCEPHALITIS. Some ticks secrete a toxin in the saliva that can cause paralysis.

Tietze's syndrome persistent inflammation of the cartilages between the ribs and the breast-bone causing pain and tenderness in the front of the chest wall, made worse by movement. There may be a tender lump at the site of the pain. The condition is treated with painkilling (ANALGESIC) drugs and nonsteroidal anti-inflammatory drugs (NSAIDs) and passes off

after a few months. (Alexander Tietze, 1864–1927, German surgeon).

Tilade a brand name for NEDOCROMIL.

Tildiem a brand name for the calcium channel blocker anti-ANGINA drug DILTIAZEM.

Tiloryth a brand name for ERYTHROMYCIN.

tiludronic acid a BISPHOSPHONATE drug used to treat PAGET'S DISEASE of bone. A brand name is Skelid.

timolol a non-cardioselective beta-blocker drug used to treat high blood pressure (HYPERTENSION), ANGINA PECTORIS, MIGRAINE and, in the form of eye drops, to treat GLAUCOMA. The drug is on the WHO official list. Brand names are Timoptol LA, Betim and Nyogel.

Timopotol a brand name for eye drops containing TIMOLOL, used to control GLAUCOMA.

Timoptol LA a brand name for an ophthalmic gel-forming solution containing TIMOLOL, used to control GLAUCOMA.

Tinacidin a brand name for TOLNAFTATE.

Tinaderm-M a brand name for a mixture of the antifungal drugs NYSTATIN and TOLNAFTATE, used to treat skin fungus infections.

tincture an alcoholic solution of a drug.

tinea infection of the skin by fungi, especially *Microsporum*, *Trichophyton* and *Epidermophyton* species. These parasitize the dead outer layer of the skin (epidermis), the hair and the nails. Common sites of infection are the feet (tinea pedis), the groin (tinea cruris), the trunk (tinea corporis), the scalp (tinea capitis) and the nails (tinea unguium). The infection causes intense itching and a raised, scaly, inflammatory linear rash that tends to move outwards from its start point. Tinea of the nails is very persistent and the affected nail is often lost. Tinea is treated with the drug GRISEOFULVIN, taken by mouth, or by local applications of IMIDAZOLES, TERBINAFINE or other fungicides. The condition is often called 'ringworm'.

tinea capitis TINEA of the scalp. Also known as kerion.

tinea cruris TINEA affecting the groin, that tends to spread to the upper thighs and the lower abdomen.

Tineaderm a brand name for TOLNAFTATE.

Tineafax a brand name for TOLNAFTATE.

tinea pedis involvement of the skin between

the toes and, sometimes, the remainder of the skin of the foot, with the fungus infection TINEA.

tinea versicolor infection of the skin of the trunk, neck and sometimes the face, with the yeast fungus *Pityrosporon orbiculare*. This causes multiple, slightly scaly patches varying in colour from white to brown. It is usually treated with a selenium preparation.

tine test a disposable TUBERCULIN TEST unit similar to the Heaf test.

tinidazole an antibacterial and antiprotozoal drug similar to METRONIDAZOLE but with a longer duration of action. It is used to treat AMOEBIASIS, TRICHOMONIASIS and GINGIVITIS. A brand name is Fastigyn.

tinnitus any sound originating in the head and perceptible by the person concerned. Tinnitus may be a hissing, whistling, clicking or ringing sound, appearing to come from one or both ears, or from the centre of the head. It is usually associated with deafness and may be caused by anything that damages the hearing mechanism of the inner ear, such as loud noise, drugs toxic to the ear, MÉNIERÈ'S DISEASE, OTOSCLEROSIS and PRESBYACUSIS. Tinnitus is best ignored, as a preoccupation with the symptom can be disabling. White noise tinnitus maskers are sometimes helpful.

tinzaparin a LOW MOLECULAR WEIGHT HEPARIN drug that interferes with the action of Factor Xa in the blood coagulation cascade and can be used to prevent blood clotting within the blood vessels in people undergoing surgery. A brand name is Innohep.

tioconazole an IMIDAZOLE antifungal drug used externally to treat nail infections with TINEA and CANDIDA ALBICANS fungi. A brand name is Trosyl.

tiotropium bromide a long-acting muscarinic receptor antagonist used to treat chronic obstructive pulmonary disease (COPD). A brand name is Spiriva.

tirofiban an anticoagulant drug with the brand name Aggrastat. See SAW-SCALED VIPER VENOM.

tissue any aggregation of joined cells and their connections that perform a particular function. Body tissues include bone, muscle, nerve tissue, nerve supporting glial tissue, epithelium, fat, fibrous and elastic tissue.

tissue adhesives cyanoacrylate glues used to close minor skin wounds without stitching. Examples are octylcyanacrylate (Dermabond),

enbucrilate (Histoacryl) and N-butylcyanoacrylate (Indermil, Liquiband).

tissue fluid the fluid occupying the spaces between body cells by way of which oxygen, carbon dioxide and dissolved substances are passed to and from the cells. Also known as interstitial fluid.

tissue culture the artificial growth of sheets of human tissue in the laboratory. Tumour cells are readily cultured and some appear to be immortal. These are widely used for laboratory purposes. Normal skin cells (keratinocytes) can be cultured and used for grafting in the same person. Three-layered arteries have been grown as have sheets of urethral endothelium for purposes of urethral reconstitution in hypospadias. It has even been possible to grow a new ear around a mould of polymer mesh.

tissue plasminogen activator (TPA) a natural body ENZYME involved in the breakdown of blood clots. TPA is a small molecure protease that activates the conversion of plasminogen to plasmin. Plasmin is an enzyme that can convert fibrin strands in the blood clot to soluble products so that the blood clot can be dissolved. TPA has been produced synthetically, as alteplase and is used in the treatment of conditions, such as heart attacks, caused by blockage of arteries by clotted blood.

tissue proteinase one of a range of enzymes that bring about controlled protein breakdown in a wide range of developmental, physiological and pathological processes. These enzymes are active in such processes as embryogenesis, angiogenesis, blood coagulation, fibrinolysis and inflammation. Over-expression of some of the proteinases has been implicated in a range of pathologies, especially connective tissue disorders such as rheumatoid arthritis in which collagen breakdown is an important factor.

tissue typing the identification of particular chemical groups present on the surface of all body cells and specific to the individual. These groups are called the histocompatibility antigens and include the human leukocyte antigens (HLAs) which are short chains of linked amino acids unique to each person except that they are shared by identical twins. Tissue typing is important in organ donation to reduce the risk of rejection. See also MAJOR HISTOCOMPATIBILITY COMPLEX.

titre a measure of the concentration and

strength of a substance, such as an antiserum or antibody, in solution. Titre is estimated by the highest dilution that still allows a detectable effect.

tizanidine a muscle relaxant drug used to treat muscle spasm in multiple sclerosis or spinal injury. This drug is said to reduce spasm without reducing strength. A brand name is Zanaflex.

TMJ syndrome *abbrev. for* TEMPORO-MANDIBULAR JOINT SYNDROME.

tobacco dried leaves of the plant Nicotina tabacum. Tobacco contains the drug NICOTINE for the effects of which it is smoked, chewed or inhaled as a powder (snuff). All these activities are dangerous. Cigarette smoking, in particular, is responsible for a greatly increased risk of cancer of the lung, mouth, bladder and pancreas and for an increased likelihood of chronic BRONCHITIS, EMPHYSEMA, coronary artery disease and disease of the leg arteries. Smoking is also harmful during pregnancy, leading to smaller and less healthy babies.

tobacco-free social norm the concept that the avoidance of smoking should be generally regarded as natural and normal and that smoking is harmful and undesirable. The establishment of such a norm is especially important as a means of discouraging young people from smoking.

tobramycin an antibiotic drug similar in use to Gentamicin, but useful in the treatment of gentamicin-resistant infections. A brand name is Nebcin.

tocography a procedure for recording contractions of the muscle of the womb during childbirth.

tocopherol one of the group of substances constituting vitamin E.

Todd's paralysis loss of power in part of the body affected by an epileptic seizure and lasting for periods of from a few minutes to a few days. (Robert Bentley Todd, 1809–60, Irish-born English physician).

toe disorders see BUNION, HALLUX VALGUS, HAMMER TOE, INGROWN TOENAIL.

Tofranil a brand name for IMIPRAMINE.

togavirus one of the group of viruses that contains the RUBELLA virus and most of the ARBOVIRUSES.

tolbutamide a drug used in the treatment of maturity-onset, non-insulin-dependent DIABETES. A brand name is Rastinon.

tolfenamic acid a NON-STEROIDAL ANTI-INFLAMMATORY DRUG used to treat MIGRAINE. A brand name is Clotam Rapid.

tolnaftate an antifungal drug used to treat TINEA. A brand name is Tinaderm-M.

tomography X-ray examination performed so as to produce an image of a slice of tissue. In tomography, a narrow beam and a detector, fixed relative to each other, move in a rotary manner around the patient. CT scanning is a form of (computer-assisted) tomography.

Tomudex a brand name for RALTITREXED.

-tomy *suffix denoting* a cutting or making an incision into.

tone the degree of tension maintained in a muscle when not actively contracting. In health, this is slight. Tone is abolished in certain forms of paralysis and greatly increased in others.

tongue the muscular, mucous membrane-covered, highly flexible organ that is attached to the lower jaw (mandible) and the HYOID BONE in the neck, and forms part of the floor of the mouth. The mucous membrane contains numerous small projections called papillae. On the edges and base of the tongue are many special nerve endings subserving taste and called taste buds.

tongue disorders see GLOSSITIS, LEUKOPLAKIA and TONGUE TIE.

tongue depressor a flat wooden or metal spatula used to press the tongue gently downwards so as to expose the back of the throat for examination.

tongue tie a rare condition in which the mucous membrane partition under the tongue (the FRENULUM) is so tight as to limit tongue movement and even affect speech. The condition is easily corrected by snipping the frenulum.

tonic a mythical remedy commonly prescribed by doctors as a PLACEBO.

tono- *combining form denoting* pressure or tension.

tonometer an instrument used to measure the hydrostatic pressure within the eye. Raised pressure is an important feature of GLAUCOMA.

tonometry measurement of the pressure of the fluid within the eye.

tonsil 1 an oval mass of lymphoid tissue, of variable size, situated on the back of the throat on either side of the soft palate.

2 any bodily structure resembling the palatine tonsil.

tonsillectomy surgical removal of the tonsils. This may be done using forceps and blunt dissection with minimal cutting, or by means of a wire snare that is tightened with a rachet. General anaesthesia is needed.

tonsillitis inflammation of the TONSILS as a result of infection with one of a range of organisms. The tonsils are swollen and red and pus may be seen exuding from the tonsillar pits (crypts). There is pain in the throat, especially on swallowing, and often fever and headache. The lymph nodes in the neck are enlarged and may be tender. Tonsillitis responds well to antibiotic treatment.

tonsil test for CJD prion the identification of rogue prion protein in a small biopsy sample of tonsil from a suspected victim of new-variant CJD. The protein is digested with an enzyme proteinase K and the fragments subjected to electrophoresis. The resulting banding pattern in new-variant CJD differs from that of other forms of CJD.

tooth see TEETH.

tooth abscess inflammation and local tissue destruction, with pus formation, around the tip of the root of a tooth (apex). This is a late complication of neglected tooth decay (dental caries). There is pain, especially on biting and the adjacent gum is inflamed and swollen. The tooth can sometimes be saved by ROOT CANAL TREATMENT but may have to be extracted.

toothache pain in or around a tooth, usually from TOOTH DECAY or a TOOTH ABSCESS.

tooth decay local destruction of the enamel and underlying dentine of a tooth so that cavities form and infection can gain access to the pulp. Such infection can destroy the internal blood vessels and nerves and kill the tooth. Tooth decay is caused by acids formed by bacterial action on dental PLAQUE and can be prevented by regular brushing and flossing. Also known as dental caries.

toothpaste a tooth-cleaning preparation containing a fine abrasive powder, such as chalk, a little soap or detergent, some flavouring, often peppermint, and some sweetening agent and, ideally, a fluoride salt. Many dentifrices also contain a chemical to coagulate protein in the tooth tubules and desensitize them to acids and temperature changes.

Topal a brand name for a mixture of ALUMINIUM HYDROXIDE, ALGINIC ACID and MAGNESIUM CARBONATE, used to treat DYSPEPSIA.

Topamax a brand name for TOPIRAMATE.

tophi crystals of monosodium urate that may appear as chalky outcroppings on the skin of the ear, or may occur in tendons or joints in GOUT.

topical pertaining to something, usually medication, applied to a surface on or in the body, rather than taken internally or injected. Examples of topical applications are skin ointments or creams, eye and ear drops or ointments and vaginal pessaries.

Topicycline a brand name for TETRACYCLINE for external use,

topiramate a drug that reduced the sensitivity to firing of nerve cells and is used to prevent epileptic seizures. A brand name is Topamax.

topoisomerases enzymes that assist in the topological manipulation of DNA. Before DNA can replicate it must be unwound. This occurs in short segments and is achieved by a Type I topoisomerase that cuts one strand so that the free end can be rotated around the unbroken strand. Topoisomerase 1 then re-ligates the broken strand. Type II topoisomerases cut both strands. The term is pronounced 'topo – isomerase'. The derivation is Greek, *topos*, a place; *iso*, equal; *meros*, a part; with the -ase suffix denoting an enzyme.

topoisomerase 1 inhibitor drugs a range of drugs that interfere with DNA replication by inhibiting the action of the topoisomerase enzymes that allow the uncoiling of the double helix – a necessary preliminary to replication. They are used as anticancer drugs and, by local application, to treat warts. Examples are topotecan (Hycamtin) and irinotecan (Campto).

topological isomers of DNA DNA molecules that are identical except for the number of times one strand of the double helix crosses over the other in a given length. Any change in this number (the linking number) requires that at least one strand must be broken. This process to change the linking number is catalyzed by a TOPOISOMERASE.

topotecan the first of the CAMPOTHECIN analogue drugs to be approved for clinical use. Topotecan is a TOPOISOMERASE inhibitor drug used to treat cancer of the ovary and small cell cancer of the lung. (see CYTOTOXIC DRUGS). A brand name is Hycamtin.

torasemide a LOOP DIURETIC drug used to treat high blood pressure (HYPERTENSION) or oedema from any cause. A brand name is Torem.

Toradol a brand name for KETOROLAC.

TORCH *acronym for* Toxoplasmosis, Rubella, Cytomegalovirus and Herpes simplex virus infections. This group of infections is often routinely looked for in investigating ill infants, especially if there is a possibility of CONGENITAL infection. The practice has been criticized as being wasteful and inefficient.

Torem a brand name for TORACEMIDE.

toremifene an anti-oestrogen drug used to treat oestrogen-dependent breast cancers that have spread. Most breast cancers are oestrogen-dependent. A brand name is Fareston.

torsion twisting or rotation, especially of a part that hangs loosely on a narrow support. Torsion may affect a loop of bowel or other organ and commonly results in dangerous obstruction to the blood supply of the part. Urgent surgical correction may be needed.

torsion of testis twisting of the SPERMATIC CORD within, or just above, the scrotum. This causes occlusion of the veins so that return of blood is obstructed and there is great swelling, pain, tenderness and bruising. Early surgical correction is necessary to preserve the fertility of the affected testicle.

torticollis a permanent, intermittent or spasmodic twisting of the head or neck to one side. Causes of torticollis include birth injury to one of the long neck muscles, scarring and shortening of the neck skin, spasm of the neck muscles, WHIPLASH INJURY, TICS and vertical imbalance of the eye muscles. Treatment depends on the cause. Also known as wry neck.

totipotentiality, totipotency the ability of a cell to differentiate to form any kind of fully differentiated body cell. In stem cell research totipotentiality is taken to be a property of the cells of the embryo, the zygote and the immediate descendants of the first two cell divisions. Compare PLURIPOTENTIALITY and UNIPOTENTIALITY.

Tourette's syndrome see GILLES DE LA TOURETTE'S SYNDROME.

tourniquet an encircling band placed around a limb and tightened enough to compress blood vessels and prevent blood flow. Tourniquets are used in surgery or in the emergency control of severe bleeding from an artery or a large vein, but are dangerous if left in place for more than an hour or so. A forgotten tourniquet inevitably causes GANGRENE and loss of the limb beyond the point of application.

toxaemia the presence of bacterial or other poisons (toxins) in the blood. Compare SEPTICAEMIA.

toxaemia of pregnancy see PRE-ECLAMPSIA and ECLAMPSIA.

toxi-, toxico- *combining form denoting* poison or toxin.

toxic epidermal necrolysis a severe skin disorder featuring redness, peeling, blistering and loosening and shedding of large sheets of the EPIDERMIS. In children it was believed to be usually due to a circulating staphylococcal toxin and is often called the staphylococcal scalded skin syndrome (SSSS). It is now thought that the condition is almost always a severe reaction to a drug. The condition is also known as Lyell disease after the dermatologist Alan Lyell who first described it in 1956.

toxicity the quality or degree of poisonousness.

toxicology the study of the nature, properties and identification of poisons, of their biological effects on living organisms and of the treatment of these effects.

toxic megacolon a gaseous ballooning or dilatation of the colon occurring as a complication of inflammatory bowel disease such as ulcerative colitis or Crohn's disease. The danger is of perforation which carries a high mortality. The condition can often be relieved by turning the patient into the prone position.

toxic psychosis a mental disorder caused by the effect on the brain of any poison or drug. Possible causes include alcohol, lead, mercury, cocaine, amphetamine (amfetamine), cannabis and hallucinogenic drugs.

toxic shock syndrome a rare but dangerous condition caused by the damaging effect of toxins of *Staphylococcus aureus* and *Streptococcus* species on the lining of blood vessels. One form of the condition has been associated with the use of high-absorbency vaginal tampons and a rise in the numbers of staphylococci in the vagina, with local inflammation. There is high fever, a scaly rash, vomiting and diarrhoea, muscle pain, liver damage, disorientation and an acute and sometimes fatal drop in blood pressure. Blood transfusion and antibiotics are given. In toxic shock, staphylococcal ENTEROTOXINS can act as SUPERANTIGENS which react directly with T cells causing massive release of CYTOKINES. In streptococcal toxic shock, the M PROTEINS of the streptococcal wall are involved. See also SEPTIC SHOCK.

toxin any substance produced by a living organism that is poisonous to other organisms. Bacterial disease is largely the result of poisoning by the toxins they produce. Some bacteria release soluble exotoxins that act remotely. Others produce only endotoxins which operate only locally. Some bacterial toxins are among the most poisonous substances known.

toxo- *combining form denoting* bow-shaped.

toxocariasis infection, via the mouth, with the juvenile forms of the common bow-shaped puppy worm *Toxocara canis*. This is a frequent event in children in contact with puppy fur and contaminated soil. Infection causes a transient illness with fever, lassitude, loss of appetite, pallor and often coughing and wheezing. Rarely, a juvenile worm may lodge in an eye and cause a tumour-like mass on the retina that may damage vision and may be mistaken for the highly malignant RETINOBLASTOMA. Puppies are often infected before birth and should be de-wormed regularly.

toxoid a bacterial toxin that has been chemically changed so as to lose its poisonous properties but retain its ability to stimulate antibody production. Toxoids make excellent vaccines against infections characterized by exotoxin production, such as DIPHTHERIA and TETANUS.

toxoplasmosis infection with the single-celled, bow-shaped, microscopic organism *Toxoplasma gondii*, often acquired before birth or from domestic cats. Severe congenital infection may damage the nervous system and other organs and cause stillbirth, but most infections are symptomless. The organism may damage the RETINA and this damage may be progressive calling for treatment with steroid drugs and PYRIMETHAMINE. Toxoplasmosis is common in people with immune deficiency, as in AIDS.

TPHA test *abbrev. for* Treponema pallidum haemagglutination assay, a test for SYPHILIS.

TPA *abbrev. for* TISSUE-PLASMINOGEN ACTIVATOR.

trabecula supporting strands of connective tissue constituting part of the framework of an organ.

trabeculation the formation of ridges on a surface.

trabeculectomy an eye operation to treat cases of GLAUCOMA that cannot be controlled by medication. Trabeculectomy provides a new outlet route for the aqueous humour which is under excessive pressure.

trace elements dietary minerals required only in tiny amounts to maintain health. They include zinc, copper, chromium and selenium, and are rarely deficient except under unusual circumstances such as artificial feeding.

tracer 1 a biochemical that has been tagged with a radioactive atom so that its destination can be determined.

2 a length of nucleic acid tagged with a radioactive atom that can be used to find and identify samples of its complementary strand.

trach-, tracheo- *combining form denoting* trachea.

trachea the windpipe. A cylindrical tube of mucous membrane and muscle reinforced by rings of CARTILAGE, that extends downwards into the chest from the bottom of the LARYNX for about 10 cm. The trachea terminates when it branches into two main bronchi.

tracheitis inflammation of the lining of the windpipe (trachea), usually from infections originating in the throat or BRONCHI. There is pain, made worse by coughing, hoarseness and wheezing. In young children breathing is noisy and crowing (CROUP) and in very small children there may be a risk of asphyxia. Treatment depends on the cause and may include antibiotics, soothing inhalations and drugs to control coughing.

tracheo-oesophageal fistula an abnormal connection between the windpipe (trachea) and the gullet (oesophagus), present at birth. This results from failure of full differentiation of the two structures in early fetal life. The baby cannot swallow normally and milk may enter the trachea causing choking and the risk of asphyxia, pneumonia and collapse of the lungs. Early surgical correction is necessary.

tracheostomy an operation to make an artificial opening through the front of the neck into the windpipe (trachea). A tube is then inserted to maintain the opening and allow breathing. Tracheostomy is necessary when life is threatened by obstruction to the airway or when breathing must be maintained artificially for long periods by an air pump.

trach- *combining form denoting* rough.

trachoma an eye infection with the organism *Chlamydia trachomatis*, common in under-developed countries and responsible for millions of cases of blindness each year. The organism is spread by contact and by flies and causes severe inflammation of the CONJUNCTIVA, inturning of the upper lids, and secondary damage to the CORNEA, with opacification, ulceration and often perforation. Treatment with antibiotic ointments is effective.

tract 1 an associated group of organs forming a pathway along which liquids, solids or gases are moved. Examples are the digestive tract, the urinary tract and the respiratory tract.
2 a bundle of nerve fibres with a common function.

Tracleer a brand name for BOSENTAN.

traction the process of exerting a sustained pull on a part of the body, to achieve and maintain proper alignment of parts, as in the treatment of fractures. Spinal traction is used to reduce the tendency for soft tissue to be squeezed out of INTERVERTEBRAL DISCS.

Tractocile a brand name for ATOSIBAN.

tragus the small projection of skin-covered cartilage lying in front of the external ear opening (meatus).

training the inculcation of skills and abilities and of improved muscular bulk, power and performance by repetitive action in applying a force. Physical training alters muscle in several ways, some as subtle as mitochondrial changes, and improves the efficiency of the heart and the respiratory system. Other forms of training involve psychological or sensory modification.

trait 1 any inheritable characteristic.
2 a mild form of a recessive genetic disorder.

tramadol a centrally-acting synthetic opiate pain-killing drug. It is less likely to cause respiratory depression, constipation, euphoria and addiction than many of the ipioid agonists. It is currently the fourth most commonly prescribed analgesic in the world. Brand names are Tramake, Zamadol and Zydol.

Tramake a brand name for TRAMADOL.

Tramazoline a SYMPATHOMIMETIC drug used to treat hay fever. A brand name of a preparation of tramazoline combined with DEXAMETHASONE

and NEOMYCIN is Dexa-Rhinaspray.

TRAM flap *abbrev. for* transverse rectus abdominis mycocutaneous flap. This is a layered piece of tissue, consisting of skin, muscle, and fat, taken from the abdomen of a woman and used in the reconstruction of her breast after mastectomy.

trance a state of reduced consciousness with diminished voluntary action. Trances may occur in some forms of EPILEPSY, in CATALEPSY, in HYSTERIA and in HYPNOSIS.

TRANCE *acronym for* tumour-necrosis-factor-related activation-induced CYTOKINE. This cytokine stimulates osteoclast differentiation and offers the possibility of developing new control over bone loss in osteoporosis.

Trandate a brand name for the beta-blocker drug LABETALOL.

trandolapril an ANGIOTENSIN-CONVERTING ENZYME inhibitor drug used to treat high blood pressure (HYPERTENSION) and weak function of the left ventricle following a heart attack. Brand names are Gopten and Odrik.

tranexamic acid a drug that interferes with the dissolution of blood clot (fibrinolysis) and can be used to prevent bleeding during minor operations such as tooth extraction in people with HAEMOPHILIA. A brand name is Cyklokapron.

tranquillizer drugs drugs used to relieve anxiety or to treat psychotic illness.

trans in chemistry, of two groups having the configuration of being on opposite sides of a ring or a double bond.

trans- *prefix denoting* across, through or beyond. In stereochemistry, indicating that two groups are in the TRANS configuration. The prefix is usually italicized.

transactional analysis a psychological interpretation of behaviour based on a study of social interactions in which the individual is perceived as adopting one of three roles – 'adult', 'parent' or 'child'. Relationships are said to be satisfactory if the choice of role is appropriate and complementary, but are disruptive if the people concerned refuse to play the game. Transactional analysis explores the way people play these life games and identifies bad play which may damage the quality of life.

transaminase any enzyme that catalyses the transfer of amino groups in the metabolism of amino acids (transamination). Also known as aminotransferase.

transcervical endometrial ablation
see ENDOMETRIAL ABLATION.

transcervical endometrial resection
see ENDOMETRIAL RESECTION.

transcranial Doppler ultrasonography
ultrasonography, using the DOPPLER EFFECT, of the arteries supplying the brain with blood. This allows monitoring during neurosurgery and the detection of abnormal arterial narrowing or of dangerous arterial spasm after subarachnoid haemorrhage. The method has been used to investigate mood disorders and has identified abnormalities in the limbic system in severe depression.

transcriptase any enzyme that catalyses transcription of a molecule, as in the process of producing a copy of RNA from DNA. Reverse transcriptase is an enzyme found in viruses, such as HIV, that catalyses DNA from an RNA template – the reverse of the usual procedure.

transcription the synthesis of RNA on a DNA template.

transduction 1 the conversion of energy in one form into energy in another.
2 the transfer of a gene from one bacterial host to another by means of a phage.
3 the transfer of a gene from one cell host to another by a retrovirus.

transfection gene transfer by infection of a cell with nucleic acid by a virus, followed by viral replication in the affected cell.

transferase any enzyme that catalyses the movement of atoms or groups of atoms from one molecule to another. A kinase adds a phosphate group to a substrate such as an amino acid.

transference the transfer of emotional wishes or thoughts experienced in relation to one person, to another person, especially a psychotherapist. Freud regarded transference in psychoanalysis as essential to success.

transfer factor a LYMPHOKINE released by T cells that activates MACROPHAGES and prompts them to attack fungi.

transferrin a blood protein (beta globulin) that can combine reversibly with iron and transport it to the cells.

transfer RNA a short-chain RIBONUCLEIC ACID molecule present in cells in at least 20 different varieties, each capable of combining with a specific amino acid and positioning it

appropriately in a polypeptide chain that is being synthesized in a ribosome. Transfer RNA is a four-armed, clover-leaf-like structure. At the end of one arm is an ANTICODON, complementary to the codon for an amino acid in MESSENGER RNA. At the end of the opposite arm is a site to which the appropriate amino acid can be covalently linked. When a molecule of transfer RNA is linked to the amino acid corresponding to its anticodon it becomes aminoacyl-tRNA. The identity of the passenger on a particular tRNA molecule is determined by its anticodon rather than by its attached amino acid.

transfusion the replacement of lost blood by blood, or blood products, usually donated by another person. Blood transfusion is given in cases of shock or severe anaemia and is often life-saving. Blood must be of a compatible group and is invariably checked by CROSS-MATCHING before being given.

transgenic animal an animal that has had a new DNA sequence introduced into its germ line by insertion into a fertilized egg or an early embryo. All subsequent offspring will carry the new genetic material in their genomes and will show its effects.

Transiderm-Nitro a brand name for GLYCERYL TRINITRATE.

transient global amnesia a state, lasting for less than 24 hours, in which there is inability to form new memories and in which there is loss of memory for periods of up to years (retrograde amnesia) prior to the attack. After the attack there is permanent memory loss for the period of the attack. The condition may be brought on by emotional upset, physical exertion, sexual intercourse or the Valsalva manoeuvre.

transient ischaemic attacks disturbances of body function lasting for less than 24 hours and caused by localized nervous system defects. These occur because of temporary interruption or reduction of the blood supply to part of the brain. There may be visual loss, weakness in an arm or leg, numbness, speech difficulty or confusion. Transient ischaemic attacks are a warning of the danger of STROKE and should always be investigated.

transillumination a method of examination in which a bright light is shone through tissue to try to determine whether it contains abnormal structures such as a solid tumour.

translation a final stage in the expression of a gene; the synthesis of a polypeptide on a ribosome by means of TRANSFER RNA. Translation requires several enzymes.

translocation 1 a form of chromosome mutation in which a detached part of a CHROMOSOME becomes attached to another chromosome or parts of two chromosomes may be joined. Translocations may be inherited or acquired. In many cases they cause no effect on the body because all the normal chromosomal material is present. But if a translocation results in a deficiency or excess of chromosomal material the results are serious.
2 of a gene when a new copy of the gene appears at a location on the genome remote from the original location.
3 the movement of a RIBOSOME along a MESSENGER RNA molecule from one CODON to the next.
4 of the movement of a protein across a membrane.

transmembrane crossing a membrane.

transmissible able to be passed from one person or organism to another, as in the case of infectious disease or genetic disorder.

transplacental passing across the PLACENTA.

transplantation 1 the grafting of donated organs or tissues into the body (homograft). Except in the case of identical twins, this process can succeed only if the rejection processes of the immune system are artificially suppressed.
2 the movement of tissue from one site to another in the same person (autograft). See also CTLA4-IG.

transposition in genetics, the movement of a length of genetic material from one point in a DNA molecule to another.

transposition of the great vessels one of the types of congenital heart disease. In this condition, the AORTA, the main supply artery of the body, is wrongly connected to the right ventricle, which normally pumps blood returning from the body to the lungs. The pulmonary artery is connected to the left ventricle. As a result, the lungs are effectively bypassed and the blood supplied to the body is insufficiently oxygenated. There is blueness of the skin (cyanosis), breathlessness and failure to thrive. Heart surgery is usually necessary.

transposons discrete mobile sequences in the genome that can transport themselves directly from one part of the genome to another without the use of a vehicle such as a phage or plasmid DNA. They are able to move by making DNA copies of their RNA transcripts which are then incorporated into the genome at a new site. Sometimes called 'jumping genes'.

transsexualism a persistent conviction that the true gender is the opposite of the actual anatomical sex. This may cause depression and anxiety. Transsexualism is mainly experienced by men, and SEX-REASSIGNMENT SURGERY is often sought.

transtracheal oxygen catheterization maintenance of the oxygen supply to the body by means of a fine tube passed through a TRACHEOSTOMY opening in the front of the neck into the trachea. The method has substantial advantages over nasal cannulas or facemasks and is preferred by most patients but is appropriate only if supplementary oxygen is a long-term requirement.

transudate 1 a fluid that has passed through a membrane.
2 a collection of fluid resulting from increased capillary pressure in capillary beds or decreased osmosis from reduced blood protein.

transvaginal ultrasound a method of ultrasound imaging of pelvic structures in women in which the transducer is placed in the vagina. Transvaginal imaging of the lining of the womb (endometrium) can provide useful information about thickness and texture in women with abnormal bleeding. Unduly thick endometrium suggests cancer or hyperplasia.

Transvasin a brand name for TETRAHYDROFURYL SALICYLATE.

transverse colon the middle third of the colon that loops across the upper part of the ABDOMEN.

transverse process a bony protuberance on each side of a vertebra to which muscles are attached.

transvestism male desire to wear women's clothing often for reasons of sexual gratification. The reciprocal phenomenon is not normally referred to as transvestism as it is not usually related to sexual pleasure. Transvestites are not usually transsexuals.

Tranxene a brand name for the benzodiazepine anti-anxiety drug CLORAZEPATE.

tranylcypromine a MONOAMINE-OXIDASE INHIBITOR (MAO) antidepressant drug. It is formulated in combination with TRIFLUOPERAZINE under the brand name Parstelin.

trapezius muscle a large, triangular back muscle extending from the lower part of the back of the skull (occiput) almost to the lumbar region of the spine on each side. Each muscle extends outward from the rear processes of the vertebral column to the spine of the shoulder blade and the outer tip of the collar bone (clavicle). The trapezius muscle braces the shoulder blade and rotate it outwards when the arm is raised.

Trasicor a brand name for the beta-blocker drug OXPRENOLOL.

trastuzumab a monoclonal antibody drug used to treat breast cancers that over-express the HER2 growth factor receptor. A brand name is Herceptin.

Trasylol a brand name for APROTININ.

trauma 1 any injury caused by a mechanical or physical agent.
2 any event having an adverse psychological effect.

traumatology the study and practice of the management of patients suffering from recent physical injury, as from traffic or other accidents or assault.

Travatan a brand name for TRAVOPROST.

travellers' diarrhoea a popular term for GASTROENTERITIS usually caused by faecal contamination of food or water. The organisms most commonly involved are *Escherichia coli*, *Campylobacter jejuni*, *Salmonella* species, and *Shigella* species.

travel sickness see MOTION SICKNESS.

travoprost a PROSTAGLANDIN analogue drug used in eye drops to control intraocular pressure in open angle GLAUCOMA. A brand name is Travatan.

Traxam a brand name for FELBINAC.

T-rays tetrahertz radiation, electromagnetic radiation of wavelength lying between the infrared and microwave radio waves. A method of generating T-waves has recently been developed and this radiation has been shown to be effective in detecting the precise extent of cancers lying immediately below the surface of the skin.

trazodone an antidepressant drug. A brand name is Molipaxin.

Treacher Collins syndrome an autosomal dominant disorder also known as incomplete mandibulo-facial dysostosis or the Collins-Franceschetti syndrome. It features down-sloping eyes, notches (colobomas) in the eyelids, small mouth and lower jaw, small distorted external ears and often hearing loss. The mutated gene and its protein product were identified in 1996. It is on the long arm of chromosome 5. Over 20 different mutations have been found. (Edward Treacher Collins, 1862–1932, British eye surgeon).

trematode any of the large number of parasitic flatworms, of the class *Trematoda*, that are equipped with suckers by which they attach themselves to host tissue. This class includes the *Schistosome* species and the liver flukes.

trematodiasis infection by a TREMATODE fluke parasite.

tremor rhythmical oscillation of any part of the body, especially the hands, the head, the jaw or the tongue. Tremor does not necessarily imply disease but is a feature of conditions such as CEREBELLAR ATAXIA, ENCEPHALITIS, ESSENTIAL-FAMILIAL TREMOR, LIVER FAILURE, MERCURY POISONING, MULTIPLE SCLEROSIS, PARKINSON'S DISEASE, THYROTOXICOSIS and WILSON'S DISEASE. It is also a side effect of many antipsychotic and other drugs.

trench fever a louse-borne infection caused by *Rickettsia quintana* that was prevalent in World War I but is now rare. It features headache, fever, severe pain in the legs and back, and a tendency to relapse at intervals of 5 or 6 days.

trench foot see IMMERSION FOOT.

trench mouth see VINCENT'S DISEASE.

Trental a brand name for OXPENTIFYLLINE (pentoxifylline).

trephine a hollow, cylindrical cutting instrument with the edge at one end sharpened or saw-toothed, used to cut a circular hole in bone or other tissue by pressure and rotation.

treponematosis infection caused by *Treponema* species of SPIROCHAETES.

tretinoin a RETINOID drug used to treat ACNE, scaly skin conditions such as ICHTHYOSIS, skin ageing and certain forms of LEUKAEMIA. Brand names are Retin-A, Retinova and Vesanoid.

TRH *abbrev. for* THYROTROPHIN RELEASING HORMONE.

Triadene a brand name for ETHINYLOESTRADIOL (ethinylestradiol) formulated with a PROGESTOGEN drug as an oral contraceptive.

triage a selection process, used in war or disaster, to divide casualties into three groups so as to maximize resources and avoid wastage of essential surgical skills on hopeless cases. In triage, an experienced surgeon sorts cases rapidly into those needing urgent treatment, those that will survive without immediate treatment, and those beyond hope of benefit from treatment. Triage is also used to assign treatment in the event of the appearance of a number of men suffering acute chest pain.

triamcinolone a CORTICOSTEROID drug used to treat inflammatory disorders, ASTHMA, THROMBOCYTOPENIA and some forms of LEUKAEMIA. Brand names are Adcortyl, Adcortyl in Orabase, Kenalog, Lederspan and Nasacort. Triamcinolone is also an ingredient is a range of preparations for external use.

Triam-Co a brand name for TRIAMTERENE formulated with HYDROCHLOROTHIAZIDE.

triamterene a potassium-sparing diuretic drug used to relieve the body of excess water and to treat mildly raised blood pressure. Triamterene is formulated with another diuretic drug under the brand names Diazide, Dytide, Frusene, Kalspare and Triam-Co.

triazines a class of anticonvulsant drugs. An example is lamotrigine (Lamictal).

triazole antifungals drugs used to treat skin, oral, vaginal and internal fungal infections. Examples are fluconazole (Diflucan), itraconazole (Sporanox) and voticonazole (Vfend).

Trib a brand name for CO-TRIMOXAZOLE.

tribavirin ribavirin, a drug used to treat severe respiratory syncytial virus infections. A brand name is Virazole.

triceps muscle a three-headed muscle attached to the back up the upper arm bone (humerus) and to the outer edge of the shoulder-blade (scapula) and running down the back of the arm to be inserted by a strong TENDON into the curved process (olecranon process) on the back of one of the two forearm bones (the ulna). The triceps muscle straightens the elbow in opposition to the biceps muscle, which bends it.

trich-, tricho- *combining form denoting* hair or eyelash.

trichiasis inturning or ingrowing of the eyelashes so that they rub against the CORNEA of the eye causing severe discomfort and possible abrasion, infection and ulceration. Trichiasis is a

feature of TRACHOMA. Removal of lashes affords relief but definitive treatment involves plastic procedures to evert the lid margins. See also ENTROPION.

trichinosis infection with the roundworm *Trichinella spiralis* usually from eating undercooked pork containing the tiny cysts of the dormant forms of the worm. Digestion releases the larvae which attach to the intestinal lining, reproduce, and spread throughout the body settling in the muscles to form cysts. During this migration there may be fever, swelling of the face, cough, and pain, stiffness and tenderness in the muscles. Large infections may be fatal.

trichobezoar a ball of swallowed hair in the stomach or intestine, usually of a mentally retarded or psychotic person.

trichomoniasis infection with the single-celled, flagellated PROTOZOON *Trichomonas vaginalis*, most commonly in the vagina but sometimes in the URETHRA or the PROSTATE gland in men. Trichomoniasis causes irritation, burning and itching and a frothy, yellowish, offensive discharge. Treatment is with the drug metronidazole (Flagyl). Both partners must be treated.

trichosis disease of the hair.

trichotillomania an apparent compulsion to pull out one's own hair, sometimes manifested by people with psychotic disorders or severe mental retardation. Anxious or frustrated children sometimes pull out hair.

Trichozole a brand name for METRONIDAZOLE.

trichuriasis infection of the large intestine with whipworms.

triclosan a disinfectant drug used externally in staphylococcal and other skin infections. Brand names are Aquasept, Manusept, Ster-Zac Bath Concentrate.

tricuspid 1 having three cusps or points, as on a molar tooth.
2 pertaining to the three-cusped heart valve that separates the chambers on the right side.

tricuspid incompetence leakiness of the TRICUSPID VALVE of the heart, usually as a result of stretching from a rise of pressure in the blood passing through the lungs (pulmonary hypertension). Tricuspid incompetence causes a rise in the pressure in the veins with fluid retention (oedema) and an enlarged liver. Surgery may be necessary.

tricuspid stenosis narrowing of the aperture of the TRICUSPID VALVE, usually resulting from rheumatic fever. The effects are similar to those of TRICUSPID INCOMPETENCE.

tricuspid valve the valve lying between the upper and lower chambers of the right side of the heart.

tricyclic antidepressant drug one of a group of drugs whose structure is based on three six-carbon rings. The tricyclics produce an elevation of mood but this does not occur until the drugs have been taken for two to three weeks (an important point as depressed people may commit suicide during this period). These drugs have an anticholinergic effect and may cause dry mouth, constipation, urinary retention and blurred vision. The tricyclic antidepressants are the most widely used group for depression. They act by blocking the re-uptake of noradrenaline and serotonin at synapses thus allowing these stimulatory neurotransmitters to act for longer. With use, actual changes occur in the synapses that are of benefit. FLUOXETINE (Prozac) is not a tricyclic. It has only two rings and is a selective re-uptake inhibitor of serotonin only. Other tricyclic atidepressant drugs are AMITRIPTYLINE, DOXEPIN, IMIPRAMINE, NORTRIPTYLINE and TRIMIPRAMINE. Up to 50% of patients have genetic variations that prevent them from responding to these drugs.

Tridil a brand name for GLYCERYL TRINITRATE.

trifluoperazine an antipsychotic drug used mainly to treat SCHIZOPHRENIA. A brand name is Stelazine. The drug is also formulated with TRANYLCYPROMINE under the brand name Parstelin.

trifocal 1 having three focal lengths.
2 distance-viewing spectacles having additional segments for intermediate and close ranges.

trigeminal nerve the 5th of the 12 pairs of cranial nerves and the sensory nerve of the face. Each trigeminal nerve divides into three main branches, the ophthalmic, the maxillary and the mandibular nerves, which then branch to supply the corresponding parts of the face.

trigeminal neuralgia a disorder of the sensory nerve of the face, the trigeminal nerve, on one side in which sudden episodes of excruciating stabbing pain occur in the cheek, lips, gums, chin or tongue. These attacks last for only a few seconds or minutes and may be precipitated by a light touch to the face. The drug carbamazepine (Tegretol) is often effective.

trigger finger an effect of a localized swelling in the tendon that bends a finger. The flexor tendon runs partially in a fibrous sheath and although the swelling can easily slip out of the end of the sheath, when the finger is bent, it cannot easily slip back in again. As a result, the finger remains bent until straightened passively, often with an audible click. Treatment is by opening the sheath surgically.

Triglycerides see FATS.

Trilafon a brand name for PERPHENAZINE.

trilostane a drug that interferes with the natural synthesis of steroids and is used to treat breast cancer in post-menopausal women. A brand name is Modrenal.

trimeprazine alimemazine, an antihistamine drug used to relieve itching in allergic conditions and as a sedative for children. A brand name is Vallergan.

trimethoprim an antibacterial drug used to treat urinary and other infections. The drug is on the WHO official list. Brand names are Ipral, Monotrim and Trimopan. Combined with sulphamethoxazole it is sold as co-trimoxazole (Septrin) and Chemotrim.

trimetrexate an inhibitor of the enzyme DIHYDROFOLATE REDUCTASE. It is used to treat *Pneumocystis carinii* pneumonia in people with AIDS. A brand name is Neutrexin.

Tri-Minulet a brand name for ETHINYLOESTRADIOL (ethinylestradiol) formulated with a PROGESTOGEN drug GESTODENE as an oral contraceptive.

Trinordiol a brand name for ETHINYLOESTRADIOL (ethinylestradiol) formulated with LEVONORGESTREL as an oral contraceptive.

trimipramine a tricyclic antidepressant drug with a strong sedative effect. A brand name is Surmontil.

Trimopan a brand name for TRIMETHOPRIM.

Trinovum a brand name for ETHINYLOESTRADIOL (ethinylestradiol) formulated with a PROGESTOGEN drug as an oral contraceptive.

triple vaccine a combined vaccine against DIPHTHERIA, WHOOPING COUGH (pertussis) and TETANUS.

triploblastic of an embryo, having three

primitive germ layers from each of which particular parts of the body develop.

triploid having three HAPLOID sets of chromosomes in each nucleus. The normal state of a body cell is DIPLOID.

tri-potassium di-citrato bismuthate a drug, used to treat stomach and duodenal ulcers, that reacts with the gastric secretions to provide a protective barrier for the bowel lining. A cytoprotectant drug. A brand name is DeNoltab.

triprolidine an antihistamine drug used to treat allergy and to relieve the symptoms of colds. A brand name of a preparation combined with PSEUDOEPHEDRINE is Sudafed Plus.

Triprim a brand name for TRIMETHOPRIM.

Triptafen a brand name for the tricyclic antidepressant drug amitryptyline and the antipsychotic and antiemetic drug PERPHENAZINE.

triptans a group of drugs, known as selective serotonin agonists, with effects similar to those of the neurotransmitter SEROTONIN. Their action is uncertain, but they are thought to act by tightening the branches of the carotid arteries that supply the scalp and brain. They may also act on the main sensory nerve of the face and head. They are effective in controlling the symptoms of MIGRAINE. The group includes almotriptan (Almogran), frovatriptan (Migard), naratriptan (Naramig), rizatriptan (Maxalt), sumatriptan (Imigran), zolmitriptan (Zomig).

triptorelin a synthetic gonadotrophin-releasing hormone used to treat advances cancer o fhte PROSTATE GLAND. A brand name is Decapeptyl SR.

trisodium edetate a CHELATING AGENT used to reduce excess body calcium and treat calcareous deposits in the corneas. A brand name is Limclair.

trismus lockjaw. Tight closure of the mouth from uncontrollable spasm of the chewing muscles. Causes include TETANUS, disorders of the jaw joint, TONSILLITIS, QUINSY, MUMPS, tooth decay, PARKINSON'S DISEASE or ANOREXIA NERVOSA. Treatment is the correction of the cause.

trisomy the occurrence of an extra chromosome in one of the 23 matched and identifiable pairs so that there are three, instead of two, of a particular chromosome. This anomaly may cause a wide range of structural abnormalities or even early death of the fetus.

Trisomy of chromosome 21 (trisomy 21) is the cause of DOWN'S SYNDROME.

trisomy 13 the presence of three copies of chromosome 13. Patau syndrome. There is microcephaly, cleft lip or palate, deafness, blindness, extra fingers and finger deformity. Such infants rarely survive for more than a few weeks

trisomy 18 syndrome the effect of TRISOMY of chromosome 18. Edwards syndrome. There is failure to thrive, severe mental deficiency, persistent contraction of muscles with clenching of the hands and anomalies of the face, hands, breastbone and pelvis. Survival beyond a few months is uncommon. This trisomy leads to spontaneous abortion in nine cases out of ten.

trisomy 21 syndrome see DOWN'S SYNDROME.

tritanopia unable to appreciate the colour blue. This is a rare defect of colour perception.

tRNA TRANSFER RNA.

trocar a sharp-pointed surgical stilette normally used within a CANNULA to allow its insertion into a body cavity. After the trocar and cannula have been inserted into the body, the trocar is withdrawn, leaving the cannula in place.

trochanter one of two major bony processes, the greater and lesser trochanters, on the upper part of the FEMUR. Muscle tendons are attached to the trochanters.

troche a small, medicinal lozenge.

trochlea a body structure that resembles a pulley, especially that for the tendon of the superior oblique eye muscle.

trochlear nerve the 4th of the 12 pairs of cranial nerves. The trochlear nerve supplies one of the muscles that moves the eye – the superior oblique muscle. Contraction of this muscle turns the eye downwards and outwards.

-trophic *combining form denoting* nutrition or nourishment.

tropho- *combining form denoting* nutrition or food.

trophoblastic tumours tumours derived from the early embryonic tissue that develops into the PLACENTA. Trophoblastic tumours may be BENIGN (hydatidiform mole) or MALIGNANT (choriocarcinoma). The former can develop into the latter.

trophozoite the active growing stage of a protozoan parasite, as distinct from the dormant encysted stage. In the malarial parasite, the asexual, vegetative stage before the development of the mature schizont.

-tropic *combining form denoting* moving, turning or changing in response to the stimulus specified.

tropical medicine the study of diseases and medical conditions found in tropical climates. The list that follows highlights the key entries related to tropical medicine in the dictionary: amoebiasis, cholera, diphtheria, hookworm, leishmaniasis, malaria, malnutrition, onchocerciasis, plague, rabies, schistosomiasis, shigellosis, strongyloidiasis, tapeworm, tropical sprue, tropical ulcer, trypanosomiasis, tuberculosis, typhoid, typhus, yellow fever.

tropical ulcer persistent local loss of skin and underlying tissue from one of a number of infections, including LEISHMANIASIS, DIPHTHERIA or YAWS. Tropical ulcer is common in malnourished people.

tropical sprue a disorder of food absorption, of unknown cause, occurring in people living in or visiting the tropics or developing months or years after residence in the tropics. There is loss of appetite and weight, distention of the abdomen, anaemia and fatty diarrhoea. The condition responds well to treatment with antibiotics, vitamin B_{12} and folate.

tropicamide a drug used in the form of eye drops to widen (dilate) the pupil so that the inside of the eye can more easily be examined or operated upon. The drug is on the WHO official list. Brand names are Minims tropicamide and Mydriacyl.

tropisetron a SEROTONIN receptor blocker drug used to treat severe nausea and vomiting, especially that induced by anticancer chemotherapy. A brand name is Navoban.

tropism an automatic movement made by an organism towards or away from a source of stimulation.

-tropism *combining form denoting* TROPISM in relation to the stated stimulus, as in phototropism.

Tropium a brand name for the benzodiazepine anti-anxiety drug chlordiazepoxide.

Trosyl a brand name for TIOCONAZOLE.

Trousseau's sign a sign of latent TETANY. A SPHYGMOMANOMETER cuff is applied to the upper arm and inflated. Within 4 minutes the

forearm muscles go into spasm. (Armand Trousseau, 1801–67, French physician).

Trusopt a brand name for DORZOLAMIDE.

truss a belt-like appliance with a pad that exerts pressure over the orifice of a HERNIA so as to prevent protrusion of the bowel. This is an unsatisfactory substitute for surgical repair.

trypanosome a member of the genus *Trypanosoma*, one of several hundred species of flagellated blood parasite PROTOZOA that cause disease in animals and man. See also TRYPANOSOMIASIS and CHAGAS DISEASE.

trypanosomiasis in Africa, a disease of the nervous system caused by infection with the single-celled parasite *Trypanosoma brucei*. Commonly known as 'sleeping sickness' African trypanosomiasis features extensive brain inflammation with headache, loss of concentration, lassitude, a vacant expression, drooping eyelids and finally loss of all motivation so that the affected person may starve to death. Unless treated, the condition ends in seizures, coma and death. See also TSETSE FLY and CHAGAS' DISEASE (South American trypanosomiasis).

trypanosomiasis, South American see CHAGAS' DISEASE.

trypsin one of the digestive enzymes secreted by the pancreas that breaks down protein to polypeptide fragments. These are then split further to amino acids by carboxypeptidase from the pancreas and aminopeptidase from the small intestine.

trypsinogen the precursor of TRYPSIN produced by the pancreas that is converted into the active form, trypsin, when acted upon by the enzyme enterokinase in the small intestine.

Tryptanol a brand name for AMITRIPTYLINE.

tryptophan an antidepressant drug. L-tryptophan, sold in USA as a non-prescription food additive was withdrawn by the American Food and Drugs Administration (FDA) because of reports of a severe muscle disorder apparently caused by an unidentified contaminant. It is used only by hospital specialists who are aware of the risks. A brand name is Optimax.

tsetse fly a fiercely biting fly, the vector of sleeping sickness (African trypanosomiasis) that renders large areas of the continent almost uninhabitable.

Tsutsugamushi disease scrub TYPHUS,

a disease caused by *Rickettsia tsutsugamushi*, and transmitted by larval mites. It features headache, high fever and a rash.

tubal ligation tying of the Fallopian (uterine) tubes as a method of female sterilization.

tubal pregnancy the commonest type of ECTOPIC PREGNANCY.

tubercle 1 a small nodular mass of tubercular tissue.

2 an informal term for TUBERCULOSIS.

3 any small, rounded protrusion on a bone.

tuberculin test a skin test used to assess the degree of a person's immunity to TUBERCULOSIS. The result depends mainly on whether the individual has had the usual harmless primary tuberculous infection. A small injection of tuberculin, a substance derived from tubercle bacilli, is injected into the skin (Mantoux test) or pricked in with a multi-needle gun (Heaf test). In positive cases a hard swelling develops in three days. People who react negatively can be given normal immunity by BCG vaccination. A strongly positive reaction may indicate a current tuberculosis infection.

tuberculosis infection with the organism *Mycobacterium tuberculosis*, either in the lungs (pulmonary tuberculosis) or in the LYMPH NODES (tuberculous ADENITIS), the skin (SCROFULA), the bones or in other organs. Pulmonary tuberculosis is usually acquired by aerosol spread from other people, while general (systemic) tuberculosis is transmitted in milk from cows with bovine tuberculosis. Pulmonary tuberculosis causes fever, fatigue, loss of appetite and weight, night sweats and persistent cough often with blood-streaked sputum and may spread to cause tubercular MENINGITIS or generalized (miliary) tuberculosis. Systemic tuberculosis causes areas of local tissue destruction often with SINUSES that discharge pus to the exterior. Tuberculosis is treated with a range of drugs used in various combinations for periods of up to a year. Antituberculous drugs include streptomycin, isoniazid, para-aminosalicylic acid (PAS), rifampicin, ethambutol and pyrazinamide.

tuberculous pertaining to, or affected by, TUBERCULOSIS.

tuberosity any prominence on a bone to which tendons are attached.

tuberous sclerosis see BOURNEVILLE'S DISEASE.

tuboplasty an operation on a scarred and

occluded Fallopian tube to restore continuity (patency) and improve the chances of conception.

tubule a small tube or tubular structure.

tubulin a contractile protein that forms microtubules. These form the spindle fibres in MITOSIS that draw chromosomes apart is the course of cell division.

tularaemia a disease of wild animals, caused by the organism *Francisella tularensis*, and occurring in the USA, Japan and most European countries other than Britain. It may, rarely, be contracted by humans, by contact with infected animals, by inhalation of infected material or by the bite of infected flies or ticks. The disease features an ulcer at the site of the bite, enlargement and suppuration of the local lymph nodes, and many, scattered, small localized areas of tissue death in all parts of the body. Pneumonic and ocular forms occur, depending on the route of entry. Tularaemic SEPTICAEMIA is highly dangerous. Treatment is with antibiotic drugs such as streptomycin or gentamicin.

tum-, tume- *combining form denoting* swelling.

tumbu fly an African fly that can cause skin infestation with its larvae (myiasis).

tumefacient producing or tending to produce swelling.

tumescence 1 a swelling or enlarging of a part.

2 a swollen condition.

3 a penile erection.

tumour a swelling. The term usually refers to any mass of cells resulting from abnormal degree of multiplication. Tumours may be BENIGN or MALIGNANT. Benign tumours enlarge locally, and are often enclosed in capsules, but do not invade tissue or spread remotely. Malignant tumours infiltrate locally and also seed off into lymphatic vessels and the bloodstream to establish secondary growths (metastases) elsewhere in the body.

tumour lysis syndrome the release of cellular breakdown products that occurs when tumour cells are killed by effective anticancer treatment. There is a rise in blood potassium, uric acid and phosphates and a drop in calcium. The effect may be a severe metabolic disturbance that can cause prolonged illness and may prove fatal. Severe kidney damage may occur from urate crystal deposition.

tumour markers substances in the blood or

urine that indicate, often by abnormal levels, the presence of a malignant tumour in the body. They include proteins such as thyroglobulin and immunoglobulins; glycoproteins such as the prostate-specific antigen (PSI) and CA-125; hormonal peptides such as beta-human chorionic gonadotrophin and adrenocorticotrophic hormone; enzymes such as lactate dehydrogenase and prostatic acid phosphatase; tumour-associated carbohydrate antigens; neuromediators such as catecholamines; oncogenes; oncofetal antigens such as alpha-fetoprotein and carcinoembryonic antigen; and cytogenic markers such as the Philadelphia chromosome.

tumour necrosis factor one of two related CYTOKINES capable of killing certain cancer cells and which also have regulatory functions on the immune system. Tumour necrosis factor is implicated in various inflammatory diseases including RHEUMATOID ARTHRITIS.

tumour necrosis factor antagonist a fusion protein, produced by recombinant DNA technology, consisting of the tumour necrosis factor receptor (p75) linked to the antibody IgG.

tumour-specific antigens substances produced by specific kinds of tumours that can be detected in the blood and may act as indicators or markers of the presence of tumours or of recurrences of tumours. The method is not wholly reliable because these substances can sometimes occur in the body apart from tumours.

tungiasis infestation with the jigger flea Tunga penetrans, which burrows into the skin of the feet and grows to pea size with eggs which are then discharged.

tunica a covering or investing membrane or layer of tissue.

tunnel vision a narrowing of the extent to which peripheral visual perception is possible while looking straight ahead. Such loss of the visual fields may be caused by damage to the RETINAS, OPTIC NERVES, the nerve connections with the brain or to the visual cortex of the brain itself. Causes of such damage include GLAUCOMA, RETINITIS PIGMENTOSA, tumour of the PITUITARY GLAND, STROKE, head injury or MULTIPLE SCLEROSIS.

turbinate bones three pairs of small, curled bony processes, the upper two pairs being parts of the ETHMOID BONES and the lower pair of the MAXILLAS, that extends horizontally along the outer walls of the nasal passage. The turbinates are covered with mucous membrane which warms and moistens the incoming air. Also known as conchae.

Turcot's syndrome a rare genetic disorder featuring the association a primary brain tumour and multiple adenomas of the colon and rectum. J. Turcot was a Canadian surgeon who worked at Hôtel Dieu de Quebec Hospital and Laval University.

turgid swollen and congested.

Turner's syndrome a genetic disorder affecting females and caused by the absence of one of the two X (sex) chromosomes (monosomy). This may be the case in all body cells or only in some of them (mosaicism). Turner's syndrome features short stature, webbed skin on each side of the neck, misshapen ears, absent pubic and armpit hair and failure of development of the vagina, womb and breasts with absent menstruation. There are also abnormalities of the eyes and the bones and an area of narrowing of the largest artery in the body (coarctation of the aorta). Some degree of mental retardation is usual. (Henry Hubert Turner, 1892–1970, American physician).

TURP abbrev. for transurethral resection of the prostate, the commonest type of operation for enlargement of the PROSTATE GLAND.

Tussinol a brand name for PHOLCODINE.

twilight sleep a popular term formerly used for a state of relative insensitivity to pain and partial consciousness, induced by drugs such as morphine and scopolamine, to ease the pains of childbirth.

twins two offspring from a single pregnancy. Twins may be derived from a single fertilized egg that separates into two after the first division. Such monozygotic twins are genetically identical. Alternatively, twins may be derived from two eggs fertilized at the same time. Such twins are dizygotic and non-identical and in about half the cases are of different sex. The rate of monozygotic twinning in humans is fairly stable at 0.35%, while the rate of dizygotic twinning varies more widely around an average of 1% of pregnancies.

twitch a brief muscular contraction resulting

from a sudden spontaneous impulse in a nerve supplying a group of muscle fibres. Twitching is common and is seldom of any medical significance.

tylectomy LUMPECTOMY.

Tylex a brand name for a mixture of the painkilling drugs CODEINE and PARACETAMOL.

tympan-, tympano- *combining form denoting* eardrum or middle ear auditory bones, or both.

tympanites a drum-like distention of the abdomen caused by gas or air in the intestine or the peritoneal cavity.

tympanometry measurement of the air pressure in the middle ear and of the stiffness of movement of the eardrum and the AUDITORY OSSICLES. Tympanometry may be used as part of the assessment of hearing defect.

tympanoplasty an operation to reconstitute a severed linkage in the chain of tiny bones (auditory ossicles) lying between the eardrum and the oval window of the inner ear, so as to restore hearing.

tympanum 1 the ear drum and the middle ear cavity.

2 the middle ear and its contents.

type genus any taxonomic genus selected as being representative of the family to which it belongs.

typh-, typho- *combining form denoting* typhus or typhoid.

typhoid carrier a person who has recovered from TYPHOID FEVER but who continues to culture *Salmonella typhi* organisms in the gall bladder and to excrete them in the stools. If such a person handles food, the disease is liable to be transmitted to others. Typhoid carriers can be rendered innocuous by having the gall bladder removed.

typhoid fever an infectious disease caused by the organism *Salmonella typhi* which is acquired in fecally contaminated food or water. The disease varies in severity from a mild upset, lasting for a week, to a major illness. There is severe headache, fever, loss of appetite, abdominal discomfort, bloating and constipation. The fever rises higher each day and there may be delirium. The constipation later gives way to diarrhoea. During the acute illness, the organisms accumulate and multiply in the gall bladder and are released into the bowel to appear in the faeces. In the second week of the disease a rash of small, raised red

spots (rose spots) appears on the chest and upper abdomen. The liver and spleen enlarge and the abdomen is tender. Perforation of the bowel and PERITONITIS may occur. Typhoid responds well to antibiotic treatment and can usually be controlled in a matter of days, with the antibiotics chloramphenicol or ampicillin.

typhus a range of infectious diseases caused by Rickettsial organisms, transmitted by different insects and featuring sudden headache, pain in the back and limbs, shivering, cough, constipation, a mottled rash, delirium, prostration, weakness of heart action, stupor and sometimes coma and death. Epidemic (louse-borne) typhus is caused by *Rickettsia prowazeki* and is common in conditions of civil breakdown and population migration. Rocky Mountain Spotted Fever is spread by ticks, Scrub typhus by mites and endemic typhus by fleas. Q fever may be spread by ticks or by inhalation of infected material. Antibiotics, such as tetracycline, are effective and life-saving in typhus.

typing a procedures to establish the group or classification of blood or tissues. See also BLOOD GROUPS and TISSUE TYPING.

Tyrosets a brand name for throat lozenges containing TYROTHRICIN and the local anaesthetic drug benzocaine.

tyrosinaemia a genetic AUTOSOMAL RECESSIVE metabolic disorder due to a deficiency of the enzyme tyrosine aminotransferase. This causes abnormally high blood levels of tyrosine and leads to disturbance of brain function with mental retardation.

tyrosinase a copper-containing enzyme that occurs in melanocytes and catalyses the production of MELANIN from TYROSINE. Also known as monophenol mono-oxygenase.

tyrosine the AMINO ACID 4-hydroxyphenyl-alanine. This is one of the 20 amino acids that are incorporated into protein.

tyrosine hydroxylase inhibitors drugs used to treat PHAEOCHROMOCYTOMA or to maintain patients awaiting surgery for phaeochromocytoma. An example is metirosine (Demser).

tyrosinosis a genetic disorder featuring excessive levels of TYROSINE, methionine and other amino acids in the blood. There is liver and kidney damage and a form of RICKETS that does not respond to treatment with vitamin D. Death may occur in infancy from liver failure. Liver transplantation is curative.

tyrothricin an antibiotic obtained from the soil bacterium *Bacillus brevis* and used by local application to treat GRAM POSITIVE infections and mouth and throat infections. It is too toxic for systemic use. It is formulated with BENZOCAINE as lozenges under the brand name Tyrozets.

u

ubiquitin a small 76-residue protein found in all animal cells and known to have altered minimally throughout evolutionary history. Ubiquitin is linked by covalent bonds to proteins destined for destruction by PROTEASOMES.

Ubretid a brand name for DISTIGMINE.

Ukidan a brand name for UROKINASE.

ulcer a local loss of surface covering (EPITHELIUM) and sometimes deeper tissue in skin or MUCOUS MEMBRANE. An open sore. Loss of surface leads to infection and further tissue damage. Ulcers may be caused by physical or chemical damage, by loss of blood supply or by local infection. Ulcers of the STOMACH or DUODENUM are called peptic ulcers. See also BEDSORES, VARICOSE ULCERS and TROPICAL ULCERS.

ulceration 1 an ULCER.
2 the development of an ulcer.

ulcerative colitis a disease of early adult life and of unknown cause in which the lining of the large intestine (the colon) becomes inflamed, swollen and extensively ulcerated. The bowel may become dangerously thinned and may perforate. There are recurrent attacks of diarrhoea, with blood, mucus and pus in the stools, and a constant desire to empty the bowels (tenesmus). The condition predisposes to cancer. Treatment is with corticosteroid drugs, given in suppositories, enemas or by mouth. Surgical removal of affected lengths of bowel is sometimes necessary.

Ulcol a brand name for SULPHASALAZINE.

ulna one of the pair of forearm long bones. The ulna is on the little finger side. At its upper end it has a hook-like process, the olecranon, that fits into a hollow at the back of the lower end of the upper arm bone (the humerus) and prevents the elbow from over-extending. When the hand is turned on the long axis of the arm, the radius bone rotates around the ulna.

ulnar nerve one of the main nerves of the arm that supplies some of the muscles of the forearm and all the small muscles of the hand. It also provides sensation to the skin of the third of the hand on the little finger side. It is near the surface at the back of the elbow where it is liable to be painfully struck. This is the basis for the notion of the 'funny bone'.

ultra- *prefix denoting* beyond or on the other side of.

ultracentrifuge a device for rotating small containers at extremely high speed so as to expose the liquid contents to powerful centrifugal force, of the order of 100,000 g. Ultracentrifuges are used to separate particles of molecular size and determine molecular weights.

ultrafiltration filtration through a SEMIPERMEABLE MEMBRANE that allows only the passage of small molecules, such as those smaller than protein molecules.

ultramicroscopic too small to be resolved by an ordinary optical microscope but visible when illuminated by light from the side agaist a dark background.

ultramicrotome a MICROTOME for cutting very thin slices of specimens to be examined by electron microscopy.

ultrasonic pertaining to sound waves above the upper limit of audibility, that is above about 20,000 Hz.

ultrasonic angioplasty the use of ultrasound energy delivered via a fine catheter to break down a thrombotic occlusion in an artery such as a coronary artery. Such methods suffer from the danger that solid particles will be carried by the blood flow to occlude smaller vessels and further damage the heart.

ultrasonography the use of ultrasonic waves to image body structures for diagnostic purposes. See ULTRASOUND SCANNING.

ultrasound scanning a method of body imaging based on the reflectivity of sound. By using very high frequency (ultrasonic) sound the wavelengths are brought down to the necessary small dimensions. Piezo-electric transducers are used both to generate the waves and to pick up the reflected sound. Ultrasound scanning is believed to be completely safe and is widely used in obstetrics as well as in other disciplines. It can show the position of the placenta, reveal twins at an early stage, show the size and sex of the fetus and detect major fetal abnormalities such as ANENCEPHALY and SPINA BIFIDA. It can measure rates of blood flow in the fetus and can detect certain forms of congenital heart disease. Ultrasound is also widely used to scan fluid-filled organs, especially the heart. Echocardiography can reveal the heart's action in detail. Doppler ultrasound provides essential information on blood flow. Intravenously-injected microbubble agents increase the reflectivity of blood many times and greatly widen the scope of ultrasound scanning.

ultrasound treatment the use of high frequency sound waves to achieve deep heating of inflamed soft tissues such as muscles, tendons and ligaments.

Ultratard a brand name for a long-acting form of INSULIN.

ultraviolet light electromagnetic radiation of shorter wavelengths than visible light but longer wavelength than X-rays. Ultraviolet light is divided into three zones – UVA with wavelengths from 380 to 320 nanometres (billionth of a metre), UVB from 320 nm down to 290 nm and UVC from 290 nm down to one tenth of a nanometre. UVC and most of UVB are absorbed by the ozone layer in the earth's stratosphere. Ultraviolet light causes sunburning and damages the skin's elastic protein, collagen. It is also a major factor in the development of the skin cancers rodent ulcer (BASAL CELL CARCINOMA), MALIGNANT MELANOMA and SQUAMOUS CELL CARCINOMA. It causes PINGUECULA and PTERYGIUM in the eyes.

umbilical cord the nutritional, hormonal and immunological link between the mother and the fetus during pregnancy. The umbilical cord arises from the PLACENTA and enters the fetus at the site of the future navel. It carries two arteries and a vein that connect to the fetal circulation.

umbilical hernia protrusion of a loop of bowel through a weakness in the abdominal wall at the navel.

umbilicus the scar formed by the healing at the exit site of the UMBILICAL CORD after this has been tied and cut and the tissues have died and dropped off.

Uncinaria a genus of hookworms.

uncinate hooked (in the literal sense). Hook-shaped.

uncircumcized in possession of a FORESKIN (prepuce). Anatomically complete.

unconditioned response an automatic or instinctive response produced by a stimulus without any prior learning or conditioning process.

unconditioned stimulus the stimulus that evokes an UNCONDITIONED RESPONSE.

unconscious 1 pertaining to a person lacking awareness or to mental processes that proceed outside consciousness.

2 A person's total memory store, whether immediately accessible or not.

3 the domain of the psyche, characterized by Freud (see FREUDIAN THEORY) as having a content that was not accessible because it was unacceptable and thus repressed. Compare CONSCIOUS, SUBCONSCIOUS.

unconsciousness a state of unrousability caused by brain damage and associated with reduced activity in part of the BRAINSTEM called the reticular formation. Unconsciousness varies in depth from a light state, in which the unconscious person responds to stimuli by moving or protesting, to a state of profound coma in which even the strongest stimuli evoke no response. Causes include head injury, inadequate blood supply to the brain, fainting, asphyxia, poisoning, near drowning, starvation, low blood sugar (HYPOGLYCAEMIA) and severe KETOSIS.

uncus a hook-shaped part near the front of the temporal lobe of the brain that is concerned with the senses of smell and taste. Disease in this area may produce hallucinations of foul smells.

undecenoates a range of drugs used to treat external fungal infections. Brand names are Monophytol paint and Mycota cream.

undescended testicle a testicle that has remained in the abdomen, where testicles normally develop, or in the inguinal canal by which they normally descended to the SCROTUM. Undescended testicles do not become fertile and are more than normally prone to cancer later in life. For these reasons it is wise to have an undescended testicle brought down in childhood.

undulant fever see BRUCELLOSIS.

ungual pertaining to a fingernail or toenail. Subungual means 'under a nail'.

unguent, unguentum an ointment.

uni- *prefix denoting* single or one.

uniarticular pertaining to only one joint. Monoarticular.

UNICEF *acronym for* United Nations Children's Fund (formerly United Nations International Children's Emergency Fund). UNICEF is a UN agency responsible for the administration of programmes to improve child and maternal health as well as education.

unicellular consisting of a single cell, as in a unicellular organism.

unilateral on or affecting one side only. One-sided. From Latin *unus*, one and *latus*, a side or flank.

uniovular originating from one egg, as in the case of monozygotic twins.

unipara a woman who has had only one baby. Primipara.

unipolar having one pole or process as in the case of a nerve cell with one AXON. As applied to an electrode, the term is something of a misnomer. A second electrode is needed to complete the circuit, but this is often attached at a remote point from the point of application of the electrode.

unipotentiality the full limitation of the ability of cells to differentiate. For example, basal epidermal cells in the skin cannot differentiate to form other types of cells; they can only produce keratinised squames. See also PLURIPOTENTIALITY and TOTIPOTENTIALITY.

Uniroid-HC a brand name for an ointment or suppository of CINCHOCAINE and HYDROCORTISONE.

Unisomnia a brand name for NITRAZEPAM.

Univer a brand name for the calcium channel blocker drug VERAPAMIL.

unmedullated see UNMYELINATED.

unmyelinated of a nerve fibre, lacking a MYELIN SHEATH.

unofficial of medication not listed in a pharmacopoeia.

unsaturated pertaining to a compound, especially of carbon, in which atoms are linked by double or triple valence bonds. A saturated compound has only single bonds. In general, unsaturated compounds are less stable than saturated compounds and can undergo a wider variety of reactions.

unstable angina a severe and dangerous form of ANGINA PECTORIS due to breakdown of atherosclerotic plaque in the coronary arteries and the formation of blood clot (thrombosis). There may also be coronary artery spasm from products derived from blood platelets. Pain becomes more frequent and prolonged and may occur at rest. The accurate predictability of pain in terms of its relation to a given amount of exertion is lost. The risk of a heart attack is high.

upper respiratory tract infection any infection of the nose, throat, sinuses or LARYNX such as the common cold, sore throat (pharyngitis), tonsillitis, sinusitis, laryngitis and croup. The cumbersome phrase is often abbreviated to URTI.

upstream in genetics, at a stage in the sequence of processes in the expression of a gene that is further away from the final protein product. The term is also used to mean in the direction of the 5´-end of a chain of bases in DNA (see PHOSPHODIESTER BOND). In both cases the opposite sense is called 'downstream'.

urachus a primitive structure in the embryo from which the bladder develops. Later it is represented by a fibrous cord that extends from the top of the bladder to the UMBILICUS.

uracil one of the four bases that form the nucleotide code in RNA.

uraemia accumulation of the nitrogenous waste products of METABOLISM in the blood as a result of failure of the kidneys to excrete them (kidney failure). The effects include nausea, vomiting, OEDEMA, itching, spontaneous bleeding, anaemia, apathy, confusion, muscle twitching, seizures, drowsiness, coma and death.

uranium 235 the isotope of uranium used to produce a fission chain reaction in atomic weapons by establishing a critical mass.

Urantoin a brand name for the antibacterial drug nitrofurantoin.

urate a salt of uric acid.

ur-defence a belief, such as a conviction of personal immortality, or of the inherent goodness of man, considered by some to be essential to psychic well-being.

urea a substance formed in the liver from the excess of nitrogenous material derived from amino acids and excreted in solution in the urine. Urea can be used as an osmotic diuretic and as a cream for ICTHYOSIS and other hyperkeratotic skin disorders. The drug is on the WHO official list. See also URAEMIA.

urease an enzyme that breaks down urea to ammonia and carbon dioxide.

Uremide a brand name for FRUSEMIDE (furosemide).

-uresis *combining form denoting* excreted in the urine or the excretion of urine.

ureter a tube that carries urine downwards from each kidney to the urinary bladder for temporary storage. The ureters have muscular walls that can contract to assist in the propulsion of the urine.

ureteric pertaining to the URETER.

ureteric colic see RENAL COLIC.

ureterolithotomy surgical removal of a stone from the URETER. Stones may be removed by open operation or by crushing them so that the gravel may be washed out. The commonest method, however, is by shock wave LITHOTRIPSY.

urethra the tube that carries urine from the bladder to the exterior. In the male, the urethra runs along the penis and opens at the tip. In addition to urine it carries seminal fluid during ejaculation. In the female, the urethra is shorter and runs directly downwards from the bladder in front of the VAGINA, opening between the vaginal orifice and the CLITORIS.

urethral pertaining to the URETHRA.

urethral discharge an outflow of PUS, MUCUS or mucus and pus from the URETHRA. A urethral discharge suggests, but does not necessarily imply, a SEXUALLY TRANSMITTED DISEASE such as GONORRHOEA or chlamydial non-specific urethritis. Sexual excitement promotes a crystal-clear discharge of lubricating mucus from the urethra in the male. This normal effect is not usually described as a urethral discharge.

urethral stricture a local narrowing of the URETHRA. This was formerly a common sequel to untreated GONORRHOEA but is now uncommon. Stricture can block the outflow of urine, and back-pressure effects can damage the kidneys. It may be treated by repeated widening (dilatation) with an instrument called a bougie or by a plastic operation.

urethral syndrome a condition, affecting mainly females, in which symptoms suggesting CYSTITIS or URETHRITIS occur but in which no infecting organisms can be found in the urine. There are several possible causes including local allergies and congestion of the urethra from sexual intercourse.

urethritis inflammation of the lining of the URETHRA. This is usually caused by a SEXUALLY TRANSMITTED DISEASE.

urethro- *combining form denoting* URETHRA.

urethroplasty plastic surgical repair of the URETHRA.

urethroscope an instrument for examining the inner lining of the URETHRA.

Urex a brand name for FRUSEMIDE (furosemide).

-uria *combining form denoting* the presence in the urine of a specified substance or specifying the state or quantity of the urine, usually implying abnormality. Examples are HAEMATURIA and OLIGURIA.

Uriben a brand name for the antibacterial drug NALIDIXIC ACID.

uric acid the main end product of PURINE metabolism. Uric acid is derived from ADENINE and GUANINE, two of the purines in DNA and RNA (nucleic acids). An excess of uric acid salts in the body can cause GOUT and kidney stones.

uricosuric any drug that promotes the excretion of URIC ACID or urates.

uridine the nucleoside of URACIL found in RNA and other NUCELOTIDES.

urinal a container into which bedridden men may urinate.

urinalysis urine testing, especially if a battery of tests is applied.

urinary bladder the muscular bag for the temporary storage of urine situated in the midline of the pelvis at the lowest point in the abdomen, immediately behind the pubic bone. The bladder wall relaxes at intervals to allow filling but as the internal pressure rises the intervals become shorter and the urgency to empty the bladder becomes more frequent and then continuous. Unless emptied voluntarily, the bladder will eventually empty spontaneously.

urinary bladder disorders see BLADDER STONE, BLADDER CANCER, CYSTITIS and INCONTINENCE.

urinary calculus any stone or concretion of mineral or organic substances that forms within the kidney or urine collecting system. Urinary stone formation is encouraged by reduced urinary output with highly concentrated urine, infection, and various metabolic conditions in which abnormal quantities of substances occur in the urine.

urinary catheterization the passage of a blunt-ended, rubber or plastic tube along the URETHRA into the bladder so as to release urine in cases of obstruction to outflow or inability to pass urine voluntarily for other reasons (URINARY RETENTION).

urinary diversion provision of an alternative exit route for urine or of an alternative temporary urine store in the body, after surgical removal of the URINARY BLADDER. The ureters may be brought out on to the surface of the abdomen, implanted into the COLON or RECTUM or implanted into a substitute bladder, formed from a loop of small bowel, with an outlet through the skin or the anus.

urinary infection see CYSTITIS and PYELONEPHRITIS.

urine the fluid excretion of the kidneys, a solution in water of organic and inorganic substances, most of which are waste products of METABOLISM. Normal urine is clear, of varying colour, of specific gravity between 1.017 and 1.020 and slightly acid. It contains UREA, URIC ACID, creatinine, ammonia, sodium, chloride, calcium, potassium, phosphates and sulphates.

urine retention the inability to urinate voluntarily or to empty a full bladder. Urine retention affects predominantly males because of the frequency with which enlargement of the PROSTATE GLAND causes obstruction to the outflow of urine. The condition can also be caused by disorder of the neurological control of the bladder function. There is constant discomfort or pain in the lower abdomen and a swelling above the pubis. Emergency treatment involves passage of a CATHETER or drainage of the bladder by way of a CANNULA passed

through the wall of the abdomen. The cause of the obstruction must then be removed.

Urispas a brand name for the urinary ANTISPASMODIC drug flavoxate.

uro- *combining form denoting* urine or the urinary system.

urobilinogen a pigment formed from BILIRUBIN in the intestine by bacterial action that is absorbed into the bloodstream and excreted in the urine. Excess is found in the urine in HAEMOLYTIC ANAEMIA and certain liver disorders. None is found in complete obstruction to the the outflow of bile from the liver.

uricosurics drugs used to treat GOUT. An example is sulfinpyrazone (Anturan).

urodynamics functioning of the urinary bladder, urethral sphincter and pelvic floor muscles. Urodynamic studies, which may be made in various ways, involve measurement, over a period, of such parameters as urine flow rates; total bladder capacity; bladder urine volume before voiding; residual urine volume; bladder pressure before and during voiding; bladder contractability; urethral sphincter pressure; patient's perception of bladder fullness; and ability to inhibit voiding. Urodynamics has been described as the 'gold standard investigation' in the management of all forms of urinary incontinence.

urogenital, urinogenital pertaining to both urinary and genital structures or functions.

urography X-ray examination of the urinary system using a CONTRAST MEDIUM to show the outline of the interior of the urinary drainage system and the bladder. The contrast medium is usually an iodine-containing solution given either by way of a vein (intravenous urography) or passed back up the URETERS using a fine tube inserted through a CYSTOSCOPE (retrograde urography).

urokinase an enzyme found in human urine that is used as a drug to dissolve blood clots occurring within blood vessels. A PLASMINOGEN activator.

urolith a URINARY CALCULUS.

urolithiasis the presence or formation of urinary stones (calculi).

urologist a doctor who specializes in the diagnosis and treatment of disorders of the KIDNEYS, the URETERS, the URINARY BLADDER and the URETHRA.

urology the scientific study of the disorders of the kidneys and the urine drainage system. The list that follows highlights the key entries related to urology in the dictionary: bladder, bladder cancer, catheterization, cystoscopy, kidney, lithotripsy, prostate, prostate cancer, prostatectomy, prostate gland, prostate-specific antigen (PSA), prostatic hyperplasia, prostatitis pyelitis, intravenous pyelography, Peyronie's disease, priapism, renal calculus, renal colic, renal failure, renal transplant, retrograde ejaculation, ureter, urethra, urinalysis, urinary stones, vesicoureteric reflux, renal calculus, urinary diversion.

Uromitexan a brand name for MESNA.

uroprotectants drugs used to minimise damage to the epithelium of the urinary tract in patients under treatment with cyclophosphamide or ifosfamide. An example is Uromitexan.

Uro-Tainer a brand name for a fluid containing the antiseptic MANDELIC ACID.

ursodeoxycholic acid a drug that helps to dissolve cholesterol gallstones.

Ursofalk a brand name for URSODEOXYCHOLIC ACID.

URTI *acronym for* UPPER RESPIRATORY TRACT INFECTION.

urticant 1 causing itching.
2 a substance that causes itching.

urticaria an allergic skin condition featuring itchy, raised, pink areas surrounded by pale skin. These patches persist for periods of half an hour to several days and then resolve. Urticaria may result from sunlight, cold, food or drug allergy, insect bites, scabies, jelly fish stings or contact with plants. Treatment is with antihistamine drugs or corticosteroids.
Also known popularly as nettle rash or hives.

uterine 1 pertaining to the UTERUS.
2 having the same mother but not the same father.

uterine dystocia weak and uncoordinated contractions of the womb during childbirth.

Dystocia affects about 4% of all births and is one of the commonest indications for emergency caesarean section. Often the cause remains obscure.

uterotropics drugs used to induce or stimulate labour by causing uterine contractions. Examples are synthetic oxytocin (Syntocinon) and ergometrine with synthetic oxytocin (Syntometrine).

uterus the female organ in which the fetus grows and is nourished until birth. The uterus is a hollow, muscular organ, about 8 cm long in the non-pregnant state, situated at the upper end of the VAGINA and lying behind and above the URINARY BLADDER and in front of the RECTUM. It is suspended by LIGAMENTS from the walls of the pelvis. The lining of the uterus is called the endometrium. Under the influence of hormones from the ovaries this thickens progressively until shed during menstruation. In pregnancy, the uterus expands considerably with the growth of the fetus until it rises almost to the top of the abdominal cavity.

uterus disorders see CERVICAL EROSION, CERVICITIS, ENDOMETRIOSIS, FIBROIDS, PROLAPSE and RETROVERTED UTERUS.

Utinor a brand name for NORFLOZACIN.

utricle a small sac or pocket.

uvea the coat of the eye lying immediately under the outer SCLERA (the CHOROID), together with its continuum, the CILIARY BODY and the IRIS. The uvea contains many blood vessels and a variable quantity of pigment. From the Greek word *uvea*, a grape, because of the resemblance of the uvea to a peeled black grape). See also UVEITIS.

uveitis inflammation of the UVEA. Uveitis of the front part of the uvea is called IRIDOCYCLITIS or anterior uveitis, inflammation of the rear part is called CHOROIDITIS or posterior uveitis.

uvula the small fleshy protuberance that hangs from the middle of the free edge of the soft PALATE. Like the rest of the soft palate, the uvula is composed of muscle and connective tissue covered by MUCOUS MEMBRANE.

V

vaccination see IMMUNIZATION.

vaccination encephalitis inflammation of the brain following vaccination. This has occurred after whooping cough immunization but no causal relationship has been proved. The risks of whooping cough are much greater than the risks of immunization. Mumps immunization very rarely causes encephalitis.

vaccinal pertaining to VACCINE or IMMUNIZATION.

vaccine a suspension of microorganisms of one particular type that have been killed or modified so as to be safe, given to promote the production of specific ANTIBODIES to the organism for purposes of future protection against infection.

vaccinia a mild disease, acquired from the udders of cows, that causes blisters on the hands but no significant general upset. The disease is of historic importance. From knowledge of it, Edward Jenner developed vaccination against SMALLPOX. Also known as cowpox.

vacuole a small, clear region in the CYTOPLASM of a cell, sometimes surrounded by a membrane. Vacuoles may be used to store cell products or may serve an excretory function.

vacuum extraction a method of assisting childbirth used as an alternative to FORCEPS DELIVERY. A cup-like device is applied to the baby's scalp and firmly secured by suction. Traction can then be applied via a short chain and handle. The equipment is known as a ventouse.

vagal pertaining to the VAGUS NERVE.

Vagifem a brand name for OESTRADIOL (estradiol).

vagina literally a sheath. In the female it acts as a receptacle for the penis in coitus and as the birth canal. The vagina is a fibromuscular tube, 8–10 cm long lying behind the URINARY BLADDER and URETHRA and in front of the RECTUM. The cervix of the UTERUS projects into it upper part. The vagina is highly elastic and has a thickened and folded mucous membrane lining that can stretch readily.

vaginal pertaining to the VAGINA or to a sheath.

vaginal disorders see GONORRHOEA, THRUSH, TRICHOMONIASIS, VAGINAL DISCHARGE, VAGINISMUS, VAGINITIS and VULVOVAGINITIS.

vaginal discharge the release from the VAGINA of a clear or creamy fluid which may or may not be offensive. Some degree of discharge, compounded of mucus from the glands in the CERVIX and cast-off cells from the vaginal lining, is normal. Profuse, offensive discharge may be caused by a retained tampon or by infection with *Candida albicans* or *Trichomonas vaginalis*.

vaginal evisceration a rare event in which loops of bowel herniate downwards through the vagina. Vaginal evisceration may occur as a result of injury or following uterine or vaginal surgery or it may occur spontaneously as a result of the rise in intra-abdominal pressure caused by straining at stool or coughing.

vaginal hysterectomy an operation to remove the womb, performed by way of the VAGINA so that no external scar is visible. The operation, however, leaves more extensive scars in the wall of the vagina than in the case of an ABDOMINAL HYSTERECTOMY.

vaginal ultrasound see TRANSVAGINAL ULTRASOUND.

vaginismus apparently involuntary rejection, by a woman, of attempted sexual intercourse or gynaecological examination. The legs are straightened, the thighs pressed together and the muscles of the pelvic floor, that surround the vagina, tighten. Sexual desire may appear normal until penetration is tried. Treatment involves full explanation and instruction in the insertion of vaginal dilators of gradually increasing size.

vaginitis inflammation of the vagina from any cause, such as chlamydial infection, GONORRHOEA, THRUSH or TRICHOMONIASIS. Also known as colpitis.

vaginosonography a form of ULTRASOUND SCANNING adapted to examination of the womb and capable of showing thickening of the womb lining characteristic of cancer of the ENDOMETRIUM. It can be used as a screening test, especially in postmenopausal women.

vagotomy an operation to cut some or all of the branches of the VAGUS NERVE to the stomach so as to reduce its effect in promoting acid and PEPSIN secretion. As a result of advances in drug treatment with H_2 receptor blockers such as Ranitidine (Zantac) and the discovery of the role of the organism *Helicobacter pylori* in causing peptic ulceration, this operation has almost been abandoned.

vagus nerves the 10th of the 12 pairs of cranial nerves that arise directly from the brain. The vagus nerves arise from the sides of the MEDULLA OBLONGATA and pass down the neck to supply and control the throat, LARYNX, BRONCHI, lungs, OESOPHAGUS and heart. They then enter the abdomen on the front and back of the oesophagus and supply the stomach and the intestines as far as the descending COLON. The vagus is an important part of the AUTONOMIC NERVOUS SYSTEM. From the Latin *vagus*, wandering or straying.

valaciclovir an antiviral drug used to treat genital herpes and SHINGLES. Like ACICLOVIR, the drug is a DNA polymerase inhibitor. Research has shown that a daily dose of 500 mg of this drug reduces the risk of transmission of genital herpes by 75%. A brand name for valaciclovir is Valtrex.

Valcite a brand name for VALGANCICLOVIR.

valdecoxib a COX-2 INHIBITOR drug used to treat OSTEOARTHRITIS, RHEUMATOID ARTHRITIS and DYSMENORRHOEA. A brand name is Bextra. In late 2004 the drug was shown to have cardiotoxic properties similar to those of rofecoxib and it was recommended that the drug should be withdrawn.

valence, valency the property of an atom or group of atoms to combine with other atoms or groups of atoms in specific proportions. The number of atoms of hydrogen with which an atom can combine or displace in forming compounds. An atom may be monovalent, divalent, trivalent or tetravalent.

Valclair a brand name for DIAZEPAM.

valetudinarian 1 a person constantly suffering from one illness or another, especially one deeply preoccupied with ill health. 2 a HYPOCHONDRIAC.

valganciclovir a pro-drug of GANCICLOVIR used to treat CYTOMEGALOVIRUS INFECTION especially with retinitis. A brand name is Valcyte.

valgus, valgum, valga abnormal displacement of a part in a direction away from the midline of the body. Hallux valgus is the condition in which the big toe is bent outwards so as to point towards the little toe. Compare VARUS.

valine one of the ESSENTIAL AMINO ACIDS, a constituent of protein.

Valium a now abandoned brand name for DIAZEPAM. It would appear that the name has become too well known.

vallate surrounded by a rimmed depression.

vallecula a small hollow, groove or depression on the surface of an organ.

Vallergan a brand name for the antihistamine drug TRIMEPRAZINE (alimemazine).

Valoid a brand name for the ANTIEMETIC antihistamine drug cyclizine.

valproic acid an ANTICONVULSANT drug used to prevent all kinds of epileptic seizures. The drug is on the WHO official list. A brand name is Convulex.

valsalva manoeuvre the effort to breathe out forcibly while the mouth and nose are firmly closed or the vocal cords pressed together. The valsalva manoeuvre is employed while straining at stool and in other circumstances. It causes a rise in blood pressure followed by a sharp drop and then a second sharp rise in blood pressure. This may be dangerous in people with heart disease and should be avoided. (Antonio Maria Valsalva, 1666–1723, Italian anatomist).

valsartan a drug that interferes with the action of ANGIOTENSIN II and is used to treat high blood pressure (HYPERTENSION). A brand name is Diovan.

Valtrex a brand name for VALACICLOVIR.

valve a structure that allows movement in a predetermined direction only. There are valves in the heart, the veins, the lymphatics, the urethra and elsewhere.

valvotomy cutting or breaking open adhesions that have formed between the cusps of a valve, especially in the heart.

valvular pertaining to, or possessing, a VALVE or valves.

valvulitis inflammation of a VALVE, especially a heart valve.

Vancocin a brand name for the antibiotic VANCOMYCIN.

vancomycin an antibiotic drug effective against many GRAM POSITIVE bacteria. It is toxic and its use is limited to infections that fail to respond to the common antibiotics. The drug is on the WHO official list. A brand name is Vancocin.

vardenafil a selective inhibitor of phosphodiesterase type 5, the enzyme in the penis that limits the action of nitric oxide in promoting erection. (See SILDENAFIL CITRATE for fuller account). The drug is said to be effective more rapidly than Viagra. A brand name, presumably selected with the irresistible necessity for humour, is Levitra.

variable region the part of an ANTIBODY at the tip of each arm (N-terminal region) that varies considerably in its AMINO ACID sequence from one antibody to another. The remaining parts of the structure of antibodies are fixed and almost identical. This region is coded for by the V gene.

varicella see CHICKENPOX.

varices varicosities. Swollen, twisted and distorted lengths of vessels, usually veins. Veins affected by varices are called VARICOSE VEINS and these are commonest in the legs. Oesophageal varices are the varicosities of the veins at the lower end of the OESOPHAGUS that occur when the portal vein drainage through the liver is impeded by CIRRHOSIS. They are liable to cause dangerous bleeding. The singular form of the word is varix.

varico- *combining form denoting* VARICES *or* varicosity.

varicocele VARICES in the plexus of veins that surrounds the testicle, usually on the left side, forming an irregular swelling in the scrotum. This is usually of no significance but may cause a dragging ache and may affect fertility. In these cases surgical correction is needed.

varicose pertaining to VARICES.

varicose ulcer a breakdown of the skin overlying an area of poor local nutrition from blood stagnation in varicose veins. Varicose ulcers often start following a minor injury to an area of skin already prejudiced by a poor blood supply. They tend to be very persistent unless the underlying cause is treated.

varicose veins enlarged, twisted and distorted veins, occurring in the legs, at the lower end of the gullet (see VARICES) or in the scrotum (see VARICOCOELE). Leg varicosities are due to a constitutional or acquired failure of the vein valves so that deep vein pressure is transmitted to the surface veins. They cause stagnation of blood, inadequacy in local tissue nutrition and tissue staining and breakdown to form varicose ulcers. Deep veins, if healthy, afford adequate blood drainage so varicose veins of the legs can safely be removed or obstructed by injections of sclerosing substances. Support from firm elastic hosiery is also helpful. Exercise is beneficial.

Varidase a brand name for a mixture of STREPTOKINASE and STREPTODORNASE used locally to remove blood clots and organic debris from wounds.

variola an alternative term for SMALLPOX.

varix see VARICES.

varus, varum, vara displaced or angulated towards the midline of the body. Coxa vara is a deformity at the upper end of the thigh bone (femur) in which the angle between the neck and the shaft is decreased.

vas a vessel or channel conveying fluid. See VAS DEFERENS.

Vascace a brand name for CILAZAPRIL.

Vascardin a brand name for the nitrate VASODILATOR drug, isosorbide dinitrate, used to treat ANGINA PECTORIS.

vascular endothelial growth factor (VEGF) a naturally-occurring POLYPEPTIDE of between 121 and 206 amino acids. It occurs in four forms, the commonest of which has 165 amino acids. VEGF promotes the production of tiny new blood vessels by stimulating the growth, migration and proliferation of endothelial cells. It increases permeability of existing vessels and causes widening of blood vessels through the mediation of NITRIC OXIDE. Local shortage of blood supply (ischaemia) increases the gene expression of VEGF. Chronic lymphocytic leulkaemia B cells resist APOPTOSIS by secreting and binding VEGF. VEGF in retinal ischaemia is believed to be the basis of one kind of AGE-RELATED MACULAR DEGENERATION (ARMD). The drug pegaptanib that opposes VEGF has achieved some success in treating ARMD.

vascularization the process of forming new blood vessels.

vascular naevus a birthmark caused by a non-malignant tumour of skin blood vessels. See also PORT-WINE STAIN and HAEMANGIOMA.

vascular retinopathy abnormalities in the RETINA caused by blood vessel disease or high blood pressure (HYPERTENSION).

vasculature any system of blood vessels supplying an organ, an area of the body or the whole body.

vasculitis widespread inflammation of blood vessels occurring as the principal feature of a range of conditions including ERYTHEMA NODOSUM, POLYARTERITIS NODOSA, some forms of PURPURA, RHEUMATOID ARTHRITIS, TEMPORAL ARTERITIS and THROMBOANGIITIS OBLITERANS. In many cases vasculitis is caused by combinations of ANTIGENS and ANTIBODIES (immune complexes) that circulate in the blood until they settle on the wall of a small artery and excite a severe inflammatory response. Vasculitis is often treated with corticosteroid and other immunosuppressive drugs.

vas deferens the fine tube that runs up in the SPERMATIC CORD on each side from the EPIDIDYMIS of the TESTICLE, over the pubic bone and alongside the bladder to end by joining the seminal vesicle near its entry to the PROSTATE GLAND. The vas deferens conveys spermatozoa from the testicle to the seminal vesicle. See also VASECTOMY.

vasectomy the common operation for male sterilization. The VAS DEFERENS is exposed on each side through a short incision, just below the root of the penis, and is cut through and the ends tied off and secured well apart. Following this no newly produced spermatozoa can reach the exterior. The operation can be reversed but fertility is not always restored.

vaso- *combining form denoting* a vessel, especially a blood vessel.

vasoactive affecting blood vessels.

vasoconstriction active narrowing of small arteries as a result of contraction of the circular smooth muscle fibres in their walls. This severely reduces the flow of blood through them. Compare VASODILATATION.

vasodilatation widening of blood vessels as a result of relaxation of the muscles in the walls. This allows a greater volume of blood to pass through in a given time. Compare VASOCONSTRICTION.

vasodilation see VASODILATATION.

vasogenic shock a dangerous condition in which the small arteries of the body widen so much that the volume of the blood is insufficient to maintain the circulation. Urgent measures to constrict the vessels or to increase the blood volume by fluid infusion are necessary.

vasomotor pertaining to the control of the muscles in the walls of blood vessels and hence the rate of blood flow.

vasopressin a hormone secreted in the HYPOTHALAMUS and stored in and released from the PITUITARY GLAND. Vasopressin controls water retention by the kidneys and thus the water content of the body. Deficiency of vasopressin causes DIABETES INSIPIDUS.

vasospasm tightening or spasm of blood vessels.

vasovagal pertaining to the VAGUS NERVE and to its effects on blood vessels.

vCJD *abbrev. for* new variant CREUTZFELDT-JAKOB DISEASE.

vasovagal syncope see FAINTING.

Vasoxine a brand name for METHOXAMINE.

VD *abbrev. for* venereal disease, now, for reasons of political correctness, largely obsolete. See SEXUALLY TRANSMITTED DISEASES.

VDRL *abbrev. for* Venereal Disease Research Laboratory (test). This is a standard test for SYPHILIS.

vector an animal such as an insect, capable of transmitting an infectious disease from one person to another. The disease organism develops and multiplies in the vector and may pass through various stages, or may even be transmitted through one or more generations of the vector, before being passed on to a human host. From the Latin *vectus*, one who carries.

vecuronium a non-DEPOLARIZING muscle relaxant used in general anaesthesia. A brand name is Norcuron.

Veganin a brand name for a mixture of the painkilling drugs ASPIRIN, CODEINE and PARACETAMOL.

vegetarianism the policy of deliberate exclusion of animal muscle protein and sometimes of other animal products, such as eggs and milk, from the diet. Strict vegetarians, such as Vegans (who avoid eggs and dairy products), must exercise care to ensure that all essential elements are present in the diet.

vegetation a fungus-like excrescence, especially that caused by abnormal blood clotting on heart valves and on the lining membranes of the heart chambers in infective ENDOCARDITIS.

vegetative state see PERSISTENT VEGETATIVE STATE.

VEGF *abbrev. for* VASCULAR ENDOTHELIAL GROWTH FACTOR.

veins thin-walled blood vessels containing blood at low pressure which is being returned to the heart from tissues that have been perfused by arteries.

veins disorders see HAEMORRHOIDS, PHLEBITIS, THROMBOPHLEBITIS, VARICES, VARICOCELE and VARICOSE VEINS.

Velbe a brand name for the anticancer drug VINBLASTIN.

Velcade a brand name for BORTEZOMIB.

Velosulin a brand name for a neutral INSULIN.

vena cavae the largest veins in the body. The superior vena cava drains blood from all parts of the body above the level of the heart, the inferior vena cava from all parts below the heart. The two veins empty into the right atrium of the heart.

vena caval filter a wire mesh filtering device that is inserted into the lower of the two major veins of the body (the inferior vena cava) to prevent the passage of dangerous blood clots from the leg veins and elsewhere to the lungs, via the heart (pulmonary embolism). If large, such emboli are very dangerous and are a common cause of death. Vena caval filters can be inserted by way of a vein in the groin.

venene a mixture of snake venoms used to produce a general antidote (antivenin).

venereal pertaining to love. The term is seldom, if ever, used in its strict sense and has come to be indissolubly associated with disease spread during coitus. Today, however, even in this context the word has a very old-fashioned, even archaic, ring and has been almost universally replaced by the less emotive 'sexually-transmitted'. From the Latin *Venus*, the Roman goddess of love.

venereal diseases see SEXUALLY TRANSMITTED DISEASES.

venereal warts warts growing on the penis or vulva, usually pink and fleshy. Venereal warts are almost always multiple and are ordinary warts modified by their situation and caused by papillomaviruses spread during sexual intercourse.

venereology the medical speciality concerned with the sexually transmitted diseases. Now usually known, for purposes of euphemism, as genitourinary medicine.

venepuncture entry into a vein, usually with a hollow needle so as to gain access to the bloodstream for the purpose of obtaining a sample of blood or giving an injection directly into it.

venesection cutting of a vein for the purposes of removing blood. This is done to obtain blood for transfusion, or, rarely, to treat conditions, such as POLYCYTHAEMIA, HAEMOCHROMATOSIS and PORPHYRIA.

venlafaxine a SEROTONIN and NORADRENALINE re-uptake inhibitor drug used to treat depression. Brand names are Efexor and Efexor XL.

venogram an X-ray of a vein or veins, using a CONTRAST MEDIUM.

venom poison produced by scorpions, some jellyfish, some fish, a few snakes, some toads, the Gila monster, some spiders and a few insects such as bees, wasps or hornets. Venoms act in various ways and may affect either the nervous system, to cause paralysis, or the blood to cause either widespread clotting or bleeding. Venoms are seldom fatal except in very young or debilitated people.

veno-occlusive causing veins to be closed by flattening or other means.

veno-occlusive disease a liver disorder in which the small branches of the hepatic vein within the liver become obliterated, but not by blood clotting. The condition can be caused by drinking 'bush tea' containing pyrrolizidine alkaloids, and in other ways. The effects are almost identical to those of the BUDD-CHIARI SYNDROME.

venous stasis syndrome post-thrombotic syndrome, a disabling, dangerous and cosmetically disfiguring complication of deep vein thrombosis. The syndrome features chronic leg swelling, dermatitis, hard cellulitis, skin pigmentation and chronic ulceration, and a tendency to recurrent thrombosis and embolism.

Ventavis a brand name for ILOPROST TROMETAMOL.

ventilator a mechanical air or oxygen pump used to maintain breathing in a paralysed, deeply anaesthetized or brain-damaged person unable to breathe spontaneously. Ventilators provide an intermittent flow of air or oxygen under pressure and are connected to the patient by a tube inserted into the windpipe (trachea) either through the mouth or nose or through an opening in the neck (a tracheostomy).

ventimask an oxygen mask that provides oxygen enrichment of the inspired air while eliminating rebreathing of the expired carbon dioxide. Various models are available providing different concentrations of oxygen.

Ventmax SR a brand name for SALBUTAMOL.

Ventodisks a brand name for SALBUTAMOL.

Ventolin a brand name for the bronchodilator drug SALBUTAMOL.

ventouse the suction equipment used for assisting in childbirth. See VACUUM EXTRACTION.

ventral pertaining to the front of the body. From the Latin *venter*, the belly. Compare DORSAL.

ventral hernia a HERNIA through the abdominal wall but not through the commoner UMBILICAL, INGUINAL or FEMORAL routes.

ventricle a cavity or chamber filled with fluid, especially the two lower pumping chambers of the heart and the four fluid-filled spaces in the brain.

ventricular pertaining to a VENTRICLE.

ventricular ectopy a recent term for ventricular ectopic (premature) beats, also known as EXTRASYSTOLES. There are indications that ventricular ectopy during exercise may be due to perfusion defects in the heart muscle, and that frequent ectopic beats after exercise may be more significant indications of risk than when they occur during exercise.

ventricular fibrillation a rapid fluttering, or twitching motion of the heart muscle which has replaced the normal forceful contraction and which is ineffective in moving blood. Ventricular fibrillation is a form of cardiac arrest and causes irremediable brain damage within a matter of minutes and unless reversed by DEFIBRILLATION is soon fatal. The drug

bretylium tosylate (Bretylate) can be used when electrical defibrillation fails.

ventricular tachycardia a dangerous disorder of heart rhythm in which the contraction of the lower main pumping chambers is initiated from uncontrolled electrical impulses arising in the ventricles instead of in the SINOATRIAL NODE. The heart rate is abnormally fast – between 140 and 220 beats per minute and this may persist for hours or days and progress to severe HEART FAILURE and death. Treatment is by the use of drugs such as lignocaine (lidocaine) to regulate the rate or by electrical DEFIBRILLATION.

venule a very small VEIN.

Vepeside a brand name for ETOPOSIDE.

Veractil a brand name for the antipsychotic drug methotrimeprazine (levomepromazine).

verapamil a calcium channel blocker drug used to correct irregularities in the heart beat. There is evidence that verapamil and other calcium channel blockers are anti-atherogenic and can prevent recurrent narrowing of arteries, such as the coronary arteries after these have been widened by CORONARY ANGIOPLASTY. The drug is on the WHO official list. Brand names are Cordilox, Securon, Univer and Vertab SR. Formulated with trandolapril it is marketed as Tarka.

vecuronium a non-polarizing muscle relaxant used with light general anaesthesia to achieve muscle relaxation for operations lasting for 20 to 30 minutes. The drug is on the WHO official list.

vergence 1 movement of one or both eyes so that the visual axes converge or diverge. 2 the effect caused on a parallel beam of light by a convex (converging) or concave (diverging) lens.

vermi- *combining form denoting* worm.

vermicide a drug that kills worms.

vermiform appendix see APPENDIX.

vermifuge a drug that drives out intestinal worms.

verminous infected with worms or infested with ectoparasites (vermin).

Vermox a brand name for the anthelmintic drug MEBENDAZOLE.

vernal pertaining to the spring.

vernal conjunctivitis an allergic form of inflammation of the CONJUNCTIVA probably caused by contact with spring pollens.

vernix an abbreviation of vernix caseosa, a layer

of greasy material, skin scales and fine hairs with which fetuses and new-born babies are covered. Vernix is easily washed off after birth.

verruca a WART on any part of the skin.

verruca peruviana a benign form of BARTONELLOSIS with persistent skin spots.

verrucose, verrucous covered with warts or wart-like protrusions.

verrucous endocarditis small, non-infective, wartlike collections of clotted blood (thromboses) occurring on the heart valves and the lining of the heart chambers in SYSTEMIC LUPUS ERYTHEMATOSUS.

versicolor of various colours.

version 1 a procedure in obstetrics to turn the fetus in the womb into a position more suitable for delivery.
2 rotation of both eyes simultaneously in the same direction.

vertebra one of the 24 bones of the VERTEBRAL COLUMN.

vertebral column the bony spine. A curved column of bones, called vertebrae, of the same general shape but increasing progressively in size from the top of the column to the bottom. Each vertebra has a stout, roughly circular body behind which is an arch that encloses an opening to accommodate the spinal cord. The arch bears bony protuberances on either side and at the back and facets for articulation with the vertebrae above and below. The vertebral bodies are fixed together by cushioning intervertebral discs and strong longitudinal ligaments. There are 7 neck vertebrae, 12 in the back and 5 in the lumbar region. The 5th lumbar vertebra sits on top of the sacrum, which is formed from the fusion of five vertebrae. The coccyx, hanging from the lower tip of the sacrum, is the fused remnant of the tail.

vertebral column disorders see ANKYLOSING SPONDYLITIS, KYPHOSIS, LORDOSIS, OSTEOPOROSIS, SCOLIOSIS, SLIPPED DISC, SPINA BIFIDA, SPONDYLOLISTHESIS and SPONDYLOLYSIS.

vertebrobasilar insufficiency an inadequacy in the supply of blood to the brainstem and lower part of the brain as a result of disease in the pair of vertebral arteries that run up through holes in the side processes of the bones of the neck. This causes VERTIGO and loss of balance, double vision, weakness or paralysis on one side of the body, speech disturbances and sometimes loss of consciousness.

vertex 1 the top of the head.
2 any apex or highest point on a body structure.

vertical transmission transmission, as of a hereditary characteristic or of a disease, from parent to offspring. Horizontal transmission is transmission between contemporaries or individuals of the same generation.

vertigo the illusion that the environment, or the body, is rotating. Severe vertigo causes the sufferer to fall. It may be due to TRAVEL SICKNESS, fear of heights, anxiety, alcohol, drugs or HYPERVENTILATION. Some cases of the most severe and persistent vertigo may be caused by disorders of the balancing mechanisms in the inner ears, such as MÉNIÈRE'S DISEASE or LABYRINTHITIS, or to disease of the CEREBELLUM or its connections from VERTEBROBASILAR INSUFFICIENCY, TUMOUR or MULTIPLE SCLEROSIS.

Vertigon a brand name for the phenothiazine antiemetic drug prochlorperazine.

Vesanoid a brand name for TRETINOIN.

vesical pertaining to a bladder, especially the URINARY BLADDER.

vesication blistering.

vesicle 1 a small blister.
2 any small pouch, as the SEMINAL VESICLES, the small bladders which store semen. From the Latin *vesiculum*, the diminutive of vesica, a bladder or bag.

vesicoureteric reflux backward passage of urine from the bladder up into the URETERS during voiding. This occurs, mainly in children, because of failure of the valve-like effect of the oblique entry of the ureters through the bladder wall. Organisms from the bladder are able to gain access to the kidneys and set up an acute PYELONEPHRITIS.

vessel any closed channel for conveying fluid.

vestibule a space or cavity forming the entrance to another cavity.

vestige a body structure with no current apparent function which appears to have had a function at a previous evolutionary stage.

vestigial pertaining to a VESTIGE.

Vfend a brand name for VORICONAZOLE.

V gene a gene that codes for the main part of the VARIABLE REGION of an antibody.

Viagra a brand name for the oral drug SILDENAFIL CITRATE. The drug, which is made by the firm Pfizer, has been dubbed 'the Pfizer riser'.

Viazem XL a brand name for DILTIAZEM.

Vibramycin a brand name for the tetracycline antibiotic DOXYCYCLINE.

vibration-induced disorders a range of disorders that includes deafness, vibration-induced neuropathy, Raynaud's phenomenon ('white finger'), and, in the case of whole body vibration, motion sickness, low-back pain, visual disturbances and insomnia. The hand-arm vibration syndrome (HAVS) features spasm of blood vessels with white fingers, sensory and motor nerve damage and even muscle, bone and joint changes. This syndrome was recognized by international agreement in 1985.

vibration white finger one of the VIBRATION-INDUCED DISORDERS.

vibrator an electrically driven reciprocating device used to apply low-frequency repetitive force for the purpose of massaging any part of the body.

vibratory saw an electrically driven saw with a circular blade that does not rotate but oscillates through a small arc. The vibratory saw cannot cut soft tissue such as skin or muscle which move with the blade but readily cuts through unyielding material such as bone or a plaster cast.

Vibrio a genus of curved, motile, GRAM NEGATIVE organisms that contains the bacillus, *Vibrio cholerae* that causes CHOLERA.

vidarabine a drug that inhibits DNA synthesis and is used to treat Herpes simplex infections.

video game epilepsy epileptic attacks triggered by playing video games on a TV set or in an amusement arcade. The stimulus may be regularly changing lights (intermittent photic stimulation) or pattern alone. Children should view the TV screen from a distance of 2 metres.

videoscopic surgery see LAPAROSCOPIC SURGERY.

Videx, Videx EC a brand name for DIDANOSINE.

vigabatrin a drug that simulates the action of the NEUROTRANSMITTER GABA and is used to treat EPILEPSY resistant to other controlling agents. A brand name is Sabril.

villous 1 pertaining to villi (see VILLUS).
2 featuring numerous fingerlike processes.

villous adenoma a benign, finger-like tumour of the COLON that often secretes excessive quantities of mucus and may develop into a cancer.

villous atrophy flattening and disappearance of the finger-like absorptive processes of the

small intestine that is a feature of COELIAC DISEASE. Villous atrophy is associated with an increased density of LYMPHOCYTES in the bowel lining (intraepithelial lymphocytes), but whether they cause it is uncertain.

villi small finger-like processes on a surface, as in the small intestine, the PLACENTA, the tongue and the CHOROID PLEXUSES of the brain.

villin an actin-binding, severing and bundling protein found in the MICROVILLI of the apical membranes of certain cells, including the canalicular microvilli of hepatocytes. Abnormalities in the expression of the gene for villin, resulting in the absence of this protein are thought to be a cause of such liver disorders as biliary atresia.

vinblastine an anticancer drug used mainly in the treatment of HODGKIN'S DISEASE and other LYMPHOMAS. The drug is on the WHO official list. A brand name is Velbe.

vinca alkaloids a class of cytotoxic drugs used to treat various cancers. Examples are vindesine (Eldisine), vincristine (Oncovin) and vinblastine (Velbe).

Vincent's angina see VINCENT'S DISEASE.

Vincent's disease painful inflammation of the mouth caused by two organisms, *Bacillus fusiformis* and *Borrelia vincenti*. These are commonly present in the mouth and cause infection only if some other factor, such as immune deficiency or vitamin B deficiency, operates. Vincent's disease features painful ulcers and an acute destructive inflammation of the gums called necrotizing gingivitis. It is treated with the antibacterial drug metronidazole, an antiseptic mouthwash and dental scaling to remove calculus. Also known as trench mouth. (Jean-Hyacinthe Vincent, 1862–1950, French bacteriologist).

vincristine a vinca alkaloid anticancer drug used to treat LEUKAEMIA. The drug is on the WHO official list. A brand name is Oncovin.

vinculum a slender connecting band.

vindesine a vinca alkaloid anticancer drug (see CYTOTOXIC DRUGS) used to treat LEUKAEMIA. A brand name is Eldisine.

vinorelbine a vinca alkaloid anticancer drug (see CYTOTOXIC DRUGS) used to treat lung and breast cancer. A brand name is Navelbine.

Vioform a brand name for the antibacterial drug CLINOQUINOL. Vioform is usually formulated with other drugs, such as

Viokase a brand name for PANCREATIN.

violaceous of a violet or purple colour.

viomycin an antibiotic drug used in cases of TUBERCULOSIS that resist standard treatment.

Vioxx a brand name for ROFECOXIB.

VIPoma a neuroendocrine tumour of tissue that stains for chromogranin A and is rich in vasoactive intestinal peptide, hence the name. The condition features persistent large-volume watery diarrhoea.

viraginity 1 male-like psychology in a woman. 2 a violent, ill-tempered personality in a woman (a virago).

viraemia the presence of viruses in the blood.

Viraferon a brand name for INTERFERON ALFA-2b.

viral pneumonia inflammation of the lung (PNEUMONIA) caused by a virus infection.

Virazole a brand name for TRIBAVIRIN (ribavirin).

Viread a brand name for TENOFOVIR DIOPROXIL.

virgin a person who has never had sexual intercourse. From the Latin *virgo*, a maiden, so should, strictly, apply only to a female. The claimed physical sign of virginity, an intact HYMEN, cannot always be relied upon because the part is subject to wide anatomical variations and to trauma. Both the term and the importance placed on an intact hymen are residua of a male-dominated past.

virgin birth conception and child-bearing by a woman who has never had sexual intercourse, as a result of artificial insemination with donated semen.

viricidal capable of killing VIRUSES.

Viridal Duo a brand name for ALPROSTADIL.

virilism masculinization in the female. This may occur in tumours of the adrenal glands or ovaries which secrete abnormal quantities of the male hormones, the androsterones, or in the condition of congenital adrenal hyperplasia. There is increased growth of body hair, balding at the temples, acne, absence of menstruation, enlargement of the clitoris, increased muscular development and deepening of the voice. The treatment involves removal of the cause.

virility the quality of sexual maleness, strength, vigour and energy.

virion a complete virus particle, as found outside cells, and consisting of the genetic material and the surrounding capsid.

virology the study of viruses of medical importance and the diseases they produce.

Virormone a brand name for the male sex hormone drug TESTOSTERONE.

virotherapy a new treatment modality in which viruses are used to detect cancerous cells, invade them, and replicate in them in such a way as to kill them. Viruses that bind only to proteins found on tumour cells may be used, or they may be modified so that their genes will transcribe only in tumour cells. Virotherapy may also involve the transport of cytotoxic drugs selectively into tumour cells. It has produced hopeful results in animals and clinical trials on humans have begun.

virtual patient a highly complex software model consisting of representations of the hundreds of different metabolic or immunological states that occur in the organs of human patients with a particular disease. In theory, and perhaps soon in practice, the method can be used to test new drugs by applying the detailed technical description of the drug to the program and observing its effect. Simulation of diabetes has already been achieved and tested for its validity.

virucidal-anhidrotics drugs used to remove warts. An example is glutaraldehyde (Glutarol).

virulence the capacity of any infective organism to cause disease and to injure or kill a susceptible host.

viruses infectious agents of very small size and structural simplicity, all of which are smaller than the smallest bacterium. They consist of a core of nucleic acid, either DNA or RNA encased in a protein shell. Viruses can maintain a life-cycle and reproduce only by entering a living cell and taking over part of the cell function. All living cells are believed to be susceptible to virus infection. The most important virus diseases are AIDS, ARTHROPOD-BORNE FEVERS, ASEPTIC MENINGITIS, BURKITT'S LYMPHOMA, CHICKENPOX, COLD SORES, the COMMON COLD, CYTOMEGALOVIRUS INCLUSION DISEASE, EPIDEMIC KERATOCONJUNCTIVITIS, EQUINE ENCEPHALITIS, some forms of GASTROENTERITIS, GLANDULAR FEVER, INFLUENZA, LASSA FEVER, MEASLES, MOLLUSCUM CONTAGIOSUM, MUMPS, ORF, PARAINFLUENZA, POLIOMYELITIS, PROGRESSIVE MULTIFOCAL LEUCOENCEPHALOPATHY, RABIES, SARS, SHINGLES, VACCINIA, WARTS and YELLOW FEVER.

virus interference protection of cells against

virus infection, as a result of prior virus infection of neighbouring cells. This stimulates the production of proteins, called INTERFERONS, which become attached to the membranes of other cells and prompt them to produce enzymes which interfere with replication of subsequent viral invaders. Interferons also stimulate killer LYMPHOCYTES to attack and destroy cells which have been invaded with viruses.

viscera organs within a body cavity, especially digestive organs. The singular form of the word is viscus.

visceral leishmaniasis see KALA AZAR.

visceroptosis downward displacement or sagging of an organ or organs within a body cavity, especially the intestines, due to loss of support.

Viscotears a brand name for CARBOMER (POLYACRYLIC ACID).

viscous of a liquid substance, thick and sticky so that there is resistance to flow.

vision disorders see ASTIGMATISM, CATARACT, CORNEAL ULCERATION, DIABETIC RETINOPATHY, GLAUCOMA, HYPERMETROPIA, HYPHAEMA, KERATOCONUS, MACULAR DEGENERATION, MYOPIA, OPTIC NEURITIS, PRESBYOPIA, RETINOPATHY, TRACHOMA and TRANSIENT ISCHAEMIC ATTACKS.

Visken a brand name for the beta blocker drug pindolol.

visual acuity the extent to which an eye is capable of resolving fine detail. Visual acuity is measured by means of a SNELLEN'S CHART TEST.

visual aids optical devices, often of a telescopic type, used by the visually handicapped to assist vision. Also known as low visual aids.

visual evoked responses a method of modifying the ELECTROENCEPHALOGRAM by exposing the subject to visual stimuli. The most useful is a reversing chessboard pattern in black and white. The time taken after each reversal for the change to occur on the EEG is affected by defects of conduction along the optic nerves, tracts and radiations, such as may be caused by MULTIPLE SCLEROSIS. Unlike visual acuity tests, the method is purely objective.

visual fields the area over which some form of visual perception is possible while the subject looks straight ahead. The visual fields normally extend outwards to about 90 on either side but are more resticted below and above. Parts of the fields may be lost as a result of GLAUCOMA, retinal damage, optic nerve disease and brain disease.

visual purple rhodopsin. A light-sensitive pigment in the rods of the retina that is chemically changed on exposure to light and in the process stimulates production of a nerve impulse. Visual purple is reformed in the dark.

visuscope an instrument used in ORTHOPTICS to determine whether or not a patient is using the central macular region of the RETINA. The device projects an image on to the retina and the relationship of this to the FOVEA can be observed.

vital capacity the volume of air that can be expelled from the lungs by a full effort following a maximal inspiration.

vital signs indications that a person is still alive. Vital signs include breathing, sounds of the heart beat, a pulse that can be felt, a reduction in the size of the pupils in response to bright light, movement in response to a painful stimulus and signs of electrical activity in the brain on the ELECTROENCEPHALOGRAM.

vital statistics figures of births, marriages and deaths in a population, from which the rate of natural increase or decrease in the population can be calculated. Vital statistics also indicate life expectancy at birth and the main causes of death.

vitamin D analogues drugs used to treat nutritional malabsorption and rickets and osteomalacia resistant to vitamin D treatment. Examples are alfacalcidol (Alfad, One Alpha), calcitriol (Calcijex, Rocaltrol), calcipotriol (Dovonex) and tacalcitol (Curatoderm).

vitamins chemical compounds necessary for normal body function. Vitamins are needed for the proper synthesis of body building material, HORMONES and other chemical regulators; for the biochemical processes involved in energy production and nerve and muscle function; and for the breakdown of waste products and toxic substances. The B group of vitamins are COENZYMES without which many body ENZYMES cannot function normally. The amounts of vitamins needed for health are very small and are almost always present in adequate amounts in normal, well-balanced diets. Excess intake of vitamins A and D is dangerous. Vitamins C and E are antioxidants and may be valuable, in doses many times the minimum requirement, in combating the damaging effect of FREE RADICALS. Folic acid supplements are valuable in preventing NEURAL TUBE DEFECTS. Vitamins are conventionally divided into the fat-soluble group A,D,E and K, and the water-soluble group, vitamin C (ascorbic acid) and the B vitamins – B1 (thiamine), B2 (riboflavine, riboflavin), nicotinic acid, B6 (pyridoxine), pantothenic acid, biotin, folic acid and B12. The term was derived from the belief that vitamins were 'vital amines'.

vitamin K dilemma the conflicting requirements to protect small babies from dangerous internal, often intracranial, bleeding resulting from vitamin K deficiency (which is readily avoided by an injection of the vitamin) and the increased risk of cancer in children who have received an intramuscular injection of the vitamin early in life. It was hoped that an oral preparation of the vitamin would eliminate this risk, but cases have occurred in which the oral vitamin has failed to prevent intracranial bleeding.

vitamin S a proposed term for the dietary content of salicylates (SEE ASPIRIN) which are becoming recognized as micronutrients because of their wide range of actions in maintaining health.

vitiligo a skin disorder that features white patches, of variable size and shape, especially on the face, the backs of the hands, the armpits and around the anus. Vitiligo is inconspicuous in white people in winter but very obvious in black people or tanned whites. The affected areas of skin are deficient in pigment cells called melanocytes, but the cause of this is unclear. An immunological process is thought to be involved. Repigmentation can be achieved by taking a melanin precursor, L-phenylalanine, and then exposing the skin to ULTRAVIOLET LIGHT.

vitrectomy an ophthalmic operation to remove part or all of the VITREOUS BODY of the eye.

vitreous body the transparent gel that occupies the main cavity of the eye between the back of the CRYSTALLINE LENS and the RETINA.

vitreous detachment separation of the rear part of the VITREOUS BODY from the retina as a result of the natural shrinkage that occurs in the elderly. Perception of floating specks or moving clouds may be a conspicuous, but often temporary, feature of the process.

vitreous haemorrhage bleeding into the VITREOUS HUMOUR of the eye. This occurs most commonly from RETINOPATHY caused by DIABETES. Vision may be severely affected and bleeding tends to recur. Vitreous haemorrhage may lead to extension of blood vessels and fibrous tissue from the RETINA into the vitreous (proliferative retinopathy) and subsequent detachment of the retina. Treatment of diabetic retinopathy can prevent vitreous haemorrhage.

vivax malaria MALARIA caused by *Plasmodium vivax* and causing bouts of fever on alternate days.

vivisection 1 experiments performed on living animals involving surgery.
2 any scientific work in which live animals are used.

vocal cords a pair of pearly-white shelves of thin mucous membrane stretched across the interior of the LARYNX and capable of being tensioned to a widely varying degree by small laryngeal muscles. The vocal cords are caused to vibrate by the outwards passage of air from the lungs and the sound so produced is modulated by changes in the shape and volume of the mouth cavity to produce speech and song.

vocal cord disorders see LARYNGITIS, RECURRENT LARYNGEAL NERVES and SINGER'S NODES.

Volsaid Retard a brand name for DICLOFENAC.

Voltarol, Voltarol Rapid a brand name for DICLOFENAC.

voluntary muscle striped muscle normally contracted in the course of volitional activity.

volar pertaining to the palm of the hand or the sole of the foot.

Volkmann's ischaemic contracture shortening, weakening and FIBROSIS of forearm muscles as a result of loss of blood supply, usually following a fracture of the upper arm bone or an elbow injury. The effect is a fixed and disabling deformity with bending of the wrist and fingers. Treatment is difficult and involves major surgery. (Richard von Volkmann, 1830–89, German surgeon).

Volsaid Retard a brand name for DICLOFENAC.

volsella forceps a long grasping instrument with sharp teeth, used especially in gynaecological surgery to grasp and pull or rotate tissue.

Voltarol a brand name for DICLOFENAC.

volvulus twisting of a loop of intestine.

Volvulus causes obstruction to the flow of contents and threatens occlusion of the supplying blood vessels. This will inevitably lead to GANGRENE of the affected segment of bowel unless quickly relieved by surgery. This may involve removing the affected loop of bowel and joining up the free ends.

vomer a thin, flat plate of bone that forms the rear part of the partition of the nose (the nasal septum).

vomiting involuntary upward expulsion of the stomach contents. Vomiting is prompted by the presence of vomit-stimulating substances in the blood and effected by sudden, forceful downward movement of the DIAPHRAGM and inward movement of the abdominal wall. The stomach wall muscle plays no part.

vomitus material vomited.

von Gierke's disease a form of glycogen storage disease caused by a genetically induced deficiency of the enzyme glucose-6-phosphatase. The condition features obesity, enlargement of the liver and kidneys, poor muscles, OSTEOPOROSIS, stunted growth and a round, doll-like face. Attacks of HYPOGLYCAEMIA occur and these may be fatal. Treatment is necessary from birth and involves a special diet to maintain the level of blood sugar. (Edgar Otto Conrad von Gierke, 1877–1945, German pathologist).

von Hippel-Lindau disease an autosomal dominant genetic disorder with incomplete penetrance due to a mutation on chromosome 3. The principal feature is a single or multiple tumour of blood-forming tissue (haemangioblastoma) in the retina, the cerebellum, the brainstem or the spinal cord. These are highly vascular lesions that may grow dangerously at puberty or during pregnancy. Some secrete erythropoietin that leads to a large over-production of red blood cells. (Eugen von Hippel, 1867–1939, German ophthalmologist; and Arvid Lindau, b. 1892, Swedish pathologist).

von Recklinghausen's disease see NEUROFIBROMATOSIS.

von Willebrand's disease a rare group of hereditary bleeding disorders, similar to HAEMOPHILIA but usually less severe, due to deficiency of a clotting factor necessary for PLATELET adhesion to blood vessel walls and as a carrier for Factor VIII. The condition is usually inherited as an autosomal dominant and, unlike haemophilia, occurs equally in both sexes. Some cases are autosomal recessive. The mutations, which are many, are on the short arm of chromosome 12. The von Willebrand factor (vWF) is a protein, the levels of which are raised in pregnancy. (E. A. von Willebrand, 1870–1949, Swedish physician).

voriconazole a second-generation triazole antifungal drug used to treat invasive ASPERGILLOSIS and other fungal infections resistant to FLUCONAZOLE. A brand name is Vfend.

vorticose veins four veins in the CHOROID coat of the eye, the branches of which have a whorled appearance.

voyeurism covertly observing people undressing or engaging in sexual intercourse, so as to obtain sexual stimulation. Voyeurism is a male activity, engaged in by the lonely and the socially inadequate, and is usually accompanied by MASTURBATION.

vulva the female external genitalia, comprising the mons pubis, the two pairs of LABIA, the area between the labia minora, and the entrance to the VAGINA.

vulval disorders see BARTHOLINITIS, CHANCRE, GENITAL HERPES, KRAUROSIS VULVAE, SEXUALLY TRANSMITTED DISEASES, THRUSH, TRICHOMONIASIS and VULVOVAGINITIS.

vulvitis inflammation of the VULVA.

vulvodynia chronic pain or burning sensation in the vulva in the absence of any objective physical cause. The condition is associated with depression and diminished or absent libido. The condition has been successfully treated with the anticonvulsant drug gabapentin.

vulvovaginitis inflammation of the VULVA and the VAGINA. The condition is commonest in childhood as a result of poor hygiene, a foreign body in the vagina or sexual assault. There is soreness on urination, redness and sometimes a slight discharge. Daily washing is often all that is necessary.

waist the part of the trunk between the lower ribs and the pelvis.

waist circumference a measurement that has been shown to be a valid index identifying people who need weight management if they are to avoid a significant risk of heart attacks. Waist circumferences of more than 94 cm in men and more than 80 cm in women indicate danger.

Waldenström's macroglobulinaemia a rare disease of elderly people in which a MONOCLONAL immunoglobulin, IgM, is present in excessive quantities in the blood. This is caused by a cancerous overgrowth of B LYMPHOCYTES in the bone marrow. The condition progresses to immune deficiency. Treatment is by PLASMAPHERESIS and the use of the drug CHLORAMBUCIL. (Jan Waldenström, Swedish physician, b. 1906).

walking aids supports for people with muscle weakness, joint disease or balancing problems. They include plain walking sticks, sticks with three or four small feet, light alloy Zimmer frame 'walkers', elbow crutches and walking calipers.

wall-eyed having a divergent squint (STRABISMUS) or a large, white scar on the cornea.

wan unnaturally pale.

warfarin an ANTICOAGULANT drug used to prevent blood from clotting in the blood vessels. The drug is on the WHO official list. A brand name is Marevan.

Warticon a brand name for PODOPHYLLOTOXIN.

warts verrucas, non-malignant, localized skin excrescences caused by different strains of the more than 130 human papilloma viruses. These stimulate overgrowth of the prickle cell layer at the base of the EPIDERMIS of the skin, resulting in excessive local production of the horny material KERATIN. Warts on the soles (plantar warts) are forced into the skin by the weight of the body. Most warts resolve without treatment but may be removed by cutting, electric cautery, freezing with liquid nitrogen or by applications of SALICYLIC ACID or formalin. A recent treatment, said to be highly effective, is the use of a molecular complex derived from human milk called ALPHA-LACTALBUMIN which is compounded with oleic acid.

WASP gene see WISKOTT-ALDRICH SYNDROME.

Wassermann reaction a now obsolescent COMPLEMENT-FIXATION test for SYPHILIS. The Wassermann test is not entirely specific for syphilis and, for a positive diagnosis, tests such as the *Treponema pallidum* haemagglutination assay (TPHA) or a fluorescein-labelled antibody test (FTA-ABS) are used. See also VDRL. (August Paul von Wassermann, 1866–1925, German pathologist).

water the oxide of hydrogen. Water is essential for life and provides about 70% of the body weight in lean people and about 50% in the obese. The body of the average 70 kg man contains about 40 l of water. Just over half the total body water is within the cells and the remainder is outside, partly in the blood, but mainly in the tissue spaces surrounding the cells. Water molecules are very small and move freely across cell membranes. Water is lost from the body in the urine, in evaporation from the skin, in the expired air and in the faeces. Losses are reduced automatically if there is reduced intake. Restricting water intake is dangerous especially in hot conditions.

water-borne infection diseases spread by

bacterial and other organismal contamination of water. Those spread by drinking water include TYPHOID FEVER and other SALMONELLA infections, CHOLERA, HEPATITIS A, AMOEBIC DYSENTERY and worm parasite infestations. Those acquired by contact with water include LEPTOSPIROSIS, SCHISTOSOMIASIS and GUINEA WORM infection.

waterbrash sudden, unexpected secretion of a quantity of saliva into the mouth as a reflex response to symptoms of DYSPEPSIA.

water for injection sterile water provided in sealed glass ampoules ranging in volumes from 1 ml to 100 ml. It is on the WHO official list.

water-hammer pulse a pulse of high amplitude that seems to collapse suddenly. This is characteristic of regurgitation from leakage (incompetence) of the heart valve at the outlet of the main pumping chamber – the aortic valve. Also known as collapsing pulse or Corrigan's pulse.

Waterhouse-Friderichsen syndrome a rare disorder caused by invasion of the blood by meningococcus organisms often in the course of an attack of MENINGITIS. There is bleeding into the ADRENAL GLANDS causing adrenal failure and SHOCK. Enlarging purple spots appear on the skin and there is rapid collapse and coma. Death is inevitable unless effective antibiotic and supportive treatment is quickly given. (Rupert Waterhouse, 1873–1958, English physician; and Carl Friderichsen, b. 1886, Danish paediatrician).

water intoxication the effect of excessive water retention in the brain in the course of any disorder causing general OEDEMA. The condition features headache, dizziness, confusion, nausea and sometimes seizures and coma. Treatment is the correction of the cause and measures to withdraw water from the brain into the blood.

watermelon stomach a malformation of the blood vessels in the stomach lining resulting in an appearance on endoscopic examination resembling the inside of a watermelon. The longitudinal folds of the lining (rugae) contain convoluted columns of blood vessels like the stripes of a watermelon. The condition mainly affects elderly women and results in blood loss into the stools and iron-deficiency ANAEMIA. Surgery or corticosteroid treatment may be necessary.

water on the brain see HYDROCEPHALUS.

water on the knee a common term for an accumulation of SYNOVIAL FLUID within the knee joint. Such an accumulation is called an effusion and results from inflammation caused by injury or disease.

Watson-Crick model the double helix concept of the DNA molecule, proposed by two workers in Cambridge in 1953, which triggered off a revolution in biology and medicine and led to an explosive succession of advances in genetics. (James D. Watson, b. 1928, American molecular biologist; and Francis H. C. Crick, 1916–2004, English biochemist and neurophysiologist).

wax bath a form of local heat treatment using hot molten wax into which the affected part is dipped.

wax, ear see EAR WAX.

Waxsol a brand name for DOCUSATE SODIUM.

WBC *abbrev. for* white blood cell.

weakness a state of debility caused by prolonged bed rest, muscle disease or wasting, severe infection, anaemia, starvation or psychological disorder with loss of motivation. Once causes have been removed, the only cure for weakness is activity. See also FATIGUE, MYALGIC ENCEPHALOMYELITIS.

weaning substitution of solid foods for milk in an infant's diet.

webbing edge-to edge joining of the fingers or toes by flaps of skin. This is a common congenital abnormality and is easily corrected by surgery. Webbing of the neck may occur in TURNER'S SYNDROME.

web eye a popular term for PTERYGIUM.

web-fingered see WEBBING.

Wegener's granulomatosis a form of AUTOIMMUNE small blood vessel disease in which local masses of cells, blood capillaries and fibrous tissue (granulation tissue) form in the nose, the kidneys, the lungs and the heart. These masses cause local damage and become gangrenous. Symptoms include nose-bleeds, blood in the urine (haematuria) and chest pain. The condition may progress to kidney failure. Treatment is with cyclophosphamide. (F. Wegener, German pathologist, b. 1907).

weight, inability to perceive see ABAROGNOSIS.

weight loss the effect of an absorbed CALORIE intake that is smaller than the calorie expenditure. Weight loss is a feature of

ANOREXIA NERVOSA, CANCER, DEPRESSION, DIABETES, persistent DIARRHOEA, deliberate dieting, MALABSORPTION, starvation, THYROTOXICOSIS, TUBERCULOSIS and persistent VOMITING. Unexplained weight loss is a warning sign of possible serious disease and should never be disregarded.

Weil-Felix reaction a test for rickettsial infections such as Q FEVER, RICKETTSIAL POX, ROCKY MOUNTAIN SPOTTED FEVER, TRENCH FEVER and SCRUB TYPHUS. The test does not use rickettsial ANTIGENS but strains of the organisms Proteus OK 19 and OXK which happen to react with antibodies to rickettsiae. (Edmund Weil, 1880–1922, Austrian physician; and Arthur Felix, 1887–1956, Czechoslovakian bacteriologist).

Weil's disease see LEPTOSPIROSIS.

welder's eye an acute CONJUNCTIVITIS occurring a few hours after unprotected exposure to the intense ULTRAVIOLET LIGHT output from an electric welding or cutting arc. The eyes are markedly inflamed and the outer layer of the CORNEAS strips off exposing the corneal nerves. There is acute pain, tearing and uncontrollable spasm of the muscles that close the eye. Regeneration of EPITHELIUM occurs in a few days. Antibiotic eye drops are used to prevent infection.

Welldorm a brand name for the sleeping drug CHLORAL BETAINE (cloral betaine).

Welldorm Elixir a brand name for CHLORAL HYDRATE.

Wellferon a brand name for INTERFERON ALFA.

well-man a healthy man who attends a clinic or surgery to ensure that his general health, lifestyle, and sexual performance are satisfactory.

Wellvone a brand name for ATOVAQUONE.

wen see SEBACEOUS CYST.

Werdnig-Hoffman disease spinal muscular atrophy of infants. This is one of the causes of the FLOPPY INFANT SYNDROME. There is profound loss of muscle TONE, absence of reflexes, weakness of the muscles of respiration and twitching of the tongue. The diagnosis can be confirmed by muscle BIOPSY. There is no known treatment and the outlook is grave. (Guido Werdnig, 1844–1919, Austrian neurologist; and Johann Hoffman, 1857–1919, German neurologist).

Werner's syndrome a hereditary, probably autosomal recessive, condition featuring dwarfism, premature ageing, atrophy of the skin, CATARACTS, severe arterial disease, OSTEOPOROSIS, atrophy of the testicles and DIABETES. (C. W. Otto Werner, b. 1879, German physician).

Wernicke-Korsakoff syndrome a late form of brain damage occurring in long-term alcoholics who rely mainly on alcohol for nutrition and who are severely deficient in the B vitamin thiamine. One form, Wernicke's encephalopathy, starts suddenly with incoordination, staggering, paralysis of eye movements and mental confusion progressing to stupor and death. Patients can be saved by a timely injection of a large dose of thiamine. The other form, Korsakoff's psychosis, features severe memory loss with inability to store new data and a process of confabulation, in which the affected person makes up stories to fill in the gaps in the memory. Korsakoff's psychosis is usually irreversible and proceeds to profound DEMENTIA. (Karl Wernicke, 1848–1904, German neurologist; and Sergei Sergeivitch Korsakov, 1853–1900, Russian psychiatrist and neurologist).

Wernicke's encephalopathy see WERNICKE-KORSAKOFF SYNDROME.

Wernicke's sign a physical sign demonstrating damage to the nerve pathways subserving vision. This commonly causes loss of half the field of vision in each eye. When a narrow beam of light is projected on to the blind half of one retina, the pupils do not constrict. Light shone on the normal half, however, causes the pupils to constrict.

Western blotting a method of detecting very small quantities of a protein of interest in a cell or body fluid. The sample is spread by ELECTROPHORESIS on a block of polyacrylamide gel. The separated proteins are then transferred, by blotting, to a thin plastic sheet to make them more accessible for reaction with an antibody specific for the protein of interest. The antibody-antigen complex can then be detected by rinsing the sheet with a second, radioactive, antibody that recognises the first. The sheet will now produce a dark band on X-ray film. See also SOUTHERN BLOTTING.

West's syndrome an epileptic brain disorder featuring clusters of tonic spasms and characteristic findings on electroencephalography that affects young children between 3 and 6 months of age, causing psychomotor regression. See also INFANTILE SPASMS. W.J. West was a British doctor who described the syndrome in a letter to *The Lancet* in 1840.

West Nile fever a flavivirus arthropod-borne (arboviral) infection endemic mainly in birds and spread by culicine mosquitoes. The disease causes a feverish illness mainly affecting young children. There is headache, muscle pain, enlarged lymph nodes and a rash of slightly raised spots. Widespread epidemics in the USA in 2002 – the first reported in the Western hemisphere – featured a high percentage of cases of encephalitis, especially in elderly patients, with a mortality of about 9%. New features were noted, including a poliomyelitis-like involvement of anterior horn cells with muscle paralysis.

wet dream a popular term for an erotic dream culminating in a spontaneous orgasm and ejaculation of semen.

wet nurse a woman who breast feeds another woman's child.

whiff test a semi-humourous term applied to the test for GARDNERELLA VAGINALIS organisms. A drop of 10% potassium hydroxide is added to a drop of vaginal discharge on a microscope slide. If the test is positive a distinct fishy smell, from the production of amines, becomes apparent. The test is not completely specific but is quick and of practical value.

whiplash injury a neck injury caused by the application of sudden accelerative or decelerative forces to the body so that the neck bends acutely in a direction opposite to the direction of the force. This results in immediate reflex contraction of the stretched muscles so that the head is jerked in the other direction. Neck ligaments may be stretched or torn or a neck VERTEBRAE may be fractured. There is pain and disability, often for weeks, and an orthopaedic collar may be needed.

Whipple's disease a rare MALABSORPTION disorder in which the VILLI of the intestine are stubby or absent and fatty masses occur in the bowel, the local lymph nodes and elsewhere in the body. Enormous numbers of MACROPHAGES containing foamy material are found in the intestine and elsewhere and with them many bacteria that can be identified by POLYMERASE CHAIN REACTION as *Tropheryma whipplei*.

Symptoms are numerous and include arthritis, fever, loss of weight, abdominal pain, diarrhoea, ANAEMIA, abnormal skin colouring, PLEURISY, ENDOCARDITIS, OEDEMA and FINGER CLUBBING. The joint problems often precede the intestinal disorder by months or years. The condition responds well to prolonged antibacterial treatment with co-trimoxazole. Also known as intestinal lipodystrophy. (George Hoyt Whipple, 1878–1976, American pathologist).

whipworm infection infection with *Trichuris trichiura*, a 2–5 cm intestinal parasitic worm that inhabits the lower bowel of many people living in underdeveloped areas. The infection is acquired by ingestion of the microscopic worm eggs found in damp soil contaminated with faeces. Usually the infections are symptomless but large numbers of worms may cause wasting diarrhoea in children and this may be serious if there is malnutrition. The worms can be expelled with mebendazole.

white blood cell see LEUKOCYTE.

white coat hypertension a rise in blood pressure induced by the act of measuring it. People who react in this way show a higher pressure when it is measured by a doctor or nurse than they show on 24-hour ambulatory monitoring measurements that are recorded on a cassette. Assuming the latter method shows acceptable levels, white coat hypertension will usually not require treatment, but close follow-up is required as affected people may develop later complications such as kidney impairment or enlargement of the left ventricle of the heart.

whitlow infection of the pulp of the finger-tip usually from a deep prick. There is dull pain, redness and swelling of the finger, throbbing and severe tenderness. At this stage, the condition may often be controlled with antibiotics. If untreated the condition often proceeds to abscess formation necessitating surgical drainage. The term whitlow is also applied to an infection of the skin in the region of the nail by herpes simplex viruses. Also known as a felon.

WHO *abbrev. for* WORLD HEALTH ORGANIZATION.

WHO essential medicines list (EML) a list, first published in 1977 and regularly revised thereafter, of drugs considered more important than the generality of medication and that, ideally, should be accessible to all populations. Currently, the EML contains 309 drugs, as follows: abacavir; acetazolamide; acetylcysteine; acetylsalicylic acid; aciclovir; albendazole; alcuronium; allopurinol; aluminium diacetate; aluminium hydroxide; amidotrizoate; amikacin; amiloride; aminophylline; amitriptyline; amoxicillin; amoxicillin + clavulanic acid; amphotericin B; ampicillin; anti-D immunoglobulin (human); antitetanus immunoglobulin (human); antivenom sera; artemether; artemether + lumefantrine; artesunate; ascorbic acid; asparaginase; atenolol; atropine; atropine; azathioprine; barium sulfate; BCG vaccine (dried); beclometasone; benzathine benzylpenicillin; benznidazole; benzoic acid + salicylic acid; benzoyl peroxide; benzyl benzoate; benzylpenicillin; betamethasone; biperiden; bleomycin; bupivacaine; calamine lotion; calcium folinate; calcium gluconate; capreomycin; captopril; carbamazepine; ceftazidime; ceftriaxone; charcoal activated; chloral hydrate; chlorambucil; chloramphenicol; chlorhexidine; chlorine base compound; chlormethine; chloroquine; chloroxylenol; chlorphenamine; chlorpromazine; ciclosporin; cimetidine; ciprofloxacin; cisplatin; clindamycin; clofazimine; clomifene; clomipramine; clonazepam; cloxacillin; coal tar; codeine; colchicine; copper-containing intrauterine device; cromoglicic acid; cyclophosphamide; cycloserine; cytarabine; dacarbazine; dactinomycin; dapsone; daunorubicin; deferoxamine; desmopressin; dexamethasone; dextran 70; dextromethorphan; diaphragms with spermicide (nonoxinol); diazepam; didanosine; diethylcarbamazine; diethyltoluamide; digoxin; diloxanide; dimercaprol; diphteria-pertussis-tetanus vaccine; diphtheria antitoxin; diphtheria-tetanus vaccine; dithranol; DL-methionine; dopamine; doxorubicin; doxycycline; efavirenz; eflornithine; ephedrine; epinephrine; epinephrine; ergocalciferol; ergometrine; ergotamine; erythromycin; ethambutol; ethanol; ether, anaesthetic; eEthinylestradiol; ethionamide; ethosuximide; etoposide; Factor IX complex (coagulation Factors II, VII, IX, X) concentrate; Factor VIII concentrate; ferrous salt + folic acid; fluconazole; flucytosine; fludrocortisone; fluorescein; fluorouracil; fluphenazine; folic acid; furosemide;

gentamicin; gentamicin; glibenclamide; glucose with sodium chloride; glucose; glutaral; glyceryl trinitrate; griseofulvin; haloperidol; halothane; heparin sodium; hepatitis B vaccine; hydralazine; hydrochlorothiazide; hydrocortisone; hydrocortisone; hydrocortisone; hydroxocobalamin; ibuprofen; idoxuridine; imipenem + cilastatin; immunoglobulin, normal human; indinavir; influenza vaccines; insulin injection, soluble; insulin, intermediate-acting; intraperitoneal dialysis solution; iodine; iohexol; iopanoic acid; ipecacuanha; ipratropium bromide; iron dextran; isoniazid; isoniazid + ethambutol; isoprenaline; isosorbide dinitrate; ivermectin; kanamycin; ketamine; lamivudine; levamisole; levodopa + carbidopa; levofloxacin; levonorgestrel; levonorgestrel + ethinylestradiol; levothyroxine; lidocaine; lidocaine; lithium carbonate; magnesium hydroxide; magnesium sulfate; mannitol; measles-mumps-rubella vaccine; mebendazole; medroxyprogesterone acetate (depot); mefloquine; meglumine antimonite; meglumine iotroxate; melarsoprol; meningococcal vaccines; mercaptopurine; metformin; methotrexate; methyldopa; methylrosanilinium chloride (gentian violet); methylthioninium chloride (methylene blue); metoclopramide; metronidazole; metronidazole; miconazole; morphine; nalidixic acid; naloxone; nelfinavir; neomycin + bacitracin; neostigmine; nevirapine; niclosamide; nicotinamide; nifedipine; nifurtimox; nitrofurantoin; nitrous oxide; norethisterone; norethisterone + ethinylestradiol; norethisterone enantate; nystatin; nystatin; nystatin; ofloxacin; oral rehydration salt formulations; oxamniquine; oxygen; oxytocin; p-aminosalicylic acid; paracetamol; penicillamine; pentamidine; permethrin; pethidine; phenobarbital; phenoxymethylpenicillin; phenytoin; phytomenadione; pilocarpine; podophyllum resin; poliomyelitis vaccines; polygeline; polyvidone-iodine; potassium chloride; potassium ferric hexacyanoferrate (Prussian blue); potassium iodide; praziquantel; prazosin; prednisolone; prednisolone; primaquine; procainamide; procaine benzylpenicillin; procarbazine; proguanil; promethazine; propranolol; propyliodone; propylthiouracil;

protamine sulfate; pyrantel; pyrazinamide; pyridostigmine; pyridoxine; pyrimethamine; quinidine; quinine; rabies immunoglobulin; rabies vaccines; reserpine; rRetinal; riboflavin; rifampicin; rifampicin + isoniazid + pyrazinamide; rifampicin + isoniazid + pyrazinamide + ethambutol; rifampicin + isoniazid; ritonavir; ritonavir + lopinavir; rubella vaccines; salbutamol; salbutamol; salicylic acid; saquinavir; selenium sulphide; senna; silver nitrate; silver sulfadiazine; sodium calcium edetate; sodium chloride; sodium fluoride; sodium hydrogen carbonate; sodium lactate, compound solution; sodium nitrite; sodium nitroprusside; sodium thiosulfate; spectinomycin; spironolactone; stavudine; streptokinase; streptomycin; sulfadiazine; sulfadoxine + pyrimethamine; sulfamethoxazole + trimethoprim; sulfasalazine; sun protection agent with activity against ultraviolet A and ultraviolet B; suramin sodium; suxamethonium; tamoxifen; testosterone; tetracaine; tetracycline; theophylline; thiamine; thioacetazone + isoniazid; thiopental; timolol; trimethoprim; tropicamide; tuberculin, purified protein derivative (PPD); Typhoid vaccines; urea; valproic acid; vancomycin; vecuronium; verapamil; vinblastine; vincristine; warfarin; water for injection; yellow fever vaccines; zidovudine.

whole blood blood, usually for transfusion, from which no constituent has been removed.

whole body MRI the scanning of the entire body as a single event by magnetic resonance imaging. The technique has been found valuable for detecting skeletal and other cancer metastasis, as a means of whole body fat measurement and as an acceptable alternative to conventional autopsy.

whooping cough an acute, highly infectious, disease of early childhood acquired by droplet infection and caused by the organism *Bordetella pertussis*. For the first 2 weeks the infection resembles a common cold but then a characteristic cough develops. There is a succession of short, rapid coughs with no time to draw breath between them. This is followed by a long, inspiration with a whooping sound. From 3 to 50 paroxysms of coughing may occur and these are very exhausting. The final paroxysm in a series is often followed by

vomiting. The cough may persist for weeks. Whooping cough may be complicated by OTITIS MEDIA, PNEUMONIA, collapse of part of a lung or seizures from lack of oxygen to the brain. Vomiting may interfere with nutrition. Antibiotics are of no value once the cough has developed but if given earlier reduce the severity of the disease. All babies should be immunized against whooping cough unless there is a sound medical objection. Also known as pertussis.

Widal test a serological agglutination reaction of Salmonella typhi and similar organisms by the patient's serum, used to diagnose typhoid and paratyphoid fevers. (George Fernand Isadore Widal, 1862–1929, Algerian born French pathologist).

wild relating to an entity, such as a virus, bacterium or gene that arises naturally or that comes from a natural environment, rather than that originates in a laboratory or as a result of artificial circumstances.

Will-Ironside syndrome new variant CREUTZFELDT-JAKOB DISEASE. (R.G. Will and J.W. Ironside who reported this condition in *The Lancet* in 1996).

Wilms' tumour see NEPHROBLASTOMA. (Max Wilms, 1867–1918, German pathologist and surgeon).

Wilson's disease a rare genetic disorder in which copper accumulates in the body, especially in the liver and brain, causing CIRRHOSIS and brain damage. There are behaviour abnormalities and personality changes, writhing movements of the limbs (athetoid movements), muscle rigidity and shortening, dementia and, in untreated cases, death. If diagnosed early, often by the observation of a ring of greenish-brown discoloration in each cornea (KAYSER-FLEISCHER RING), the condition may be controlled with a diet low in copper and the use of the drug d-penicillamine, which binds copper into a form which is excreted in the urine. Also known as hepatolenticular degeneration. (Samuel Alexander Kinnier Wilson, 1878–1937, American-born English neurologist).

wind a popular term for the result of air swallowing by greedy babies. Air swallowed along with a feed becomes compressed by PERISTALSIS and may cause COLIC and much crying. Slower feeding, dill water and silicone polymer oils, to reduce surface tension and form froth, are helpful.

windburn inflammation of the skin caused by exposure to hot dry wind. The condition can be prevented by covering exposed areas of skin.

wind chill the cooling effect of wind at low temperatures. This is greater than the effect of ambient cold alone and may cause rapid heat loss, adding to the risk of HYPOTHERMIA.

windpipe see TRACHEA.

wisdom tooth a popular term for the rearmost tooth in each of the four quadrants of the jaws. The 3rd molar. Usually, the 3rd molars do not erupt until the ages of 17 to 21, but often one or more is unable to emerge fully from the gum because of overcrowding. This is called an impacted wisdom tooth.

Wiskott-Aldrich syndrome an X-linked recessive immune deficiency disorder featuring recurrent infections, eczema and bleeding because of small platelets present in inadequate numbers. The affected gene, the product of which has been cloned, is on the short arm of the X chromosome. Like other X-linked recessive diseases the condition is almost confined to males. In female carriers the unmutated chromosome is preferentially selected in haematoipoietic cells. (Arthur Wiskott, German-born American paediatrician; and Robert Anderson Aldrich, b. 1917, American professor of paediatrics and preventice medicine).

witches' milk brief milk production from the breasts of newborn babies of either sex due to the presence of the hormone PROLACTIN in the mother's blood. This passes through the placenta to the fetus before birth. The effect is harmless and soon wears off.

withdrawal bleeding bleeding from the lining of the womb (UTERUS) caused by withdrawal of the female sex hormones progesterone or oestrogen. This occurs naturally in menstruation, but is a feature of cessation of any treatment with these hormones, for any purpose, including contraception.

withdrawal syndrome the complex of symptoms experienced on withdrawal of a drug on which a person is physically dependent. Symptoms of heroin withdrawal include craving for the drug, restlessness, depression, running nose, yawning, pain in the abdomen, vomiting, diarrhoea, loss of appetite, sweating

and gooseflesh ('cold turkey'). Those caused by withdrawal of other narcotic drugs are similar but less intense. See also DETOXIFICATION UNDER ANAESTHESIA.

Wolff-Parkinson-White syndrome a heart disorder caused by an abnormal band of conductive tissue that can by-pass the controlling node, the atrio-ventricular node, between the upper and lower chambers. The result can be a kind of feed-back oscillator that may produce fatally rapid heart rates. Treatment is by drugs, such as AMIODARONE or DISOPYRAMIDE to slow the heart. (Louis Wolff, American cardiologist, b. 1898, Sir John Parkinson, b. 1885, English cardiologist; and Paul Dudley White, 1886–1973, American cardiologist).

womb see UTERUS.

woody leg a feature of severe vitamin C deficiency (SCURVY) resulting from repeated bleeding into the tissues of the leg. The appearance is that of OEDEMA but the tissues are hard to the touch.

woolsorter's disease ANTHRAX of the lungs resulting from inhalation of spores of *Bacillus anthracis* from contaminated sheep's wool.

word blindness see DYSLEXIA.

World Health Organization an organization of major importance established in 1948 as an agency of the United Nations to promote the health of all peoples. The Headquarters of WHO is in Geneva and there are regional offices for all continents. WHO organizes campaigns against infectious diseases and sponsors research in medical laboratories all over the world. It provides expert advice on all matters directly or indirectly concerned with physical or mental health to all its member states. The eradication of SMALLPOX was a major achievement of WHO and in 1981 the organization adopted a policy of health for all by the year 2000. This is an unrealistic goal since so much depends on economic factors, but WHO has formulated specific targets for the provision of such fundamental public health needs as clean drinking water, sewage disposal, adequate nutrition, universal immunization programs and assaults on the major health hazard of smoking.

worried well people who do not need medical treatment, but who visit the doctor to be reassured.

wound any injury involving a break in the surface of the skin or an organ by any means including surgical incision.

wrist the complex, many-boned joint between the hand and the arm. The eight wrist bones, or carpals, are arranged in two rows, the nearer row, which articulates with the forearm bones, containing the scaphoid, lunate, triquetral, and pisiform bones, and the farther row the trapezium, trapezoid, capitate, and hamate. These are connected to the bones of the palm, the metacarpals. Many tendons, connecting forearm muscles to the fingers and thumb, run through the wrist. These pass under ligamentous straps (retinacula) which prevents them from springing away from the wrist.

Arteries and nerves also pass through the wrist.

wrist disorders see CARPAL TUNNEL SYNDROME, COLLES' FRACTURE, SCAPHOID FRACTURE and TENOSYNOVITIS.

writer's cramp a psychological disorder causing spasm of the muscles involved in holding a pen or pencil so writing becomes impossible. Other activities using the same muscles are usually unaffected. The condition is probably due to a mistaken vocation. Writers using word processors may develop a REPETITIVE STRAIN INJURY.

wryneck see TORTICOLLIS.

Wuchereriasis infection with parasitic worms of the genus *Wuchereria*. See FILARIASIS. (Otto Wucherer, 1820–73, German physician).

X

Xanaltan a brand name for LATANOPROST.

xamoterol a now-withdrawn beta-adrenergic stimulant drug that was used to treat mild degrees of HEART FAILURE. The drug has been used as a stimulant by athletes to try to improve performance and is on the International Olympic Committee's list of banned substances. A brand name was Corwin.

Xanax a brand name for the benzodiazepine antianxiety drug ALPRAZOLAM.

xanth-, xantho- *combining form denoting* yellow.

xanthelasma cholesterol deposits in the eyelid skin, near the inner corner of the eye, appearing as unsightly, raised, yellow plaques that enlarge slowly. Xanthelasma does not necessarily imply raised blood cholesterol, but this should be checked to eliminate the dangerous condition of familial hypercholesterolaemia, of which it is a feature. Plaques of xanthelasma can easily be removed but tend to recur.

xanthine oxidase inhibitors drugs used to treat gout and to prevent the development of uric acid and oxalate stones. An example is allopurinol (Zyloric).

xanthoma a yellowish or orange mass of fat-filled cells occurring in the skin of people with various disorders of fat metabolism. Also known as generalized XANTHELASMA.

xanthomatosis a condition occurring in various, often hereditary, disorders of fat metabolism, in which cholesterol-containing fatty nodules (xanthomas) occur in different parts of the body, including the tendons, arteries, the skin, the corneas, the crystalline lenses, the internal organs and the brain. The effects depend on the site of the deposits and may include mental deficit. Treatment with

CHENODEOXYCHOLIC ACID, to inhibit synthesis of bile acids, may help.

xanthopsia yellow vision. This sometimes occurs in JAUNDICE or in poisoning with DIGITALIS.

Xatral, Xatral XL a brand name for ALFUZOSIN.

X chromosome the CHROMOSOME which, with the Y chromosome, determines the sex of the individual. About 50% of sperms carry an X chromosome and 50% a Y. The sex of the future child is determined by whether an X-carrying or a Y-carrying sperm happens to fertilize the ovum. The ovum carries only an X chromosome. Females have two X chromosomes in each body cell, males have one X and one Y. The X chromosome is large and contains about 6% of the genomic DNA. The Y is about half the size. Well over a hundred disorders are known to be determined by genes on the X chromosome. These are called X-linked conditions. See also X-INACTIVATION.

xeno- *combining form* denoting foreign or strange.

xenogeneic pertaining to the genetic differences between different species.

xenograft a tissue graft taken from an animal of a different species from the host. Xenografts include pig heart valves and pig kidneys. Catgut, made from sheep intestine, is not a graft as it is intended to be absorbed. Also known as heterograft. From Greek *xenos*, a stranger or guest.

xeno-oestrogens substances with oestrogenic properties derived from other than biological sources. A number of organochloride compounds, for instance, have been found to be sufficiently oestrogenic to cause a rise in the incidence of breast cancer in groups of women exposed to them. The insecticide dieldrin is a case in point.

Xenopsylla a genus of fleas of which the species *X. cheopis*, the oriental rat flea, is the VECTOR of PLAGUE and murine TYPHUS.

xenorexia see PICA.

xenotransplantation transplantation of organs from animals, usually TRANSGENIC animals, especially pigs, specifically engineered for the purpose. Until recently, no transplanted pig organ had survived for more than a month. But advances in the development of new immunosuppressive agents against xenografts and the identification of the main target for human xenoreactive (anti-pig) antibodies have extended this period to an average of 76 days. Precautions can also be taken against virus transmission. The future for xenotransplantation seems bright.

xero- *combining form denoting* dry.

xeroderma dryness of the skin.

xeroderma pigmentosum a group of rare AUTOSOMAL RECESSIVE genetic skin diseases featuring excessive sensitivity to sunlight, which causes premature ageing of the skin, PIGMENTATION and the development of skin cancers. Victims are condemned to an almost wholly indoor existence and have to use protective coverings and skin sunscreen creams out of doors.

xerophthalmia dryness of the eyes with thickening of the CONJUNCTIVA, occurring in vitamin A deficiency, PEMPHIGUS and autoimmune disorders such as SJÖGREN'S SYNDROME. Artificial tears must be used constantly to maintain the essential film of water over the cornea.

xeroradiography a form of X-ray screening for breast cancer in which the image is formed on special photographic paper instead of on transparent film. Xeroradiographs can be viewed directly without special lighting. Also known as xeromammography.

xerosis dryness, especially of the eyes, mouth, vagina or skin.

xerostomia dry mouth.

ximelagatran an oral direct thrombin inhibitor drug used as an anticoagulant alternative to warfarin in the management of thromboembolism. In late 2004 the American FDA rejected an application for approval of this drug on the grounds of liver toxicity.

xipamide a thiazide DIURETIC drug. A brand name is Diurexan.

xiphisternum the flat, leaf-like process hanging down from the lower end of the breastbone (sternum). The xiphisternum is cartilaginous in childhood, partly bony (ossified) in adult life and wholly ossified and fused to the sternum in old age. Also known as the xiphoid process.

X-linked pertaining to genes, or to the effect of genes, situated on the X CHROMOSOME. X-linked disorders are those caused by mutated genes on the X chromosome. They include AGAMMAGLOBULINAEMIA, ALBINISM, ALPORT SYNDROME, Charcot–Marie–Tooth peroneal muscular atrophy, COLOUR BLINDNESS, DIABETES INSIPIDUS, ectodermal dysplasia, glucose-6-phosphate dehydrogenase deficiency, FABRY DISEASE, glycogen storage disease VIII, gonadal dysgenesis, HAEMOPHILIA A, one form of HYDROCEPHALUS, HYPOPHOSPHATAEMIA, ICHTHYOSIS, TURNER'S SYNDROME, one form of mental retardation, Becker and Duchesse MUSCULAR DYSTROPHY, one form of RETINITIS PIGMENTOSA and the TESTICULAR FEMINIZATION SYNDROME.

X-inactivation the normal failure of expression of one of the two X chromosomes in females. Early in development some cells switch off the paternal X chromosome, other cells switch off the maternal one. Inactivated chromosomes remains so in all subsequent daughter cells. Most women have a mixture of two different cells populations each expressing a different X chromosome. The inactivated chromosome is visible microscopically as the Barr body. This effect, sometimes called Lyonization after the British geneticism Mary Frances Lyon (1925–), who proposed it in 1961, accounts for a number of observed phenomena in genetics.

X-linked recessive pertaining to a gene situated on an X chromosome which is expressed if the chromosome is carried on both X chromosomes in a female (which is necessarily rare). In males, however, the Y chromosome carries little or no genetic material and does not contain the normal ALLELE, so the gene on the X chromosome will always manifest itself. An X-linked recessive condition will thus usually occur only in males (who have one X and one Y chromosome) but cannot be transmitted by a father to his son because the son receives only the Y chromosome. The characteristic is, however, transmitted via the daughters, who are carriers. Their sons have a 50/50 chance of acquiring the X chromosome and manifesting the characteristic.

XO configuration the state of the CHROMOSOMES when only one sex chromosome, an X, is present. This is the sex chromosome abnormality most commonly found in TURNER'S SYNDROME. Also known as monosomy X.

X-ray a form of electromagnetic radiation produced when a beam of high-speed electrons, accelerated by a high voltage, strikes a metal, such as copper or tungsten. X-radiation penetrates matter to a degree depending on the voltage used to produce it and the density of the matter. It acts on normal photographic film in much the same way as does visible light, but can also produce an image on a fluorescing screen. These properties make X-radiation valuable in medical diagnosis. X-rays are damaging to tissue, especially rapidly reproducing tissues, and can be used to treat various cancers (see RADIOTHERAPY).

X-ray therapy see RADIOTHERAPY.

XXX configuration the state of the body cells when an additional X CHROMOSOME is present. Females possessing this chromosome configuration are often mentally retarded but their children, if any, are usually normal.

xylitol a polyol sugar alcohol found in plums, strawberries, raspberries, and birch trees that reduces the growth of *Streptococcus mutans* and the resulting acid production which is the most important cause of dental caries. Xylitol-sweetened chewing gum has also been found effective in preventing OTITIS MEDIA.

Xylocaine, Xylocard brand names for the local anaesthetic drug lignocaine (lidocaine).

xylol the solvent xylene used to dissolve wax from slices of tissue that have been cut from a wax block and mounted on a slide for staining and microscopic examination.

xylometazoline a decongestant drug used to relieve a blocked nose.

XYY configuration a male chromosome abnormality in which an additional male sex chromosome is present in every body cell. This configuration has been found in normal men, but is often associated with mental retardation and criminal tendencies.

y

Yasmin a brand name for a combined oral contraceptive containing ETHINYLOESTRADIOL (ethinylestradiol) and DROSPERINONE. (The origin of the term is obscure, but Yasmin was the beautiful but heartless temptress of James Elroy Flecker's play *Hassan*.)

yawning an involuntary and often infectious act of slow, deep inspiration accompanied by an almost uncontrollable desire to open the mouth widely. The purpose of yawning remains a matter of speculation but it stretches and opens the air sacs of the lungs and helps to improve the return of blood to the heart, reducing blood stagnation and increasing its oxygen content.

yaws a disease of underdeveloped areas caused by a SPIROCHAETE of the genus *Treponema* identical to that causing SYPHILIS. Yaws is not, however, a sexually transmitted disease. It is acquired in childhood and is spread by direct contact. Initially, an itchy, red, warty patch appears at the site of infection. This is teeming with spirochaetes and scratching leads to further patches arising elsewhere on the skin. These, and secondarily appearing patches, heal, but, as in syphilis, a more serious tertiary stage occurs several years later. This features deep skin ulcers with much tissue destruction, bone changes and leprosy-like deformity. Yaws is easily treated with antibiotics such as penicillin or tetracycline. Mass treatment campaigns have been effective but have been followed by a sharp rise in the incidence of venereal syphilis, possibly reflecting a general decline in immunity.

year-and-a-day rule the long-established legal principle that a person cannot be held criminally liable for a death that occurs more than a year and a day after the commission of the act alleged to be its cause.

yeasts single-celled nucleated fungi that produce enzymes capable of fermenting carbohydrates. The yeasts of chief medical interest are those of the *Candida* and *Monilia* species which cause THRUSH. Yeasts are rich in B vitamins.

yellow fever an acute infectious disease of tropical America and Africa, caused by a flavivirus of the togavirus family transmitted between humans by the bite of the *Aedes aegypti* mosquito and from monkeys by various jungle mosquitoes. The disease may be mild and brief but is often severe with high fever, severe headache, muscle aches, nosebleeds and vomiting of blood. The liver is often severely damaged and jaundice is a major feature, hence the name. The kidneys, too may be damaged. Severe bleeding from the bowel and the womb are grave signs, often followed by delirium, coma and death. There is no specific treatment.

yellow fever vaccine a suspension of a live, attenuated yellow fever virus (17D strain). Immunity conferred by this vaccine probably persists for life but is officially accepted as being for ten years. The vaccine is on the WHO official list.

yellow jack 1 YELLOW FEVER.
2 a yellow nautical flag formerly hoisted to warn of disease on board.

yellow spot the MACULA LUTEA of the RETINA.

Yersinia a genus of GRAM NEGATIVE rod-shaped organisms that includes the bacillus *Y. pestis* responsible for PLAGUE. Formerly classified as *Pasteurella*, *Yersinia* have been reclassified as *Enterobacteriaceae* and the genus renamed. Louis Pasteur, although nominal head of the Institute, was not entitled to the credit or the discovery of the plague bacillus. (Alexandre Émile Jean Yersin, 1862–1943, French bacteriologist, working in Hong Kong.)

yin and yang the opposite but complementary principles of Chinese philosophy incorporated into traditional Chinese medicine. Yin is feminine, dark and negative, Yang masculine, bright and positive. Their interaction and balance is believed to maintain the harmony of the body.

yoga one of the six orthodox systems of Indian philosophy. In Hatha Yoga the emphasis is on physical preparation for spiritual development. It incorporates a series of poses, known as asanas, by which, it is claimed, one may retain youthful flexibility and control of the body and achieve relaxation and peace of mind.

yogurt a mildly acid milk product produced by fermentation by enzymes produced by the *Lactobacillus bulgaricus*. Yogurt has no special nutritional value, nor is it likely to produce any advantageous change in the intestinal organisms as has been claimed. It has been used as a vaginal cream to restore the normal acidity and help in the treatment of THRUSH.

yohimbin an alkaloid adrenoreceptor antagonist derived from the yohimbe tree. It lowers blood pressure and controls arousal and anxiety and has been used to treat both physical and psychogenic IMPOTENCE.

yolk sac a tiny bag attached to the embryo that provides early nourishment before the PLACENTA is formed.

Yomesan a brand name for the ANTHELMINTIC drug niclosamide.

yoni a symbol for the VULVA, as a source of pleasure, in Indian religion.

Yutopar a brand name for the womb-relaxing drug RITODINE.

Z

Zaditen a brand name for KETOTIFEN.

zalcitabine a REVERSE TRANSCRIPTASE inhibitor drug used in combination with other drugs to treat AIDS. A brand name is Hivid.

Zamadol a brand name for TRAMADOL.

Zanaflex a brand name for the muscle relaxing drug TIZANIDINE.

zanamivir a neuraminidase inhibitor antiviral drug used for the treatment of influenza A and influenza B. To be effective, the drug must be taken within 48 hours of the onset of symptoms. It is liable to cause tightening of the bronchial tubes and this may be dangerous in people with ASTHMA. A brand name is Relenza.

Zanidip a brand name for LERCANIDIPINE.

Zantac, Zantac 75 a brand name for the stomach acid reducing drug RANITIDINE.

ZAP-70 a tyrosine kinase normally expressed in T cells and NK cells. The gene for ZAP-70 is differentially expressed in patients with or without mutations of the gene for IgVH. This provides a valuable prognostic guide as to whether chronic lymphocytic leukaemia is likely to have a good or a poor outcome. ZAP-70 protein levels are can be measured much more easily than the mutational state of the IgVH gene. Zap-70 is a strong predictor of the need for treatment in B-cell chronic lymphocytic leukaemia.

Zarontin a brand name for the ANTIEPILEPSY drug ETHOSUXIMIDE.

Zavedos a brand name for IDARUBICIN.

Z DNA an uncommon configuration for DNA. It is a left-hand helix with about 12 bases per turn.

Zenker's degeneration death of segments of muscle cells that sometimes occurs in prolonged fevers such as TYPHOID or in HEPATITIS. Also known as hyaline necrosis. (Friedrich Albert von Zenker, German pathologist, 1825–89).

Zestoretic a brand name for the ANGIOTENSIN CONVERTING ENZYME inhibitor LISINOPRIL formulated in conjunction with the diuretic drug HYDROCHLOROTHIAZIDE.

Zestril a brand name for LISINOPRIL.

Zidoval a brand name for METRONIDAZOLE.

zidovudine an antiviral drug used to try to retard the progress of AIDS. Also known as azidothymidine or AZT. The drug is on the WHO official list. A brand name is Retrovir.

zinc a metallic element required in small quantities for health. Deficiency is rare but may occur in people with certain MALABSORPTION conditions, with ANOREXIA NERVOSA, DIABETES, severe burns, prolonged feverish illness, severe malnutrition in childhood and in alcoholics. Zinc deficiency is associated with atrophy of the thymus gland and depressed cell-mediated immunity, skin atrophy, poor wound healing, loss of appetite, persistent diarrhoea, apathy and loss of hair. A normal diet contains plenty of zinc but a small zinc supplement is said to shorten the duration of the common cold.

Zincfrin a brand name for eye drops containing ZINC sulphate and PHENYLEPHRINE.

zinc oxide a white powder with mild ASTRINGENT properties used as a dusting powder or incorporated into creams or ointments and used as a bland skin application. Mixed with oil of cloves, zinc oxide forms an effective and pain-relieving temporary dressing for a tooth cavity. Zinc oxide is an ingredient in numerous proprietary medical preparations.

zinc sulphate a drug used as a source of zinc in zinc deficiency states. Brand names are

Solvazinc and Zincfrin.

Zinga a brand name for NIZATIDINE.

Zinnat a brand name for the cephalosporin antibiotic CEFUROXIME.

Zirtek Allergy a brand name for CETIRIZINE.

Zispin a brand name for MIRTAZAPINE.

Zithromax a brand name for AZITHROMYCIN.

Zocor a brand name for SIMVASTATIN.

Zofran a brand name for ONDANSETRON.

Zoladex a brand name for GOSERELIN.

Zollinger-Ellison syndrome a severe form of stomach and duodenal ulceration caused by an excessive production of acid by the stomach. This is stimulated by one or more tumours of the pancreas, known as gastrinomas, that secrete a powerful hormone acting on the stomach. Gastrinomas are often malignant, although slow-growing. Complete surgical removal is not always possible and drugs in the H-2 receptor antagonist group, such as cimetidine, or the more recent proton pump blocking drugs, such as OMEPRAZOLE, are often used. Removal of the stomach (gastrectomy) may be necessary. (Robert Milton Zollinger, b. 1903, American surgeon; and Edwin Horner Ellison, 1918–70, American professor of Surgery).

zolmitriptan a drug that stimulates SEROTONIN receptors and is used to treat MIGRAINE. A brand name is Zomig.

Zomig a brand name for ZOLMITRIPTAN.

zolpidem an imidazopyridine HYPNOTIC drug used for the short-term treatment of INSOMNIA. A brand name is Stilnoct.

Zomacton a brand name for SOMATOTROPIN (somatropin).

zombification the purported conversion by magic means to a state in which the awareness of an individual is retained by a sorcerer in a bottle or jar while the body, lacking will or agency, becomes the slave of the sorcerer. Zombification is deemed to be murder in Haiti even if the victim is manifestly still alive. The state is either induced by various poisons or by strong suggestion in a context of powerful superstitious belief. Some zombis have been found to be schizophrenics.

Zomorph a brand name for MORPHINE.

zonule the delicate suspensory ligament of the CRYSTALLINE LENS of the eye.

Zonulysin a brand name for the protein-splitting enzyme alpha-chymotrypsin that was made up in a solution for the purposes of dissolving the ZONULE as a preliminary to the now-obsolete INTRACAPSULAR method of removal of a cataractous lens. This technique is now rarely used in developed countries.

zoo blot the use of SOUTHERN BLOTTING to check whether a DNA probe from one species can hybridize with the DNA of other species.

Zoomastigophorea a class of flagellated PROTOZOA many of which cause diseases such as LEISHMANIASIS, TRICHOMONIASIS and TRYPANOSOMIASIS.

zoonoses diseases of animals that can affect people. The zoonoses do not include human diseases transmitted from person to person by animal vectors. The zoonoses include ANTHRAX from cattle, BRUCELLOSIS and Q FEVER from goats and sheep, GLANDERS from horses, LEPTOSPIROSIS and PLAGUE from rats, PSITTACOSIS from birds, RABIES from any mammal, ROCKY MOUNTAIN SPOTTED FEVER from small mammals, TOXOCARIASIS from dogs, TOXOPLASMOSIS from cats, TUBERCULOSIS from cows and YELLOW FEVER from monkeys.

zoophobia irrational fear of animals.

zoster 1 SHINGLES.

2 the herpes zoster virus that causes shingles and CHICKEN POX. From the Greek *zoster*, a girdle, reflecting the position of the typical skin eruption in shingles.

Zoton a brand name for LANSOPRAZOLE.

Zovirax a brand name for the antiviral drug ACICLOVIR.

Z-plasty a plastic surgical technique for relieving skin tension or releasing scar contracture. Adjacent, V-shaped flaps, pointing in opposite directions are cut, undermined, freed and their points transposed.

zuclopenthixol a thioxanthene antipsychotic drug used to treat SCHIZOPHRENIA and other psychotic disorders. A brand name is Clopixol.

Zumenon a brand name for OESTRADIOL (estradiol).

zwitterions the dipolar ions that form from amino acids when they are in solution at a neutral pH.

Zyban a brand name for BUPROPION.

Zydol SR, Zydol XL brand names for TRAMADOL.

zygoma the cheek bone.

zygomatic pertaining to the ZYGOMA.

zygomatic arch the bony arch extending below

and to the outer side of the eye socket (the orbit) andforming the prominence of the cheek.

zygomatic process any of the three processes that make up the ZYGOMATIC ARCH.

zygote an egg (ovum) that has been fertilized but has not yet undergone the first cleavage division. A zygote contains a complete (DIPLOID) set of chromosomes, half from ovum and half from the fertilizing sperm, and thus all the genetic code for a new individual.

zygomycosis a fungus infection in which masses of various fungi form in the nasal sinuses, under the skin of the face and in other parts of the body especially in people with immune deficiency.

Zyloric a brand name for the drug ALLOPURINOL.

zymogen the inactive protein precursor of an ENZYME.

zymogenesis the conversion of an ENZYME precursor to the active state.

Zyprexa a brand name for OLANZAPINE.

Illustrations

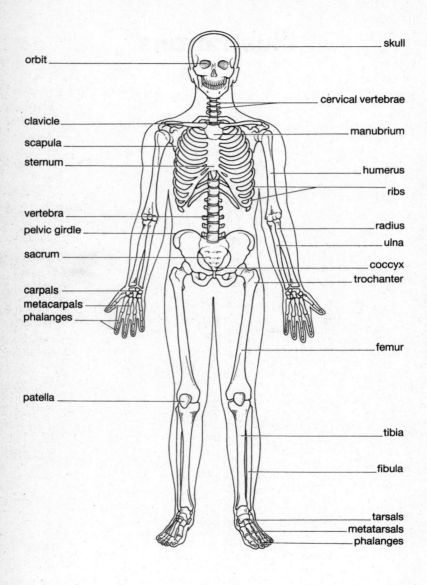

orbit

skull

clavicle

cervical vertebrae

scapula

manubrium

sternum

humerus

ribs

vertebra

radius

pelvic girdle

ulna

sacrum

coccyx

trochanter

carpals

metacarpals

phalanges

femur

patella

tibia

fibula

tarsals

metatarsals

phalanges

Fig. 1 **Skeleton**

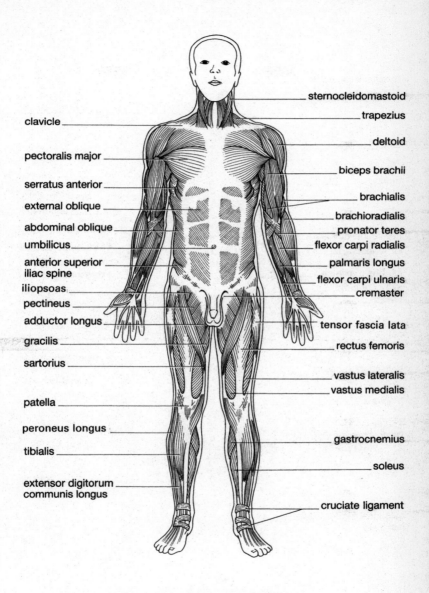

clavicle

pectoralis major

serratus anterior

external oblique

abdominal oblique

umbilicus

anterior superior
iliac spine

iliopsoas

pectineus

adductor longus

gracilis

sartorius

patella

peroneus longus

tibialis

extensor digitorum
communis longus

sternocleidomastoid

trapezius

deltoid

biceps brachii

brachialis

brachioradialis

pronator teres

flexor carpi radialis

palmaris longus

flexor carpi ulnaris

cremaster

tensor fascia lata

rectus femoris

vastus lateralis
vastus medialis

gastrocnemius

soleus

cruciate ligament

Fig. 2 **The muscle system (front view)**

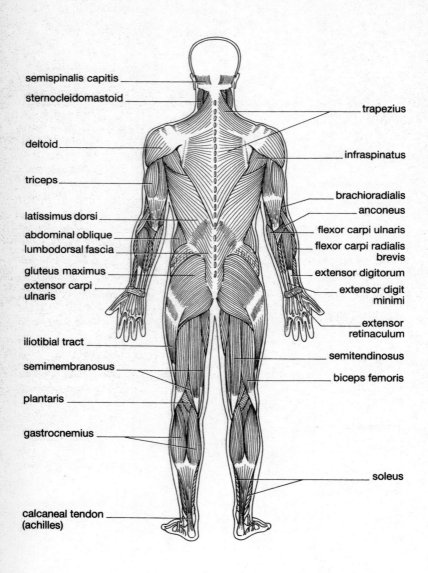

semispinalis capitis

sternocleidomastoid

trapezius

deltoid

infraspinatus

triceps

brachioradialis

anconeus

latissimus dorsi

flexor carpi ulnaris

abdominal oblique

flexor carpi radialis brevis

lumbodorsal fascia

gluteus maximus

extensor digitorum

extensor carpi ulnaris

extensor digit minimi

extensor retinaculum

iliotibial tract

semitendinosus

semimembranosus

biceps femoris

plantaris

gastrocnemius

soleus

calcaneal tendon (achilles)

Fig. 3 **The muscle system (rear view)**

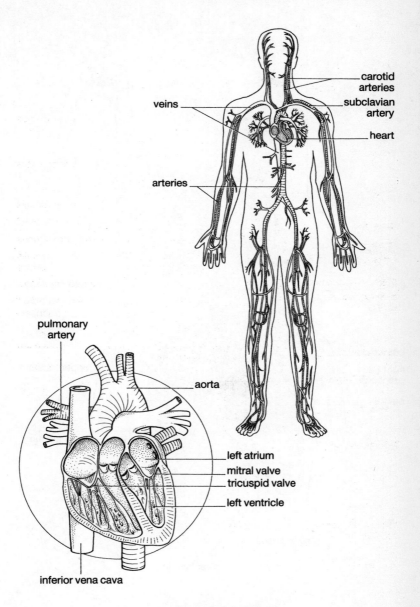

Fig. 4 **The circulatory system**

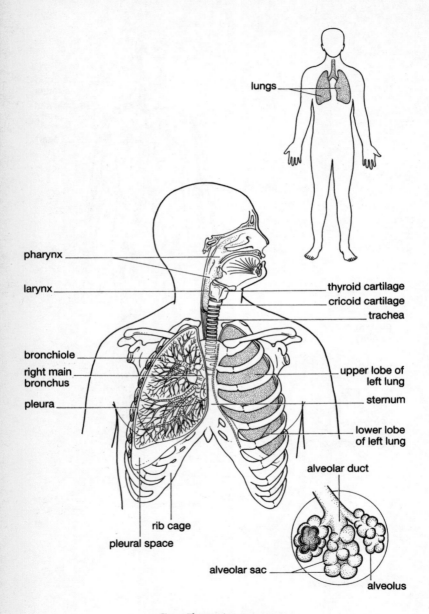

Fig. 5 **The respiratory system**

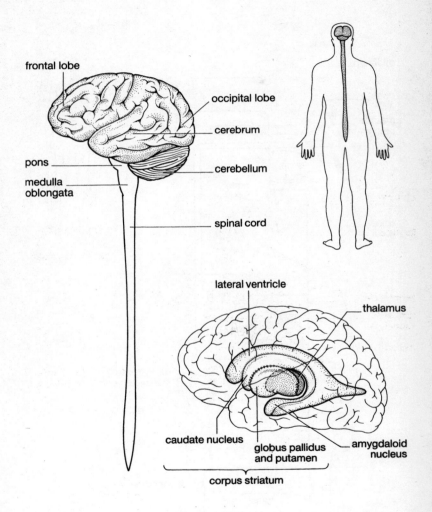

frontal lobe

occipital lobe

cerebrum

pons

cerebellum

medulla
oblongata

spinal cord

lateral ventricle

thalamus

caudate nucleus

globus pallidus
and putamen

amygdaloid
nucleus

corpus striatum

Fig. 6 **The brain and spinal cord**

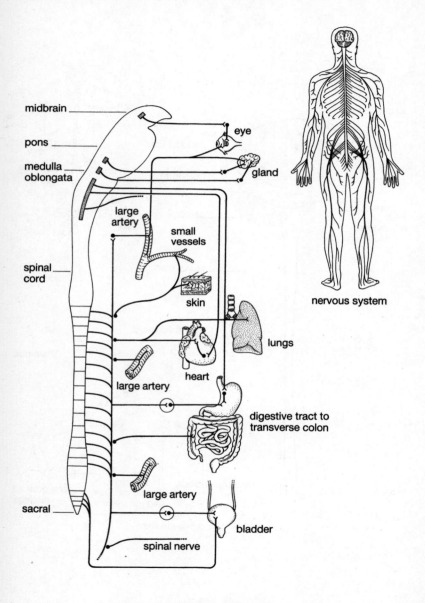

midbrain

pons

medulla oblongata

spinal cord

large artery

small vessels

skin

large artery

heart

sacral

large artery

spinal nerve

eye

gland

lungs

digestive tract to transverse colon

bladder

nervous system

Fig. 7 **The autonomic nervous system**

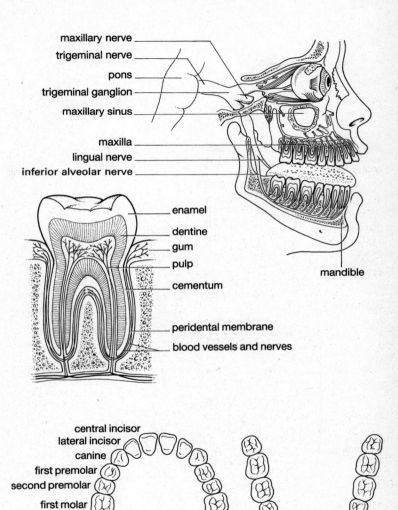

maxillary nerve
trigeminal nerve
pons
trigeminal ganglion
maxillary sinus

maxilla
lingual nerve
inferior alveolar nerve

mandible

enamel
dentine
gum
pulp
cementum

peridental membrane
blood vessels and nerves

central incisor
lateral incisor
canine
first premolar
second premolar
first molar
second molar
third molar
(wisdom tooth)

Fig. 8 **The dental system**

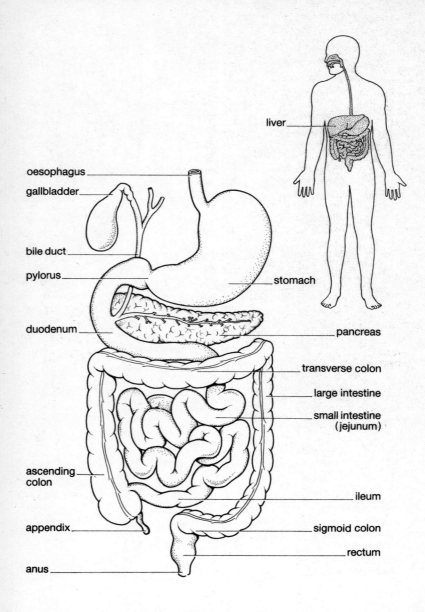

Fig. 9 **The digestive system**

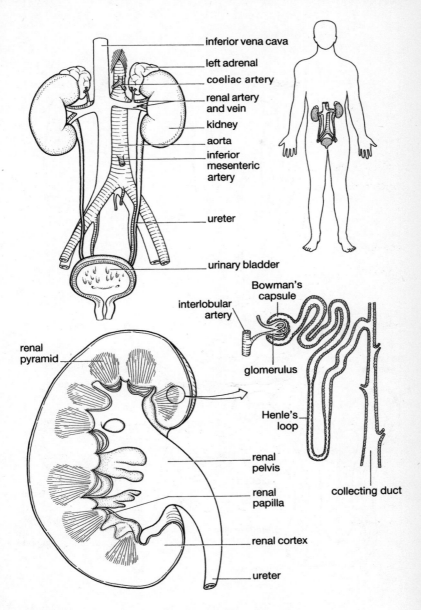

inferior vena cava

left adrenal

coeliac artery

renal artery
and vein

kidney

aorta

inferior
mesenteric
artery

ureter

urinary bladder

Bowman's
capsule

interlobular
artery

glomerulus

renal
pyramid

Henle's
loop

renal
pelvis

renal
papilla

collecting duct

renal cortex

ureter

Fig. 10 **The urinary system**

669

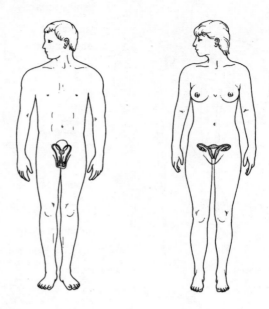

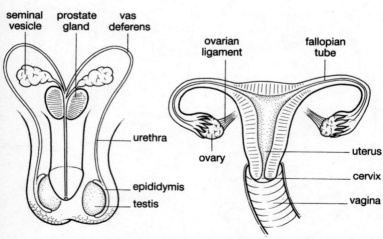

Fig. 11 **The reproductive system**

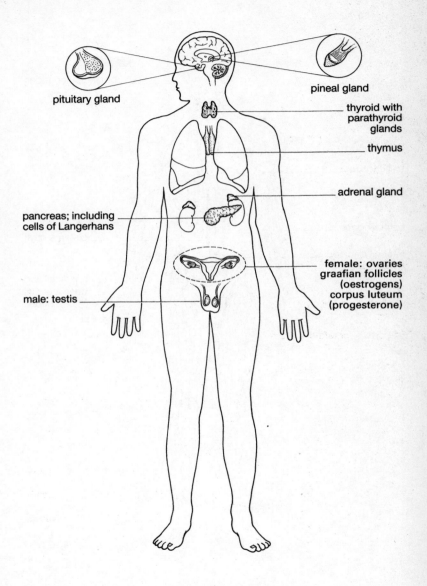

pituitary gland

pineal gland

thyroid with
parathyroid
glands

thymus

adrenal gland

pancreas; including
cells of Langerhans

female: ovaries
graafian follicles
(oestrogens)
corpus luteum
(progesterone)

male: testis

Fig. 12 **The endocrine system**

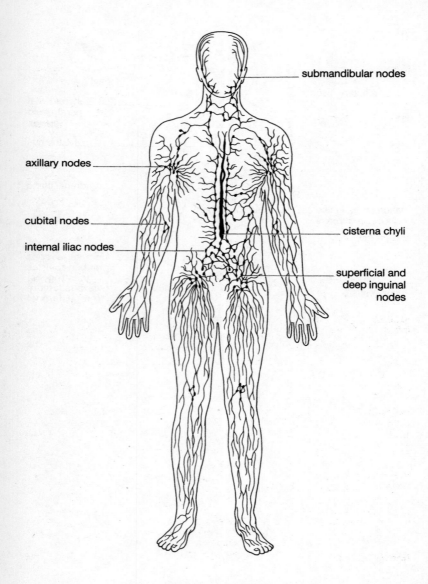

submandibular nodes

axillary nodes

cubital nodes

internal iliac nodes

cisterna chyli

superficial and
deep inguinal
nodes

Fig. 13 **The lymphatic system**

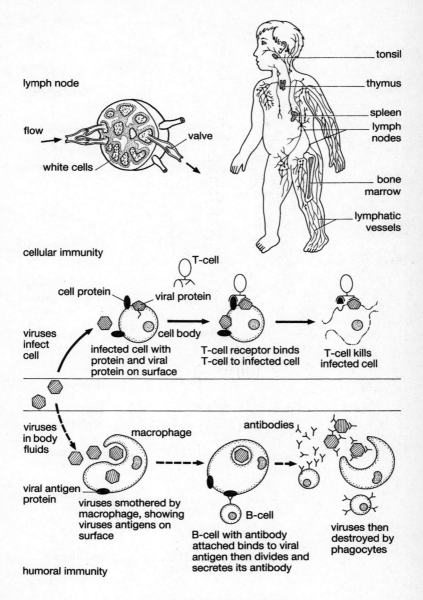

lymph node

flow

valve

white cells

tonsil

thymus

spleen
lymph
nodes

bone
marrow

lymphatic
vessels

cellular immunity

T-cell

cell protein

viral protein

viruses
infect
cell

cell body

infected cell with
protein and viral
protein on surface

T-cell receptor binds
T-cell to infected cell

T-cell kills
infected cell

viruses
in body
fluids

macrophage

antibodies

viral antigen
protein

viruses smothered by
macrophage, showing
viruses antigens on
surface

B-cell

B-cell with antibody
attached binds to viral
antigen then divides and
secretes its antibody

viruses then
destroyed by
phagocytes

humoral immunity

Fig. 14 **The immune system**

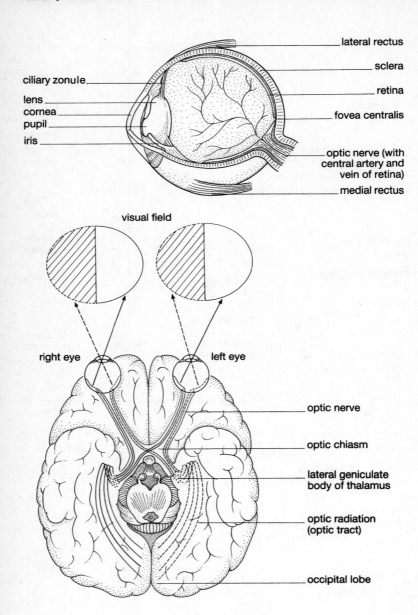

Fig. 15 **The visual system**

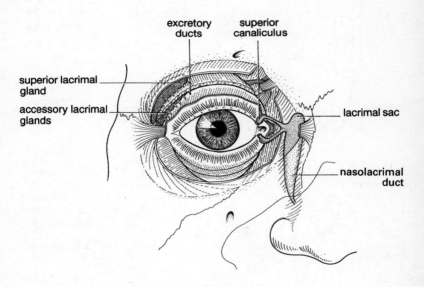

Fig. 16 **The lacrimal system**

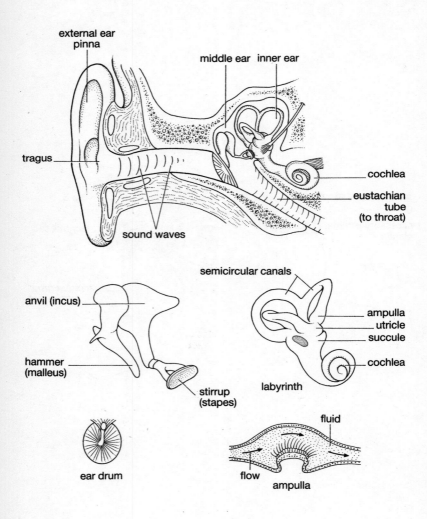

Fig. 17 **The auditory system**

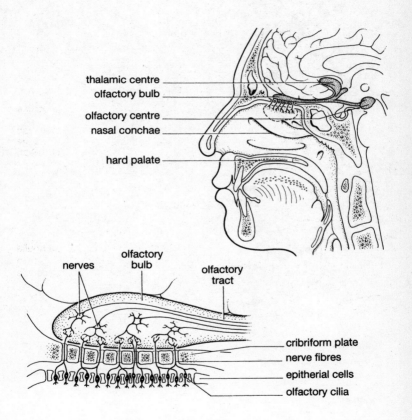

thalamic centre

olfactory bulb

olfactory centre

nasal conchae

hard palate

nerves

olfactory bulb

olfactory tract

cribriform plate

nerve fibres

epitherial cells

olfactory cilia

Fig. 18 **The olfactory system**

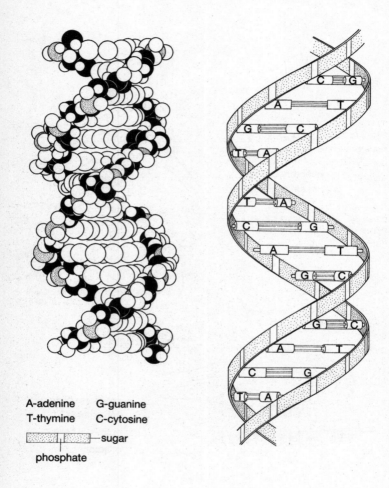

A-adenine   G-guanine
T-thymine   C-cytosine
—sugar
phosphate

Fig. 19 **DNA structure**

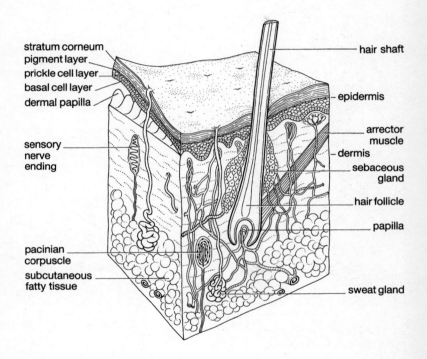

stratum corneum
pigment layer
prickle cell layer
basal cell layer
dermal papilla

hair shaft

epidermis

arrector
muscle

dermis

sensory
nerve
ending

sebaceous
gland

hair follicle

papilla

pacinian
corpuscle

subcutaneous
fatty tissue

sweat gland

Fig. 20 **Skin structure**

Internet Links

There is a wealth of medical resources on the internet. The web addresses below provide you with key references to particular topics and to the main medical organizations, and there is also a selection of websites specifically for Personal Digital Assistants. These details can also be found at www.collins.co.uk

abortion clinics
www.gynpages.com

access to essential medicines
www.accessmed-msf.org/index.asp

Action on Smoking and Health
ash.org

acupuncture
www.acupuncturewashington.org

addiction
www.clearinghouse.net/cgi-bin/chadmin/viewcat

ageing
www.asaging.org

AIDS
www.aids.org
www.clearinghouse.net/cgi-bin/chadmin/viewcat/Health_Medicine
www.hivpositive.com

AIDS, drugs and treatments
www.acrc.org/drugglos.htm

AIDS, frequently asked questions
www.aids.org/info/FAQs.html

AIDS Information
www.ashastd.org/hotlines/index.html#

AIDS Research
www.amfar.org

alcohol and drug problems
www.adpana.com

Alcoholics Anonymous
www.alcoholics-anonymous.org

allergies
www.sig.net/~allergy/welcome.html

allergy and infectious disease
www.niaid.nih.gov/default.htm

allergy, asthma and immunology
www.aaaai.org

Alliance for the Mentally Ill
www.nami.org

Alzheimer's Association
www.alz.org

American Academy of Pediatrics
www.aap.org

American Academy of Dermatology
www.aad.org

American Academy of Family Physicians
www.familydoctor.org

American Association for World Health
www.thebody.com/aawh/aawhpage.html

American College of Medical Informatics
www.amia.org/acmi/acmi.html

American College of Dentists
www.acdentists.org

American College of Rheumatology
www.rheumatology.org

American College of Surgeons
www.facs.org

American Diabetes Association
www.diabetes.org

American Foundation for the Blind
www.afb.org

American Geriatrics Society
www.americangeriatrics.org

American Health Care Association
www.ahca.org

American Health Foundation
www.ahf.org

American Heart Association
www.americanheart.org

American Liver Foundation
www.liverfoundation.org

American Lung Association
www.lungusa.org

American Medical Association
www.ama-assn.org

American Osteopathic Association
www.aoa-net.org

American Pain Society
www.ampainsoc.org

American Pharmaceutical Association
www.aphanet.org

American Prostate Society
www.ameripros.org

American Psychiatric Association
www.psych.org

American Psychological Association
www.apa.org

American Red Cross
www.redcross.org

American Urological Association
www.auanet.org/index_hi.cfm

American Yoga Association
www.americanyogaassociation.org

anatomy
www.nlm.nih.gov/research/visible/visible_human.html
www.innerbody.com
www.medtropolis.com/VBody.asp

antibiotics
www.intmed.mcw.edu/AntibioticGuide.html

anxiety disorders
www.adaa.org

arthritis
www.arthritis.org

Association for Addiction Professionals
www.naadac.org

Association of the Deaf
www.nad.org

Association of Asthma Educators
www.asthmaeducators.org

asthma control
www.controlasthma.com

Asthma and Allergy Foundation of America
www.aafa.org

attention deficit hyperactivity disorder
www.mhsanctuary.com/add

Attention deficit disorder
www.seas.upen.edu/~mengwong/add

Australasian anaesthesia web site
www.usyd.edu.au/su/anaes/anaes.html

Australian College of Health Informatics
www.achi.org.au

Autism Society of America
www.autism-society.org/site/PageServer

bad breath (halitosis)
www.seattle-dentist.com/halitosis.htm

biomedical and health informatics
www.dbhi.washington.edu

biomedical informatics
www.umdnj.edu/shrp/gpbi.html

biomedical internet directory
www.yahoo.com/Health/tree.html

bipolar disorder
www.mhsanctuary.com/bipolar

blindness links
www.seidata.com/%7Emarriage/rblind.html

blindness prevention
www.preventblindness.org

blood glucose
www.lifescan.com

bone marrow transplants
www.ai.mit.edu/people/laurel/Bmt-talk/maillist.html

borderline personality disorder
www.mhsanctuary.com/borderline

breast cancer
www.breastcancercare.org.uk/splash

breast cancer answers
www.canceranswers.org

British Medical Council
www.bma.org.uk

British Medical Journal
www.bmj.com

Cancer Care Inc
www.cancercare.org

cancer control tools
cancercontrolplanet.cancer.gov

cancer education
www.aaceonline.com/index.asp

cancer guide
cancerguide.org

cancer help
www.rwneill.com/cancerhelp.htm

cancer network
www.cancernetwork.com

cancer news
members.aol.com/abiaca/cancerwire.htm

cancer of pancreas
www.healthyfoundations.com/Pancreaticlinks.html

cancer rates and risks
rex.nci.nih.gov/NCI_Pub_Interface/raterisk/index.html

cancer survivorship
www.access.diges.net/~mkragen/cansearch.html

CancerNet
www.cancernet.com

cataract
www.nei.nih.gov/health/cataract/cataract_facts.htm

CDC Morbidity and Mortality reports
www2.cdc.gov/mmwr

Center for Biomedical Informatics
www.cbmi.pitt.edu

Centers for Disease Control
www.cdc.gov/pcd

Centre for eHealth and Learning
www.ihi.aber.ac.uk

Center for Infectious Diseases
www.cdc.gov/ncidod/ncid.htm

child and adolescent psychology
www.aacap.org

childbirth
www.childbirth.org

childbirth myths
efn.org/~djz/birth/obmyth/epis.html

child growth and nutrition
www.who.int/nutgrowthdb

Christopher Reeve Paralysis Foundation
www.apacure.com

chronic fatigue syndrome
chronicfatigue.miningco.com/mbody.htm

chronic Pain
www.theacpa.org

clinical trials
www.centerwatch.com

Coalition on Smoking or Health
tobaccodocuments.org

**Cognitive Science Branch, National Library of Medicine/
National Institutes of Health**
wwwetb.nlm.nih.gov

College of Health Sciences
cfprod.imt.uwm.edu/chs/ugp/hs/hciccurr.htm

Communicable Disease Surveillance Centre
www.open.gov.uk/cdsc/cdschome.htm

Computer Vision & Media Technology Laboratory
www.vision.auc.dk

Cooperative Cardiovascular Project
www.usccp.org

cosmetic dentistry
www.seattle-dentist.com/cosmeticdentist.htm

Council for Responsible Nutrition
www.crnusa.org

Council on Aging
www.ncoa.org

Crohn's and Colitis Foundation of America
www.ccfa.org
Cystic Fibrosis Foundation
www.cff.org

Deafness Research Foundation
www.drf.org

deafness
www.agbell.org

death education and counselling
www.adec.org

dengue
www.paho.org/dengue

dental advice
www.seattle-dentist.com/dental-advice.htm

dentistry
www.moderndentalconcepts.com

depression in men
menanddepression.nimh.nih.gov

dermatology
www.vh.org/adult/provider/dermatology/PietteDermatology

Diabetes, American Diabetes Association
www.diabetes.org/home.jsp

diabetes care
www.diabetes.org/DiabetesCare

Diabetes Foundation
www.nlm.nih.gov/medlineplus/diabetes.html

diabetes in childhood
www.childrenwithdiabetes.com

Digestive Diseases Information Clearinghouse
www.niddk.nih.gov

Digestive Disorders Foundation
www.digestivedisorders.org.uk

drowsy driving
www.drowsydriving.org

Down Syndrome Association
www.nads.org

Down Syndrome Society
www.ndss.org

drug abuse
www.nida.nih.gov/NIDAHome.html

drug addiction
www.well.com/user/woa

dry mouth
www.seattle-dentist.com/xerostomia.htm

Duke University Division of Clinical Informatics
dmi-www.mc.duke.edu

Duke University Medical Informatics
dmi-www.mc.duke.edu/DCMWeb/index.htm

E-Drug Forum
www.essentialdrugs.org/edrug/about.php

eating disorders referral
edreferral.com

Epilepsy Foundation of America
www.apa.org/science/efa.html

ethics in long-term care
www.who.int/chronic_conditions/ethical_choices.pdf

European Federation for Medical Informatics
www.efmi.org/efmi/default.asp

evidence-based medicine
www.uic.edu/depts/lib/lhsp/resources/ebm.shtml

Eye Care Foundation
www.eyecarefoundation.org

eye diseases
www.stlukeseye.com/Conditions
www.mic.ki.se/Diseases/C11.html

facial and plastic surgery
www.facial-plastic-surgery.org
Federation of the Blind
www.nfb.org

flossing teeth
www.seattle-dentist.com/flossing.htm

Foundation for Children with AIDS
www.caaf4kids.org

Gastroenterological Society of Australia
www.gesa.org.au/about/index.htm

gastrointestinal disorders
www.gastrosite.com

Gastrointestinal Research Foundation
www.girf.org

Genetic Alliance
www.geneticalliance.org

genetics research
history.nih.gov/exhibits/genetics

Harvard University Biomedical Informatics
www.mi-boston.org/fellowship

headache
www.headaches.org

heart structure and function
www.fi.edu/biosci/heart.html

health A to Z
www.healthatoz.com

health acronyms
www.geocities.com/~mlshams/acronym/acr.htm

Health and Medical Informatics Digest
www.son.wisc.edu/hmid/home.htm

health articles
www.mayoclinic.com/index.cfm?

health, consumer information
www.healthfinder.gov

health informatics education
www.healthcare-informatics.info

health informatics
203.147.217.77/ACS/chapter_sigs/health.htm
www.otago.ac.nz/subjects/hein.html

Health Informatics Society of Australia Ltd
www.hisa.org.au

Health Information Center
nhic-nt.health.org

health information management
www.ahima.org

health link
www.healthlinkplus.org

healthy lives
www.imgw.com/healthylives_splash

health politics
www.liv.ac.uk/PublicHealth/Publications/publications01.html

Health Web
healthweb.org

Heart, Lung, and Blood Institute
www.nhlbi.nih.gov/index.htm

helicobacter pylori
www.helico.com

help for carers
www.netofcare.org

Hemophilia Foundation
www.hemophilia.org

Herpes help
www.herpeshelp.com

herpes recurrences
www.herpes.com/Recurrences.html

high blood pressure
www.ugrad.cs.jhu.edu/~baker/bp.html
HIV/AIDS Education Program
www.ipfw.edu/ce/catalog/health/hea2003su03w.htm

Huntington's Disease Society of America
www.hdsa.org

Institute for Genomics and Bioinformatics
www.igb.uci.edu/index.htm

Institute of Arthritis
www.niams.nih.gov

internet clinical medicine resources
www.kumc.edu:8o/mmatrix

in-vitro diagnostic devices
www.fda.gov/cdrh/oivd/index.html

International Cancer Research Database
www.cancerportfolio.org

International Childbirth Education Association
www.icea.org

International Council on Disability
www.disabilityworld.org

International Diabetic Athletes Association
www.diabetes-exercise.org

International Journal of Medical Informatics
www.elsevier.nl/inca/publications

Internet Clinical Medicine Resources
www.kumc.edu:8o/mmatrix

Internet in Medicine
www.epub.org.br/intermedic

ISABEL
www.isabel.org.uk

James Watson
library.cshl.edu/honestjim

Japanese encephalitis resources
www.childrensvaccine.org/html/v_enceph_id.htm

Johns Hopkins, School of Medicine Division of Health Sciences Informatics
dhsi.med.jhmi.edu

Journal of the American Medical Association
pubs.ama-assn.org

Juvenile Diabetes Foundation International
www.jdf.org

kidney dialysis
www.kdf.org.sg/indexkdf.htm

Kidney Foundation
www.kidney.org

Leukemia and Lymphoma Society of America
www.leukemia.org

Library of Medicine
www.nlm.nih.gov

Linus Pauling and DNA
osulibrary.orst.edu/specialcollections/coll/pauling/dna/index.html

liver diseases
www.aasld.org

loose teeth
www.seattle-dentist.com/Smoking-Periodontitis.htm

lupus erythematosus
www.hamline.edu/lupus/index.html

Lyme disease
www.geocities.com/HotSprings/Oasis/6455/lyme-links.html
www.lymediseaseaudio.com/lymechat.htm

lymphoma
www.lymphoma.org/site/PageServer

macular diseases
www.macula.org

Madrid University Medical Informatics
www.infomed.dia.fi.upm.es/index.html

maternal health
www.hsph.harvard.edu/Organizations/healthnet/maternal/info.html
maternal and newborn health
www.who.int/reproductive-health/MNBH/index.htm

medical acupuncture
www.medicalacupuncture.org

medical biochemistry
www.kumc.edu/research/medicine/biochemistry

Medical Education Information Center
medic.med.uth.tmc.edu

medical ethics education
www.ama-assn.org/go/Step

Medical Help International
telemedical.com/~drcarr

medical informatics
www.eur.nl/FGG/MI
www-informatics.ucdmc.ucdavis.edu
www.ohsu.edu/bicc-informatics

medical metasearch engine for health care providers
SUMSearch.uthscsa.edu

medical toxicology resources
www.pitt.edu/~martint

Med Nexus
www.mednexus.com

Medicine (biosciences)
golgi.harvard.edu/biopages/medicine.html

Medscape
www.medscape.com

mental health
www.coil.com/~grohol

Mental Health Consumer Self-Help Clearinghouse
www.mhselfhelp.org

Mental Health Association
www.nmha.org

mental illness
www.mentalhealth.com

Microsoft Healthcare Users Group
www.mshug.org

migraine
www.migrainehelp.com
www.neurologist.com/migraines.html

migraine diagnosis and treatment
www.uib.no/isf/sats/quality/quality3.htm

Multimedia Medical Reference Library
www.tiac.net/users/jtward

multiple sclerosis
www.suite101.com/welcome.cfm/multiple_sclerosis

Myasthenia Gravis Foundation
www.myasthenia.org

National Cancer Institute
cancer.gov

National Institutes of Health
www.nih.gov

New England Journal of Medicine
content.nejm.org

NHS Direct
www.nhsdirect.nhs.uk

Nursing Index on the Internet
allnurses.com

nutrition
navigator.tufts.edu

obesity
www.obesity-news.com

older drivers
www.ama-assn.org/amapub/category/10791.html

oncolink
cancer.med.upenn.edu
organ donors
www.multiline.com.au/~donor

Organization for Rare Disorders
www.w2.com/nord1.html

orthopaedics
www.dundee.ac.uk/orthopaedics/link/welcome.htm

osteopathic medicine
www.aacom.org

paediatrics
www.uab.edu/pedinfo/index.html

pain in labour
www.painfreebirthing.com

pain management
www.aapainmanage.org
www.aapainmanage.org

parenteral and enteral nutrition
www.nutritioncare.org

Parkinson's Disease Foundation
www.parkinson.org

Patient's Guide to the Internet
www3.bc.sympatico.ca/me/patientsguide

Pediatric AIDS Foundation
www.pedaids.org

periodontitis
www.seattle-dentist.com/Smoking-Periodontitis.htm

placebo effect
www.pbs.org/saf/1307

pollen allergies
www.allegra.com

porphyria
www.prophyria-europe.com

pregnancy
www.babyhopes.com/pregnancytests.html
www.amazingpregnancy.com
Pregnancy and Infant Loss Center
www.bloomington.in.us/socserv/mit

prescription drugs
pharminfo.com/pin_hp.html

prescription drug list
www.rxlist.com

Prevent Blindness America
www.preventblindness.org

Primary Health Care Specialist Group, British Computer Society
www.phcsg.org.uk

psychiatry
www.psychiatry.com/index.php

quackery
www.cl.utoledo.edu/canaday/quackery/quack-index.html

rare disorders (Europe)
www.eurordis.org

rare disorders (International)
www.raredisorders.com

rare disorders (UK)
www.cafamily.org

rare disorders (US)
www.rarediseases.org

Regenstrief Institute Medical Informatics Fellowship
informatics.regenstrief.org

Renal Physicians Association
www.renalmd.org

reproductive health
www.reproline.jhu.edu
www.cdc.gov/nccdphp/drh

reproductive health gateway
www.rhgateway.org

reproductive medicine
www.infertilityprofessionals.com/clinical/asrm.html
www.asrm.org
retarded mental development in children
www.iacny.org/manhatta.htm

Rochester University, Division of Medical Informatics
www.urmc.rochester.edu/smd/MedInfo/index.html

Royal College of Surgeons of Edinburgh – Diploma in Medical Informatics
www.diploma.rcsed.ac.uk

schizophrenia
www.schizophrenia.com

scientific gateways
www.bmn.com

Sex Information and Education Council of the United States
www.siecus.org

Sickle Cell Anemia Research Foundation
www.ascaa.org/support.asp

Sickle Cell Disease Association of America
www.sicklecelldisease.org/default.htm

sleep
www.sleepnet.com

Sleep, American Sleep Disorders Foundation
www.asda.org

Sleep Foundation
www.sleepfoundation.org

sleep medicine
www.users.cloud9.net/~thorpy

sleep research
www.sleepfor science.org

smallpox pathology
www.afip.org/Departments/infectious/sp/text/1_1.htm

snoring
www.seattle-dentist.com/sleep-apnea.htm

speech development
www.vocaldevelopment.com

spina bifida
www.waisman.wisc.edu/~rowley/sb-kids

Spinal Cord Injury Association
www.spinalcord.org

sports medicine
www.acsm.org/index.asp

Stanford Medical Informatics
www.smi.stanford.edu

STD & AIDS Hotlines
www.ashastd.org

Stroke Association
209.107.44.93/NationalStroke/default.htm

sudden infant death syndrome
www.sids.org

suicide information and education
www.suicideinfo.ca

Tay-Sachs disease
www.tay-sachs.org

The Medical Algorithms Project
www.medal.org

travellers' health
healthlink.mcw.edu/travel-links.html

UCLA – Medical Informatics
www.itmedicine.net/informatics/page-home.html

United Ostomy Association
www.uoa.org

United Cerebral Palsy Association
www.ucpa.org

veins
www.veins1.com

vital signs
www.vitalsigns.com

wellness
www.wellweb.com

World Health Organization (WHO)
www.who.ch

women's health
www.mindspring.com/~mperloe
www.ibiblio.org/cheryb/women/
www.nytimes.com/pages/health/womenshealth/index.html
www.spwomenshealth.com/genhelthlinks.html
www.anesthesiology.com/links/women.htm

Woman's Hospital
www.womans.com

WHO World Health Report 2003
www.who.int/whr/2003/en

Yale University, Center for Medical Informatics
ycmi.med.yale.edu

Handheld Computers, Personal Digital Assistant (PDA) websites

access to medical literature
www.avantgo.com

American College of Physicians
www.acc.org/clinical/palm_download.htm

American Academy of Family Physicians
www.aafp.org/x433.xml

American Medical Student Association
www.amsa.org/resource/pda.cfm

American College of Physicians
www.acponline.org/pda/index.html

Anatomy and Microbiology flashcards
kaplan.pdaverticals.com

Arizona Health Sciences Library
educ.ahsl.arizona.edu/pda/index.htm

clinical predictions
www.medicaltoolbox.com

clinical prediction rules
pbrain.hypermart.net/medrules.html

collection of medical books for Palm and Windows
www.handheldmed.com

customized drug databases
www.skyscape.com

customized extensive drug database
www.lexi.com

Dalhousie University
www.medicine.dal.ca/palm

drug databases
www.epocrates.com

electronic medical record for Windows CE
www.gemedicalsystems.com

electronic medical record for Pocket PC
www.digital-doc.com

General Medical PDA Websites
www.pdamd.com

handhelds for palliative care and anesthesia
www.portablehealth.com/quail

health sciences resources for PDA
www.library.ualberta.ca/subject/oncology/pdahealth/index.cfm

immunization schedule
www.immunizationed.org

infectious diseases
hopkins-abxguide.org

links to Clinical Practice Guidelines for handheld computers
www.guideline.gov/resources/pda.aspx

literature searches
www.ovid.com

MedCalc
medcalc.med-ia.net

medical textbooks for Palm and Windows
www.skyscape.com

medical statistics calculator
www.cebm.utoronto.ca/practise/ca/statscal

medical publishers
www.franklin.com

medical software collections
www.healthypalmpilot.com

medical calculators
smi-web.stanford.edu/people/pcheng/medmath

medical mnemonics
www.medicalmnemonics.com

Mount Sinai Hospital, Toronto
www.medtau.org

New York University School of Medicine
endeavor.med.nyu.edu/research/pda/pilot

pediatric critical care
www.mverive.com

pharmaceutical information
www.healthprolink.com

Physicians' Desk Reference
www.pdr.net

reviews of medical handheld applications
ect.downstate.edu/support/palm

Riley Hospital for Children
kidometer.com

student's guide to the medical literature
denison.uchsc.edu/SG/index.html

University of Connecticut Healthcare Centre
library.uchc.edu/pda